The Scientific Basis of Urology

The Scientific Basis of Urology

Second Edition

Edited by

Anthony R Mundy MS FRCP FRCS
Professor of Urology
The Institute of Urology and Nephrology
London UK

John M Fitzpatrick MCh FRCSI FRC(Urol) FRCSGlas FRCS
Professor and Chairman
Department of Surgery
University College Dublin
Dublin 7 Ireland

David E Neal FMed Sci MS FRCS
Professor of Surgical Oncology
Department of Oncology
Addenbrooke's Hospital
Cambridge UK

Nicholas J R George MD FRCS
Senior Lecturer/Consultant Urologist
Department of Urology
University Hospitals of South Manchester
Manchester UK

Taylor & Francis
Taylor & Francis Group
LONDON AND NEW YORK

First published in the United Kingdom in 1999 by Isis Medical Media Ltd

Second edition published in the United Kingdom in 2004
by Taylor & Francis, an imprint of the Taylor & Francis Group,
11 New Fetter Lane, London EC4P 4EE

Tel.: +44 (0) 20 7583 9855
Fax.: +44 (0) 20 7842 2298
E-mail: info@dunitz.co.uk
Website: http://www.dunitz.co.uk

A CIP record for this book is available from the British Library.

Library of Congress Cataloging-in-Publication Data
Data available on application

ISBN 1 90186 513 4

Distributed in North and South America by
Taylor & Francis
2000 NW Corporate Blvd
Boca Raton, FL 33431, USA

Within Continental USA
Tel.: 800 272 7737; Fax.: 800 374 3401
Outside Continental USA
Tel.: 561 994 0555; Fax.: 561 361 6018
E-mail: orders@crcpress.com

Distributed in the rest of the world by
Thomson Publishing Services
Cheriton House
North Way
Andover, Hampshire SP10 5BE, UK
Tel.: +44 (0)1264 332424
E-mail: salesorder.tandf@thomsonpublishingservices.co.uk

Composition by J&L Composition, Filey, North Yorkshire

Printed and bound in Spain by Grafos SA Arte Sobre Papel

Contents

Contributors

Ken M Anson MBBS FRCS MS FRCS(Urol)
Consultant Urologist
Department of Urology
St George's Hospital
London, UK

David A Brealey BSc MRCP
Clinical Lecturer
Bloomsbury Institute of Intensive Care Medicine
University College London
London, UK

John A Bridgewater PhD MRCP
Honorary Consultant in Medical Oncology
Royal Free & University College
School of Medicine
University College London
London, UK

Richard SD Brown MRCP FRCF
Department of Oncology
Middlesex Hospital
London, UK

Steven C Clifford PhD
Lecturer in Molecular Oncology
Northern Institute for Cancer Research
University of Newcastle upon Tyne
Newcastle upon Tyne, UK

Michael Craggs FRCS
Professor and Director of Spiral Research
Institute of Urology
Royal National Orthopaedic Hospital Stanmore
Middlesex
London, UK

AC Cunningham
Sunderland Pharmacy School
University of Sunderland
Fleming Building
Sunderland, UK

Jeremy Elkabir MBBS FRCS FRCS(Urol) FEBU
Consultant Urological Surgeon
Northwick Park & St Mark's Hospitals
Harrow
London, UK

Mark Emberton FRCS FRCS(Urol) MD
Institute of Urology
Middlesex Hospital
London, UK

John M Fitzpatrick MCh FRCSI FRC(Urol) FRCSGlas FRCS
Professor and Chairman
Department of Surgery
University College Dublin
Dublin 7, Ireland

Alex Freeman
Department of Histopathology
University College London
London, UK

Christopher H Fry FRCS
Institute of Urology & Nephrology
University College London
London, UK

Judith Gaffan
Royal Free & University College
School of Medicine
University College London
London, UK

Nicholas J R George MD FRCS
Senior Lecturer/Consultant Urologist
Department of Urology
University Hospital of South Manchester
Manchester, UK

TR Leyshon Griffiths
Senior Lecturer in Urological Surgery
Department of Urology
Leicester General Hospital
Leicester, UK

Suresh K Gupta
Department of Urology
Wrexham Maelor Hospital
Croesnewydd Road
Wrexham, UK

Freddie C Hamdy MD FRCSEd (Urol)
Professor and Head of Urology
Academic Urology Unit
University of Sheffield
Royal Hallamshire Hospital
Sheffield, UK

Stephen J Harland MD MSc FRCP
Consultant
Institute of Urology
University College London
Middlesex Hospital
London, UK

George B Haycock MB BChir FRCP FRCPCH
Professor
Department of Paediatrics
Guy's Hospital
London, UK

NJ Hegarty
Department of Surgery
Mater Misericordiae Hospital
Conway Institute of Biomolecular and Biomedical Research
University College Dublin
Dublin, Ireland

Mark I Johnson MD FRCS (Urol)
Department of Urology
University of Sheffield
Royal Hallamshire Hospital
Sheffield, UK

John A Kirby DPhil FRCS
Professor of Immunobiology and
Postgraduate Tutor Applied Immunobiology Group
Department of Surgery
University of Newcastle
Newcastle upon Tyne, UK

Sarah Knight MA PhD
Clinical Scientist
Institute of Urology
Royal National Orthopaedic Hospital Stanmore
Middlesex
London, UK

Eamonn R Maher
Section of Medical and Molecular Genetics
Department of Paediatrics and Child Health
University of Birmingham
Birmingham, UK

Marie E Mathers
Department of Cellular Pathology
Royal Victoria Infirmary
Newcastle upon Tyne, UK

Mary McCormack PhD FRCR
Department of Oncology
Middlesex Hospital
London, UK

J Kilian Mellon MD FRCS (Urol)
Professor of Urology
Department of Urology
Leicester Warwick Medical School
Leicester General Hospital
Leicester, UK

Suks Minhas
Institute of Urology
University College London
London, UK

Julie A Morris
Head of Medical Statistics
Education and Research Building
Wythenshawe Hospital
Southmoor Road
Manchester, UK

Anthony R Mundy MS FRCP FRCS
Professor of Urology
The Institute of Urology and Nephrology
London, UK

David E Neal FMed Sci MS FRCS
Professor of Surgical Oncology
Department of Oncology
Addenbrooke's Hospital
Cambridge, UK

Guy H Neild FRCP
Professor
Institute of Urology and Nephrology
Middlesex Hospital
London, UK

Marie O'Donnell
Department of Histopathology
Sunderland Royal Hospital
Sunderland, UK

Uday Patel MBChB MRCP(UK) FRCR
Consultant and Hon. Senior Lecturer
Department of Radiology
St George's Hospital and Medical School
London, UK

Heather A Payne MBBS MRCP FRCR
Department of Oncology
Middlesex Hospital
London, UK

John P Pryor MBBS MS FRCS
Consultant
The Lister Hospital
London, UK

David J Ralph BSc MS FRCS(Urol)
Middlesex Hospital
London, UK

William G Robertson FRCS
Institute of Urology and Nephrology
University College London
London, UK

Craig N Robson PhD
Department of Urology
University of Sheffield
Royal Hallamshire Hospital
Sheffield, UK

David W Ryan MBChB FRCA
Consultant Clinical Physiologist
Department of Perioperative and Critical Care
The Freeman Hospital
Newcastle upon Tyne, UK

Naeem A Soomro MBBS FRCS(Urol)
Consultant Urologist
Department of Urology
Freeman Hospital
Newcastle upon Tyne, UK

David Talbot MD FRCS PhD
Consultant and Senior Lecturer in Transplant and Hepatobiliary Surgery
The Freeman Hospital
Newcastle upon Tyne, UK

David FM Thomas FRCP FRCS
Consultant Paediatric Urologist
Department of Paediatric Urology
Clinical Sciences Building
St James' University Hospital
Leeds, UK

SN Venn
Institute of Urology and Nephrology
University College London
London, UK

R William G Watson
Department of Surgery
Mater Misericordiae Hospital
Conway Institute of Biomolecular and Biomedical Research
University College Dublin
Dublin, Ireland

Andrew R Webb MD FRCP
Medical Director (Clinical Services)
UCL Hospitals NHS Trust
London, UK

Hugh N Whitfield MA FRCS MChir FEBU
Harold Hopkins Department of Urology
Royal Berkshire Hospital
Reading, UK

Neville Woolf
Professor
Medical School Administration
University College London
London, UK

Preface to the first edition

For even the most junior urological trainee learning the basic medical sciences is all but a distant memory. Since then the sciences have changed as knowledge has advanced and whole new disciplines have developed. The focus of a urological trainee is, in any case, fundamentally different from a student just beginning his or her medical education who must have a grounding in order to be equipped to comprehend the whole field of medicine and surgery in the ensuing few years of undergraduate medical training. So, even discounting all that a trainee urologist has forgotten, there is a great deal of new knowledge to acquire and a specifically urological perspective from which to view that knowledge.

Five years ago the Editors were asked to organise an annual course on 'The Scientific Basis of Urology'. The aim was to address basic science in urology from just this perspective and to take account of the recent changes in the scope and format of medical and surgical undergraduate and postgraduate examinations, as a result of which the student and subsequently the trainee is no longer expected to have such a detailed knowledge of these subjects as used to be expected. This annual course is sponsored by the *British Association of Urological Surgeons* and the *British Journal of Urology* and is regarded nowadays as mandatory for all urological trainees during the first two years of training. It is evidence of how highly we regard the importance of a grounding in basic science for training in clinical urology.

This book arose from the course, although some of the authors have not taught on the course, some of the course teachers are not authors here, and the titles of the chapters in this book do not match closely with the titles of the lectures on the course. This is because we have tried to make the scientific material more clinically relevant with a wider audience in mind. In this way we hope to make this book interesting to all practising urologists, although we should stress that although many of the chapters address specific disease conditions the authors cover only the scientific aspects. Details of diagnosis and treatment will have to be sought elsewhere. Equally, this book does not aim to be comprehensive. We have tried to keep it to a size that a reader, with an average attention span, might expect to read in its entirety rather than let the book expand to a size that would confine it to a dusty shelf. Indeed some of the more basic 'basic sciences' have been skated over to a degree that the purist might find objectionable. We have aimed the text, however, at the specifically urological audience who, we think, wants to be able to understand these particular topics without necessarily acquiring any great depth of knowledge.

Hence, also, the use of recommended reading lists in such chapters rather than the more traditional list of references.

The Editors have all learnt a great deal from the exercise of preparing the annual courses and now from the preparation of this book. For those who have attended the courses and have nagged us (incessantly) for the book during its preparation – here it is, and thank you for giving us the opportunity to benefit from the whole teaching process as well.

A. R. Mundy
London, 1998

Preface to the second edition

We were pleased with the reception that greeted the first edition of this book. We were, however, a little more critical and felt that although the course, on which the book is based, is fairly comprehensive, the written version did not do it full justice. We have therefore expanded the number of chapters to include those topics, such as *Inflammation, shock, detrusor smooth muscle physiology, pathophysiology of bladder dysfunction, urodynamics, biology of cancer and metastasis, molecular genetics and pathology of renal cell carcinoma, principles of chemotherapy, urological and biochemical aspects of transplantation biology, perioperative care of the urological patient*, that we thought were missing. We are grateful to both new contributors and also previous ones for reviving their manuscripts.

The scientific basis of urology is changing frighteningly quickly, with new developments in molecular biology and pathophysiology. This makes the task to keep such a book as this up-to-date an increasingly difficult one. We hope that the reader will find this interesting whether he or she is a new reader or someone who read the first edition.

A. R. Mundy
London, 2004

1

An introduction to cell biology

Anthony R Mundy

INTRODUCTION

For many urologists, the mere mention of the words cell and molecular biology is sufficient to induce a state of anxiety. It is a recent and changing science with an unfamiliar and often confusing jargon. Nonetheless, even these same urologists appreciate that it is impossible to escape the subject altogether if one is to understand many of the recent developments in urology, especially in the field of urological oncology.

The aim of this chapter is to present the subject from a specifically urological viewpoint so that the reader might be better able to understand some of the discussion in later chapters of this volume. Some of the more important or key terms are highlighted in italic to draw attention to them as they may be unfamiliar to some. Also, suggested reading material is given at the end of the chapter, rather than using specific references in the text as is usual as these are unlikely to be helpful to the clinical urologist.

This first chapter deals with events outside the nucleus while Chapter 2 deals with the nucleus and cell division. The purpose of this chapter is to describe the mechanisms that hold cells, and therefore tissues, together and how cells communicate, and so provide the basis for understanding, for example, how organs can distend and collapse as the bladder does during filling and emptying; how the mechanisms that hold cells together can be broken down in tumour invasion; and how different cells communicate at a local level as in the stromal–epithelial interaction in benign prostatic hyperplasia or in the development of neoplasia. In essence, the purpose is to outline those aspects of cellular structure and function that are important when considering the relationship between one cell and another and between cells and the extracellular matrix. The interface in both instances is the cell membrane.

THE CELL MEMBRANE

The cell membrane and the membranes of intracellular organelles all have a very similar structure (Figure 1.1), although there is considerable variation in detail from cell to cell in different tissues. The principal components are lipids and proteins. Forty per cent to 80% of the cell membrane is lipid and 50% is phospholipid. The protein content is much more variable – anything from a 0.2 : 1 protein to lipid ratio in cells in the central nervous system, in which electrical insulation is important, to a 3.2 : 1 ratio in mitochondrial membranes, where metabolic activity is particularly high. Cell membranes essentially depend on lipids for their structure and on proteins for their function. These proteins are of two types. There are integral proteins that span the full thickness of the cell membrane from the exterior to the cytosol, such as the transmembrane signalling proteins; and there are peripheral proteins that are adherent to the cytosolic aspect of the cell membrane, such as the structural proteins related to the cytoskeleton.

The phospholipids that form the cell membrane are arranged in two layers, with a hydrophilic head and a hydrophobic tail. The hydrophilic head faces outwards to the exterior on the outer leaflet and inwards to the cytosol on the inner leaflet, and the hydrophobic tails of the phospholipids of both leaflets face inwards to the centre of the membrane.

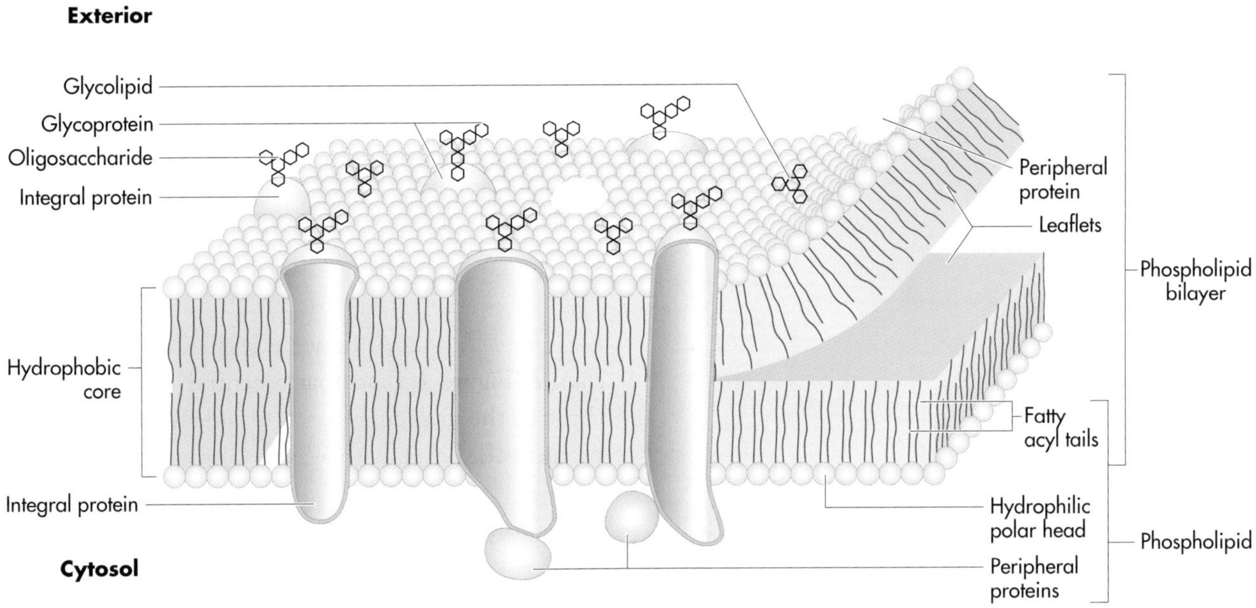

Figure 1.1 *A typical biological membrane. Two leaflets of phospholipids are orientated with their hydrophilic polar heads like the bread of a sandwich and the fatty acyl tails like the filling of a sandwich. Integral proteins span the full thickness of the lipid bilayer and peripheral proteins attach onto them (generally) on the cytosolic aspect of the cell membrane. Sugars are generally located as oligosaccharide glycoproteins or glycolipids bound to the external aspect of the integral proteins. (Modified from Darnell J, Lodish H, Baltimore D. Molecular cell biology, second edition. New York: Scientific American Books, 1990.)*

This orientation in the form of a 'lipid sandwich' is particularly important when considering transmembrane signalling and membrane transport in general – How do molecules get through the lipid layer?

It is important to appreciate that the membrane is fluid – it is a viscous gel. This means that the proteins and phospholipids can move around within the membrane gel; indeed, they can move very rapidly in some instances.

The phospholipids of the cell membrane are variable and numerous, but the principal ones in most cell membranes are: phosphatidylcholine, phosphatidylinositol, phosphatidylethanolamine and phosphatidylserine. Although principally subserving a structural role, some of these molecules take part in important functional activities, as described below. Not all metabolic function is related to the protein component.

The sugar component of the cell membrane is small. The vast majority of sugars are related to the external aspect of the cell membrane or to the internal aspect of organelles. Outside the cell, these are mostly oligosaccharides, glycoproteins or glycolipids (which are discussed in more detail below).

MEMBRANE TRANSPORT

Transport may be passive or active. Passive transport processes do not require energy; examples include the diffusion of gases such as oxygen and carbon dioxide and of small uncharged molecules down a concentration gradient, and of water down an osmotic gradient.

Diffusion of specific molecules such as glucose and certain amino acids – molecules that either are too big to diffuse or for which a speedier process is needed – may be *facilitated* by *multipass transmembrane proteins*.

Sometimes, the transport of one molecule across a membrane by a facilitator molecule is linked, or *coupled*, to the movement of another (Figure 1.2). If both molecules move in the same direction, the co-transport molecule is known as a *symport*; if the movement of the two molecules is in opposite directions, the co-transport molecule is called an *antiport*.

Active transport consumes energy, usually generated by the hydrolysis of adenosine triphosphate (ATP). Sodium–potassium adenosine triphosphatase (ATPase) is a multipass transmembrane protein (Figure 1.3) enzyme that exchanges sodium for potassium so as to maintain intracellular potassium at 20 to 40 times its extracellular concentration and extracellular sodium at 10 to 20 times its intracellular concentration (Figure 1.4). Similar ATPases pump calcium out of cells or into intracellular stores.

The hydrophobic phospholipid membrane is virtually impermeable to ions in aqueous solution. Various systems exist to allow ionic movement to occur. These include *permeases* such as the ATPase enzymes described above. An important mechanism is provided by transmembrane proteins that form aqueous ion channels across the lipid bilayer. They allow ion transport at high speed without expending energy, but although they influence the speed of flow, they do not affect the direction of flow, which is always down a concentration gradient. These transmembrane ion channels are important in transmitting nerve impulses and in muscle contraction. They are all glycoproteins and they all work such that when they are stimulated they undergo a *conformational change* (Figure 1.5) so that a central pore is created through the molecule from one side of the cell membrane to the other, with a hydrophilic lining to allow the passage of water-soluble ions (Figure 1.6).

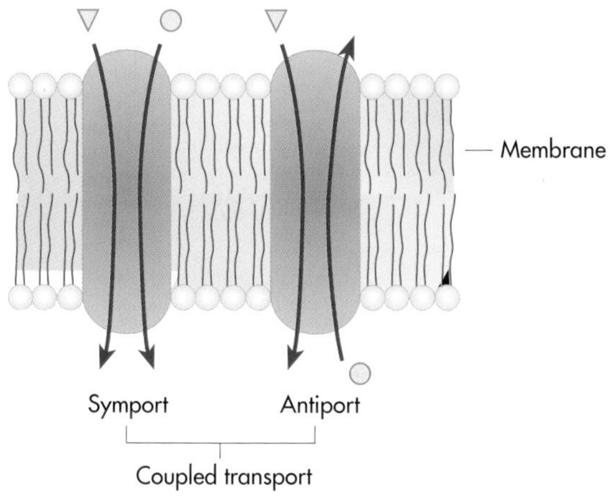

Figure 1.2 *Coupled transport. (Modified from Darnell J, Lodish H, Baltimore D. Molecular cell biology, second edition. New York: Scientific American Books, 1990.)*

Stimuli for the conformational change include:

- a change in voltage
- the binding of another molecule – known as a *ligand* – to the original molecule
- mechanical deformation (in some cells)
- gap junction activation (described below).

Opening and closing the protein channel is called *gating* (Figure 1.7) and so there are *voltage-gated channels*, *ligand-gated channels* and *mechanically gated channels* and different channels exist both for different stimuli and for different ions.

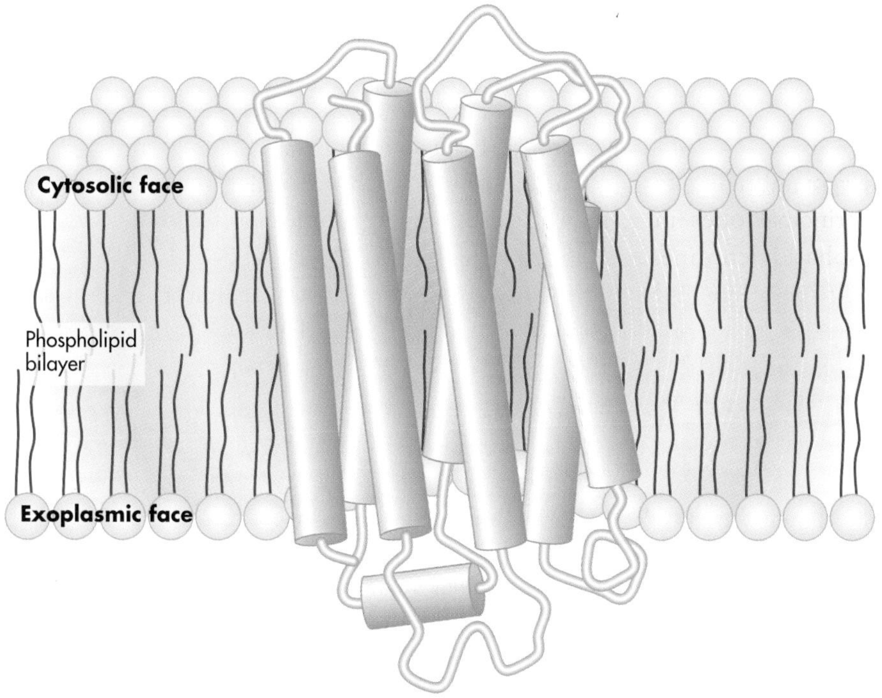

Figure 1.3 *The general structure of a multipass transmembrane protein. The transmembrane helices are here represented as cylinders spanning the phospholipid bilayer. (Modified from Darnell J, Lodish H, Baltimore D. Molecular cell biology, second edition. New York: Scientific American Books, 1990.)*

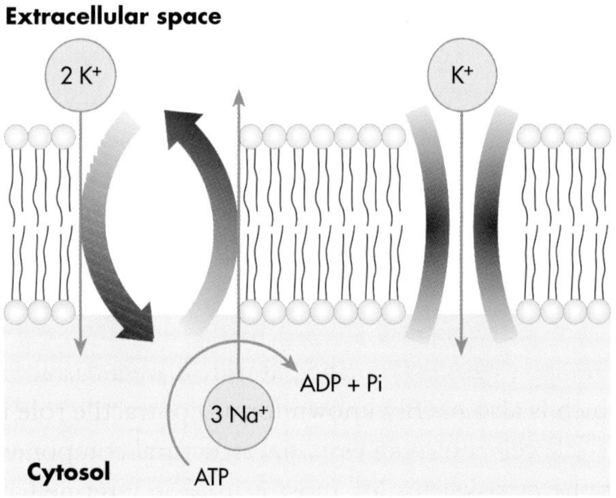

Figure 1.4 *Two classes of membrane transport proteins. On the left, active transport mediated by sodium/potassium ATPase; on the right, passive transport through potassium channel-forming proteins. (Modified from Goodman SR. Medical cell biology. Philadelphia: JB Lippincott Company, 1994.)*

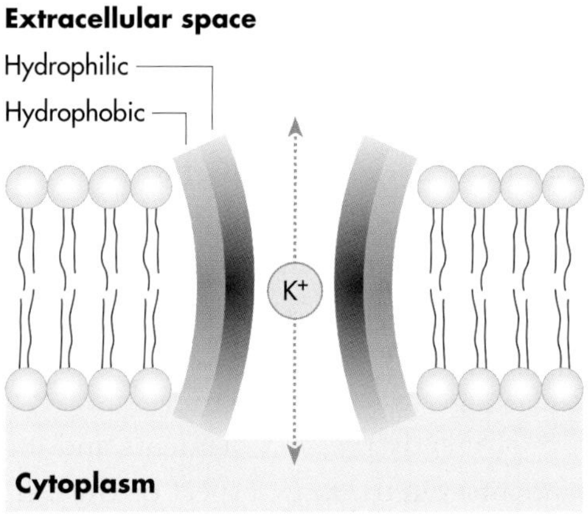

Figure 1.6 *An aqueous channel-forming protein. The hydrophilic portion of the molecule lines the pore and the hydrophobic portion is interposed between the hydrophilic lining and the surrounding membrane lipid. (Modified from Goodman SR. Medical cell biology. Philadelphia: JB Lippincott Company, 1994.)*

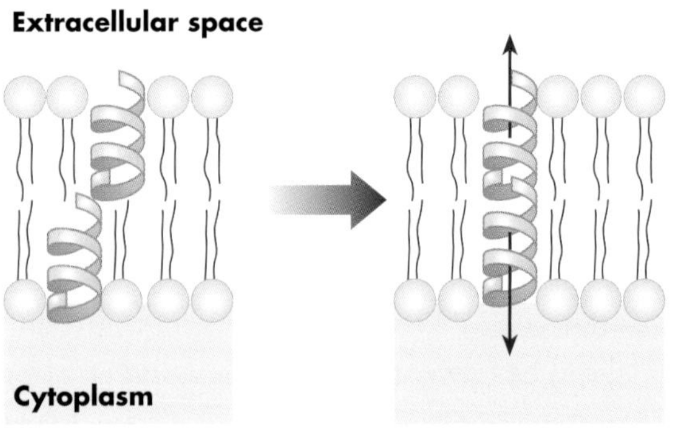

Figure 1.5 *A transmembrane channel developing as two peptides dimerize head to head (in this case) to span the lipid bilayer. (Modified from Sawyer DB, Koepp ER, Andersen O. Biochemistry 1989; 28: 6571.)*

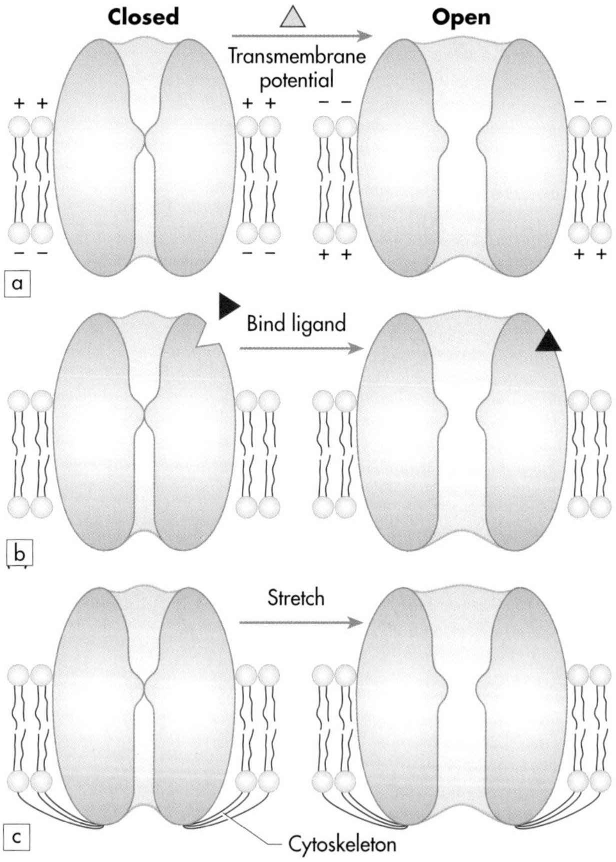

Figure 1.7 *Diagrammatic view of three different types of ion channels stimulated by different gating mechanisms. (a) Voltage-gated ion channel. (b) Ligand-gated receptor. (c) Mechanically gated channel. (Modified from Kandel ER, Schwartz JH, Jessell TM. Principles of neural science, third edition. New York: Elsevier, 1991.)*

These ion channels make cells electrically excitable. Cells maintain slightly more negative than positive ions in the cytosol and slightly more positive than negative ions in the extracellular fluid. This causes a voltage difference across the lipid membrane, which is a poor conductor because of its lipid content and therefore allows the voltage difference to exist. This *resting membrane potential* – largely caused by sodium–potassium ATPase – is the driving force for many biochemical processes.

THE CYTOSKELETON

The cytoskeleton has an important role in maintaining the integrity of the cell membrane and is also involved in cell–cell and cell–matrix adhesions. It stops major deformation of the cell membrane when contraction of the cell pulls on the inner aspect of the cell membrane or when distension, adhesion and other forces pull on the outside of the cell membrane.

Within the cell there is a meshwork of filaments of different types that run from one side of the cell to the other, mainly the thin filaments and intermediate filaments. On the inner aspect of the cell membrane there is a scaffolding of proteins that supports the cell membrane in the way that rafters support a roof or poles support the canvas of a tent (Figure 1.8). This scaffolding is called the *spectrin membrane skeleton* as spectrin is its principal component. It maintains the shape and stability of the cell membrane and was first identified in red blood cells, where it is most elaborately developed. It is now known to be ubiquitous.

There are three main types of filaments involved in the cytoskeleton: microtubules, thin filaments and intermediate filaments. Thick filaments, which are principally myosin, are contractile rather than structural and are only found in significant concentrations in muscle cells. The principal thin filament is actin, which is also mainly known for its contractile role in muscle cells but is an essential structural component of the cytoskeleton of most cells. The intermediate filaments are the most variable in composition, with different types in smooth muscle, fibroblasts and epithelia. Microtubules that are composed of tubulin are principally important in intracellular transport, especially in neurons and in the activity of villi and cilia.

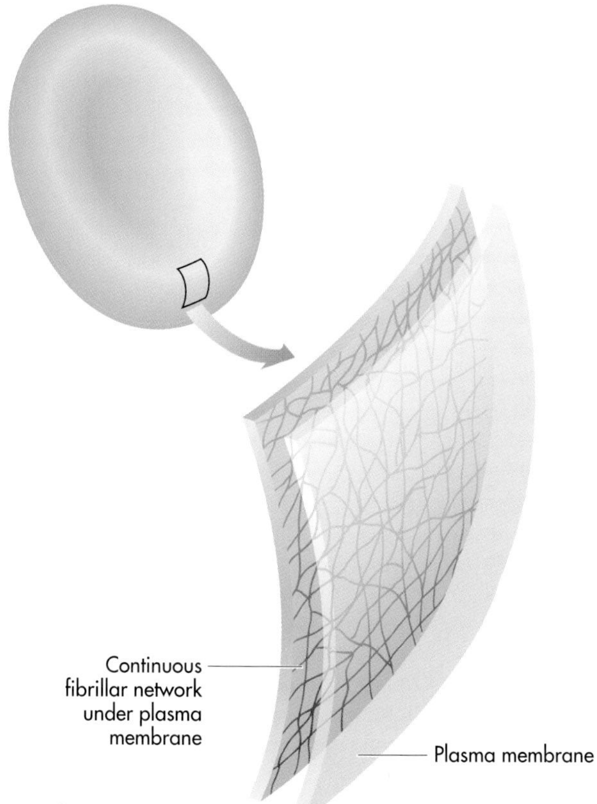

Figure 1.8 *The membrane cytoskeleton in relation to the plasma membrane, in this case in a red blood cell. A continuous fibrillar network of spectrin molecules links to integral membrane proteins on the under aspect of the plasma membrane. (Modified from Darnell J, Lodish H, Baltimore D. Molecular cell biology, second edition. New York: Scientific American Books, 1990.)*

Microfilaments

Microfilaments include actin, tropomyosin and caldesmon. The most important is actin, which forms 5% to 30% of the total protein content of non-muscle cells. It is a globular and contractile protein component of the cytoskeleton and its role in the cell can be compared to the muscular element of the musculoskeletal system of the body as a whole. It links to the membrane scaffolding system and to adjacent cells or extracellular proteins, as described below; it forms the contraction ring that separates the two daughter cells in cell division; and it controls the gel–sol state of cytoplasm and so allows cells to change their shape or move.

Intermediate filaments

These, by comparison, correspond to the ligaments in the musculoskeletal system of the human body. They are heterogeneous fibrous proteins that bind one cell to another or to the extracellular membrane (as do the microfilaments) by means of transmembrane *linker* proteins or protein complexes. The best known of the intermediate filaments are keratin in epithelial cells, vimentin in fibroblasts, and desmin which coexists with vimentin in smooth muscle cells.

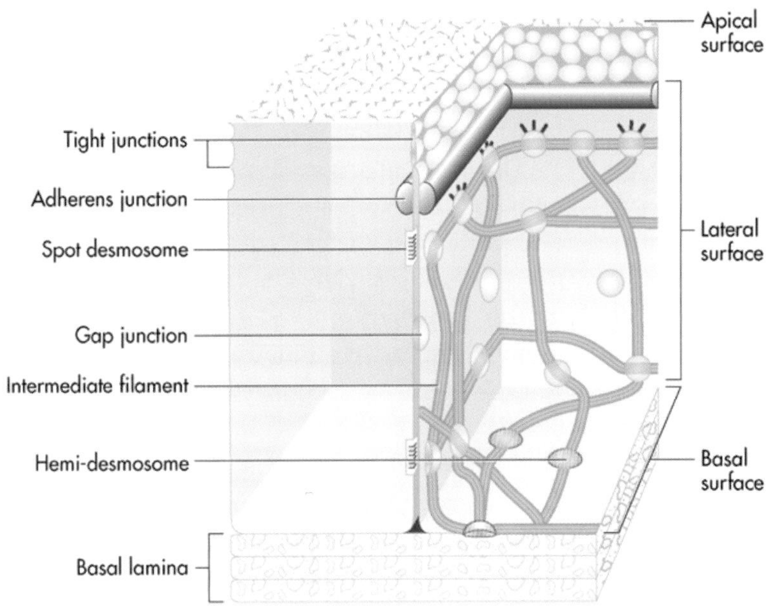

Figure 1.9 *The principal types of cell junctions: tight junctions at the apices of cells, adherens junctions below, spot desmosomes between cells, and desmosomes between cells and the basal lamina, all interlinked by intermediate filaments. Gap junctions join adjacent cells. (Modified from Darnell J, Lodish H, Baltimore D. Molecular cell biology, second edition. New York: Scientific American Books, 1990.)*

CELL TO CELL ADHESION

Cell to cell adhesion is mediated by different types of *junctions*. The main ones are: tight junctions, anchoring junctions (or desmosomes) and communicating (or gap) junctions (Figure 1.9). These junctions are usually proteinaceous and their integrity is commonly calcium dependent. There are various *adhesion molecules*, which again are mainly proteinaceous and calcium dependent in their action, of which the best known are the *cadherins*. These are the glue that holds the junctions together. In epithelia, the principal adhesion molecule is *E-cadherin* (also known as uvomorulin). In different cell types there are different cadherins and there are also adhesion molecules that are not calcium dependent in their action, but proteinaceous and calcium-dependent adhesion is the general rule in the urinary tract.

Tight junctions

At a tight junction, adjacent cell membranes actually fuse together (Figure 1.10). Tight junctions are usually close to the apex of cells, particularly in epithelial cell layers, where they form and maintain a watertight seal. They are therefore prominent in a system such as bladder epithelium, where they help avoid backward flux of urinary constituents into the blood stream thereby reversing the effects of

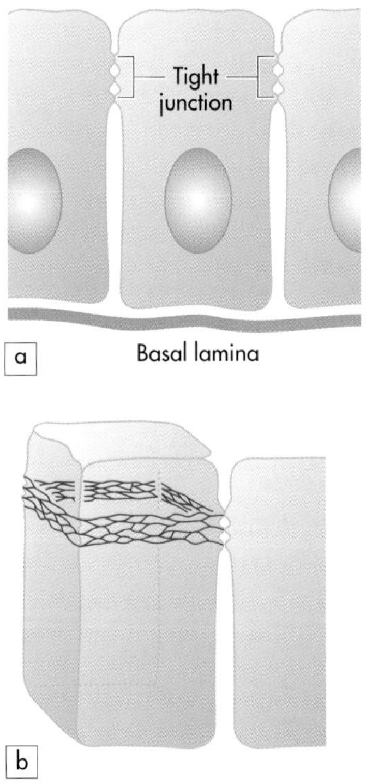

Figure 1.10 *A tight junction. (a) The cross-sectional appearance. (b) The circumferential disposition of a tight junction. (Modified from Goodman SR. Medical cell biology. Philadelphia: JB Lippincott Company, 1994.)*

renal function. Equally important is the integrity of the intestinal epithelium, for similar reasons, and here tight junctions are also prominent. Tight junctions are formed by calcium-dependent, single-span, transmembrane linker glycoproteins, like cadherins, and the more there are, the more impermeable the junction.

Anchoring junctions

Anchoring junctions are the means by which the cytoskeleton connects, via transmembrane linker proteins and calcium-dependent adhesive molecules, to the cytoskeleton of other cells or to the extracellular matrix. There are two main types of anchoring junctions: one is related to the microfilaments of the cytoskeleton and the other to the intermediate filaments of the cytoskeleton. In each main type there are two subtypes, depending on whether the junctional complex relates to another cell or to the extracellular matrix (Figures 1.11 and 1.12 and Table 1.1).

Microfilamentous junctions with adjacent cells

The microfilament actin commonly produces a band of adhesion around the inside of epithelial cells, close to the apex of the cell and just below the tight junctions mentioned above. This belt of actin filaments circling the periphery of the inside of the cell membrane is commonly known as a *belt desmosome* and depends on cadherins to anchor it to the adjacent cell.

Microfilamentous junctions with the extracellular matrix

Actin links to the extracellular matrix by means of a system of linker proteins that connects the actin to extracellular *fibronectin*, which is an important adhesive glycoprotein in the extracellular matrix (Figure 1.13). In this linker protein complex is another type

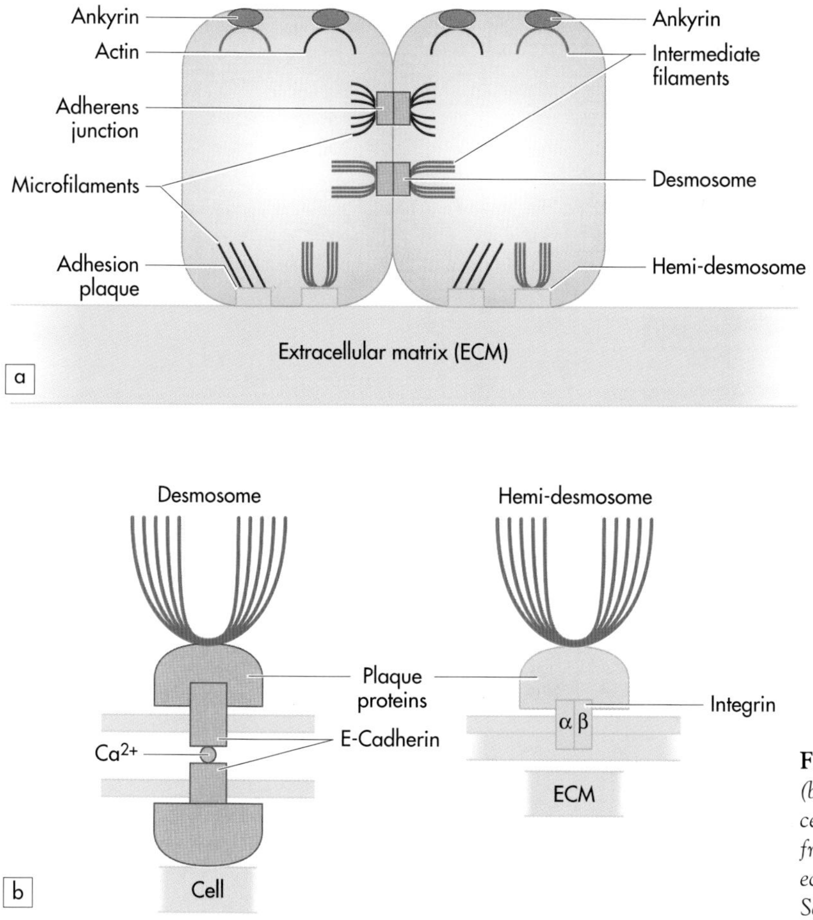

Figure 1.11 *(a,b) The features of desmosomes (between cells) and hemi-desmosomes (between cells and the basement membrane). (Modified from Darnell J, Lodish H, Baltimore D. Molecular cell biology, second edition. New York: Scientific American Books, 1990.)*

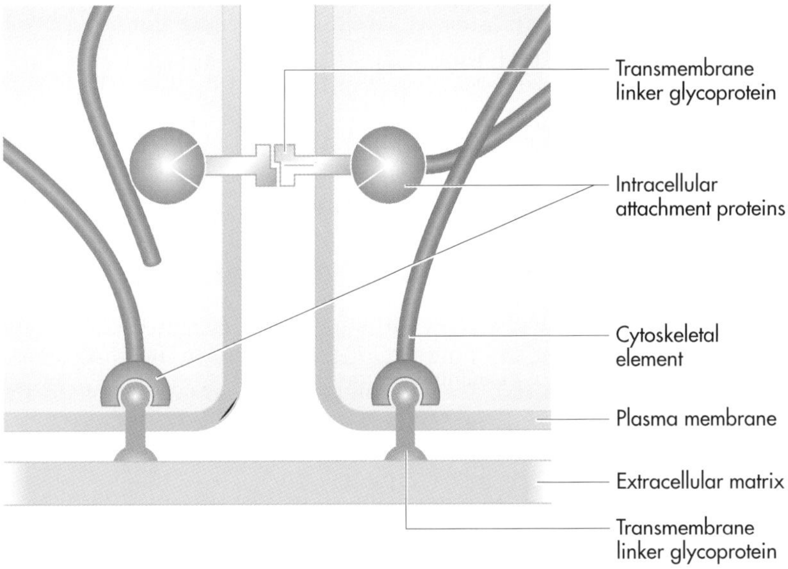

Figure 1.12 *The principal features of adherens junctions: their morphological disposition. (Modified from Goodman SR. Medical cell biology. Philadelphia: JB Lippincott Company, 1994.)*

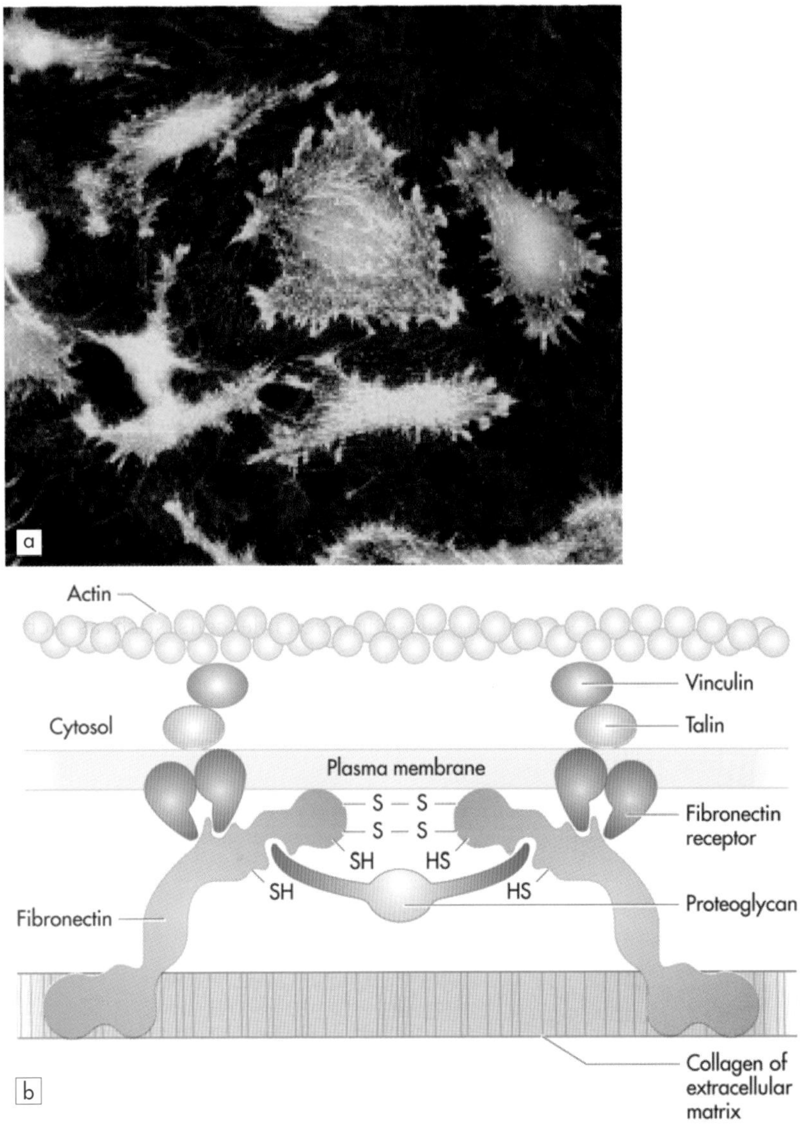

Figure 1.13 *(a) Histochemical illustration of the interrelationship between intracellular actin (stained yellow) and extracellular fibronectin (stained red). (b) The transmembrane linker protein complex. (Modified from Darnell J, Lodish H, Baltimore D. Molecular cell biology, second edition. New York: Scientific American Books, 1990.)*

Table 1.1 The principal features of adherens junctions for each of the main types.

Junctional complex	Type	Cytoskeletal element	Transmembrane linker glycoprotein	Intracellular attachment protein
Adhesion belt/ zonula adherens	Cell–cell	Microfilament	Cadherins	Catenins
Focal contacts/ adhesion plaques	Cell–matrix	Microfilament	Fibronectin receptor	Viniculin, talin, and α-actinin
Desmosome/ macula adherens	Cell–cell	Intermediate filament	Desmocollins and desmogleins	Plakoglobin and desmoplakins
Hemi-desmosome	Cell–matrix	Intermediate filament	Laminin receptor	?

Modified from Goodman SR. Medical cell biology. Philadelphia: JB Lippincott Company, 1994.

of cell adhesion molecule, which – like the cadherins – is calcium dependent, called an *integrin*. The integrins are a family of cell adhesion molecules of which one type helps bind cytoskeletal actin to matrix fibronectin. Another type is involved in the binding of intermediate filaments to other protein fibres in the extracellular matrix.

Intermediate filamentous junctions with adjacent cells

Intermediate filaments communicate with the intermediate filaments of adjacent cells by means of *spot desmosomes*. These have been likened to 'spot welds' or rivets and are relatively fixed, as are belt desmosomes and tight junctions.

Intermediate filamentous junctions with the extracellular matrix

Intermediate filamentous anchoring junctions to the extracellular matrix are called *hemi-desmosomes*. Here, the linker protein that joins the intermediate filament to the extracellular matrix is called *laminin*, and the specific protein in the extracellular matrix that laminin links to is type IV collagen in the basement membrane. The laminin receptor complex is another integrin. These anchoring junctions to the basement membrane and to the other proteins of the extracellular matrix are less fixed than anchoring junctions or spot desmosomes between adjacent cells, and the microfilamentous junctions to fibronectin are particularly mobile to allow cell movement in growth and repair and during inflammatory and immune responses. Adhesions should not be thought of as producing rigidity.

Communicating junctions

These are sometimes called *gap junctions*. Gap junctions are composed of protein subunits that connect the inside of one cell, across an 'intercellular gap', to the inside of the adjacent cell across both cell membranes (Figure 1.14). They behave as transmembrane ion channels, which undergo conformational change with the appropriate stimulus to give a central pore (Figure 1.14b), as described above. In this way, small molecules can move between cells and allow them to communicate with each other. This may also account for so-called 'cable properties' in the transmission of electrical impulses in excitable cells such as nerve and smooth muscle.

Because most of these adhesions are proteinaceous and calcium dependent, they are vulnerable to fluctuating extracellular calcium and to proteases – hence the importance of proteases and metalloproteases (which bind a metal as a catalyst), and collagenases in tumour invasion.

THE EXTRACELLULAR MATRIX

The extracellular matrix used to be thought of as an essentially inert ground substance in which cells lay, connecting one cell type to another and one tissue to

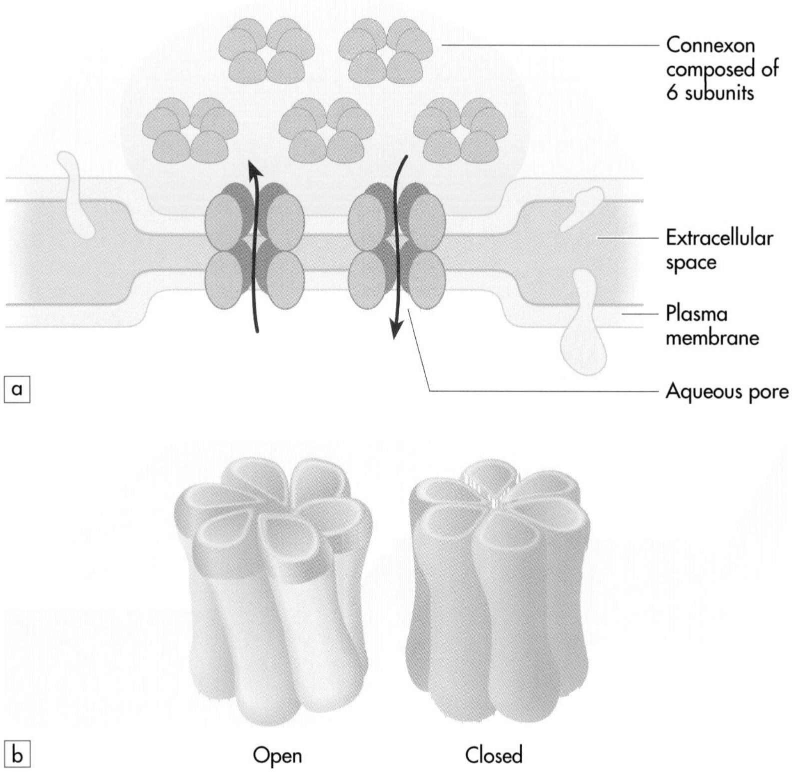

Figure 1.14 *A gap junction: (a) to show the general format, and (b) to show how conformational change of the connexon subunits allows the formation of a transcellular porous channel between neighbouring cells. (Modified from Darnell J, Lodish H, Baltimore D. Molecular cell biology, second edition. New York: Scientific American Books, 1990.)*

the next. It is nothing of the sort. Other than providing structural support, it is extremely important in growth, differentiation, nutrition and repair.

There are three principal components of the extracellular matrix: fibrous proteins, especially collagen; the glycosaminoglycans and proteoglycans; and the adhesive glycoproteins, especially laminin and fibronectin, mentioned above.

Collagen

Collagen gives the extracellular matrix tensile strength to resist stretch. It is the single most abundant protein in the animal kingdom and there are at least 12 types, all of which, except type IV, are fibrous and generally disposed in a cable structure. Types I, II and III are the most abundant. Type II is a particularly important component of cartilage. Types I and III go together and are almost ubiquitous as the main interstitial types in general connective tissue.

Type IV collagen is the main component of the basal lamina. It forms a mesh, which looks like chicken wire and which gives the basal lamina its structure (Figure 1.15). The basal lamina acts as a sheet to which epithelial cells are fixed by means of the specific receptor protein laminin and to which the fibrous proteins and other components of the underlying connective tissue are connected (Figure 1.16).

Glycosaminoglycans and proteoglycans

The principal glycosaminoglycan is *hyaluronic acid*. This is a very long compound composed of repeating disaccharide molecules. Although the most widespread of the glycosaminoglycans, it is different from the remainder, which are sulphated and linked to proteins to form the proteoglycans. These other glycosaminoglycans are chondroitin sulphate, dermatan sulphate, keratan sulphate, heparan sulphate and heparin. Like hyaluronic acid, the other glycosaminoglycans consist of repeating disaccharide molecules, but they are also highly negatively charged. This means that they tend to attract water and can thereby fill a lot of space in comparison with their actual size. Proteoglycans have the appearance

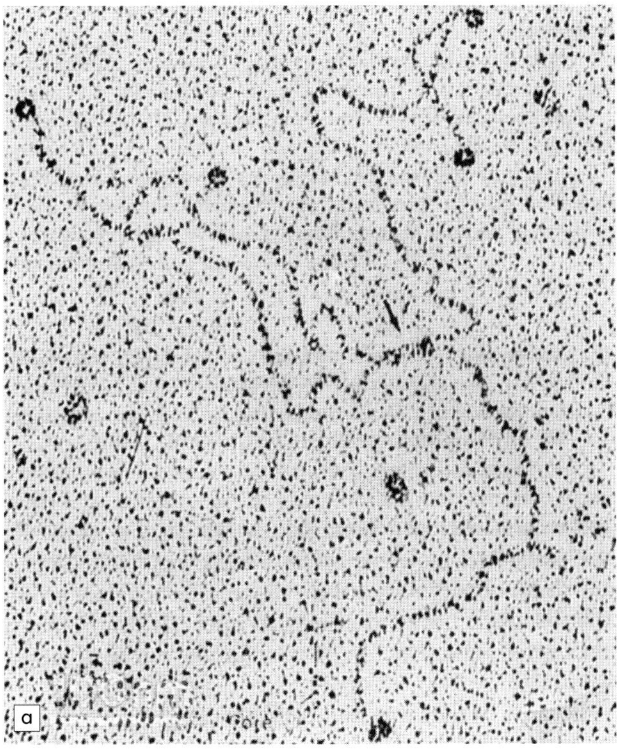
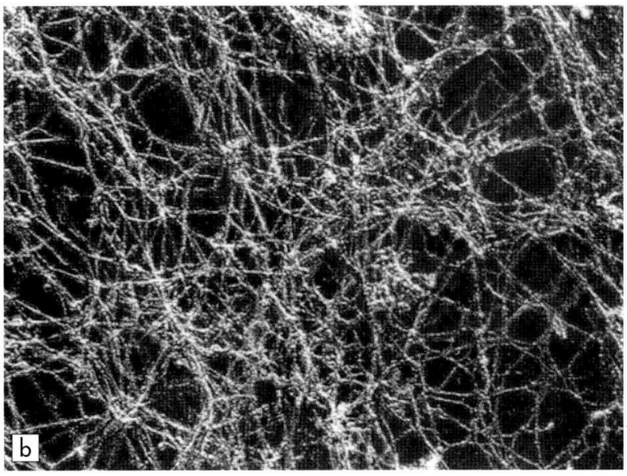

Figure 1.15 *(a) The general appearance of a type IV collagen molecule. (b) The general appearance of type IV collagen molecules bound together – like a chicken-wire mesh – to form basement membrane. (Modified from Darnell J, Lodish H, Baltimore D. Molecular cell biology, second edition. New York: Scientific American Books, 1990.)*

of a bottlebrush in which the core protein is the handle and the glycosaminoglycans are the bristles. They help to anchor cells to matrix fibres, binding to types I and II collagen and to fibronectin. In turn, proteoglycans often bind to hyaluronic acid, also 'bottlebrush' fashion, giving two levels of organization of these molecules (Figure 1.17).

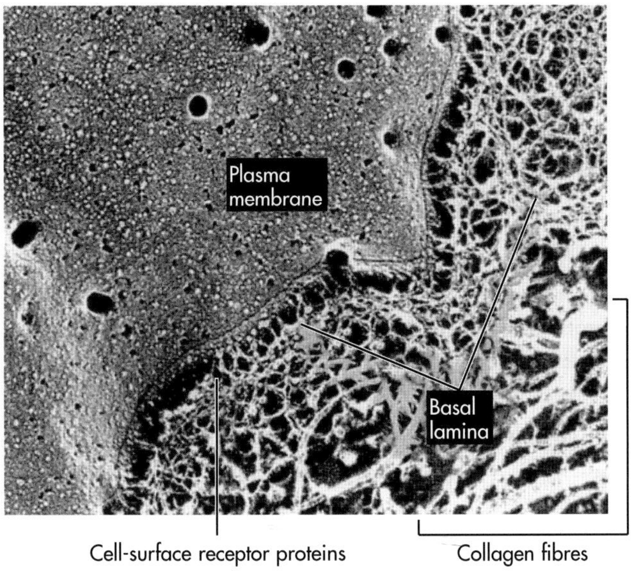

Figure 1.16 *The relationship between a cell and the type IV collagen fibres of the basal lamina. (Modified from Darnell J, Lodish H, Baltimore D. Molecular cell biology, second edition. New York: Scientific American Books, 1990.)*

Like collagen, the glycosaminoglycans provide structural support to the extracellular matrix, but whereas collagen gives tensile strength to resist stretch, the glycosaminoglycans help resist shearing strains and compression. Cartilage is obviously the best example. The glycosaminoglycans tend to keep cells apart and, by virtue of this and their lattice-like structure, they allow the rapid diffusion of nutrients, waste products and signalling molecules through the extracellular matrix. This filtering role is particularly prominent in the kidney, where those of the extracellular matrix are largely responsible for glomerular filtration. Many of them, particularly heparan sulphate and heparin, bind and activate various growth factors (see below), especially *fibroblast growth factor*. In this role, they act both to protect the so-called *heparin binding growth factors* (of which fibroblast growth factor is the best example) against degradation by sequestering them away from the reach of proteolytic enzymes, and also as co-factors to facilitate binding to high-affinity receptors on the cell membrane.

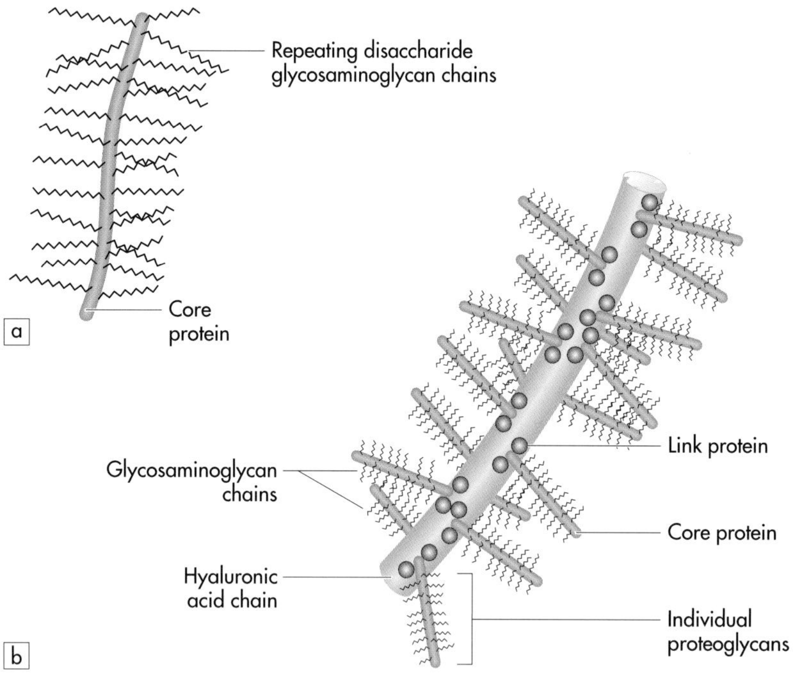

Figure 1.17 *A proteoglycan showing (a) the 'bottlebrush' structure, with glycosaminoglycan chains as the 'bristles' attached to the core protein, and (b) the further 'bottlebrush' structure with individual proteoglycans, as in (a), attached to the central hyaluronic acid chain. (Modified from Alberts B, Bray D, Lewis J et al. Molecular biology of the cell, second edition. New York: Garland Publishing, 1989.)*

Adhesive glycoproteins

The two main adhesive glycoproteins are laminin and fibronectin. Laminin binds type IV collagen of the basal lamina to the plasma membrane and to the intermediate filaments of the cytoskeleton through cell-surface laminin receptors and also by means of receptors on both components for heparan sulphate. Fibronectin binds to everything except type IV collagen, principally to actin in the cytoskeleton using cell-surface fibronectin receptors and transmembrane linker proteins as an intermediary. Fibronectin also binds to fibrous collagen and other extracellular matrix proteins.

Both these glycoproteins help maintain the structural integrity of the extracellular matrix, but they also facilitate the movement of nutrients and waste products and in addition allow cell movement in growth, repair and during inflammatory and immune responses. The fibronectin receptor, in particular, allows mobility so that inflammatory and immune cells (for example) can reach out pseudopodia to make contact with fibronectin and then pull themselves along fibronectin fibres to reach their destination by virtue of the mobility of connections made both on the cell membrane and on the fibronectin fibre. In a similar way, fibronectin promotes cell migration during embryogenesis and healing by providing tracks along which the cells can migrate.

Glycoproteins on the cell surface are also important in immune reactivity (described in Chapter 24).

THE BASEMENT MEMBRANE

Viewed under the electron microscope, the basal lamina consists of two layers: the lamina rara, which consists of laminin and the proteoglycans that are interposed between the cell membrane itself; and the lamina densa, which is the two-dimensional reticulum of type IV collagen. The lamina lucida (or rara) and lamina densa together form the basal lamina, but in many circumstances there is a third layer – the lamina reticularis – which is the underlying connective tissue component. These three laminae together constitute the basement membrane (Figure 1.18).

The basement membrane, in addition to providing a means by which nutrient, waste and signalling molecules can be transported and cell migration can occur (as described above), is also important in cellular differentiation. In embryogenesis in particular, the mesenchyme – the basal lamina, extracellular

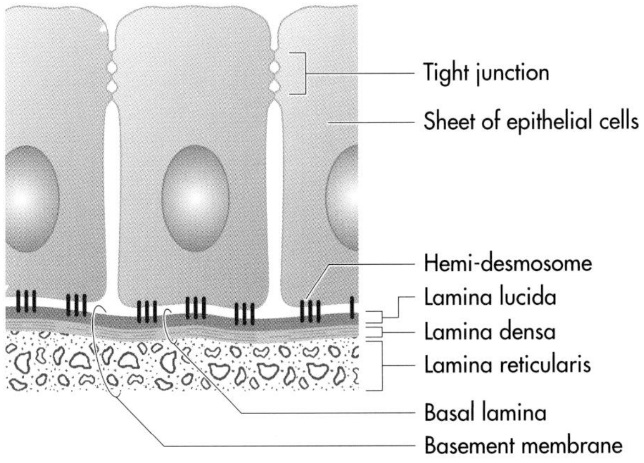

Figure 1.18 *The structural organization of the basal lamina and the basement membrane. (Modified from Alberts B, Bray D, Lewis J et al. Molecular biology of the cell, second edition. New York: Garland Publishing, 1989.)*

matrix and mesodermal cells – is essential. Without the underlying dermal mesenchyme, the overlying 'skin' cannot differentiate into nails, hairs or the cornea, nor can it simply differentiate into thin skin or thick skin. Cunha's studies on prostatic epithelium show that even differentiated epithelium can be 'redifferentiated' in the presence of embryonic mesenchyme; in his experiments, mature bladder epithelium in the presence of male urogenital sinus mesenchyme developed into prostatic epithelium (Figure 1.19).

Similarly, without attachment to fibronectin, smooth muscle cells change from their differentiated phenotype, which contracts, to an undifferentiated proliferative phenotype. For similar reasons, explanted cells grown in vitro tend to group together so that a mixed group of kidney cells, liver cells and other cells will separate out into groups of specific types even when the cell types come from different species. In part, this is because of growth factor binding to the basal lamina and other components of the extracellular matrix, but there are undoubtedly other factors and the details are as yet unknown.

CELL TO CELL COMMUNICATION

Reference has been made already to cellular adhesion mechanisms and, through the medium of the extracellular matrix, to some of the mechanisms of cell migration. Reference has also been made to the possibility of cell to cell communication through gap (communicating) junctions. Cells also communicate together, locally, by so-called *autocrine* or *paracrine* mechanisms (Figure 1.20). In autocrine

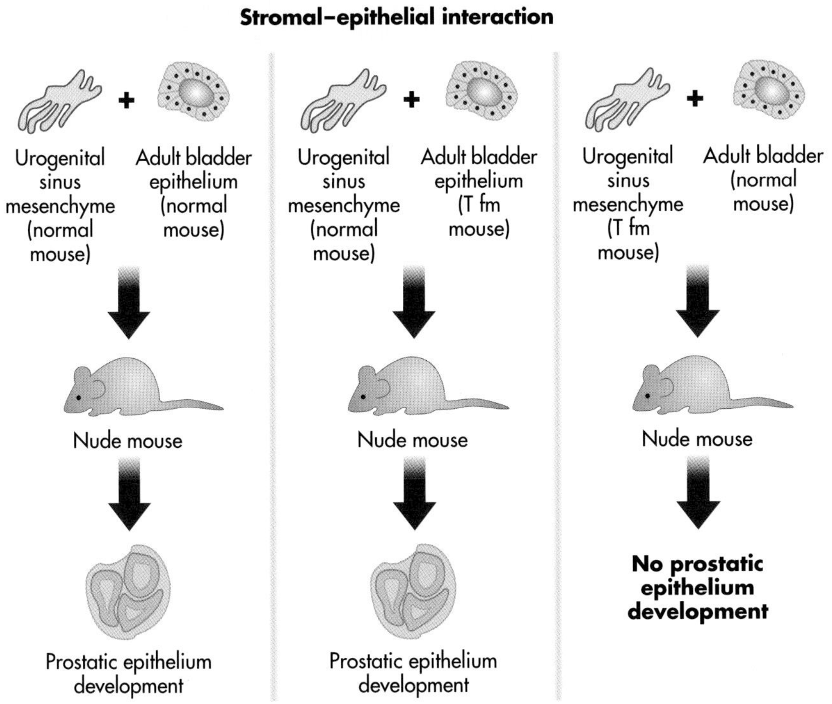

Figure 1.19 *Cunha's experiments. Three experiments are illustrated to show that normally functioning urogenital sinus mesenchyme induces the differentiation or redifferentiation of epithelium so that it develops into prostatic epithelium. Tfm = testicular feminization syndrome (mice with androgen receptor deficiency).*

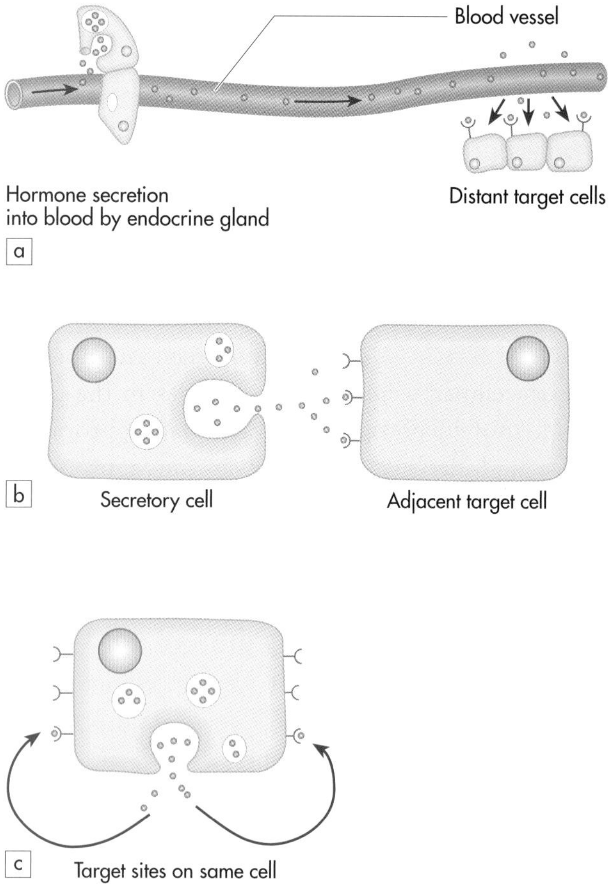

Figure 1.20 *The differences between (a) endocrine, (b) paracrine and (c) autocrine signalling.* ∘ *Extracellular signal;* Y *receptor.*

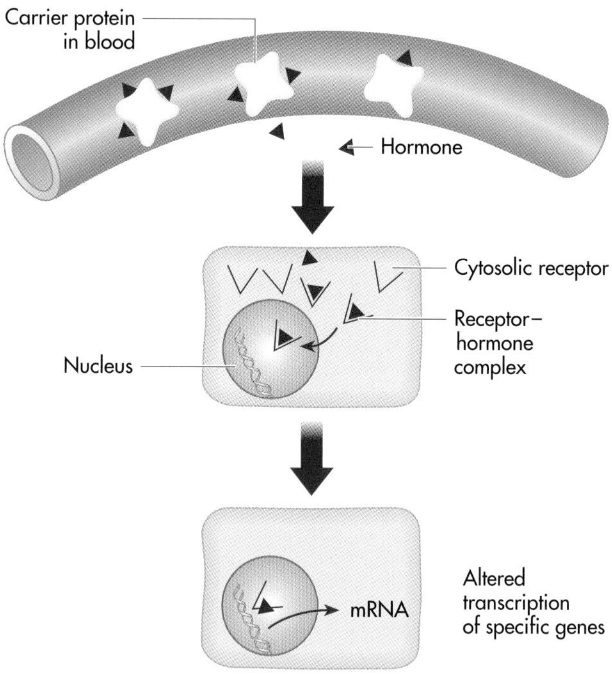

Figure 1.21 *The transport mechanism for small lipid-soluble molecules with intracellular receptors. Being lipophilic, these small molecules require transport by carrier proteins in the blood but, at their target site, dissociate from these carriers and diffuse across the cell membrane with ease. In the cytosol they bind to their specific receptors and the receptor–hormone complex then acts on nuclear DNA. (Modified from Darnell J, Lodish H, Baltimore D. Molecular cell biology, second edition. New York: Scientific American Books, 1990.)*

signalling, a cell is stimulated through receptors on its cell membrane by signalling molecules it has produced and secreted itself. In paracrine signalling, the same molecules diffuse out into the extracellular space and extracellular matrix and act on cell surface receptors of the cells close by. The best and most specialized example of paracrine signalling is across the neuromuscular junction, but in general the features are very similar to those of endocrine signalling but over very much smaller distances and by means of compounds produced by all cells rather than by highly specialized 'glands'.

CELL TO CELL SIGNALLING

Gap junctions and adhesive junctions are not considered any further here and only brief reference is made to neurotransmission as this is discussed in a later chapter. The main point of this section is to discuss how the huge range of extracellular stimuli act across the cell membrane to regulate enzymes or genes with a similarly wide range of outcomes. The mechanism is surprisingly simple. The very numerous extracellular stimuli have an equally large range of receptors on the cell surface but the transmembrane signalling and intracellular transmission systems of these signals are very much fewer in number. With the exception of the steroid hormones and a few other substances that are lipid soluble and can therefore cross the cell membrane with ease (Figure 1.21), most of the remaining signals are transmitted by water-soluble molecules that bind to very specific receptors on the cell surface. There are thousands of these specific receptors, but they transmit their signals through to the interior of the cell by only a few transmembrane signalling mechanisms, which in turn activate just a few intracellular second messenger systems (Figure 1.22). These

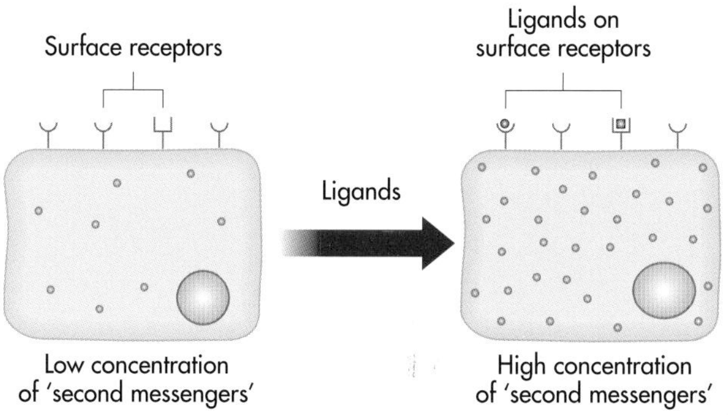

Figure 1.22 *The transport mechanism for large water-soluble molecules by means of cell surface receptors and second messenger systems. These do not need carrier proteins in the blood because they are water soluble, but for the same reason cannot cross the cell membrane – hence the need for the surface receptor/second messenger system. (Modified from Darnell J, Lodish H, Baltimore D. Molecular cell biology, second edition. New York: Scientific American Books, 1990.)*

second messenger systems activate proteins, most of which are enzymes, generally by a process of *phosphorylation*. Phosphorylation involves the activity of protein *kinases* that transfer phosphate groups (usually from ATP) onto the substrate protein, thereby activating it. This activity is in turn 'switched off' by specific *phosphatases* that remove the phosphate group, thereby greatly reducing the activity of the protein/enzyme. Whether the end result of an extracellular signal is gene activation in the nucleus or extracellular secretion from vesicles in the cytoplasm, protein phosphorylation by an appropriate kinase and dephosphorylation by an appropriate phosphatase are the most common end result of signal transduction (Figure 1.23).

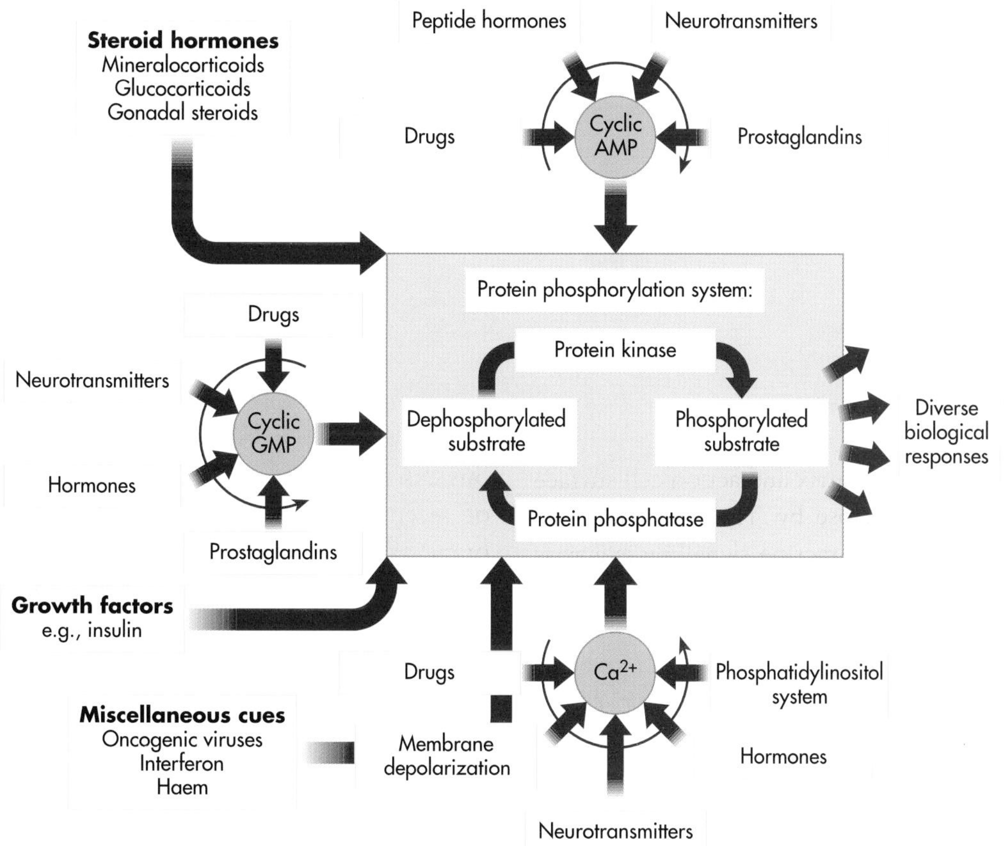

Figure 1.23 *The importance of phosphorylation and dephosphorylation in cellular mechanisms. (Modified from Goodman SR. Medical cell biology. Philadelphia: JB Lippincott Company, 1994.)*

EXTRACELLULAR STIMULI

There is a vast range of extracellular stimuli that excite human cells, from light falling on the retina to a sperm cell penetrating an ovum, but the majority fall into one of two types. The commonest are large, hydrophilic molecules that react directly and with high affinity to cell surface receptors, which in turn activate second messengers in the cytosol, which in turn leads to the intracellular changes characteristic of that particular stimulus.

Secondly, there are small, lipophilic molecules, typically the steroid hormones, that diffuse through the plasma membrane and bind to receptors within the cytosol or the nucleus. These molecules generally act to control the transcription of DNA or the stability of mRNA. Typically, the steroid receptor molecule is in two parts that are hinged so that the receptor becomes folded in on itself, thus concealing the DNA-binding *domain* of the receptor (Figure 1.24). This closed-hinge position is maintained by a steroid inhibitor protein such as a heat shock protein. When the relevant steroid binds to the hormone binding site on the hormone binding domain of the receptor, this causes the steroid inhibitor protein to be displaced and the hinge opens (i.e. there is a conformational change), so that the receptor molecule opens up, exposing the DNA-binding domain so that it can bind to DNA – to the so-called hormone-responsive element – to initiate transcription (Figure 1.25).

CELL SURFACE RECEPTORS

Much more commonly, extracellular stimuli are in the form of larger hydrophilic molecules that, because they are hydrophilic, cannot cross the lipid cell membrane in the way that steroid hormones can. These need to have a system for transmembrane signal transduction to the interior; this system begins with the cell surface receptor.

Receptors come in two main types. The first and simpler type is a single molecule with three functional components or *domains*. The first, or external, domain is an outward-facing recognition site; the second is the transmembrane domain in the middle, which traverses the cell membrane; and the third, or cytosolic, domain is the inward-facing component of the molecule on the interior of the cell, which initiates a mechanism for the onward transmission of the stimulus to the interior (Figure 1.26). This

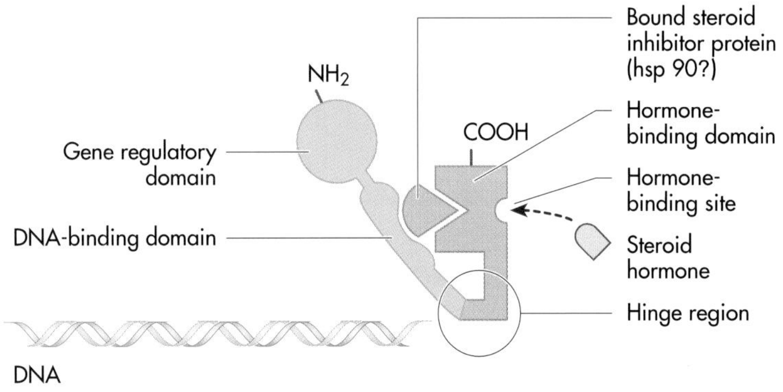

Figure 1.24 *A steroid hormone receptor and receptor activation (i). (Modified from Goodman SR. Medical cell biology. Philadelphia: JB Lippincott Company, 1994.)*

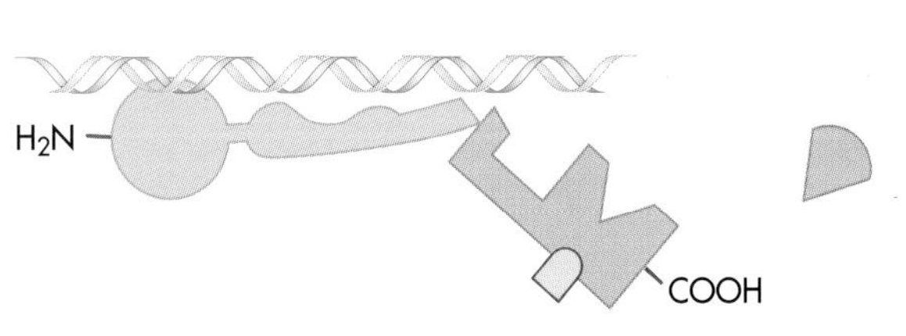

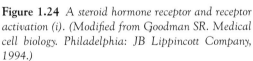

Figure 1.25 *A steroid hormone receptor and receptor activation (ii). Binding of the steroid hormone causes the receptor to 'open up' at its hinge region, allowing it to bind to its appropriate DNA binding site. (Modified from Goodman SR. Medical cell biology. Philadelphia: JB Lippincott Company, 1994.)*

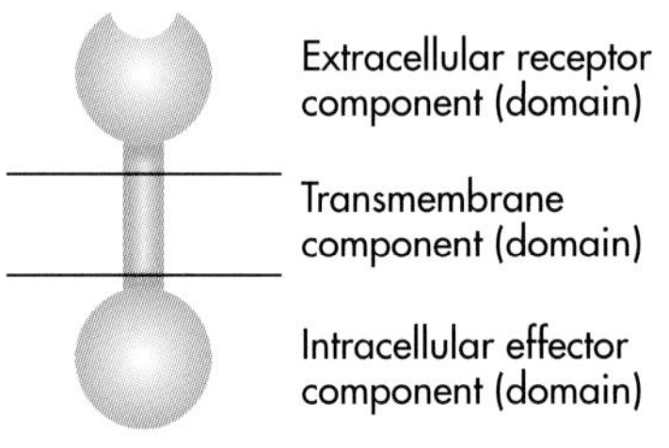

Figure 1.26 *Stylized form of a simple type of transmembrane receptor. (Modified from Darnell J, Lodish H, Baltimore D. Molecular cell biology, second edition. New York: Scientific American Books, 1990.)*

mechanism for onward transmission may be to open a channel for ions to pass through to the interior, as in the case of a *ligand-gated ion channel* like the nicotinic acetylcholine receptor (Figure 1.27), or it may be a kinase (referred to above), which acts by phosphorylating a substrate protein. An example of this latter type of receptor is one with *tyrosine kinase* activity such as the *epidermal growth factor receptor* (Figure 1.28).

The other main type of receptor system is a relay system in which, rather than having a single receptor molecule to change the extracellular stimulus to an intracellular stimulus, there is a relay consisting of a receptor protein molecule, a coupling protein and an effector protein (Figure 1.29) These receptor proteins, many of the coupling proteins and some of the effector proteins are integral cell membrane proteins referred to earlier in this chapter. In effect, each of the three domains of the simpler receptor system described in the last paragraph is here represented by a separate protein molecule.

In this type of system, the receptor protein is in an inactive state until it binds its highly specific stimulatory molecule (the ligand), which it binds with high affinity. Ligand binding activates the receptor, which allows it to activate its specific coupling protein (Figure 1.30). Because the plasma membrane is a fluid gel and because the integral proteins of the cell membrane, including receptor proteins, are mobile, the ligand–receptor complex can activate several coupling proteins. This is the first step in amplifying the stimulus. Many of the coupling proteins are known as *G-proteins* because they have guanosine triphosphatase (GTPase) enzymic activity. The G-protein has three

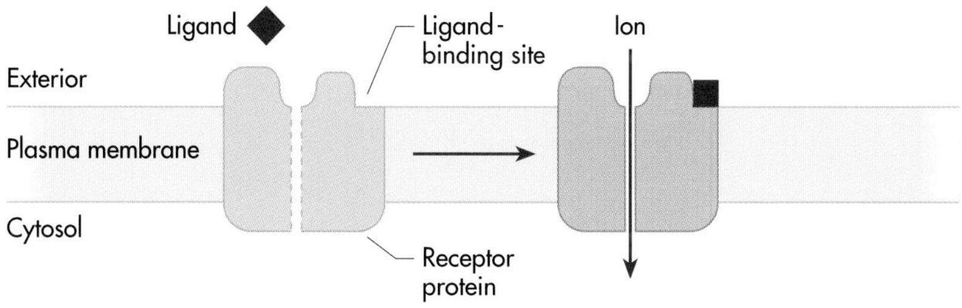

Figure 1.27 *A ligand-gated ion channel such as the nicotinic acetylcholine receptor at a nerve–muscle junction. (Modified from Darnell J, Lodish H, Baltimore D. Molecular cell biology, second edition. New York: Scientific American Books, 1990.)*

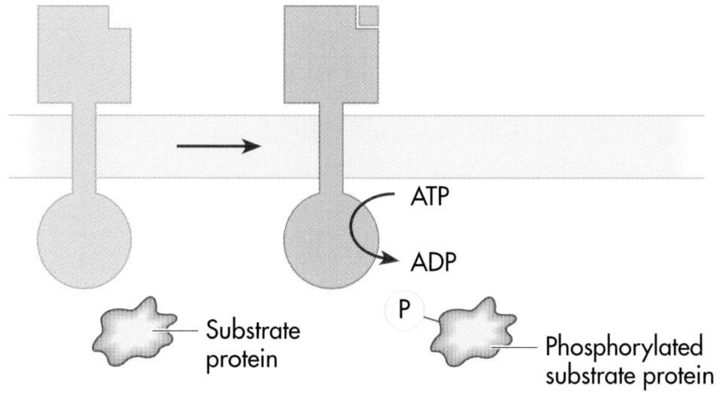

Figure 1.28 *A ligand-gated tyrosine kinase receptor such as the epidermal growth factor receptor. (Modified from Darnell J, Lodish H, Baltimore D. Molecular cell biology, second edition. New York: Scientific American Books, 1990.)*

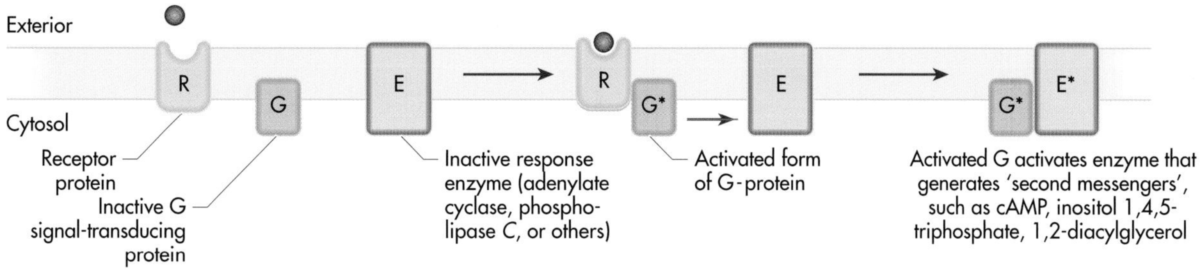

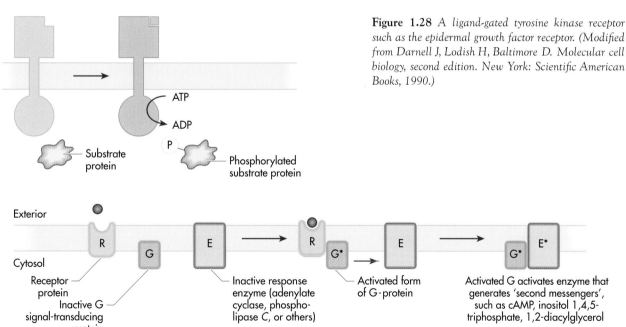

Figure 1.29 *A G-protein-linked receptor. (Modified from Darnell J, Lodish H, Baltimore D. Molecular cell biology, second edition. New York: Scientific American Books, 1990.)*

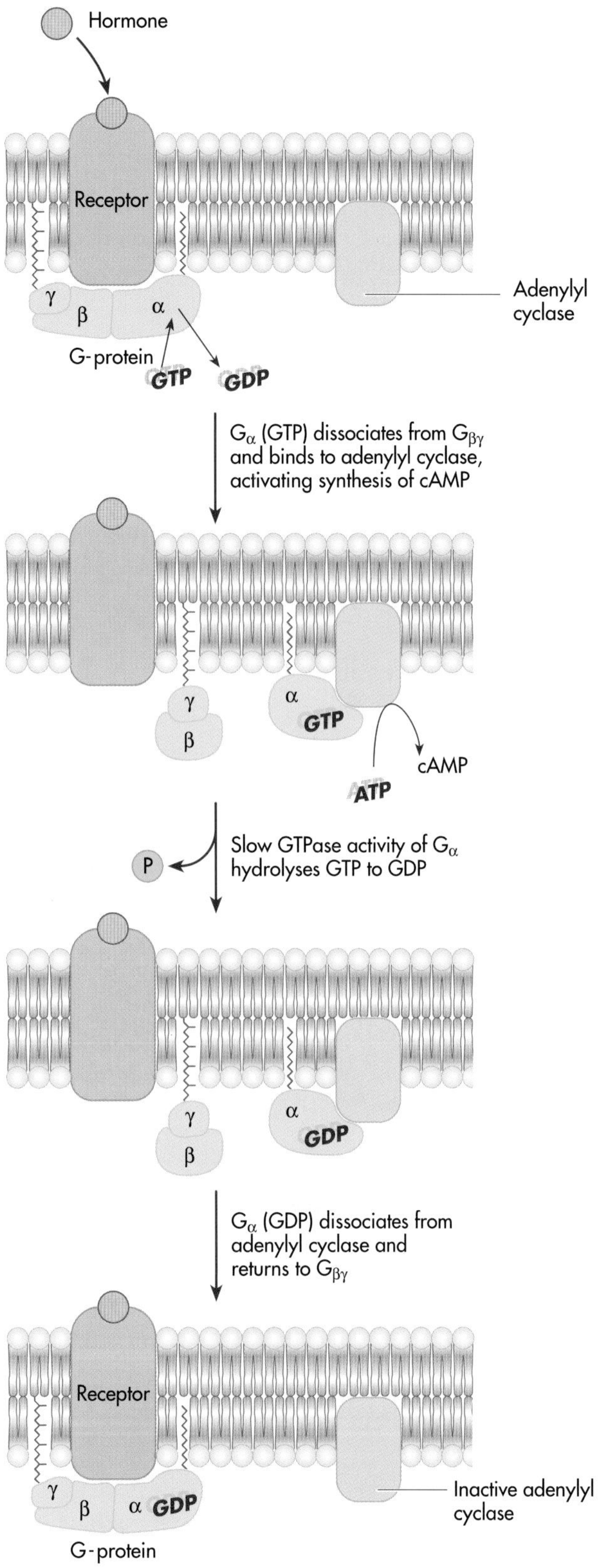

Figure 1.30 *Activation of a G-protein-linked receptor, in this case an adrenoceptor in which the effector is adenylyl cyclase. (Garrett RH, Grisham CM. Molecular aspects of cell biology. Fort Worth: Harcourt Brace College Publishers, 1995.)*

subunits, one of which – the alpha subunit – has a guanosine diphosphate (GDP) molecule bound to it in the inactive state. Binding (coupling) of the ligand–receptor complex to the G-protein catalyses the conversion of intracellular guanosine triphosphate (GTP) to GDP. This enzymatic conversion of GTP to GDP transfers a phosphate molecule from the intracellular GTP molecule onto the GDP molecule of the alpha subunit of the G-protein, which activates this alpha subunit by converting its own GDP molecule to GTP, thus causing it to separate off from the combined beta-gamma subunit of the G-protein and bind to the effector protein, to which it remains bound until its GTP molecule is hydrolysed back to GDP. When this happens, the alpha subunit of the G-protein dissociates from the effector molecule and recombines with the beta-gamma subunit to restore the G-protein to its unified, inactive state. It is this latter phenomenon that gives this relay system the additional feature of self-limiting duration. The system is only active in stimulating the effector protein for the short period that the alpha subunit of the G-protein is activated by having its GDP molecule phosphorylated to GTP. As soon as the GTP reverts to GDP, the system switches itself off.

To recapitulate, the three features of this system are:

1. as with all types of receptor, there exists a common system for onward transmission of a stimulus in which only the receptor molecule needs to be specialized for its own particular ligand
2. there is an in-built mechanism for amplification of the signal to guarantee a significant cellular response to the initiating signal
3. there is a mechanism for switching the signal off so that the whole process is self-limiting.

From these observations, one can readily extrapolate the three ways in which the mechanism can break down in a disease such as cancer:

1. if the ligand-binding process goes wrong, becoming persistent rather than transient
2. if the amplification process goes wrong, again becoming persistent rather than transient
3. if the switch-off mechanism goes wrong, so that it remains switched on.

There are various different types of *G-protein-coupled receptors*. In some, the effector protein is the enzyme *adenylyl cyclase*. When this is the case, the G-protein may be stimulatory, activating the adenylyl cyclase enzyme, or inhibitory, having the opposite effect (Figure 1.31). In such cases, we have the same effector molecule – adenylyl cyclase – but a different type of G-protein switching it on and off. Examples of receptors that activate adenylyl cyclase are the beta-1 and beta-2 adrenergic receptors. The alpha-2 adrenergic receptor inhibits it. The action of the adenylyl cyclase enzyme is to break down ATP to cyclic adenosine monophosphate (cyclic AMP or cAMP). Cyclic AMP in turn initiates chemical reactions that are specific to the cell type, in which role it is functioning as a second messenger molecule.

Sometimes, the effector protein in a G-protein-coupled receptor is an ion channel such as the hyperpolarizing potassium channel opened by the M2 muscarinic receptor. In this circumstance, the alpha subunit of the activated G-protein binds to the effector molecule, which then undergoes a conformational change so that it develops a central pore through which potassium ions flow from one side of the cell membrane to the other.

Many receptors, including the muscarinic receptor, have several simultaneous and complementary effects (Figure 1.32).

Another important effector molecule is the enzyme *phospholipase* C (Figure 1.33). This molecule breaks down phosphatidylinositol 4,5-biphosphate (PIP_2), which is derived from one of the membrane phospholipids, phosphatidylinositol, referred to at the beginning of this chapter. Splitting PIP_2 liberates

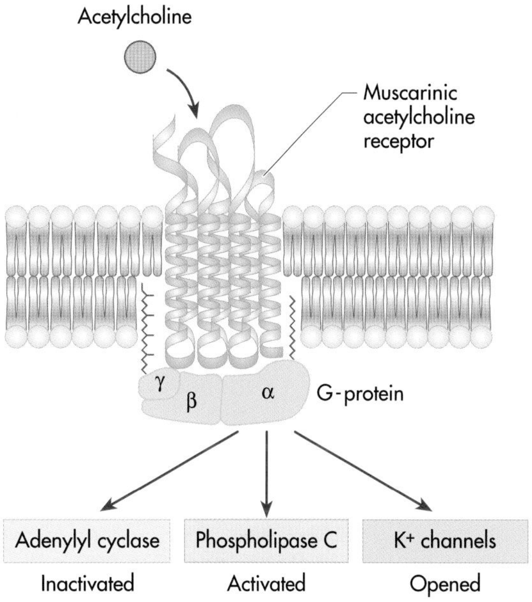

Figure 1.32 *Various actions of the muscarinic acetylcholine receptor. (Garrett RH, Grisham CM. Molecular aspects of cell biology. Fort Worth: Harcourt Brace College Publishers, 1995.)*

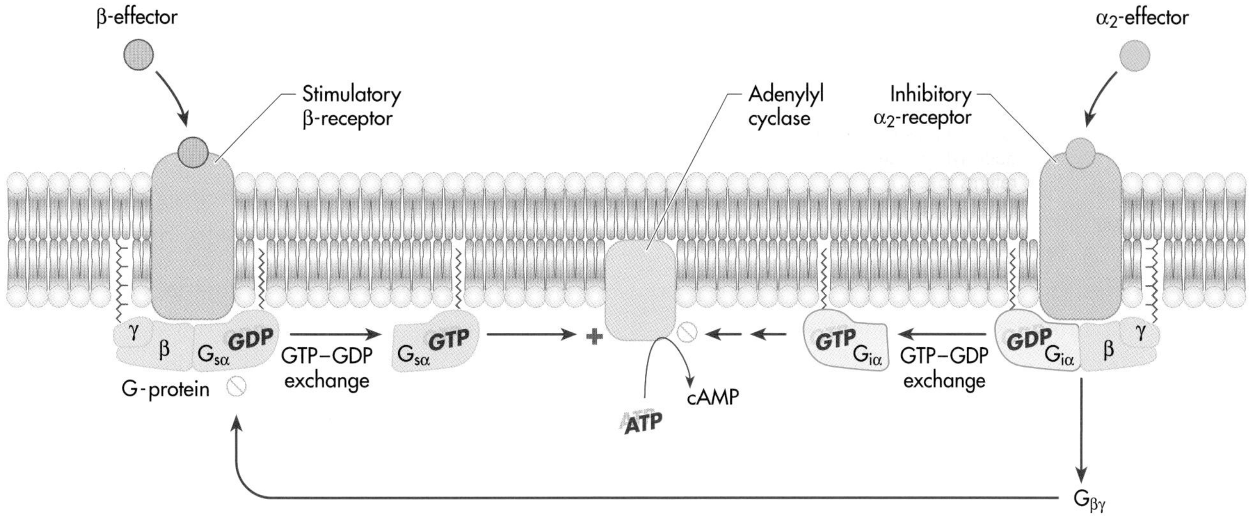

Figure 1.31 *Effector activity – in this case adenylyl cyclase activity – can be modulated by the interplay of stimulatory (Gs) and inhibitory (Gi) G-proteins, in this case the β-receptor and α_2-receptor, respectively. (Garrett RH, Grisham CM. Molecular aspects of cell biology. Fort Worth: Harcourt Brace College Publishers, 1995.)*

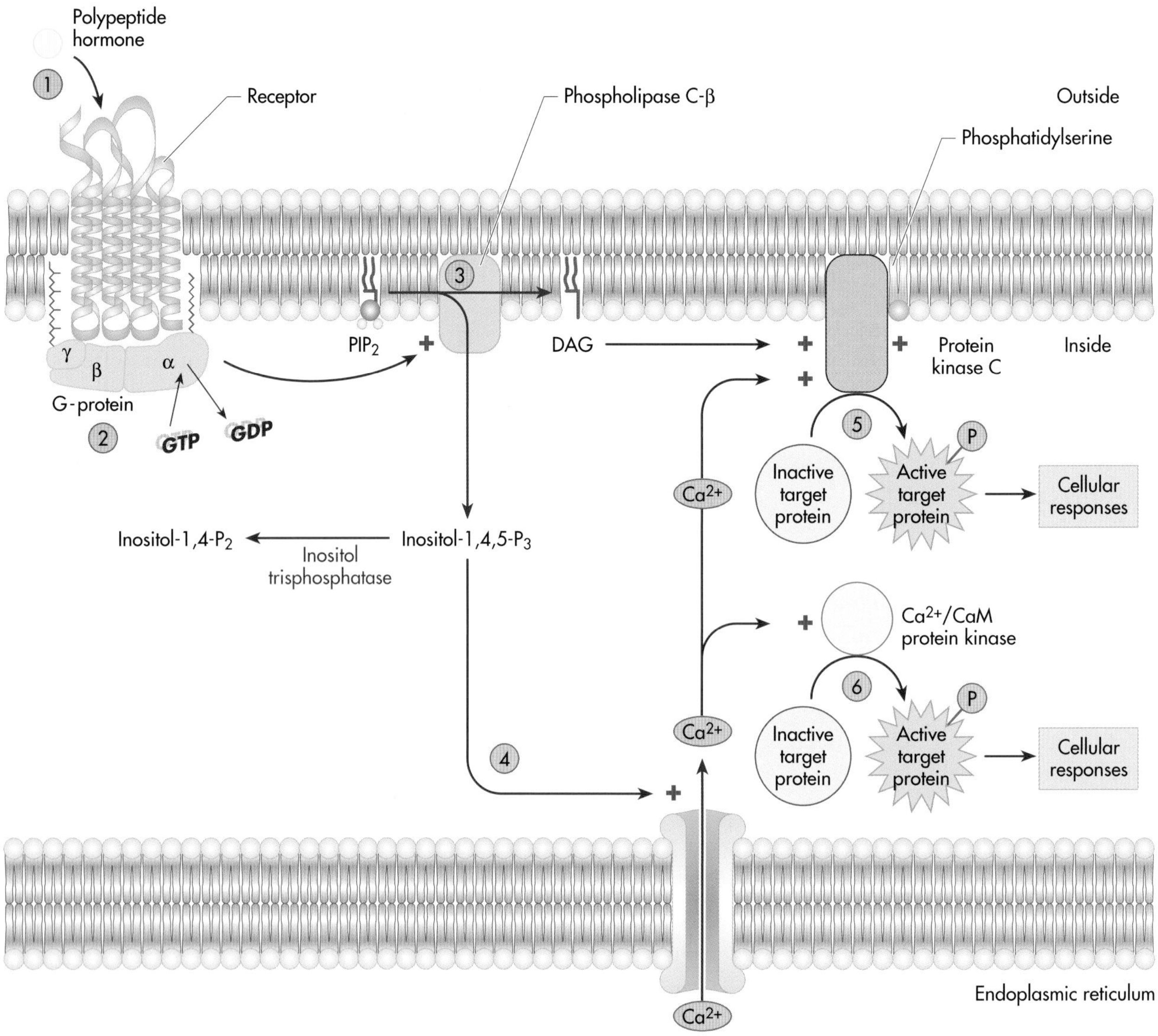

Figure 1.33 *IP_3-mediated signal transduction pathway and the central role of phospholipase C-β. (Modified from Garrett RH, Grisham CM. Molecular aspects of cell biology. Fort Worth: Harcourt Brace College Publishers, 1995.) (1) The receptor is activated by ligand binding. (2) This activates its G-protein, which in turn activates (3) phospholipase C-β. This has two effects: firstly (4), the production of inositol-1,4,5-triphosphate which binds to calcium channel receptors on the endoplasmic reticulum to cause the liberation of calcium (Ca^{2+}). The second action of phospholipase C-β is to stimulate by means of diacylglycerol (DAG), in conjunction with calcium. (5) Protein kinase C activates its particular target proteins, and calcium bound with calmodulin activates its own target proteins (6), and both produce appropriate cellular responses.*

two molecules, both of which are second messengers. The first is *inositol 1,4,5-triphosphate* (IP_3), which is active within the cytosol as a second messenger, and the second is *1,2-diacylglycerol* (DAG), which remains membrane bound in its role as a second messenger. IP_3 acts to release calcium, which is itself a second messenger, from intracellular stores.

All of these second messenger systems – cyclic AMP, cyclic guanosine monophosphate (GMP), DAG, IP_3, and calcium – have many different effects but in any particular system those effects are governed by the type of cell that is stimulated. Calcium, for example, will make muscle cells contract, the epithelial cells of the salivary glands secrete, and the cells of the islets of Langerhans in the pancreas produce insulin, to give but a few examples. Cyclic AMP will cause the breakdown of glycogen in liver cells, where its action is stimulatory, and will cause smooth muscle cells to relax, in which case its action is inhibitory. Thus, a very small number of second messenger systems can produce different effects according to the cell type that they are being generated in.

The reader should also bear in mind that examples are largely being chosen to illustrate the subject from a urological perspective. In a book with a different readership in mind, different examples would be given and the emphasis would be placed on the second messengers, receptor types and extracellular stimuli appropriate to that alternative perspective.

INOSITOL TRIPHOSPHATE AND CALCIUM

These are two very important second messengers, particularly with respect to detrusor smooth muscle as rises in intracellular calcium are the basis of detrusor smooth muscle contraction. The liberation of IP_3 from PIP_2 in the cell membrane by the action of phospholipase C following activation of phospholipase C by its appropriate G-protein in response to ligand binding of the receptor molecule has already been described. In the case of detrusor contraction, the ligand is acetylcholine and the receptor molecule is the M3 muscarinic receptor. The IP_3 thus liberated binds to receptor proteins on intracellular calcium stores. These receptors are ligand-gated ion channels that release stored intracellular calcium into the cytosol. As with other second messenger systems, the binding of IP_3 to its receptor is highly specific but of short duration and lasts only until the IP_3 is metabolized to inactive IP_2. Whilst the IP_3 is bound to its receptor, calcium is released from intracellular stores into the cytoplasm. When IP_3 is converted to IP_2, the calcium channel closes off and the IP_2 is recycled to IP_3.

To replenish intracellular calcium stores and also further to increase intracellular calcium, some IP_3 is metabolized to IP_4, which opens cell membrane calcium channels from the inside. These let calcium in from outside the cell.

In addition to its own actions, calcium activates the DAG liberated in the same chemical reaction that produced its 'parent' IP_3 but which has been left in the cell membrane. DAG in turn activates a protein kinase – protein kinase C – which produces an array of intracellular responses by phosphorylating various substrate proteins (see below and also Figure 1.33).

The calcium liberated into the cytosol is bound to a protein called *calmodulin* and it is the calcium–calmodulin complex, thereby activated (Figure 1.34), that produces the effect rather than calcium itself in most instances. In smooth muscle, calcium–calmodulin produces contraction, but the reader should remember that in other systems calcium–calmodulin produces other effects, as referred to above.

The system of smooth muscle contraction is described in Chapter 6 (Figure 1.35). It should be noted at this stage that this excitatory system that starts with IP_3 in smooth muscle is inhibited by adenylyl cyclase and cAMP in the same system, and so we see another feature of the second messenger system – that almost all of the second messengers are interrelated to modulate the final response of the

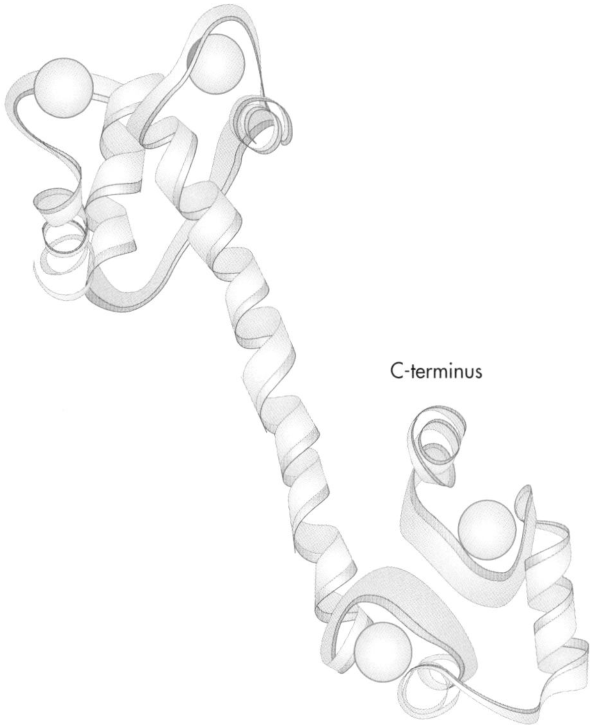

Figure 1.34 *Structure of calmodulin as deduced from crystallographic analysis of the calcium–calmodulin complex. The blue spheres are bound calcium ions. (Modified from Darnell J, Lodish H, Baltimore D. Molecular cell biology, second edition. New York: Scientific American Books, 1990.)*

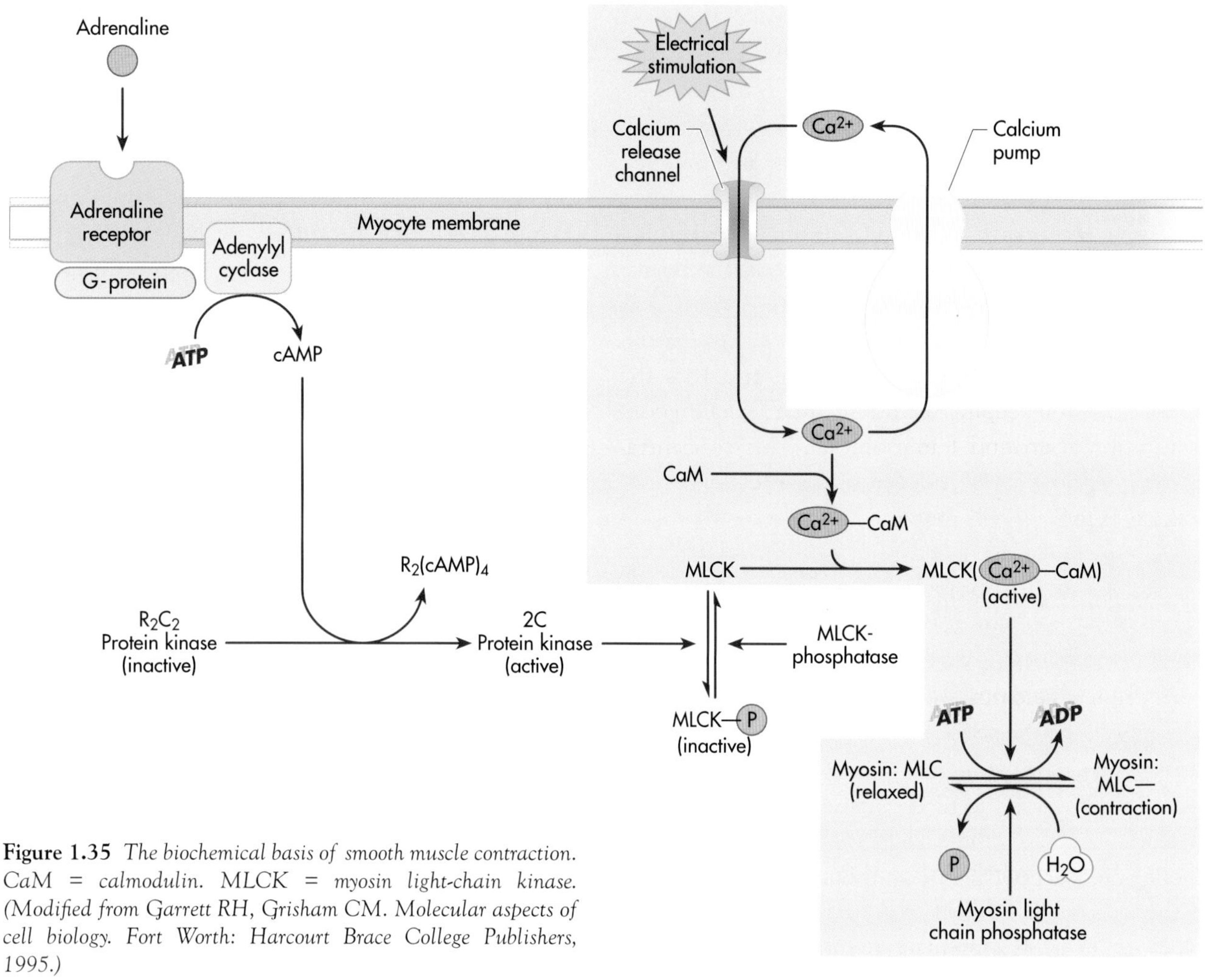

Figure 1.35 *The biochemical basis of smooth muscle contraction. CaM = calmodulin. MLCK = myosin light-chain kinase. (Modified from Garrett RH, Grisham CM. Molecular aspects of cell biology. Fort Worth: Harcourt Brace College Publishers, 1995.)*

cell. Not only is each signal transduction system specific, amplifying and self-regulatory, but stimulatory and inhibitory systems interact at several points to produce a finely tuned response. A description or illustration in a book is two dimensional and generally shows just one reaction taking place. In real life, most reactions depend upon a critical amount of stimulus producing the appropriate response by producing the relevant intracellular changes at the right time and for the correct duration. The system described here does just this. To recapitulate with an example: when a single neuronal impulse travels down a terminal nerve ending to the detrusor, an aliquot of about 5000 acetylcholine molecules is liberated from the axonal terminus at each neuromuscular junction to bind with the same number of receptor molecules on the smooth muscle cell membrane. This process is repeated as long as nerve impulses are being generated. Because the muscarinic receptor protein is mobile within the cell membrane, each ligand–receptor complex within the neuromuscular junction activates several G-proteins, maybe a dozen or so, before the acetylcholine is displaced or metabolized. Each activated G-protein probably only activates one phospholipase C molecule, but until the alpha subunit of the G-protein is deactivated again, each phospholipase C molecule will catalyse the breakdown of several molecules of PIP_2 – again, maybe a dozen or more. Each PIP_2 molecule liberates a molecule of IP_3 (and a molecule of DAG) which in turn liberate a considerable number of calcium ions and activate several molecules of protein kinase C, respectively. The calcium liberated in the former reaction helps to potentiate the activation of the protein kinase C in the latter reaction and the liberation of calcium not only produces its own effect –

contraction – through further intracellular activity, but also opens membrane calcium channels to let more calcium in, to potentiate the response and to refurbish the intracellular calcium stores.

One factor that makes calcium so important as an intracellular ion is its presence in the cytosol in such low concentrations. Whereas there are ten-fold to 20-fold differences in sodium concentration and 30-fold to 40-fold differences in potassium concentration across the cell membrane, there is a 10 000-fold difference in calcium ion concentration across the cell membrane keeping the intracellular calcium concentration at around 1 micromolar. This concentration is so low that even a few calcium ions released into the cytosol will make a large difference in the concentration. The calcium concentration is kept so low by active pumping of calcium either out of the cytosol and out of the cell altogether through the cell membrane, or out of the cytosol and into intracellular calcium stores where it is sequestered and bound to the sequestering protein *caldesmon* (as described above).

OTHER COMPOUNDS DERIVED FROM MEMBRANE PHOSPHOLIPIDS

The reader will appreciate the importance of the enzyme phospholipase C and the products of its reaction with the membrane phospholipid phosphatidylinositol. Another important phospholipase enzyme – phospholipase A_2 – also acts on membrane phospholipids, in response to a wide range of stimuli, to produce the *eicosanoids*. The eicosanoids are three groups of compounds: the *prostaglandins*, the *thromboxanes* and the *leukotrienes* (Figure 1.36). The parent molecule produced by the action of phospholipase A2 is *arachidonic acid*, which is a polyunsaturated fatty acid. The eicosanoids are all lipid-soluble, freely diffusible, oxygenated molecules with effects, in general terms, that are associated with inflammation, injury and nociception.

The prostaglandins are the best-known products of the arachidonic acid cascade. They are lipid-soluble molecules that are unusual in that they bind to cell surface receptors rather than diffuse through the cell membrane like other small, lipophilic molecules such as the steroid hormones. There are 16

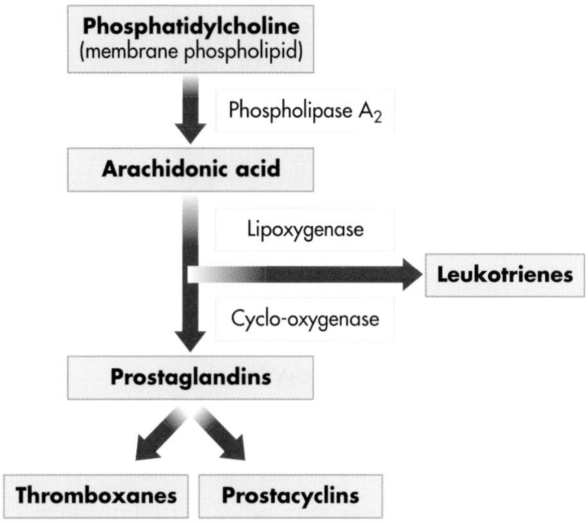

Figure 1.36 *The eicosanoids and their derivation from arachidonic acid.*

prostaglandins in nine classes designated PGA to PGI, although the latter are generally known as the prostacyclins. The prostaglandins and thromboxanes, which are prostaglandin derivatives, are synthesized and secreted continuously by many cells. They act locally in both an autocrine and a paracrine fashion and are broken down by enzymes in the extracellular fluid.

TYROSINE KINASE RECEPTORS

These have already been referred to as a fairly simple form of signal transduction system in which the same molecule has an extracellular domain for receptor binding, a transmembrane component and an intracellular domain that acts as a tyrosine kinase to phosphorylate tyrosine residues on substrate protein. These are very unusual: most residues on intracellular proteins that generate a second messenger response are either serine or threonine residues; tyrosine residues are unusual. They are of particular interest, though, because they are the principal receptors for the so-called *growth factors*. The intracellular response to the tyrosine kinase receptors is not entirely clear but involves the *ras* protein, which is a sort of G-protein, and *raf* protein, which is activated by reaction with the *ras* protein to activate intermediaries which in turn activate the so-called *mitogen-activated protein kinase* (MAP kinase), which phosphorylates a number of transcription factors including the *fos*, *myc* and *jun* proteins to initiate gene transcription (see below).

Thus, whereas most of the other receptors described produce an intracytoplasmic response appropriate to the cell type, such as contraction or secretion, the tyrosine kinase receptors tend to lead to cell division – they are *mitogenic*.

GROWTH FACTORS

There is a large number of known growth factors and this number has been growing exponentially in recent years. There is a wide variety of different chemical types of growth factors, all of which include among their actions the ability to stimulate cell proliferation, which may be the only feature they have in common. It is important to appreciate that all growth factors have other effects besides stimulation of cell proliferation and that they are no more related than members of a football team who put on the same shirt once a week when they actually play football.

Growth factors were initially identified in serum as the factors necessary to grow cells in culture – hence their collective name – where growth refers to expansion of number rather than increase in size. It has always been known that serum is necessary to allow cells to replicate in culture rather than just survive, and because plasma does not have the same effect, it was assumed that the relevant factor(s) was liberated from platelets during the process of clotting. As a result, one of the first growth factors to be identified was called *platelet-derived growth factor* (PDGF). Insulin was also known to be necessary for the growth of cells in culture. Slowly, other factors were identified so that it is now possible to grow certain cell types with individual growth factor ingredients specific to that cell type rather than adding whole serum (although this is much cheaper and simpler).

The various growth factors are wildly dissimilar in many ways, but it was observed that groups of two or three or more often produced a similar sort of response, and so growth factors became grouped into families. Most growth factors in a family have molecules which are three-dimensionally similar and it is thought that this three-dimensional similarity means that there are chemical or physico-chemical regions on the molecules that produce the functional effect and give similarity in action to members of the same family group. Thus, in the *epidermal growth factor* (EGF) family (EGF being one of the first growth factors to be identified), *transforming growth factor alpha* (TGFα) has similar actions and a similar three-dimensional structure to EGF (Figure 1.37).

It should also be noted that the names given to these growth factors relate to the effect originally observed rather than to their current family grouping or to any other effects that they may have. Thus, for example, it was observed that two factors were acting in a particular experiment to cause cells to grow in the centre of an agar gel without any physical attachment, a condition which hitherto had been thought to be necessary for cell growth. Because the factors had caused the cells to be 'transformed' in this way, they were called TGFα and TGFβ. It later became clear that TGFα and TGFβ had completely different properties, and are accordingly classified in completely different families, but together shared the common factor of causing transformation in that particular experimental design. Hence, some of the confusion about growth factors.

One of the other confusing points about the subject of growth factors is that in a normal individual we tend to regard tissues as essentially static and fail

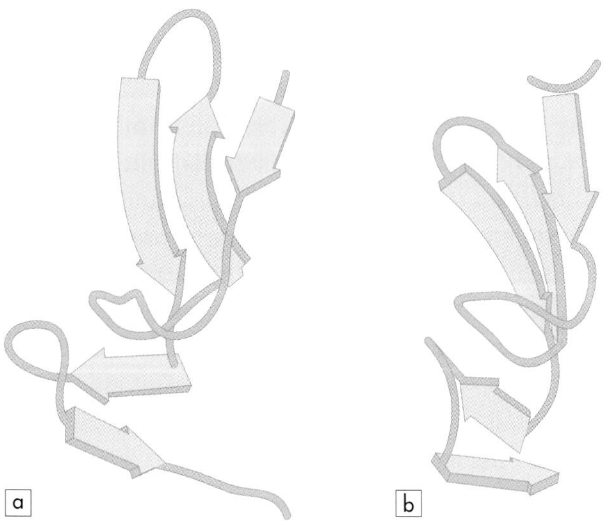

Figure 1.37 *The three-dimensional similarity of (a) epidermal growth factor (EFG) and (b) transforming growth factor alpha (TGFα). (Redrawn from Heath JK. Growth factors. Oxford: IRL Press, 1993.)*

sometimes to appreciate that there is cell death and cell division producing a net turnover of zero to achieve that static effect. Cell growth is not necessarily associated with neoplasia. Growth factors are therefore important in health. They are, of course, particularly important in healing, inflammation, the immune response and more so still in embryogenesis, in which they have been particularly widely studied, especially in the nervous system.

The growth factor families that are discussed later on in this volume include the EGF family, the fibroblast growth factor (FGF) family, the TGFβ family, the insulin-like growth factor (IGF) family and the PDGF family. The characteristic feature of all of these is that they are polypeptides that are produced locally in tiny concentrations and act in an autocrine fashion on the cells that produced them or in a paracrine fashion on their neighbouring cells. Different growth factors may be produced by different cells in a tissue or by the same cells under differing circumstances, and another characteristic feature is that there tend to be several factors that act to limit their release or the response to their release and thereby control their actions.

A final problem is that we understand comparatively little about them. Our knowledge is largely based on a collection of isolated facts in experimental models. To give the best idea of how growth factors work, one has to slip from urology to haematology and observe haemopoiesis, in which a number of growth factors act to produce a co-ordinated proliferation of multiple cell types derived from a set of common precursor cells in a series of steps. The system of haemopoiesis is itself by no means fully understood, but it is clear that specificity of action on each cell type is the key to the system as different growth factors act at different stages to produce the different responses that end up in a perfectly co-ordinated system. Presumably, other organs are subject to equally complex and possibly hierarchical controls involving a large number of growth factors released in sequence to act in specific ways at specific times to produce the required end result. In this way, the apparently multiple and seemingly unrelated actions of many of the growth factors in vitro may be carefully controlled in vivo in terms of their release, effects and duration of response.

It is clearly important that mechanisms exist to control the release and effect of these potent agents. EGF and TGFα are localized in their effects because their precursor molecules are transmembrane proteins that are therefore fixed in position. EGF is still more localized in its action because it is only produced in a very small number of organs, principally the submaxillary gland and the kidney, although once secreted it can have effects elsewhere such as, in the case of renal EGF, in the remainder of the urinary tract. TGFα, which is from the same family and has very similar effects, is more widely distributed.

The activity of the FGF family is restricted in its effects in a different way. Some members of the FGF family are not secreted and can only be released by cell death, so although they are almost ubiquitous, their effects are tightly controlled by circumstances. Even then, basic FGF is only active when bound to heparin in the extracellular matrix, which thereby not only activates it but also sequesters it from enzymic degradation. Furthermore, the effects of various members of the FGF family are different at different times of life – acidic FGF is active in early life and basic FGF later on.

Whereas most growth factors stimulate cellular proliferation, the members of the TGFβ family are different. They are secreted in an inactive or 'latent' form that must be activated – another example of growth factor control. They generally modulate the activity of other growth factors and are often inhibitory, but are nonetheless capable of inducing anchorage-independent growth – the property known as transformation referred to above, which gives the family its name.

The receptors for the various growth factors confer cell-type specificity on the growth factors and their intracellular effects. Tyrosine kinase receptors have been referred to already and the EGF, PDGF, FGF and IGF receptors are all of this type. They stimulate transcription through the *ras* and *raf* proteins, mitogen-activated protein kinase and the various nuclear transcription factors such as the fos, jun and myc proteins, which activate genes in a time-dependent sequence leading to the synthesis of DNA and the passage of the cell through the cell cycle, ultimately to cell division (see below). The mechanism by which this happens is important to understand because it illustrates how precisely the system has to function to produce its intended effects and so illustrates how it might be therapeutically manipulated – for example, in the treatment of cancer.

Using the EGF receptor as an example, the first step is the binding of the ligand (EGF) to the receptor (Figure 1.38), which in the inactive state is a monomer, causing adjacent monomers to *dimerize*, that is, to form pairs. Dimerization of the receptor monomers causes autophosphorylation of tyrosine residues on the cytosolic domain of the receptor molecule, thereby activating the molecule. The next step is the activation of the *ras* protein, which requires two events: firstly the GDP on the inactive

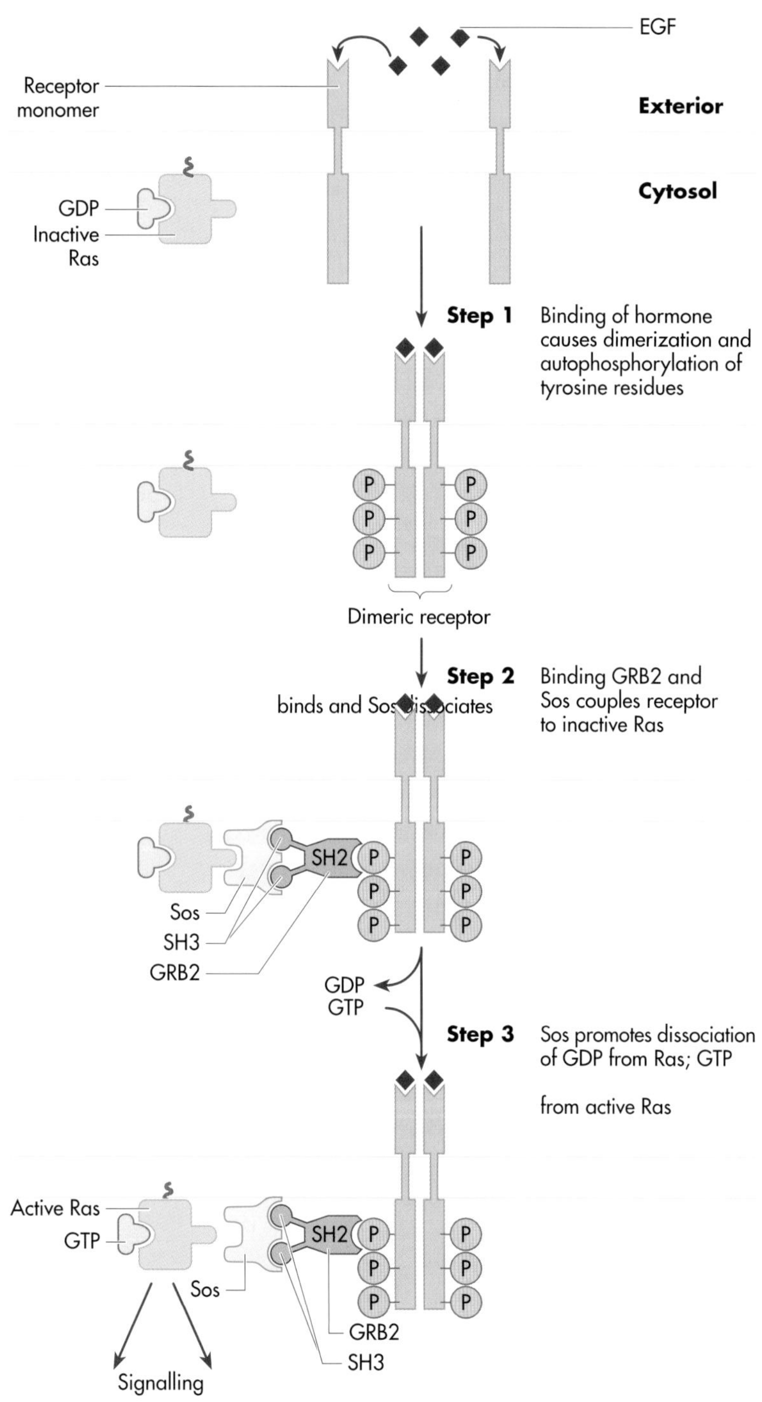

Figure 1.38 *The activation of ras following the binding of EGF by means of the intermediates GRB2 and Sos. (Modified from Darnell J, Lodish H, Baltimore D. Molecular cell biology, second edition. New York: Scientific American Books, 1990.)*

ras molecule must be replaced by GTP, which is done by a guanine nucleotide exchange factor, in this case a molecule called Sos, which itself requires an adapter protein (GRB2) to bind it to the cystosolic domain of the EGF receptor; and, secondly, the *ras* molecule must be bound to the inner aspect of the cell membrane by a biochemical bonding to membrane phospholipids called *farnesylation*. If farnesylation could be inhibited, preventing the localization of *ras* to the inner aspect of the cell membrane, then activation of *ras* and its mitogenic effects could be inhibited.

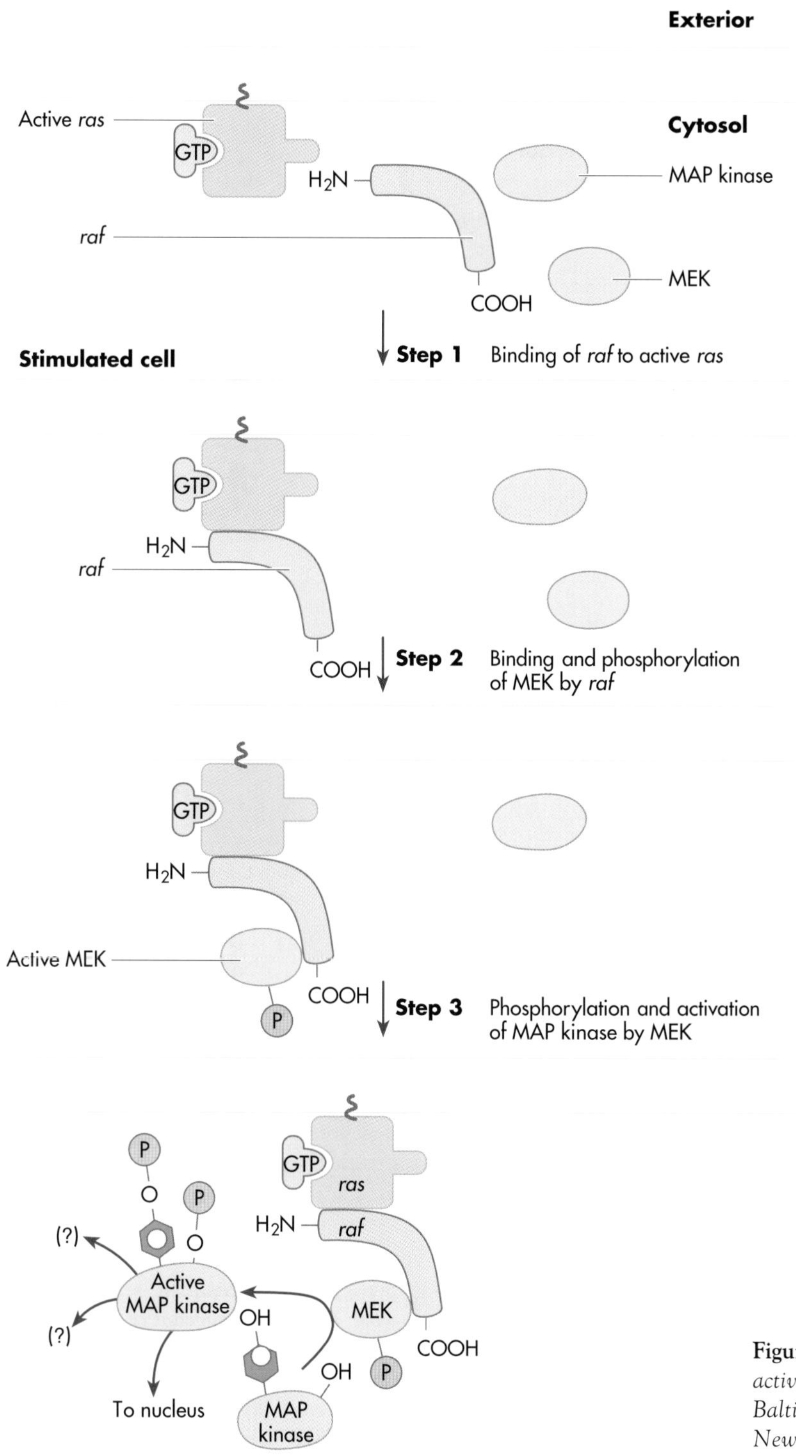

Figure 1.39 *Activation of* raf *and MAP kinase by activated* ras. *(Modified from Darnell J, Lodish H, Baltimore D. Molecular cell biology, second edition. New York: Scientific American Books, 1990.)*

The activated *ras* molecule then binds and thereby activates *raf*, which must also occur in relation to the cell membrane. *raf* then binds and phosphorylates a mitogen-activated protein (MAP) kinase called MEK, which in turn activates another mitogen-activation protein kinase that is actually called MAP kinase (Figure 1.39). MAP kinase is a serine/threonine kinase that phosphorylates transcription factors in the nucleus such as *fos*, *jun* and *myc*, which in turn leads to gene transcription, as described in the next chapter (Figure 1.40 and Table 1.2).

Another substrate of tyrosine kinase, other than the G-protein-like *ras* protein, is a particular type of phospholipase C that generates inositol triphosphate and diacylglycerol leading to the activation of protein kinase C. Protein kinase C is a serine/threonine kinase and a potent mitogen, although its substrates and mode of action are unclear. It is also not clear what part, if any, inositol triphosphate has in the mitogenic process.

Specific growth factors are discussed in later chapters with regard to specific circumstances.

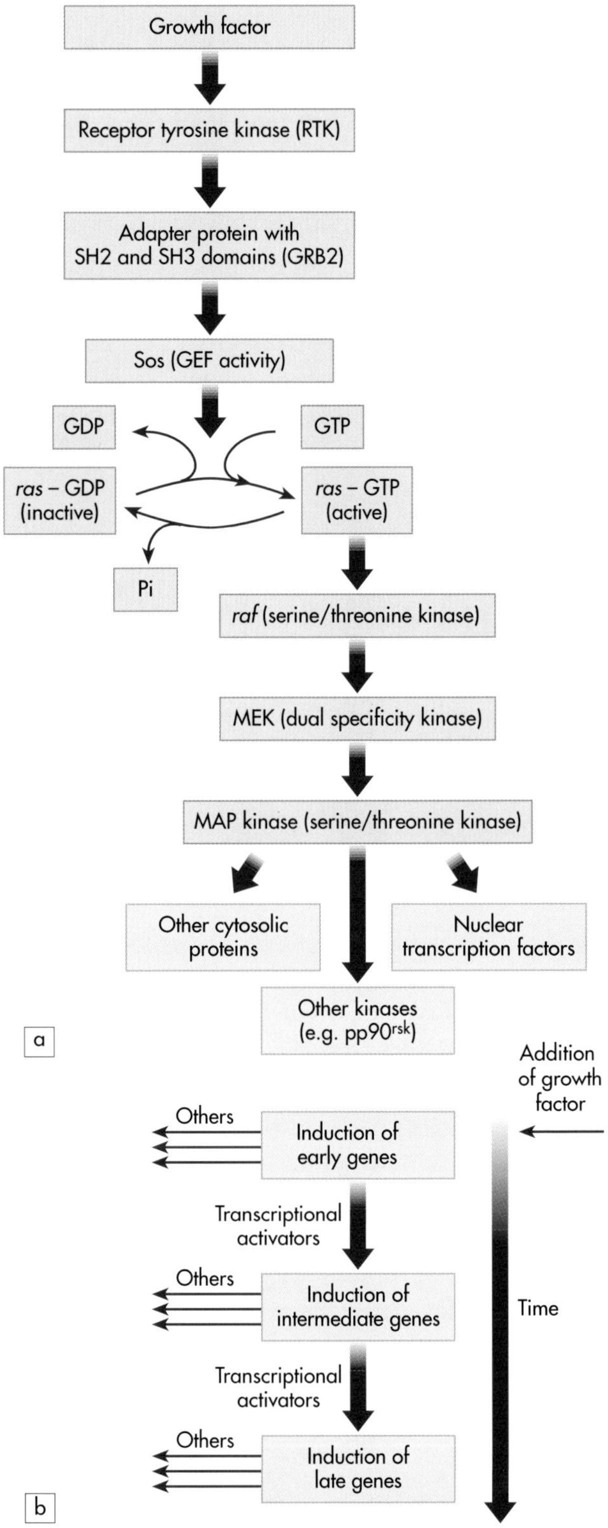

Figure 1.40 *(a) An overview of the growth factor/tyrosine kinase cascade. (Modified from Darnell J, Lodish H, Baltimore D. Molecular cell biology, second edition. New York: Scientific American Books, 1990.) (b) Activation of nuclear transcription factors illustrating the sequence of activation. (Taken from Heath JK. Growth factors. Oxford: IRL Press, 1993.)*

Table 1.2 The growth factor/tyrosine kinase cascade: the relevant genes activated and their function.

Genes	Function
Early	
c-fos	
Krox-20	
Krox-24	Transcription factors
Fra-1	
c-myc	
Intermediate	
Collagenase	Metalloprotease
JE	Cytokine
Cathespin L	Protease
Osteopontin	Extracellular matrix protein
Fibronectin	Extracellular matrix protein
TIMP	Protease inhibitor
Late	
Dihydrofolate reductase	Nucleotide metabolism
Histone H4	Chromatin structure
Thymidine kinase	Nucleotide metabolism

From Heath JK. Growth factors. Oxford: IRL Press, 1993.

APOPTOSIS

Finally, after considering cell growth, we turn to a consideration of cell death and of 'programmed cell death' in particular. This is one of the four ways in which a cell can respond to an appropriate signal; the other three being proliferation, differentiation and hypertrophy. The role of apoptosis in health is principally in modelling and re-modelling tissues in various different ways throughout life.

The process originally referred to as programmed cell death was first observed in fetal life. Although fetal and emobryonic life are largely characterized by enormous cell growth it has always been clear that cell death was necessary at selected times and in response to specific stimuli to account for the breakdown of various membranes for the canalization of solid cords of cells to form tubes and for the regression of whole tubular systems such as the Mullerian or Wolffian duct systems. The need for tissue re-modelling in post natal and adult life is not nearly so striking but nonetheless evident. Perhaps the most striking urological example is the shrinkage of the prostate in response to castration and in surgery in general in the re-modelling of surgical wounds during healing.

This process of programmed cell death has distinct morphological features that distinguish it from the other main type of cell death – necrosis. Further characterization of this pathological process was associated with the development of the new name 'apoptosis' which is the Greek term to describe a leaf falling off a tree in autumn.

In necrosis the characteristic feature is the disruption of the cell membrane, associated with swelling of the cell and swelling and disintegration of the intracellular organelles. Leakage of cytosolic material into the surrounding tissue then sets up an inflammatory reaction. In apoptosis there is cellular shrinking rather than cellular swelling and this occurs as a consequence of a process rather like exocytosis (called 'blebbing') in which small amounts of cytosole are extruded through the cell membrane which remains intact throughout the process. There is no local inflammatory response. Intracellular organelles condense and fragment and finally the cell detaches from its neighbours by degrading its adhesive molecules until all that remains is a so-called 'apoptotic body' which is disposed of either by extrusion into the lumen if it is within a tubular structure or by phagocytosis if it is part of a solid organ.

The process of apoptosis is regulated by both gene products that promote it and other gene products that suppress it. The mechanism is not entirely clear and is the subject of intense scrutiny at the moment but it appears that the main pro-apoptotic regulator is *p53*. This was one of the first tumour suppressor genes to be characterized and acts as a transcription factor that controls the expression of other factors that block cell cycle progression in the G1 phase (see Chapter 2). It is also an important factor in promoting apoptosis in response to certain stimuli. The exact role it has is not clear but it may be by activating bax (see below) and a cell surface protein called fas and other similar molecules. The final executors of the apoptotic process appear to be a family of catalytic enzymes called caspases.

The main anti-apoptotic factor appears to be bcl-2. This appears to act by binding bax which is a closely related protein. bax, which we have already mentioned is a promoter of apoptosis, acts to disrupt the mitochondrial membrane and bcl-2 therefore stabilizes mitochondrial membrane by binding bax.

By preventing apoptosis bcl-2 may be very important in, for example, prostate cancer progression in the hormone-resistant state and in other aspects of oncogenesis and in benign prostatic hyperplasia as well.

FURTHER READING

Garrett RH, Grisham CM. Molecular aspects of cell biology. Fort Worth: Harcourt Brace College Publishers, 1995

Goodman SR. Medical cell biology. Philadelphia: JB Lippincott Company, 1994

Heath JK. Growth factors. Oxford: IRL Press, 1993

Lodish H, Baltimore D, Berk A, Zipursky SL, et al. Molecular cell biology. New York: Scientific American Books, 1995

2

The cell and cell division

David E Neal

STRUCTURE OF THE CELL

Cell membrane

The cell membrane confines the contents of the cell. It consists of a continuous bilayer of phospholipid with the polar hydrophilic ends forming the outer and inner layers and the hydrophobic tails forming the central core of the bilayer. The hydrophilic heads on the two sides of the cell membrane are of different composition, those on the outside often being modified by glycosylation: a process that involves the addition of various sugar residues. Embedded in this lipid bilayer are proteins whose function can be classified as follows:

- Signal transduction (mediating the action of external ligands such as growth factors and neurotransmitters). These receptor proteins cross the cell membrane and may have intrinsic enzyme functions (such as the tyrosine kinase activity of the receptor for epidermal growth factor) or may be linked to other proteins such as G proteins (for example, the muscarinic acetylcholine receptor) (Figure 2.1).
- Cell–cell or cell–matrix contact. Specialized junctions between cells and between cells and the intercellular matrix occur, involving transmembrane proteins such as integrins and cadherins that interact on the outside with molecules such as fibronectin, and on the inside with molecules such as catenin, talin and vinculin that act as intermediate links to the cell skeleton, which is made of actin fibres. These

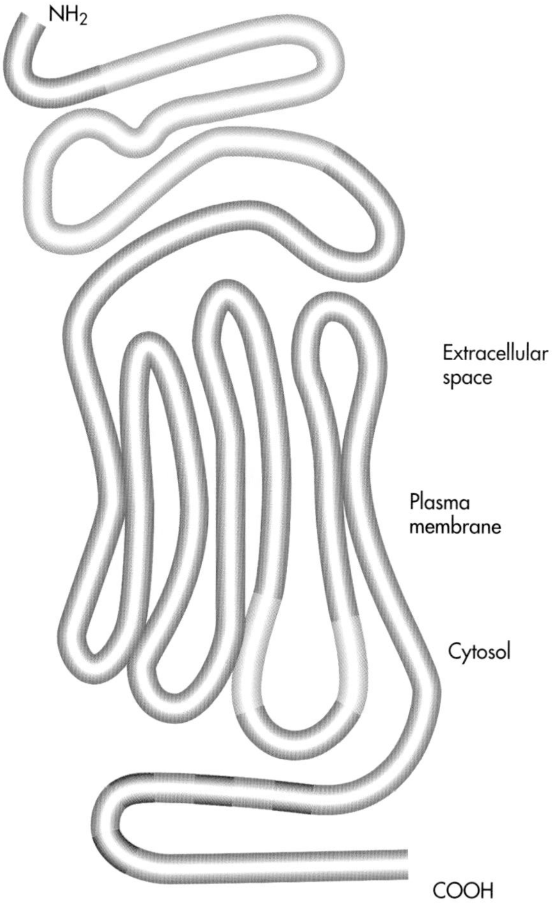

Figure 2.1 *A schematic drawing of a G-protein-linked receptor. Receptors that bind protein ligands have a large, extracellular, ligand-binding domain formed by the part of the polypeptide chain shown in* light green. *Receptors for small ligands such as adrenaline (epinephrine) have small extracellular domains, and the ligand-binding site is usually deep within the plane of the membrane, formed by amino acids from several of the transmembrane segments. The parts of the intracellular domains that are mainly responsible for binding to trimeric G proteins are shown in* orange, *while those that become phosphorylated during receptor desensitization (discussed later) are shown in* red.

proteins form specialized cellular contacts, such as desmosomes and tight junctions.

- Carrier proteins. These are involved in the transport of small molecules and ions across the cell membrane, as in glucose, the Na^+/K^+ pump or the multidrug resistance [MDR] pump). These proteins may be energy dependent or passive – if they are active, they usually utilize ATP. These carrier proteins often transport other molecules at the same time in the opposite direction (Figure 2.2).
- Channel proteins. These are involved in the transport of ions across the cell membrane. These function in a passive way and effectively are hydrophilic pores; they function more efficiently than carrier proteins and can carry ions more than 1000-fold faster. They are selective for certain ions and may be closed or open. The stimuli for opening these channels may be electrical current, ligand binding (as with nicotinic acetylcholine) or mechanical deformation.
- Intracellular organelles (rough and smooth endoplasmic reticulum [ER], Golgi apparatus, nuclear membranes). These membranes compartmentalize the cell into functionally distinct units (Figure 2.3). They are extensive, having a surface area 10–25-fold greater than the cell membrane itself.

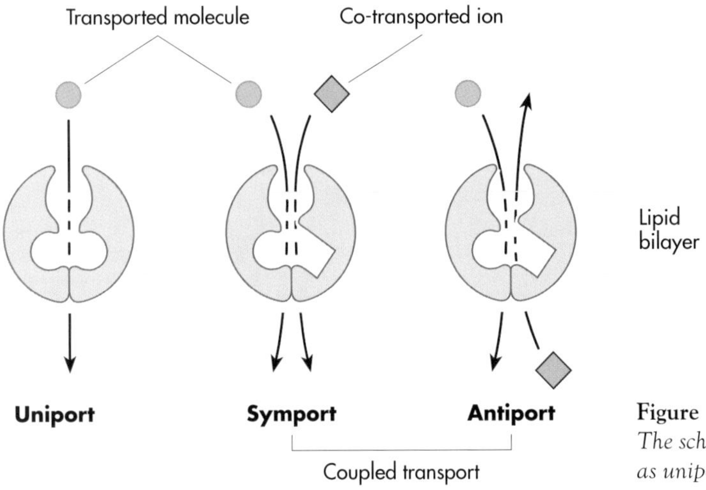

Figure 2.2 *Three types of carrier-mediated transport. The schematic diagram shows carrier proteins functioning as uniports, symports and antiports.*

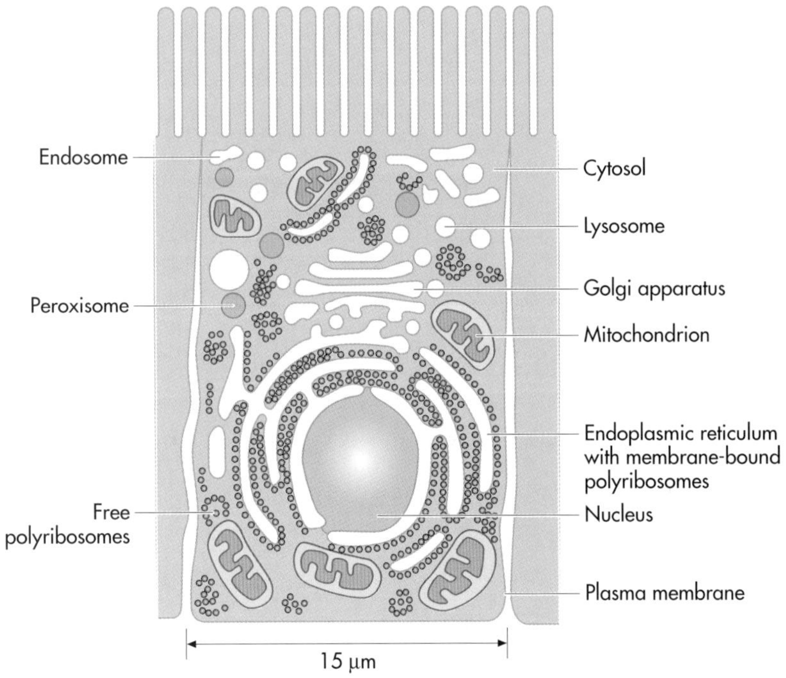

Figure 2.3 *The major intracellular compartments of an animal cell. The cytosol (grey), ER, Golgi apparatus, nucleus, mitochondrion, endosome, lysosome and peroxisome are distinct compartments isolated from the rest of the cell by at least one selectively permeable membrane.*

Intracellular proteins are synthesized on free cytosolic ribosomes and remain in the cytoplasm. Proteins for export begin their life by being synthesized on ribosomes that have special signalling molecules that dock with receptors on the endoplasmic reticulum (ER), Golgi apparatus, lysosomes, etc., which mediate transport to their final destination.

Endoplasmic reticulum (ER)

The ER is convoluted and may occupy up to 10% of the cell volume; it plays a central role in protein and lipid biosynthesis and is the site for synthesis of proteins and lipids that are destined to be incorporated in other cell organelles such as mitochondria (Figure 2.4).

Ribosomes are found free in the cytosol or attached to the ER (rough ER) when a ribosome is making a protein destined for export. In the latter circumstance, a signalling molecule targets the ribosome with its mRNA to the ER, into which it secretes its protein (Figure 2.5).

Smooth ER is abundant in some cells. It is involved in the storage of calcium and has a role in the contraction of smooth muscle cells brought about by intracellular calcium release (as well as transmembrane influx); together with the Golgi apparatus, it is involved in the synthesis of lipoproteins. In liver and some other cells, it contains the cytochrome p450 enzymes, which detoxify lipid-soluble drugs by converting them into water-soluble forms.

Golgi apparatus

This system of flattened sacs, which lie in continuity with the ER, is involved in sorting, packaging and modifying macromolecules for secretion or for delivery to other intracellular organelles (Figure 2.6). It consists of a stack of four to six flattened cisternae with an entry (cis-) and exit (trans-) surface. Glycosylation of proteins such as mucin takes place in the Golgi apparatus. Other proteins are sorted for

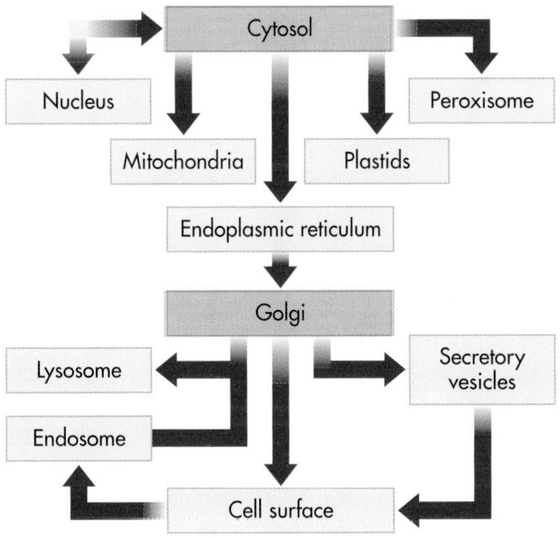

Figure 2.4 *The intracellular compartments of the eukaryotic cell involved in the biosynthetic-secretory and endocytic pathways. Each compartment encloses a space that is topologically equivalent to the outside of the cell, and they all communicate with one another by means of transport vesicles. In the biosynthetic-secretory pathway, protein molecules are transported from the ER to the plasma membrane or (via late endosomes) to lysosomes. In the endocytic pathway, molecules are ingested in vesicles derived from the plasma membrane and delivered to early endosomes and then (via late endosomes) to lysosomes. Many endocytosed molecules are retrieved from early endosomes and returned to the cell surface for reuse; similarly, some molecules are retrieved from the late endosome and returned to the Golgi apparatus, and some are retrieved from the Golgi apparatus and returned to the ER. All of these retrieval pathways are shown with* blue arrows.

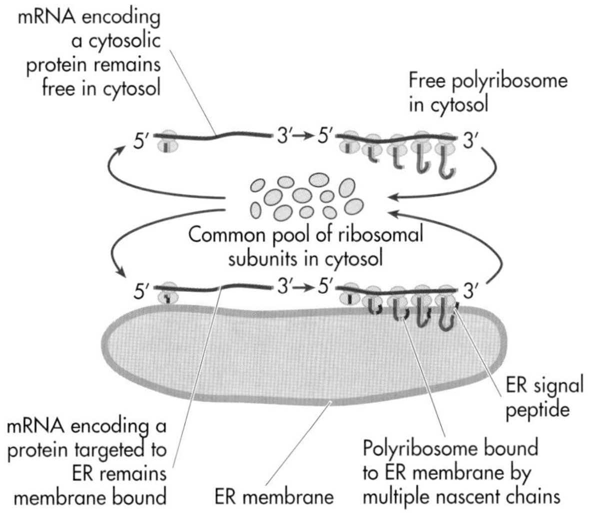

Figure 2.5 *Free and membrane-bound ribosomes. A common pool of ribosomes is used to synthesize both the proteins that stay in the cytosol and those that are transported into the ER. It is the ER signal peptide on a newly formed polypeptide chain that directs the engaged ribosome to the ER membrane. The mRNA molecule may remain permanently bound to the ER as part of a polyribosome, while the ribosomes that move along it are recycled; at the end of each round of protein synthesis, the ribosomal subunits are released and rejoin the common pool in the cytosol.*

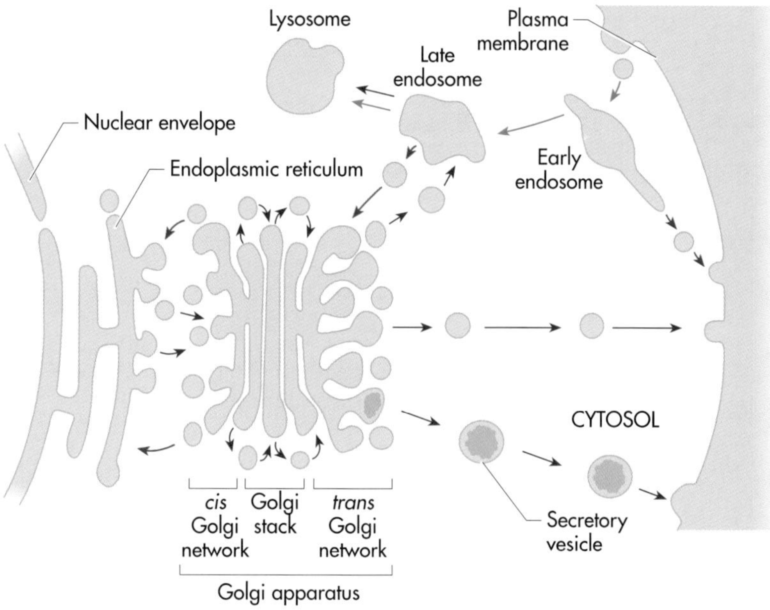

Figure 2.6 *The major intracellular compartments of an animal cell. The cytosol (grey), ER, Golgi apparatus, nucleus, mitochondrion, endosome, lysosome and peroxisome are distinct compartments isolated from the rest of the cell by at least one selectively permeable membrane.*

differential transport to certain organelles; for instance, acid hydrolase is transported from here to the lysosomes, and if the cell synthesizes hormones or neurotransmitters, these are excreted by small, smooth vesicles budding off from the Golgi apparatus before transport to the cell membrane, where exocytosis takes place.

Mitochondria

These are the powerhouse of the cell and are responsible for the production of most of the high-energy phosphate intermediates, such as ATP. They are present in virtually all cells and mediate oxidative respiration, in which pyruvate is converted to carbon dioxide and water with the production of about 30 molecules of ATP. Mitochondria consist of an outer membrane and a convoluted inner membrane containing the inner space or matrix, which is packed with hundreds of enzymes. Acetyl coenzyme A is the central intermediate produced by fatty acid oxidation and glycolysis (Figure 2.7), and the citric acid cycle takes place in the mitochondria (Figure 2.8). In the mitochondria, high-energy electrons from NADH and FADH2 are passed to oxygen during oxidative phosphorylation by the respiratory chain, which is situated on the inner membrane of the mitochondria (Figure 2.9). There are three large enzyme groups embedded in the inner membrane (Figure 2.10):

1. the NADH dehydrogenase complex, which contains a flavin and ubiquinone
2. the cytochrome b–c_1 complex, which contains three haemes and iron–sulphur protein
3. the cytochrome oxidase complex, which contains two cytochromes and copper.

It is thought that ATP is formed by a process of chemiosmotic coupling. The passage of electrons down each of the three parts of the respiratory chain results in H^+ being pumped into the intermembrane space of the mitochondria to set up an electrochemical proton gradient. The subsequent back-flow of H^+ into the matrix provides the energy to drive the enzyme ATP synthase. Mitochondria are actively involved in the induction of caspases during the process of apoptosis (Figure 2.11).

Mitochondrial DNA

Mitochondria and chloroplasts contain the DNA that encodes the structural and functional proteins permitting the mitochondria to divide during cell division. Mitochondrial DNA utilizes biochemically distinct pathways from those of nuclear DNA. For instance, protein synthesis mediated by nuclear DNA in the cytoplasm is blocked by cyclohexidine, whereas that in the mitochondrion is blocked by chloramphenicol, erythromycin and tetracycline. Mitochondria are not synthesized de novo, but arise

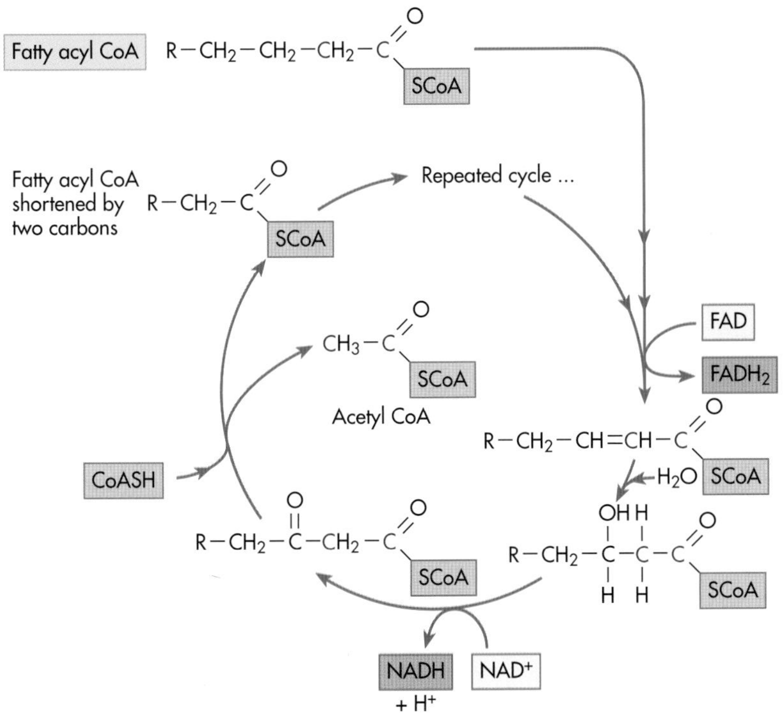

Figure 2.7 *The fatty acid oxidation cycle. The cycle is catalysed by a series of four enzymes in the mitochondrial matrix. Each turn of the cycle shortens the fatty acid chain by two carbons (shown in red), as indicated, and generates one molecule of acetyl CoA and one molecule each of NADH and $FADH_2$. The NADH is freely soluble in the matrix. The $FADH_2$, in contrast, remains tightly bound to the enzyme fatty acyl-CoA dehydrogenase; its two electrons will be rapidly transferred to the respiratory chain in the mitochondrial inner membrane, regenerating FAD.*

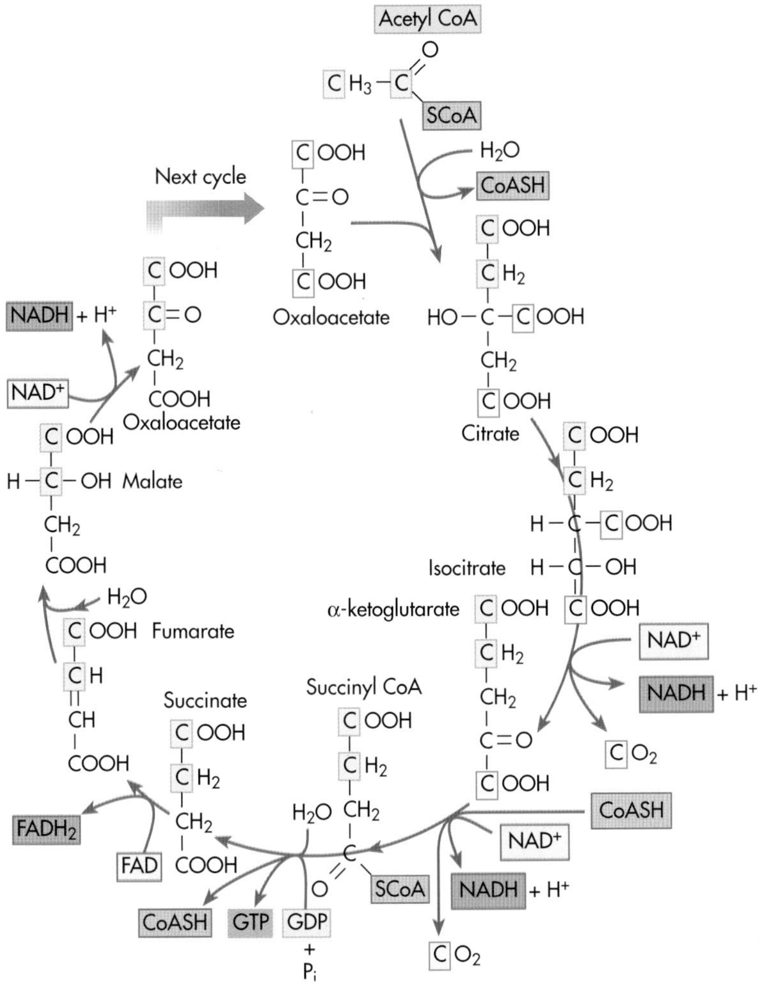

Figure 2.8 *The citric acid cycle. The intermediates are shown as their free acids, although the carboxyl groups are actually ionized. Each of the indicated steps is catalysed by a different enzyme located in the mitochondrial matrix. The two carbons from acetyl CoA that enter this turn of the cycle (shadowed in red) will be converted to CO_2 in subsequent turns of the cycle: it is the two carbons shadowed in blue that are converted to CO_2 in this cycle. Three molecules of NADH are formed. The GTP molecule produced can be converted to ATP by the exchange reaction GTP + ADP $\rightarrow$ GDP + ATP. The molecule of $FADH_2$ formed remains protein-bound as part of the succinate dehydrogenase complex in the mitochondrial inner membrane; this complex feeds the electrons acquired by $FADH_2$ directly to ubiquinone (see below).*

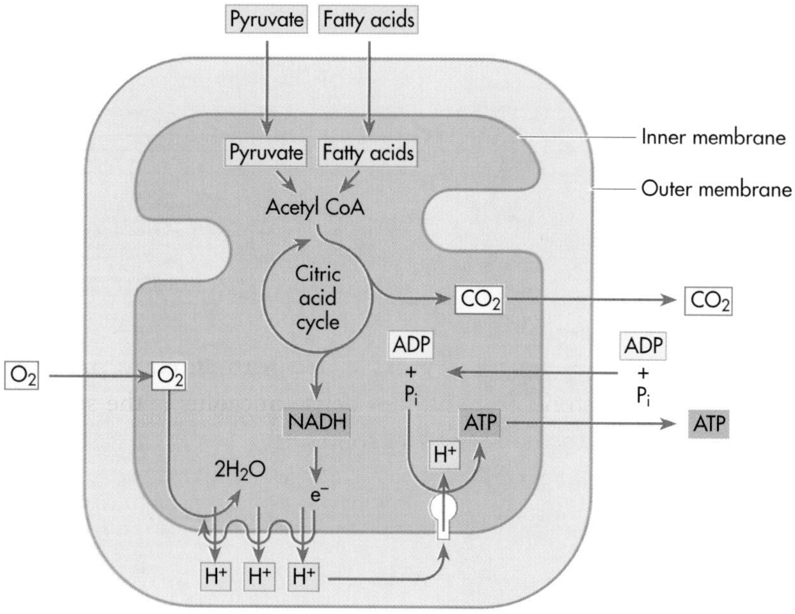

Figure 2.9 *A summary of mitochondrial energy metabolism. Pyruvate and fatty acids enter the mitochondrion, are broken down to acetyl CoA, and are then metabolized by the citric acid cycle, which produces NADH (and $FADH_2$, which is not shown). In the process of oxidative phosphorylation, high-energy electrons from NADH (and $FADH_2$) are then passed to oxygen by means of the respiratory chain in the inner membrane, producing ATP by a chemiosmotic mechanism. NADH generated by glycolysis in the cytosol also passes electrons to the respiratory chain (not shown). Since NADH cannot pass across the mitochondrial inner membrane, the electron transfer from cytosolic NADH must be accomplished indirectly by means of one of several 'shuttle' systems that transport another reduced compound into the mitochondrion; after being oxidized, this compound is returned to the cytosol, where it is reduced by NADH again.*

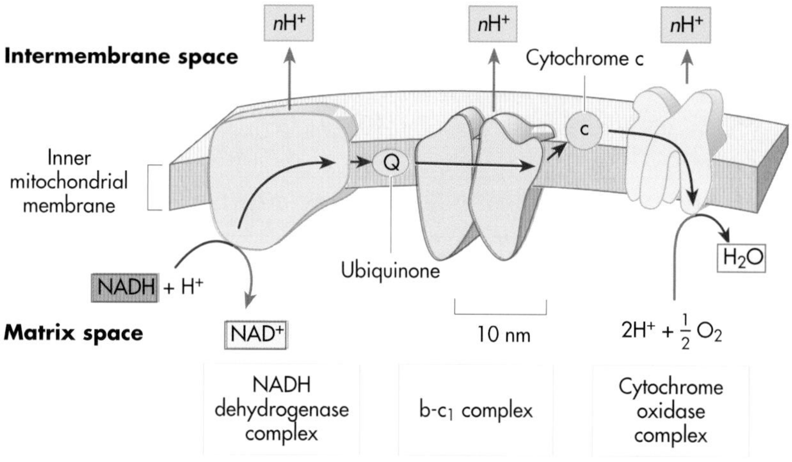

Figure 2.10 *The path of electrons through the three respiratory enzyme complexes. The size and shape of each complex is shown, as determined from images of two-dimensional crystals (crystalline sheets) viewed in the electron microscope at various tilt angles. During the transfer of two electrons from NADH to oxygen (red lines), ubiquinone and cytochrome c serve as carriers between the complexes.*

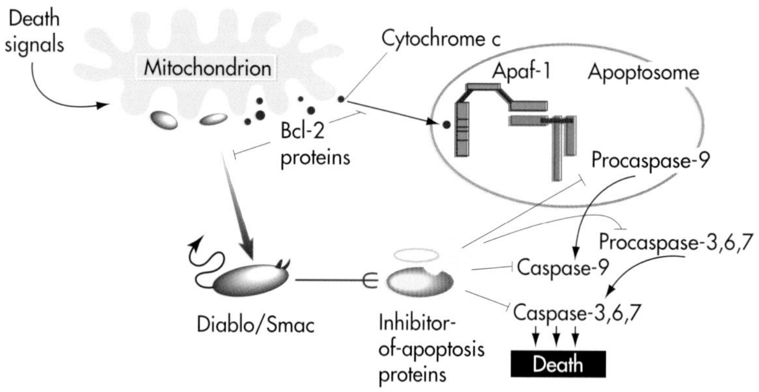

Figure 2.11 *Factors in apoptosis. This diagram shows that DNA-damaging agents result in induction of apoptosis through release of cytochrome c from mitochondria.*

from division of the organelle, which occurs during mitosis and is driven by mitochondrial DNA. Mitochondrial DNA is a circular structure like that of bacteria; in mammalian cells, it contains around 16.5 kbp. It synthesizes two ribosomal RNAs, 22 transfer RNAs (tRNAs) and 13 peptides. Unlike nuclear DNA, most of the nucleotides are direct coding sequences with little or no space left for regulatory codons. Analysis of the genetic code shows that the codon sequence is relaxed, allowing many transfer RNA (tRNA) molecules to recognize any one of four nucleotides in the third or 'wobble' position. In addition, in man, three of the 64 codons have different meanings from the standard codons.

Because mitochondrial inheritance is cytoplasmic, one would expect mitochondria to be inherited from the maternal side, as the sperm has little cytoplasm. It is thought that both mitochondria and chloroplasts evolved from endosymbiotic bacteria more than a billion years ago. However, over time, some mitochondrial genes have been transferred to nuclear DNA; for instance, lipoproteins in the mitochondrial membranes are synthesized from nuclear genes and modified in the cell's Golgi apparatus.

THE NUCLEUS

This is the most striking organelle in the cell. It is separated from the rest of the cell by the nuclear membrane, which consists of a lipid bilayer fenestrated by multiple nuclear pores. Inside the nucleus is the nucleolus, which is the factory that produces ribosomes. All chromosomal DNA is held in the nucleus, but it is associated with an equal mass of histone proteins. The dense nuceolus is the site for the assembly of ribosomes.

Table 2.1 Differences between nuclear and mitochondrial coding.

Codon	Standard	Mitochondrial
UGA	STOP	Trp (tryptophan)
AUA	Ile (isoleucine)	Met (methionine)
AGA/AGG	Arg (arginine)	STOP

Arrangement of DNA

Each DNA molecule in the nucleus is packaged as a chromosome, which, in essence, is an enormously long molecule arranged as two strands of a double helix. There are 23 pairs of chromosomes (22 autosomes and one sex chromosome: X or Y), which contain about 6×10^9 nucleotide pairs. Each DNA molecule not only has to be able to code for many different proteins (Figure 2.12), but also has to be able to replicate itself reliably during mitosis and to be able to repair itself when damaged by chemicals or radiation. At the ends of each chromosome are

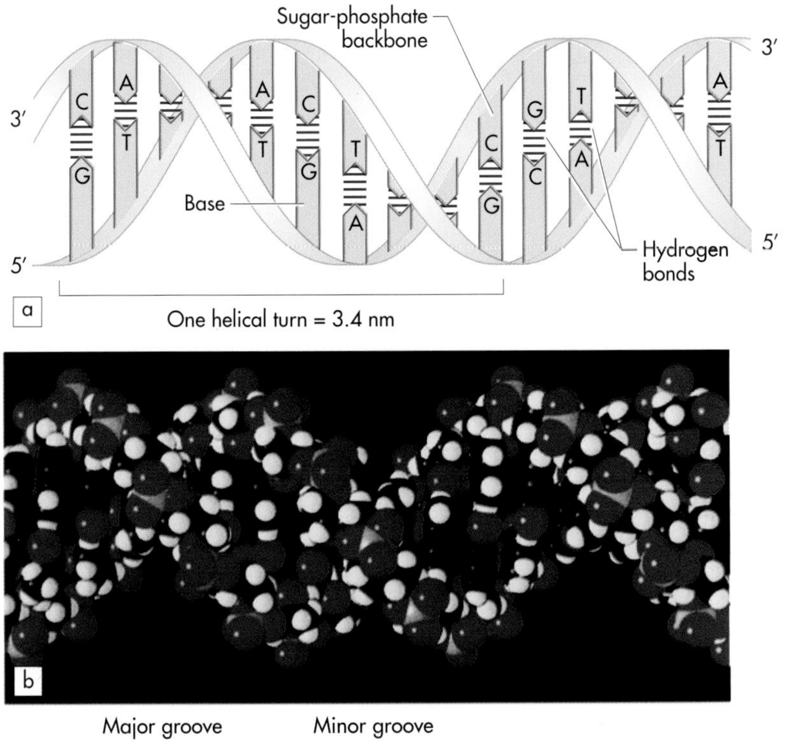

Figure 2.12 *DNA double helix. In a DNA molecule, two antiparallel strands that are complementary in their nucleotide sequence are paired in a right-handed double helix with about 10 nucleotide pairs per helical turn. A schematic representation (top) and a space-filling model (bottom) are illustrated here.*

the telomeres and at the centre is the centromere, which serves to anchor the chromosome via the kinetochore to the mitotic spindle during cell division. Not all DNA in the chromosomes is used to produce mRNA; indeed most of it is arranged into regulatory elements (non-coding sequences), introns or material called 'junk DNA' because its function is not yet understood.

Histone proteins

These proteins allow formal packaging of DNA in the nucleus; without them, DNA in mammalian cells would not be arranged in a regular way, and cell division and gene transcription would not be possible. They are small proteins with a large amount of dibasic amino acids, such as arginine and lysine, which bind to DNA because of their positive charges. There are five types: the H1 histones and the nucleosomal histones (H2A, H2B, H3 and H4), which are highly evolutionarily conserved. The nucleosomal histones are responsible for the coiling of DNA into nucleosomes (Figure 2.13), which are essential to the accommodation of DNA in the nucleus. It is thought that nucleosome histones are preferentially bound to areas of DNA that are Adenine/Thymine (AT) rich; these proteins can be prevented from binding by the attachment of inhibitory proteins. Nucleosomes are themselves packed together even more tightly by H1 histone proteins.

Figure 2.14 shows how DNA within chromosomes is ordered. DNA that is actively being transcribed into mRNA is unfolded, but is at its most condensed during mitosis, when individual chromosomes can be recognized by their specific banded structure. Histone acetylases are crucial to the process of transcription, as acetylation allows unwinding of the chromatin and access to general and specific transcription factors (Figure 2.15).

DNA replication

Replication of DNA requires that it is unwound at so-called replication forks, each strand acting as a template for synthesis. DNA polymerase α is used on the lagging strand and DNA polymerase δ on the leading strand (Figure 2.16). Both sections are synthesized in the 5′ to the 3′ direction (on the new strand), and the lagging strand is initially synthesized as short segments called Okazaki segments. In man, each molecule of DNA (the full length of the chromosome) is so long that several replication forks are required; these are often clustered together in areas of DNA that are transcriptionally active. For instance, in women whose second X chromosome is condensed as heterochromatin (Barr body), the active X chromosome replicates throughout each S phase, which lasts for about 8 hours, whereas the heterochromatin replicates only late in the S phase. During mitosis, a huge amount of histone protein has to be synthesized (histone protein forms an equal mass to DNA), and in man there are 20 replicated sets of histone protein genes arranged as tandem repeats on several chromosomes, each set of which contains all five histone proteins.

DNA replication errors

Errors can arise during DNA replication owing to insertion of the wrong base or the insertion of a run of microsatellite repeats (replication errors). These are normally repaired by nucleotide excision enzymes or replication error repair enzymes (RER), respectively.

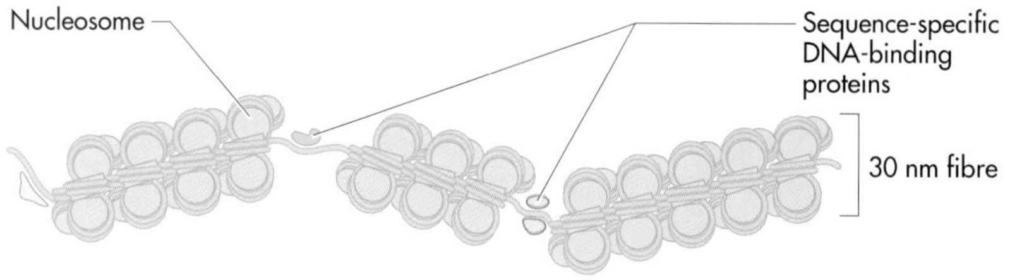

Figure 2.13 *Nucleosome-free regions in 30-nm fibres. A schematic section of chromatin illustrating the interruption of its regular nucleosomal structure by short regions where the chromosomal DNA is unusually vulnerable to digestion by DNase I. At each of these nuclease-hypersensitive sites, a nucleosome appears to have been excluded from the DNA by one or more sequence-specific DNA-binding proteins.*

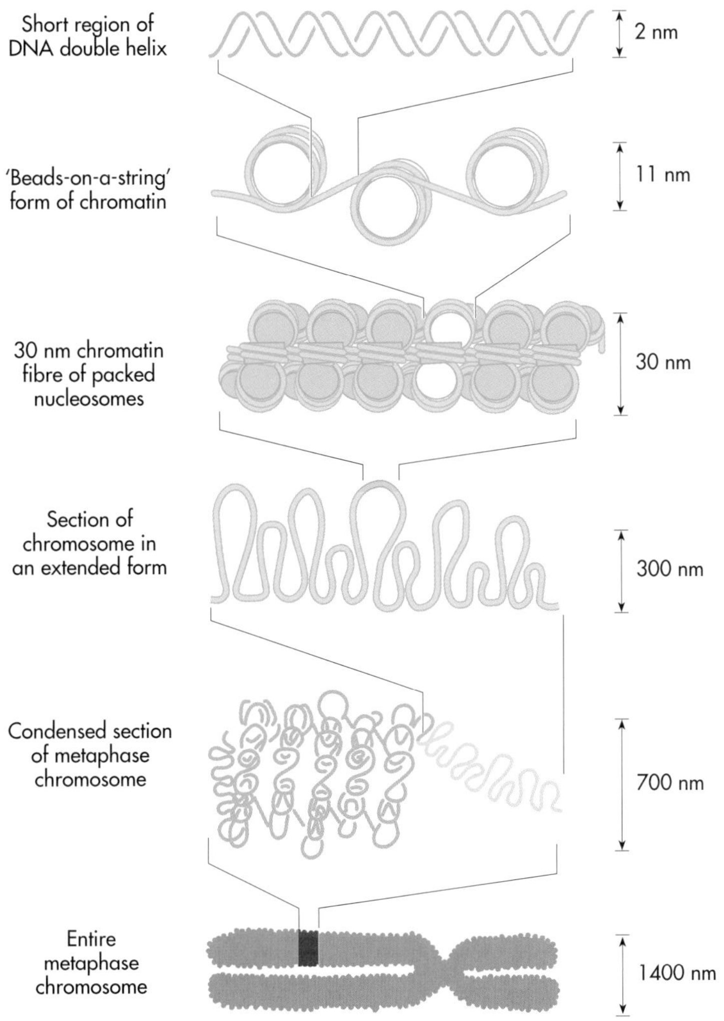

Figure 2.14 *Model of chromatin packing. This schematic drawing shows some of the many orders of chromatin packing postulated to give rise to the highly condensed mitotic chromosome.*

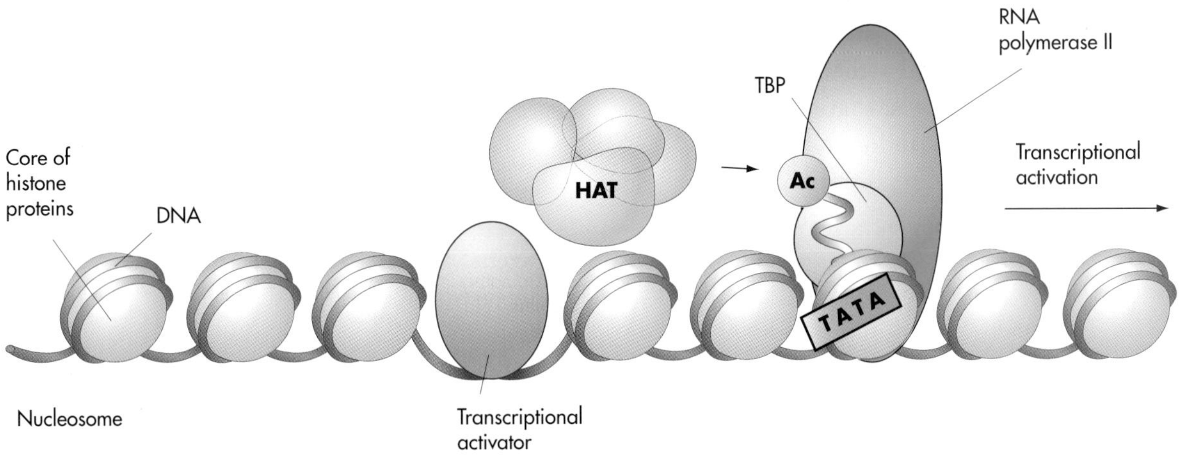

Figure 2.15 *Conventional view of how histone acetylases interact with DNA. This cartoon shows how the acetylation of histone residues 'opens up' the DNA by release of histone proteins. A more dynamic process is the current view.*

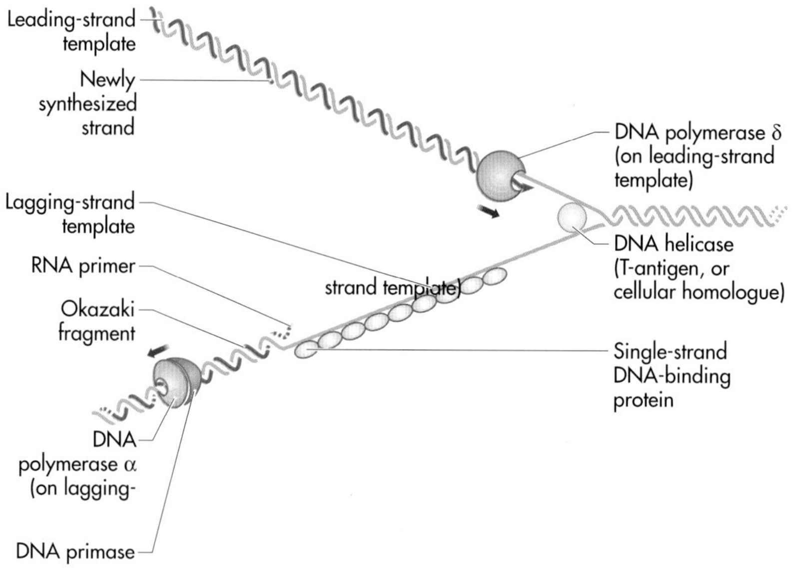

Figure 2.16 *A mammalian replication fork. The mammalian replication fork is important in several respects. First, it makes use of two DNA polymerases, one for the leading strand and one for the lagging strand. It seems likely that the leading-strand polymerase is designed to keep a tight hold on the DNA, whereas that on the lagging strand must be able to release the template and then rebind each time that a new Okazaki fragment is synthesized. Second, the mammalian DNA primase is a subunit of the lagging-strand DNA polymerase, while that of bacteria is associated with the DNA helicase.*

Telomeres and telomerase

Because of its structure and the way that it synthesizes nucleotides, DNA polymerase cannot replicate the very ends of chromosomes, which are modified into special regions called telomeres. In many species, these consist of tandem repeats rich in G (in man, GGGTTA). This region is replicated by a special enzyme called telomerase, which recognizes the GGGTTA sequence. Because there is no complementary DNA strand to replicate, telomerase uses an RNA template, which is structurally part of the telomerase, as a temporary extension for replication of the other strand. After several rounds of extension, one strand is longer and therefore can be used in turn as a template for replication of the second strand by DNA polymerase. It is thought that the telomeres shorten after each round of cell division and that this may limit the lifespan of a cell (senescence). Some malignant tumours are known to have high levels of telomerase, a feature which may mean that the cell can divide without the lengths of the telomeres being a limiting factor.

This rather simplistic view has been replaced by one in which 'capping' of the telomeres is important. It is true that during ageing of the cell, the telomeres become shorter, but while the telomeres are capped, cell division can carry on. If the capping process fails, senescence and apoptosis can occur, but, more importantly, fusion of chromosomes can occur. This process is thought to be important in carcinogenesis (Figure 2.17).

CELL DIVISION AND SENESCENCE

Senescence

Normal human cells cannot go on dividing forever in tissue culture; eventually, they senesce and will not divide further in response to mitogens. This process is accompanied by loss of telomerase, failure to phosphorylate the retinoblastoma protein in response to mitogens, and high levels of p21 (WAF1) and p16, which are cyclin-dependent kinase inhibitors that profoundly inhibit cell division.

Cell division (Figure 2.18)

Cell division involves duplication of DNA, mitosis (nuclear division) and cytokinesis (division of the

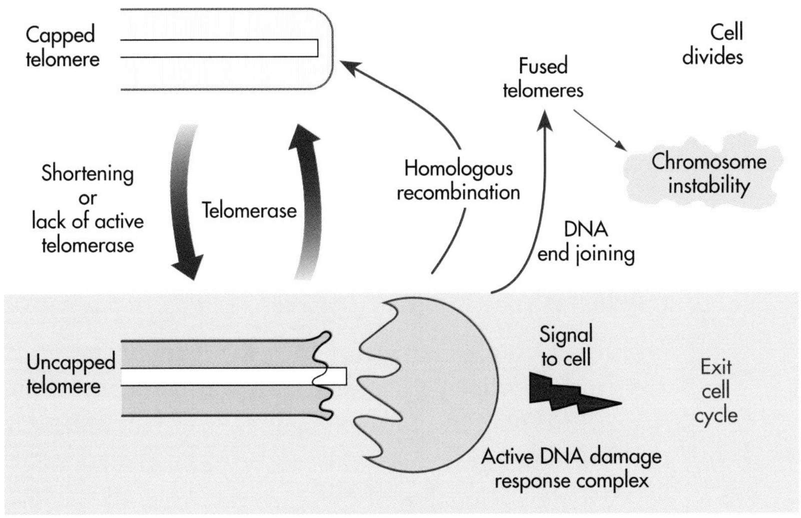

Figure 2.17 *Telomeres. Telomeres are normally capped. Even shortened telomeres can be associated with normal cell cycling – provided they are capped. If the capping is lost, cells either undergo apoptosis or may be prone to chromosome fusion and malignancy.*

cytoplasm). Following replication of DNA, the centrosome divides to form the mitotic spindle, and the chromosomes condense and align in the centre of the cell, where they are pulled apart by the mitotic spindle.

Mitosis – the 'M' phase

Prophase

The chromatin condenses into chromosomes that have duplicated and hence are formed of sister chromatids held together by the centromere. The centrosome divides to form the mitotic spindle. The nucleolus disperses.

Prometaphase

The nuclear membrane disrupts. The kinetochores begin to form. These are specialized proteins attached to the centromere to which the microtubule proteins of the spindle pole bind. Patients with scleroderma form autoantibodies to kinetochore protein.

Metaphase

The chromosomes are aligned at the metaphase plate at the centre of the cell.

Anaphase

The paired kinetochores suddenly separate, allowing the chromosomes to separate and to be pulled towards each spindle pole in a matter of minutes.

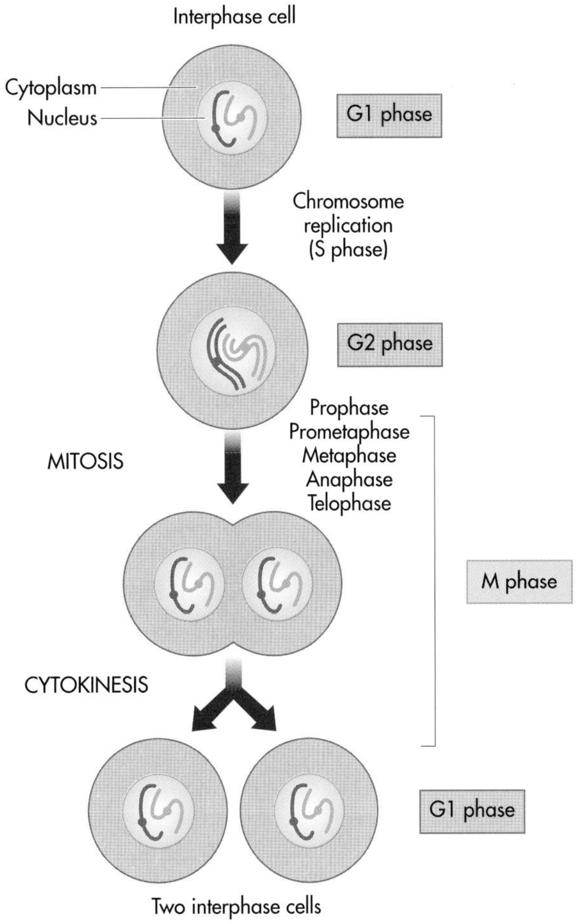

Figure 2.18 *The four successive phases of a standard eukaryotic cell cycle. During interphase, the cell grows continuously; during M phase, it divides. DNA replication is confined to the part of interphase known as S phase. G1 phase is the gap between M phase and S phase; G2 is the gap between S phase and M phase.*

Contraction of the microtubules pulls the chromosomes towards the spindle pole.

Telophase
The nuclear membrane begins to reform and the microtubules disappear. The nucleolus reappears.

Cytokinesis
The cytoplasm separates at a specialized contractile ring situated in the centre of the cell, actively cutting the cytoplasm into two parts.

THE CELL CYCLE

In the adult human, cells are continuously being lost by the process of planned, programmed cell death (apoptosis). Some cells do not divide at all, although they can be destroyed (neurons and skeletal muscle fibres); some divide slowly; and others have to divide rapidly (such as cells in the bone marrow and lining of the gut). During cell division, DNA is replicated and reproduction of intracellular organelles takes place. Replication of DNA takes place during a specific part of mitosis known as the S phase. G2 is the period of rest before the prophase part of the M phase starts. The G1 phase occupies the period between the completion of the previous mitosis and the S phase; some mature cells, however, enter a specialized period of rest, G0, which can last for months or years.

The proportion of dividing cells can be measured by a number of different tests. Administration of radiolabelled thymidine or bromodeoxyuridine (BrdU) can allow labelling of cells in the S phase to be demonstrated by the use of photographic plates or monoclonal antibodies, respectively. Other antibodies can be used to measure the Ki67 antigen (Ki67 or MIB1) or proliferating cell nuclear antigen (PCNA), which are expressed during particular parts of the cell cycle; these are useful in measuring cell proliferation within tumours. The amount of DNA

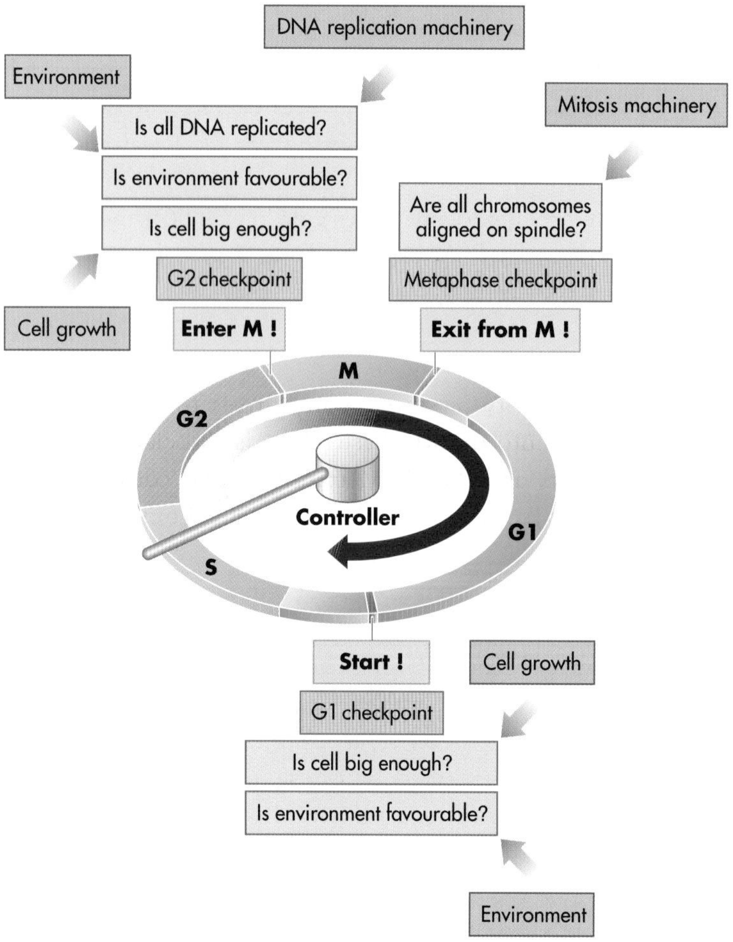

Figure 2.19 *Checkpoints and inputs of regulatory information to the cell-cycle control system. Feedback from downstream processes and signals from the environment can prevent the control system from passing through certain specific checkpoints. The most prominent checkpoints are where the control system activate the triggers shown in* yellow *boxes.*

within a population of cells can be estimated by the use of fluorescent stains such as ethidium bromide with the fluorescence-activated cell sorter.

The control of cell division

This process is tightly controlled at certain critical points of the cell cycle, which are known as cell-cycle checkpoints, at which certain brakes can be applied to stop the process if conditions are unfavourable (Figure 2.20). Checkpoints are found at the G1/S transition (the *Start* checkpoint); another is found at G2/M. Most studies have concentrated on the G2/M transition (the mitosis checkpoint). This cell-cycle control mechanism is based on two series of proteins: the cyclin-dependent protein kinases (Cdks), which phosphorylate a series of downstream proteins on serine and threonine residues, and the cyclins, which along with other regulatory proteins bind to Cdks to inhibit their activity. Different cyclins are synthesized during different parts of the cell cycle (mitotic cyclins and G1 cyclins) (Figure 2.20). In mammalian cells, there are at least six types of cyclin (A, B, C, D, E and F). Entry into mitosis is stimulated by activation of a Cdk by mitotic cyclin; in amphibians, this is known as maturation promotion factor (MPF) and consists of cyclin and a cyclin-dependent kinase called cdc2 – another is known as cdc4. Repetitive synthesis and degradation of cyclins is associated with the cell cycle. Activation of MPF drives mitosis, and degradation of cyclin then allows the cell to enter the S phase. As we shall see later, there is a set of proteins that can inhibit Cdk known as cyclin-dependent kinase inhibitors (Cdki, or inhibitors of cyclin-dependent kinases – INKs). The activity of the Cdk can therefore be abruptly switched on and off during different parts of the cell cycle.

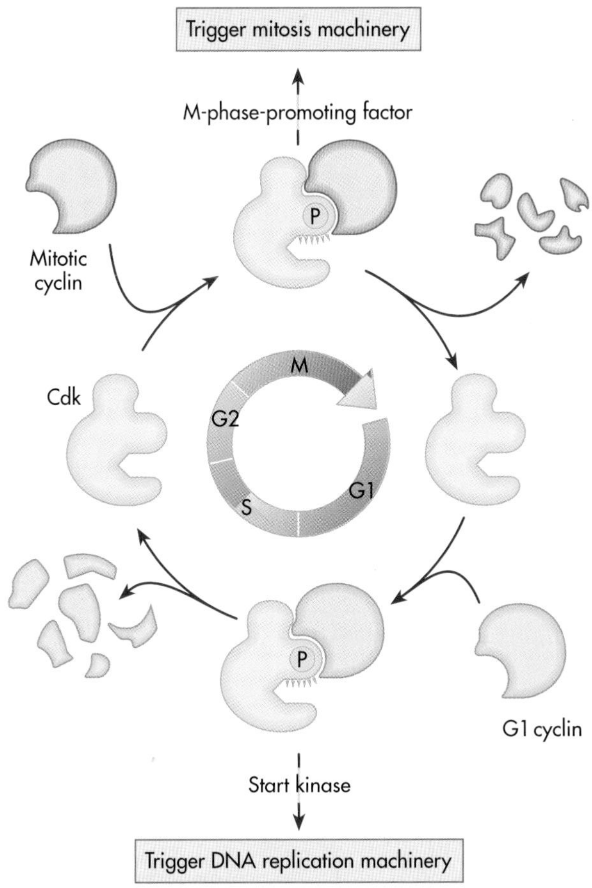

Figure 2.20 *The core of the cell-cycle control system. Cdk is thought to associate successively with different cyclins to trigger downstream processes of the cycle. Cdk activity is terminated by cyclin degradation.*

In part, this is controlled by the synthesis and degradation of the cyclins, but it is also affected by phosphorylation of the Cdk on two sites (Figure 2.21), which is controlled by two phosphatases known as Weel and MO15. Removal of one of the phosphate residues by means of another phosphatase – Cdc25 – is then needed for activation of MPF. It is thought that the MPF autocatalytically activates itself, resulting in a steady rise in MPF levels during the cell cycle until the critical point when an explosive increase in activity takes place and drives the cell irretrievably into the M phase. Cdc2 is associated with the G1/S, and the G2/M transition and cdc4 and cdc6 are associated with *Start*, but are bound to different cyclins (cyclin B at *mitosis* and cyclin E and A at *Start* at G1/S). The Kip/cip family of cyclin-dependent kinases, which include p21, p27 and p57, are capable of binding to and inhibiting most cyclin/cdk complexes. The expression of these cdk inhibitors is often dependent on upstream events that are activated by physiological signals, such as DNA damage, serum deprivation or contact inhibition. In contrast, the INK4 family of cdk inhibitors, including p15, p16, p18 and p19, bind to and inactivate D-type cyclins.

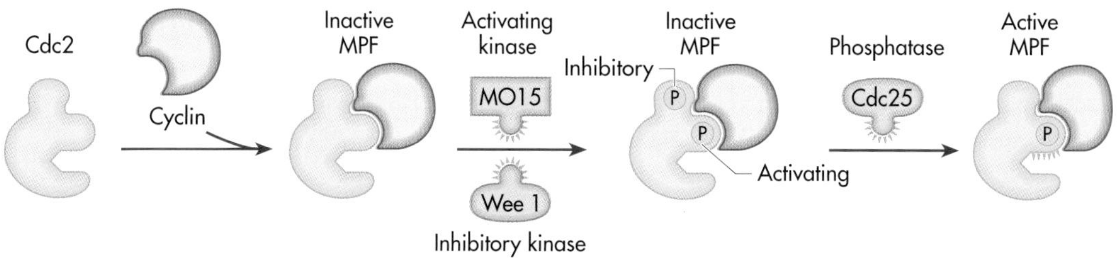

Figure 2.21 *Genesis of MPF activity. Cdc2 becomes associated with cyclin as the level of cyclin gradually increases; this enables Cdc2 to be phosphorylated by an activating kinase on an 'activating' site, as well as by Wee1 kinase on Cdc2's catalytic site. The latter phosphorylation inhibits Cdc2 activity until this phosphate group is removed by the Cdc25 phosphatase. Active MPF is thought to stimulate its own activation by activating Cdc25 and inhibiting Wee1, either directly or indirectly.*

Growth factors and the control of the cell cycle

In mammalian cells, peptide growth factors are potent inducers of cell division. These include platelet-derived growth factor (PDGF); epidermal growth factor (EGF); insulin and insulin-like growth factors I and II (IGF-I and IGF-II); acidic and basic fibroblast growth factors (a-FGF and b-FGF); transforming growth factor α (TGF-α), which binds to the EGF receptor); and transforming growth factor β (TGF-β), which is structurally unrelated to TGF-α and is generally inhibitory. Many of these growth factors act as proto-oncogenes.

These growth factors act over very short distances and may act on the cell that produces it (autocrine action) or on neighbouring cell types (paracrine action). Many are found in serum, and that is one reason why serum is required to maintain cells in culture. High-affinity receptors for these growth factors are found on the cell membrane, and, in culture, cells compete for growth factors. As well as requiring growth factors for cell division, many cells require signals produced by intercellular contact and adherence (anchorage) mediated by means of adhesion molecules before they divide (anchorage-dependent growth).

Many growth factor receptors contain an endogenous tyrosine kinase, which is activated by ligand binding (Figure 2.22). These receptors interact with proto-oncogenes, such as G proteins (such as *ras*), because tyrosine phosphorylation of the receptors facilitates binding of intermediate proteins with so-called SH2 domains, which then link with other proteins (SOS, GRB2) that activate the *ras* pathway. Phosphorylation of downstream protein by growth factor receptors activates several early-response genes, which are stimulated within a few minutes of

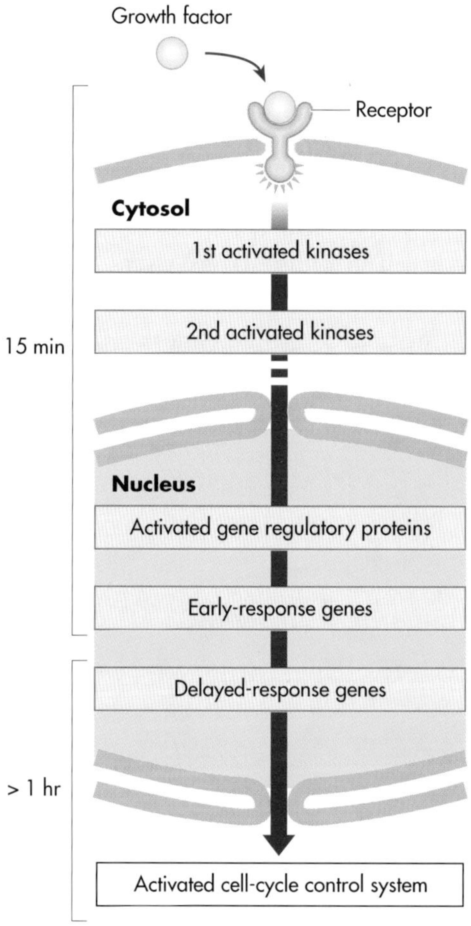

Figure 2.22 *Typical signalling pathway for stimulation of cell proliferation by a growth factor. This greatly simplified diagram shows some of the major steps. It omits many of the intermediate steps in the relay system.*

adding growth factor. In contrast, delayed-response gene activation requires protein synthesis. Many early-response genes activated by growth factor receptors control gene transcription; they include *myc*, *jun* and *fos*, which are known to be crucial for gene transcription. In particular, *myc* is thought to be closely linked to activation of cell division.

APOPTOSIS OR PROGRAMMED CELL DEATH

In many tissues, such as those of the haematopoietic system and the lining of the gut wall, proliferation and cell division are balanced by a process of planned cell death, the control of which is every bit as important as that involved in cell division. Programmed cell death also occurs in tumours, but the control of it is disrupted.

Apoptosis is a carefully orchestrated event in which the cell is programmed to die. The nucleus becomes shrunken and pyknotic, and the cytoplasm shrinks. The nucleus is sometimes extruded and may be engulfed by neighbouring cells. No inflammatory reaction is excited by the process. This process is characterized by disintegration of the nuclear envelope and marked condensation of DNA into chromatin. On electrophoresis, the DNA assumes a characteristic banding pattern, implying that it is being cut by endonuclease enzymes. Nearby macrophages recognize the apoptotic cell and begin to engulf and digest it. How this recognition process is mediated is unclear. The macrophages do not secrete inflammatory cytokines and chemokines; therefore, inflammation does not occur: apoptosis is quite different from necrosis.

Several genes are involved in this process. For instance, in thymic cells damaged by radiation, p53 is upregulated, an effect which increases the level of p21 (an inhibitor of cyclin-dependent kinase). This, in turn, slows down cell division, placing the cell in G1 arrest and allowing DNA repair to take place. It is thought that p21 is not directly concerned with the onset of apoptosis. In some cell types, such DNA damage initiates apoptosis, which is also associated with upregulation of p53. There are a number of proteins known to promote apoptosis, including the bax family. bax binds to and is inhibited by bcl2. Homo-dimers of bax, which is upregulated by p53, bring on apoptosis. The bcl-2 protein binds and inactivates bax homo-dimers, thereby preventing apoptosis. Some types of apoptosis are not activated through p53. It is thought that the end point of apoptosis is the activation of a set of ICE-like cysteine proteases. Production of activated caspases is crucial to this process and may occur as a consequence of DNA damage. Detection of DNA damage and determination of the outcome, whether repair, apoptosis or carcinogenesis, is the responsibility of several genes, including *BRCA1*, *BRCA2*, *ATM* (ataxia telangiectasia) and *p53*.

Aberrant expression of p53 and upregulation of bcl2 will decrease the rate of apoptosis (although apoptosis is often higher in tumours with mutated p53 and upregulated bcl2, because other mechanisms are activated). The point is that, in many tumours, DNA damage and the presence of mutated tumour suppressors and oncogenes will stimulate cell division, which will be in excess of the rate of apoptosis, so continued deregulated proliferation will probably lead to more DNA mutations occurring with each cell cycle.

STRUCTURE OF DNA AND RNA

The essential basis of DNA and RNA is nucleic acids. These are made of the folowing three compounds:

1. *bases*: nitrogenous ring compounds called purines (adenine and guanine) or pyrimidines (cytosine, thymine [DNA], or uracil [RNA])
2. *pentose sugars*: two types – ribose (β-D-ribose: RNA) and deoxyribose (β-D-2 deoxyribose: DNA)
3. *phosphate*: the phosphate bond is attached to the 5′ C hydroxyl group, and in a nucleic acid, it bonds to the 3′ C position of the adjacent sugar residue.

The nucleoside is defined as a base plus a sugar (adenosine, guanosine, cytidine, thymidine or uridine). The nucleotide is defined as a base plus a sugar plus a phosphate (Figure 2.23). In addition to being the building blocks of DNA and RNA, nucleotides are used:

- as high-energy intermediates (such as adenosine triphosphate – ATP)

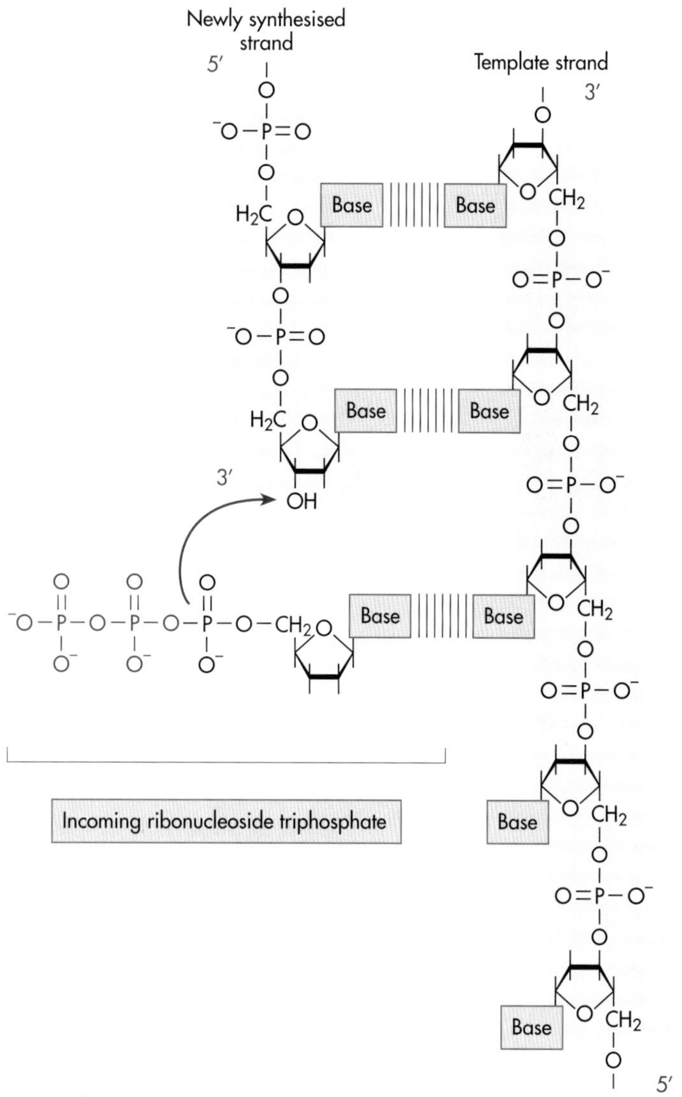

Figure 2.23 *DNA synthesis. The addition of a deoxyribonucleotide to the 3′ end of a polynucleotide chain is the fundamental reaction by which DNA is synthesized. As shown, base-pairing between this incoming deoxyribonucleotide and an existing strand of DNA (the template strand) guides the formation of a new strand of DNA with a complementary nucleotide sequence.*

- in combination with other structures to form enzymes (coenzyme A)
- as signalling molecules (such as cyclic AMP).

RNA forms a single chain, whereas DNA forms a double helix held together by hydrogen bonding between bases on opposing strands; the individual nucleotides are held together by phosphate linkages between sugar residues (Fig. 2.23), the individual bases being suspended from the other end of the sugar residue. The sequence of bases forms the basis for all genetic information and is organized as a series of triplets which code for individual amino acids. The hydrogen bonding between bases on opposing strands is not random, and on opposite sides of DNA, the following bases are always matched as complementary pairs (or Watson–Crick base pairs):

- G with C
- A with T (or A with U in RNA).

The triplet code for DNA and the corresponding amino acids are shown in Tables 2.2 and 2.3. A section of DNA can be read in a number of different 'reading frames', depending upon which particular nucleotide is the start of the reading frame.

The double helix formed by DNA occupies 3.4 nm for one complete turn, which contains 10 nucleotide pairs per turn and has a major and a minor groove. A single strand of DNA acting as a template will induce the formation of a second complementary strand if the appropriate nucleoside triphosphates and DNA polymerase are present in solution. Errors introduced by such complementary replication will induce a 'point mutation' where a single inappropriate base is inserted.

Table 2.2 The genetic code.

1st position – 5′ end	U	C	A	G	3rd position – 3′ end
U	Phe Phe Leu Leu	Sea Sea Sea Sea	Tyr Tyr STOP STOP	Cys Cys STOP Trp	U C A G
C	Leu Leu Leu Leu	Pro Pro Pro Pro	His His Gln Gln	Arg Arg Arg Arg	U C A G
A	Ile Ile Ile Met	Thr Thr Thr Thr	Asn Asn Lys Lys	Sea Sea Arg Arg	U C A G
G	Val Val Val Val	Ala Ala Ala Ala	Asp Asp Glu Glu	Gly Gly Gly Gly	U C A G

Table 2.3 Amino acids and their symbols.

Letter	Symbols	Amino acid	Codons
A	Ala	Alanine	GCA, GCC, GCG, GCU
C	Cys	Cysteine	UGC, UGU
D	Asp	Aspartic acid	GAC, GAU
E	Glu	Glutamic acid	GAA, GAU
F	Phe	Phenylalanine	UUC, UUU
G	Gly	Glycine	GGA, GGC, GGG, GGU
H	His	Histidine	CAC, CAU
I	Ile	Isoleucine	AUA, AUC, AUU
K	Lys	Lysine	AAA, AAG
L	Leu	Leucine	UUA, UUG, CUA, CUC, CUG, CUU
M	Met	Methionine	AUG
N	Asn	Asparginine	AAC, AAU
P	Pro	Proline	CCA, CCC, CCG, CCU
Q	Gln	Glutamine	CAA, CAG
R	Arg	Arginine	AGA, AGG, CGA, CGC, CGG, CGU
S	Sea	Serine	AGC, AGU, UCA, UCC, UCG, UCU
T	Thr	Threonine	ACA, ACC, ACG, ACU
V	Val	Valine	GUA, GUC, GUG, GUU
W	Trp	Tryptophan	UGG
Y	Tyr	Tryosine	UAC, UAU

BASIC GENETIC MECHANISMS

Genes

Certain sections of DNA are arranged into genes, which are defined as lengths of DNA that produce specific mRNA and protein, although this definition is not quite correct because, in some organisms, several species of RNA may be produced from one gene, and spliced variants of mRNA in higher organisms are commonly tissue specific (such as splice variants for FGF receptors and p15, which is an alternative spliced variant of p16). The size of genes varies a great deal depending partly on the size of the protein to be produced (Table 2.4). Even within a gene sequence, although all of it is transcribed as primary RNA, not all sections are exported as mature RNA (Fig. 2.24). The gene is arranged into exons, which are exported from the nucleus as mature mRNA, and introns, which are excised from the primary transcript mRNA (Figure 2.24) by means of RNA splicing and degraded in the nucleus.

Each gene produces messenger RNA (mRNA), and most genes (except those encoding ribosomes and transfer RNA) eventually produce proteins, some of which control the synthesis and modification of other compounds, such as nucleic acids, lipids and carbohydrates. Less than 1% of DNA is transcribed into mature mRNA. Proteins have myriad functions, ranging from structural proteins, such as actins, right through to those that precisely control the rate of gene transcription.

Table 2.4 The size of some human genes.

Protein	Gene size (in kb)	MRNA size (in kb)	Number of introns
β globulin	1.5	0.6	2
Insulin	1.7	0.4	2
Protein kinase C	11	1.4	7
Albumin	25	2.1	14
Catalase	34	1.6	12
LDL receptor	45	5.5	17
Factor VIII	186	9	25
Thyroglobulin	300	8.7	36
Dystrophin	> 2000	17	>50

mRNA synthesis

After the opening up of the chromatin structure that occurs as a result of acetylation of histones, the next step is the synthesis of primary or heterogeneous mRNA (hnRNA), which is initiated by RNA polymerase type II, a large multiunit enzyme (Fig. 2.25). This enzyme binds to the promoter unit of the gene that is to be transcribed in conjunction with several other proteins called transcription factors.

The promoter region contains the site at which transcription factors bind and which is rich in TATA sequences (the so-called TATA box); it is situated about 25 nucleotides upstream of the start site of the gene. An AUG codon (methionine) always represents the start of each gene. RNA polymerase opens up the double-stranded helix, and RNA is synthesized by the polymerase, moving from the 3′ to the 5′ direction of DNA (that is, the RNA is extended from the 5′ to the 3′ direction) (Figure 2.25). This elongation continues until the polymerase reaches a stop signal (UAA; UAG). Thirty nucleotides are added per second, so a chain of 5000 nucleotides will take about 3 minutes to make. Each strand of the double helix could, in theory, be used to copy into RNA, but, in any one section of DNA, only one strand is used, although, in any one chromosome, different strands are used in different parts.

There are three types of RNA polymerase (types I, II and III). Type I RNA polymerase makes large ribosomal RNA and type III makes transfer RNA (tRNA) and the small 5S ribosomal RNA. Type II RNA polymerase is responsible for synthesis of the other types of RNA. Both ends of mRNA are modified. The 5′ end is 'capped' by a methylated G nucleotide, whereas to the 3′ end a polyadenylated (poly-A) tail is added. The 5′ cap plays an important part in protein synthesis and protects the mRNA from degradation. The poly-A tail aids the export of mRNA, it may stabilize mRNA in the cytoplasm, and it serves a recognition signal for the ribosome. The primary RNA transcript from the gene is known as heterogeneous RNA (hnRNA), most of which is rapidly destroyed by removal and splicing of the

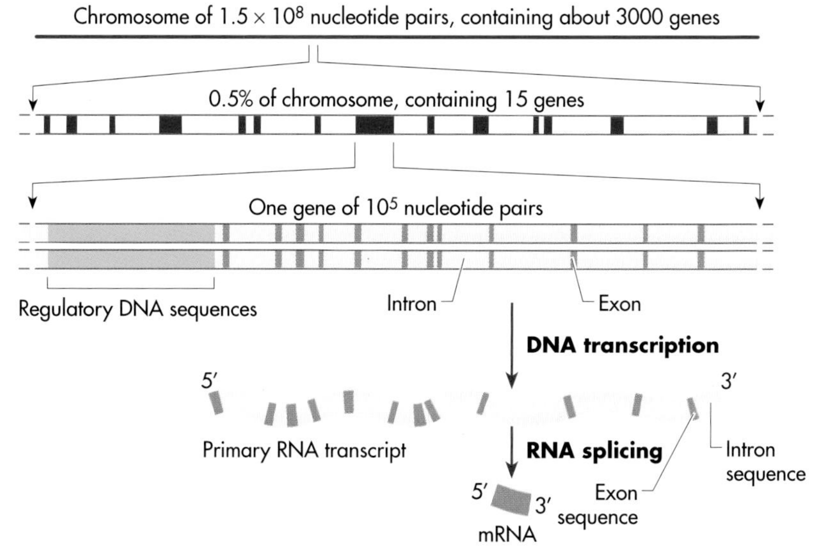

Figure 2.24 *The organization of genes on a typical vertebrate chromosome. Proteins that bind to the DNA in regulatory regions determine whether a gene is transcribed; although often located on the 5′ side of a gene, as shown here, regulatory regions can also be located in introns, in exons, or on the 3′ side of a gene. Intron sequences are removed from primary RNA transcripts to produce messenger RNA (mRNA) molecules. The figure given here for the number of genes per chromosome is a minimal estimate.*

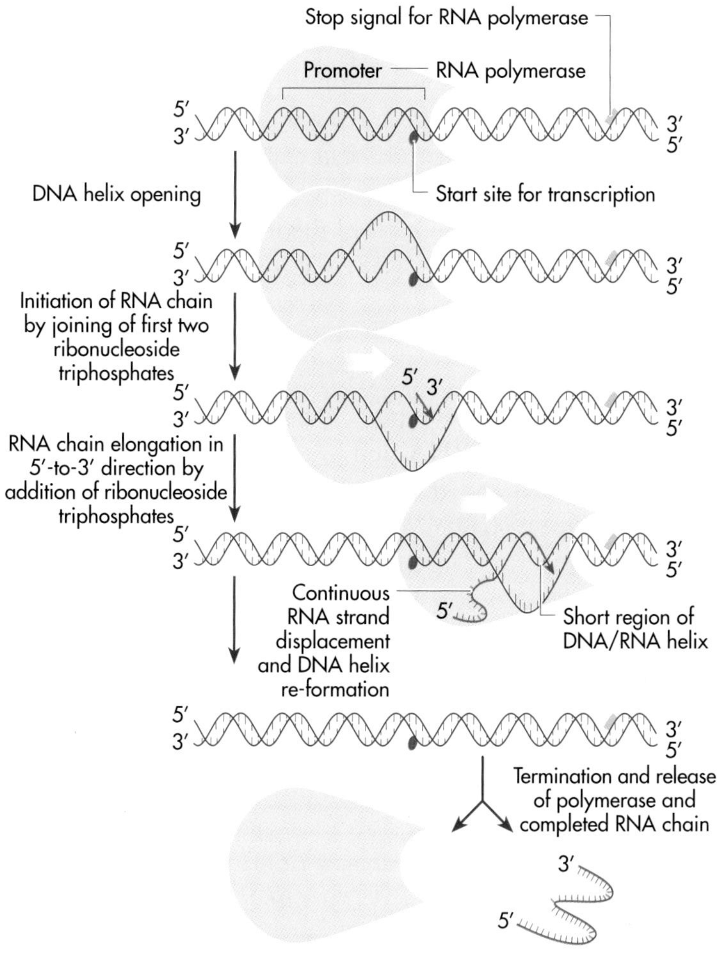

Figure 2.25 *The synthesis of an RNA molecule by RNA polymerase. The enzyme binds to the promoter sequence on the DNA and begins its synthesis at a start site within the promoter. It completes its synthesis at a stop (termination) signal, whereupon both the polymerase and its completed RNA chain are released. During RNA chain elongation, polymerization rates average about 30 nucleotides per second at 37°C. Therefore, an RNA chain of 5000 nucleotides takes about 3 minutes to complete.*

remaining mRNA. The presence of the poly-A tail allows purification of the mRNA from other types of RNA, a fact which is useful in purifying mRNA for studies.

Introns and exons: mRNA processing

Early evidence for the presence of introns was the finding that mature RNA is relatively short and when, in experiments, it was annealed to DNA containing the gene of interest, it was found that the DNA formed several large loops, only short sections of DNA being adherent to mRNA. Primary mRNA transcribed from the loops of DNA not bound to the mature mRNA does not form part of mature mRNA and is excised as introns. hnRNA, which is the primary transcript of the gene, is much longer than the mature mRNA; although it has the 5′ cap and poly-A tail, it also contains several introns. The hnRNA in the nucleus is coated with proteins and small nuclear ribonucleoproteins (snRNPs) which are somewhat similar to ribosomes, but much smaller (250 kDa compared with 4500 kDa); they are crucial to the excision of introns. Patients with systemic lupus erythematosas form autoantibodies against one or more snRNPs. As pointed out above (Table 2.4), introns form much the largest part of hnRNA and of the genome itself. Introns can accumulate several mutations without necessarily affecting protein function (that is, they comprise so-called junk DNA). However, point mutations near the exon/intron junction can have disastrous effects on protein function if they result in introns not being removed (as in thalassaemia) and in the formation of longer sections of mRNA and therefore of new types of protein. Spliceosomes are formed by aggregation of several snRNPs, ATP and other proteins onto the exon/intron junction – they remove the intron as a 'lariat' or noose-like structure (Figure 2.26). Most genes contain several introns. After excision of introns, the exons are spliced together to form mature mRNA, which is then exported from the nucleus via the nuclear pores.

In the formation of some proteins, differential RNA splicing is the norm, producing different forms of RNA and hence different proteins. This is achieved by differential binding of distinct repressors or activators to the primary RNA transcript, which can alter the splice site and therefore alter the exact structure of the final mature mRNA. This occurs with the fibroblast growth factor receptors,

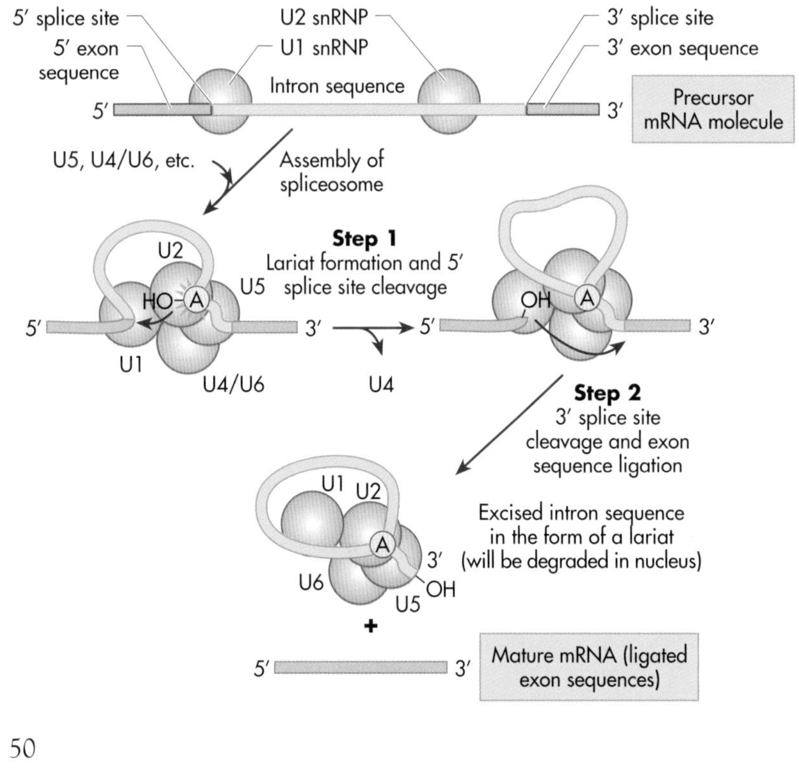

Figure 2.26 *The RNA splicing mechanism. RNA splicing is catalysed by a spliceosome formed from the assembly of U1, U2, U5 and U4/U6 snRNPs (shown as* green circles*) plus other components (not shown). After assembly of the spliceosome, the reaction occurs in two steps: in step 1, the branch-point A nucleotide in the intron sequence, which is located close to the 3′ splice site, attacks the 5′ splice site and cleaves it; the cut 5′ end of the intron sequence thereby becomes covalently linked to this A nucleotide, forming the branched nucleotide. In step 2, the 3′-OH end of the first exon sequence, which was created in the first step, adds to the beginning of the second exon sequence, cleaving the RNA molecule at 3′ splice site; the two exon sequences are thereby joined to each other and the intron sequence is released as a lariat. The spliceosome complex sediments at 60S, indicating that it is nearly as large as a ribosome. These splicing reactions occur in the nucleus and generate mRNa molecules from primary RNA transcripts (mRNA precursor molecules).*

which have several different spliced variants and different affinities for various members of the FGF family.

Control of transcription

Following histone acetylation, various proteins bind to the promoter regions of genes to act as promoters and repressors. These can be classified into the following types:

- Helix-turn-helix proteins, which are comprised solely of amino acids and have a structure that facilitates binding into the major groove of DNA – their binding may block transcription or, conversely, may force bending of the DNA molecule facilitating transcription. The homeo-domain proteins are a type of helix-turn-helix protein involved in sequential embryonic development. Each of these homeo-domain proteins contains an identical section of 60 amino acids.
- Zinc finger proteins. Some transcription factors are rich in histidine and cysteine residues which can bind zinc, thereby bending the protein into a finger-like shape. Steroid hormone receptors also contain several zinc fingers and are thought to function as transcription factors.
- Proteins with a leucine zipper motif. Certain α protein chains can form Y-shaped dimers which can attach to DNA; the two chains are held together by interactions between hydrophobic regions that are rich in leucine.
- Helix-loop-helix proteins. These form similar structures to leucine zippers.

These protein regulators of gene transcription can turn genes on or off depending on how they link with other transcription factors and RNA polymerase. It is also clear that many gene-regulatory proteins act at a distance upstream or downstream of the gene itself (Figure 2.27). These gene regulatory proteins can have their function changed by increased de novo synthesis when needed, by ligand binding, by phosphorylation or by combination with a second agent.

In addition to these specific transcription factors, general transcription factors are also required. Several proto-oncogenes are transcription factors. *Fos* and *jun* combine when phosphorylated to form the AP-1 protein, which functions as a transcription factor. Several growth factors interact through *ras* to activate MAP kinase (mitogen-activated kinase). MAP kinase phosphorylates a protein called Elk-1, which itself activates the transcription of *fos*.

Modification of DNA can alter transcription

DNA that is tightly packaged around nucleosomes or the type that is packaged into heterochromatin is not easily transcribed. Unwinding of chromatin is controlled by acetylation of histone residues (deacetylation producing chromatin condensation). Condensation of the second X chromosome in women may affect the maternal or paternal copy at random, but small zones of neighbouring cells in tissues will have the same X chromosome inactivated as a mosaic pattern. Another method of inactivating genes is heavy methylation of cytosine bases, which

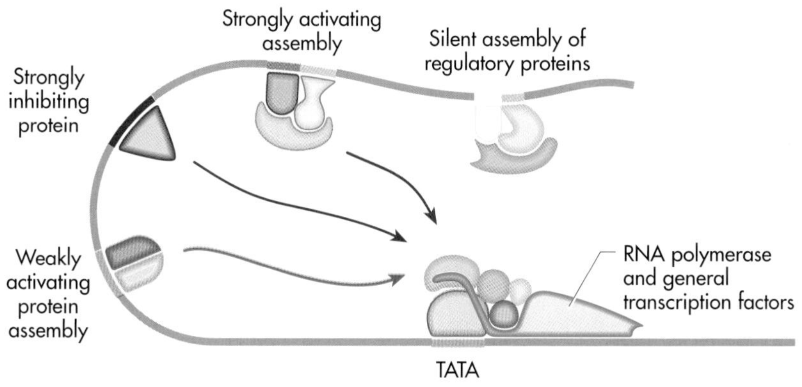

Figure 2.27 *Integration at a promoter. Multiple sets of gene regulatory proteins can work together to influence a promoter, as they do in the eve stripe 2 module. It is not yet understood in detail how the integration of multiple inputs is achieved.*

can result in inactivation of either the maternal or the paternal copies of particular genes. For instance, only the paternal insulin-like growth factor II gene is active; the maternal copy is inactivated or 'imprinted' throughout the whole body. Recent data have suggested that some tumour-suppressor genes can be inactivated – not through mutations or deletions, as in the case of retinoblastoma or p53 – but through heavy methylation (such as the *MTS* gene, which encodes the p16 protein).

Post-transcriptional modifications in mRNA stability

Another method of controlling how much protein is produced by mRNA is to alter the stability of mRNA, which is normally a nascent molecule with a half-life of around 30 minutes to 10 hours. Some mRNAs have lengths of AU-rich non-coding sequences at the 3′ end which stimulate the removal of the poly-A tail, making the mRNA more stable. Some steroid hormones also increase the stability of certain mRNA molecules. Modification of the mRNA molecule can be mediated by proteins or, in some instances, can be mediated by RNA sequences that have intrinsic enzymic activity (that is, they are RNA-ases). Post-translational modifications in peptide chains can also lead to increased protein stability and increased duration of action.

Ribosomal RNA (Figure 2.28)

During cell division, a large number of new ribosomes are required, and because the amplification process involved in protein synthesis (mRNA being translated into many protein molecules) is not available, most cells contain tandemly arranged multiple copies of ribosomal genes (around 200 per cell) on five pairs of different chromosomes. A tandem repeat is formed when duplicated DNA segments are joined head to tail. The initial ribosomal RNA (rRNA) transcript is 13 000 nucleotides long and is cut into three to form the 28S rRNA (5000 nucleotides), the 18S rRNA (2000 nucleotides) and the 5.8S rRNA (160 nucleotides) components of the ribosome. The 5S component of the large ribosomal subunit is transcribed separately by RNA polymerase III, and there are 2000 copies of the 5S rRNA genes arranged as a single cluster.

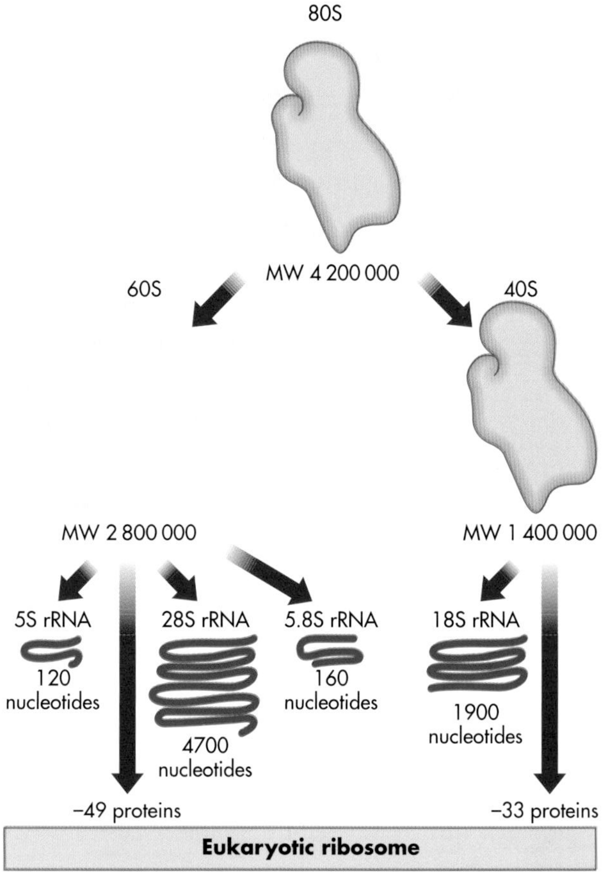

Figure 2.28 *Eukaryotic ribosomes. Ribosomal components are commonly designated by their 'S values', which indicate their rate of sedimentation in an ultracentrifuge. Despite the differences in the number and size of their rRNA and protein components, both types of ribosomes have nearly the same structure, and they function in very similar ways. Although the 18S and 28S rRNAs of the eukaryotic ribosome contain many extra nucleotides not present in their bacterial counterparts, these nucleotides are present as multiple insertions that are thought to protrude as loops and leave the basic structure of each rRNA largely unchanged.*

Packaging of ribosomal RNA occurs in the nucleolus, in which we find several large loops of DNA containing the tandem repeats for rRNA, which are known as nucleolar organizer regions. Here rRNA is transcribed by RNA polymerase I.

PROTEIN SYNTHESIS

When the mature mRNA reaches the cytoplasm after passing through the nuclear pores, it becomes

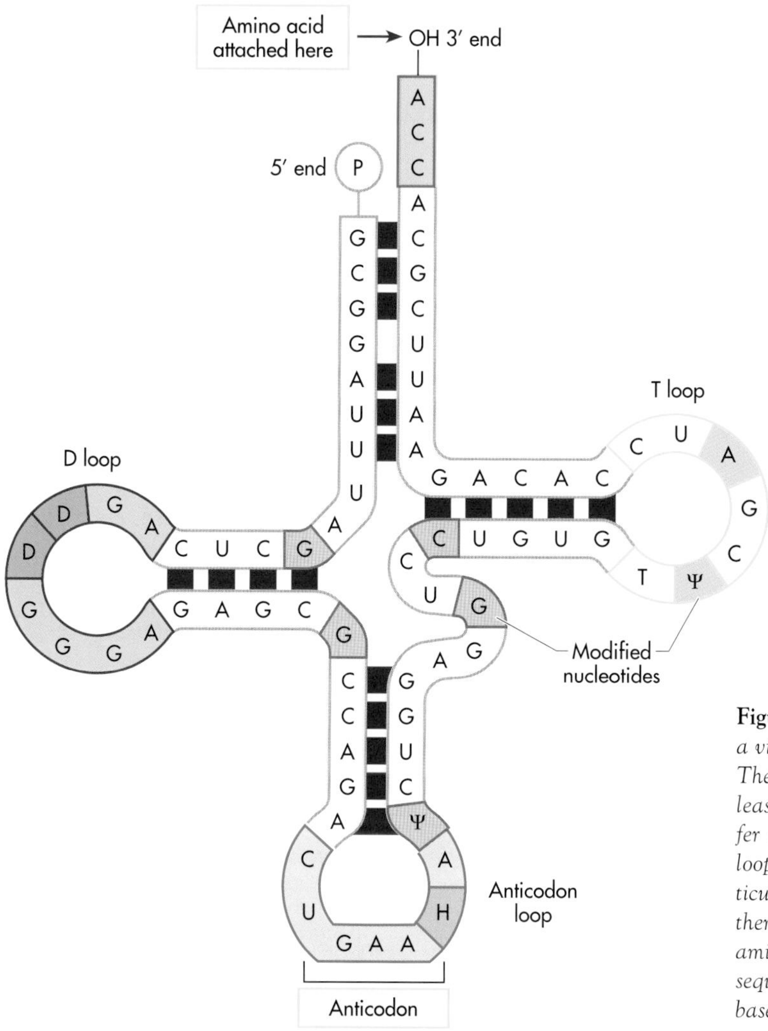

Figure 2.29 *The 'cloverleaf' structure of tRNA. This is a view of a molecule after it has been partially unfolded. There are many different tRNa molecules, including at least one for each kind of amino acid. Although they differ in nucleotide sequence, they all have the three stem loops shown plus an amino acid-accepting arm. The particular tRNA molecule shown binds phenylalanine and is therefore denoted* $tRNA^{Phe}$*. In all tRNa molecules, the amino acid is attached to the A residue of a CCA sequence at the 3′ end of the molecule. Complementary base-pairings are shown by* red bars.

attached to ribosomes which catalyse the production of a peptide chain. Each amino acid is brought to the ribosome by its own specific small molecule of RNA, the transfer RNA (tRNA: Figure 2.29) which has an 'anticodon' at its base corresponding to the codon for that particular amino acid. Specific enzymes couple specific amino acids to their particular tRNA molecule after the amino acid is activated by the attachment of AMP (an adenylated amino acid). The tRNA connected to its amino acid is referred to as an amino-acyl tRNA (transfer RNA) because of the bond between the amino acid and the tRNA. These mechanisms ensure that the right amino acid is brought by the correct tRNA to its specified position within the peptide chain. The genetic code is degenerate because most amino acids are coded for by more than one triplet, so that there is more than one tRNA for each amino acid, and a single tRNA can bind with more than one codon. Many amino acids require that the codon is accurate only in its first two positions (Table 2.2) and will tolerate 'wobble' in the third position. Each incoming amino acid is attached to the carboxy end of the growing peptide chain.

Each ribosome consists of two major parts: the 60S and 40S subunits. The large 60S subunit comprises three separate parts: a 28S rRNA, a 5.5S rRNA and a 5S rRNA (Figure 2.30). These two subunits dock separately (the small subunit attaches first) on the mRNA at the AUG start codon (Figure 2.30) and dock separately when the stop codon (UAG) is reached (Figure 2.31). Identification of the initiation site is important because, in principle, the mRNA can be read in any one of the reading frames,

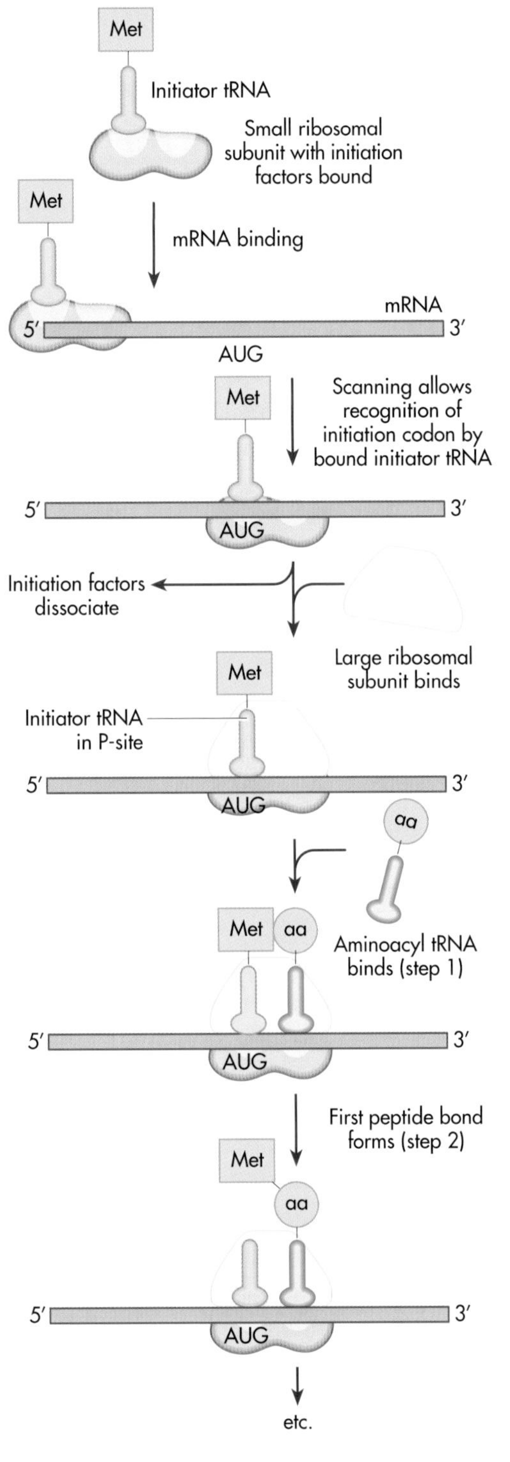

Figure 2.30 *The initiation phase of protein synthesis in eukaryotes.*

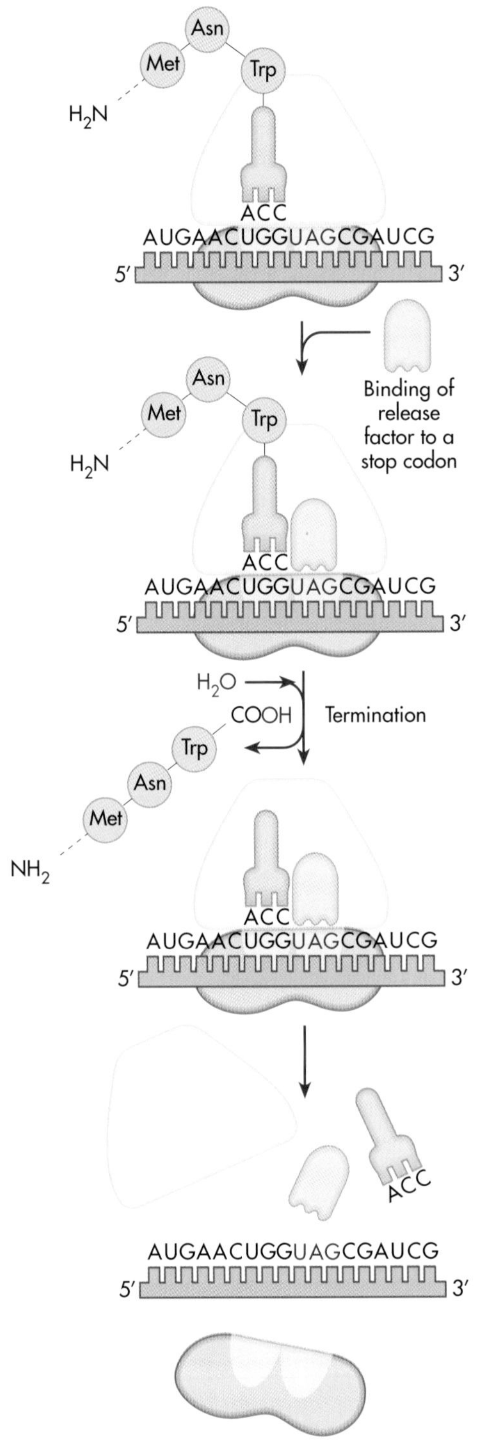

Figure 2.31 *The final phase of protein synthesis. The binding of release factor to a stop codon terminates translation. The completed polypeptide is released, and the ribosome dissociates into its two separate subunits.*

depending on the exact start site. Initiation factors assemble with the methionine tRNA at the start site before translation occurs.

Usually, there are several ribosomes attached to each mRNA molecule, so that at any one time there are several peptide chains in various stages of completion of synthesis. About 50% of the weight of the ribosome is RNA; the remainder comprises several types of proteins. Initially, it was thought that these proteins carried out the catalytic reactions of the RNA, but it is now clear that the RNA itself has these properties, and the function of the proteins is to modify these enzymatic functions. The ribosome has three binding sites for RNA; one for mRNA, one for incoming tRNA (A site) and one for outgoing tRNA and peptide chain (P site). On binding of an incoming tRNA, the amino-acyl-RNA bond is lysed, and the peptide bond is formed between the new amino acid and the peptide chain. The peptidyl-RNA in the A site is then moved to the P site by means of an energy-dependent reaction (GTP driven), freeing the A site for a new amino acid.

Obviously, recognition of the correct amino acid attached to the correct tRNA molecule is important. Firstly, the attachment of the amino acid to the tRNA is specific, and if an incorrect amino acid is bound to the amino-acyl synthetase enzyme, it is removed by hydrolysis. Secondly, the tRNA is attached to the mRNA as a complex with elongation factors which prevent the amino acid from immediately undergoing attachment to the peptide chain; there is a short delay which allows an incorrect tRNA to exit from the codon. It should be noted that the control of the levels of protein formation is achieved by the following three factors:

1. controlling over gene transcription
2. controlling the speed of mRNA degradation
3. controlling post-translational peptide and altering protein stability.

For instance, upregulation of p53 in epidermal cells following exposure to sunlight is achieved by increasing the stability of protein which has already been made.

3

Inflammation

Neville Woolf

INTRODUCTION

Inflammation is a reaction to injury in living tissue resulting in the accumulation of phagocytic cells and components of circulating plasma in the injured area. The inflammatory response is mediated via two biological pathways: the first involves changes in the calibre and permeability of the vessels constituting the microcirculation; the second is a complex series of operations leading to activation of leucocytes. Basically, the inflammatory reaction is a protective one elicited by tissue injury or by the entry into a host of non-self elements such as pathogenic micro-organisms. Inflammation acts to digest the components of dead tissue and to destroy and isolate the non-self elements just alluded to. It should not be forgotten, however, that the same functions which protect can also have devastating consequences, as, for example, when the inflammatory process becomes inappropriately activated in a systemic context, as in septic shock.

Changes in the microcirculation

Injury is followed by an increase in calibre of arterioles, capillaries and venules at the site of its application. Arterioles dilate as a result of a chemically mediated relaxation of smooth muscle; capillaries and venules do so passively as a result of the increased flow mediated by arteriolar dilatation. This increase in local blood flow leads to two of the classic signs of acute inflammation: redness and heat.

Inflammation is characterized also by an increase in permeability of the microvessels, thus allowing more water and electrolyte, derived from plasma, to escape into the interstitial tissue, as well as the escape of high-molecular-weight proteins, such as fibrinogen, not normally found in extravascular interstitial fluid. This process, termed 'exudation', causes another of the classic signs of inflammation, swelling, which may be localized, or may be the accumulation of oedema fluid within serosa-lined spaces, such as the pericardial sac or peritoneal cavity.

Leucocyte activation

This is a complex set of sequential processes, which include:

- adhesion of leucocytes to microvascular endothelium in affected areas
- migration of leucocytes through gaps between endothelial cells and across the basement membranes to reach the extravascular compartment
- attachment of phagocytes to infecting micro-organisms, to dead or injured cells or to foreign material at the site of injury
- engulfment (phagocytosis) by the leucocytes of micro-organisms or cell/tissue debris
- microbial killing or digestion of cellular debris by phagocytes
- effects on surrounding cells/tissues of chemical mediators, either secreted or otherwise released from leucocytes.

CAUSES OF INFLAMMATION

The causes of inflammation are as follows:

- mechanical trauma such as cutting or crushing
- injury caused by living organisms

- chemical injury (exogenous or endogenous)
- excess ultraviolet or X-radiation
- injury due to extremes of heat (burns) or cold (frostbite)
- ischaemia sufficiently severe to cause death or under-perfused tissues
- injury caused by excessive or inappropriate operation of the immune system.

THE FORMATION OF THE INFLAMMATORY EXUDATE

Inflammatory oedema and the formation of exudates are the expression of a net increase in the volume of water and electrolyte moving from the vascular to the extravascular compartment in the injured area, this being associated with the escape also of large-molecular-weight proteins (such as fibrinogen) that are normally held within the vascular compartment.

This process can be looked at in two ways. First, we need to consider the forces that determine the normal relationship between intra- and extravascular fluid and, second, the anatomical routes via which transfer of fluid and protein occurs.

Water, solute and protein leakage

Transport of water and solute across the microvascular endothelium shows many of the characteristics of ultrafiltration. Here, physical forces control the movement of fluid and electrolytes. The two forces normally acting (in opposition to each other) in this context are as follows:

- intravascular hydrostatic pressure, which tends to push fluid out into the extravascular compartment
- plasma oncotic pressure exerted by proteins, most notably albumin.

An increase in the first force and a decrease in the second greatly increase fluid loss from the vascular compartment, a situation that is by no means confined to the context of inflammation. Normally, the result of interaction between these opposing forces is a small net outflow of fluid from the microcirculation. This excess fluid then drains from the extravascular compartment via the lymphatics. The importance of this last step is dramatically illustrated in patients with lymphoedema.

Chemical analysis of inflammatory exudates shows a protein concentration and pattern that is simply not attainable by the mechanisms mentioned above and for which other explanations must be canvassed. Such an explanation is readily found in the many data indicating that injury is followed by an increase in the permeability of microvessels. The patterns of exudate formation that we see in mammalian inflammation are the functional expressions of the severity and duration of injury and of the effects that such injury has on microvascular endothelium.

In mild injury, such as that caused by histamine, serotonin or bradykinin, it has been proposed that plasma leakage was due to the formation of gaps between the endothelial cells of postcapillary venules. Recent studies have confirmed this and show that these gaps are coterminous with the sites of plasma leakage.

Patterns of increased vascular permeability are usually characterized in terms of two variables: the time between the injury and the first recordable changes in microvascular permeability, and the duration of the increase in such permeability. These patterns are described briefly in Table 3.1.

Neutrophil and leucocyte actions and activation in acute inflammation

One of the most important components in defence against 'non-self' elements is phagocytosis, first described by the Nobel laureate, Élie Metchnikoff. If there is a lack of phagocytic cells or if those cells cannot seek out, engulf and destroy infectious organisms, the life of the affected individual will be endangered by increased susceptibility to infection.

The pivotal cell in the early phases of any inflammatory reaction is the neutrophil, which is present in relatively high concentrations in the blood, rapidly replaceable from bone-marrow precursors and able to move more quickly than other leucocytes.

The two sets of lysosomal granules, that have led to their being called by some *granulocytes* contain enzymes such as muramidase (lysozyme), proteases, cationic proteins which act as reinforcing signals,

Table 3.1 Patterns of increased vascular permeability in acute inflammation.

	Immediate transient	Delayed persistent	Immediate persistent
Injury	Mild	Moderate	Severe
Onset	Almost immediately	Up to 24 hours	Within a few minutes
Peak time	5 minutes	4–24 hours	15–60 minutes in experimental circumstances
Site of leakage	Postcapillary venules	Capillaries (relatively early peaking); venules plus capillaries in later peaking	
Duration	± 15 minutes	Hours or days	Microvessels of all types
Mechanism	Histamine-induced interendothelial gap formation	Gap formation plus mild endothelial cell injury	Severe damage to endothelial cells and pericytes
Example	Mild type 1 hypersensitivity	Sunburn	Serious burns, major mechanical trauma

peroxidase, lactoferrin (an iron-binding protein that inhibits bacterial multiplication) and alkaline phosphatase.

The operations necessary for effective neutrophil function have been listed on page 57. Few are more intriguing than the first of these: the adhesion between neutrophils and the microvascular endothelium, without which emigration of phagocytes from the blood into areas of tissue injury cannot occur. Failure to achieve a bond between neutrophils and endothelium occurs in some rare inherited syndromes and is associated with repeated episodes of bacterial infection.

Adhesion between leucocytes and endothelium is a two-stage process. In the first of these, the neutrophils move to the periphery of the column of flowing blood, adhere momentarily to the endothelial surface and then roll along that surface. In the second phase, the cells bind to the endothelial surface and flatten out before migrating through interendothelial cell gaps.

These two phases are mediated by two distinct sets of ligands and receptors. In the rolling phase, the microvascular endothelial cells in an injured area express molecules known as selectins because of their structural resemblance to lectins, a set of proteins, widely distributed in nature, that can distinguish with exquisite sensitivity between different complex sugars. Two types of selectin are known. One, E-selectin, is synthesized and expressed only after injury. This occurs about 30 minutes after the injury and usually reaches its peak in 2–4 hours. E-selectin binds to a complex sugar on the surface of white cells known as *sialyLewisX*. Its expression is triggered by several signals, including the important cytokines interleukin-1 (IL-1) and tumour necrosis factor-α (TNF-α).

The second, P-selectin, is synthesized constitutively and is stored in organelles, the Weibel-Palade bodies, within the endothelial cytoplasm. Following stimulation by appropriate triggers, the P-selectin is translocated to the endothelial surface, where it binds to another leucocyte surface sugar, lacto-*n*-fucopentaose III.

In the second phase of leucocyte adhesion, the endothelial components in the ligand–receptor interaction belong to a set of proteins known as the immunoglobulin gene superfamily. These include heavy and light chains of immunoglobulin, the α and β chains of the T-lymphocyte receptor, major histocompatibility peptides of both classes, β_2-microglobulin, CD4 and CD8 molecules on T lymphocytes and adhesion molecules on endothelium. The last-named comprise ICAM 1 and 2 (*i*nter*c*ellular *a*dhesion *m*olecules), VCAM-1 (*v*ascular *c*ell *a*dhesion *m*olecule) and PECAM-1 (*p*latelet-*e*ndothelial *c*ellular *a*dhesion *m*olecule). ICAM 1 and 2 play a significant role in the binding of leucocytes to the endothelial surface. PECAM-1 contributes to the egress of leucocytes from the microvessels, and treatment with antibodies raised against PECAM inhibits leucocyte emigration, despite adhesion being perfectly normal. ICAM 1 and 2 are expressed constitutively on endothelium, but at very low levels. Release of the cytokines IL-1 and TNF-α upregulates IC expression, which reaches its peak about 24 hours after injury.

The leucocyte components belong to a family of two-chained transmembrane proteins known as integrins, which are expressed in many cell types. Some integrins are cell specific; this is the case with leucocytes, which express LFA-1, Mac1 and p150,95. These have a common β chain (CD18), and it is absence of this chain that underlies leucocyte adhesion syndromes.

Adhesion of leucocytes is followed by emigration from the small vessels, a process taking 2–9 minutes. Leucocyte pseudopodia are inserted into interendothelial cell gaps, and the cells then move across the vessel wall into the surrounding tissues. As already mentioned, PECAM-1 plays an important part in this process, as does C-X-C chemokine known as IL-8.

Movement of leucocytes out of the microvasculature and through the extravascular compartment uses the same mechanisms that are involved in both phagocytosis and intracellular granule movement. They involve the plasma membrane of activated leucocytes and the peripheral zone of the leucocyte cytoplasm.

As with any cell capable of movement, leucocytes move as a result of interaction between the contractile proteins actin and myosin. Stimulation of leucocytes by chemical signals results in an increasing proportion of the intracellular actin becoming arranged in a filamentous form, a process which is controlled by the expression of various proteins that can be stimulated or inhibited by calcium fluxes within the cells.

Phagocytes are stimulated not merely to move in the course of inflammatory reactions but also to move in a directed and purposive manner towards areas of tissue injury or of invasion by micro-organisms. This is termed 'chemotaxis', which, as its name implies, is controlled by a series of chemical messengers. In order for such a system to work, there must be adequate:

- generation of signals that attract leucocytes to the site of injury
- reception of these signals by protein or glycoprotein molecules on the surfaces of leucocytes
- transduction of the received signals so that the target leucocytes translate the former into action.

These signals, the chemical mediators of inflammation, are discussed in a later section of this chapter.

Reception and transduction of chemotactic signals is likely to start with the binding of the signal to a transmembrane receptor protein on the surface of the phagocyte. This is known to be true in the case of both the 5a component of the complement system and the formylated peptides released from bacteria in the course of bacterial protein synthesis. Occupation of a ligand-binding site on a surface receptor produces conformational changes that activate a G protein lying just beneath the plasma membrane and connected to the latter by a farnesyl bond. This in turn activates phospholipase, which cleaves phosphoinositol diphosphate (PIP_2). Cleavage of this molecule releases diacyglycerol and inositol triphosphate. The former activates protein kinase C, and the resulting protein cascade causes degranulation and secretion of granule contents; the latter produces calcium fluxes within the cell, which mediate chemotactic movement, and also releases arachidonic acid from cell membranes, with synthesis of prostaglandins and leukotrienes.

Cyclic nucleotides also play an important role in initiating leucocyte movement. cAMP and cGMP act in an opposing manner and may constitute a control system for regulating chemotactic movement and degranulation. cGMP enhances chemotactic movement, the release of histamine and leukotrienes from mast cells, the release of lymphokines from activated T lymphocytes and the release of granule contents from neutrophils. In this context, the main effect of the cyclic nucleotides is probably exerted on the microtubules. cGMP promotes assembly of microtubules from tubulin, and cAMP has the opposite effect. Thus, drugs (such as levamisole) that raise the intracellular content of cGMP enhance the movement of phagocytes towards the source of chemoattractant substances and reverse the depression in chemotaxis that may follow a number of viral infections.

PHAGOCYTOSIS

Phagocytosis is the biological raison d'être of neutrophils. Before it can occur, the neutrophils travelling up their chemotactic gradient must recognize the particles, living or dead, which are to be engulfed and attach to them by means of ligand–receptor interactions. It has long been known that bacteria coated with immunoglobulin or dead tissue particles that have been exposed to fresh serum are more readily phagocytosed than those that have not. This coating of particles with protein is called *opsonization*.

Opsonins are either:

- immunoglobulins of the IgG class. For successful attachment of phagocytes to take place, the Fc fragment of the immunoglobulin must be intact.
- the C3b component of complement. This is of great biological value in defence against infection since complement activation by the alternate pathway does not require interaction between bacterial antigens and specific antibody.

The apparent restriction of opsonization to these two protein classes indicates that the phagocyte plasma membrane is the site of receptors both for the Fc fragment of immunoglobulin and the C3b component of complement.

For engulfment of bacteria, non-living 'foreign' particles, or cell and tissue debris, finger-like pseudopodia project from the plasma membrane of the phagocyte and fuse on the 'far' side of the object to be engulfed, thus enclosing it within a vesicle formed of plasma membrane (the phagosome). The phagosome then buds off from the inner surface of the plasma membrane and migrates into the cytoplasm of the neutrophil or macrophage. The boundaries of the phagosome are formed of inverted plasma membrane, the inner lining of the phagosome being composed of the outer layer of the phagocyte plasma membrane.

Phagocytosis is an energy-dependent process that is inhibited by anything that interferes with ATP production. It is likely that the same mechanisms that 'power' phagocyte movement are involved in phagocytosis and substances that inhibit chemotactic movement also inhibit phagocytosis.

Lysosomal fusion and degranulation

Phagosome formation is followed by movement of the lysosomes and fusion of the phagosome/lysosome membranes, this being associated with disappearance of the intralysosomal granules. The process is extremely rapid, and, again, as is the case with phagocytosis, is inhibited by any chemical substance that interferes with phagocyte movement.

BACTERIAL KILLING

The principal method of bacterial killing is oxygen-dependent. Phagocytosis is associated with a burst of oxidative activity known as the respiratory burst. This results in a step-wise reduction of molecular oxygen, ending in the formation of hydrogen peroxide, as follows:

- The respiratory burst is associated with a 2–20-fold increase in oxygen consumption, compared with a resting phagocyte, and there is a significant increase in glucose metabolism via the hexose monophosphate shunt.
- The reduction of molecular oxygen is catalysed by a non-haem protein oxidase believed to be localized in the phagocyte plasma membrane. The presence of this oxidase is crucial for this

type of bacterial killing; its absence leads to the congenital disorder known as chronic granulomatous disease of childhood.
- The hydrogen donor for oxygen reduction is either reduced nicotinamide adenine dinucleotide (NADH) or reduced nicotinamide adenine dinucleotide phosphate (NADPH). The presence of one of these is an essential link in the chain because hydrogen peroxide formation requires regeneration of NAD to NADP. The logical correlate of this is a requirement for adequate amounts of intracellular glucose-6-phosphate dehydrogenase if bacterial killing is to proceed normally.
- The reduction of molecular oxygen involves the gain of only one electron, resulting in the formation of an oxygen free radical, the superoxide anion (O_2^-). About 90% of the molecular oxygen consumed in the respiratory burst is converted into superoxide anion.
- The reaction of two superoxide anions in the presence of water results in the formation of hydrogen peroxide and molecular oxygen. This is termed a dismutation reaction and is catalysed by the enzyme superoxide dismutase. Other highly reactive oxygen species formed in association with phagocyte activation include the highly reactive hydroxyl radical ($OH^•$), singlet oxygen and hypochlorous acid.

It is now believed that the most potent oxygen-dependent bactericidal activity in phagocytes is associated with hydrogen peroxide. This molecule, by itself, has significant bactericidal activity, but this is very markedly potentiated by a reaction occurring between hydrogen peroxide and intracytoplasmic halide ions that is catalysed by the lysosomal enzyme, myeloperoxidase. The bactericidal effect is probably mediated by halogenation or oxidation of cell-surface components.

Other mechanisms of bacterial killing

While oxygen-dependent killing is pivotal in defence against infection, it is not the only bactericidal mechanism. Some are related to the character of lysosomes and include the following:

- Low pH within the lysosome (3.5–4.0). This in itself may be bactericidal or bacteriostatic. In addition, the acid milieu promotes the production of hydrogen perioxide.
- Lysosomes containing lysozyme (muramidase), a low-molecular-weight cationic protein that attacks the mucopeptide cell walls of some bacteria.
- Lactoferrin, an iron-binding protein found within lysosomes that inhibits the growth of several micro-organisms.
- Lysosomal cationic proteins and hydrolases.

DEFECTS IN NEUTROPHIL FUNCTION

These defects may be quantitative or qualitative.

Even if all the operations described above are carried out normally, successful neutrophil defence against micro-organisms requires an adequate number of these cells. Thus, neutropaenia from any cause confers a major increment of risk of infection. This situation can occur in any form of marrow failure such as may be caused by the following:

- drugs, chemotherapeutic agents and toxins
- bone-marrow infiltration by large numbers of tumour cells
- bone marrow fibrosis.

Qualitative defects, of which there are many, can be considered most conveniently in relation to the specific functions which are defective. This is set out in Table 3.2.

CHEMICAL MEDIATORS OF ACUTE INFLAMMATION

The process involved in acute inflammation, especially those controlling the activation of neutrophils, are under the control of a very large number of chemical signals. These mediators can be broadly classified under the rubrics exogenous and endogenous.

Only one group of exogenous mediators is recognized – the formylated peptides. These are low-molecular-weight compounds produced by micro-organisms in the course of protein synthesis, and all have methionine as the N-terminal residue. The most powerfully acting of these peptides is formylated methionine-leucyl-phenylalanine (*F-Met-Leu-Phe*),

Table 3.2 Defects in neutrophil function.		
Function affected	Disorder	Characteristics
Migration and chemotaxis	'Lazy leucocyte' syndrome	Defective response to chemotactic signals; nature of defect not yet elucidated
	Job's syndrome	Typically affects fair-skinned, red-haired females; patients suffer from recurrent 'cold' staphylococcal abscesses
	Poorly controlled diabetes mellitus	Poor leucocyte movement reversed by insulin and glucose
	Chédiak-Higashi syndrome	Rare autosomal recessive syndrome occurring in humans, cattle, mink and certain strains of mouse. Characterized by partial albinism, giant lysosomal granules in neutrophils and enhanced susceptibility to infection. Believed to be related to failure of assembly of microtubules from tubulin. Can be reversed (ex vivo) by agents that increase intracellular cGMP
	Leucocyte adhesion deficiency syndrome	Due to absence of the CD18 β subunit of the integrins expressed on neutrophil surface. Affects neutrophils only since other leucocytes express and adhesion molecule binding to VCAM on endoethelium
	Drug-related inhibition of leucocyte movement	Can occur after steroids or phenylbutazone
	Deficiencies in release of chemotactic signals	Affects mainly the complement system
Disorders of phagocytosis	Opsonin deficiencies	Deficiencies in complement or IgG. Some patients with sickle-cell disease show opsonin deficiency believed to be due to failure to activate the alternate pathway of complement activation
	Failure of engulfment	Can occur in hyperosmolar states; may also be caused by drugs such as morphine analogues
	Failures in lysosomal fusion	May be caused by drugs (steroids, colchicine, certain antimalarial agents)
Disorders of bacterial killing	Chronic granulomatous diseases (CGD) of childhood	A rare disorder of childhood, sometimes X-linked and sometimes occurring as an autosomal recessive disorder. Characterized by recurrent bacterial infections involving skin, bones, lungs and lymph nodes. Lymph nodes draining infected areas are often enlarged and show sinusoids packed with mononuclear phagocytes and focal granuloma-like aggregates of mononuclear cells The functional defect is failure of the respiratory burst (see pages 61 and 62) and thus failure of oxygen-dependent killing This reflects a defect in the cytochrome b-245 oxidase system that has two subunits. The X-linked syndrome is due to a mutation in the gene encoding the larger subunit and, in most cases, no gene product at all is produced About 1/3 of patients with CGD have the autosomal recessive form, and here the defect arises as the result of a mutation in the gene encoding the smaller subunit or in the cytosolic components of the NADPH oxidase system

for which neutrophils possess a surface receptor. F-Met-Leu-Phe can also cause the expression of some adhesion molecules by microvascular endothelium.

Endogenous mediators

The endogenous mediators of inflammation are grouped as shown in Table 3.3.

While it is impossible in a chapter of this length to comment in any detail on these multiple signalling systems, a few points are worth making.

Complement

The complement system consists of about 20 different proteins, functionally interlinked to play a significant part in immune responses and inflammation. Activation of complement may be achieved in two ways. In the first, the 'classical' pathway, the union of antibody and antigen leads to the binding of a protein known as C1q. This step initiates the whole complement-activation cascade. An 'alternate' pathway exists in which no antibody/antigen union is required, and which can be triggered in many ways, including the presence of many strains of bacteria. The existence of the alternate pathway is clearly of great biological importance in the defence against infection.

Table 3.3 Endogenous mediators of inflammation.

Source	Mediators
Activated plasma protein cascades	The complement system The kinin system The intrinsic blood-clotting pathway The fibrinolytic system
Amines and proteins stored within cells and released on demand	Histamine 5-hydroxytryptamine Lysosomal enzymes and other proteins
Newly synthesized in cells and released from them on demand	**Lipids** Prostaglandins Leukotrienes Platelet-activating factor **Proteins** Cytokines such as interleukin-1 (IL-1) and tumour necrosis factor-α α and β chemokines

Whichever pathway is involved, activation of complement yields chemical species that:

- coat micro-organisms, thus functioning as opsonins
- lead to lysis of cell membranes via the formation of a membrane-attack complex
- influence both the vascular and cellular components of the inflammatory reaction.

Protein mediators – cytokines and chemokines

Activation of cells involved in inflammation and in the immune response is associated with the release of many low-molecular-weight proteins – the cytokines and chemokines. Only a few of the most important will be mentioned here.

Tumour necrosis factor-α (TNF-α)

This molecule derives its name from the fact that the serum of animals given bacterial endotoxin causes necrosis when injected into tumours. The active principle of such serum is the cytokine TNF-α. It is synthesized and secreted by activated macrophages, mast cells and T lymphocytes. At low concentrations, TNF-α upregulates the inflammatory response. It induces expression of adhesion molecules, thus promoting adhesion and migration of leucocytes from the microvessels to the extravascular compartment. It enhances the killing of intracellular organisms such as *Mycobacterium tuberculosis* and *Leishmania* and acts as a positive feedback loop for the production of a variety of cytokines.

At high concentrations (such as we may see in endotoxin shock), TNF-α acts systemically. In this context, it acts as a pyrogen, activates the clotting system, stimulates production of acute-phase proteins by the liver, inhibits myocardial contractility by stimulating nitric oxide production and causes inappropriate vasodilatation by the same mechanism.

Interleukin-1 (IL-1)

The principle sources of IL-1 are monocytes and macrophages, but other cell types, such as endothelial cells and certain epithelial cells, may also produce this cytokine. IL-1 is a potent regulator of both local inflammatory events and many systemic ones. Its synthesis is stimulated by various microbial products, most notably bacterial endotoxin, and also by various cytokines. Locally, it upregulates adhesion molecule expression by endothelial cells, thus promoting adhesion of both leucocytes and platelets. Systemically, IL-1 produces fever and promotes the release of prostaglandins, glucocorticoids and acute-phase proteins. While it shares some of the functions of TNF-α, it lacks certain others, such as the ability to produce haemorrhagic necrosis in tumours.

This commonality of some functions between two molecules as different from each other as IL-1 and TNF-α is not without interest. Many genes that are 'switched on' in inflammatory diseases have their expression induced by IL-1 and TNF-α and, in some cases, TNF-neutralizing antibodies have had a beneficial effect in certain inflammatory disorders, such as rheumatoid arthritis. The link between these two cytokines appears to be that, after binding to their individual cell-surface receptors, both TNF and IL-1 activate a cytoplasmic form of the transcription factor NF-κB. DNA-binding motifs for NF-κB are found in the promoters and enhancers of more than 50 genes that are known to be activated in inflammation.

Chemokines

Chemokines are low-molecular-weight proteins (8–11 kDa) that are important in initiating and sustaining inflammatory reactions. Some preferentially attract neutrophils; others attract monocytes. They are divided into two families: α and β.

The α family is encoded by genes located on chromosome 4. They are characterized by an amino-acid sequence in which two terminal cysteines are separated by some other amino acid, thus giving the sequence Cys-X-Cys. Included in this group are IL-8, β-thromboglobulin, *gro-α*, *-β* and *-γ*, and platelet factor 4.

The main source for the α chemokines is the monocyte, though some are produced also by T lymphocytes and endothelial cells. IL-8 mediates the rapid accumulation of neutrophils in inflamed tissues by inducing the expression of neutrophil-binding adhesion molecules on the surface of endothelial cells in the microvessels in injured areas. The chemokine *gro* acts also as a neutrophil chemoattractant as well as promoting the release of lysosomal enzymes. β thromboglobulin and platelet factor 4 are released from activated platelets and stimulate fibroblasts.

β chemokines are encoded by genes located on chromosome 17. They are potent attractants for memory T cells and monocytes.

Monocytes and macrophages in acute inflammation

The cellular component of acute inflammation includes another type of phagocyte, the mononuclear phagocyte, which exists in two forms. An intermediate form known as the monocyte circulates in the blood; after migration into the tissues, it differentiates into the macrophage.

Monocytes have a half-life of about 222 hours, three times as long as that of the neutrophil. They are derived from bone marrow, and bone-marrow destruction leads to a failure of injury to elicit a mononuclear cell response. Maturation from monocyte to macrophage within the tissues is accompanied by considerable structural and functional increase in the phagocytic, lysosomal and secretory apparatus, so that:

- The cell becomes larger.
- The plasma membrane becomes more convoluted.
- Lysosomes increase in number.
- Both the Golgi apparatus (secretion) and the endoplasmic reticulum (protein synthesis) become more prominent.

Like the neutrophil, the macrophage possesses surface receptors for the Fc component of immunoglobulin as well as for complement components. Again, like the neutrophil, the macrophage depends on anaerobic glycolysis for its energy needs during phagocytosis and has a respiratory burst after engulfment. Macrophages have certain advantages over neutrophils in that they:

- have a longer lifespan
- can synthesize and membranes and intracellular enzymes expended during phagocytosis (as the neutrophil cannot)

- can ingest particles far larger than those that can be engulfed by neutrophils
- can undergo mitotic division.

Many pathogenic micro-organisms are engulfed within macrophages. Some of these parasitize the macrophages and multiply within phagosomes. Such organisms include *Listeria*, *Brucella*, *Salmonella*, *Mycobacteria*, *Chlamydia*, *Rickettsia*, *Leishmania*, *Toxoplasma*, *Trypanosoma* and *Legionella*. This symbiotic relationship is destroyed as a result of what is effectively a dialogue between macrophages and T lymphocytes. Macrophage activation via this route leads to destruction of the 'guest' organisms.

Chemical signals that influence macrophage function

Factors chemotactic for macrophages include those already mentioned in relation to neutrophils. In addition, however, there is an important group of chemical signals that trigger a wide range of macrophage functions other than chemotaxis. These are the lymphokines, secreted by T lymphocytes activated as a consequence of encountering specific antigens. T lymphocytes synthesize and secrete many products. Noteworthy in the context of macrophage activation is interferon-γ; this is the most powerful enhancer of the ability of macrophages to kill intracellular parasites.

It should not be forgotten that macrophages also play a dominant role in the natural history of both healing and chronic inflammation. Their importance in relation to both of these processes rests on the fact that these cells have the power to:

- phagocytose living and non-living foreign material (including tissue debris, old or abnormal red blood cells, immune complexes and modified lipoprotein)
- kill many micro-organisms
- synthesize and release tissue-damaging products
- synthesize and release mediators of acute inflammation and fever
- present antigens to both T and B lymphocytes and in this way initiate immune responses
- become activated by signals released from activated lymphocytes
- release mediators that are chemoattractant for cells involved in repair and new blood vessel formation
- synthesize and release growth factors that are important in healing
- regulate their own activities to a certain extent through the operation of autocrine loops.

4

Immunology

Anne C Cunningham and John A Kirby

INTRODUCTION

The immune system is one of the largest and most complex in the body. Its primary roles are the inactivation of potentially pathogenic micro-organisms and viruses, the prevention of infestation by parasites, and the suppression of tumours. Effective functioning of the immune system is dependent upon the availability of an effective and flexible arsenal with which to fight infection. The power of immune 'effector' mechanisms is well demonstrated by the damage associated with immunopathologies seen in diseases such as glomerulonephritis, rheumatoid arthritis and the extreme vigour of acute allograft rejection. The morbidity associated with genetic or induced immunodeficiency is also indicative of the importance of immune function. Clearly, sensitive, though reliable, mechanisms must exist to regulate the numerous functions of the normal immune system.

The objective of this chapter is to describe the function and regulation of the major components of the immune system. The chapter concludes with a specific discussion of immunological examples drawn from the fields of clinical transplantation and cancer immunobiology.

INNATE IMMUNITY

Non-specific barriers to infection are the first obstacles a pathogen must overcome to achieve successful invasion of its host. These barriers are not acquired, do not change, and allow the specific immune system time to mount a response. The innate system of immune defence is therefore fast-acting but relatively non-specific and non-adaptive. However, it is increasingly clear that the type of innate response influences the quality and quantity of the subsequent specific immune response. At the simplest level, the innate immune system consists of physical and biochemical barriers such as the skin, mucus, acid in the stomach and lysozyme in many secretions, which all help to prevent the entry of micro-organisms into the body. In addition, a battery of complex mechanisms designed to eliminate microbes that have penetrated normal body tissues also exists. These mechanisms include cellular components of the reticuloendothelial system, such as phagocytic mononuclear and polymorphonuclear leucocytes, natural-killer (NK) cells, alternative-pathway activation of the complement system, and a range of acute-phase inflammatory mediators.

Phagocytes

Phagocytes engulf and digest micro-organisms and particles that are harmful to the body. Cells in this category fall into several subpopulations (polymorphonuclear; mononuclear) but are all derived from common stem cells within the bone marrow.

Neutrophils, the most common white blood cell, are generally the first cellular components to respond to tissue injury. They migrate from the blood across the endothelium and into the tissues within seconds of the recognition of a chemotactic stimulus. These stimuli may be chemicals specifically produced by bacteria, factors produced by damaged body cells, or peptides produced during the activation of complement.

Other phagocytic cells include tissue macrophages, such as mesangial cells in the kidney, Kupffer cells in the liver, alveolar macrophages in the lung, histiocytes in connective tissue and microglial cells in the nervous system. Macrophages are highly phagocytic and contain numerous lysosomes and endocytic vesicles. They possess an enhanced antimicrobicidal capacity following activation.

Phagocytes are also capable of secreting soluble agents able non-specifically to damage cells and pathogens within the microenvironment. The most active of these factors are oxygen radicals, which are produced during the 'respiratory burst' that follows cell activation.[1]

Natural-killer (NK) cells

NK cells are frequently termed large granular lymphocytes on the basis of their morphology. The key feature of NK cells is their ability to kill virally infected or transformed body cells.[2] For example, patients with defective NK cells frequently suffer severe infection by viruses such as cytomegalovirus.

In many ways, they are related to cytotoxic T cells.[3] However, their recognition of targets and control of killing is clearly different. NK cells possess receptors that can recognize class I major histocompatibility (MHC) antigens (see section below on Cancer immunotherapy; p. 79), which deliver a strong inhibitory signal to the NK cell, preventing the lysis of healthy cells.[4,5] Many tumours have defective genes or defective genetic regulation, which causes a lowering of the expression of MHC antigens. This reduces the classical immunogenicity of these cells but appears to enhance their susceptibility to NK cell-mediated cytolysis. Furthermore, infected or transformed cells express abnormal proteins, which can then be recognized by NK activating receptors, and stimulate the delivery of a lethal hit.[6]

Complement activation

The complement system consists of up to 20 serum proteins that are involved in three interrelated enzyme cascades termed the 'classical', the 'alternative' and the 'lectin' pathways. The end result of these cascades is the generation of a 'membrane attack complex', which forms a potentially lethal membrane pore and a series of proinflammatory mediators which recruit and activate other effector cells including neutrophils, macrophages and mast cells. The alternative pathway may be activated directly, but non-specifically, by a range of bacterial or yeast cell-wall components, such as lipopolysaccharide (Figure 4.1).[7] The lectin pathway is initiated by mannose-binding lectin (MBL), which recognizes repeating mannose residues in bacterial cell walls. Once bound, this associates with a family of MBL-associated serine proteases (MASP), which activate serum C4 in a similar way to the classical pathway (Figure 4.6; see later) resulting in bacterial cell lysis and the generation of inflammatory mediators (C3a, C4a and C5a).

Inflammatory mediators

The innate immune system's vast cocktail of proinflammatory substances can directly damage, or induce cells to damage, invading pathogens. Inflammation can be local, focusing effective immune responses at the site of infection by altering blood vessels (vasodilatation, increased permeability, and upregulation of adhesion molecules), and the recruitment and activation of leucocytes.

The C3a and C5a peptides released during complement activation possess wide-ranging capabilities, including the promotion of smooth muscle contraction, the retraction of endothelial cells, and the release of histamine by mast cells. Furthermore, C3a and C5a stimulate the chemotaxis and activation of phagocytic leucocytes. These cells carry C3b receptors on their surface and are able to bind specifically to C3b-coated micro-organisms prior to phagocytosis.

Families of inflammatory mediators are produced following the breakdown of membrane phospholipids to arachidonic acid and subsequently to thromboxane, prostaglandins, leukotrienes and platelet-activating factor. Significantly, the majority of anti-inflammatory drugs currently available are directed at these pathways. Other active peptides, including Hageman factor and fibrinopeptides, are released during blood clotting and also increase local vascular permeability and the recruitment of phagocytes.

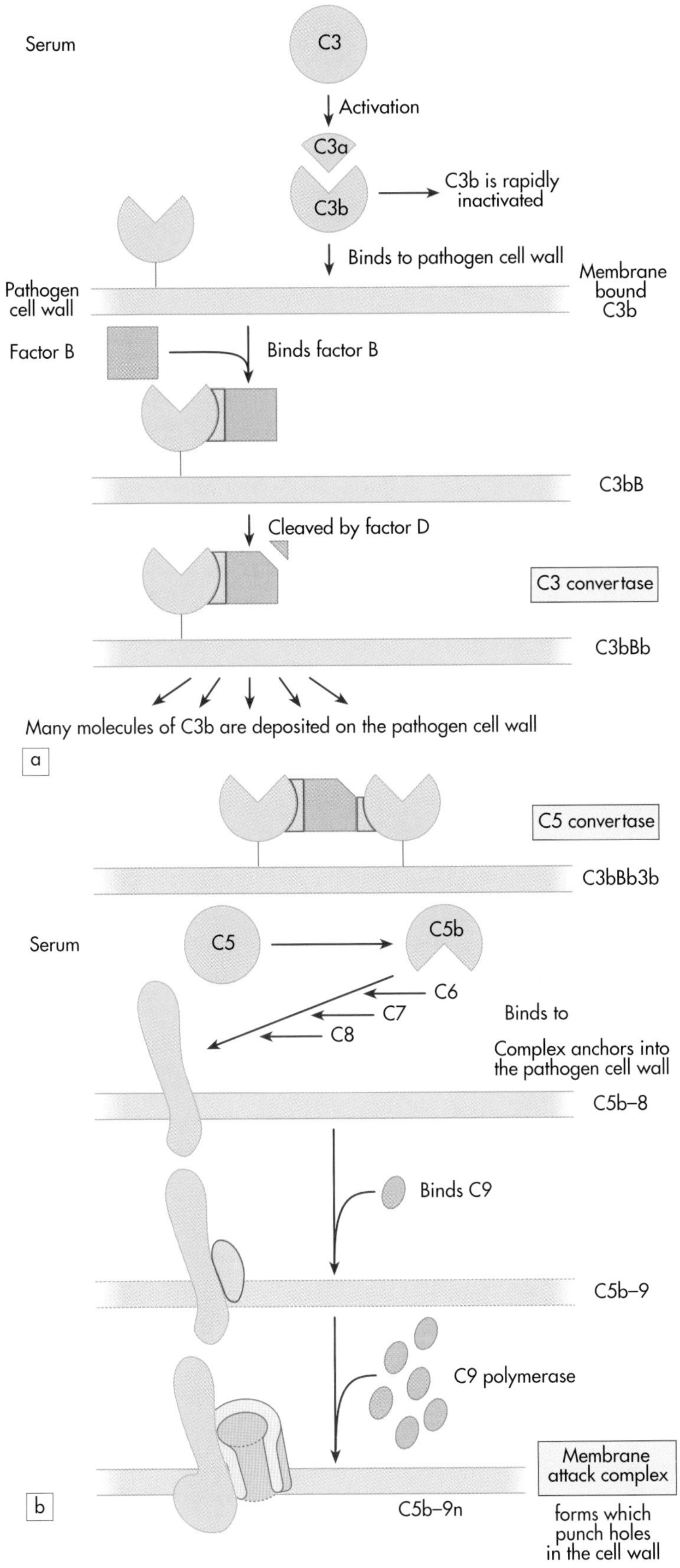

Figure 4.1 *The alternative pathway of complement (a) C3 activation; (b) lytic pathway.*

Inflammation can also be systemic, and is mediated by proinflammatory cytokines (including tumour necrosis factor-alpha (TNFα), interleukin (IL)-1β and IL-6). These lead to an increased temperature (which promotes adaptive immune responses) and increased production of leucocytes by the bone marrow. In addition, they induce acute-phase proteins, such as C-reactive protein, which are massively and rapidly upregulated during infection. These function to upregulate intracellular (phagocytosis) and extracellular (complement activation) killing mechanisms activated locally. Interferons are produced by virally infected cells and protect other cells from infection by the stimulation of mechanisms that prevent viral replication. The above-mentioned substances represent only a selection from the plethora of inflammatory mediators currently known to exist.

Dendritic cells and 'danger' signals

Innate responses play a vital role in the regulation of adaptive immunity. Dendritic cells are specialized mononuclear phagocytes which sit at the interface between these two arms of the immune system. These cells infiltrate normal body tissues and are named after the dendrite-like processes which fan out between the somatic cells. The cells are extremely phagocytic when resting and have a range of receptors which target material for removal, uptake and hydrolysis. These include mannose receptors specific for the repeating sugars found in bacterial cell walls and a receptor that binds to phosphatidyl-serine, which is expressed only on the outer membrane of apoptotic cells. In normal circumstances, dendritic cells degrade the material they phagocytose in a 'silent' manner that excites no further immune intervention, thereby minimizing the potential for autoimmunity.

However, it has become clear recently that dendritic cells also express a range of activation receptors specific for 'pathogen-associated molecular patterns' (PAMPs). The most important of these receptors are termed the 'toll-like' receptors (TLRs), which bind a wide range of molecules whose presence broadly signifies 'danger' to the organism.[8] These are typically derived from pathogenic bacteria but can also include factors such as certain heat-shock proteins, which are released from body cells during times of stress (Table 4.1).

Table 4.1 Summary of the major ligands bound by human toll-like receptors.

Toll-like receptor	Ligand
TLR2 and TLR6	Peptidoglycan (Gram +ve) Lipoarabinomannan LPS (Gram +ve) Zymosan (yeast)
TLR4 (+CD14)	LPS (Gram −ve) Lipoteichoic acids (Heat shock proteins?)
TLR-3	Double strand RNA (viral?)
TLR5	Flagellin
TLR9	Unmethylated CpG oligonucleotides (bacterial)

Following ligation, these receptors activate common pathways including mitogen-activated protein (MAP)-kinase and NF-κB, which result in cellular activation. Following activation, the cells migrate in response to chemical signals (such as chemokines) and move to draining lymph nodes. At the same time, they cease phagocytosis and prepare to present antigens acquired during recent phagocytosis to T cells, central components of the adaptive immune system.

ADAPTIVE IMMUNITY

The adaptive immune system has evolved to provide a versatile defence mechanism against infectious pathogens. The innate immune system is able to hold pathogens at bay for a time, but infectious microorganisms rapidly evolve to bypass these defences. Each process of adaptive immunity is dependent on the function of lymphocytes and is characterized by an escalating response with a high degree of specificity. Furthermore, adaptive responses are characterised by immunological memory, which enables a more vigorous reaction after secondary exposure to a specific agent.

Resting lymphocytes are small mononuclear cells with little cytoplasm. However, following exposure to an antigen, a small proportion of antigen-specific cells expand rapidly and begin to divide. This process of clonal expansion is an essential feature of adaptive immunity. Lymphocytes may be divided functionally into T and B cells.

T cells and cellular immunity

The T-cell precursor is generated within the bone marrow but migrates to the thymus before maturing and developing the ability to recognize foreign antigen. Each newly formed T cell expresses numerous copies of an identical T-cell antigen receptor (TCR). However, the receptor on each different T cell varies in sequence and antigen specificity. This seemingly random variability enables at least a few cells within the total T-cell population to respond to antigens on any given pathogen. Following antigen encounter, these few specific cells divide to generate a sufficient number of responsive cells to mount a useful immune response. Estimates show that a single antigen-specific T cell can proliferate to generate a clone of over 1000 identical cells. This mechanism is termed clonal selection.

In recent years, the process by which maturing T cells generate their enormous receptor diversity has been determined. The T-cell receptor (TCR) is a heterodimer and, for more than 90% of the cells, consists of an α and a β chain. Each chain is composed of a variable region, a constant region, a transmembrane region and a cytoplasmic tail. The initial genomic sequence of DNA encoding each chain contains a large number of possible variable sequences followed by multiple diversity and joining sequences. Each mature chain is produced after a genetic rearrangement process that involves extensive deletion of genomic DNA and the resplicing of single, variable, joining and diversity regions. It has been estimated that this process can yield a total of 10^{17} different $\alpha\beta$ T-cell receptors.[9]

A proportion of T cells, particularly those found close to the epithelial cells of the mucosa (including the genitourinary tract), express an alternative form of the T-cell antigen receptor. This consists of a γ and δ chain heterodimer. The function of these $\gamma\delta$ T cells is not clear. They appear to be less variable than $\alpha\beta$ T cells, and are thought to represent an older, more primitive lineage.[10]

Receptors expressed by each T cell are generated by a random process, and it is therefore likely that some newly formed cells will recognize antigens produced by healthy, or 'self', body cells. The capacity to discriminate between self and non-self, and to prevent a response to self, is vital for normal immune function. This important requirement is fulfilled by the thymus, which is essential for the generation of T-cell self-tolerance. Equally essential to normal immune function is the thymus' other function – to provide a microenvironment suitable for T-cell maturation.

Thymic tolerance

T-cell function is regulated by the affinity of the antigen receptor for a given ligand. The T cell will be activated by interaction with an antigen only if the affinity is sufficiently high. Essentially, the thymus selects newly formed cells that show no more than a low affinity for all self antigens but deletes any cell bearing receptors that recognize self antigens with a dangerously high affinity. It has been estimated that only 3% of newly formed T cells survive this selection process and escape the thymus to join the recirculating pool.

T-cell recirculation

T cells that have not encountered their specific antigen, and are therefore naive, migrate from the circulation across specialized high endothelial venules to secondary lymphoid sites, such as the spleen, lymph nodes, and Peyer's patches in the genitourinary tract. These sites provide the ideal environment for contact with foreign antigens, and enable antigen-specific clonal expansion and the generation of effector/memory subsets. If a naive lymphocyte is not activated after 10–20 hours, it recirculates from the lymph node, through the lymphatic system and back into the blood at the thoracic duct. However, during an immune response, the blood flow through a lymph node rises dramatically and increases the number of lymphocytes within the node. Non-specific resting cells leave the node followed, after 3–4 days, by a large number of activated antigen-specific T cells. These cells recirculate to the site of primary inflammation and to local lymphoid tissues. Finally, after a week or so, small, long-lived memory cells begin to leave the lymph node to join the recirculating pool. It has been estimated for adults that almost 50% of recirculating T cells are memory cells. These memory cells migrate differently from naive T cells and recirculate through the peripheral tissue where they first encountered their specific antigen (such as the skin, genitourinary, gastrointestinal or respiratory system).

Major histocompatibility antigens

Human cells can express two classes of MHC antigen. The class I antigens are expressed constitutively on most cells, whereas the class II antigens are generally induced by stimulation with proinflammatory cytokines such as interferon-γ or TNF-α. Class II MHC antigens are generally only expressed constitutively by specialized cells of the immune system that are adapted for antigen presentation (such as dendritic cells). MHC molecules are specialized glycoproteins that bind a diverse array of peptides and present them to T cells.

Resolution of the structure of the MHC antigens (Figure 4.2) has been one of the most significant advances in immunology during the past few years.[11,12] Class I and class II MHC antigens have a similar three-dimensional structure but a different subunit structure. Class I MHC consists of a transmembrane α-chain that has three domains and a non-covalently attached β2-microglobulin. Class II MHC is a heterodimer of two transmembranous glycoproteins. A remarkable feature of these molecules is the prominent groove on their membrane-distal surface, which is always occupied by short peptide sequences. Class I MHC molecules typically contain nine amino-acid peptides, whereas class II molecules can accommodate much larger peptides of up to 25 amino-acid residues.

The genes encoding MHC antigens are extremely polymorphic within the human population. This polymorphism is generally restricted to the region of the groove and allows different forms of the MHC molecule to bind different families of short peptides. Table 4.2 contains the number of polymorphisms for the human class I (HLA-A, HLA-B and HLA-C) and class II (HLA-DR, HLA-DP and HLA-DQ) MHC alleles.[13]

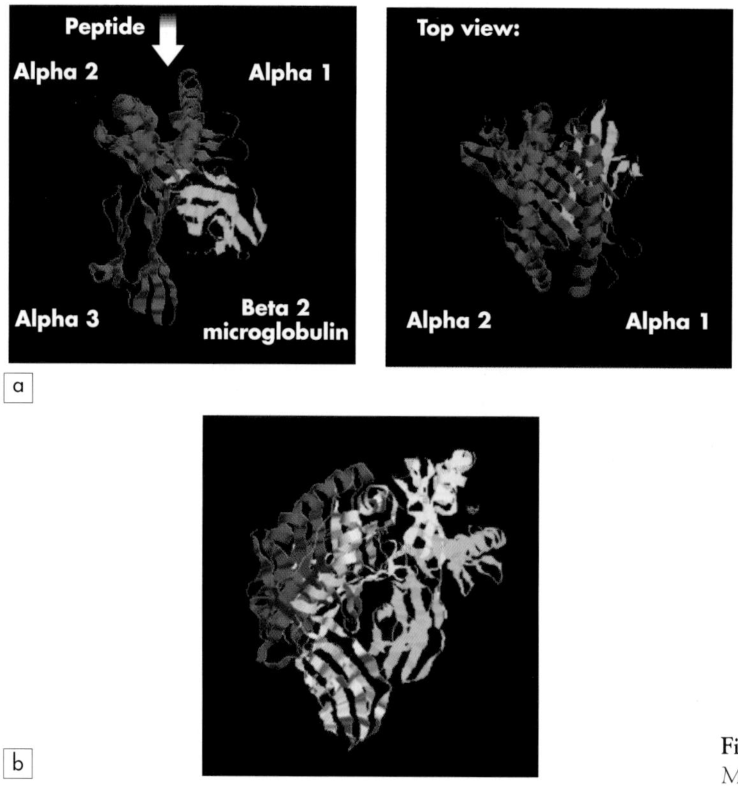

Figure 4.2 *Crystal structures of (a) class I and (b) class II MHC antigens.*

Table 4.2 Number of polymorphic variants of human MHC antigens (as assigned in January 2003).

MHC	Class I			Class II		
Name	HLA-A	HLA-B	HLA-C	HLA-DR	HLA-DP	HLA-DQ
Number of serologically identified antigens	28	61	10	24	9	6
Number of allelic variants	266	511	128	408	76	123

A complete list of HLA alleles is available at *www.anthonynolan.com/HIG/nomenc.html*

T-cell antigens

The T-cell antigen receptor can recognize only short peptide 'epitopes' bound in the groove of MHC antigens. Evidence suggests that the T-cell receptor interacts simultaneously with the MHC molecule and the peptide. In general, peptides from intracellular proteins are loaded into class I molecules, and peptides from phagocytosed extracellular proteins are loaded into class II antigens.

T-cell self-tolerance is vital given the inability of MHC molecules to discriminate between loading peptides from normal self proteins and peptides from, for example, a pathogenic organism. The lymphocyte is activated only when the T-cell receptor binds to an MHC–peptide complex with an affinity greater than a triggering level. Thus, thymic deletion of all T cells that recognize MHC–self peptide complexes with an affinity above this level will produce cells that can reach the required affinity only by interaction with complexes formed with non-self peptides.

Helper or $CD4^+$ T cells

Approximately 60% of human peripheral T cells express the CD4 antigen on their cell surface. This antigen binds to a domain on the class II MHC antigen during interaction between the T-cell receptor and the class II MHC–peptide complex. Formation of this complex plays an important role in T-cell activation and has an additional implication for the immune response. As class II MHC antigens primarily form complexes with peptides derived from extracellular proteins, it follows that $CD4^+$ T cells are activated, albeit indirectly, by extracellular antigens (Figure 4.3).

It is now clear that $CD4^+$ T cells are responsible for the regulation of most phases of the adaptive immune response. These cells are generally not directly cytotoxic, but produce a range of soluble mediators, or cytokines, able to affect other cells in the local environment. For this reason, they are often termed helper cells. Recent studies of individual

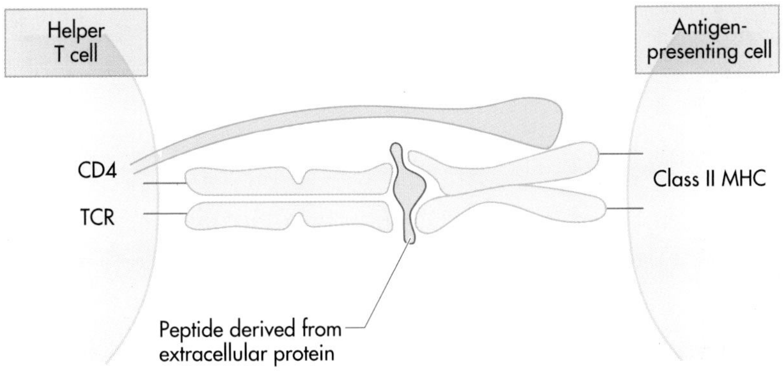

Figure 4.3 *The presentation of antigen to $CD4^+$ T cells.*

clones of activated helper cells have shown that they can be divided functionally into at least two subpopulations. These are termed Th1 and Th2 cell types and are distinguished from each other by the range of cytokines they produce.[14] However, it is increasingly clear that T cells are heterogeneous, and functionally distinct. T cells at mucosal surfaces are characterized by their production of transforming growth factor-β (TGFβ). These have been described as Th3 lymphocytes and are thought to play an important role in oral tolerance.[15]

The Th1 lymphocyte subpopulation appears to direct delayed-type hypersensitivity reactions by the production of cytokines such as interferon-γ (IFNγ), interleukin-2 (IL-2), interleukin-12 (IL-12) and tumour necrosis factor-β (TNFβ). These factors enhance the local recruitment and activation of phagocytes and stimulate the division of antigen-specific lymphocytes, including the $CD8^+$ cytotoxic cells described in the next section.

The Th2 subpopulation produces a range of cytokines that are involved in antibody responses mediated by B cells and in mast-cell proliferation,

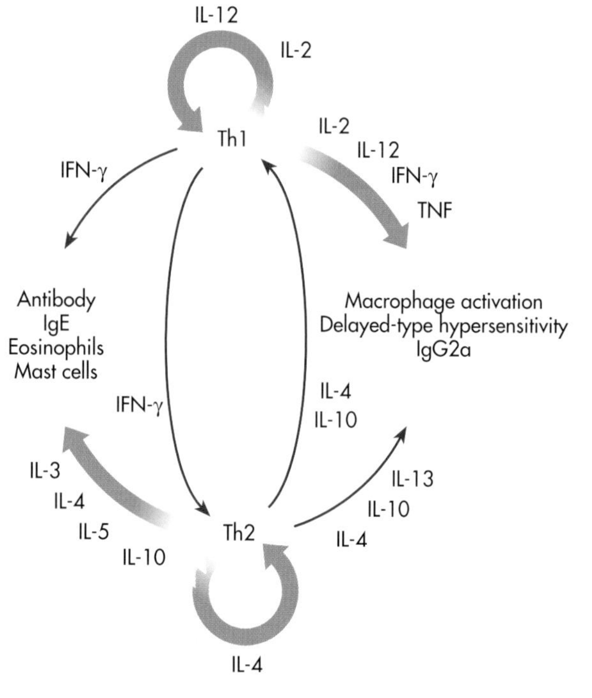

Figure 4.4 *The function and regulation of Th1 and Th2 helper T cells. Positive regulation by cytokines (broad arrows); negative regulation by cytokines (fine arrows).*

eosinophilia and granuloma formation. These cytokines include IL-3, IL-4, IL-5 and IL-10. Significantly, IL-4 stimulates B cells to produce the IgE class of antibody, and these antibodies are involved in the release of histamine by degranulating mast cells.

Th1 and Th2 cells are mutually regulated. The IFNγ produced by Th1 cells inhibits the activity of Th2 cells, whereas the IL-4 and IL-10 produced by Th2 cells inhibit Th1 lymphocytes (Figure 4.4).[16]

Cytotoxic or $CD8^+$ T cells

Approximately 40% of peripheral T cells express the CD8 antigen. This molecule binds to a domain on the class I MHC antigen during interaction between the T-cell receptor and the class I MHC–peptide complex. The formation of this complex plays an important role in the activation of $CD8^+$ T cells. As class I MHC antigens primarily form complexes with peptides derived from intracellular proteins, it follows that $CD8^+$ T cells are activated by intracellular antigens (Figure 4.5).

The $CD8^+$ lymphocyte subpopulation fulfils two roles. Its primary role is its involvement in the process of antigen-specific target cell lysis followed by cytokine secretion. Following activation, the $CD8^+$ T cell differentiates from a resting, or precursor, state to form a cytotoxic effector cell. This cell efficiently kills target cells that express the specific class I MHC–peptide complex. The direct lytic process involves lymphocyte degranulation and the secretion of agents including perforin, which forms pores in the target cell membrane, and granzymes, which induce the fragmentation of DNA within the target cell by a process termed apoptosis.

The ability of $CD8^+$ cytotoxic cells to lyse target cells containing non-self proteins is consistent with their involvement in the prevention of the spread of viruses by killing virally infected cells. Virally infected cells are recognized by the cytotoxic lymphocyte because non-self viral peptides are expressed in the peptide-binding groove of their class I MHC antigens. A similar mechanism may allow cytotoxic cells to kill class I MHC antigen-expressing tumour cells that produce novel tumour-associated antigens (see section below on Cancer immunotherapy; p. 79).

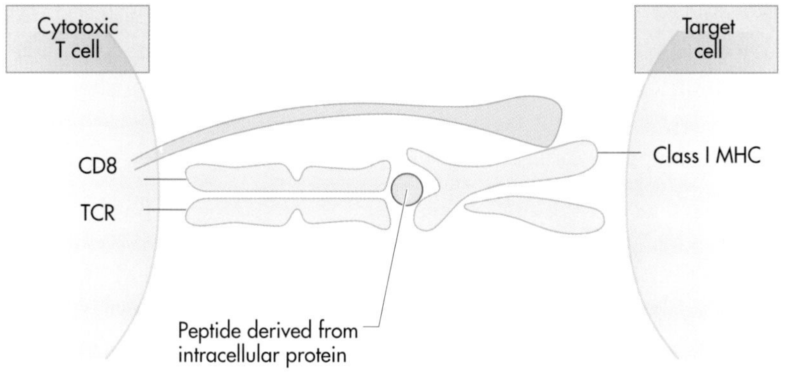

Figure 4.5 *The presentation of antigen to CD8$^+$ T cells.*

B cells and humoral immunity

In humans, B cells constitute approximately 10% of the circulating lymphocytes and are produced within the bone marrow. Resting B cells are morphologically similar to T cells despite being functionally distinct from them. B cells use a membrane-bound form of immunoglobulin to recognize antigen. The receptor can also be secreted as an immunoglobulin molecule or antibody following B-cell activation. Like T cells, B cells also have a clonal specificity for antigen, with each activated cell producing soluble immunoglobulins with a single specificity. B cells also express class II MHC antigens constitutively, and can therefore present foreign peptide to T cells.

Immunoglobulins

The immunoglobulins (Igs), or antibodies, are a group of five glycoproteins that are divided into five classes, termed IgM, IgG, IgA, IgD and IgE. These classes differ from each other in structure and molecular weight, but their functions are broadly similar. One portion of the molecule, the variable region, binds to a specific site on an antigen, whereas the constant region may interact with, and regulate the function of, additional components of the immune system, such as complement, phagocytes or cytotoxic cells. Unlike the T-cell receptor, immunoglobulins are not restricted to peptide binding and are able to bind efficiently to carbohydrates, nucleic acids, proteins and a range of chemical and biochemical compounds.

Approximately 10% of the total immunoglobulin pool consists of IgM, which is a large, pentameric structure normally restricted to the blood. After primary infection, IgM is the first immunoglobulin produced by antigen-specific B cells. It has a low affinity for antigen, but the multivalency confers a relatively high avidity of overall binding. IgM is able to activate complement efficiently. Activated helper T cells, particularly of the Th2 phenotype, produce cytokines able to stimulate B cells to class-switch from production of IgM to IgG. This smaller immunoglobulin makes up about 75% of the immunoglobulin pool, can diffuse more rapidly than IgM and, in addition to the activation of complement, can bind to a range of cellular components of the innate immune system.

IgA makes up about 15% of the total immunoglobulin pool and is generally restricted to mucosal sites. It is present in colostrum, saliva and tears. Nearly all the IgD is associated with antigen recognition on the surface of B cells, whereas IgE is found on the surface of mast cells.

Immunoglobulin diversity

The diversity of immunoglobulin specificities is generated by genetic splicing in a manner analogous to that of the rearrangement of the genes encoding the T-cell antigen receptor. In the case of human immunoglobulins, it has been estimated that this process can produce up to 10^{11} different immunoglobulin molecules. However, unlike T cells, B cells supplement this process by rearranging immunoglobulin genes after antigen recognition by 'somatic hypermutation'. The mutated B cells, which, coincidentally, have a higher affinity for the antigen than the original clone, survive. The overall immunoglobulin response tends to become more specific as the immunoglobulins produced by the mutant cells possess an increased affinity for their antigen. This process is termed affinity maturation.

Classical pathway of complement activation

The classical pathway of complement is activated by the interaction between subunit q of the complement C1 complex and the constant region of IgM or IgG molecules bound to their specific antigen. The activated C1 complex initiates the classical pathway of complement activation, in which classical C3 and C5 convertase are produced (Figure 4.6). Beyond this point, both the alternative and classical pathways are identical and cause cell damage in a similar way (see Figure 4.1b).[7]

Opsonization

Many human leucocytes express one or more of three classes of Fc receptor for domains on the constant region of IgG molecules. These cells include mononuclear phagocytes, neutrophils, eosinophils and NK cells. These Fc receptors enable the leucocytes to recognize antibody-coated antigens by a process known as opsonization. This greatly enhances the efficiency of phagocytosis and increases the specificity of cellular elements of the innate immune response.

Antibody-dependent, cell-mediated cytotoxicity

Many NK cells express a relatively low-affinity Fc receptor for IgG. This receptor enables these cells to bind to IgG-coated targets and triggers a process that

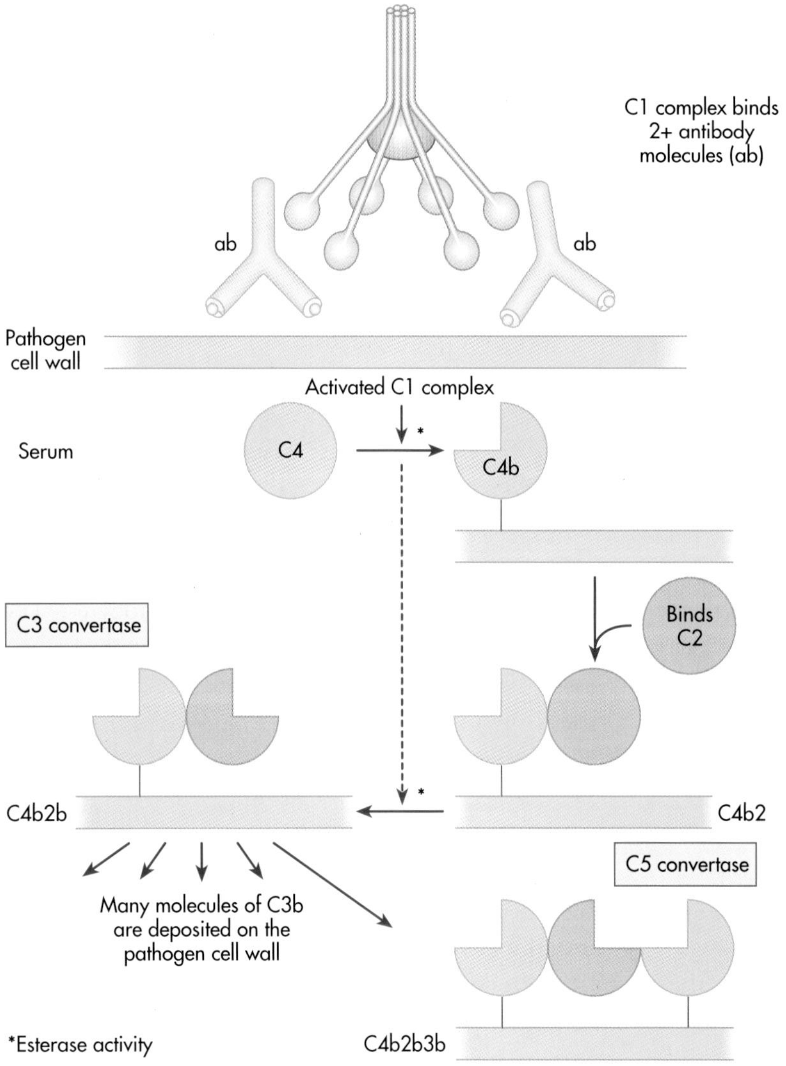

Figure 4.6 *The classical pathway of complement activation.*

results in target cell lysis. As the receptor has a low IgG affinity, it binds aggregated IgG more readily than monomeric immunoglobulin in the plasma. This appears to prevent the inappropriate activation of NK cells in the blood.

ADHESION MOLECULES

A series of specialized adhesion and signalling molecules is involved in the migration of leucocytes across vascular endothelium and into body tissues and also in the regulation of T-cell activation.[17]

Ligands and receptors

Three main families of molecules are involved in binding and supporting the migration of leucocytes. These are the selectins and members of the integrin and immunoglobulin superfamilies. The involvement of selectins is mainly restricted to an initial low-affinity interaction typified by leucocytes 'rolling' across the vascular endothelium. Members of the other two families are of importance during leucocyte stimulation, tight adhesion to endothelium, and extravasation into tissues.

Selectins

The three members of the selectin family are designated L-selectin, E-selectin and P-selectin after the lymphocyte, endothelial cell and platelet on which they were respectively identified. These molecules contain three structural regions and a cytoplasmic tail. The N-terminal domain is closely related to calcium-dependent lectins, whereas the central domain shares characteristics with an epidermal growth factor sequence. The third domain contains a number of repeating sequences homologous to a sequence found in proteins that regulate the activity of complement. Each selectin is thought to possess the ability to bind to a number of carbohydrate ligands.

Integrins

Integrins are a superfamily of transmembrane glycoproteins consisting of non-covalently linked α and, generally smaller, β subunits. They are widely expressed by cells of the body and are usually grouped by virtue of their common β chains into eight subfamilies. At least 14 discrete α subunits have been identified, and it is clear that a given α chain may associate with more than one β chain (Table 4.3). The extracellular portion of the α chain contains three or four sites that bind divalent cations essential for integrin function. Both chains generally have short cytoplasmic regions able to interact with the cytoskeleton, and these may be phosphorylated. Phosphorylation is often associated with cell activation and can enhance the affinity of adhesion to the ligand (inside-out signalling).[18]

Integrins play a key role in both cell–cell and cell–matrix adhesion. They bind to components of the extracellular matrix, such as collagen, fibronectin, laminin and vitronectin. Some integrins have affinity for specific peptide domains, such as the well-characterized arginine–glycine–aspartic acid sequence, which is present on a number of extracellular matrix components. Three subfamilies of integrins are of particular importance for leucocyte adhesion. These include a member of the β1 family of 'very late antigens', VLA-4 ($\alpha_4\beta1$), β2 integrins termed the leucocyte cell adhesion molecules (LCAM; $\alpha_L\beta2$, $\alpha_M\beta2$ and $\alpha_X\beta2$) and β7 integrins ($\alpha_4\beta7$ and $\alpha_e\beta7$).

The β1 integrin VLA-4 is expressed by many mononuclear leucocytes and binds to the immunoglobulin superfamily member vascular cell adhesion molecule-1 (VCAM-1) in addition to fibronectin. The β2 subfamily is restricted to cells of the leucocyte lineage and includes lymphocyte function-associated antigen-1 (LFA-1) and Mac-1, which both serve to anchor leucocytes to cells that express intercellular adhesion molecule-1 (ICAM-1). The β7 family is expressed by mucosal lymphocytes. The $\alpha_4\beta7$ integrin has recently been demonstrated to be the gut-homing receptor, enabling gut-trophic lymphocytes to enter the Peyer's patches. The $\alpha_e\beta7$ (CD103) integrin is expressed by nearly all lamina propria lymphocytes in the gut, and by approximately 50% of intraepithelial lymphocytes.

Immunoglobulin superfamily members

ICAM-1 is a large transmembrane glycoprotein bearing five domains containing the folded β sheet characteristic of immunoglobulins. The molecule is expressed constitutively by endothelial cells but is

Table 4.3 The integrin family.

Integrin	β subunit	Other names	α subunit	Other common names	Ligands
VLA-1	β1	CD29	α_1	CD49a	Laminin (collagen)
VLA-2		or VLAβ	α_2	CD49b	Collagen (laminin)
VLA-3		or gpIIa	α_3	CD29c	Fibronectin, laminin, collagen
VLA-4			$\boldsymbol{\alpha_4}$	**CD49d**	**VCAM-1, fibronectin**
VLA-5			α_5	CD49e	Fibronectin
VLA-6			α_6	CD49f	Laminin
$\beta1\alpha_7$			α_7		Laminin
$\beta1\alpha_8$			α_8		
$\beta1\alpha_V$			α_V	CD51	Fibronectin
LFA-1	**β2**	**CD18**	$\boldsymbol{\alpha_L}$	**CD11a**	**ICAM-1, ICAM-2, ICAM-3**
Mac-1			$\boldsymbol{\alpha_M}$	**CD11b**	**ICAM-1, C3bi, fibrinogen**
p150, 95			$\boldsymbol{\alpha_X}$	**CD11c**	**C3bi**
CD41a	β3	CD61 or	αIIb	CD41	Fibrinogen, fibronectin, vitronectin, Von Willebrand factor
$\beta3\alpha_V$		gpIIIa	α_V	CD51	As above + thrombospondin
$\beta4\alpha_6$	β4		α_6	CD49f	Laminin
$\beta5\alpha_V$	β5	β_X, β_S	α_V	CD51	Vitronectin, fibronectin
$\beta6\alpha_V$	β6		α_V	CD51	Fibronectin
LPAM-1	β7	βp	α4	**CD49d**	**VCAM-1, MadCam1, fibronectin**
CD103			αe		**E-cadherin**
$\beta8\alpha_V$	β8	α_V	CD51		

Elements in bold print are of particular importance for leucocyte adhesion.

significantly upregulated by stimulation with IL-1, TNFα and IFNγ. The cytokines TNFα and IFNγ also induce and upregulate the expression of ICAM-1 on a range of parenchymal cells, including fibroblasts and epithelial cells in the skin, lung and liver. This process enhances the adhesion of β2 integrin-expressing leucocytes.

Structural studies have shown that VCAM-1 contains seven immunoglobulin domains. The first and fourth of these regions are homologous and function during lymphocyte adhesion. VCAM-1 is constitutively expressed on endothelial cells at a low level, but expression is upregulated within 12 hours and then maintained at high levels by stimulation with the cytokines IL-1 and TNFα. Immunocytochemical studies have also demonstrated the presence of VCAM-1 on a variety of non-vascular cells, including renal epithelial cells, neural cells, and the synovial cells of inflamed joints.

Co-stimulation

Ligation of a T-cell receptor with its specific MHC–peptide ligand is insufficient to activate the T cell. This observation has generated the two-signal hypothesis for lymphocyte activation. Signal one is defined as interaction with specific MHC and peptide, and signal two is a non-specific co-stimulatory signal.

Studies have indicated that the T-cell antigen receptor has only a very modest affinity for its specific MHC–peptide ligand. This has been estimated as between 1×10^{-5} M and 5×10^{-5} M, which is considerably lower than the value for a typical IgG molecule, which is of the order of 1×10^{-9} M. This affinity is too low to allow stable conjugates to form between T-cell receptors and the 210–340 specific MHC–peptide ligands required for lymphocyte activation.[19] The multiplicity of antigen-independent adhesion molecule interactions plays a vital role in stabilizing the T-cell and antigen-presenting cell complex sufficiently to allow T-cell receptor signal transduction to take place. This adhesion is rapidly increased following T-cell receptor ligation by an increase in the affinity of LFA-1 (inside-out signalling).[17]

Appropriate ligation of the lymphocyte adhesion molecules LFA-1 and VLA-4 is known to generate co-stimulatory signals able to augment lymphocyte activation. Furthermore, monoclonal antibodies specific for LFA-1 have been shown to stimulate the proliferation of resting lymphocytes. The best characterized co-stimulatory molecule is the T-cell-surface molecule CD28, which interacts with members of the B7 ligand family (CD80, CD86) on antigen-presenting cells, leading to the generation of a signal important for the activation and proliferation of antigen-specific T cells. Expression of the B7 family of ligands is restricted to a small group of specialized mononuclear cells including dendritic cells and B cells. Other co-stimulatory molecules contribute to the response, including CD40 ligand (CD40L), which binds to CD40 on antigen-presenting cells. This leads to upregulation of B7 and therefore further T-cell stimulation. Antigen presentation in the absence of satisfactory co-stimulatory signal transduction may even produce stable lymphocyte hyporeactivity. Indeed, the therapeutic elimination of CD28 signalling by the blockade of B7 molecules with the soluble receptor-like construct CTLA4-Ig has resulted in partial cardiac allograft tolerance in a murine model.[20]

EXAMPLES OF CLINICAL IMMUNOLOGY

Acute allograft rejection

The extreme vigour of allograft rejection can be explained by the process termed alloreactivity. Although mature T cells have been selected in the thymus for specific tolerance of all potential self MHC antigen–self peptide complexes, the cells have not been selected for tolerance of the subtly different MHC molecule–peptide complexes expressed on the surface of donor cells. It has been estimated that up to 2% of all recipient T cells may respond to the allogeneic MHC molecules expressed by graft tissues. Furthermore, as this situation reflects an artificial cross-reaction, a significant proportion of the responsive lymphocytes are present as memory cells, which facilitate the rapid initiation of the rejection response.[21,22]

It is not clinically feasible to match the organ donor and recipient for identical MHC antigens, given the enormous polymorphism of MHC alleles (see Table 4.2). Consequently, it has been necessary to develop drugs to suppress the immune response. One of the most successful immunosuppressive drugs in use today is ciclosporin A. This cyclic peptide blockades the production of IL-2 during T-cell activation. The function of this cytokine is best illustrated by its original name, which was 'T-cell growth factor'. Without IL-2, the graft-specific lymphocytes are unable to divide and cannot initiate the rejection response.

Cancer immunotherapy

The prospects for successful cancer immunotherapy depend on the ability of T cells to recognize tumour antigens. During the 1950s, some chemically induced tumours were shown to express specific, 'non-self' antigens that allowed sensitized animals to reject transplanted tumour cells. More recent studies have shown that T cells are able to recognize tumour-derived peptides complexed in the groove of MHC molecules.

A range of tumour-specific antigens has been detected, including the MAGE family (MAGE-1), which is found in 37% of human melanomas, a smaller proportion of other tumours, and no normal tissues except the immunologically privileged testis.[23] Peptides from MAGE-1 associate with the class I molecules HLA-A1 and HLA-Cw16 and can be recognized by cytotoxic lymphocytes. The related molecule MAGE-3 is associated with a greater proportion of cancers and yields immunogenic peptides that complex with HLA-A1 and HLA-A2. Studies have demonstrated that up to 35% of transitional bladder cancers express MAGE antigens, with the proportion increasing to 61% of invasive tumours.

Further tumour-associated proteins have been identified, including BAGE, and GAGE-1 and GAGE-2, which also yield peptides that can be recognized by cytotoxic T cells and are expressed by 10–20% of bladder cancers. In addition to the identification of proteins expressed by a range of cancer cells, tumours also express unique peptide epitopes derived from mutated genes. Recent work has identified such mutations in murine cancers, which yield peptides recognizable by both $CD8^+$ CTL and $CD4^+$ 'helper' T cells.

It is, however, becoming increasingly clear that many cancer cells have developed a capacity to 'evade' a local immune response.[24] Not only do some cells express reduced levels of MHC molecules, the primary T-cell receptor ligand, but some also acquire a capacity actively to kill specific 'effector' T cells by the 'Fas-counterattack'. In this system, the cancer cell develops expression of Fas-ligand, which can engage the Fas receptor on local T cells, thereby initiating a proapoptotic cycle which results in T-cell death. Another potential example of an immune evasion strategy is loss of the expression of E-cadherin by many epithelial cancer cells. It is now known that this molecule is an effective adhesion receptor for intraepithelial T cells, which are thought to be responsible for normal immune surveillance of mucosal surfaces. It is possible that the acquisition of these successful phenotypic attributes (from the cancer's point of view!) is a reflection of microevolution within the developing cancer, leading to selection of phenotypic variants which can evade an otherwise cancer-clearing immune response.

BCG treatment of bladder cancer

The treatment of superficial bladder cancer by intravesical administration of BCG is almost a unique example of successful cancer 'immunotherapy'. The mechanism by which BCG can cause bladder cancer regression is not clear. However, it is known that BCG is an effective agent for the activation of dendritic cells in vitro,[25] presumably by a mechanism involving ligation of multiple PAMPs, including the TLRs. Furthermore, model systems have shown that both activated T cells and NK cells are potentially involved in the clearance of bladder cancer cells. A challenge remaining in this area is the precise definition of optimal ways to induce immunological clearance of bladder cancer cells without resorting to the administration of viable, and often harmful, BCG bacteria. Indeed, current research is focusing on methods to induce an intravesical immune response by administration of defined subfractions of BCG by ligation of an optimal repertoire of PAMPs.

REFERENCES

1. Allen LAH, Aderem A. Mechanisms of phagocytosis. Curr Opin Immunol 1996; 8: 36–40
2. Cerwenka A, Lanier LL. Natural killer cells, viruses and cancer. Nat Rev Immunol 2001; 1: 41–49
3. Obata-Onai A, Hashimoto S, Onai N, Kurachi M et al. Comprehensive gene expression analysis of human NK cells and CD8(+) T lymphocytes. Int Immunol 2002; 14: 1085–1098
4. Moretta L, Bottino C, Pende D, Mingari MC et al. Human natural killer cells: their origin, receptors and function. Eur J Immunol 2002; 32: 1205–1211
5. Ljunggren HG, Karre K. In search of the 'missing self': MHC molecules and NK cell recognition. Immunol Today 1990; 11: 237–244
6. Borrego F, Kabat J, Kim DK, Lieto L et al. Structure and function of major histocompatibility complex (MHC) class I specific receptors expressed on human natural killer (NK) cells. Mol Immunol 2002; 38: 637–660
7. Reid KBM. The complement system. In: Hames BD, Glover DM eds. Frontiers in Molecular Biology. Oxford: IRL Press, 1996: 326
8. Janeway CA Jr, Medzhitov R. Innate immune recognition. Ann Rev Immunol 2002; 20: 197–216
9. Davies MM, Chien Y-H. T cell antigen receptor genes. In: Hames BD, Glover DM, eds. Frontiers in Molecular Biology. Oxford: IRL Press, 1996; 101
10. Hayday AC. Gamma delta cells: a right time and a right place for a conserved third way of protection. Ann Rev Immunol 2000; 18: 975–1026
11. Bjorkman PJ, Saper MA, Samraoui B, Bennett WS et al. Structure of the human class-I histocompatibility antigen, HLA-A2. Nature 1987; 329: 506–512
12. Brown JH, Jardetzky TS, Gorga JC, Stern LJ et al. 3-Dimensional structure of the human class-II histocompatibility antigen HLA-DR1. Nature 1993; 364: 33–39

13. Marsh SGE, Albert ED, Bodmer WF, Bontrop RE et al. Nomenclature for factors of the HLA system, 2002. Eur J Immunogenet 2002; 29: 463–515
14. Mosmann TR, Coffman RL. Th1 and Th2-cells: different patterns of lymphokine secretion lead to different functional-properties. Ann Rev Immunol 1989; 7: 145–173
15. Weiner HL. Induction and mechanism of action of transforming growth factor-beta-secreting Th3 regulatory cells. Immunol Rev 2001; 182: 207–214
16. O'Garra A, Arai N. The molecular basis of T helper 1 and T helper 2 cell differentiation. Trends Cell Biol 2000; 10: 542–550
17. Dustin ML, Springer TA. Role of lymphocyte adhesion receptors in transient interactions and cell locomotion. Ann Rev Immunol 1991; 9: 27–66
18. Hynes RO. Integrins: bidirectional, allosteric signaling machines. Cell 2002; 110: 673–687
19. Valitutti S, Lanzavecchia A. Serial triggering of TCRs: a basis for the sensitivity and specificity of antigen recognition. Immunol Today 1997; 18: 299–304
20. Baliga P, Chavin KD, Qin LH, Woodward J et al. CTLA4Ig prolongs allograft survival while suppressing cell-mediated immunity. Transplantation 1994; 58: 1082–1090
21. Lechler RI, Lombardi G, Batchelor JR, Reinsmoen N et al. The molecular basis of alloreactivity. Immunol Today 1990; 11: 83–88
22. Wang JH, Reinherz EL. Structural basis of T cell recognition of peptides bound to MHC molecules. Mol Immunol 2002; 38: 1039–1049
23. Patard JJ, Brasseur F, Gildiez S, et al. Expression of MAGE genes in transitional-cell carcinomas of the urinary bladder. Int J Cancer 1995; 64: 60–64
24. Pettit SJ, Seymour K, O'Flaherty E, Kirby JA. Immune selection in neoplasia: towards a microevolutionary model of cancer development. Br J Cancer 2000; 82: 1900–1906
25. Pettit SJ, Neal DE, Kirby JA. Evaluation of dendritic cell immunogenicity after activation and chemical fixation: a mixed lymphocyte reaction model. J Immunother 2002; 25: 152–161

5

The nature of renal function

George B Haycock

HOMEOSTASIS

Homeostasis was originally defined as *maintenance of the constancy of the internal environment*. The 'internal environment' is the fluid that bathes the cells, the *extracellular fluid (ECF)*. Homeostasis can therefore be redefined as the *regulation of the volume and composition of the ECF*. The kidney is the pre-eminent organ of homeostasis, although the lungs, gut and skin also contribute to it. One component of homeostasis is *excretion* of products of metabolism: failure of excretion leads to accumulation of these products with progressive pollution of the ECF. A second component is *conservation* of ECF solutes (mainly nutrients) that are too valuable to be allowed to escape into the urine. The third component is constant adjustment of the urinary excretion rate of water and inorganic solutes to maintain their concentrations in the ECF within the normal range, in the face of unpredictably changing input from the diet and from other body water compartments. This last might be called homeostasis proper. In order to achieve it, the kidney must:

1. detect small changes in ECF volume, or in the concentration of any of its many constituents, before such changes become serious
2. respond by altering the volume or composition of the urine so as to correct the tendency to abnormality.

This is achieved by negative feedback: a rise in the ECF concentration of, say, potassium leads to an increase in its excretion rate with a consequent return of the ECF concentration to normal, while a fall in its concentration leads to a decrease in excretion rate, defending the ECF against hypokalaemia. The kidney's capacity to alter the volume of urine and the concentration of its constituent solutes is very large. An adult can vary daily urine volume between a minimum of about 500 ml and a maximum of more than 20 litres, while the urinary concentration of the major ECF cation, sodium, can vary by at least three orders of magnitude.

The concept of external balance

Homeostasis requires (in the non-growing organism) that net input of any substance into the ECF be exactly equal to net output from it. In health, body composition remains constant because output, mainly via the kidney, can be varied continuously in response to changes in input. The *net external balance (NEB)* for any substance is the algebraic difference between input and output over any specified period of time; that is,

Equation 1

$$NEB = input - output$$

Balance may be positive (input > output), negative (output > input) or zero (input = output). Normally, NEB for all non-metabolized substances is zero, except in growing individuals, in whom it is continuously positive. Since the main determinant of input is food intake, an obvious survival advantage enjoyed by an animal with a large reserve of renal function is the ability to eat a varied diet. As renal function is lost, dietary freedom becomes constrained. In advanced renal failure, survival is possible only on a rigorously controlled diet, reversing the normal physiological state of affairs: homeostasis is achieved by adjusting intake to match a relatively constant urinary output.

Growth and renal function

The size of the kidneys, and therefore their functional capacity, increases with growth of the body as a whole. Between the age of 2 years and maturity, glomerular filtration rate (GFR) and renal blood flow in healthy humans are approximately proportional to body surface area (BSA) at about 120 ml/min per 1.73 m^2 (range 90–150).* The association between renal function and BSA is empirical, and probably does not reflect any underlying physiological principle. Some have argued that it should be standardized to ECF volume or body weight: the latter undoubtedly gives a better fit than BSA in newborn infants (Figure 5.1).[1] GFR in healthy, term, newborn infants is about 30 ml/min per 1.73 m^2, rising to 50 ml/min per 1.73 m^2 at 1 month, 80 ml/min per 1.73 m^2 at 6 months, and 100 ml/min per 1.73 m^2 at 1 year, and attaining the adult value by 18 months–2 years.

Whatever standardizing factor is applied, renal function is low at birth and during the first few months of extrauterine life, even corrected for body size. Despite this, normal infants thrive and show no clinical or biochemical evidence of failure of excretion or homeostasis. This can be explained by the fact that the infant is growing very rapidly at this stage, increasing body weight by up to 5% per week. This results in a strongly positive NEB for most nutrients, particularly since they are supplied by the baby's normal diet (human milk) in quantities that provide only just enough energy, protein and minerals to support normal growth and activity. The residue remaining for excretion is therefore very small: growth provides the infant with a 'third kidney'.[2] A major advantage to the infant of constraining glomerular filtration at a low level is conservation of energy. Approximately 99% of filtered sodium is absorbed, with its attendant anions, in the renal tubule. This is an active process (see below) and accounts for almost all of the energy expenditure of the kidney. The additional energy cost of reabsorbing the sodium filtered at an 'adult' level of glomerular filtration would be prohibitive, given the marginal sufficiency provided by human milk, as referred to above.[3] The negative aspect of the low GFR of the newborn is its lack of reserve. If growth is interrupted for any reason (such as intercurrent infection), or if an unphysiological diet is given (such as unmodified cow's milk), the solute load presented for excretion can overwhelm the kidney, leading to a form of acute renal insufficiency with resulting metabolic imbalance. This principle is illustrated by the syndrome of late metabolic acidosis of prematurity.[4]

* In a rational world, the figure of 1.73 m^2, taken as the surface area of the 'average adult', would be discarded and physiological values would be normalized to 1 m^2. The average GFR would then be expressed as 70 ml/min per m^2 (range 50–90).

The concept of renal clearance

It follows from the above that, in a steady state, the composition of the urine is determined by dietary and metabolic input to the ECF, and not by renal function: individuals with a GFR of 100 and 10 ml/min, respectively, will produce identical urine if they are eating identical diets. Since the function of the kidneys is to regulate the ECF, one way of quantifying renal function is to measure the rate of processing of ECF (plasma). For any substance (x) present in both plasma and urine, it is simple to calculate the volume of plasma containing the quantity of x excreted in the urine in a specified period of time. This volume is the *renal clearance* of x, the volume of plasma (not urine) cleared of x per unit of time. Renal clearance is given by the formula:

Equation 2

$$C_x = \frac{U_x \times V}{P_x}$$

where C, U and P represent clearance, urine and plasma concentrations, respectively, and V is the urine flow rate. C is expressed in the same units as those chosen to express V (for example, ml/min, L/day).

In the special case of a substance which is freely filtered by the glomerulus, such that its concentration in plasma water and glomerular filtrate are the same, and which is not secreted or reabsorbed by the tubule or metabolized by the kidney, the filtration

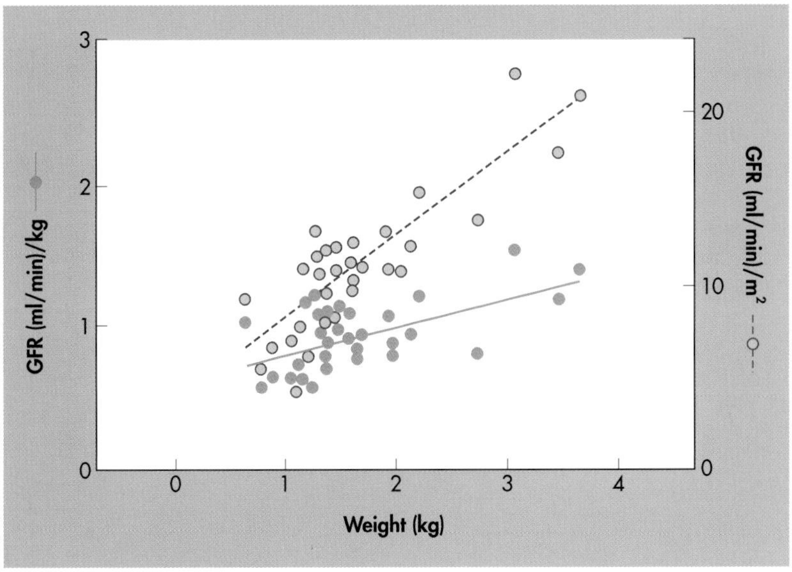

Figure 5.1 *Glomerular filtration rate (GFR) corrected for body surface area (interrupted line) and weight (continuous line) in newborn infants. Within the range studied, GFR factored by surface area increases threefold while GFR factored by weight less than doubles. (Reproduced from* Archives of Disease in Childhood *with permission.*[1]*)*

rate of x (F_x) must equal its excretion rate (E_x). The renal clearance of such a substance is equal to the GFR. No endogenous substance has been described that fulfils these criteria exactly in humans. Inulin, a starch-like polymer of fructose, does fulfil them, and is therefore an ideal marker for measurement of GFR. The chelating agents EDTA and DTPA, which can be labelled with radioisotopes for easy assay in plasma and urine, and the radio contrast chemical, sodium iothalamate, are excellent alternatives. Creatinine is an ideal marker for GFR in the dog; unfortunately, in humans, it is secreted by the tubule to a small extent when renal function is normal but to a considerably greater extent when renal function is reduced. Despite this limitation, a carefully performed creatinine clearance test is an adequate measure of GFR for most clinical purposes.[5]

Any substance whose clearance is greater than GFR must be secreted by the tubule. Conversely, any freely filtered substance with a clearance less than GFR must be reabsorbed by the tubule. Dividing C_x by GFR gives the *fractional excretion* of x (FE_x). If creatinine clearance (C_{cr}) is taken as GFR:

Equation 3

$$FE_x\,(\%) = \left(\frac{U_x \times P_{cr}}{U_{cr} \times P_x}\right) \times 100$$

Note that it is not necessary to measure V to calculate FE_x: random, simultaneously obtained blood and urine samples are all that is required.

A substance that is completely cleared by the kidney, that is, its concentration in renal venous plasma is zero, has a clearance equal to renal plasma flow (RPF). The organic anions para-aminohippurate (PAH) and ortho-aminohippurate (hippuran) are almost ideal markers for measurement of RPF in most circumstances. An exception is in the newborn, in whom renal extraction of PAH is incomplete.[6] Dividing GFR by RPF gives the *filtration fraction (FF)*, the proportion of renal arterial plasma removed from the circulation as glomerular filtrate:

Equation 4

$$FF = \frac{GFR}{RPF} = \frac{C_{inulin}}{C_{PAH}} = \frac{U:P_{inulin}}{U:P_{PAH}} = \frac{U_{inulin} \times P_{PAH}}{U_{PAH} \times P_{inulin}}$$

Typical normal values (after infancy) for GFR, RPF and FF are 120 ml/min per 1.73 m^2, 600 ml/min per 1.73 m^2, and 0.2, respectively.

FUNCTIONAL SEGMENTATION OF THE NEPHRON

Each nephron consists of a glomerulus and its attached tubule (Figure 5.2). The tubule is divided into two major segments: the *proximal* and *distal* tubules. The proximal tubule is further divided into the early (S_1) and late (S_2) proximal convoluted tubule, the proximal straight tubule (*pars recta*, S_3) and the loop of Henle. About 90% of the human

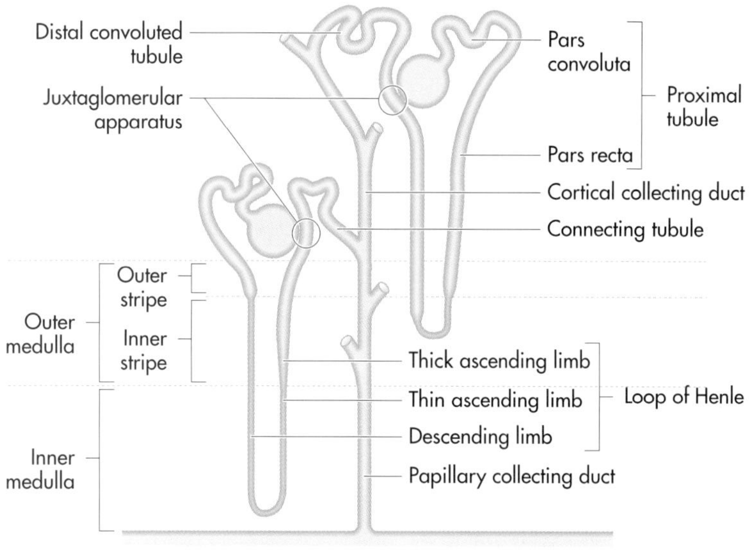

Figure 5.2 *Schematic representation of two nephrons, one of which is a juxtamedullary nephron (long loop of Henle) and one a superficial cortical nephron (short loop of Henle). The figure is not drawn to scale – the loop of Henle of the juxtamedullary nephron is actually much longer in proportion to the rest of the nephron than represented here.*

nephron population have short loops of Henle that descend only into the outer medulla before bending and returning towards the surface of the cortex. The remaining 10% have long loops of Henle that descend deep into the inner medulla and bend at or near the papillary tip. These are the tubules that arise from those glomeruli situated in the deepest layer of the cortex, the *juxtamedullary* nephrons: they form an important part of the mechanism for urinary concentration and dilution. The parts of the loop that extend into the inner medulla are thin-walled and are called the *thin descending* and *thin ascending limbs* of the loop, respectively. The cortical part of the ascending limb is relatively thick-walled and is referred to as the *thick ascending limb* (TAL). The TAL of both types of nephron passes through the vascular pole of its own glomerulus where it is intimately related to both the afferent and the efferent arteriole in a structure called the *juxtaglomerular apparatus* (JGA). The JGA marks the functional division between the proximal and distal tubules.

The distal tubule is also divided into distal convoluted tubule, connecting tubule, cortical collecting duct and medullary collecting duct. The different segments of the nephron are identifiable not only by their anatomical relationships but also by the ultrastructural and histochemical characteristics of their epithelia. Details may be found in relevant anatomical and pathological studies.[7–9]

The function of the glomerulus

The glomerulus is a microscopic network of specialized capillaries that act as a size- and electrical charge-selective ultrafilter, retaining large molecules such as proteins within the lumen while allowing the passage of small molecules (water, electrolytes and other crystalloid solutes) into Bowman's space. The concentration of these solutes in glomerular filtrate is almost identical with that in plasma, with a small correction for the Gibbs-Donnan effect (due to the fact that negatively charged proteins are in much higher concentration within the capillary lumen than in glomerular filtrate). Ultrafiltration is a passive process, and the concentrations of small solutes in glomerular filtrate depend entirely on their concentrations in plasma. Glomerular filtrate is therefore a precursor of urine, the final composition of which is extensively modified by tubular reabsorption and secretion. Some important waste products of protein metabolism, such as urea and creatinine, are mainly excreted by glomerular filtration. Although the excretion rate of these compounds is maintained at reduced levels of GFR, this is at the cost of sustained elevation of their plasma concentrations.

The function of the proximal tubule

Pars convoluta and pars recta

Two-thirds of the volume of the glomerular filtrate is reabsorbed in the proximal tubule. The nature of the reabsorptive process can be summarized as follows:

1. It is isotonic.
2. Some solutes (bicarbonate, glucose and amino acids) are preferentially reabsorbed in the initial segments of the proximal tubule, leading to their almost complete removal from the tubular fluid and a rise in the concentration of chloride (Cl^-).
3. It is energy- and oxygen-dependent.
4. Some solutes (such as inulin, creatinine and urea) are reabsorbed little or not at all, and are therefore markedly concentrated with respect to plasma by the end of the proximal tubule.

Organic anions such as PAH and penicillin are actively secreted in this segment. The fluid delivered into the loop of Henle is therefore:

1. isotonic with plasma
2. chloride-rich and bicarbonate-poor
3. at a pH lower than that of plasma
4. more concentrated than plasma with respect to those substances (urea, creatinine and inulin) excreted solely or principally by glomerular filtration. The ratio of the tubular fluid inulin concentration to the plasma inulin concentration ($TF:P_{inulin}$) at any point along the tubule is a measure of the volume of filtrate that has been absorbed at that point. Similarly, the urine-to-plasma inulin ratio ($U:P_{inulin}$) is a measure of the amount of filtered water that is reabsorbed between glomerular filtrate and the final urine (as is, approximately, $U:P_{creatinine}$).

Loop of Henle

Net reabsorption continues in the loop so that about 85% of filtered sodium and 70% of filtered water have been reabsorbed at entry into the distal tubule. The major function of the loop is concentration and dilution of urine: reabsorption in this segment is therefore no longer isotonic.

Concentration and dilution of urine are both powered by the same energy-dependent process: absorption of salt without water in the TAL. This results in the fluid entering the distal tubule being hypotonic with respect to plasma, irrespective of whether the final urine is concentrated or dilute at the time. It also generates hypertonicity in the interstitium surrounding the TAL. This hypertonicity is amplified by countercurrent exchange and multiplication in the loops of Henle and vasa recta, leading to the establishment of an osmotic gradient in the medulla with the highest osmolality at the papillary tip. In the presence of antidiuretic hormone (ADH), the collecting duct becomes permeable to water, which is osmotically extracted from the lumen by the hypertonic medulla, leading to the formation of concentrated urine.

The function of the distal tubule

The distal tubule adjusts the composition of the final urine by selectively reabsorbing or secreting individual solutes according to the need of the moment. For example, reabsorption of Na from the tubular fluid is virtually complete in Na depletion, while in Na repletion exactly sufficient Na escapes reabsorption to balance dietary input. Many substances (such as sodium, chloride, calcium and phosphate) are normally filtered in amounts greatly exceeding dietary input, and the excretion rate is regulated by varying the amount reabsorbed. Other important substances, notably hydrogen ion and potassium, generally enter the distal tubule in very small amounts, and the rate of excretion depends mainly on varying the rate of active secretion into the tubular fluid. The rate of water excretion is determined by ADH, which increases the water permeability of the collecting duct and thus regulates the rate of osmotic reabsorption of water into the hypertonic medullary and papillary interstitium.

GLOMERULAR FILTRATION

The glomerular filtration rate (GFR) is determined by the interaction of the physical forces driving filtration and the permeability of the filtration barrier (the glomerular capillary wall) to water and small solutes. The composition of the filtrate in health is that of a protein-free ultrafiltrate of plasma, due to the almost complete impermeability of the glomerular capillaries to protein.

The glomerular capillary wall

Structure

The glomerular capillary wall has three layers: a lining endothelium composed of thin, fenestrated polygonal squames, a basement membrane, and an outer epithelium consisting of cells (podocytes) each of which possesses a central body from which radiate fern-like foot processes (pedicels) that interdigitate with those of adjacent cells. In section, the transected foot processes appear as islands of cytoplasm intimately attached to the basement membrane and connected to one another by a fine membrane. The view afforded by scanning electron microscopy shows these islands to be sections through alternating processes from adjacent cells.[10] The basement membrane is a hydrated proteoglycan gel with a thickness of about 3200 Å in the adult and rather less in the infant. Ultrastructural examination reveals a central relatively electron dense *lamina densa*, sandwiched between a *lamina rara interna* and a *lamina rara externa*. The thin squames of the endothelium contain numerous *fenestrae* of 700 Å diameter. This differentiates them from the endothelium of capillaries in other tissues. All three layers take up cationic stains, indicating that they are negatively charged.

Location of the filtration barrier

All three layers of the glomerular capillary wall probably contribute to the retention of macromolecules in the capillary lumen. Ultrastructural studies using macromolecular tracers of different sizes and electrical charge suggest that very large molecules are completely excluded from the basement membrane, while smaller ones penetrate it to varying degrees.[11] Small quantities of molecules of approximately the size of albumin appear to traverse the basement membrane but are retained at the filtration slits between the epithelial foot processes.[12] The electrical charge, as well as the size, of molecules is an important determinant of their ability to cross the capillary wall into Bowman's space.[13] Proteinuric states are associated with loss of negative charge from one or more layers of the capillary wall. It is widely accepted that the escape of large amounts of protein from the plasma into the glomerular filtrate is prevented partly by the physical structure of the proteoglycan mesh of the basement membrane and partly by its electronegativity. The small amount of albumin that crosses the membrane is further contained by the polyanionic coat surrounding the epithelial cells and extending to the filtration slits between them. The relative importance of charge- and size-selectivity is still controversial. The filtration slits between foot processes are bridged by a fine membrane, the slit diaphragm, which consists mainly of a specialized membrane protein, *nephrin*.[14] Nephrin molecules from adjacent foot processes interdigitate to form a zipper-like structure which is believed to be the limiting part of the filtration membrane for albumin. Mutations in the gene for nephrin cause a particularly severe form of recessively inherited congenital nephrotic syndrome (CNS), known as CNS of the Finnish type.[15] Other specialized proteins expressed in the foot processes are also essential to the proper formation of the filtration barrier and mutations in the genes that code for them cause other, even rarer, forms of CNS. The role of these proteins, if any, in the pathogenesis of acquired forms of nephrotic syndrome is unknown.

Dynamics of glomerular filtration

Starling forces

Glomerular filtration is driven by the balance between the hydrostatic pressure gradient between capillary and Bowman's space, generated by myocardial contraction, and the oncotic pressure (colloid osmotic pressure) gradient generated by the protein concentration gradient between the same two compartments. Hydrostatic pressure favours, and oncotic pressure opposes, filtration. These forces are referred to as Starling forces. Starling forces govern the movement of fluid between the intravascular and extravascular compartments of the extracellular fluid throughout the body as a whole, glomerular filtration being a special example of their application. The net *ultrafiltration pressure* (P_{UF}) is therefore the algebraic sum of the hydrostatic (P) and oncotic (Π) pressure gradients between capillary (C) and Bowman's space (BS):

Equation 5

$$P_{UF} = (P_C - P_{BS}) - \sigma(\Pi_C - \Pi_{BS})$$

Since Π_{BS} is insignificant and σ (the reflection coefficient for albumin) has a value of unity:

Equation 6

$$P_{UF} = P_C - P_{BS} - \Pi_C$$

P must be higher at the arterial than at the venous end of the glomerular capillary plexus, or blood would not flow. The pressure drop is small, however, since the glomerular capillaries are low-resistance vessels between two high-resistance components (the afferent and efferent arterioles). As plasma passes through the glomerulus, filtration occurs and the plasma proteins are progressively concentrated towards the venous end by removal of water. The force opposing filtration (Π_C) therefore increases. The combination of falling P_C and rising Π_C causes P_{UF} to diminish towards the venous end of the capillary. These pressures have been directly measured in several species. At least in the Munich-Wistar rat and the squirrel monkey, P_{UF} at the venous end of the circuit is zero.[16] This means that filtration actually stops before the efferent arteriole is reached, a condition referred to as *filtration equilibrium*. A normalized plot of filtration pressure gradients can therefore be drawn (Figure 5.3). The mean ultrafiltration pressure is shown as the integrated area between the curves for P and Π. For technical reasons, it is not possible in filtration equilibrium to measure at what point along the notional distance between afferent and efferent arteriole equilibrium is achieved. If all other variables are held constant, and plasma flow is increased or decreased, this point will move to the right or the left, respectively: there is an infinite family of curves yielding pressure equilibrium at the efferent arteriole. Under these conditions, filtration fraction is constant, and:

Equation 7

$$GFR \propto GPF$$

that is, GFR is plasma flow dependent.[17] It is not known whether filtration equilibrium is the normal condition in humans.

The ultrafiltration coefficient

At any given P_{UF}, filtration rate is inversely proportional to the resistance offered by the filtering

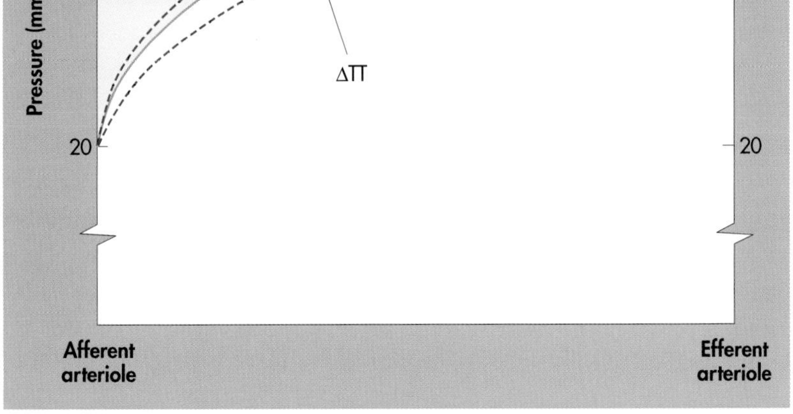

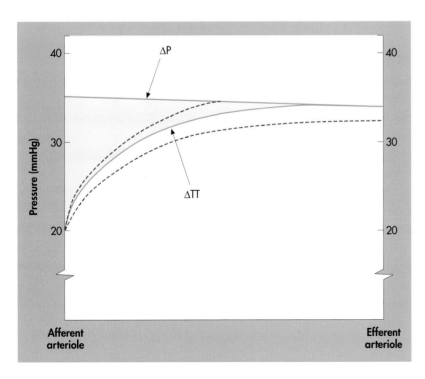

Figure 5.3 *Hydrostatic (P) and oncotic (Π) pressure profiles along an idealized glomerular capillary. ΔP and ΔΠ refer, respectively, to the hydrostatic and oncotic pressure gradients between the capillary lumen and Bowman's space. As plasma traverses the capillary bed from afferent to efferent arteriole, removal of fluid by filtration causes the plasma protein concentration to rise, with a consequent increase in ΔΠ. In filtration equilibrium (unbroken lines), ΔΠ rises to equal ΔP, and filtration stops, before the efferent arteriole is reached. An infinite number of lines (for example, upper interrupted line) can be drawn that yield filtration equilibrium: these cannot be experimentally distinguished. As flow increases, the point of intersection of ΔP and ΔΠ moves to the right, eventually producing filtration disequilibrium (lower interrupted line). In filtration disequilibrium, measurements of afferent and efferent arteriolar pressures allows a unique curve for ΔΠ to be plotted, from which Kf can be calculated (see text). The shaded area represents P_{UF}. (Reproduced from* Journal of Clinical Investigation *with permission.[18])*

membrane. The reciprocal of this resistance is the *ultrafiltration coefficient* (Kf). Kf is the product of the surface area of the membrane (S) and its hydraulic permeability or conductivity (k), the latter being expressed as rate of flow (Q) per unit S per unit P_{UF}:

Equation 8

$$k = Q \times S^{-1} \times P_{UF}^{-1}$$

Although S can be estimated morphometrically, it is difficult or impossible to measure effective S, the area participating in filtration at any given time. In the absence of a reliable value for S, k cannot be calculated. The composite term Kf is therefore preferred for most purposes. Thus:

Equation 9

$$GFR = P_{UF} \times k \times S = P_{UF} \times Kf$$

In filtration equilibrium, Kf is not limiting to GFR and cannot be calculated from experimental measurements. When filtration disequilibrium is induced by massive volume expansion, Kf becomes rate limiting, and a unique value can be calculated for it from measurements of hydrostatic and oncotic pressures in the afferent and efferent arterioles and in Bowman's space, and single nephron GFR. Identical values for single nephron Kf of 0.08 $nl.s^{-1}.mmHg^{-1}$ have been found experimentally in both rat and dog, despite the fact that filtration equilibrium does not obtain in the latter species.[18,19] Depending on the value taken for S, this yields an estimate for k in the range 25–50 $nl.s^{-1}.mmHg^{-1}.(cm^2)^{-1}$. This is 10–100 times higher than that found in capillaries from other tissues, enabling filtrate to be formed at a very high rate despite rather low values for P_{UF} (<10 mmHg). It is evident from equation 9 that GFR may change as a result of changes in factors affecting one or more of the components of P_{UF} (changes of glomerular plasma flow, and changes of plasma albumin concentration or urinary tract obstruction), changes in S (reduction of nephron numbers) or changes in k (diffuse glomerular disease). More than one of these may be involved in progressive renal disease.

Regulation of glomerular filtration

Factors affecting P_{UF}

As discussed above, GFR is plasma flow dependent if:

1. Filtration equilibrium exists.
2. $\Delta P - \Delta \Pi$ at the afferent arteriole does not change.
3. Kf is constant.

Under physiological conditions, these requirements are probably met, at least approximately. Plasma flow is determined by arterial pressure and renal vascular resistance, which resides mostly in the afferent and efferent glomerular arterioles. Angiotensin II (AII) and norepinephrine (noradrenaline, NE) constrict both afferent and efferent arterioles; these hormones are released in ECF volume contraction and other conditions in which arterial filling, and therefore renal perfusion pressure, is reduced. Efferent arteriolar constriction raises P_C, and therefore P_{UF}, more than it reduces glomerular blood flow, leading to maintenance of GFR by an increase in FF. Conversely, vasodilators such as prostaglandins E_2 and I_2 (prostacyclin) and bradykinin, despite a lowering of arterial blood pressure, cause renal plasma flow to rise due to dilatation of both afferent and efferent arterioles. Here again, GFR remains relatively constant with an associated fall in FF. It is likely that both vasodilator and vasoconstrictor hormones also affect Kf (see below). Obstruction of the flow of urine causes reduction or abolition of glomerular filtration due to a rise in P_{BS}.

Factors affecting Kf

The mesangial cells which support the glomerular capillaries are contractile.[20] Their contraction causes constriction of the capillaries, with a resulting fall in S and therefore Kf. AII, NE and prostaglandins all alter Kf to the degree necessary to offset their effects on P_{UF}; in other words, the glomerular haemodynamic response to vasoactive substances is nicely balanced by changes in Kf, maintaining GFR approximately constant. Both AII and ADH cause cultured mesangial cells to contract, and this may be a physiologically important effect in vivo.

Autoregulation

In common with other vital organs, the kidney is capable of regulating its own blood flow, even in an artificial perfusion system where systemic humoral and nervous controlling factors cannot operate. This is due to differential constriction of the afferent and efferent arterioles. Analysis of the determinants of GFR in this model system suggests that the damping effect on GFR is mediated in part by autoregulation of plasma flow and partly by compensatory changes in P_C, producing parallel changes in P_{UF}. As mentioned in the previous section, a role for mesangial cell contraction in autoregulation is likely, probably by altering Kf; locally produced AII may be involved in this process. Autoregulation fails at extremes of blood pressure. In malignant hypertension, the exposure of the kidney to excessive pressure leads acutely to disturbance of the mechanisms coupling GFR to tubular reabsorption, causing the phenomenon of pressure natriuresis. When blood pressure falls below the autoregulatory range, RPF and GFR fall and prerenal failure develops.

PROXIMAL TUBULAR FUNCTION

About two-thirds of filtered salt and water is reabsorbed in the proximal tubule. Other solutes including glucose, amino acids, bicarbonate and low molecular weight proteins are almost completely reclaimed in this tubule segment, as is about 90% of filtered inorganic phosphate. Epithelial transport of all of these is linked to sodium transport and dependent on it for its energy supply.

Salt and water reabsorption in the proximal tubule

Sodium reabsorption

The proximal tubular epithelial cells are arranged in a single layer lining the cylindrical basement membrane. They exhibit *polarity*: the membranes on opposite sides of the cells have different characteristics. The part of the cell membrane that faces the tubular lumen is called the *apical membrane*; the part that faces the basement membrane and the intercellular space is the *basolateral membrane*. Adjacent cells are attached to one another at the *tight junction*, which separates the apical from the basolateral membranes (Figure 5.4).

The enzyme sodium, potassium adenosine triphosphatase (Na^+, K^+-ATPase, commonly known as the sodium pump) is located in the basolateral membrane. Powered by energy released by the hydrolysis of ATP, it transports sodium out of the cell interior and potassium into it, with a stoichiometry of 3 Na^+:2 K^+. This process is called *primary active transport*. A consequence of the action of Na^+, K^+-ATPase is a very low intracellular sodium concentration, establishing a steep concentration gradient between the tubular fluid and the cell interior that favours sodium entry across the apical membrane. This membrane is impermeable to sodium, but contains proteins of several different types that act as specialized sodium channels. Each of these not only allows sodium entry but also transports another solute into or out of the cell. This is called *secondary active transport*, since the energy driving it is provided indirectly by Na^+, K^+-ATPase at a site remote from the transport process itself. Inhibition of Na^+, K^+-ATPase by ouabain blocks sodium reabsorption in all nephron segments.[21]

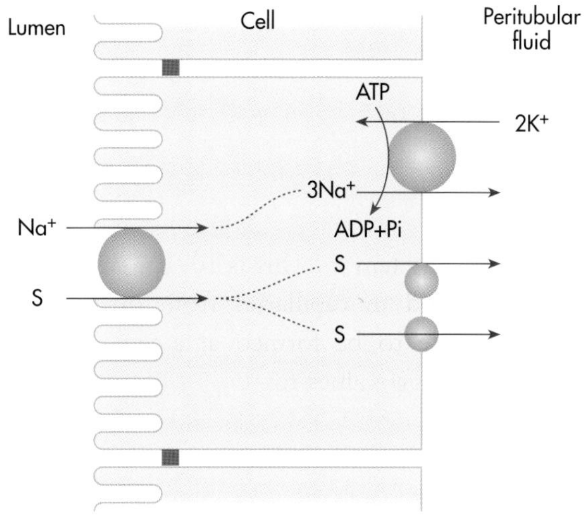

Figure 5.4 *Schematic view of a proximal tubular cell. The apical (brush border) membrane (left) is depicted as a wavy line. The basolateral membrane (right and lining the intercellular space) is separated from the apical membrance by the tight junction (dark squares). S represents any substance that enters the cell across the apical membrane by secondary active transport via a sodium-S contra–sporter. The enzyme Na^+, K^+-ATPase (upper right) maintains a steep gradient for sodium across the apical membrane by constantly extruding sodium across the basolateral membrane.*

One of these proteins is a member of a group of transporters called Na^+, H^+-*antiporters*, known as NHE3.[22] Antiporters are so called because they transport sodium and hydrogen ions (protons) in opposite directions. Sodium entry therefore leads to alkalinization of the cell interior and acidification of the tubular fluid. By an indirect process described later in this chapter, this effectively causes reabsorption of bicarbonate in an amount chemically equivalent to the amount of sodium entering via the antiporter. This takes place early in the proximal tubule, and because bicarbonate, in common with other solutes described below, is reabsorbed in preference to chloride,[23] the concentration of chloride in the tubular fluid increases to a level substantially higher than that in the peritubular fluid. Chloride therefore moves down its concentration gradient from tubular fluid to peritubular space, partly by simple diffusion across the tight junction (which is not really chemically tight) and partly via chloride channels in the apical and basolateral membranes. Diffusion across the tight junction, bypassing the cell interior, is referred to as reabsorption via the *paracellular shunt pathway*. Because chloride is an anion, its removal from the luminal to the peritubular aspects of the tubule generates an electrical voltage, lumen positive, across the epithelium that acts as a further driving force for sodium reabsorption.[24] At least some of this also occurs through the paracellular shunt pathway.

Other apical membrane proteins transport sodium and another solute (the *cotransportate*) in the same direction, and are called *cotransporters*. For example, the sodium-glucose cotransporter is activated when one sodium ion and one glucose molecule attach to specific receptors on the protein on the luminal side of the membrane. The molecule then either rotates in the membrane or alters its configuration in such a way that the sodium and glucose are transferred to the cytoplasmic side of the apical membrane, where they are released. Other cotransporters include a sodium-phosphate transporter and a whole set of specific transporters for different amino acids. The general mode of operation of secondary active transport in the apical membrane of the proximal tubule is schematized in Figure 5.4. It should be realized that both the antiporter and the cotransporters are potentially bidirectional. It is only the maintenance of the steep concentration gradient favouring sodium entry, resulting from sodium removal by Na^+, K^+-ATPase, that causes them to transport protons out of the cell and the various cotransportates in. The antiporter and several of the apical membrane cotransporter proteins have now been sequenced and the corresponding genes mapped and cloned.

Water reabsorption in the proximal tubule

Water is reabsorbed by osmosis, diffusing down the osmotic gradient established by solute reabsorption. The epithelium is sufficiently permeable to water that osmotic equilibration is virtually instantaneous, and the osmolality of the tubular fluid at all points in the proximal tubule is not measurably different from that of plasma. An unknown, but probably substantial, proportion of water reabsorption takes place through the paracellular shunt pathway and provides yet another mechanism promoting sodium reabsorption. Active transport of sodium across the basolateral membrane into the lateral intercellular spaces leads to a small, transient osmotic water gradient favouring water reabsorption across the tight junction. The resulting water flux causes salt to be transported passively by a process known as convection or solvent drag, given that the tight junction is permeable to sodium and chloride. The relative importance of transcellular and paracellular reabsorption of sodium and water is still uncertain.

Effect of physical forces on proximal tubular reabsorption

Water and solute reabsorbed from the tubular lumen is returned to the blood in the peritubular capillary plexus, which is perfused by blood draining from glomerular efferent arterioles. The peritubular capillaries are therefore *in series with* and *downstream from* the glomerulus. The rate of reabsorption of tubular fluid is governed by the Starling forces across the peritubular capillary wall.[25] The importance of the peritubular oncotic pressure in this process has been demonstrated both by micropuncture in the intact animal and by studies in the isolated, perfused rabbit proximal tubule.[26,27] The effect of changes in peritubular hydrostatic pressure is less clear. Since the protein concentration of postglomerular plasma is proportional to the filtration fraction (equation 4), it follows that changes in glomerular function may induce secondary changes in proximal tubular reabsorption rate; this may be important in maintenance of *glomerulotubular balance* (see below).

Proximal tubular reabsorption of other solutes

Glucose

Glucose is reabsorbed by cotransport with sodium, chiefly in the early proximal tubule. Glucose is not merely acting as an energy source for sodium transport, since the non-metabolized analogue α-methyl-D-glucoside can be substituted for it, but its transport is dependent on sodium reabsorption. At least two sodium-glucose cotransporters have been identified in mammalian proximal tubule; they have been named SGLT-1 and SGLT-2, respectively. SGLT-1 binds one sodium ion and one glucose molecule, while SGLT-2 has a stoichiometry of $2Na^+$:1 glucose. SGLT-2 is probably the more important of the two.[28] It is saturable, and when the filtered load of glucose exceeds its maximal transporting capacity (Tm), the excess is excreted in the urine. The relationship between glucose filtration, reabsorption and excretion is shown in Figure 5.5. Glycosuria occurs in hyperglycaemia (as in diabetes mellitus) because the filtered load of glucose exceeds the Tm of the transport system. Glycosuria due to abnormalities of the tubular glucose transport system (renal glycosuria) occurs when the renal threshold for glucose is less than the normal blood glucose concentration and is due to mutations in the gene for SGLT-2.[29]

Phosphate

The majority of filtered phosphate is reabsorbed, with sodium, in the early proximal tubule. Studies of phosphate excretion at different plasma phosphate concentrations show that the ion is handled in a manner similar to glucose, that is, by a saturable transport system with a Tm and a threshold; hence, a similar set of titration curves can be drawn (Figure 5.5). In contrast to glucose, some degree of phosphaturia is normally present, since dietary phosphate in excess of requirement must be excreted. Thus, the normal plasma phosphate concentration is just above the threshold value, and is indeed defined by it, whereas, in health, the plasma glucose concentration is always well below the renal threshold. The mechanism of proximal tubular phosphate reabsorption is discussed in more detail later in this chapter.

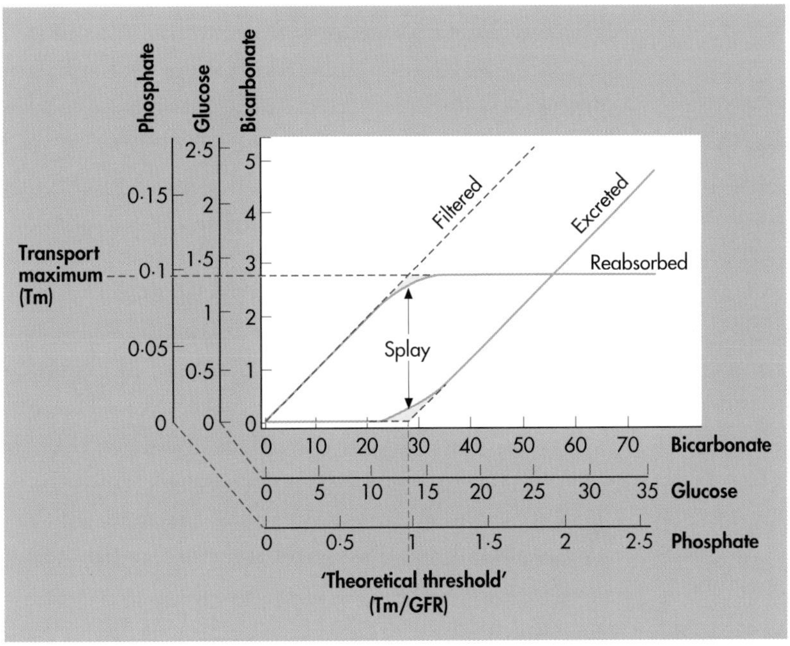

Figure 5.5 *Curves of filtration, excretion and reabsorption of three solutes reabsorbed actively from glomerular filtrate, plotted against the plasma concentration of the solute. Values plotted on the abscissa are plasma concentrations (mmol/L); those on the ordinate are the quantities filtered, excreted and reabsorbed (mmol/100 ml GFR).*

Amino acids

Amino acids are reabsorbed in the same general manner as glucose and phosphate. At least five transport proteins exist, some of which transport sodium and one of the major subclasses of amino acids with high specificity, while others operate as exchangers, transporting one group of amino acids out of the cell in exchange for entry of another.[30] The normal plasma concentrations of all the amino acids are below threshold in health, so that normal urine contains virtually no amino acids of any kind. Several inherited defects of proximal tubular amino-acid transport systems have been described. By far the commonest is cystinuria. This is caused by mutations in an apical membrane system that operates as an amino-acid exchanger. It transports cystine and the dibasic amino acids arginine, lysine and ornithine into the cell in exchange for exit of neutral amino acids. This is another form of secondary active transport. The driving force for exchange is the steep cell-to-lumen gradient for neutral amino acids generated by sodium-coupled entry of the latter, also across the apical membrane. The exchanger is a heterodimer of two components, labelled rBAT and $b^{0,+}$AT, respectively.[31] The mutations that cause cystinuria affect rBAT, and more than 60 mutations have so far been identified in different families.[32] The only clinical significance of cystinuria is the tendency to form cystine stones in the urinary tract: affected individuals are otherwise healthy.

Proteins

Several low molecular weight proteins are present in normal plasma in measurable concentrations. Examples are α-1 microglobulin, β-2 microglobulin and retinol-binding protein (RBP). Because they are smaller than the size barrier of the glomerular ultrafilter, significant amounts are present in glomerular filtrate and enter the proximal tubule, where they are reabsorbed by pinocytosis into the tubular epithelial cells where they are digested to their component amino acids and returned to the body protein pool. They are therefore virtually absent from normal urine. Proximal tubular dysfunction, however, leads to a urinary leak of these proteins and a characteristic pattern of low molecular weight proteinuria known as *tubular proteinuria*. Measurement of urinary excretion of β-2 microglobulin and RBP, usually expressed as fractional excretion rates, is a useful means of distinguishing between proteinuria of glomerular and non-glomerular (tubulo-interstitial) origin.[33]

Only very small amounts of albumin and other large plasma proteins normally pass the glomerular filter. These are essentially completely reabsorbed by a mechanism similar to that for low molecular weight proteins. At low filtered loads, the system behaves as a high-affinity, low-capacity transporter with virtually complete clearance of albumin from the tubular fluid, while at high filtered loads this mechanism becomes saturated and a high-capacity, low-affinity mode operates, so that reabsorption continues to rise with increasing load, but about one-third of the filtered albumin escapes reabsorption and appears in the urine.[34] In such conditions of glomerular proteinuria, the urinary albumin excretion rate is always considerably less than the amount filtered and catabolized. This probably explains why proteinuria of nutritionally trivial amounts (<10 g/day) may cause hypoalbuminaemia in some cases of the nephrotic syndrome.

Proximal tubular secretion of organic anions

Many organic substances, anionic at physiological pH, are actively secreted by the proximal tubule. These include endogenous substances such as hippurate and exogenous substances such as penicillin, probenecid and derivatives of hippuric acid such as ortho- and para-amino hippurate (hippuran and PAH). The renal clearance of these compounds exceeds GFR and in the case of hippuran and PAH, at least, extraction may be practically complete. The secretory site is the proximal convoluted tubule, especially the middle and late segments. The small amount of PAH that escapes secretion is accounted for by blood perfusing the deepest (juxtamedullary) nephrons, in which the post-glomerular blood flows directly into the medullary vasa recta system without passing through the cortical peritubular capillary plexus, bypassing the secretory site. In the adult, only about 10% of nephrons are of this type so the underestimation of renal plasma flow by PAH clearance is small. In the newborn infant, in contrast, the superficial cortical nephrons (the last to be formed) function little or not at all, and the juxtamedullary nephrons provide the lion's share of renal function. Clearance of PAH and similar substances is therefore an unreliable measure of renal plasma flow in babies and newborn animals. PAH secretion is saturable and Tm-limited; below the renal threshold, excretion increases in parallel with rising plasma concentration, while above this value, there is no further rise in excretion. A similar, but separate, transport system exists for the secretion of organic cations.

GLOMERULOTUBULAR BALANCE

Delivery of fluid to the distal tubule is, by definition, the difference between GFR and proximal tubular reabsorption rate. Since the rate of distal fluid delivery is an important determinant of distal tubular function, and therefore of homeostasis, it is important that glomerular and proximal tubular function are coupled together. This coupling is known as glomerulotubular balance (GTB): changes in GFR are partially offset by parallel and proportional changes in proximal tubular reabsorption.[35] GTB has been shown experimentally to exist: when GFR is manipulated by altering renal perfusion pressure, changes in proximal tubular reabsorption take place as the theory predicts. At least three mechanisms are involved.

Peritubular physical forces

The protein concentration in postglomerular plasma is determined by arterial plasma protein concentration and filtration fraction. If GFR increases without a parallel increase in plasma flow, filtration fraction rises and peritubular capillary oncotic pressure is increased. This alters the balance of Starling forces in the peritubular environment in a direction that favours reabsorption. Conversely, a fall in GFR and filtration fraction leads to a reduction in the pressure gradient for reabsorption.[36] The oncotic pressure of the peritubular capillary plasma has been shown to be a powerful, and possibly rate-limiting, factor in proximal tubular reabsorption.[26]

Filtration of preferentially reabsorbed substances

Sodium is reabsorbed in the early proximal tubule with bicarbonate, phosphate, amino acids, lactate and citrate in preference to chloride; glucose is also absorbed by cotransport. The more of these substances presented to the tubule, the more sodium (and therefore water) will be reabsorbed. At any plasma concentration, a change in GFR will produce a parallel and proportionate change in the rate of filtration of these substances, inducing a change in proximal tubular reabsorption rate in the same direction. This effect will be amplified by the secondary effect on downstream, passive sodium reabsorption described in a previous section. Thus, any random fluctuation in GFR will cause secondary changes in both active proximal tubular sodium reabsorption and in the peritubular environment, reinforcing one another in the preservation of GTB.

Tubuloglomerular feedback

The ascending limb of the loop of Henle passes through the vascular pole of its own glomerulus, where it is intimately associated with the afferent and efferent arterioles in the JGA. There is strong evidence that delivery of some solute, probably chloride, is sensed at the JGA, where it provides the afferent stimulus for regulation of GFR by negative feedback.[37] In experiments where the loop of Henle was perfused in both orthograde and retrograde directions with solutions of various NaCl concentrations and at various rates, a clear inhibitory effect was seen on RPF and GFR as concentration (or flow rate) was increased.[38] The effect is probably mediated at least in part by local production and conversion of angiotensin, producing glomerular vasoconstriction (especially of the efferent arteriole) and increasing vascular resistance. TGF may provide an emergency defence against drastic salt and water depletion in tubular injury. If proximal tubular NaCl reabsorption were severely impaired by anoxia or the action of a nephrotoxic drug, the resulting flood of sodium-rich urine would lead rapidly to fatal dehydration and electrolyte depletion unless GFR were to fall by some means. The oliguria of acute renal failure may be seen, in this light, as a life-preserving response rather than an undesirable feature of the syndrome. Recognition that the thick ascending limb (TAL) of the loop of Henle is the most vulnerable part of the nephron to ischaemic injury[39] is entirely consistent with this view, since the TAL is included in the anatomical feedback loop consisting of glomerulus–proximal tubule–loop of Henle–JGA.

SODIUM EXCRETION AND EXTRACELLULAR FLUID VOLUME

Sodium and extracellular fluid volume

The major osmotically active solute in the ECF is sodium chloride: 90% of the sodium in the body, and almost all the chloride, is located in the extracellular compartment. Since the tonicity of body fluids is held within very narrow limits by regulation of water intake and excretion, it follows that a gain or loss of total body NaCl leads to expansion or contraction of ECF volume. Conversely, ECF volume is the major determinant of sodium excretion rate. In subjects on a salt-restricted diet, a tiny increase in ECF volume is followed by an immediate natriuresis.[40] ECF volume expansion beyond a certain threshold volume is a stimulus to sodium excretion, the magnitude of the natriuresis being proportionate to the amount by which this volume is exceeded. Conversely, sodium-free urine is produced when ECF volume is below this threshold, while sodium appears in the urine as soon as this volume is even slightly exceeded. The relationship between ECF volume and sodium excretion is shown in Figure 5.6. It is evident that the stimulus producing the increase in sodium excretion cannot be plasma sodium concentration, which does not change, but ECF volume. How changes in this volume are sensed and whether it is the total ECF volume or a particular component or function of it that is important have been the subject of much investigation.

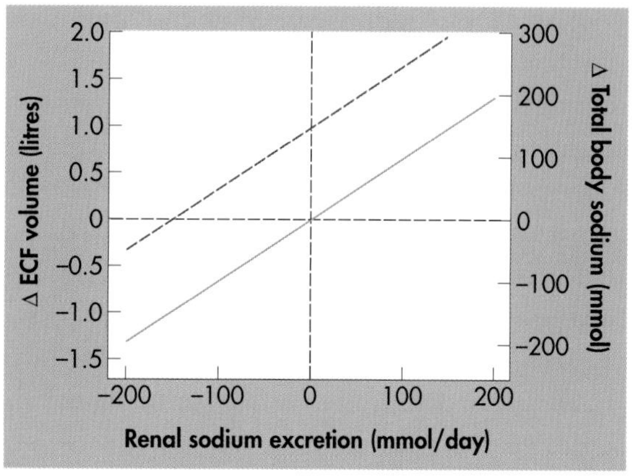

Figure 5.6 *The relationship between extracellular fluid (ECF) volume, total body sodium and urinary sodium excretion rate, assuming that a gain or loss of 1 litre of extracellular fluid corresponds to a gain or loss of 150 mmol sodium, and that the ECF sodium concentration does not change. Negative values for sodium excretion indicate the magnitude of the sodium deficit that must be made up before sodium appears in the urine, which is actually sodium free at points to the left of the vertical zero line. The solid oblique line describes the relationship as observed in recumbent subjects; in the upright position, the point of interception with the y-axis is displaced upwards, corresponding to sodium retention, but the slope of the relationship is unchanged. (Reproduced from* Archives of Internal Medicine *with permission.[40])*

Control of sodium excretion

The control system regulating sodium excretion and, therefore, ECF volume is in three parts: an afferent (sensory) component, which detects a signal indicating the need to excrete or conserve sodium; an effector organ (the kidney); and a means of transmitting the response to the afferent stimulus to the kidney, the efferent (messenger) component.

The afferent stimulus

Both acute (saline loading) and chronic (high dietary sodium intake) volume expansion are natriuretic stimuli. Manoeuvres that expand intrathoracic blood volume, such as head-out water immersion, are natriuretic even though total ECF volume becomes contracted as natriuresis continues.[41] The magnitude of the response is correlated with left atrial volume, and left atrial stretch receptors probably mediate the effect. Stimulation of carotid sinus baroreceptors by underfilling of the arterial tree, as by hypotension or vasodilatation, is antinatriuretic; observations in subjects with arteriovenous fistulae indicate that underfilling of the high-pressure (arterial) compartment overrides the effect of overfilling of the low-pressure (venous) compartment, so that the net response is antinatriuretic.[42] Volume or sodium receptors have been postulated in the liver or portal venous system, following the observation that saline infused into the portal vein or ingested orally is more natriuretic than the same amount infused into a peripheral vein. The presence of baroreceptors in the interstitial space is suggested by the differential natriuretic effects of saline infusions of different oncotic pressures; the fluid that expands intravascular volume the least and the interstitial compartment the most (isotonic saline) is much more natriuretic than an equivalent volume of plasma or hyperoncotic albumin.[43] Receptors in the pulmonary interstitium may subserve this function.

Changes in the perfusion pressure perceived by the kidney itself, in consequence of changes in arterial blood pressure, lead to changes in urinary sodium excretion both by intrarenal mechanisms and by affecting the rate of renin secretion. It is likely that most or all of these receptors play a part in determining the natriuretic status of the kidney, perhaps via a (hypothetical) integrating mechanism located in the hypothalamus or elsewhere. In general, reduction of effective arterial volume, that is, underfilling of the arterial tree in relation to its holding capacity, seems to engender a sodium-retaining response sufficient to override conflicting or interfering stimuli from elsewhere. Examples include congestive cardiac failure, the nephrotic syndrome and cirrhosis of the liver in some patients.

Renal effector responses

Theoretically, the renal sodium-excretion rate could be altered either by changing GFR without an accompanying change in tubular reabsorption, or by the reverse. In fact, changes in tubular reabsorption are undoubtedly responsible for physiological regulation of this function. Patients with chronic renal failure are able to remain in external sodium balance on a fixed sodium intake despite progressively falling GFR; an adjustment of tubular reabsorption must have taken place. It has been shown in many experimental models that the natriuretic response to volume expansion is not abolished if GFR is prevented from increasing, or even artificially decreased. Furthermore, experimental manipulations which produce large increases in GFR are not necessarily natriuretic. For example, in dogs, protein feeding, dexamethasone administration, dopamine infusion and saline infusion all increase GFR by up to 30%: of these, only saline loading is consistently natriuretic.[44]

If sodium excretion is modulated by changes in tubular reabsorption, which part of the tubule is mainly responsible? Experimental studies favour the distal nephron as the important effector. Natriuresis can be dissociated not only from GFR (see above) but also from absolute and fractional proximal tubular sodium reabsorption.[45] Humoral factors known to influence sodium reabsorption rate (such as aldosterone and atrial natriuretic peptide) act mainly on distal nephron segments. In rats, saline loading causes marked changes in sodium reabsorption in the collecting duct, resulting in apparent sodium secretion in response to extreme volume expansion. Newborn infants, in whom fractional proximal tubular sodium reabsorption is lower than that in adults, maintain sodium balance perfectly well, presumably by distal tubular compensation. Furthermore, it appears logical that the most distal part of the nephron is responsible for the final adjustment of the sodium excretion rate in that, by definition, further downstream adjustments are not possible.

It should be emphasized that the response to saline volume expansion is normally a reduction in sodium reabsorption in both proximal and distal nephron segments, and that the dissociation between these mentioned above was produced by unphysiological experimental manipulations. The fact that the distal parts of the nephron can maintain a degree of sodium homeostasis in the absence of parallel responses in the proximal tubule probably reflects the extreme importance of control of ECF volume; if proximal tubular reabsorption is impaired or abnormal, external balance for sodium can still be maintained. However, the cost of maintaining sodium balance in these circumstances may be secondary disturbances of potassium and hydrogen ion excretion, as in Bartter's syndrome.

Intrarenal control of sodium excretion

Sodium excretion is correlated with renal artery pressure. ECF volume is an important determinant of renal artery pressure, with resulting effects on intrarenal haemodynamics. The main resistance vessels in the renal microcirculation are the afferent and efferent glomerular arterioles. The latter are interposed between the glomerular and peritubular capillary plexuses. The hydrostatic pressure in the peritubular capillaries therefore varies in proportion to renal artery pressure and in inverse proportion to renal arteriolar resistance. Volume expansion directly increases perfusion pressure and, partly by inhibition of the renin-angiotensin-aldosterone system (RAAS), reduces arteriolar resistance: volume contraction has the reverse effects. Thus, volume expansion leads to an increase, and volume contraction to a decrease, in peritubular capillary pressure. The effect of angiotensin II on the renal circulation is complex. It causes both preglomerular (afferent arteriole) and postglomerular (efferent arteriole) vasoconstriction, but the postglomerular effect predominates, largely due to production of vasodilator prostaglandins in the afferent arteriole that offset the vasoconstrictor action of angiotensin II. Conditions in which the RAAS is stimulated, such as volume contraction, therefore increase glomerular capillary pressure, leading to an increase in filtration fraction and an increase in postglomerular plasma oncotic pressure. Suppression of the RAAS (volume expansion) has the opposite effect. In sum, volume expansion causes an increase in hydrostatic pressure and a decrease in oncotic pressure in the peritubular capillaries. This reduces the Starling pressure gradient for fluid reabsorption from the peritubular interstitium and hence from the proximal tubule, favouring natriuresis. Volume contraction initiates the opposite sequence of events and is therefore antinatriuretic. These processes are schematized in Figure 5.7.[46]

Although the above discussion has focused on the proximal tubule, the rate of fluid absorption in the distal nephron is also influenced by Starling forces, since the cortical part of the distal tubule is supplied by the same peritubular capillary network that supplies the proximal tubule, and the medullary part by capillaries that receive part of their blood supply from the efferent arterioles of juxtamedullary (deep cortical) nephrons. It has sometimes been argued that physical forces alone are sufficient to explain the regulation of renal sodium excretion, but this hypothesis is rendered untenable by other observations, notably the fact that saline expansion is natriuretic even if renal perfusion pressure is artificially prevented from rising or even reduced. It follows that extrarenal factors are also involved.

The efferent limb in the regulation of sodium excretion

The fact that sodium excretion is influenced by changes in the apparent volume of ECF subcompartments remote from the kidney indicates not only that

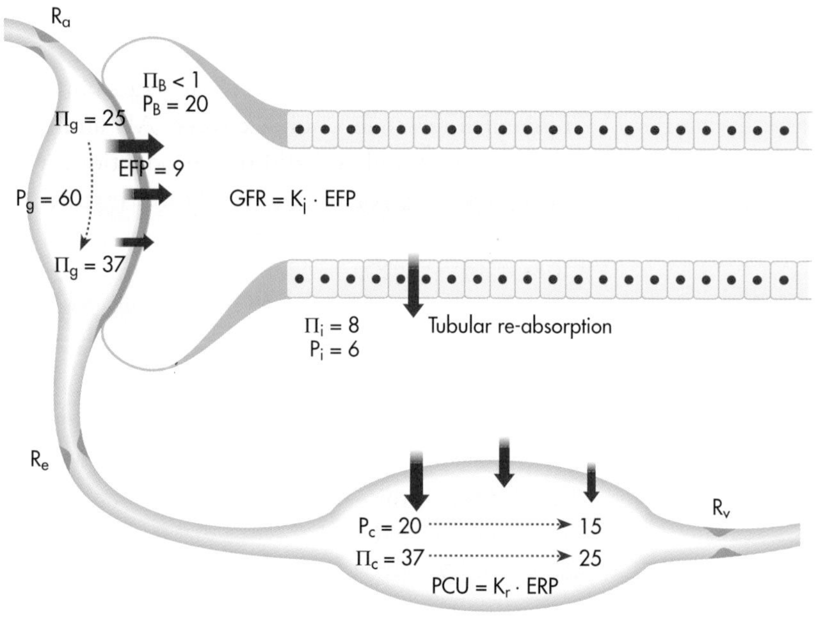

Figure 5.7 *Schematic diagram of the forces responsible for filtration of fluid from the glomerular capillaries and reabsorption of fluid into the peritubular capillaries. The forces are expressed in mmHg and are considered representative of those found in normal humans. (Reproduced by permission of Little, Brown.[46])*

volume sensors exist at those sites, but also that some means exist of altering renal sodium excretion in response to the signals they receive. This message ('increase or decrease sodium excretion') may be transmitted from sensor to effector by a number of efferent pathways. The renal nerve supply contains efferent postganglionic fibres located in the splanchnic nerves: stimulation of these is antinatriuretic while denervation is natriuretic. α-Adrenergic endings have been identified in close approximation to proximal and distal tubules as well as blood vessels; a direct effect on epithelial transport seems likely. Denervation of one kidney causes natriuresis in the ipsilateral and antinatriuresis in the contralateral kidney, suggesting a role also for the afferent fibres in the control of sodium excretion, perhaps by integrating the responses of the two kidneys via a reno-renal reflex.[47]

Aldosterone

The mineralocorticoid aldosterone is an important regulator of tubular sodium handling. Released in response to activation of the renin-angiotensin system, which in turn is stimulated by volume contraction, it acts on the distal convoluted tubule and collecting duct to stimulate sodium reabsorption, where it also promotes secretion of K^+ and H^+ (see below). Although other factors undoubtedly interact with aldosterone and can even override it in the *mineralocorticoid escape phenomenon*, its importance in sodium homeostasis is illustrated by the finding that adrenalectomized animals, on a fixed replacement dose of mineralocorticoid, achieve sodium balance only at the cost of greatly exaggerated changes in ECF volume, body weight, blood pressure and potassium concentration.[48]

Catecholamines

Catecholamines affect sodium excretion, noradrenaline (norepinephrine) being antinatriuretic and dopamine natriuretic; both α-adrenergic and dopaminergic receptors have been identified in the kidney. It has been suggested that dopamine is an important mediator of sodium excretion, particularly in chronic renal failure; however, it is likely that the major effects of these amines are mediated via their action as locally released neurotransmitters, rather than as circulating hormones proper. The fact that L-dopa, a precursor of dopamine, is natriuretic when infused into the renal artery further supports the view that local synthesis accounts for the origin of most or all of the dopamine present in the kidney. This does not exclude an important role for the amine as a second messenger, that is, a locally acting vasoactive and natriuretic factor the activity of which may be increased by other, circulating, substances.

Prostaglandins

The vasodilator prostaglandins PGE_2 and PGI_2 (prostacyclin) are synthesized within the kidney and are natriuretic. Inhibitors of prostaglandin synthetase, such as indometacin, cause RPF and GFR to fall and fractional proximal tubular sodium reabsorption to increase. These effects are partly offset by volume expansion and greatly exaggerated by volume contraction; the combination of volume contraction and a non-steroidal anti-inflammatory agent may lead to acute renal failure. Angiotensin II stimulates renal release of prostaglandins: the main physiological role of renal PGs may be to maintain glomerular plasma flow and filtration rate in volume-contracted states, when AII levels are high.

The kallikrein-kinin system

The kinins bradykinin and kallidin are another class of vasodilator and natriuretic substances produced locally within the kidney. They are formed by the action of the proteinase kallikrein, produced in the distal tubule, on a circulating precursor. The renin-angiotensin-aldosterone system, prostaglandins and kinins all interact in complex ways. AII and aldosterone both stimulate kallikrein production, while kinins promote prostaglandin synthesis. Angiotensin-converting enzyme (ACE) not only converts AI to AII but also inactivates bradykinin; it is also known as kininase II. ACE therefore causes vasoconstriction and antinatriuresis by both AII production and bradykinin degradation; ACE inhibition has the opposite effects, accounting for the fact that ACE inhibitors lower blood pressure even when the RAAS is not activated. Catecholamines, the RAAS, prostaglandins and kinins can be regarded as components of a complex intrarenal paracrine system that normally act synchronously to regulate and stabilize renal blood flow and GFR in response to changes in extrarenal influences such as ECF volume and circulating hormones.

Natriuretic hormones

Volume expansion causes natriuresis in dogs even when GFR is artificially constrained and supramaximal doses of mineralocorticoid and vasopressin are given.[49] The design of the experiments in which this was demonstrated excluded all feasible explanations for the natriuresis except the action of a natriuretic hormone. In the 1980s, a new class of peptide hormones was identified.[50] The first of these was atrial natriuretic peptide (ANP), so called because it is synthesized in the cardiac atria and released in response to atrial stretch. Related peptides are produced elsewhere in the body, including the brain, probably the anterior hypothalamus. Human ANP is composed of 28 amino acids, including a 17-amino acid ring formed by a disulphide bridge. It is formed by cleavage of a 126-amino-acid prohormone. At least three other fragments of the same prohormone have hormonal activity and are known, respectively, as long-acting natriuretic peptide (amino acids 1–30), vessel dilator hormone (31–67) and kaliuretic hormone (79–98). ANP is a systemic and renal vasodilator, and also reduces pulmonary vascular resistance. It acts directly on arteriolar smooth muscle by a pathway not involving prostaglandins or nitric oxide. Its actions on the renal vasculature include dilatation of the arcuate arteries and afferent arterioles, and antagonism of mesangial cell contraction induced by both AII and vasopressin. These effects combine to cause an increase in GFR and a reduction in fractional proximal tubular sodium reabsorption, probably due to altered physical (Starling) forces. It also has direct effects on the distal renal tubule, decreasing sodium reabsorption by inhibiting both its entry into the tubular cells through sodium channels in the apical membrane and its exit from the cell across the basolateral membrane by reducing Na^+, K^+-ATPase activity. At the cellular level, the actions of ANP are mediated by cyclic guanosine monophosphate (c-GMP) and c-GMP-dependent protein kinase.[51] Other actions of ANP include suppression of renin release, inhibition of aldosterone synthesis and antagonism of AII-mediated vasoconstriction.

There is a compelling logic in atrial distension being an important natriuretic stimulus, since in most circumstances atrial stretch is a sensitive indicator of circulating volume. The right atrium is the main source of ANP, suggesting that the observed pulmonary effects of the hormone may be physiologically important. In pathological states such as congestive heart failure, atrial distension may become dissociated from ECF and circulatory volume. It is theorized that ANP release is beneficial in heart failure both by reducing afterload and by mitigating the salt and water retention characteristic of that condition. ANP is involved, and may be pre-eminent, in the natriuresis of the syndrome of inappropriate secretion of antidiuretic hormone. The major actions of ANP are schematized in Figure 5.8.

SODIUM REABSORPTION BEYOND THE PROXIMAL TUBULE

About one-third of filtered sodium is reabsorbed distal to the proximal tubule. As in the proximal tubule, active extrusion of sodium by Na^+, K^+-ATPase across the basolateral membrane accounts for the exit step of sodium from the cell interior, and also generates a steep concentration gradient across the apical membrane. Entry from tubular fluid to cell interior takes place by secondary active transport down this gradient via a family of Na-(K)-Cl cotransporters, coded for by genes collectively named SLC12, at least three of which are expressed in different segments of the distal nephron, and an amiloride-sensitive sodium channel. In contrast to events in the proximal tubule, where reabsorption is isotonic, salt and water reabsorption are dissociated in more distal segments.

The loop of Henle

About 25% of filtered sodium is reabsorbed in the loop of Henle, all of it in the thick ascending limb (TAL). Entry into the cell here is effected by the transporter NKCC2 (the corresponding gene is SLC12A2; see above), which transports 1 Na^+, 1 K^+ and $2Cl^-$. Since the number of positively and negatively charged ions transported is equal, trans-

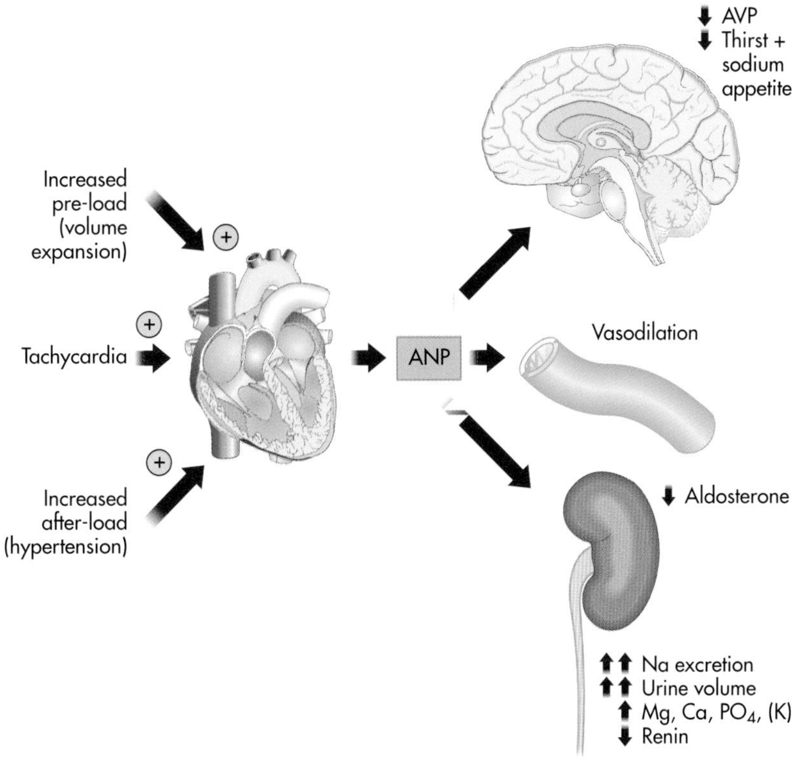

Figure 5.8 *Schematic outline of the major actions of atrial natriuretic peptide.*

port is electroneutral. Ammonia ($NH4^+$), if present in the tubular fluid, can substitute for K^+. NKCC2 is inhibited by bumetanide and furosemide (frusemide), a fact which accounts for the diuretic action of these drugs. The gene is located on chromosome 15q, and mutations of it cause one form of Bartter's syndrome of hypokalaemic alkalosis and hypercalciuria,[52] as had been predicted from the close similarity between Bartter's syndrome and the effect of chronic administration of loop diuretics. The very large amount of sodium reabsorbed by this transport system, and its relatively distal location, accounts for the great pharmacological power of furosemide (frusemide) and its congeners. The activity of NKCC2 causes large amounts of potassium and chloride, as well as sodium, to enter the cell from the tubular fluid. The absorbed potassium is recycled back into the tubule lumen via another apical membrane transporter, ROMK, and the chloride leaves the cell across the basolateral membrane via a chloride channel, ClC-Kb. Mutations in both ROMK and ClC-Kb can also cause forms of Bartter's syndrome[53,54] since NKCC2 can operate efficiently only if the absorbed potassium and chloride are prevented from accumulating within the cell. The relationship between the various transporters in the TAL cell is shown in Figure 5.9.

The distal convoluted tubule (DCT)

About 5–8% of filtered sodium is reabsorbed in the DCT. Apical sodium entry in this segment takes place via an electroneutral, thiazide-sensitive Na^+-Cl^- cotransporter (TSC). The gene is SLC12A3, located at 16q12–13. Mutations of this gene cause Gitelman's syndrome, a variant of Bartter's syndrome distinguished from the classical forms by milder clinical course, hypocalciuria and hypomagnesaemia.[55] As would be expected, inhibition of the TSC by thiazide diuretics mimics the features of Gitelman's syndrome precisely. Because much less sodium is reabsorbed by the TSC than by NKCC2, thiazides are much weaker diuretics than loop diuretics. However, if a loop diuretic (such as furosemide [frusemide]) and a thiazide (such as metolazone) are used together, the two effects reinforce one another and massive diuresis results.

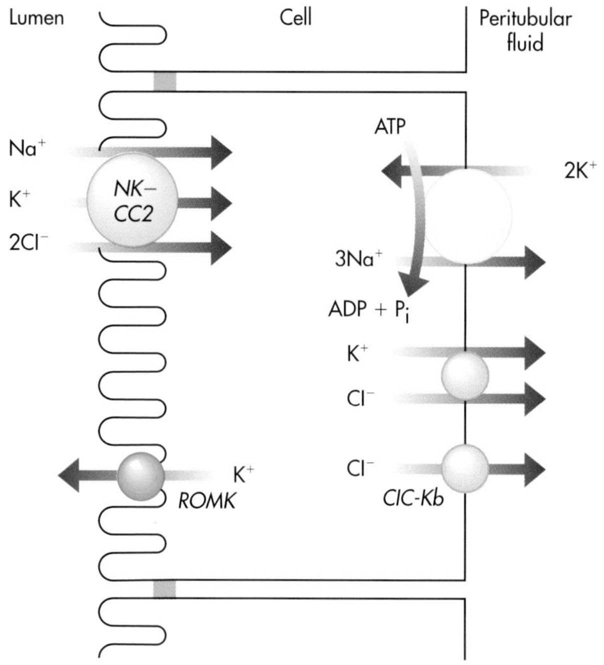

Figure 5.9 *Membrane transporters in the thick ascending limb (TAL) of the loop of Henle. Orientation as in Figure 4.4. Sodium, potassium and chloride enter the cell via NKCC-2 (upper left). Sodium is then returned to the peritubular fluid by the action of Na^+, K^+-ATPase (upper right); chloride is returned to the peritubular fluid by C1C-Kb (lower right) and potassium is recycled to the lumen via the potassium channel ROMK (lower left). Mutations in any of these three transport proteins (NKCC-2, ROMK or C1C-Kb) cause Bartter's syndrome (see text for further details).*

The collecting duct

Only 3–5% of filtered sodium enters the cortical collecting duct in most circumstances. However, the filtered load of sodium is so large that this amounts to 750–1250 mmol/day, several times the normal daily intake. Regulation of sodium reabsorption in this terminal nephron segment is therefore crucial to homeostasis, since no further adjustment of urine composition can occur at a more distal site. Sodium enters the cell in this segment via a highly sodium-selective, low-conductance, amiloride-sensitive sodium channel located in the apical membrane of the principal cells, commonly abbreviated to ENaC (epithelial sodium channel). Opening of ENaC is under the control of aldosterone, and therefore volume contraction promotes, and volume expansion inhibits, sodium reabsorption through it. Entry of sodium across the apical membrane, without an accompanying anion, creates a lumen-negative voltage across the epithelium which promotes the movement of H^+ and K^+ in the opposite direction. Blockade of this channel with amiloride therefore leads to H^+ and K^+ retention, as does aldosterone deficiency. The channel consists of three subunits, designated α-, β- and γ-ENaC, respectively, coded for by three separate genes. The gene for α-ENaC is on chromosome 12, while those for β- and γ-ENaC are close together on 16p. Two distinct hereditary diseases are caused by mutations in ENaC genes. Liddle's syndrome, a form of dominantly inherited hypertension with hypokalaemia and suppression of renin and aldosterone, was first shown to be due to mutations in the β-ENaC gene that cause the channel to be constitutively open even in the absence of mineralocorticoid.[56] The consequence is overabsorption of sodium, volume expansion and increased potassium excretion. It was subsequently shown that the syndrome could also be caused by mutations in the gene for γ-ENaC. The rare disorder pseudohypoaldosteronism type 1 (PHA1) is physiologically the mirror image of Liddle's syndrome with salt wasting, hyperkalaemia and acidosis despite high levels of renin and aldosterone. It is due to mutations that render ENaC ineffective as a sodium channel.[57] The inheritance of PHA1 is recessive in some pedigrees and dominant in others. Some families with PHA1 have mutations in the α-ENaC gene; others, in that for β-ENaC. The three subunits of ENaC have considerable sequence homology and structural similarity, suggesting descent from a common ancestor gene.

RENAL CONTROL OF POTASSIUM AND HYDROGEN ION SECRETION

Potassium excretion

On a normal diet and at normal levels of renal function, the rate of potassium filtration exceeds that of potassium excretion five- to tenfold. At first sight, this might suggest that excretion is controlled by varying the rate of tubular reabsorption of filtered potassium, as is the case for sodium. In fact, almost all the filtered potassium is reabsorbed in the proximal tubule; potassium excretion depends on distal tubular secretion of the ion.

Proximal tubular potassium reabsorption

Potassium is reabsorbed isotonically throughout the length of the proximal convoluted tubule, a process apparently continued in the proximal straight tubule. As described above, it is absorbed by NKCC2 in the TAL but recycled to the lumen via ROMK; the loop of Henle probably makes little or no net contribution to potassium reabsorption or secretion. The fluid issuing from the loop into the early distal convoluted tubule contains relatively little potassium (5–15% of the filtered load); this fraction remains constant while urinary potassium excretion varies from minimum to maximum, a 200-fold range. It is therefore logically necessary that changes in potassium excretion are effected at a more distal site.

Potassium transport in the distal tubule and collecting duct

Potassium is secreted in the distal tubule in potassium repletion and reabsorbed in potassium depletion; the latter case is unusual. The major site of potassium secretion is the late distal convoluted tubule and cortical collecting duct (CCD), corresponding to the location of ENaC (see *sodium reabsorption in the collecting duct*, above). There are two major cell types in the CCD: principal cells and intercalated cells. Potassium secretion is a function of the former; reabsorption, of the latter. The driving force for potassium secretion is the lumen-negative voltage resulting from sodium reabsorption. Although perhaps 90% of this potential difference is effaced by secondary, passive chloride reabsorption, the remaining 10% or so is associated with countermovement of potassium and H^+. Electrophysiological studies indicate that epithelial potassium transport is a complex process involving several component steps.

Intracellular potassium concentration is an important modulator of potassium secretion into the tubular lumen. Like all cells, distal tubular cells transport sodium out and potassium in across both basolateral and apical membranes. The apical (luminal) membrane of principal cells, however, allows potassium to leave the cell down its electrochemical gradient by two mechanisms: one is the potassium channel ROMK and the other a potassium-chloride symporter (cotransporter). A rise in the peritubular (ECF) potassium concentration stimulates Na^+, K^+-ATPase in the basolateral membrane, thus increasing potassium entry. The net force driving potassium secretion is therefore made up of two components: a *concentration gradient*, resulting mainly from intracellular potassium concentration, and an *electrical potential gradient*, resulting from sodium reabsorption, as described above. The electrical driving force is proportional to the rate of sodium reabsorption. This is determined by two main factors. The first is the rate of sodium entry into the CCD: anything that increases distal sodium delivery, such as inhibition of its reabsorption in more proximal segments, stimulates sodium entry into principal cells and hence potassium secretion. The second is aldosterone, which increases both sodium entry across the apical membrane via ENaC and sodium–potassium exchange across the basolateral membrane by upregulating Na^+, K^+-ATPase.[58,59]

The interaction between distal sodium delivery and aldosterone is crucially important in the normal control of potassium excretion in response to changes in ECF volume. Volume expansion increases distal sodium delivery by inhibition of reabsorption at more proximal sites, and suppresses activity of the RAAS. The resulting effects on distal sodium reabsorption, and thus on potassium secretion, are mutually opposed and cancel one another. Volume contraction produces opposite effects (↓ distal Na delivery, ↑ aldosterone). Therefore, physiological changes in sodium excretion rate due to changes in ECF volume do not cause inappropriate secondary effects on potassium excretion. Conditions in which the normal relationship between distal sodium delivery and aldosterone release are disrupted, however, cause predictable disturbances of potassium balance: some examples are given in Table 5.1.

Acute and chronic changes in acid–base status exert important effects on potassium balance. Acute metabolic alkalosis enhances, and metabolic acidosis inhibits, tubular potassium secretion, leading to hypokalaemia and hyperkalaemia, respectively. This is probably secondary to changes in intracellular potassium concentration: alkalosis promotes potassium entry into cells, thus increasing the cell-to-tubular lumen potassium gradient, while acidosis has the opposite effect. The rate of secretion of H^+ may have a further effect on potassium secretion: in

Table 5.1 The effects of various conditions on the factors determining renal potassium excretion.

Condition	Δ distal sodium delivery	Δ aldosterone	Δ intracellular [K^+]	Δ U_KV	Δ P_K
Volume expansion	↑	↓	–	–	–
Volume contraction	↓	↑	–	–	–
K^+ loading	–	–	↑	↑	↓[1]
K^+ depletion	–	–	↓	↓	↑[1]
Acute metabolic acidosis	–	–	↓	↓	↑
Chronic metabolic acidosis	↑	–	–	↑	↓
Metabolic alkalosis	–	–	↑	↑	↓
Mineralocorticoid deficiency	↓	↓	?↓	↓	↑
Mineralocorticoid excess	↑	↑	?↑	↑	↓
Proximal tubulopathies	↑	↑	?↑	↑	↓
Loop diuretucs, thiazides	↑	↑	–	↑	↓
K^+-sparing diuretucs	↓	↑	?↓	↓	↑

U_KV = urinary potassium excretion rate; P_K = plasma potassium concentration.
↓ Direction of change in U_KV produced in order to restore P_K to normal.
Data from references cited in the text.

acidosis, increased H^+ flux attenuates the potential difference between cell and tubular fluid, reducing the driving force for potassium extrusion. Chronic metabolic acidosis, in contrast to acute, is accompanied by increased potassium secretion and eventual potassium depletion. This is probably due to increased distal delivery of sodium secondary to hyperchloraemia: bicarbonate deficiency inhibits proximal sodium reabsorption by mechanisms discussed in an earlier section. The fact that chronic respiratory acidosis, in which bicarbonate levels are elevated, is not accompanied by potassium wasting lends support to this view. Diuretics that inhibit sodium reabsorption at sites proximal to the CCT cause urinary potassium wasting due to the simultaneous induction of increased distal sodium delivery and hyperaldosteronism secondary to volume contraction. These include loop diuretics such as mercurials, furosemide (frusemide) and ethacrynic acid, as well as thiazides, carbonic anhydrase inhibitors and osmotic diuretics. Diuretics such as spironolactone, triamterene and amiloride, which work by inhibiting sodium reabsorption at the potassium-secreting site, cause potassium retention and hyperkalaemia.

Hydrogen ion excretion

Volatile and non-volatile acid

The pH of the ECF is regulated within a very narrow range (7.40 ± 0.04) despite a number of perturbing influences. By far the largest of these is the continuous generation of carbonic acid as the end product of carbohydrate metabolism. Because carbonic acid can be dehydrated to CO_2 and water by the enzyme carbonic anhydrase (CA) in the lung, and the resulting CO_2 excreted in expired air, it is known as volatile acid (VA). Regulation of CO_2 excretion therefore depends on pulmonary function, and its retention or excessive loss result in respiratory acidosis and alkalosis, respectively. In addition, a much smaller amount of non-volatile acid (NVA), acid that cannot be dehydrated to anhydrides in the lung, is generated from other metabolic pathways. The principal components of NVA are as follows:

1. sulphuric acid, from combustion of sulphur-containing amino acids
2. phosphoric acid, mainly from dietary organic phosphate

3. organic acids (OA), such as lactic and aceto-acetic acids, from incomplete combustion of carbohydrate and fat, respectively.

Organic acids usually form only a small component of NVA but may become important in disease states (diabetic ketoacidosis, lactic acidosis and hereditary organic acidaemias). The amount of sulphuric acid produced depends on the intake of animal protein: strict vegetarians (vegans), who eat no animal products at all, generate predominantly alkaline products of metabolism and therefore excrete alkaline urine. Since, by definition, NVA cannot be excreted via the lungs it must be excreted by the kidney if the pH of the ECF is not to become progressively, and eventually fatally, lowered. The disproportion between the production rates of VA and NVA is enormous. An adult human on a mixed Western diet produces about 14 000 mmol of carbonic acid daily but only about 50–100 mmol of NVA. This fact is dramatically illustrated by the difference in the rate of development of acidosis following total obstruction of the trachea, as opposed to total obstruction of the urinary tract.

ECF buffers

A quantity of acid added to plasma or whole blood lowers the pH far less than it would if added to a similar volume of water. This is due to the presence of powerful buffer systems in both plasma and red cells. The most important of the ECF buffers is the carbonic acid–bicarbonate buffer system:

Equation 10

$$pH = 6.1 + \log \frac{[HCO_3^-]}{[H_2CO_3]}$$

Addition of H^+ depletes $[HCO_3^-]$ by titrating it to H_2CO_3 with a consequent fall in pH. The role of the kidney is to regenerate HCO_3^- (buffer base) by excreting H^+, thus back-titrating or recharging the buffer system. Addition of 1 mol of HCO_3 (as $NaHCO_3$) is equivalent to the excretion of 1 mmol of H^+; loss of 1 mmol of HCO_3^- (as in diarrhoea or bicarbonaturia) causes metabolic acidosis quantitatively equivalent to the addition of 1 mol of H^+ (for example, as HCl) to the ECF.

Reabsorption of filtered bicarbonate

The bicarbonate concentration in glomerular filtrate is the same as that in plasma. At normal GFR (180 litres/day) and normal plasma bicarbonate (26 mmol/litre) this represents a potential daily loss of more than 4500 mmol of bicarbonate, equivalent to adding 4500 mmol of acid to the ECF. All, or very nearly all, of this filtered bicarbonate must be reabsorbed to prevent severe acidosis. This takes place almost entirely in the proximal tubule,[60] according to the scheme shown in Figure 5.10. Note (a) that bicarbonate reabsorption is dependent on H^+ secretion, (b) that it is accompanied by reabsorption of an equivalent amount of sodium, and (c) that the HCO_3^- ion restored to the ECF is synthesized in the proximal tubular cell, and is not the same one that is titrated by secreted H^+ in the tubular lumen. The process is dependent on intracellular CA to provide a source of H^+ and HCO_3^- ions by hydration of CO_2, and intraluminal CA (derived from the brush border of the apical cell membrane) to remove the H_2CO_3 formed there by dehydration to CO_2; the high diffusibility of CO_2 leads to its rapid movement down its concentration into the cell, completing the cycle and preventing the intraluminal reaction from coming to equilibrium and stopping.

Titration curves similar to those for glucose and phosphate (Figure 5.5) can be plotted for bicarbonate and a Tm and threshold value identified. An abnormally low threshold defines proximal renal tubular acidosis (RTA), in which urinary acidification capacity is normal but only when the plasma bicarbonate has fallen below the (low) threshold value; that is, at the cost of sustained metabolic acidosis (Figure 5.11). Proximal RTA is most commonly seen as part of a generalized disorder of proximal tubular function (the Fanconi syndrome), but has been described as an isolated tubular defect in at least two forms.[61,62]

Distal tubular H^+ secretion

Proximal reabsorption of filtered HCO_3^- does not contribute to the excretion of ingested or endogenously formed NVA and is therefore irrelevant to external H^+ balance: it merely prevents acidosis due to renal HCO_3^- wasting. To achieve acid balance, H^+ must be secreted into the urine in a quantity exactly

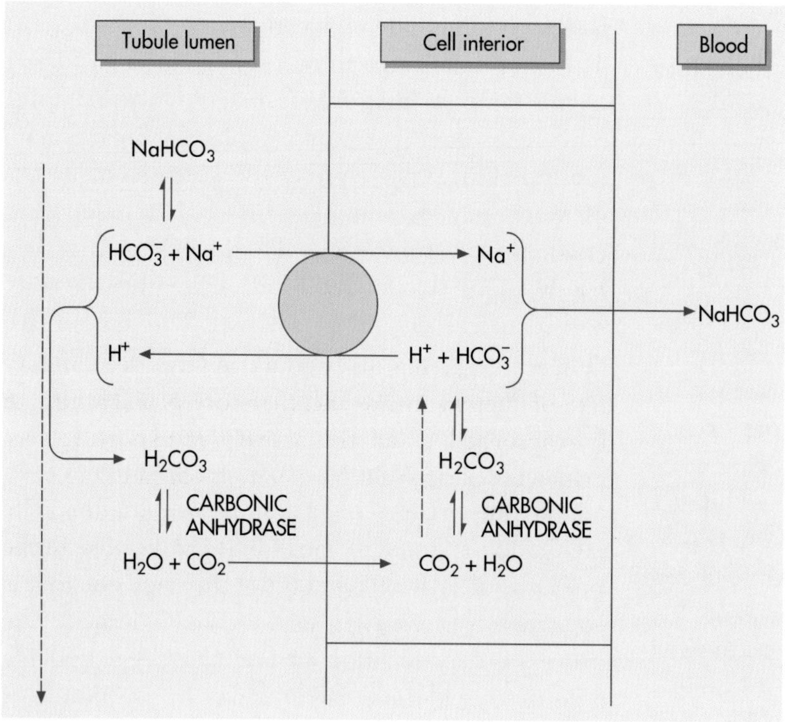

Figure 5.10 *Proximal tubular bicarbonate reabsorption. The process is dependent on intraluminal carbonic anhydrase, present in the proximal but not the distal tubule.*

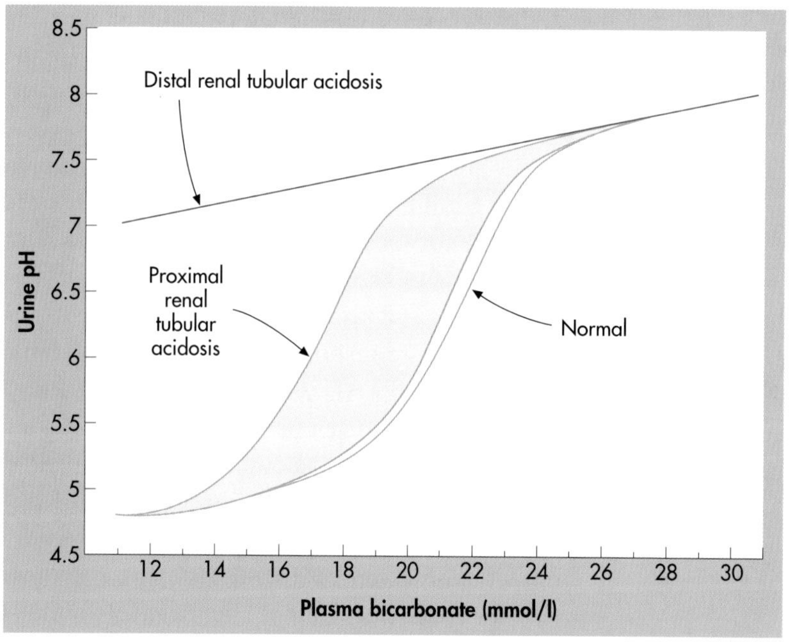

Figure 5.11 *Urine pH plotted against plasma bicarbonate concentration in normal subjects and patients with proximal and distal renal tubular acidosis (RTA). In distal RTA, urine pH does not fall significantly below that of plasma, even in severe metabolic acidosis. In proximal RTA, normal urine acidification is achieved but only at abnormally low plasma bicarbonate concentrations. The curve of the relationship in proximal RTA shows the same sigmoid form as in normals but is shifted to the left to varying degrees depending on the severity of the condition, passing through the shaded area. (Reproduced from* Pediatric Research *with permission.[61])*

equivalent to dietary and metabolic input or NVA, typically 50–100 mmol/day for an adult. This requires that the pH of the urine be lowered below that of ECF; that is, the tubule must pump hydrogen ions 'uphill' from high pH (low $[H^+]$) to low pH (high $[H^+]$). This takes place in the distal nephron, particularly the collecting duct. The reaction whereby H^+ is secreted into the lumen in exchange for Na^+, and HCO_3^- returned to the ECF, is the same as that operating in the proximal tubule: intracellular synthesis and ionization of H_2CO_3 from CO_2 and water. The tubular H^+ pump can sustain a maximum pH gradient of about 10^3 (ECF pH 7.4, urine pH 4.4). One litre of water at pH 4.4 contains only about 0.4 mmol H^+: at a daily urine flow rate of 2–3 litres, this is clearly inadequate to achieve H^+ balance. The ability to do so depends on the presence of urinary buffers.

Urinary buffers
The principal buffer in normal urine is inorganic phosphate. The buffering reaction is as follows:

Equation 11

$$H^+ + Na_2HPO_4 \leftrightarrow Na^+ + NaH_2PO_4$$

The pK of this reaction is 6.8, leading to the following version of the Henderson-Hasselbalch equation:

Equation 12

$$pH = 6.8 + \log \frac{[NaHPO_4^-]}{[Na_2HPO_4]}$$

The pK of 6.8 is well suited to the normal ECF pH of 7.4, since maximal buffering will take place within one pH unit of 7.4, that is, well within the capacity of the H^+ pump.

The other important means of accommodating a large amount of secreted H^+ within the available range of urinary pH is by the formation of ammonium (NH_4^+). This is formed in the urine from secreted pH and ammonia (NH_3), the latter being synthesized from glutamine by the tubular cells. Thus:

Equation 13

$$NH_3 + H^+ + NaCl \rightarrow NH_4Cl + Na^+$$

The Na^+ ion is reabsorbed in exchange for the secreted H^+ and restored to the ECF as $NaHCO_3$. The reactions between secreted H^+ and urinary phosphate and ammonia are illustrated in Figure 5.12. Unlike urinary phosphate excretion, ammonia synthesis can be stepped up in response to increased need to secrete H^+; this is a very important adaptive response to chronic acidosis. The classical (distal) type of RTA is due to inability to lower urinary pH significantly below that of plasma; an acquired form of distal RTA may be seen in obstructive uropathy.[63]

Relationship between H^+ secretion and Na^+ reabsorption
As discussed above, H^+ secretion requires the reabsorption of an equivalent amount of sodium. Conversely, failure of H^+ secretion is associated with impairment of Na^+ reabsorption: patients with proximal and distal RTA have proximal and distal Na^+ wasting, respectively. Control of H^+ secretion is fundamentally dependent on changes in Na^+ reabsorption at different nephron sites.[64]

DIVALENT CATIONS, PHOSPHATE AND VITAMIN D

Renal handling of calcium

Calcium is filtered in amounts greatly exceeding its rate of dietary intake and therefore of excretion; it is reabsorbed in all the actively transporting segments of the tubule by a variety of mechanisms. Reabsorption occurring in the distal tubule is responsive to changes in calcium intake and to other factors known to influence calcium excretion; that in more proximal segments is not.

Glomerular filtration
Calcium is present in plasma in three forms: protein bound, complexed to anions (principally phosphate) and ionized. The last two together form ultrafilterable calcium (Ca_{UF}). The concentration of calcium in glomerular filtrate is the same as that of plasma Ca_{UF}, approximately 1.58 mmol/litre (6.3 mg/dl).

Proximal tubule
Calcium is reabsorbed approximately isotonically in the proximal tubule: a slight rise in tubular fluid concentration occurs in the initial (S1) segment, with little or no change in the remainder of the proximal tubule. Reabsorption is partly passive and dependent on sodium transport, but an active transport system also exists in the basolateral membrane probably involving sodium-calcium countertransport; that is, calcium is extruded from the cell as sodium enters. The interdependence of proximal sodium and calcium reabsorption is very close: factors such as changes in ECF volume that affect sodium absorption produce proportionate and parallel changes in calcium absorption. As with sodium, about 60% of filtered calcium is reabsorbed in the proximal tubule.[65]

Loop of Henle
Calcium reabsorption continues in parallel with that of sodium in the TAL; factors affecting the delivery

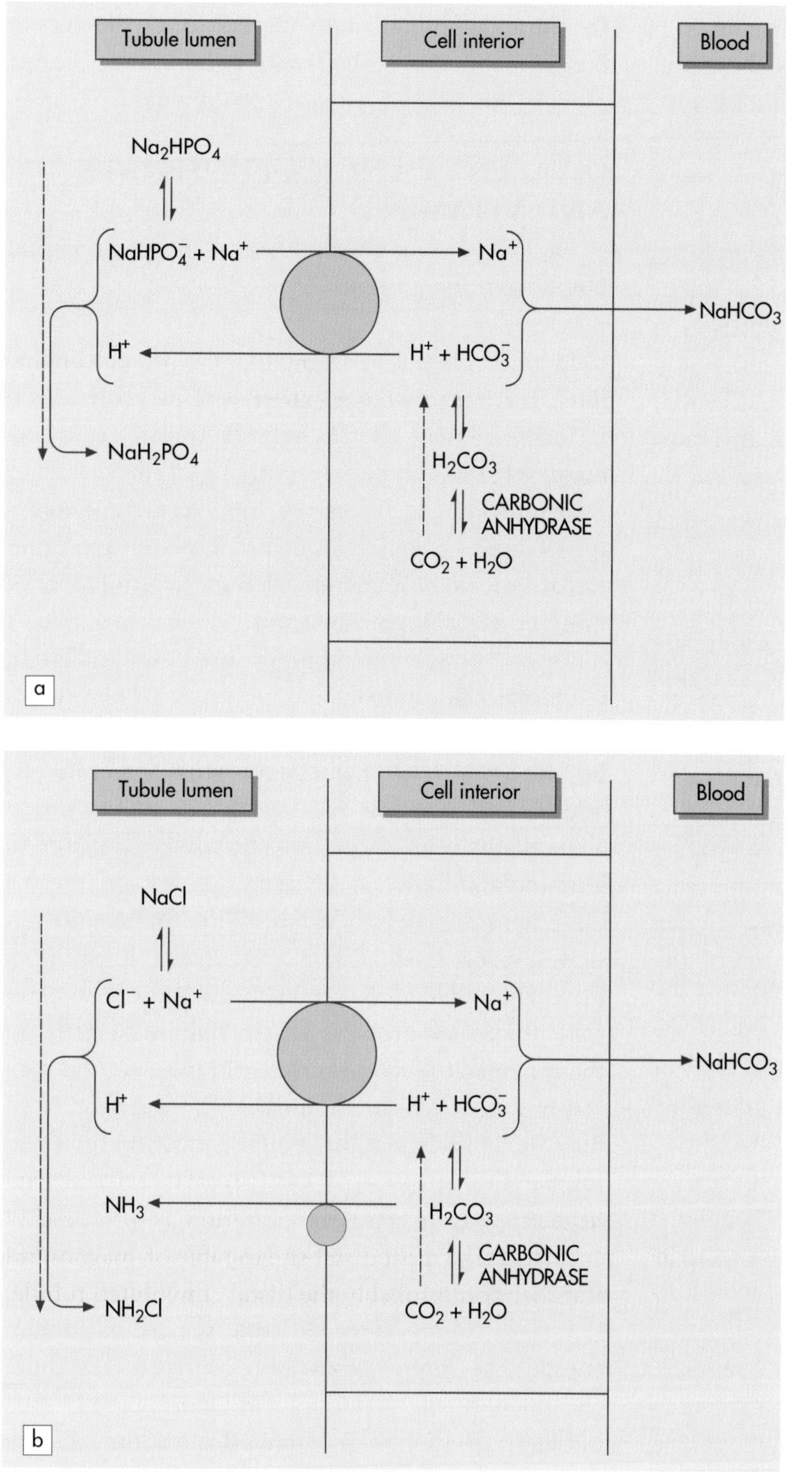

Figure 5.12 *Distal tubular hydrogen ion secretion (urinary acidification). (a) Titration of urinary phosphate buffer. (b) Buffering by secreted ammonia. See text for further details.*

of sodium out of the loop produce proportionate changes in calcium delivery. The reabsorption of both is markedly inhibited by furosemide (frusemide).[66] As previously explained, the NKCC2 transporter is electroneutral, but back-leak of potassium into the tubular fluid takes place through specific potassium channels in the apical membrane. This recycling of potassium creates a lumen-positive voltage across the epithelium which drives other positively charged ions, including calcium, into the peritubular space via the paracellular shunt pathway, accounting for calcium reabsorption in this part of the tubule.

Distal tubule

Calcium ions are actively reabsorbed in the distal convoluted tubule and collecting duct. Transport in this segment varies independently of sodium reabsorption: it is probable that homeostatic changes in calcium excretion are effected here. Factors increasing calcium reabsorption include parathyroid hormone, hypocalcaemia (probably by PTH-independent mechanisms as well as by promoting PTH release), metabolic alkalosis and hyperphosphataemia. Hypoparathyroidism, hypercalcaemia, chronic metabolic acidosis and phosphate depletion are inhibitory (that is, they increase calcium excretion). Vitamin D has been reported to have both enhancing and inhibiting effects on calcium excretion: a physiologically important role for vitamin D in renal calcium excretion has not been demonstrated in man. The apparent discrepancies among these reports may be due to species differences. Calcium enters distal tubular cells across the apical membrane through nifedipine-sensitive calcium channels. The driving force appears to be the electrical polarization of the membrane, which is strongly influenced by intracellular chloride concentration. Measures that decrease intracellular chloride (such as thiazide diuretics) cause hyperpolarization of the membrane and enhance calcium uptake, thus decreasing its excretion. This explains why thiazides decrease calcium excretion while increasing sodium excretion.[67]

Renal handling of magnesium

Magnesium is processed by the kidney in a manner similar, but not identical, to calcium. The major difference is that the proximal tubule is proportionately less important and Henle's loop more important in the case of magnesium. Moreover, unlike calcium, overall renal magnesium handling is of the Tm-threshold type (Figure 5.5).

Glomerular filtration

Like calcium, magnesium is present in plasma in protein-bound, complexed and ionized forms. Mg_{UF} is about 80% of total plasma magnesium, a rather higher fraction than for calcium.

Proximal tubule

Magnesium is absorbed less avidly in the proximal tubule than sodium and calcium, so that its concentration rises along the length of the segment to a value about 1.6 times that in glomerular filtrate. This probably reflects a lower epithelial permeability to magnesium than to calcium, the forces driving reabsorption of the two being similar. Proximal magnesium reabsorption changes in parallel with that of sodium in response to changes in factors influencing the latter, but to a lesser extent.

Loop of Henle

Eighty per cent of the magnesium delivered into the loop is reabsorbed there; this segment therefore accounts for quantitatively the most important fraction of magnesium reabsorption. To what extent active and passive (voltage-dependent) transport are responsible is not known. Furosemide (frusemide) strongly inhibits magnesium reabsorption, suggesting that the same mechanism that accounts for calcium reabsorption in the loop is involved.

Distal tubule

Only a small proportion (<5%) of filtered magnesium is reabsorbed in the distal tubule and collecting duct. The mechanism responsible has not been identified. Although it is tempting to dismiss distal tubular reabsorption as unimportant because the amount involved is small, this is misleading because 5% of the filtered load represents a large quantity of magnesium in relation to dietary intake, and the final regulation of magnesium excretion is presumably effected at the most distal site capable of magnesium reabsorption, probably the distal convoluted tubule.

Renal handling of phosphate

Inorganic phosphate (P) is filtered and reabsorbed by a Tm-limited transport system (Figure 5.5). Although FEP can be calculated by Equation 3, marked variability in TmP secondary to changes in GFR makes FEP an imprecise way of describing tubular P reabsorption. The quotient TmP/GFR defines the theoretical P threshold, that is, the intercept on the *x*-axis of Figure 5.5 obtained by extending the P excretion curve and ignoring the splay. It is this quantity that is altered by changes in circulating PTH and other modulators of tubular P transport. TmP/GFR can be calculated from the equation:[68]

Equation 14

$$\frac{TmP}{GFR} = P_P - \left(\frac{U_P \times P_{creatinine}}{U_{creatinine}}\right)$$

Segmental tubular phosphate reabsorption

The bulk of filtered P is reabsorbed in the proximal tubule, where it is responsive to influences such as changes in ECF volume which alter sodium reabsorption. Entry into the cell is via sodium-phosphate cotransporters in the apical membrane. Two families of such transporters have now been characterized in renal cortex from several species, including man. Designated as type I and type II transporters, respectively, both are present in proximal tubular apical membranes. All relevant evidence indicates that the type IIa transporter (NPT2a) is the physiologically important regulator of P reabsorption. It is a protein of 635 amino acids, probably has eight transmembrane-spanning domains and has sites for protein phosphorylation which probably regulate transporter activity via protein kinase C. It transports with a stoichiometry of 3Na:1P. The gene is located on chromosome 5 (that for the type I transporter is on chromosome 6).

PTH and phosphate reabsorption

PTH inhibits P reabsorption in both proximal and distal segments. Changes in proximal P reabsorption are paralleled by changes in sodium reabsorption, as would be expected from the nature of the transport process, whereas, in the distal tubule, PTH has no effect on sodium transport. PTH binds to proximal tubular cell receptors that activate the adenylate cyclase and protein kinase C pathways. Acute changes in transporter activity are mediated by activation of protein kinase C, which reduces activity of the sodium-phosphate cotransporter (NPT2a). Chronic changes probably involve alterations in gene transcription and translation. PTH release is controlled directly and indirectly by phosphate intake. Increasing P intake leads to transient hyperphosphataemia, which causes in turn hypocalcaemia. Hypocalcaemia stimulates PTH release both directly and by altering vitamin D metabolism (see below). The increased level of PTH inhibits P reabsorption, leading to phosphaturia that compensates for the increase in dietary P.

Phosphatonin, PHEX and phosphate reabsorption

The activity of NPT2a is inhibited not only by PTH, but also by a recently described protein of the fibroblast growth factor family, FGF23. This substance is secreted by some tumours that cause *tumour-induced osteomalacia*, a paraneoplastic syndrome leading to renal phosphate wasting, hypophosphataemia and rickets/osteomalacia. FGF23 is cleaved in turn by a neutral endopeptidase, PHEX, which thus exerts an indirect permissive effect on NPT2a function by inactivating its inhibitor. Mutations in PHEX are responsible for a fairly common form of inherited rickets, familial X-linked hypophosphataemia or vitamin D-resistant rickets. Mutations in FGF23 itself, rendering the molecule resistant to cleavage by PHEX, cause a much rarer, autosomal dominant, form of hypophosphataemic rickets. PHEX and FGF have only recently been described, and their role in normal phosphate homeostasis is not yet known.[69]

Renal metabolism of vitamin D

The active end product of vitamin D metabolism is the hormone 1,25-dihydroxycholecalciferol (1,25-DHCC, 1,25-dihydroxyvitamin D_3). It is produced from vitamin D by 25-hydroxylation, which takes place in the liver, and subsequent 1α-hydroxylation, which takes place in the mitochondria of the proximal tubular cells. In conditions of 1,25-DHCC repletion, 1α-hydroxylation is suppressed and the inactive metabolite 24,25-DHCC is produced instead.[70] The kidney is thus an endocrine organ producing a hormone under negative feedback control: according to need, conversion of 25-HCC oscillates between 1α- and 24-hydroxylation. Apart from the circulating concentration of 1,25-DHCC, other factors promoting 1α-hydroxylation include, in descending order of power, hypocalcaemia, hypophosphataemia and PTH. As well as regulating the production of 1,25-DHCC, the kidney is one of its target organs, along with intestine and bone. Localization of the hormone to the nuclei of distal tubular cells occurs[71] and presumably mediates its renal action, which is to enhance tubular calcium reabsorption, reinforcing the elevation of ECF Ca and P concentrations mediated by its other major actions: stimulation of intestinal Ca and P transport and mobilization of bone mineral. Failure of renal 1α-hydroxylation of vitamin D is one of the two main processes involved in the causation of the bone disease of chronic renal failure, the other being secondary hyperparathyroidism.

CONCENTRATION AND DILUTION OF URINE

Tonicity of body fluids

The tonicity, or effective osmolality, of body fluids is controlled within narrow limits (291 ± 4 mosmol/kg H_2O) by regulation of water intake and excretion. Changes in ECF tonicity are sensed by osmoreceptors located in the anterior hypothalamus. ECF hypertonicity produces thirst, leading to increased water intake (providing the subject has access to water), and release of antidiuretic hormone (ADH), leading to a reduction in water excretion: hypotonicity has the opposite effects. Mammals in the wild state drink in response to thirst: they therefore oscillate between isotonicity, the point at which thirst disappears, and marginal hypertonicity, which stimulates further water intake. They rarely, if ever, need to excrete dilute urine but may need to excrete highly concentrated urine if water is not available in response to the thirst stimulus. Civilized man, in contrast, frequently drinks in excess of biological need for social and cultural reasons and due to the availability of flavoured (and otherwise adulterated) drinks. The ability to excrete urine more dilute than ECF is therefore essential to the avoidance of dilutional hypotonicity.

The diluting segment

As previously discussed, proximal tubular fluid reabsorption is isotonic. The dissociation between water and solute reabsorption necessary for the production of urine with osmolality different from that of ECF takes place in more distal parts of the nephron. Micropuncture studies showed that the fluid in the early distal convoluted tubule was hypotonic to plasma (about 100 mosmol/kg H_2O) irrespective of whether the final urine was concentrated or dilute at the time.[72] Solute is therefore actively reabsorbed without water in this segment. This is now known to be via the Na^+-K^+-$2Cl^-$ transporter NKCC2 (see above). The TAL and early distal convoluted tubule therefore comprise the obligate diluting segment. When maximally dilute urine is being produced, the late distal tubule and collecting ducts also become water impermeable in the absence of ADH, and continuing solute (NaCl) reabsorption in the late distal convoluted tubule and the collecting duct leads to the elaboration of urine of osmolality about 40 mosmol/kg H_2O. The production of concentrated urine depends on the establishment of interstitial hypertonicity in the medulla, a process that ingeniously utilizes the same transporting process that is responsible for dilution, that is, active electrolyte reabsorption in the TAL.

Countercurrent multiplication and exchange

The processes of countercurrent multiplication and exchange convert the hyperosmolality of the interstitium surrounding the TAL, and resulting from NaCl reabsorption, into an axial concentration gradient maximal at the papillary tip. The elements of the countercurrent system are the loops of Henle (multipliers) and the vasa recta (exchangers), the collecting duct being the site of final osmotic water reabsorption. The mechanism was described in principle many years ago, but a more detailed understanding of the process required methods of investigation not available until much later. A general description of the medullary countercurrent system is beyond the scope of this chapter: the reader is referred to an authoritative symposium published in 1983.[73] A recurring difficulty has been to account for concentration of solute in the inner medullary and papillary interstitium (where the tonicity is highest) in the apparent absence of active solute reabsorption in the thin (inner medullary) segment of the ascending limb (Figure 5.2). This probably depends on passive recycling of urea through facilitated diffusion in the medulla. Various models have been constructed to account for the observed hypertonicity in the inner medulla without the need to postulate active solute reabsorption in the thin ascending limb, but none has been unequivocally validated to date.

The antidiuretic hormone

The human antidiuretic hormone is the cyclic nonapeptide arginine vasopressin (AVP):

Cys – Tyr – Phe – Glu – Asp – Cys – Pro – Arg – Gly – NH_2

A ring structure is formed by a disulphide bridge between the two cystine residues. It is synthesized in cells whose bodies lie in the supraoptic and paraventricular nuclei of the anterior hypothalamus, and released from their axonal endings in the posterior pituitary. It is released in response both to osmoreceptor stimulation and carotid sinus and aortic arch baroreceptor stimulation.[74] The former is responsible for maintaining tonicity of body fluids in the normal range, while the latter causes renal water retention in the face of underfilling of the high-pressure compartment of the circulation due to, for example, volume depletion, vasodilatation or left ventricular failure. Baroreceptor-mediated AVP release is not suppressible by hypotonicity, and so hyponatraemia is commonly seen in conditions associated with it. A much larger proportional volume change is needed than osmolar change to initiate an AVP response (Figure 5.13). An increase of only 1–2% in plasma osmolality suffices to elicit a maximally antidiuretic plasma level (5 pg/ml), while a reduction in blood volume or pressure of about 8% is needed before a significant AVP response is seen.[75] However, very high AVP levels are produced when hypovolaemia or hypotension become more severe than this.

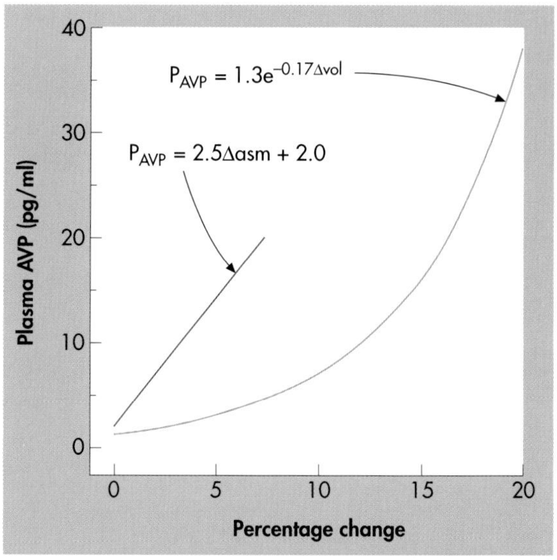

Figure 5.13 *The antidiuretic response to isovolaemic increase in plasma osmolality (linear relationship) and isotonic depletion of plasma volume (exponential relationship). The minus value of the exponent of the equation relating P_{AVP} to volume arises from the fact that the volume change (Δvol) is in a negative direction. (Reproduced from* Journal of Clinical Investigation *with permission.*[75]*)*

Antidiuretic hormone receptors

AVP binds to specific receptors (V_2 receptors) on the collecting duct cells, causing activation of adenylate cyclase and conversion of ATP to cyclic AMP. This initiates a chain of intracellular events that culminate in the insertion of water channels in the apical membrane of the cell, rendering it permeable to water. The gene for the V_2 receptor is on the long arm of the X chromosome: mutations in it are responsible for the disease X-linked diabetes insipidus.[76]

Aquaporins

The water channels referred to in the previous paragraph belong to a family of proteins known as *aquaporins*, of which different members are expressed in different cell types. The human collecting duct aquaporin is aquaporin 2, and the gene that codes for it is located on chromosome 12 in the region 12q13. Mutations in the gene for aquaporin 2 cause a form of diabetes insipidus clinically indistinguishable from that caused by mutations in the V_2 receptor gene except that, as would be expected, it is inherited as an autosomal recessive condition and affects both sexes equally.[77]

Free water clearance and reabsorption

The urinary solute excretion rate is determined by dietary and metabolic factors, but is usually in the region of 500–1500 mosmol/day for an adult on an average diet. Taking a notional value of 580 mosmol/day, and assuming a plasma osmolality of 290 mosmol/kg H_2O, it is evident that 2 litres of isotonic urine would suffice to excrete this amount of solute. Any additional water excretion will render the urine hypotonic to plasma: such additional water excretion is called free water clearance, CH_2O. Osmolar clearance can be calculated by the following equation:

Equation 15

$$C_{OSM} = \frac{U_{OSM} \times V}{P_{OSM}}$$

When urine is isotonic, $U_{OSM} = P_{OSM}$ (by definition), and therefore $C_{OSM} = V$. When urine is hypotonic to plasma, $C_{OSM} < V$, and:

Equation 16

$$C_{H_2O} = V - C_{OSM}$$

When urine is hypertonic, $C_{OSM} > V$, and therefore the calculated value for CH_2O is negative. Reversing the sign, negative free water clearance becomes free water reabsorption, usually designated TcH_2O:

Equation 17

$$TcH_2O = C_{OSM} - V$$

CH_2O and TcH_2O define the limiting values for renal water excretion, and therefore for tolerated water ingestion. At a solute excretion rate of 580 mosmol/day, C_{OSM} is 2 litres a day. Rearranging equation 16:

Equation 18

$$V = \frac{C_{OSM} \times P_{OSM}}{U_{OSM}}$$

and taking values of 40 and 1200 mosmol/kg H_2O as minimal and maximal U_{OSM}, respectively, yields limiting values for V of 14.5 and 0.48 litres daily. Corresponding maximum values for CH_2O and TcH_2O are 12.5 and 1.52 litres/day. Thus, at any given solute excretion rate, the defence against overhydration and dilution (CH_2O) is much more effective than that against dehydration and concentration (TcH_2O), a conclusion borne out by clinical experience. This huge capacity to protect the body fluids from dilution may be an evolutionary inheritance from our fishy and amphibian ancestors, to whom (in fresh water) osmotic dilution is a constant threat.

REFERENCES

1. Coulthard MG, Hey EN. Weight as the best standard for glomerular filtration in the newborn. Arch Dis Child 1984; 59: 373–375
2. McCance RA. The maintenance of stability in the newly born. I. Chemical exchange. Arch Dis Child 1959; 34: 361–370
3. Dugdale AE. Evolution and infant feeding. Lancet 1986; 1: 1441–1442
4. Kildeberg P. Disturbances of hydrogen ion balance occurring in premature infants. II. Late metabolic acidosis. Acta Paediatr 1964; 53: 517–526
5. Arant BS, Jr, Edelmann CM, Jr, Spitzer A. The congruence of creatinine and inulin clearances in children: use of the Technicon AutoAnalyzer. J Pediatr 1972; 81: 559–561
6. Calcagno PL, Rubin MI. Renal extraction of para-aminohippurate in infants and children. J Clin Invest 1963; 42: 1632–1639
7. Tisher CC, Bulger RE, Trump BF. Human renal ultrastructure. I. Proximal tubule of healthy individuals. Lab Invest 1966; 15: 1357–1394
8. Bulger RE, Tisher CC, Myers CH, Trump BF. Human renal ultrastructure. II. The thin limb of Henle's loop and the interstitium in healthy individuals. Lab Invest 1967; 16: 124–141
9. Tisher CC, Bulger RE, Trump BF. Human renal ultrastructure. III. The distal tubule in healthy individuals. Lab Invest 1968; 18: 655–668
10. Arakawa M. A scanning electron microscopic study of the human glomerulus. Am J Pathol 1970; 64: 457–466
11. Kanwar YS, Farquar MG. Anionic sites in the glomerular basement membrane. In vivo and in vitro localization in the laminae rarae by cationic probes. J Cell Biol 1979; 81: 137–153
12. Venkatachalam MA, Karnovsky MJ, Fahimi HD, Cotran RS. An ultrastructural study of glomerular permeability using catalase and peroxidase as tracer proteins. J Exp Med 1970; 132: 1153–1167
13. Brenner BM, Hostetter TH, Humes HD. Glomerular permselectivity: barrier function based on discrimination of molecular size and charge. Am J Physiol 1978; 234: F455-F460
14. Ruotsalainen V, Ljungberg P, Wartiovaara J, Lenkkeri U et al. Nephrin is specifically located at the slit diaphragm of glomerular podocytes. Proc Natl Acad Sci USA 1999; 96: 7962–7967
15. Tryggvason K, Ruotsalainen V, Wartiovaara J. Discovery of the congenital nephrotic syndrome gene

discloses the structure of the mysterious molecular sieve of the kidney. Int J Dev Biol 1999; 43: 445–451
16. Maddox DA, Deen WM, Brenner BM. Dynamics of glomerular filtration. VI. Studies in the primate. Kidney Int 1974; 5: 271–278
17. Brenner BM, Troy JL, Daugherty TM, Deen WM et al. Dynamics of glomerular ultrafiltration in the rat. II. Plasma flow dependence of GFR. Am J Physiol 1972; 223: 1184–1190
18. Deen WM, Troy JL, Robertson CR, Brenner BM. Dynamics of glomerular filtration in the rat. IV. Determination of the ultrafiltration coefficient. J Clin Invest 1973; 52: 1500–1508
19. Navar LG, Bell PD, White RW, Watts RL et al. Evaluation of the single nephron glomerular filtration coefficient in the dog. Kidney Int 1977; 12: 137–149
20. Ausiello DA, Kreisberg JJ, Roy C, Karnovsky MJ. Contraction of cultured rat glomerular mesangial cells after stimulation with angiotensin II and arginine vasopressin. J Clin Invest 1980; 65: 754–760
21. Burg MB, Orloff J. Electrical potential difference across proximal convoluted tubules. Am J Physiol 1970; 219: 1714–1716
22. Brant SR, Yun CH, Donowitz M, Tse CM. Cloning, tissue distribution, and functional analysis of the human Na^+/H^+ exchanger isoform, NHE3. Am J Physiol 1995; 269: C198–C206
23. Burg MB, Green N. Bicarbonate transport by isolated perfused rabbit proximal convoluted tubules. Am J Physiol 1977; 233: F307–F314
24. Kokko J. Proximal tubule potential difference. Dependence on glucose, HCO_3 and amino acids. J Clin Invest 1973; 52: 1362–1367
25. Martino JA, Earley LE. Relationship between intrarenal hydrostatic pressure and hemodynamically induced changes in sodium excretion. Circ Res 1968; 23: 371–386
26. Spitzer A, Windhager E. Effect of peritubular oncotic pressure changes on proximal tubular fluid reabsorption. Am J Physiol 1970; 218: 1188–1193
27. Berry CA, Cogan MG. Influence of peritubular protein on solute reabsorption in the rabbit proximal tubule. J Clin Invest 1981; 68: 506–516
28. Mackenzie B, Loo DD, Panayotova-Heiermann M, Wright EM. Biophysical characteristics of the pig kidney Na^+/glucose cotransporter SGLT2 reveal a common mechanism for SGLT1 and SGLT2. J Biol Chem 1996; 271: 32678–32683
29. Wright EM, Martin MG, Turk E. Familial glucose-galactose malabsorption and hereditary renal glycosuria. In: Scriver CR, Beaudet AL, Sly WS, Valle D, eds. The Metabolic and Molecular Bases of Inherited Disease. 8th edn. New York: McGraw-Hill, 2001: 4891–4908
30. Silbernagl S. The renal handling of amino acids and oligopeptides. Physiol Rev 1988; 68: 911–1007
31. Palacín M, Estevez R, Bertran J, Zorzano A. Molecular biology of mammalian plasma membrane amino acid transporters. Physiol Rev 1998; 78: 969–1054
32. Palacín M, Goodyer P, Nunes V, Gasparini P. Cystinuria. In: Scriver CR, Beaudet AL, Sly WS, Valle D, eds. The Metabolic and Molecular Bases of Inherited Disease. 8th edn. New York: McGraw-Hill, 2001: 4909–4932
33. Waldmann TA, Strober W, Mogielnicki BP. The renal handling of low molecular weight proteins. II. Disorders of serum protein catabolism in patients with tubular proteinuria, the nephrotic syndrome, or uremia. J Clin Invest 1972; 51: 2162–2174
34. Park CH, Maack T. Albumin absorption and catabolism by isolated perfused proximal convoluted tubules of the rabbit. J Clin Invest 1984; 73: 767–777
35. de Wardener HF. The control of sodium excretion. In: Handbook of Physiology. Washington, DC: American Physiological Society, 1973: 677–720
36. Ichikawa I, Hoyer JR, Seiler MW, Brenner BM. Mechanism of glomerulotubular balance in the setting of heterogeneous glomerular injury. Preservation of a close functional linkage between individual nephrons and surrounding microvasculature. J Clin Invest 1982; 69: 185–198
37. Wright FS, Briggs P. Feedback regulation of glomerular filtration rate. Am J Physiol 1977; 233: F1–7
38. Schnaper HW. The immune system in minimal change nephrotic syndrome. Pediatr Nephrol 1989; 3: 101–110
39. Brezis M, Rosen S, Silva P, Epstein FH. Selective vulnerability of the medullary thick ascending limb to anoxia in the isolated perfused rat kidney. J Clin Invest 1984; 73: 182–190
40. Strauss MB, Lamdin E, Smith WP, Bleifer DJ. Surfeit and deficit of sodium: a kinetic concept of sodium excretion. Arch Intern Med 1958; 102: 527–536
41. Epstein M. Cardiovascular and renal effects of head-out water immersion in man. Circ Res 1976; 39: 619–628
42. Epstein FH, Post RS, McDowell M. Effects of an arteriovenous fistula on renal hemodynamics and electrolyte excretion. J Clin Invest 1953; 32: 233–241

43. Martino JA, Earley LE. Demonstration of the role of physical factors as determinants of natriuretic response to volume expansion. J Clin Invest 1967; 46: 1963–1978
44. Lindheimer MD, Lalone RC, Levinsky NG. Evidence that an acute increase in glomerular filtration rate has little effect on sodium excretion in the dog unless extracellular volume is expanded. J Clin Invest 1967; 46: 256–265
45. Howards SS, Davis BB, Knox FB, Wright FS et al. Depression of fractional sodium reabsorption by the proximal tubule of the dog without sodium diuresis. J Clin Invest 1968; 47: 1561–1572
46. Arendshorst WJ, Navar LG. Renal circulation and glomerular hemodynamics. In: Schrier RW, Gottschalk CW, eds. Diseases of the Kidney. Boston, MA: Little, Brown, 1993: 75
47. Moss NG. Renal function and renal afferent and efferent nerve activity. Am J Physiol 1982; 243: F425–433
48. Young DB, Guyton AC. Steady state aldosterone dose–response relationships. Circ Res 1977; 40: 138–142
49. de Wardener HE, Mills IH, Clapham WF, Hayter CJ. Studies on the efferent mechanism of the sodium diuresis which follows the administration of intravenous saline in the dog. Clin Sci 1961; 21: 249–258
50. Flynn TG, Davies PL. The biochemistry and molecular biology of atrial natriuretic factor. Biochem J 1985; 232: 313–321
51. Brenner BM, Ballermann BJ, Gunning ME, Zeidel ML. Diverse biological actions of atrial natriuretic peptide. Physiol Rev 1990; 70: 665–699
52. Simon DB, Karet FE, Hamdan JM, Di Pietro A et al. Bartter's syndrome, hypokalemic alkalosis with hypercalciuria, is caused by mutations in the Na-K-2Cl transporter NKCC2. Nat Genet 1996; 13: 183–188
53. Simon DB, Karet FE, Rodriguez-Soriano J, Hamdan JH et al. Genetic heterogeneity of Bartter's syndrome revealed by mutations in the K^+ channel, ROMK. Nat Genet 1996; 14: 152–156
54. Simon DB, Bindra RS, Mansfield TA et al. Mutations in the chloride channel gene, CLCNKB, cause Bartter's syndrome type III. Nat Genet 1997; 17: 171–178
55. Simon DB, Nelson-Williams C, Bia MJ, Ellison D et al Gitelman's variant of Bartter's syndrome, inherited hypokalaemic alkalosis, is caused by mutations in the thiazide-sensitive Na-Cl cotransporter. Nat Genet 1996; 12: 24–30
56. Shimkets RA, Warnock DG, Bositis CM, Nelson-Williams C et al. Liddle's syndrome: heritable human hypertension caused by mutations in the beta subunit of the epithelial sodium channel. Cell 1994; 79: 407–414
57. Chang SS, Grunder S, Hanukoglu A, Rosler A et al. Mutations in subunits of the epithelial sodium channel cause salt wasting with hyperkalaemic acidosis, pseudohypoaldosteronism type 1. Nat Genet 1996; 12: 248–253
58. Rossier BC, Palmer LG. Mechanism of aldosterone action on sodium and potassium transport. In: Seldin DW, Giebisch G, eds. The Kidney, Physiology and Pathophysiology. New York: Raven Press, 1992: 1373–1409
59. Feldman D, Funder JW, Edelman IS. Subcellular mechanisms in the action of adrenal steroids. Am J Med 1972; 53: 545–560
60. Gottschalk CW, Lassiter WE, Mylle M. Localisation of urine adidification in the mammalian kidney. Am J Physiol 1960; 198: 581–585
61. Rodriguez Soriano J, Boichis H, Stark H, Edelmann CM, Jr. Proximal renal tubular acidosis. A defect in bicarbonate reabsorption with normal urinary acidification. Pediatr Res 1967; 1: 81–98
62. Brenes LG, Brenes JN, Hernandez MM. Familial proximal renal tubular acidosis: a distinct clinical entity. Am J Med 1977; 63: 244–252
63. Hutcheon RA, Kaplan BS, Drummond KS. Distal renal tubular acidosis in children with chronic hydronephrosis. J Pediatr 1976; 89: 372–376
64. Schwartz WB, Cohen JJ. The nature of the renal response to chronic disorders of acid–base equilibrium. Am J Med 1978; 64: 417–428
65. Lassiter WE, Gottschalk CW, Myolle M. Micropuncture study of renal tubular reabsorption of calcium in normal rodents. Am J Physiol 1963; 205: 771–775
66. Burg MB, Stoner L, Cardinal J, Breen N. Furosemide effect on isolated perfused tubules. Am J Physiol 1973; 225: 119–124
67. Gesek FA, Friedman PA. Mechanism of calcium transport stimulated by chlorothiazide in mouse distal convoluted tubule cells. J Clin Invest 1992; 90: 429–438
68. Brodehl J, Krause A, Hoyer PF. Assessment of maximal tubular phosphate reabsorption: comparison of direct measurement with the nomogram of Bijvoet. Pediatr Nephrol 1988; 2: 183–189
69. Kronenberg HM. NPT2a—the key to phosphate homeostasis. N Engl J Med 2002; 347: 1022–1024

70. DeLuca HF, Schnoes HK. Metabolism and actions of vitamin D. Annu Rev Biochem 1976; 45: 631–666
71. Stumpf WE, Sar M, Reid FA, DeLuca HF. Target cells for 1,25-dihydroxyvitamin D. Science 1979; 206: 1188–1190
72. Gottschalk CW, Mylle M. Micropuncture study of the mammalian urinary concentrating mechanism: evidence for the countercurrent hypothesis. Am J Physiol 1959; 196: 927–936
73. Stephenson JL, Kriz W, Jamison RL, March DJ et al. Symposium on the renal concentrating mechanism. Fed Proc 1983; 42: 2377–2405
74. Schrier RW, Bichet DG. Osmotic and nonosmotic control of vasopressin release and the pathogenesis of impaired water excretion in adrenal, thyroid and edematous disorders. J Lab Clin Med 1981; 98: 1–15
75. Dunn FL, Brennan TJ, Nelson AE, Robertson GL. The role of blood osmolality and volume in regulating vasopressin secretion in the rat. J Clin Invest 1973; 52: 3212–3219
76. Knoers N, van den Ouweland A, Dreesen J, Verdijk M et al. Nephrogenic diabetes insipidus: identification of the genetic defect. Pediatr Nephrol 1993; 7: 685–688
77. van Lieburg AF, Verdijk MA, Knoers VV, van Essen AJ et al. Patients with autosomal nephrogenic diabetes insipidus homozygous for mutations in the aquaporin 2 water-channel gene. Am J Hum Genet 1994; 55: 648–652

6

Principles of radiological imaging of the urinary tract

Uday Patel

INTRODUCTION

This chapter outlines the principles of those radiological modalities used to image the urinary tract, except nuclear medicine, which is covered elsewhere. The various modalities exploit a number of body tissue–energy interactions, and the fundamental basis of these is explained below. Of the newer developments, technological refinements have greatly improved anatomical resolution, but the ability to analyse information rapidly involves also the possibility of physiological/functional studies, multimedia presentation and electronic transmission of images.

PLAIN AND CONTRAST RADIOGRAPHY

Plain radiography

After over a century of clinical use and though increasingly challenged, this remains the workhorse radiological study. The physics behind the generation of an X-ray image are relatively simple. X-radiation (electromagnetic radiation of short wavelength – 10 nm to 0.01 pm) is produced when an electron beam bombards tungsten. Interaction between electrons and tungsten atoms releases energy, principally as heat, but a minor fraction (<1%) of the energy is dissipated as an electromagnetic wave, or X-rays.

The radiograph is produced when X-radiation falls on a silver halide radiographic plate (the X-ray film), converting silver ions into stable, dense and visible silver atoms. As the beam travels through human tissues, it undergoes attenuation proportionate to the atomic number, and the density and thickness of the tissue; thus, the radiograph is an accurate representation of the intervening body tissues. As calcium attenuates greatly, a calcium-containing renal calculus permits transmission of very few photons, and its presence is revealed as an unexposed white area on a darker background. These principles are illustrated in Figure 6.1. Fluoroscopy is essentially the same, except the final image is viewed on a monitor in real time as a dynamic image. Although fluoroscopic images are of a lower radiating dose to the patient, image definition is poorer compared to the plain radiograph.

Digital radiography and PACS

The plain radiograph is being increasingly replaced by digital radiography (DR), where the image is acquired electronically – chemical or electronic detectors replace the conventional radiographic plate. Unlike a conventional film, a digital radiograph can be manipulated at will and viewed either on a screen or as a hard copy. However, digital radiographs have poorer spatial resolution – *the ability to distinguish two adjacent structures as separate entities* – than conventional radiographs, although this is partly compensated for by a superior contrast resolution – *the ability to distinguish adjacent areas of differing opacity* – as a wider grey scale may be employed. In practical terms, this means that certain fine abnormality, such as the punctate calcification of nephrocalcinosis, is still best seen on conventional radiographs.

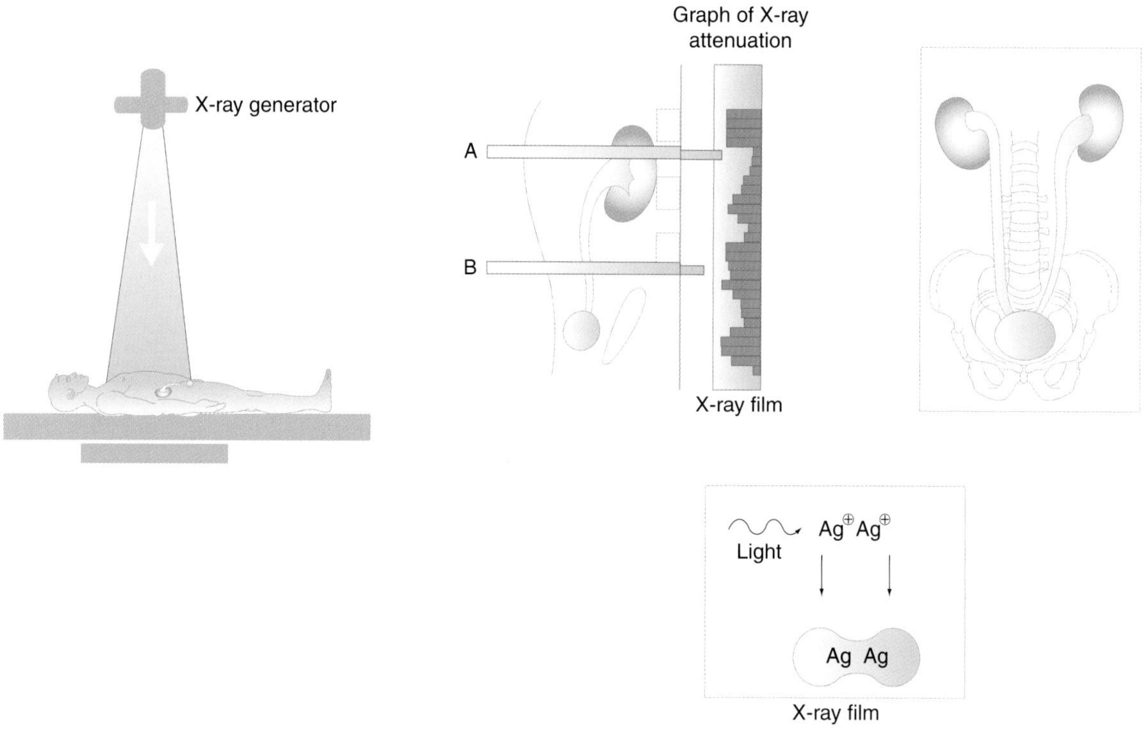

Figure 6.1 *Basics of X-radiograph production. Body tissues attenuate the beam by variable amounts, depending on tissue density, tissue thickness and atomic number. Conversion of silver ions to atoms by X-rays produces the permanent radiographic image.*

The fundamentals of image formation still apply (Figure 6.1); but DR promises a future of filmless departments with rapid dissemination of images through electronic links – the so-called PACS (picture archiving and communication systems). Multimodality images may be recalled from memory banks and displayed on a single monitor with image incorporation for surgical planning. Departments are becoming digital at a rapid pace, as unit costs decline and the necessary cultural change takes place such that radiologists and clinicians feel comfortable using monitors alone to view 'hard copy'. The promise is not necessarily cost-saving, but may mean more efficient patient management – 'lost films' may become a thing of the past, and the complete imaging history is instantly available at any point inside, or even outside, the hospital at any time of day or night. The technology is still incapable of all these demands, but progress is accelerating.

Iodinated contrast media

The inherently low density of soft tissues and the internal structures of organs limit their visibility on plain radiography and fluoroscopy. Only a sufficient density gradient between adjacent tissues will confer radiographic visibility; thus, calcium-containing stones or bones are easily seen, but the fluid-containing renal calyces and pelvis cannot be distinguished from surrounding renal parenchyma. Radiographic contrast media (CM) are oral or intravenous agents able to accentuate the natural tissue-density gradients, and so enhance radiographic visibility. The currently used intravenous contrast agents are, and have been for nearly 70 years, iodine (atomic weight 127)-containing compounds, and no novel chemicals are under active clinical evaluation. Contrast media are designed to be hydrophilic, with low lipid solubility or protein binding; and with mol-

Table 6.1 Adverse reactions to iodinated radiographic contrast media.

- Nausea and vomiting
- Rigors
- Sneezing
- Urticaria
- Bronchospasm
- Vagal reactions
- Contrast media nephrotoxicity
- Anaphylactoid reactions (angio-oedema, laryngeal oedema, bronchospasm, circulatory collapse)

Notes:
- Severe drug reactions – bronchospasm, angio-oedema, circulatory collapse – are more common in those with a previous history of asthma/ allergy, previous reactions to contrast media, renal disease and diabetes mellitus
- The incidence of severe adverse drug reactions after non-ionic, low osmolar contrast media is between 0.03 to 0.23%[1]
- Steroid prophylaxis is commonly used but the evidence that they reduce allergic reactions is still disputed
- Nephrotoxicity is uncommon in patients with no pre-existing renal disease (<1%)[2]

ecular weights of <2000. This ensures brisk dissemination into the extravascular, extracellular space and rapid excretion. All body soft tissues enhance, and the kidneys particularly so, as they are the principal source of excretion (99%) with a half-life of 2 hours. Renal excretion is by free glomerular filtration without tubular reabsorption, and in the urine, CM further undergoes 50–100-fold concentration. This makes it an ideal agent for the intravenous urogram.

Adverse effects of contrast media

The adverse effects of CM are due to idiosyncratic anaphylactoid reactions or non-idiosyncratic causes[1] (Table 6.1). Many of the latter are due to the high osmolarity of CM or direct chemotoxicity. The chemotoxic factors are still unclear, but in the kidney, tubular and vasospastic renal toxicity, mediated by endothelin, has been proposed.[2] The relative risks of CM toxicity are given in Table 6.1. The most modern agents are now iso-osmolar and of lower toxicity, but these are also more expensive.

RADIATION HAZARDS

Soon after Roentgen's discovery of X-rays in December 1885, their harmful effects became increasingly evident. In 1896, the first case of radiodermatitis was reported, followed soon after by cases of radiation-induced malignancy. The harmful effects arise from the ionizing effect of X-rays on human tissue, with genetic and somatic consequences (Figure 6.2). Terminologically, there are two broad groups of ionizing hazards – stochastic and non-stochastic effects. Stochastic effects have no threshold level – '*stochastic*' means '*governed by the laws of probability*' – and the probability of the effect increases linearly with the radiation dose. These have important population consequences, as even small increments in radiation burden increase the risk of radiation-induced disease: cancers are induced and there are risks to the fetus during the period of organogenesis (8–15 weeks). In contrast, non-stochastic effects are not seen unless a threshold dose is crossed, but, once it is reached, the severity of the effect is dose dependent. Examples of the received dose due to various investigations are given (Table 6.2). In comparison, the average annual effective dose received by the UK population is 2.2 mSv per head, of which 11% is due to medical exposure, and the risk of induction of fatal cancer is 1 in 10^5/mSv.

Table 6.2 Effective radiation dose for patients undergoing radiological investigations.

	Effective dose (mSv)	Approx. of natural background radiation
Chest X-ray	0.02	3 days
Lumbar spine X-ray	1.3	7 months
IVU	2.5	14 months
Bone scan	4.0	1.8 years
CT Head	2.3	1 year
Abdomen	10	4.5 years
(Renal stone protocol)	(4.7)	
Renal scan DTPA	1.0	6 months
Mag 3	1.0	6 months
Barium enema	7.0	3.2 years
Average effective dose in UK (87% natural sources, 13% from artificial sources of which 11% is medical sources)	2.2	

* Extracted from Making the Best use of a Dept. of Clinical Radiology (4th Edn). Royal College of Radiologists (1998)

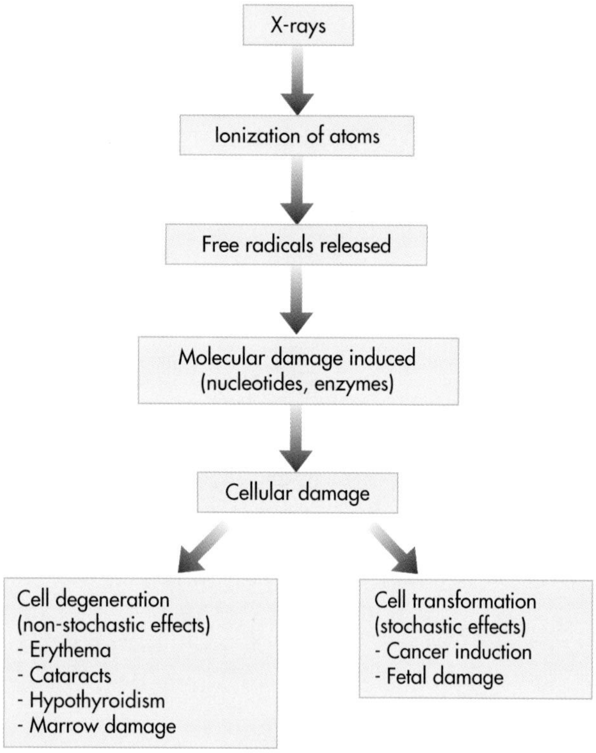

Figure 6.2 *The damaging ionizing action of X-rays has cellular and genetic consequences (see text for further explanation of stochastic and non-stochastic effects).*

Note that radiation due to a standard intravenous urogram is just over the annual effective dose, while a computerized tomography (CT) scan of the kidneys is 2–4 times this amount depending on the type of study. For the benefits of both the individual, whether patient or practitioner, and society as a whole, radiation exposure should be used only if justified and prudently.

CROSS-SECTIONAL IMAGING

Plain and contrast radiography is limited to a two-dimensional format with no perception of depth. But if the source of an energy–tissue interaction can be precisely located in the three perpendicular planes, this digitized information can be used to build a slice-by-slice sectional image, or, increasingly, a 3-D solid model. This is an oversimplification of cross-sectional imaging, and it has made possible the non-invasive imaging of those internal tissues and organs beyond resolution by conventional radiography. CT, ultrasound (US) and magnetic resonance imaging (MRI) are all examples. CT uses X-radiation while US and MRI exploit novel energies and tissue–energy interactions.

Computerized tomography (CT)

CT is now nearly 30 years old and has matured from a slow and cumbersome examination limited to the head to a modality of choice when fast, precise diagnosis is required – for example, it is indispensable in major trauma management. Figure 6.3 illustrates its principles. CT also uses ionizing radiation, and the fundamental physics of X-ray/tissue interaction – the density-related attenuation of an X-ray beam, as explained above under plain radiography – still applies, but CT is very much more sensitive than conventional radiography, recording a 10-fold greater density range.

For CT, the X-ray beam is generated as a precise, pencil-thin beam, which is detected by similarly small detectors, positioned diametrically opposite. The beam rotates through a 360° circle, at each cross-section of the body – a section being 1–10 mm thick (Figure 6.3). Data are acquired with great anatomical precision, and after further heavy post-processing, are divided into pixels: '*pixel*' means '*picture element*'. Each pixel represents a sum density of tissue at that point in the body, and each pixel is assigned a grey-scale value proportionate to this density: the CT or Hounsfield number, after Sir Godfrey Hounsfield, the pioneer of CT.[3] By lining up adjacent picture elements, one can format a 'grey-scale' pixellated CT slice. Figure 6.4 represents the 'CT numbers' of a variety of common body tissues. By convention, water is assigned a neutral density at 0; air is −1000, fat −100, and bone above +200. Kidneys are in the soft tissue range of +40 to +60, rising to around 150 units after intravenous contrast. Renal calculi are near the bone range and readily seen.

Iodinated contrast media are used commonly in CT as well. After contrast injection, the CT numbers of all soft tissues increase as the medium distributes within the extracellular space. This further increases the density gradient between normal and abnormal tissues, broadly improving diagnostic accuracy, but the kidneys show particular enhancement, as the contrast is further concentrated in the collecting ducts.

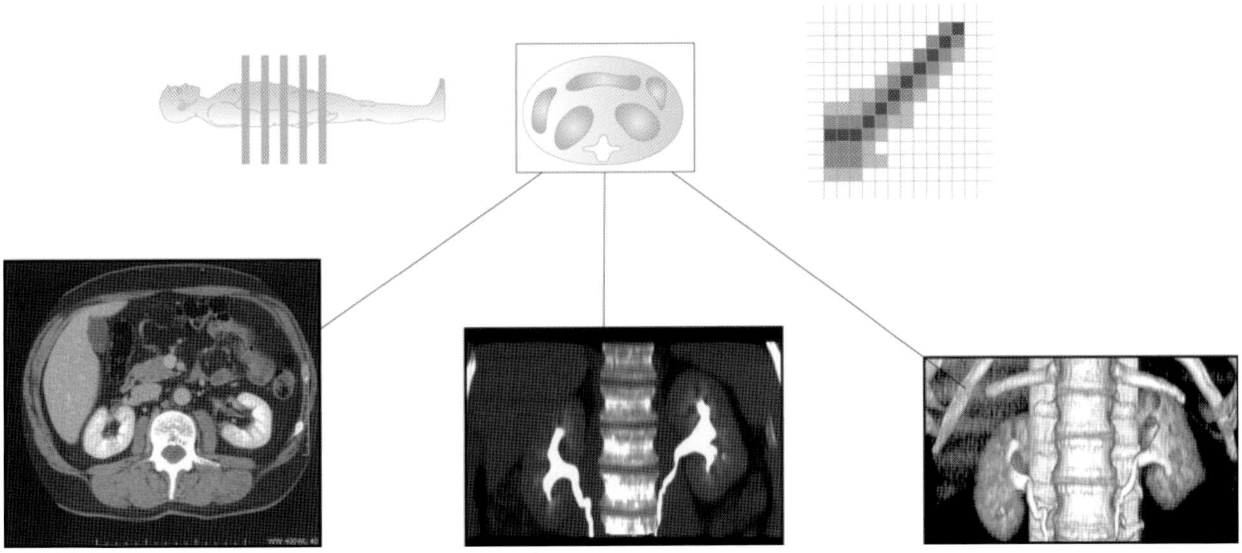

Figure 6.3 *Principles of computerized tomography (CT). The magnified portion of the CT image shows the individual pixels (picture elements) assigned a grey-scale darkness/lightness according to the sum density of the tissues in each pixel of the renal capsule (top right). The images at the bottom represent the variety of formats used in modern CT (conventional axial view on the left, coronol reformats in the middle and volume-reconstructed 3-D image on the right).*

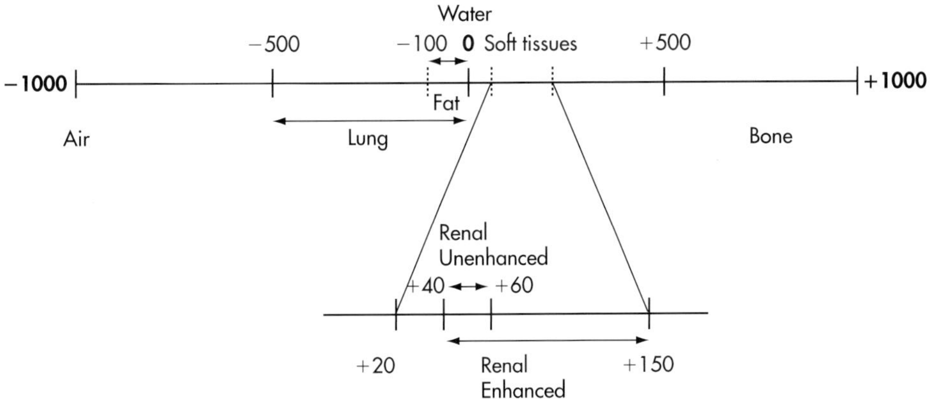

Figure 6.4 *A scale showing the CT (or Hounsfield) numbers of various body tissues. Water is conventionally graded as zero units, air as −1000 and soft tissues, such as kidneys, are +40–60 units.*

Spiral CT and volume or 3-D reconstruction

Modern machines are capable of fast scanning – the whole kidney can now be scanned in less than 10 seconds. Speed is achieved by spiraling through the area of interest rather than traversing as a step-by-step slice – a smooth, seamless spiral can be completed quicker than the stop–start motion of conventional sectional CT. The most modern machines are faster still, as they are capable of multilevel spirals.

Continuous data acquisition minimizes movement artefact, but, in addition, the speed and volume information of spiral or multislice CT lends itself to physiological studies. The study of enhancement patterns after contrast-enhanced CT has had a major impact in the non-invasive diagnosis and characterization of renal masses, as shown in Figure 6.5. For kidneys, after rapid contrast injection, an early corticomedullary phase and a later nephrographic phase can be identified by following density changes (or CT numbers). Focal renal pathology generally demonstrates reduced function and is seen as a poorly enhancing island (Figure 6.5). Rapid, fine section volume information allows the detection of acute ureteric calculous obstruction, and this is more reliable than conventional IVU.

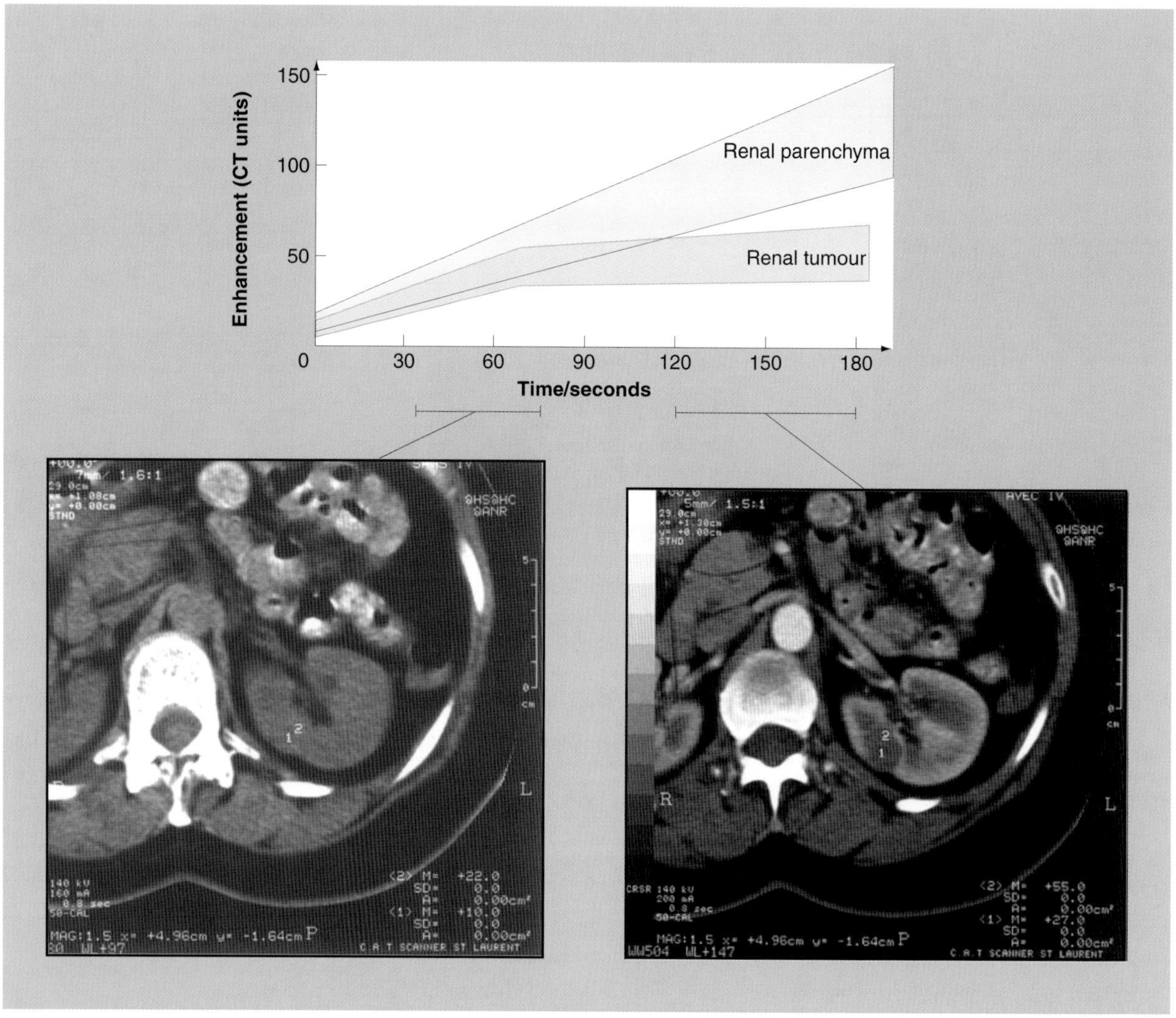

Figure 6.5 *Enhancement pattern of kidney after intravenous injection of iodinated contrast media. Examples of early (cortico-medullary)-phase and late (nephrographic)-phase renal patterns are shown. Abnormal renal tissue enhances less, as in this example of a renal cell carcinoma.*

Volume acquisition is also a prerequisite for 3-D anatomical modeling (Figure 6.3), which is, subjectively at least, helpful in surgical planning. A variety of methods are used in 3-D reconstruction (CT, MRI or US), of which 'surface-shaded' display is the most intuitive and readily grasped, as it presents the surface of the organ or structures of interest with the extra tissues or other features selectively cut out or subtracted from the image. Additionally, different shading of the pixels provides depth perception – those pixels closer to the surface are shaded lighter and so perceived to be closer to the surface. Virtual endoscopy or cystoscopy is a further example of the kind of 3-D rendering increasingly feasible. Although not fully exploited yet, fast-sequence CT may also be used to calculate renal cortical perfusion and regional glomerular filtration rate.[4]

With further improvement in the speed of acquisition, a 'snapshot' CT view of the kidneys may be feasible in the future and with continuing improvements in hard- and software, ever finer imaging can be predicted. At the time of writing, an upper level to improvement in CT is difficult to envisage, as the

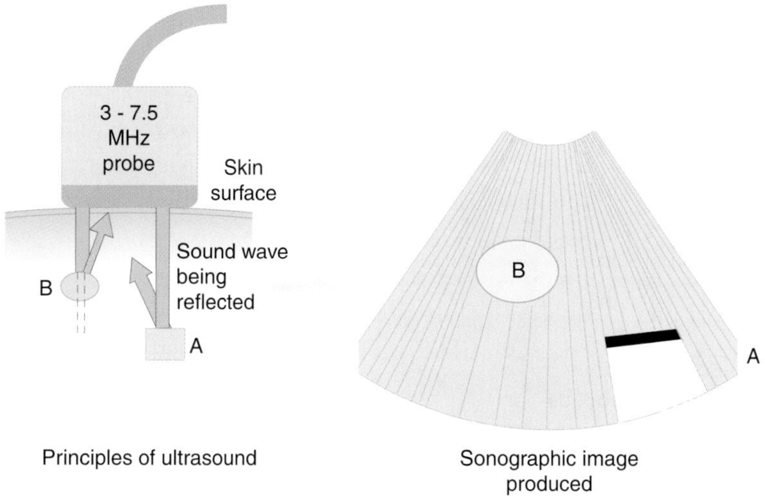

Figure 6.6 *Principles of medical ultrasound. Tissue A is deeper and, because it is a dense renal calculus, more sound reflecting than tissue B, which is a cyst. Therefore, on the sonogram, tissue B is depicted as nearer the skin surface and as less dense – spatial localization is calculated from the time delay before sound is received and density of image from the percentage of sound reflected back.*

pace of change seems to be accelerating; however, CT carries a high radiation burden (Table 6.1) and this will always be a limiting factor.

Ultrasound (US)

The safest, cheapest and most versatile of the cross-sectional modalities, medical US exploits inaudible sound waves of short wavelength, in the 3–12 MHz frequency range, which are non-ionizing with, so far, no proven serious tissue consequences. In this range, sound waves will transmit through the body but are altered in many ways by the intervening tissues and tissue–tissue interfaces. Of the numerous alterations, only three are commonly exploited for imaging – the absorption of sound by tissue, the reflection of sound at static interfaces and the apparent change in frequency of sound at moving interfaces (the Doppler effect). The first two are used to build the familiar 'grey-scale' ultrasound image, and the last allows 'vascular sonography' or duplex/colour Doppler.

Grey-scale ultrasound

The amount of sound absorbed by a given tissue is calculated by analysis of the reflected echo, and this is used to build a pixellated image. The factors that influence absorption and reflection are given in Figure 6.6. The weaker the reflection, the more 'grey' or darker the pixel value; and the varying shades of greys from different points in an organ are used to build a digital image that can be viewed on a television monitor. As water is a good sound transmitter and poor reflector, a renal cyst is seen as black; while fat, a good reflector, is seen as white. Bone and calcium are highly sound attenuating and reflective, and demonstrate a sharp interface with a shadow beyond (Figure 6.7). Unlike the other cross-sectional modalities, this is a real-time, interactive technique and ideally suited for biopsy and percutaneous intervention of soft tissues.

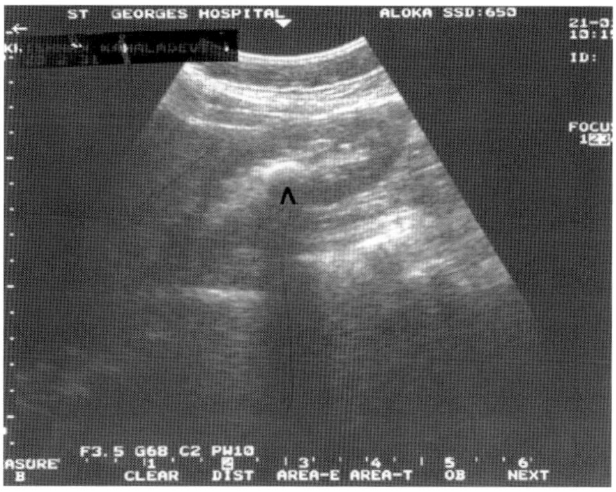

Figure 6.7 *A sonogram demonstrating the powerful beam reflection that occurs when sound encounters a dense material such as a renal calculus (seen in the centre of the kidney – arrowed).*

The Doppler effect

In 1843, Christian Doppler described the change in perceived frequency of sound emitted by a moving source: an everyday example is the crescendo/decrescendo sound of the train whistle as it hurtles past the station platform. Medical ultrasound is also subject to this Doppler shift effect, and the frequency change can be recalculated to give the velocity of the moving interface – the equation for this Doppler effect is given in Figure 6.8. The common dynamic interface in human tissues is the red blood cell, and blood flow and tissue haemodynamics can be studied easily. Calculated velocities can be presented quantitatively as a continuous, time-framed trace of true velocity (the 'Doppler or spectral waveform') or semiquantitatively/qualitatively as a 'colour Doppler' image.

Spectral or duplex Doppler

Spectral Doppler represents the full spectrum of recorded velocities in a given time period. Spectral Doppler can be used to diagnose and to grade arterial stenosis, using the velocity gradient across a narrowing. This is of some value in the assessment of renal artery stenosis. As well as velocity information, the shape of a spectral waveform encodes further qualitative or semiquantitative data about tissue character. The peripheral resistance (PR) or 'stiffness' of the tissue bed alters the waveform. Increased PR, as seen immediately after acute ureteric obstruction, restricts flow during diastole with reduced diastolic velocities. These waveform alterations can be quantified by calculating so-called waveform indices, such as the resistive index (Figure 6.8). Resistive index (RI) analysis is of some value in evaluation of

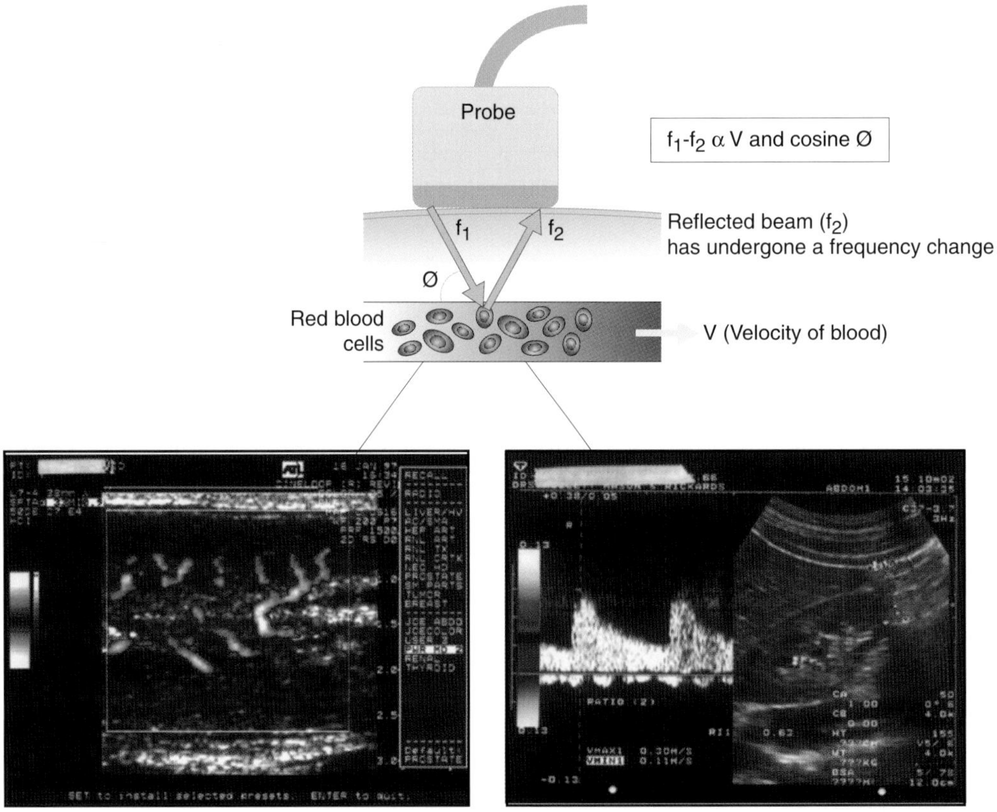

Figure 6.8 *Principles of Doppler ultrasound. The Doppler effect is used to calculate the velocity of a moving substance, such as blood. The velocity can be presented as a continuous Doppler or spectral waveform or can be superimposed on the grey-scale ultrasound image as a 'colour Doppler' image. The left-hand image is a power Doppler image showing the fine details of the penile vasculature. The right-hand image is a montage showing a colour and spectral Doppler image – a waveform has been measured with a resistive index (RI) of 0.63, indicating normal peripheral resistance in this non-obstructed kidney.*

renal dilatation. However, the diagnostic specificity of RI is modest, as adaptive physiological responses after obstruction counteract the elevated PR. Conversely, tumours have a low RI and elevated diastolic flows – because of intratumoural arteriovenous shunts and the lack of a complete smooth muscle wall in tumoural neovessels. This improves the diagnostic specificity in tumour diagnosis.

Colour Doppler

With colour Doppler, the peak velocity in a given time frame is assigned a value on a colour scale, and this is superimposed on the grey-scale image – conventionally, red represents flow towards the probe and blue away. Conveniently, renal arterial flow is usually towards and venous flow away from the probe, and so the grey and colour Doppler findings are easily assimilated by the observer. Simultaneous assessment of morphology/anatomy and vascularity adds a qualitative or functional element to the grey-scale ultrasound image. Most disease processes have some alteration of the blood flow, and colour Doppler assists diagnostic evaluation. Tumours such as renal cell carcinoma or testicular cancer are seen as 'hypervascular' areas (Figure 6.9) because of the increased vessel density as well as the higher mean velocity within microvessels resulting from the reduced peripheral resistance in the tumour.

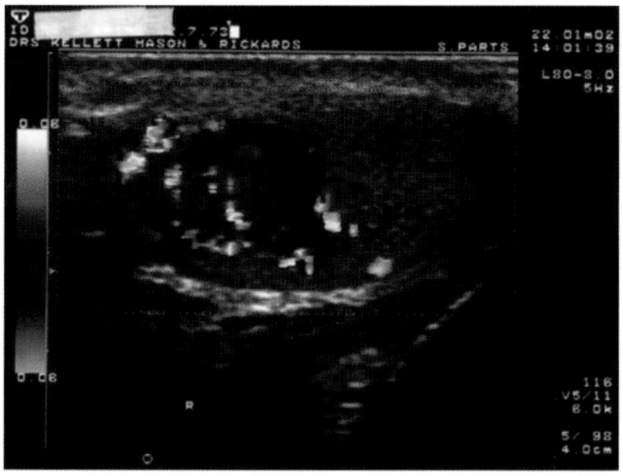

Figure 6.9 *A sonogram demonstrating tumour neovascularity, seen as a halo of increased 'colour flow' in a case of testicular cancer.*

Ultrasound contrast media

As with radiographic contrast media, certain injected agents can be used to enhance the signal/noise ratio of ultrasound imaging. Essentially, these agents are stabilized microbubbles (2–10 μm range), which are sonovisible. Only intravascular agents are available at the moment with no soft-tissue distribution. These are useful for vascular studies as they improve the strength of the Doppler effect and allow more detailed vascular analysis. They can also, under some circumstances, return a signal of a specific frequency (or harmonic) that can be individually isolated and analysed. Such harmonic imaging is currently being evaluated, and with the development of more refined agents with a tissue distribution, harmonic imaging of soft-tissue abnormalities may expand the diagnostic range of grey-scale ultrasound.

Many of the recent developments in medical ultrasound are to do with improved transducer design and post-processing. This has improved the quality of the US image significantly, but some disease processes remain frustratingly beyond current sonographic visibility. Prostate cancer is a germane example – the prostate gland is ideally suited for ultrasound examination, as with a high-frequency transrectal probe, it is very close to the probe surface, with few intervening tissues to degrade the sound, and yet many biopsy-proven prostate cancers are not visible. This highlights the limitation of current grey-scale ultrasound. Early or small volume disease, in the prostate gland and elsewhere, is poorly resolved by even the most modern scanners and probes. To overcome this limitation, other fundamental properties of tissue–sound interaction are being investigated. These include the imaging of harmonic frequencies (as above) and tissue sonoelasticity.[5]

Therapeutic medical ultrasound

After over 30 years of constant use, there has not been even one convincing report of harm attributable to clinical ultrasound, although there are theoretical risks due to local heating or microcavitation in tissues. With current transducers, these are not of clinical concern, but they may prove to be of therapeutic value. Direct local heating effect is being explored as a non-invasive means of tissue

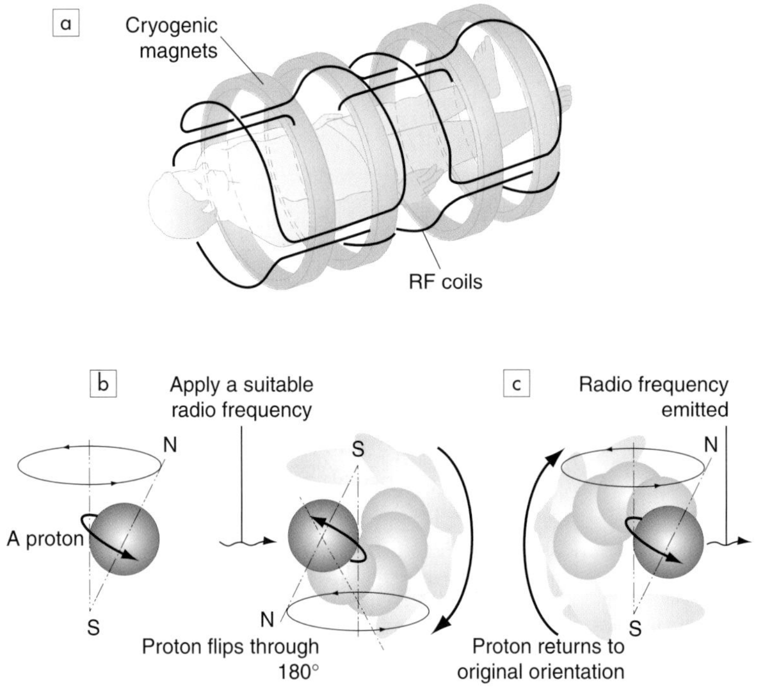

Figure 6.10 *Principles of magnetic resonance imaging. (a) The permanent magnet aligns protons in the direction of the main field. (b) The second radio-frequency coil temporarily changes the phase and rotation of the protons. (c) On recovery, these displaced protons emit a signal, from which the proton density and the T1 and T2 relaxation times are calculated (see text for definition of T1 and T2 times). Adapted from Fundamentals of Radiographic Photography, Vol 4. Published by Kodak Ltd. ISBN 0-901023-27-2.*

ablation – high-frequency ultrasound ablation or HIFU. Another promising area is the use of US beams to destabilize injected microbubbles to release therapeutic agents precisely within the organ of disease.[5]

Magnetic resonance imaging (MRI)

Some mobile elements – hydrogen being a good example – are naturally paramagnetic, and their behaviour in a strong magnetic field can be used to image body tissues. Water and fat, both rich in hydrogen nuclei (or protons), are principally exploited for current MRI. The physics of MRI is complex, but an oversimplified version is given in Figure 6.10.

A strong permanent magnet (typically 0.5–1.5 tesla) lies at the heart of the technique and aligns protons and other paramagnetic substances in the line of the magnetic field. Aligned protons also spin (or 'precess') around the axis of the magnetic field – like a child's spinning top. As it is positively charged, the proton's spin around the axis induces a magnetic moment, which can be resolved into a longitudinal and transverse magnetic vector (Figure 6.10). When a short-lived, second magnetic pulse is applied in another plane – of a particular frequency: the resonant frequency of the element being studied or the 'R' in MRI – many of these spinning protons temporarily change their alignment and rotation. Once the second pulse is switched off, the protons recover to their baseline position and orientation. This slow recovery generates three signals – *proton density (PD), T1 relaxation and T2 relaxation*. PD represents the number of spinning protons per predetermined volume – the greater the spinning density, the brighter the signal. T1 represents the time taken for the longitudinal component of the magnetization vector to recover to 63% of its maximum value, and T2 is the time until the transverse magnetization reduces by 37% of its maximum level.

The T1 and T2 times vary between tissues, and unlike the other modalities discussed so far, these signals are independent of tissue density. Study conditions can be further manipulated to enhance selectively either T1 or T2 information (Figure 6.11), and this accounts for the unique tissue contrast and diagnostic information of MRI. Heavily T2-weighted images (water and urine are seen 'bright' or white) are being evaluated as the emerging modality of MR urography, a technique of particular promise in the pregnant woman. At the moment, CT and MRI are comparable in terms of overall diagnostic contribution in urology, but

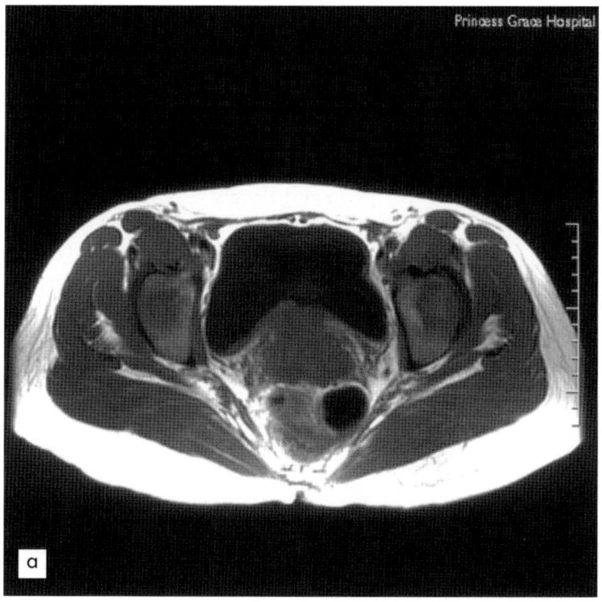

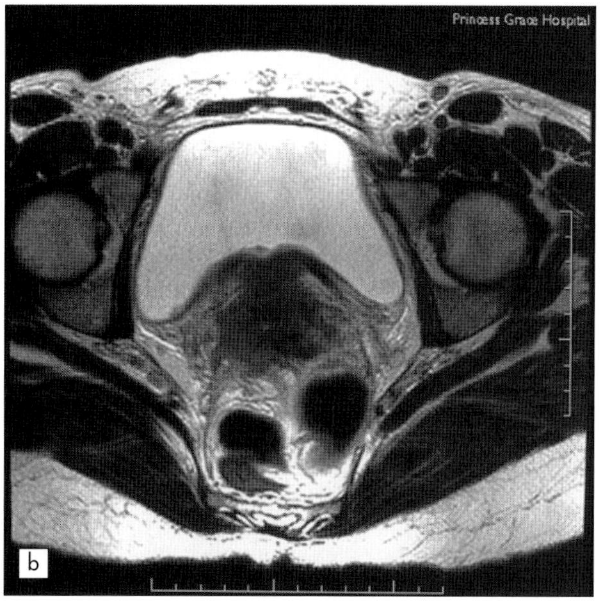

Figure 6.11 *Magnetic resonance images of the bladder and pelvic anatomy – (a) T1 image; (b) T2. The naturally high T2 relaxation times of urine mean the bladder is well seen in the T2-weighted study.*

there are specific areas of superiority – for stones/colic and fine definition, CT is better, while for renal cancer and prostate cancer, staging MRI is more accurate.

MR contrast agents

MRI-specific contrast media are also available. These are paramagnetic agents, which, in common with all other radiological CM, improve the signal to noise ratio. Gadolinium citrate is an example; the pharmacokinetics of gadolinium citrate and other agents in general clinical use are broadly similar to conventional iodinated CM, being short-lived intravascular, extracellular agents excreted by kidneys, but as with iodinated and ultrasonic media, tissue-specific agents are under development. Such agents may herald a new era of renal specific anatomical and physiological imaging. Liver-specific agents are already available, and further agents are being explored.

MR angiography and spectroscopy

The physics behind MR angiography is still more complex, and the interested reader is referred to standard MRI textbooks (see below, under suggestions for further reading). The important consideration is fast acquisition of heavily T1-weighted images, enhanced with gadolinium. This requires very specific MRI sequences, but this non-invasive technique is replacing standard catheter angiography (Figure 6.12).

Elements other than hydrogen also possess a magnetic moment and can be used for MRI, but their signals are much lower, too low for current MRI machines. Future, high-strength machines may overcome this limitation. A further area of promise is magnetic resonance spectroscopy or the non-invasive study of specific tissue metabolites. This has been evaluated in the prostate gland to study the

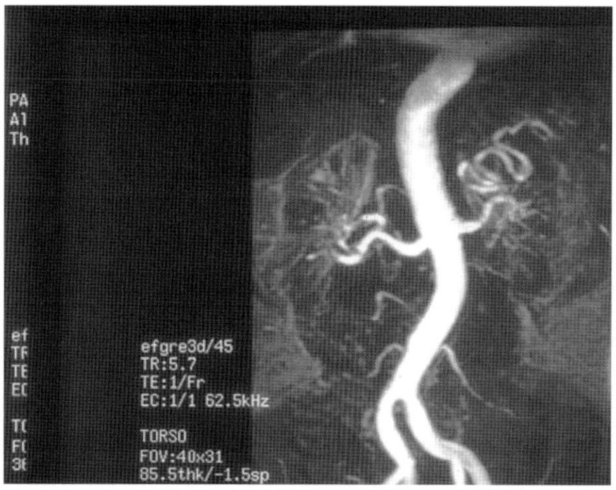

Figure 6.12 *A magnetic resonance angiogram showing single normal renal arteries on both sides.*

ratio of citrate/choline levels in the normal and the cancerous prostate gland[6] but is not yet used in routine imaging.

SUMMARY

The principles of the various tissue–energy interactions that are exploited in current uroradiological imaging, and their hazards and future potential, are summarized. As this is a vast topic, suggestions for further reading follow, as many simplifications – some oversimplifications – were necessary for the sake of brevity.

REFERENCES

1. Katayama H, Yamaguchi K, Kozuka T, Tashima T et al. Adverse reactions to ionic and non-ionic contrast media. Radiology 1990; 175: 621–628
2. Morcos SK. Contrast media induced nephrotoxicity – questions and answers. Br J Radiol 1998; 71: 357–365
3. Ambrose J, Hounsfield G. Computerized axial tomography. Br J Radiol 1973; 46: 148–149
4. Dawson P, Blomley MJK, Cosgrove DO. Functional and physiological imaging. In: Grainger RG, Allison DJ, eds. Diagnostic Radiology – A Textbook of Medical Imaging. London: Churchill Livingstone, 1997: 137–146
5. Kremkau FW, Merritt CR, Carson PL, van der Graaf I et al. The American Institute of Ultrasound in Medicine and the Society of Radiologists in Ultrasound – future directions in diagnostic US. Radiology 1998; 209: 305–311
6. Heerschap A, Jager GJ, van der Graaf I et al. In vivo proton MR spectroscopy reveals altered metabolite content in malignant prostate tissue. Anticancer Res 1997; 17: 1455–1460

FURTHER READING

Baxter GM, Allan PLP, Morley P. Clinical Diagnostic Ultrasound. Oxford: Blackwell Science, 1999

Farr RF, Allisy-Roberts PJ. Physics for Medical Imaging. London: WB Saunders, 1997

Lee JKT, Sagel SS, Stanley RJ, Heiken JP. Computed Tomography with MRI Correlation. 3rd edn. New York: Raven Press, 1998

Taylor KJW, Burns PN, Wells PNT. Clinical Applications of Doppler Ultrasound. New York: Raven Press, 1988

7

Upper urinary tract obstruction

Nicholas J Hegarty, R William G Watson and John M Fitzpatrick

AETIOLOGY

Ureteric obstruction (UO) can arise from disease of the ureter, the retroperitoneum or the abdomen, or as ureteric involvement in systemic disease. It can also arise as a consequence of bladder outflow obstruction. Obstruction can be unilateral or bilateral, acute or chronic, partial or complete, constant or intermittent. The causes of obstruction can be classified as congenital or acquired, luminal or extraluminal (see Table 7.1).

INCIDENCE

Evidence of obstruction is present in 3.9% of autopsies.[1] The true incidence is considerably higher, as many of the causes are successfully treated or resolve without treatment. UO presents at all ages, though there is a bimodal peak in its distribution: congenital causes typically present in childhood and acquired conditions present in mid- to late-adult life. Currently, the widespread use of antenatal scanning is highlighting increasing numbers of potential cases of UO.

Table 7.1a Congenital upper tract obstruction.

Intraluminal	Extraluminal
PUJ obstruction	Ureterocele Ectopic
Ureteric atresia	Orthotopic
Ureteric valves	Bladder diverticulum
Ureteric folds	Vascular
Congenital stricture	Retrocaval ureter
Vesico-ureteric reflux	Retroiliac ureter
Megaureter	Lower pole renal vessels
	Persistent umbilical artery
	? Gonadal vessels

CLINICAL PRESENTATION

The clinical presentation depends largely on the speed of onset, on the presence of a functioning contralateral kidney or bilateral involvement and, to a lesser extent, on the degree of obstruction. Bilateral obstruction, or obstruction in a solitary kidney, results in anuria and a rapid deterioration in renal function. This is a surgical emergency and requires urgent relief of obstruction. The clinical importance of UO therefore comprises physical

Table 7.1b Acquired upper tract obstruction.

Intraluminal	Extraluminal
Calculus	Pelvic malignancy – prostate, colorectal, ovarian, uterine, cervical Retroperitoneal malignancy – lymphoma, sarcoma, mesothelioma, secondary
Stricture	Gastrointestinal – pancreatitis, appendicitis, diverticulitis, Crohn's disease
Urothelial tumour	Vascular – abdominal aortic aneurysm, iliac artery aneurysm
Blood clot	Pregnancy
Sloughed papilla	Gynaecological – fibroids, endometriosis
Benign polyp	Retroperitoneal fibrosis – idiopathic, secondary
Fungal ball	Iatrogenic injury
Foreign body	

discomfort, impairment of renal function, complications such as stone formation or infection, and loss of renal tissue mass.

DIAGNOSIS

Along with the history and physical examination, basic investigations include urinalysis and microscopy. Investigations may include some or all of the following: intravenous pyelogram, ultrasound, computerized tomography (CT), isotope renography, retrograde pyelography and magnetic resonance imaging (MRI). Ureteroscopy may be both diagnostic and therapeutic. Percutaneous pressure studies (the Whitaker test) may be required where the diagnosis remains uncertain, and the details of this and other investigations are described elsewhere in this text.

TREATMENT

Interventional

The approach to ureteric obstruction is guided by the cause of the obstruction, the remaining function in the obstructed kidney and overall renal function. Obstruction can be quickly relieved by the insertion of percutaneous nephrostomy under ultrasound or CT guidance, or by retrograde (endoscopic) insertion of a ureteric stent. Stents also facilitate future endoscopy by dilating the ureter, but they probably slow the natural clearance of an obstructing calculus by reducing ureteric peristalsis.[2] Advances in rigid and flexible ureteroscope design allow a broader range of diagnostic and therapeutic manoeuvres to be performed with higher success rates and probably fewer complications.[3] Similarly, upper tract obstruction can often be relieved by percutaneous procedures. Laparoscopy for ureteric obstruction can be performed transperitoneally with mobilization of the overlying colon or by a retroperitoneal approach. Stone extraction, pyeloplasty, ureterolysis and nephrectomy for end-stage obstructive uropathy have all been described by this means. Extracorporeal shock wave lithotripsy (ESWL) is another minimally invasive technology that has revolutionized the treatment of renal and ureteric calculi, with immediate stone fragmentation rates of 90% achievable.[4] The development of these less invasive techniques has reduced the need for open surgery in UO. Surgery does, however, retain a significant role in the treatment of ureteric injuries, tumours and most non-urological causes of obstruction.

Medical

The main focus of medical treatment in UO is the relief of the associated pain. Non-steroidal anti-inflammatories (NSAIDs) are widely used in UO and provide remarkable pain relief in many cases. However, concerns over the potential detrimental effects of prostaglandin and thromboxane inhibition on blood flow and renal function raise questions as to their use in UO.[5] Antispasmodics and calcium channel blockers have limited efficacy in controlling pain.[6] While both morphine and pethidine are potent analgesics, pethidine is recommended for pain relief in UO, as morphine results in prolonged spasm of the ureter.[7]

Medical strategies to safeguard the kidney against the injurious effects of UO provide an interesting avenue of exploration as an adjunct to drainage procedures or operative removal of the obstruction. These have focused on vascular and inflammatory processes: inhibition of prostaglandin synthesis,[8] manipulation of the renin-angiotensin system,[9] nitric oxide and endothelin activity[10,11] and inflammatory cytokines[12] all being shown to lessen the detrimental effects of UO on renal blood flow in the experimental animal. To date, these studies have been principally confined to the experimental setting, and few human data are available on their efficacy.

PATHOLOGICAL CHANGES IN UO

Macroscopic changes

The main features visible in ureteric obstruction are dilatation of the ureter and the renal pelvis and calyces proximal to the obstruction (see Figure 7.1). The papillae are flattened and there is thinning of the renal parenchyma. Changes occur diffusely throughout the kidney, and the extent of these changes is largely dependent on the degree and duration of obstruction.

Microscopic changes

The earliest change observed is dilatation of the renal collecting ducts and distal tubules. Dilatation is accompanied by flattening of the tubular epithelial cells. As obstruction persists, dilatation extends to the proximal tubules and tubular atrophy occurs. Changes are often patchy in man, with areas of tubular loss being interspersed with histologically normal tissue. As obstruction persists, the proximal tubular brush border membrane becomes thinned. Interdigitations of cells become more broadly spaced, intercellular space in the collecting duct widens and, in some areas, tubular epithelial cells lift off the basement membrane, initially leaving the basement membrane intact.[13] Accompanying these changes is an inflammatory cell infiltrate and deposition of collagen matrix in the tubulointerstitium. Urine leaves the obstructed tubules to enter the interstitium and from there pass into dilated renal lymphatics or go directly through polyps that project into the renal veins (termed tubulovenous anastamoses). There is initially expansion of the interstitium despite tubular atrophy occurring. The renal vasculature remains well preserved and glomerular hyalinization occurs only as a late event.[14]

PHYSIOLOGICAL CHANGES

Acute complete unilateral UO is accompanied by a well-defined series of changes in ureteric pressure and renal blood flow. These are divided into three phases (see Table 7.2):[15]

Phase 1 (0–90 minutes): increase in ipsilateral renal blood flow and collecting system pressure.

Phase 2 (90 minutes–4 hours):
- Blood flow decreases to below control levels.
- Collecting system pressure remains elevated.

Phase 3 (4–18 hours):
- Blood flow continues to decrease.
- Collecting system pressure decreases.

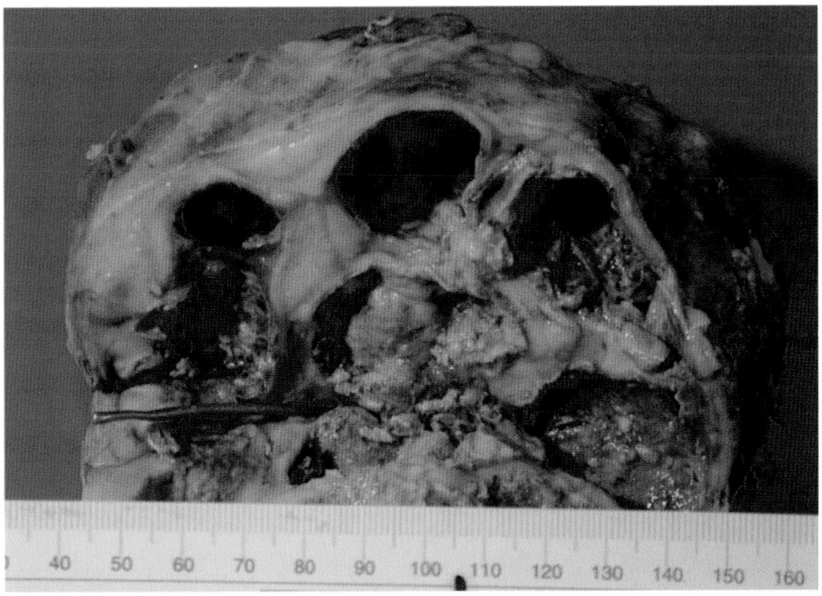

Figure 7.1 *Chronically obstructed kidney, demonstrating marked, hydronephrosis and renal parenchymal loss.*

Table 7.2 Triphasic blood-flow and pressure response in unilateral ureteric obstruction.

		Collecting system pressure	Renal blood flow
Phase 1	0–90 mins	↑	↑
Phase 2	90 mins–4 hours	↔ (remains elevated)	↓ (below resting blood flow)
Phase 3	4–18 hours	↓ (toward resting)	↓ (continued decrease)

Pressure changes

Shortly after the onset of UO, the intrapelvic pressure rises from a resting value of 6.5 mmHg[16] to values of 50–70 mmHg.[17] This pressure is transmitted to the renal tubules, with similar values being recorded in renal tubules 1–3 hours after the onset of obstruction.[18,19] Compensatory mechanisms, including dilatation of the renal pelvis and collecting system, afferent vasoconstriction, pyelotubular and tubulovenous reflux, and dilatation of pelvic lymphatics with increased shunting of urine into the perirenal lymphatics (see Figure 7.2),[20] result in collecting system pressure decreasing to approximately half these levels (30 mmHg) after 24 hours of obstruction, with gradual resolution over the subsequent 4–6 weeks.[21]

Blood-flow and GFR changes

Following the onset of unilateral ureteric obstruction (UUO), there is an abrupt increase in blood flow to the obstructed kidney. This is mediated by afferent glomerular arteriolar dilatation and results in maintenance of GFR, despite the increased pressure in Bowman's space transmitted from the obstructed tubule.[22] With ongoing obstruction, vasodilatation gives way to vasoconstriction, resulting in a decrease in GFR. Both the renin-angiotensin and prostaglandin-thromboxane systems show increased activity during UUO. Angiotensin-converting enzyme (ACE) inhibitors abolish the initial hyperaemic response to UO[23] and ameliorate the effects of chronic UO on blood flow and GFR.[24] Inhibition of prostaglandin/thromboxane synthesis

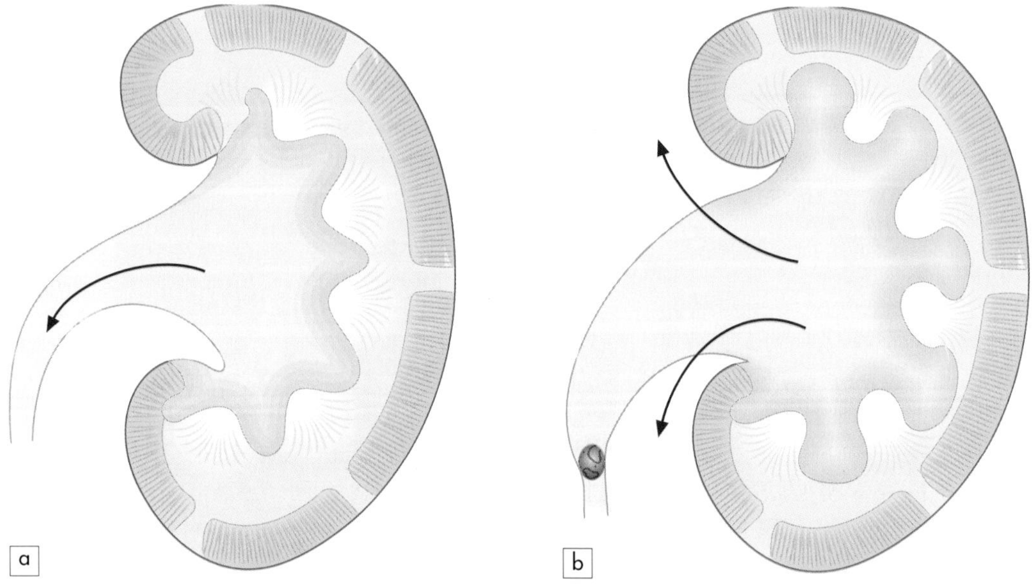

Figure 7.2 *Dilatation of perirenal lymphatics allows urine output to be maintained while lowering collecting system pressure in the obstructed kidney. (a) Antegrade flow of urine in non-obstructed kidney; (b) obstructed kidney with dilated collecting system and pyelolymphatic back flow of urine.*

has similar effects.[25,26] Reversal of the blood flow changes of UO has also been demonstrated, with either augmentation of nitric oxide[27] or inhibition of endothelin.[28]

Tubular function

As it is difficult to study functional changes in the kidney in the presence of ongoing obstruction, most studies assess renal function immediately after the release of obstruction. This does not allow assessment of the contribution of obstruction away from any injury that may be associated with its release. Whether there is a significant reperfusion injury with the release of UO remains a topic of debate. It is clear, however, that significant injury does occur prior to the release of obstruction, and it is by limiting the damage in the obstructed phase that the optimum outcome is likely to be achieved.

Evidence of renal injury is reflected by impairment of renal tubular function, which can also be used as a marker of the degree of renal tubular injury.

Sodium excretion

Even in the absence of ultrastructural damage, the cellular mechanisms of active transport are impaired in UO.[29,30] Levels of natriuretic substances are seen to be elevated in the obstructed kidney.[31,32] Therefore, despite a decrease in GFR, sodium excretion (and urine volume) is maintained or even slightly increased in UO.

Potassium excretion

The excretion of potassium in unilateral UO (UUO) decreases in proportion to the decrease in GFR.[33] Proximal tubular potassium reabsorption remains normal in bilateral obstruction, but there is further potassium added in the collecting duct in response to the increased delivery of sodium and volume.[34]

Urine concentration

UO results in impairment of both renal urinary concentration and dilution capabilities, with urine osmolarity approaching that of plasma. The medullary thick ascending limb loses the ability to remove solute without water, resulting in a decrease in the normal osmotic gradient and a reduced capability to concentrate urine. There is also a failure of the collecting duct to increase water permeability in response to antidiuretic hormone and cyclic adenosine monophosphate,[35,36] impairing the kidneys' ability to dilute urine.

Urine acidification

There is a relative preservation of proximal tubule bicarbonate reabsorption. There is, however, a reduced ability to lower urine pH in response to acid loading, suggesting a defect in the ability of the distal nephron to acidify urine after release of the obstruction.[37,38] A reduced capacity to generate ammonia in the proximal tubule also contributes to decreased acid excretion in obstruction.[39,40]

Enzyme function

The spectrum of tubular injury in UO ranges from mild impairment to increased apoptosis and occasionally necrosis. Sublethal injury is associated with loss of brush border in renal tubules and impairment of tubular enzyme function. Impairment of several enzymes has been described. Decreased Na-H ATPase and Na-K ATPase activity[41,42] results in tubular swelling and a reduced capacity to acidify urine. Alterations in prostaglandin synthesis contribute to the observed alterations in renal blood flow in UO.[8] There is decreased tubular cell arginase activity, resulting in a relative L-arginine deficiency and thus a reduced capacity for nitric oxide production.[43] Other enzymes that show alterations in activity include a significant reduction in alkaline phosphatase and alanineaminopeptidase,[44] and these can be used as a marker for the severity of damage in UO.[45]

INFLAMMATORY RESPONSE IN UO

An inflammatory cell infiltrate is seen in the kidney within 4 hours of the onset of UO. This is predominantly macrophage (both resident and circulating), but also contains cytotoxic T lymphocytes. It peaks 24 hours after the onset of obstruction,[46] at which stage expansion of the interstitial space is seen, with interstitial fibroblasts and extravasated red blood cells being the principal cell types alongside the mononuclear cells. Recruitment of neutrophils is seen, with increased neutrophil counts after 24 hours of UO. Associated with this is an increase in myeloperoxidase activity at 24 hours, reflecting increased neutrophil activity. Persistence of macrophage activity is seen in chronic UO, while neutrophil activity is seen to have returned to baseline within 1 week of obstruction.[47] The inflammatory cell infiltrate is most apparent in the tubulointerstitium. Renal tubules and peritubular capillaries disappear, to be replaced by fibroblasts, mononuclear cells and matrix protein deposition in a process termed 'interstitial fibrosis'.

Interstitial fibrosis

Inflammatory changes occurring in UO of short duration are probably reversible. Cortical thinning with mature scar formation in chronic obstruction represents irreversible change, and part of the goal of unravelling the fibrotic processes in UO is to develop treatments to prevent these changes. Fibronectin deposition commences soon after the onset of obstruction and acts as a scaffold as well as a chemoattractant for fibroblasts.[48] Deposition of collagen types I, II and IV in the tubulointerstitium with sparing of the cortex is seen to occur in the interstitium within 3 days of the onset of obstruction.[49] Type IV collagen is also deposited within the basement membrane of renal tubules, resulting in impaired tubular function (see Figure 7.3).

Other studies suggest that the net increase in matrix protein in UO is the result of decrease in the breakdown of collagen rather than increased synthesis.[50] Tissue inhibitor metalloproteinase-1 (TIMP-1), which inhibits collagen breakdown by metalloproteinases, is expressed by tubular cells and interstitial cells.[51] During UO, there is a 13-fold increase in its expression,[52,53] with only a transient increase in metalloproteinase mRNA expression.[52] Similarly, there is increased expression of plasminogen activator inhibitor-1 (PAI-1) in interstitial fibrosis,[54] resulting in decreased activation of plasmin with consequent decreased activation of collagenase.

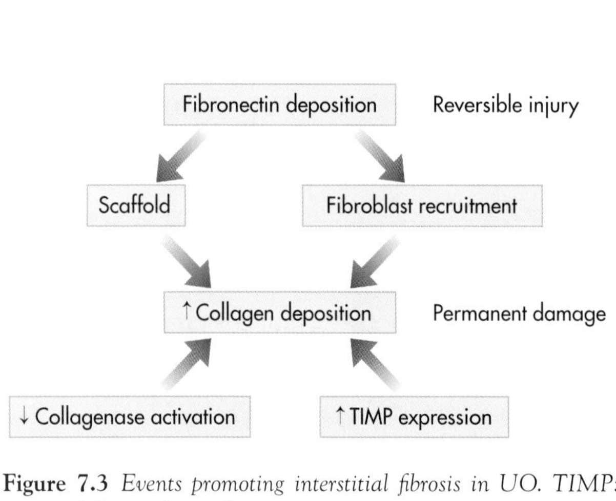

Figure 7.3 *Events promoting interstitial fibrosis in UO. TIMP: tissue inhibitor of metalloproteinase.*

Origin of the inflammatory response in UO

The factors underlying the inflammatory response in UO have not been delineated fully, and there is debate as to whether renal tubular cells or the inflammatory cell infiltrate are the main source of cytokines and mediators of inflammation in UO. Renal cortex extracts from obstructed kidneys show increased chemotactic activity when compared to those from the contralateral kidney.[55] Increased expression of monocyte chemoattractant peptide 1 (MCP-1) is detected in tubular cells within 12 hours of the onset of obstruction.[56] Other substances with chemotactic properties, including TGF-β,[57] TNF-α,[58] osteopontin,[59] intercellular adhesion molecule-1 (ICAM-1)[60] and vascular cell adhesion molecule-1 (VCAM-1),[61] are all seen to be upregulated in renal tubules within 24 hours of the onset of obstruction.

Strategies to abolish the inflammatory cell infiltrate in UO, including total body irradiation (TBI), do not blunt the increase in expression of TNFα occurring with UO.[58] Similarly, there is a partial but incomplete reversal of the reduced GFR and plasma flow of UO,[62] implying a role for both local inflammatory responses and the influx of inflammatory cells. More recent data suggest that the inflammatory changes are independent of lymphocyte infiltration[63] and that the initiating stimuli are more likely to reflect the effects of pressure, stretch and relative hypoperfusion of the renal tubules.

Role of individual cytokines in UO

In the context of UO, TGFβ-1 has been the cytokine studied in the most detail. The TGFβ family comprises at least three isomers (TGFβ-1,

TGFβ-2 and TGFβ-3). These are secreted in an inactive form and are cleaved to their active state by serine proteases or an acidic medium. TGFβ isomers bind type II TGFβ receptors on the cell surface. Type I receptors are recruited, and phosphorylation of the type I receptor leads to activation of intracellular signalling pathways.[64] TGFβ has been shown to have an important role in inflammatory processes and neoplasia.[65,66] In UO, it has been shown to increase matrix protein synthesis, inhibit matrix degradation and upregulate matrix adhesion molecule expression, and to be chemoattractant for fibroblasts and monocytes (see Table 7.3).[66,67] Anti-TGFβ-1 antibodies have been shown to reduce the renal injury in glomerulonephritis,[68,69] diabetic nephropathy[70,71] and cyclosporine nephrotoxicity,[72] but these have not been studied in UO. In renal tubule cells, TGFβ-1 expression has been shown to be stimulated by angiotensin II.[73] ACE inhibitors and angiotensin II receptor blockers decrease TGFβ-1 expression and collagen IV mRNA in UO[9,49,74] with preservation of the renal interstitium. However, this results in incomplete blockade, conversely, mice deficient in angiotensin II receptor develop mild interstitial fibrosis and elevation in TGFβ-1 expression by 3 weeks.[75] Though a central role has been proposed for TGFβ, other inflammatory mediators have been shown to operate independently of it in UO: platelet derived growth factor (PDGF) can stimulate interstitial fibrosis without any elevation in TGFβ-1.[76] TGFβ is also expressed by regenerating renal tubules;[77] thus, strategies aimed at inhibition may also impair healing processes. Other inflammatory mediators are discussed below in relation to their functions in cellular injury in UO.

Table 7.3 Inflammatory role of the TGFβ in UO.

TGFβ in UO
↑ matrix protein synthesis
↓ matrix degradation
↑ matrix-adhesion molecule expression
Chemoattractant for fibroblasts and monocytes
Inhibition of TGFβ-1 expression reduces interstitial fibrosis

MECHANISMS OF CELLULAR INJURY

Cell death is described as occurring by two pathways: necrosis and apoptosis. Necrosis results from severe energy (ATP) depletion and the consequent rapid, uncoordinated collapse of cellular homeostasis. In UO, apoptosis, rather than necrosis, is the principal mechanism of cell death.[78] In contrast to necrosis, apoptosis is an energy-dependent genetically controlled process whereby individual cells are eliminated from tissue.[79] There is rapid uptake of apoptotic bodies by surrounding cells, without exciting an inflammatory response unless extremely high rates of apoptosis are occurring.

Cell signalling in apoptosis

Apoptosis involves three main steps. Firstly, the cell is given a signal to undergo apoptosis. The cell then integrates this message with other internal stimuli and 'decides' to enter the apoptotic pathway. Finally, the cascade of protein digestion and cell destruction occurs. Cell surface receptors involved in apoptotic signalling include Fas, tumour necrosis factor receptor-1 (TNFR-1) and TNF receptor apoptosis-inducing ligand receptor (TRAIL). These in turn bind or recruit other membrane or intracellular adapter molecules, including Fas-associated death domain (FADD), TNF receptor-associated death domain (TRADD), Fas-associated phosphatase (FAP) and Fas-associated factor (FAF), thereby activating them. Fas expression is increased in the obstructed kidney,[80] as are FADD and FAP levels.[81] Distal tubular cells that do not express functional Fas on their cell surface appear to be less susceptible to apoptosis in UO.[82] The activated adapter molecules then trigger a family of proteolytic enzymes named the caspases. These are a 13-member family of cysteine proteases. They specifically cleave proteins after an aspartate residue. Upstream caspases (caspases 10, 8 and 7) are termed 'initiator caspases', as they exert their effects at a pre-mitochondrial level. Upstream caspases can be bypassed by noxious chemicals and irradiation, which act directly on the mitochondrion. The resultant membrane disruption causes cytochrome c release and apoptosis. The downstream caspases (caspase 3) are termed 'effector caspases', and these represent the final step in the apoptotic pathway.

Increased mRNA and immunohistochemistry staining for caspases is seen in the obstructed kidney, paralleling alterations in the rate of tubular cell apoptosis.[83]

Apoptotic signalling in UO

Acting in conjunction with the caspases are a number of apoptosis-regulating proteins. The Bcl-2 family, growth factors, adhesion molecules and repair genes, such as p53, all interact to influence cell proliferation and apoptosis, thus regulating cell turnover.

Bcl-2 family

Some of these block apoptosis and others promote apoptosis, and the balance in expression of the various Bcl-2 family members determines their effect on apoptosis. In UO, Bcl-2 expression increases in both the adult and the fetal kidney,[84] while Bax expression decreases.[85] Expression is seen to localize to tubules undergoing apoptosis, with little change seen in non-apoptotic tubules.[86] Treatments that reduce interstitial fibrosis and apoptosis in UUO are also associated with increased Bcl-2 expression.[12]

Adhesion molecules

Loss of cell adhesion leads to disconnection from the basement membrane and apoptosis – a process termed 'anoikis'.[87] Cell adhesion is maintained by integrins, which are associated with cell–cell communication and the production of survival factors. Intercellular adhesion molecule-1 (ICAM-1) expression increases within 3 hours of the onset of obstruction[88] and may remain elevated for several weeks following the relief of obstruction.[60] Experimental manipulation of ICAM-1 expression is seen to reduce tubulointerstitial fibrosis in UO.[89] In clinical practice, elevated serum ICAM-1 levels are seen in patients with obstructing ureteric calculi.[45] Other adhesion molecules are thought to play important roles in the inflammatory processes of UO, but have been less studied than ICAM. Selectins, a family of three adhesion molecules, are associated with macrophage infiltration in UUO.[90] P-selectin levels are elevated within 1 hour of the onset of UO and remain elevated for 96 hours.[91] A gradual increase in vascular cell adhesion molecule-1 (VCAM-1) expression is also seen within the interstitium, but not tubules during UO.[88] Understanding the role of adhesion molecules in UO is likely to increase with the development of models of applying mechanical strain and distortion to renal tubules in vitro.[92]

Growth factors in UO

The role of transforming growth factor-beta (TGFβ) as a modulator of interstitial injury has been described above. Like TGFβ, platelet-derived growth factor (PDGF) expression is increased in UO. This is seen particularly in the interstitium where it is likely to enhance proliferation of interstitial fibroblasts.[93] Epidermal growth factor (EGF) expression is reduced in UO. Administration of EGF reduces apoptosis, increases tubular proliferation and decreases interstitial fibrosis in the obstructed kidney.[94] Hepatocyte growth factor (HGF) expression is also reduced in UO.[95] Neutralizing HGF worsens interstitial fibrosis, while exogenous HGF attenuates the progression of interstitial fibrosis,[95] decreasing the transition of renal tubular cells to myofibroblasts.[96] Expression of insulin-like growth factor-1 (IGF-1) and IGF receptor (IGFR) are unchanged in UO. However, the administration of IGF-1 is associated with a reduction in tubular apoptosis and interstitial collagen deposition,[97] suggesting this as a potential treatment in UO. Like adhesion molecules, the range of growth factors and their role in apoptotic, proliferative and inflammatory processes in UO continues to be elucidated. They hold considerable potential as targets for treatment and for monitoring the effects of therapeutic intervention in UO.

Clusterin

Clusterin is a glycoprotein that participates in a number of biological processes. It is involved in membrane lipid recycling, in apoptosis, and acts as a stress-induced chaperone protein.[98] In UUO, its expression is seen to increase in parallel with the changes in apoptotic rate in the obstructed kidney: increased expression is evident within 12 hours of obstruction, and a 10-fold increase on control is seen within 3 days. Expression is localized to the collecting ducts and tubules and remains elevated after 2 months UO.[99] The increase in clusterin expression is reversed by administration of an angiotensin II receptor inhibitor, which is also associated with a reduction in the rate of apoptosis in the obstructed kidney.[100] A transient increase in clusterin expression is also seen in the contralateral kidney in UUO, but this returns to control values within 24 hours of the onset of obstruction.[99]

Osteopontin

Osteopontin is a macrophage-adhesive protein with chemoattractant properties. In UO, increased osteopontin expression is seen in tubular cells within 4 hours of obstruction.[59] The increased expression is localized to non-dilated tubules of UUO.[101] This expression would appear to be renal in origin rather than systemic, as it is not altered by total body irradiation[59] and may play an important role in stimulating the inflammatory cell response of UO.

p53

p53 is important in repairing functional genes. It is involved in G1 cell-cycle arrest and apoptosis.[102] p53 knockout mice display less apoptosis in tubular and interstitial cells in chronic UUO than wild-type mice.[103] Similarly, treatments that decrease apoptosis as well as decrease proliferation in interstitial cells result in a reduction in p53 and p21 expression.[104] Thus, p53 has potential as both a marker of tissue injury and a target for treatment in UO.

It is clear that much data are accruing on the various cell signalling pathways in the apoptotic and proliferative responses to UO (summarized in Table 7.4). The importance of this cannot be overstated with regard to elucidating the mechanisms by which renal tissue destruction occurs. It is also likely to contribute significantly to planning and monitoring means by which the kidney may be protected in the face of ongoing obstruction.

Table 7.4 Cell signalling pathways in UO.

Mediator	Expression in UO	Role in UO	Alteration in expression
Fas	↑	↑ susceptibility to apoptosis	
Caspases	↑	Reflect rate of apoptosis	
Bcl family			
Bcl-2	↑	↑ apoptosis	Renoprotective treatments → ↓ Bcl-2 expression
Bax	↓	↓ apoptosis	
Adhesion molecules			
ICAM-1	↑	↑ TIF	↓ expression → ↓ fibrosis
VCAM-1	↑	↑ TIF	
P-selectin	↑	Chemoattractant	
Growth factors			
TGFβ	↑	↑ TIF	Inhibition → ↓ TIF
PDGF	↑	↑ TIF	
EGF	↓	↓ apoptosis and ↓ TIF	
HGF	↓		Exogenous HGF → ↓TIF
IGF-1	↔		Administration → ↓ tubular apoptosis and ↓ TIF
Clusterin	↑	Reflects rate of apoptosis	
Osteopontin	↑	↑ inflammatory cell response	
p53		↓ tubular apoptosis	↓ with treatments that ↓ TIF

TIF: tubulointerstitial fibrosis; ICAM-1: intercellular adhesion molecule-1; VCAM-1: vascular adhesion molecule-1; TGFβ: transforming growth factor-β; PDGF: platelet derived growth factor; EGF: epidermal growth factor; HGF: hepatocyte growth factor; IGF-1: insulin-like growth factor-1.

RELIEF OF OBSTRUCTION

Following relief of obstruction, the recovery of function in the post-obstructed kidney is inversely proportional to the duration and the degree of obstruction.[105] Immediately following the relief of obstruction, there is an increase in blood flow,[15,18,106] which soon decreases to a level below preobstruction values.

The recovery of function is divided into two phases – the first phase has been termed the 'tubular phase' and approximates to the first 2 weeks following relief of obstruction. This initial response reflects a gradual reversal of the tubular changes that had occurred during obstruction. Increased fractional excretion of sodium and water results in a diuresis, alleviating the fluid retention associated with BUO and thus improving the associated hypertension, peripheral oedema and pulmonary oedema.[107] The second phase is more gradual and is termed the 'glomerular phase'. The ability to concentrate and acidify urine increases; however, the osmolality of urine remains lower than normal at 2-month follow up.[108] There is also an impaired ability to lower urinary pH in response to acid loading.[109] Potassium excretion also improves but may not increase sufficiently to eliminate the accumulated potassium entirely. Thus, it is common for patients to remain slightly hyperkalaemic, a condition which is perhaps due to impaired responsiveness of the distal tubule to aldosterone post-obstruction.[110] Tubular recovery is probably maximal at 3 months, with no further significant recovery of function at 6 months.[111]

The mechanism of recovery of function would appear to be predominantly hyperplasia in the post-obstructed kidney. Similarly, with ongoing obstruction, the contralateral kidney undergoes hyperplasia more than hypertrophy.[111] This response increases with the duration of obstruction, to maintain roughly equal total function for several weeks. As a result of compensatory changes in the non-obstructed kidney, functional changes following the release of unilateral obstruction are less dramatic than in bilateral obstruction. There is an increase in free water excretion associated with a concentrating defect; however, significant post-obstructive diuresis is extremely rare.

Estimating the duration of obstruction after which function will not return is often difficult. In the experimental animal, after a period of obstruction of 2 months, there is no improvement in function:[112] however, case reports describe recovery following relief of obstruction of 10 years' duration.[113] It is clear that permanent damage can occur after a much shorter duration of obstruction. Predicting recovery has been described in children using isotope renography,[114] but has not been successfully achieved in adults.

THE CONTRALATERAL KIDNEY

In unrelieved chronic UUO, there is compensatory growth in the contralateral kidney. The response of the non-obstructed kidney is proportional to the degree of injury to the obstructed kidney – a process termed 'counterbalance'.[115] This process is similar to that seen following nephrectomy.[116,117] Following nephrectomy, increased RNA/DNA ratio can be seen in the contralateral kidney within 12 hours.[118] There is even evidence to suggest that increased cell synthesis in the remnant kidney begins within 5 minutes of uninephrectomy.[119] In UUO, an increase in cell number is seen in both kidneys within 48 hours.[120] The capacity for compensatory renal growth (CRG) following nephrectomy is age-dependent in both the experimental animal and humans.[121,122] It would appear that the initial rates of CRG are similar in the neonate and adult, but that it is sustained for a considerably longer period in the young, resulting in a greater amount of total growth.[123] Similar age-dependence is seen in partial UUO,[124] where the degree of CRG in the contralateral kidney is seen to decrease as obstruction occurs later in life.

Changes in blood flow and GFR in the contralateral kidney occur in parallel with CRG in UUO.[124] Though the initial blood flow response is vasoconstrictive,[21] mediated by renal nerves,[125] this soon gives way to an increase in renal blood flow, with compensatory trophic changes.[8] There is some evidence to implicate vasoactive mediators in these later changes. During UUO, increased endothelin (ET) RNA is seen in the obstructed kidney with a decrease in the contralateral kidney.[28] Similarly,

Table 7.5 Comparison between obstructed and contralateral kidneys in unilateral ureteric obstruction.

	Obstructed	Contralateral
Apoptosis	Increased	Unchanged
Cell proliferation	Increased	Increased
Initial response	Vasodilatory	Vasoconstrictive
Prolonged obstruction	Vasoconstrictive	Vasodilatory
Endothelin excretion	Increased	Reduced

while urinary ET excretion is elevated in the obstructed kidney, contralateral excretion is reduced.[126] This suggests that an imbalance in ET expression between the obstructed and contralateral kidney contributes to the observed blood-flow and trophic changes (see Table 7.5).

BILATERAL OBSTRUCTION

Bilateral obstruction is frequently encountered in the setting of functional or mechanical infravesical obstruction. It may also occur when disease processes extend to involve both upper tracts simultaneously. Presentation tends to be gradual, with renal impairment or symptoms of the primary condition being the usual presenting features. There is considerable overlap between the physiological changes occurring in bilateral as well as unilateral UO. A few notable differences are that the renal function is globally affected and there is no compensatory response possible when both kidneys are obstructed. Similar blood-flow changes to those in the unilaterally obstructed kidney are seen;[126] however, the initial hyperaemic response is absent or markedly decreased,[125] while the subsequent decrease in renal blood flow is more pronounced than in UUO.[106,127] Collecting system and intratubular pressures show greater elevations in bilateral obstruction[127] and remain elevated for a considerably longer period.[128] Single nephron GFR is reduced by a similar degree as in UUO, though the mechanisms are slightly different: in UUO, the decrease in glomerular filtration pressure is largely due to afferent arteriolar vasoconstriction, with intratubular pressures being relatively lower;[106] in bilateral obstruction, vasoconstriction is less pronounced, but elevated intratubular pressures lower the glomerular filtration pressure.[127] There is identical impairment of tubular function in unilateral and bilateral obstruction.[29,30] Impaired function in the medullary thick ascending limb (mTAL) results in an impaired ability to actively absorb sodium without water (therefore impairing urinary diluting capacity). The decrease in sodium absorption also leads to impairment of the ability to maintain a high osmolality in the medullary interstitium and therefore to concentrate urine. There is also impaired ability of the collecting duct to increase water permeability to ADH and cAMP, which is similar in both unilateral and bilateral obstruction.[29,30] Na-H ATPase and Na-K ATPase pump mechanisms are affected in BUO as in UOO, with resultant defect in acidification of urine.[129]

Release of bilateral obstruction results in a reversal of the urinary concentrating and acidification defects that have occurred during obstruction as described above. Unlike UUO, where compensation by the contralateral kidney has been possible during obstruction, a profound diuresis may occur.

POST-OBSTRUCTIVE DIURESIS

Though a transient increase in output may be seen from the relief of obstruction in UUO (as seen by high output from nephrostomy tube), this is rarely, if ever, of clinical significance. Release of bilateral obstruction or obstruction in a solitary kidney, however, frequently produces post-obstructive diuresis. It is probably multifactorial in origin. Theories that have been advanced include excretion of fluid retained during UO, persistence of the tubular concentrating defect initiated during UO or the accumulation of natriuretic substances or urea (though diuresis may occur in those with a normal blood urea).[130] Over-aggressive replacement of fluid output contributes to prolongation of diuresis in many cases. In the conscious patient with free access to water, thirst mechanisms alone are usually sufficient to guide appropriate fluid replacement.[131]

Serial electrolyte measurements as well as weighing, and erect and supine blood pressure measurements are used to monitor the small proportion of patients that will require intravenous fluid and electrolyte replacement. This is usually confined to those with a sustained urine output of >200 ml/hour. Even then, tubular function will usually return to normal over the first 3–7 days after release of obstruction; however, persistence of diuresis with copious salt loss is a rare form of tubular defect that may require prolonged and stringent fluid and electrolyte replacement.[132]

PARTIAL OBSTRUCTION

Partial obstruction is the form of UO most frequently encountered in clinical practice. It can present acutely, with renal calculi or injury to the ureter, or more insidiously, as occurs with gradually stenosing benign and malignant strictures. The problems associated with conclusively diagnosing ureteric obstruction are even more apparent in the setting of partial obstruction. When standard radiological tests fail to confirm partial obstruction, antegrade nephrostogram through a nephrostomy tube, in combination with a Whitaker test, may be required to confirm the presence of partial obstruction.[8,133]

Reproducing partial obstruction in the experimental animal is not without difficulty either. Experimental models that rely upon burying the ureter are of limited value in attaining a particular degree of partial obstruction, and a sizeable proportion of cases studied by this technique need to be excluded, as it often results in complete obstruction, or conversely, in no obstruction at all.[134] A more reliable method is one in which a portion of ureter is replaced with a narrow bore tube.[135] Much information as to the physiological changes associated with partial obstruction and its release has been attained by this method.[112,136,137] As in complete UO, there is dilatation of the collecting system proximal to the obstruction and decreased renal perfusion, with impaired renal function and loss of renal parenchyma. Histological changes in partial obstruction are similar to those in complete obstruction. Gross appearance shows cortical thinning. Dilatation of renal tubules is seen with interstitial fibrosis.[138] Tubular apoptosis is seen to increase in rate with duration of partial obstruction to values approaching those of complete obstruction. The expression of fibrogenic proteins such as TGFβ is elevated, while protective growth factors, such as EGF, show a gradual decline in expression.[139] Growth of the developing kidney remains possible in the presence of partial obstruction but does lag behind that of the non-obstructed contralateral kidney.[140]

Physiological changes in partial obstruction mirror those in complete obstruction. Decreased blood flow is seen in the obstructed kidney with segmental renal arterial constriction.[136] Blood flow is redistributed from the outer to the inner cortex. In the contralateral kidney, there is a compensatory increase in blood flow with similar shunting from outer to inner renal cortex.[137,140] The rise in renal pelvis pressure is lower and more gradual than in complete obstruction, reaching a maximum of 15–20 mmHg at 1 week. It reverts to normal by 2 weeks,[136] but provoked renal pelvis pressures remain elevated at values of 40–50 mmHg with ongoing partial obstruction.[8,137] Following release of partial obstruction, the blood flow in the contralateral kidney returns toward baseline; however, the ability to recover in the obstructed kidney is often compromised. The severity of renal injury and the ability to recover in partial obstruction have been shown to differ with the degree of obstruction[136] and its duration.[112] While there is no change in creatinine clearance after 14 days' partial obstruction, there is a profound decrease after 28 days' obstruction. Some recovery is seen in those obstructed for 28 days, but no recovery is seen 28 days after release of partial obstruction of 60 days' duration.[112] This has obvious implications in timing intervention in patients with UO, particularly those who are symptomless.

CONCLUSIONS

UO covers a broad range of clinical settings, resulting in significant clinical burden in terms of patient discomfort, impairment of renal function and threat to the integrity of the kidney in both acute and chronic settings. Considerable overlap exists in physiological changes between partial and complete, unilateral and bilateral obstruction. Understanding of the vascular and molecular mechanisms underlying cellular injury continues to evolve. This is likely to aid in answering fundamental questions such as how soon intervention is required in UO and how these mechanisms might be exploited to minimize renal injury in UO.

REFERENCES

1. Bell E. Renal Diseases. Philadelphia: Lea & Febiger, 1946
2. Ryan PC, Lennon GM, McLean PA, Fitzpatrick JM. The effects of acute and chronic JJ stent placement on upper urinary tract motility and calculus transit. Br J Urol 1994; 74: 434–439
3. Harmon WJ, Sershon PD, Blute ML, Patterson DE et al. Ureteroscopy: current practice and complications. J Urol 1997; 157: 28–32
4. Grace PA, Gillen P, Smith JM, Fitzpatrick JM. Extracorporeal shock wave lithotripsy with the Lithostar lithotriptor. Br J Urol 1989; 64: 117–121
5. Montini G, Sacchetto E, Murer L, DallAmico R et al. Renal glomerular response to the inhibition of prostaglandin E_2 synthesis and protein loading after the relief of unilateral ureteropelvic junction obstruction. J Urol 2000; 163: 556–560
6. Basar I, Bircan K, Tasar C et al. Diclofenac sodium and spasmolytic drugs in the treatment of ureteral colic: a comparative study. Int Urol Nephrol 1991; 3: 227–230
7. Lennon GM, Bourke J, Ryan PC, Fitzpatrick JM. Pharmacological options for the treatment of ureteric colic. Br J Urol 1993; 71: 401–407
8. Sheehan SJ, Moran KT, Dowsett DJ, Fitzpatrick JM. Renal haemodynamics and prostaglandin synthesis in partial unilateral ureteric obstruction. Urol Res 1994; 22: 279–285
9. Ishidoya S, Morrissey J, McCracken R, Reyes A et al. Angiotensin II receptor antagonist ameliorates renal tubulointerstitial fibrosis caused by unilateral ureteral obstruction. Kidney Int 1995; 47: 1285–1294
10. Hegarty NJ, Young LS, Kirwan CN, O'Neill AJ et al. Nitric oxide in unilateral ureteral obstruction: effect on regional renal blood flow. Kidney Int 2001; 59: 1059–1065
11. Young LS, Hegarty NJ, Fitzpatrick JM. Mechanisms of regional renal blood flow during ureteric obstruction. Surg Forum 1998; 49: 689–690
12. Miyajima A, Chen J, Lawrence C, Ledbetter S et al. Antibody to transforming growth factor-beta ameliorates tubular apoptosis in unilateral ureteral obstruction. Kidney Int 2000; 58: 2301–2313
13. Nagle RB, Bulger RE, Cutler RE, Jervis HR et al. Unilateral obstructive nephropathy in the rabbit. I. Early morphologic, physiologic and histochemical changes. Lab Invest 1973; 28: 456–467
14. Nagle RB, Bulger RE. Unilateral obstructive nephropathy in the rabbit. I. Late morphologic changes. Lab Invest 1978; 38: 270–278
15. Vaughan ED, Sorensen EJ, Gillenwater JY. The renal hemodynamic response to chronic unilateral complete ureteral occlusion. Invest Urol 1970; 8: 78–90
16. Michaelson G. Percutaneous puncture of the renal pelvis, intrapelvic pressure and the concentrating capacity of the kidney in hydronephrosis. Acta Med Scand Suppl 1974; 559: 1–26
17. Backlund L, Nordgren L. Pressure variations in the upper urinary tract and kidney at total ureteric occlusion. Acta Soc Med Ups 1996; 71: 285–301
18. Yarger WE, Griffith LD. Intrarenal hemodynamics following chronic unilateral obstruction in the dog. Am J Physiol 1974; 227: 816–826
19. Moody TE, Vaughan ED, Gillenwater JY. Relationship between renal blood flow and ureteral pressure during 18 hours of total unilateral ureteral occlusion. Invest Urol 1975; 13: 246–251
20. Naber KG, Madsen PO. Renal function in chronic hydronephrosis with and without infection and the role of lymphatics: an experimental study on dogs. Urol Res 1974; 2: 1–9
21. Vaughan ED, Sweet RE, Gillenwater JY. Mechanism of acute hemodynamic response to ureteral occlusion. Invest Urol 1971; 9: 109–118
22. Gaudio KM, Siegel NJ, Hayslett JP, Kashgarian M. Renal perfusion and intratubular pressure during ureteral occlusion in the rat. Am J Physiol 1980; 238: F205–F209
23. Frokiaer J, Djurhuus J, Neilsen M, Pedersen E. Renal haemodynamic response to ureteral obstruction during converting enzyme inhibition. Urol Res 1996; 24: 217–227
24. Wahlberg J, Stenberg A, Wilson DR, Persson AE. Tubuloglomerular feedback and interstitial pressure in obstructive nephropathy. Kidney Int 1984; 26: 294–301
25. Allen JT, Vaughan ED, Gillenwater JY. The effect of indomethacin on renal blood flow and ureteral pressure in unilateral ureteral obstruction in awake dogs. Invest Urol 1978; 15: 324–327
26. Klotman PE, Smith SR, Volpp BD, Coffman TM et al. Thromboxane synthetase inhibition improves function of hydronephrotic rat kidneys. Am J Physiol 1986; 250: F282–F287

27. Hegarty NJ, Young LS, Fitzpatrick JM. Renal vascular changes in chronic ureteric obstruction are mediated by inducible nitric oxide synthase. Surg Forum 1998; 49: 688–689
28. Hegarty NJ, Young LS, O'Neill AJ, Watson RWG et al. Endothelin in unilateral ureteral obstruction – vascular and cellular effects. J Urol 2003; 169: 740–744
29. Hanley MJ, Davidson K. Isolated nephron segments from the rabbit models of obstructive nephropathy. J Clin Invest 1982; 69: 165–174
30. Campbell HT, Bello-Reuss E, Klahr S. Hydraulic water permeability and transepithelial voltage in the isolated perfused rabbit cortical collecting tubule following acute unilateral obstruction. J Clin Invest 1985; 75: 219–225
31. Lear S, Silva P, Kelley VE, Epstein FH. Prostaglandin E_2 inhibits oxygen consumption in rabbit medullary thick ascending limb. Am J Physiol 1990; 258: F1372–F1378
32. Stokes JB, Kokko JP. Inhibition of sodium transport by prostaglandin E_2 across isolated perfused rabbit collecting tubule. J Clin Invest 1977; 59: 1099–1104
33. Buerkert J, Martin D, Head M. Effect of acute ureteral obstruction on terminal collecting duct function in the weanling rat. Am J Physiol 1979; 236: F260–F267
34. Buerkert J, Head M, Klahr S. Effect of acute bilateral ureteral obstruction on deep nephron and terminal collecting duct function in the young rat. J Clin Invest 1977; 59: 1055–1065
35. Zeidel ML, Strange K, Emma F, Harris HW Jr. Mechanisms and regulation of water transport in the kidney. Semin Nephrol 1993; 13: 155–167
36. Harris HW Jr, Strange K, Zeidel ML. Current understanding of the cellular biology and molecular structure of the antidiuretic hormone-stimulated water transport pathway. J Clin Invest 1991; 81: 1–8
37. Ribiero C, Suki WN. Acidification in the medullary collecting duct following ureteral obstruction. Kidney Int 1986; 29: 1167–1171
38. Laski ME, Kurtzman NA. Site of the acidification defect in the perfused postobstructed collecting tubule. Miner Electrolyte Metab 1989; 15: 195–200
39. Blondin J, Purkerson ML, Rolf D, Schoolwerth AC et al. Renal function and metabolism after relief of unilateral ureteral obstruction. Proc Soc Exp Biol Med 1975; 150: 71–76
40. Klahr S, Schwab SJ, Stokes TJ. Metabolic adaptations of the nephron in renal disease. Kidney Int 1986; 29: 80–89
41. Eaim-Ong S, Dafnis E, Spohn M, Kurtzman NA, et al. H-K-ATPase in distal renal tubular acidosis: urinary tract obstruction, lithium, and amiloride. Am J Physiol 1993; 265: F875–F880
42. Sabatini S, Kurtzman NA. Enzyme activity in obstructive uropathy: basis for salt wastage and the acidification defect. Kidney Int 1990; 37: 79–84
43. Reyes AA, Karl IE, Yates J, Klahr S. Low plasma and renal tissue levels of L-arginine in rats with obstructive nephropathy. Kidney Int 1994; 45: 782–787
44. Heinert GG, Rauh W, Scherberich JE, Mondorf WA et al. Quantitative enzymatic histophotometry of morphologic alterations caused by urologically relevant tubular kidney damages using computed image analysis device technique. Urol Int 1981; 36: 178–193
45. Huang H, Chen J, Chen C. Circulating adhesion molecules and neutral endopeptidase enzymuria in patients with urolithiasis and hydronephrosis. Urology 2000; 55: 961–965
46. Schreiner GF, Harris KPG, Purkerson ML, Klahr S. Immunological aspects of acute ureteral obstruction: immune cell infiltrate in the kidney. Kidney Int 1988; 34: 487–493
47. Bouchier-Hayes DM, Young LS, Fitzpatrick JM. Role of the activated neutrophil and nitric oxide in ureteric obstruction. Surg Forum 1997; 48: 778–790
48. Walker PD. Alterations in renal tubular extracellular matrix components after ischemia-reperfusion injury to the kidney. Lab Invest 1994; 70: 339–346
49. Kaneto H, Morrissey J, McCracken R, Reyes A et al. Enalapril reduces collagen type IV synthesis and expansion of the interstitium in the obstructed rat kidney. Kidney Int 1994; 45: 1637–1647
50. Gonzáalez-Avila G, Vadillo-Ortega F, Pérez-Tamayo R. Experimental diffuse interstitial renal fibrosis. A biochemical approach. Lab Invest 1988; 59: 245–252
51. Norman JT, Gatti L, Wilson PD, Lewis M. Matrix metalloproteinases and tissue inhibitor of matrix metalloproteinases expression by tubular epithelia and interstitial fibroblasts in the normal kidney and in fibrosis. Exper Nephrol 1995; 3: 88–89
52. Sharma AK, Mauer SM, Kim Y, Michael AF. Altered expression of matrix metalloproteinase-2, TIMP, and TIMP-2 in obstructive nephropathy. J Lab Clin Med 1995; 125: 754–761
53. Engelmyer E, van Goor H, Edwards DR, Diamond JR. Differential mRNA expression of renal cortical tissue inhibitor of metalloproteinase-1, -2 and -3 in experimental hydronephrosis. J Am Soc Nephrol 1995; 5: 1675–1683

54. Eddy AA, Giachelli CM. Renal expression of genes that promote interstitial inflammation and fibrosis in rats with protein-overload proteinuria. Kidney Int 1995; 47: 1546–1557
55. Rovin BH, Harris KG, Morrison A, Klahr S et al. Renal cortical release of a specific macrophage chemoattractant in response to ureteral obstruction. Lab Invest 1990; 63: 213–220
56. Diamond JR, Kees-Folts D, Ding G, Frye JE et al. Macrophages, monocyte peptide-1 and TGF-β1 in experimental hydronephrosis. Am J Physiol 1994; 266: F926–F993
57. Kaneto H, Morrissey J, Klahr S. Increased expression of TGF-β1 mRNA in the obstructed kidney of rats with unilateral ligation. Kidney Int 1994; 44: 313–321
58. Kaneto H, Morrissey J, McCracken R, Ishidoya S et al. The expression of mRNA for tumor necrosis factor α increases in the obstructed kidney of rats soon after unilateral ureteral ligation. Nephrology 1996; 2: 161–166
59. Diamond JR, Kees-Folts D, Ricardo SD, Pruznak A et al. Early and persistent up-regulated expression of renal cortical osteopontin in experimental hydronephrosis. Am J Pathol 1995; 136: 1455–1466
60. Ricardo SD, Levinson ME, DeJoseph MR, Diamond JR. Expression of adhesion molecules in rat renal cortex during experimental hydronephrosis. Kidney Int 1996; 50: 2002–2010
61. Duan L, Morrissey J, McCracken R, Klahr S. Regulation of MCP-1, ICAM-1 and VCAM-1 during unilateral ureteral obstruction [abstract]. J Am Soc Nephrol 1996; 7: 1697
62. Harris KPG, Schreiner GF, Klahr S. Effect of leukocyte depletion on the function of the post-obstructed kidney in the rat. Kidney Int 1989; 36: 210–215
63. Shappell SB, Gurpinar T, Lechago J, Suki WN et al. Chronic obstructive uropathy in severe combined immunodeficient (SCID) mice: lymphocyte infiltration is not required for progressive tubulointerstitial injury. J Am Soc Nephrol 1998; 9: 1008–1017
64. Wrana JL, Attisano L, Wiieser R, Ventura F et al. Mechanism of activation of the TGF-beta receptor. Nature 1994; 370: 341–347
65. Markowitz SD, Roberts AB. Tumor suppressor activity of the TGF-beta pathway in human cancers. Cytokine Growth Factor Rev 1996; 7: 93–102
66. Border WA, Noble NA. Transforming growth factor β in tissue fibrosis. N Engl J Med 1994; 331: 1286–1292
67. Sharma K, Ziyadeh FN. The emerging role of transforming growth factor-β in kidney diseases. Am J Physiol 1994; 266: F829–F842
68. Border WA, Okuda S, Languino LR, Sporn MB et al. Suppression of experimental glomerulonephritis by antiserum against growth factor beta 1. Nature 1990; 346: 371–374
69. Kasuga H, Ito Y, Sakamoto S, Kawachi H et al. Effects of anti-TGF-beta type II receptor antibody on experimental glomerulonephritis. Kidney Int 2001; 60: 1745–1755
70. Hill C, Flyvbjerg A, Rasch R, Bak M et al. Transforming growth factor-beta 2 antibody attenuates fibrosis in the experimental diabetic rat kidney. J Endocrinol 2001; 170: 647–651
71. Chen S, Hong SW, Iglesias-de la Cruz MC, Isono M et al. The key role of transforming growth factor-beta system in the pathogenesis of diabetic nephropathy. Ren Fail 2001; 23: 471–481
72. Islam M, Burke JF, Jr, McGowan TA, Zhu Y et al. Effects of anti-transforming growth factor-beta antibodies in cyclosporine-induced renal dysfunction. Kidney Int 2001; 59: 498–506
73. Wolf G, Mueller E, Stahl RAK, Ziyadeh FN. Angiotensin II-induced hypertrophy of cultured murine proximal tubular cells is mediated by endogenous transforming growth factor-β. J Clin Invest 1993; 92: 1366–1372
74. Pimental JL, Jr, Sundell CL, Wang S, Kopp JB et al. Role of angiotensin II in the expression and regulation of transforming growth factor-β in obstructive nephropathy. Kidney Int 1995; 48: 1233–1246
75. Niimura F, Labosky PA, Kakuchi J, Okuba S et al. Gene targetting in mice reveals a requirement for angiotensin in the development and maintenance of kidney morphology and growth factor regulation. J Clin Invest 1995; 96: 2947–2954
76. Tang WW, Ulich TR, Lacey DL, Hill DC et al. Platelet-derived growth factor-BB induces renal tubulointerstitial myofibroblast formation and tubulointerstitial fibrosis. Am J Pathol 1996; 148: 1169–1180
77. Basile DP, Liapis H, Hammerman MR. Increased transforming growth factor-β1 expression in regenerating rat tubules following ischemic injury. Am J Physiol 1997; 272: F640–F647
78. Gobe GC, Axelsen RA. Genesis of renal tubular atrophy in experimental hydronephrosis in the rat. Role of apoptosis. Lab Invest 1987; 56: 273–281

79. Wyllie AH, Kerr JFR, Currie AR. Cell death: the significance of apoptosis. Int Rev Cytol 1980; 68: 251–305
80. Jones EA, Shahed A, Shoskes DA. Modulation of apoptotic and inflammatory genes by bioflavonoids and angiotensin II inhibition in ureteral obstruction. Urology 2000; 56: 346–351
81. Choi YJ, Baranowska-Daca E, Nguyen V, Koji T et al. Mechanism of chronic obstructive uropathy: increased expression of apoptosis-promoting molecules. Kidney Int 2000; 58: 1481–1491
82. Hughes J, Johnson RJ. Role of Fas (CD95) in tubulointerstitial disease induced by unilateral ureteric obstruction. Am J Physiol 1999; 277: F26–F32
83. Truong LD, Choi YJ, Tsao CC, Ayala G et al. Renal cell apoptosis in chronic obstructive uropathy: the roles of caspases. Kidney Int 2001; 60: 924–934
84. Liapis H, Yu H, Steinhardt GF. Cell proliferation, apoptosis, Bcl-2 and Bax expression in obstructed opossum early metanephroi. J Urol 2000; 164: 511–517
85. Zhang G, Oldroyd SD, Huang LH, Yang B et al. Role of apoptosis and Bcl-2/Bax in the development of tubulointerstitial fibrosis during experimental obstructive nephropathy. Exp Nephrol 2001; 9: 71–80
86. Chevalier RL, Smith CD, Wolstenholme J, Krajewski S et al. Chronic ureteral obstruction in the rat suppresses renal tubular Bcl-2 and stimulates apoptosis. Exp Nephrol 2000; 8: 115–122
87. Frisch SM, Francis H. Disruption of epithelial cell–matrix interactions induces apoptosis. J Cell Biol 1994; 124: 619–626
88. Shappell SB, Mendoza LH, Gurpinar T, Smith CW et al. Expression of adhesion molecules in kidney with experimental chronic obstructive uropathy: the pathogenic role of ICAM-1 and VCAM-1. Nephron 2000; 85: 156–166
89. Cheng QL, Chen XM, Li F, Lin HL et al. Effects of ICAM-1 antisense oligonucleotide on the tubulointerstitium in mice with unilateral ureteral obstruction. Kidney Int 2000; 57: 183–190
90. Lange-Sperandio B, Cachat F, Thornhill BA, Chevalier RL. Selectins mediate macrophage infiltration in obstructive nephropathy in newborn mice. Kidney Int 2002; 61: 516–524
91. Naruse T, Yuzawa Y, Akahori T, Mizuno M et al. P-selectin-dependent macrophage migration into the tubulointerstitium in unilateral ureteral obstruction. Kidney Int 2002; 62: 94–105
92. Hegarty NJ, Watson RWG, Young LS, O'Neill AJ et al. Cytoprotective effects of nitrates in a cellular model of hydronephrosis. Kidney Int 2002; 62: 70–77
93. Sommer M, Eismann U, Deuther-Conrad W, Wendt T et al. Time course of cytokine mRNA expression in kidneys of rats with unilateral ureteral obstruction. Nephron 2000; 84: 49–57
94. Kennedy WA 2nd, Buttyan R, Garcia-Montes E, D'Agati V et al. Epidermal growth factor suppresses renal tubular apoptosis following ureteral obstruction. Urology 1997; 49: 973–980
95. Mizuno S, Matsumoto K, Nakamura T. Hepatocyte growth factor suppresses interstitial fibrosis in a mouse model of obstructive nephropathy. Kidney Int 2001; 59: 1304–1314
96. Yang J, Liu Y. Blockage of tubular epithelial to myofibroblast transition by hepatocyte growth factor prevents renal interstitial fibrosis. J Am Soc Nephrol 2002; 13: 96–107
97. Chevalier RL, Goyal S, Kim A, Chang AY et al. Renal tubulointerstitial injury from ureteral obstruction in the neonatal rat is attenuated by IGF-1. Kidney Int 2000; 57: 882–890
98. Jones SE, Jomary C. Clusterin. Int J Biochem Cell Biol 2002; 34: 427–431
99. Schlegel PN, Matthews GJ, Cichon Z, Aulitzky WK et al. Clusterin production in the obstructed rabbit kidney: correlations with loss of renal function. J Am Soc Nephrol 1992; 3: 1163–1171
100. Chung KH, Gomez RA, Chevalier RL. Regulation of renal growth factors and clusterin by AT1 receptors during neonatal ureteral obstruction. Am J Physiol 1995; 268: F1117–1123
101. Sakai T, Tanaka H, Shirasawa T. Two distinct epithelial responses may compensate for the ureteral obstruction in early and late phase of unilateral ureteral obstruction-treated rat: cellular proliferation in acute phase and osteopontin expression in chronic phase. Nephron 1997; 77: 340–345
102. Levine AJ, Momand J, Finlay CA. The p53 tumour suppressor gene. Nature 1991; 351: 453–456
103. Choi YJ, Mendoza L, Rha SJ, Sheikh-Hamad D et al. Role of p53-dependent activation of caspases in chronic obstructive uropathy: evidence from p53 null mutant mice. J Am Soc Nephrol 2001; 12: 983–992
104. Morrissey JJ, Ishidoya S, McCracken R, Klahr S. Control of p53 and p21 (WAF1) expression during unilateral ureteral obstruction. Kidney Int Suppl 1996; 57: S84–S92

105. Vaughan ED, Gillenwater JY. Recovery following complete chronic unilateral ureteral occlusion: functional, radiographic and pathologic alteration. J Urol 1971; 106: 27–35
106. Dal Canton A, Corradi A, Stanziale R, Maruccio G et al. Effects of 24-hour unilateral ureteral obstruction on glomerular haemodynamics in rat kidney. Kidney Int 1979; 15: 457–462
107. Jones DA, George NJ, O'Reilly PH, Barnard RJ. The biphasic nature of renal functional recovery following relief of chronic obstructive uropathy. Br J Urol 1988; 61: 192–197
108. Bander SJ, Buerkert JE, Martin D, Klahr S. Long-term effects of 24-hr unilateral ureteral obstruction on renal function in the rat. Kidney Int 1985; 28: 614–620
109. Thirakomen K, Kozlov N, Arruda JA, Kurtzman NA. Renal hydrogen ion secretion after release of unilateral ureteral obstruction. Am J Physiol 1976; 231: 1233–1239
110. Rodriguez-Soriano J, Vallo A, Oliveros R, Castillo G. Transient pseudohypoaldosteronism secondary to obstructive uropathy in infancy. J Pediatr 1983; 103: 375–380
111. Castle WN, McDougal WS. Contralateral renal hyperplasia and increased renal function after relief of chronic unilateral ureteral obstruction. J Urol 1984; 132: 1016–1020
112. Leahy AL, Ryan PC, McEntee GM, Nelson AC et al. Renal injury and recovery in partial ureteric obstruction. J Urol 1989; 142: 199–203
113. Morozumi M, Ogawa Y, Fujime M, Kitagawa R. Distal ureteral atresia associated with crossed renal ectopia with fusion: recovery of renal function after a release of a 10-year ureteral obstruction. Int J Urol 1997; 4: 512–515
114. Upsdell SM, Gupta S, Gough DC. The radionuclide assessment of prenatally diagnosed hydronephrosis. Br J Urol 1994; 74: 31–34
115. Hinman F. Renal counterbalance. An experimental and clinical study with reference to the significance of disuse atrophy. Trans Am Assoc Genitourin Surg 1922; 15: 241–385
116. Paulson DF, Frawley EE. Compensatory renal growth after unilateral ureteral obstruction. Kidney Int 1973; 4: 22–27
117. Northrup RE, Malvin RL. Cellular hypertrophy and function during compensatory regrowth. Am J Physiol 1976; 231: 1191–1195
118. Halliburton IW, Thomson RY. Chemical aspects of compensatory renal hypertrophy. Cancer Res 1965; 25: 1882–1887
119. Toback FG, Smith PD, Lowenstein L. Phospholipid metabolism in the initiation of renal compensatory growth after acute reduction of renal mass. J Clin Invest 1974; 54: 91–97
120. Goss RJ, Rankin M. Physiological factors affecting compensatory renal hyperplasia in the rat. J Exp Zool 1960; 45: 209–216
121. Ogden DA. Donor and recipient function 2 to 4 years after renal homotransplantations. Ann Intern Med 1967; 67: 998–1006
122. Hayslett JP. Effect of age on compensatory renal growth. Kidney Int 1983; 23: 599–602
123. Galla JH, Klein-Robbenhaar T, Hayslett JP. Influence of age on the compensatory response in growth and function to unilateral nephrectomy. Yale J Biol Med 1974; 47: 218–226
124. Taki M, Goldsmith DI, Spitzer A. Impact of age on effects of ureteral obstruction on renal function. Kidney Int 1983; 24: 602–609
125. Francisco LL, Hoversten LG, DiBona GF. Renal nerves in the compensatory adaptation to ureteral occlusion. Am J Physiol 1980; 238: F229–F234
126. Kelleher JP, Shah V, Godley ML, Wakefield AJ et al. Urinary endothelin (ET-1) in complete ureteric obstruction in the miniature pig. Urol Res 1992; 20: 63–65
127. Dal Canton A, Corradi A, Stanziale R, Maruccio G et al. Glomerular haemodynamics before and after release of 24-hour bilateral ureteral obstruction. Kidney Int 1980; 17: 491–496
128. Moody TE, Vaughan ED Jr, Gillenwater JY. Comparison of the renal hemodynamic response to unilateral and bilateral ureteral occlusion. Invest Urol 1977; 14: 455–459
129. Mujais SK. Transport enzymes and renal tubular acidosis. Semin Nephrol 1998; 18: 74–82
130. Peterson LJ, Yarger WE, Schocken DD, Glenn JF. Post-obstructive diuresis: a varied syndrome. J Urol 1975; 113: 190–194
131. Muldowney FP, Duffy GJ, Kelly DG, Duff FA et al. Sodium diuresis after relief of obstructive uropathy. N Engl J Med 1966; 274: 1294–1298
132. Howards SS. Post-obstructive diuresis: a misunderstood phenomenon. J Urol 1973; 110: 537–540
133. Whitaker RH. Methods of assessing obstruction in dilated ureters. Br J Urol 1973; 45: 15–22

134. Ulm A, Miller F. An operation to produce experimental, reversible hydronephrosis in dogs. J Urol 1962; 88: 337–341
135. Ryan PC, Fitzpatrick JM. Partial ureteric obstruction: a new variable canine model. J Urol 1987; 137: 1034–1038
136. Ryan PC, Maher KP, Murphy B, Hurley GD et al. Experimental partial ureteric obstruction: pathophysiological changes in upper tract pressures and renal blood flow. J Urol 1987; 138: 674–678
137. Grace PA, Gillen P, Dowsett DJ, Fitzpatrick JM. Partial unilateral ureteral obstruction alters regional renal blood flow. World J Urol 1990; 8: 170–174
138. Chevalier RL, Sturgill BC, Jones CE, Kaiser DL. Morphologic correlates of renal growth arrest in neonatal partial ureteral obstruction. Pediatr Res 1987; 21: 338–346
139. Kennedy WA, Stenberg A, Lackgren G, Hensle TW et al. Renal tubular apoptosis after partial ureteral obstruction. J Urol 1994; 152: 658–664
140. Nguyen HT, Kogan BA. Renal haemodynamic changes after complete and partial unilateral obstruction in the foetal lamb. J Urol 1998; 160: 1063–1069

8

Interactive obstructive uropathy: Observations and conclusions from studies on humans

Nicholas J R George

It has been known for many years that dysfunctional abnormalities of the lower urinary tract may affect the performance of the upper urinary tract in several respects. Typical examples of such bladder dysfunction include those associated with benign prostatic hypertrophy and the changes which are observed after neurological damage to the spinal cord – the neuropathic bladder. It is recognized that the renal damage caused by such interaction between the lower and upper tract may be *severe*, *silent* and *progressive*, leading to terminal renal failure if the abnormalities are not recognized and corrected.

In this chapter, the basis of our physiological understanding of the mechanisms involved in the interactive urinary tract dysfunctional states will be explored. Animal studies of such abnormalities have been few, partially because of the difficulties with complex animal experimentation and partly because natural models of lower/upper tract dysfunction do not exist. This account therefore deals with human subjects found to have a particular form of bladder dysfunction (high-pressure chronic retention) which is particularly appropriate to demonstrate the physiological changes that occur synchronously within the lower and upper tract. Naturally, all subjects gave informed consent for the procedures, which, being undertaken without any form of anaesthesia, benefited additionally from the ability of the patient to speak and comment throughout on the test procedures. Before I describe the observations and discuss the conclusions of these studies, it is pertinent first to review the historical perspective relating to interactive dysfunction; such an appreciation explains previous misunderstandings and lays a more secure foundation for a rational understanding of the interactive disorder.

HISTORICAL PERSPECTIVE

In the 1840s dissections by Guthrie in Britain and Civiale in France identified a number of abnormalities in the region of the bladder neck (Figure 8.1). Clearly visible in many cases were large lateral lobes of the prostate with a bladder showing trabeculation and sacculation. However, in a number of cases, there was equivalent detrusor hypertrophy, trabeculation, etc., but little to be seen in the way of prostatic hypertrophy, a thickened median bar at the bladder neck being the only possible source of obstruction (Figure 8.1b). A short while later, again in Paris at the Necker hospital, Professor Guyon described a third type of dysfunctional bladder which was essentially thin-walled yet still associated with typical 'prostatic' symptoms. He called this entity 'prostatisme vesicale'. At the time, the relationship between these three apparently discrete forms of bladder dysfunction was far from clear, and the situation was not assisted by the very high prevalence of lower urinary tract stones and infection (urgency, frequency and incontinence) in both middle-aged and older men.

A hypothesis was however, formed, which in the next 70–100 years became known as 'the three-stage theory of prostatism' (Figure 8.2). In this theory, the bladder first becomes trabeculated and hypertrophied because of outflow tract obstruction, usually

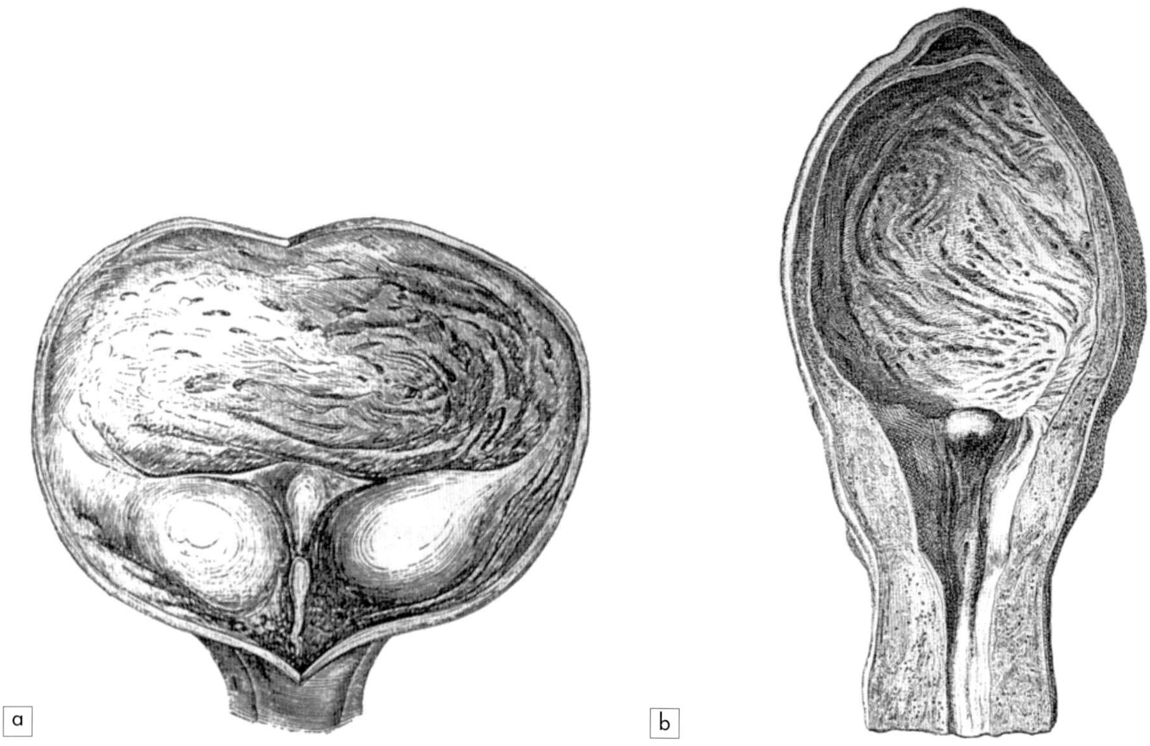

Figure 8.1 *Drawings of original dissections by early investigators.*

as a result of an easily palpable and enlarged prostate. As obstruction develops, sacculation and diverticulum formation take place, and with 'increased pressure' the ureters and subsequently upper tracts dilate, leading to hydronephrosis and eventual renal failure. In the third phase of the classically described course of events, the bladder becomes decompensated – flaccid, large and overdistended. Overflow incontinence was said to occur.

The three-stage theory of prostatism was widely accepted in the latter part of the 19th century and first half of the 20th century, and typical accounts are to be found in urological texts published as late as the 1980s. Examination of the theory, however, revealed inconsistencies which were impossible to explain on a rational basis. In particular, it was not clear why a detrusor muscle that in stage two had developed hypertrophy, trabeculation and sacculation should suddenly give way into a thin-walled atonic bag associated with overflow incontinence and upper tract hydronephrosis.

In fact, an explanation of this dilemma had been offered by some careful observational studies undertaken after World War II. In 1948, Badenoch studied

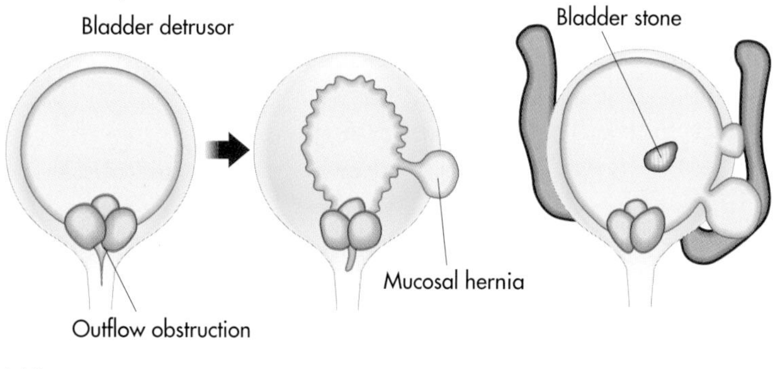

Figure 8.2 *The classically described 'three-stage theory of prostatism'.*

26 patients with bladder neck obstruction (similar to Figure 8.1b) whose mean age was 43, 16 of the patients being under 50 years. He noted no prostatic enlargement whatever in these cases but made the highly significant observation that 25 of the 26 cases had diverticulum formation and bilateral hydroureter with hydronephrosis in the majority. In 1951, Wallace complemented this study. He looked at the association between lateral lobe enlargement, median lobe enlargement, and normal and dilated upper tracts. He found that 89% of patients with large prostatic lateral lobes had no upper tract dilatation, but 72% of patients with bladder neck hypertrophy alone demonstrated clear hydronephrosis with hydroureter.

These studies showed clearly that while upper tract dilatation was indeed related to obstruction, this relatively rarely involved the expected prostatic hypertrophy but was much more strongly correlated with pure bladder neck obstruction. These and other studies eventually led to the conclusion that the unifying three-stage theory of prostatism was unlikely to be correct, and that individual or discrete disorders of the lower urinary tract (that is, bladder neck obstruction or primary atonic/thin-walled bladder) offered a more plausible explanation for the observed clinical symptom complexes. The particular group of patients with upper tract dilatation associated with bladder neck hypertrophy originally described and clarified by Badenoch were subsequently investigated in greater detail, and the advent of sophisticated urodynamic measuring equipment enabled precise recordings of this dysfunctional state – high-pressure chronic retention – to be made for the first time. Simultaneous advances in uroradiology and nephrostomy placement in particular finally made possible for sophisticated simultaneous urodynamic and radiological studies of both upper and lower urinary tracts. This chapter therefore describes and illustrates the physiological interactive changes in both lower and upper tract, using records obtained by the author and colleagues from such studies on patients with uncomplicated (sterile urine) high-pressure chronic retention.

THE MICTURITION CYCLE

It is important to consider the bladder in terms of the micturition cycle. Traditionally, the terms 'obstruction' and 'blockage' have been associated with difficulty in passing urine, and the idea of blockage has somehow become extended to the upper tracts – rather as in the three-stage theory of prostatism. However a moment's consideration of the micturition cycle (Figure 8.3) shows that the bladder spends very little time indeed on micturition and that the vast percentage of its functional existence is spent in *storage* mode. A normal 70-kg adult will micturate four times in 24 hours passing approximately 1500 ml of urine. Assuming that each micturition takes approximately 1 minute to complete, it is clear that the bladder is contracting for only 0.3% of 24 hours; more emphatically, the bladder is in *storage* phase for 23 hours and 56 minutes of the day. Even in a case severe enough to cause the patient to spend 5 minutes micturating every hour, the bladder still spends 92% of its time in the filling phase.

These simple calculations show that if there is to be any effect of the lower tract on the upper tract, any abnormality thought to be responsible must act chiefly *during the filling phase*. An abnormality during the micturition phase – however severe – would not have sufficient time to act and lead to permanent change in the ureters or renal pelvis. Hence, the state of the bladder during filling is of critical importance to a concept of interactive urinary tract dysfunction, and in this respect the mechanical and physical properties of the bladder wall (bladder compliance) require detailed consideration.

70 kg
1.86 m
Temperate climate
1 ml min^{-1}
1500–1800 ml/24 h

Day/night = 450 ml × 4/0 ml   Each void approx. 1 min

Fill phase	23 h 56 min	99.7%	
Void phase	0.3%	Worst possible case 5/60 min	8%

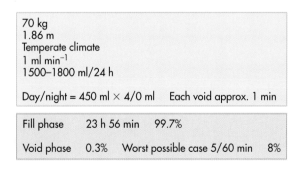

Figure 8.3 *Volumes and events during the micturition cycle.*

THE BLADDER WALL IN HIGH-PRESSURE RETENTION

The bladder wall in patients with high-pressure chronic retention is characteristically thick with massive detrusor hypertrophy. Endoscopically, bars of trabecular muscle stand out, often described as a cathedral roof appearance (Figure 8.4). Histological examination and analysis of sections taken from such trabecular bars (Figure 8.5a and b) show degeneration of the smooth muscle bundles into collagen, as illustrated with the Masson trichrome stain. It is not difficult to imagine that the course of the ureter to the vesicoureteric junction (VUJ) through the wall of such a bladder may well become obstructed. The normal co-apting process of ureteric peristalsis may be lost (Figure 8.6 top); indeed, obstruction at the VUJ may become worse as the bladder empties (Figure 8.6 bottom left). The situation is well illustrated by occasional whole mounts of such bladders (Figure 8.7). Massive trabeculation and hypertrophy may well cause intramural obstruction to the ureter, as seen in Figure 8.7, with a wire probe emerging from the ureteric orifice.

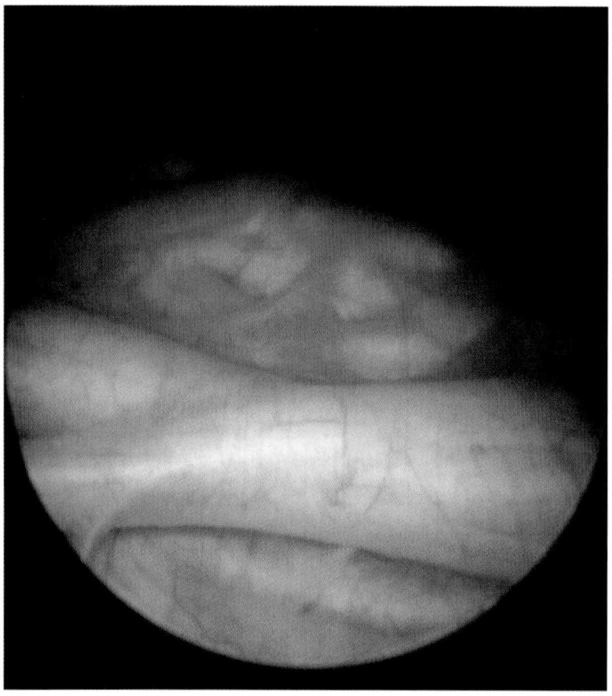

Figure 8.4 *Endoscopic appearance in high-pressure chronic retention.*

EFFECT OF BLADDER WALL HYPERTROPHY

As might be expected, the increase in detrusor muscle mass together with the collagen infiltration illustrated above fundamentally alters the urodynamic characteristics of the bladder as a storage organ. Furthermore, in high-pressure, chronic retention, an intrinsic detrusor pressure remains within the bladder after micturition has been completed, and accurate recording of this intrinsic 'end void' pressure is critical with regard to the analysis of associated renal dysfunction. It is not known at the present time (and it is extremely difficult to determine by experimental means) whether the upper tract dilatation develops as a result of the bladder wall hypertrophy illustrated in Figure 8.6 or as a result of the

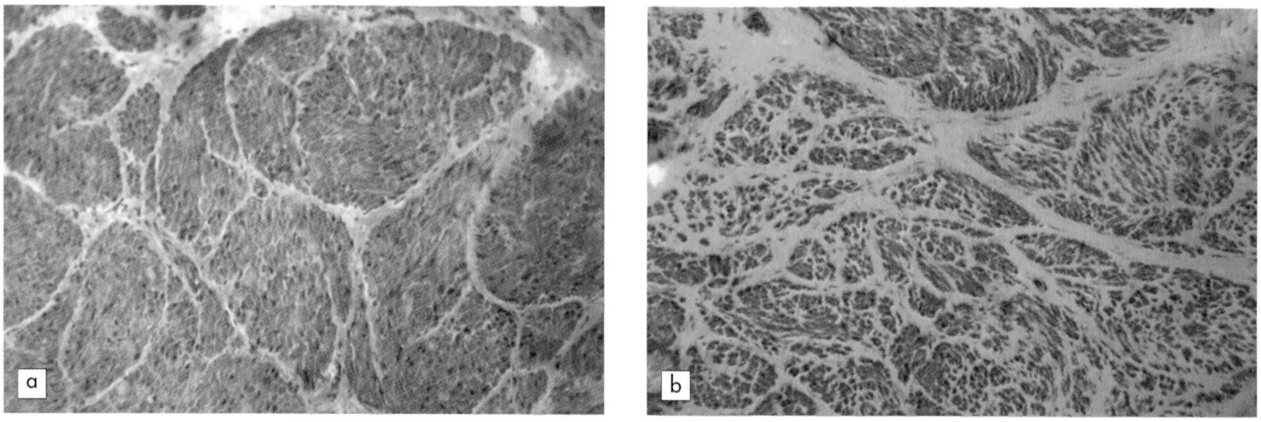

Figure 8.5 *Histological appearances of detrusor muscle in high-pressure chronic retention. Muscle hypertrophy (a) may degenerate (b) with collagen infiltration (green stain).*

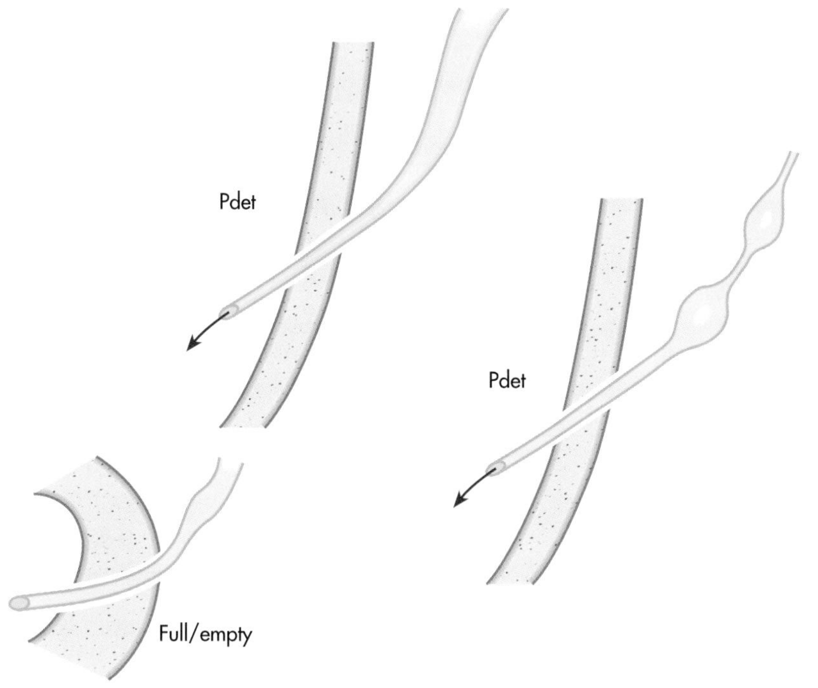

Figure 8.6 *Ureteric passage through thickened detrusor wall. Right, normal; centre, loss of peristalsis; left, increasing wall thickness after micturition.*

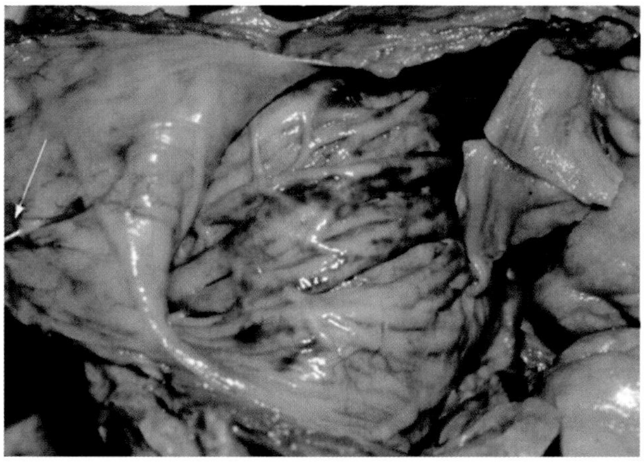

Figure 8.7 *Whole mount bladder from case of high-pressure retention. Note the wire in the ureteric orifice (arrow).*

intrinsic detrusor post-void pressure remaining within the bladder after micturition. This is perhaps a slightly academic point, as regardless of whether pressure precedes hypertrophy or vice versa, the end result – progressive upper tract dilatation – remains the same.

MEASUREMENT OF END VOID PRESSURE

As noted above, the accurate recording of end void pressure is an important measurement which correlates with renal dysfunction. Figure 8.8 illustrates such a measurement taking place. The typical patient with high-pressure retention (painless protuberant bladder) micturates in an entirely normal fashion in private and without any Valsalva manoeuvre (artificial pushing). Following the void, the patient lies on the table, and under local anaesthetic a small needle is placed suprapubically through the abdominal and bladder wall. Fluid rises up the tube as illustrated, clearly demonstrating the end void intrinsic detrusor pressure remaining within the bladder – this can easily be measured with reference to the pubic bone, as is standard practice, and is responsible for the 'high-pressure' name applied to this form of chronic retention.

This simple procedure is important because it exactly mimics the patient's natural state. On occasion, investigators have attempted to obtain such measures following urodynamic investigation of the bladder, during which the organ has almost invariably been filled at supranormal rates. Such abnormal filling rates significantly disrupt the normal working of

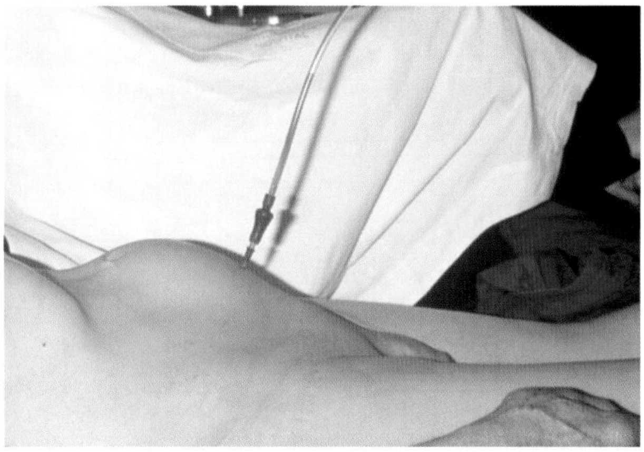

Figure 8.8 *Direct measurements of intrinsic detrusor after void pressure by suprapubic puncture.*

high-pressure bladders, and false recordings are invariably obtained. The measurement of end-void pressure as described above is the simplest and the best method of obtaining the critical pressure which relates to renal dysfunction.

SUMMARY OF URODYNAMIC DATA RELATING TO BLADDERS WITH HIGH-PRESSURE RETENTION

Figure 8.9 illustrates the important concept of the 'pressure cycle' that occurs within the bladder of patients with high-pressure chronic retention. Following micturition (end void point [EVP]), the pressure within the bladder rises as filling takes place from the upper tracts. Eventually, the end fill pressure (EFP) is reached, at which point the patient is experiencing the normal desire to void. A detrusor contraction takes place (over and above the intrinsic pressure within the bladder), and urine is expelled in the usual fashion. At the end of micturition, the pressure returns once again to the EVP, thus completing the pressure 'loop'.

It can thus be seen that in the state of high-pressure chronic retention the bladder fills and empties in cyclical fashion at an abnormally raised pressure *throughout the 24 hours*. Micturition may occur with apparent normality, but at no time are the upper tracts able freely to empty into the bladder storage organ. Thus, it might be predicted that within the upper tracts a similar cycle might be observed – reduced pressure when urine was able to drain easily into the bladder but rising pressure as the bladder filled and passage of urine distally through the vesicoureteric junction became more difficult. This hypothesis is tested by the experiment described below.

Patients with high-pressure retention never drain their bladder below the EVP unless urine is removed artificially. If a catheter is placed in the bladder and urine withdrawn (dashed line), pressure will drop towards zero, and, of course, the suprapubic mass will disappear. As already noted, measurements taken under these circumstances are highly misleading and do not give useful prognostic information regarding renal function.

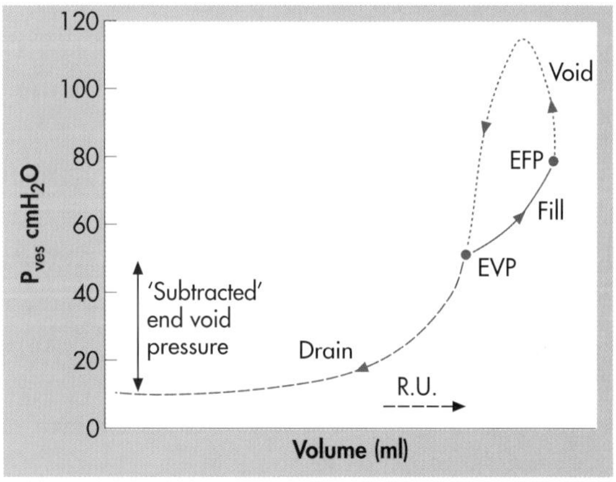

Figure 8.9 *Pressure–volume relationship in high-pressure chronic retention. EFP: end fill pressure; EVP: end void pressure; RU: residual urine.*

SUMMARY OF FILLING-PHASE ABNORMALITIES

The broad categories of filling-phase abnormality that may be seen in the human bladder are noted in Figure 8.10. Normal patients with normal inflow phases have a pressure rise to the physiological bladder capacity (approximately 500 ml) of less than 5 cm water. Cases of *poor compliance* are those in which the bladder pressure rises during filling. This can be easily understood when the bladder wall has been replaced by fibrous tissue such as occurs in interstitial cystitis or tuberculosis, or after radiation therapy. In high-pressure retention, the reduced compliance during filling is related to a

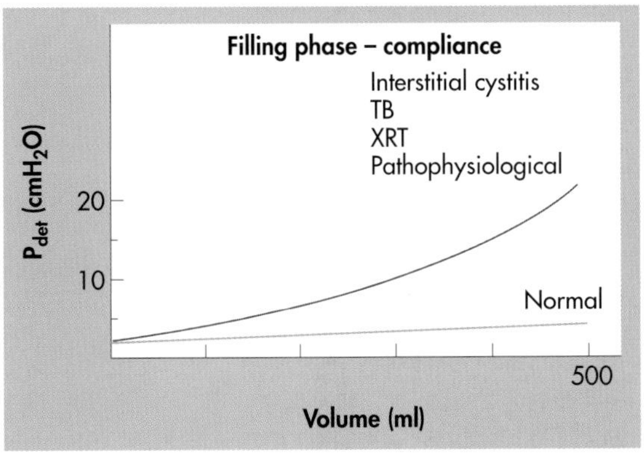

Figure 8.10 *Types of abnormal bladder compliance.*

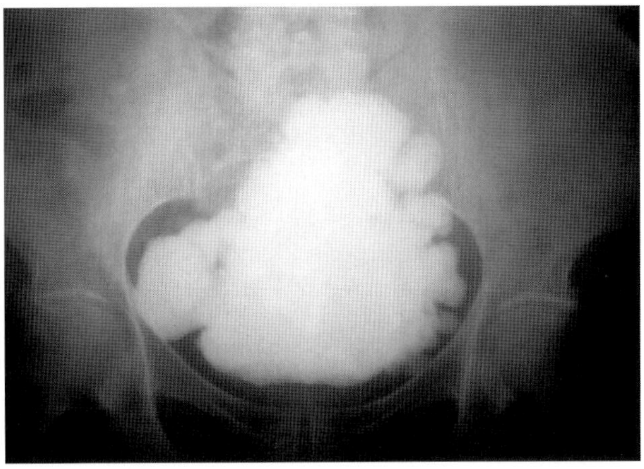

Figure 8.11 *Reflex cystogram in high-pressure retention, demonstrating competent vesicoureteric junction.*

pathophysiological abnormality of smooth muscle – detrusor hypertrophy and associated collagen formation, as illustrated earlier. It is important to note that the depiction of poor compliance in Figure 8.10 is related to abnormal (urodynamic) filling of an initially empty bladder during the test. By contrast, the abnormal pressure relationships seen in Figure 8.9 are purely the result of *natural* filling and voiding characteristics.

The reason for the development of the high-pressure obstructed characteristic remains unknown. Undoubtedly, this detrusor reaction to obstruction may occur with any form of distal urethral lesion, such as dense phimosis, urethral stricture or, in children, urethral valves. Obstruction that involves the prostate rarely seems to lead to the high-pressure type of change (as noted in the historical series). This may be related to the irritation caused by prostatic obstruction, such detrusor instability perhaps protecting against the development of painless retention.

RADIOLOGICAL ASSESSMENT OF HIGH-PRESSURE BLADDERS

Reflux cystograms (Figure 8.10) show, as might be expected, a trabeculated, sacculated picture entirely consistent with the cystoscopic appearance. It might also be expected that reflux would not be seen when one considers the oblique path of the ureter through the massively hypertrophied bladder wall (Figure 8.11). Naturally, for the purpose of these human studies into interactive dysfunction, all patients received cystograms to exclude the possibility of reflux, which would be expected to lead to unrelated and entirely different changes within the upper tracts. In the patients studied, urine was always sterile and reflux never present.

Intravenous urography demonstrates the typical picture of well-preserved renal parenchyma with general distension of the collecting system from the calyces to the vesicoureteric junction (Figure 8.12). Figure 8.12a particularly well illustrates the typical 'snake's head' appearance of high-pressure retention at the lower end of the left ureter – a near certain sign of raised intravesical pressure and a warning, if not otherwise suspected, that renal function might be at risk. Such appearances allow a relatively easy target for a skilled nephrostomist, and the placement of such a tube at last allows the synchronous measurement of upper and lower urinary tract pressures to be contemplated.

INTERACTIVE PRESSURE RECORDINGS IN PATIENTS WITH HIGH-PRESSURE CHRONIC RETENTION AND HYDROURETER/ HYDRONEPHROSIS

Following careful screening to exclude default conditions such as prostate cancer or urinary tract infection, consenting patients underwent the investigation protocol illustrated in Figure 8.13. A nephrostomy tube was placed in the renal pelvis (via

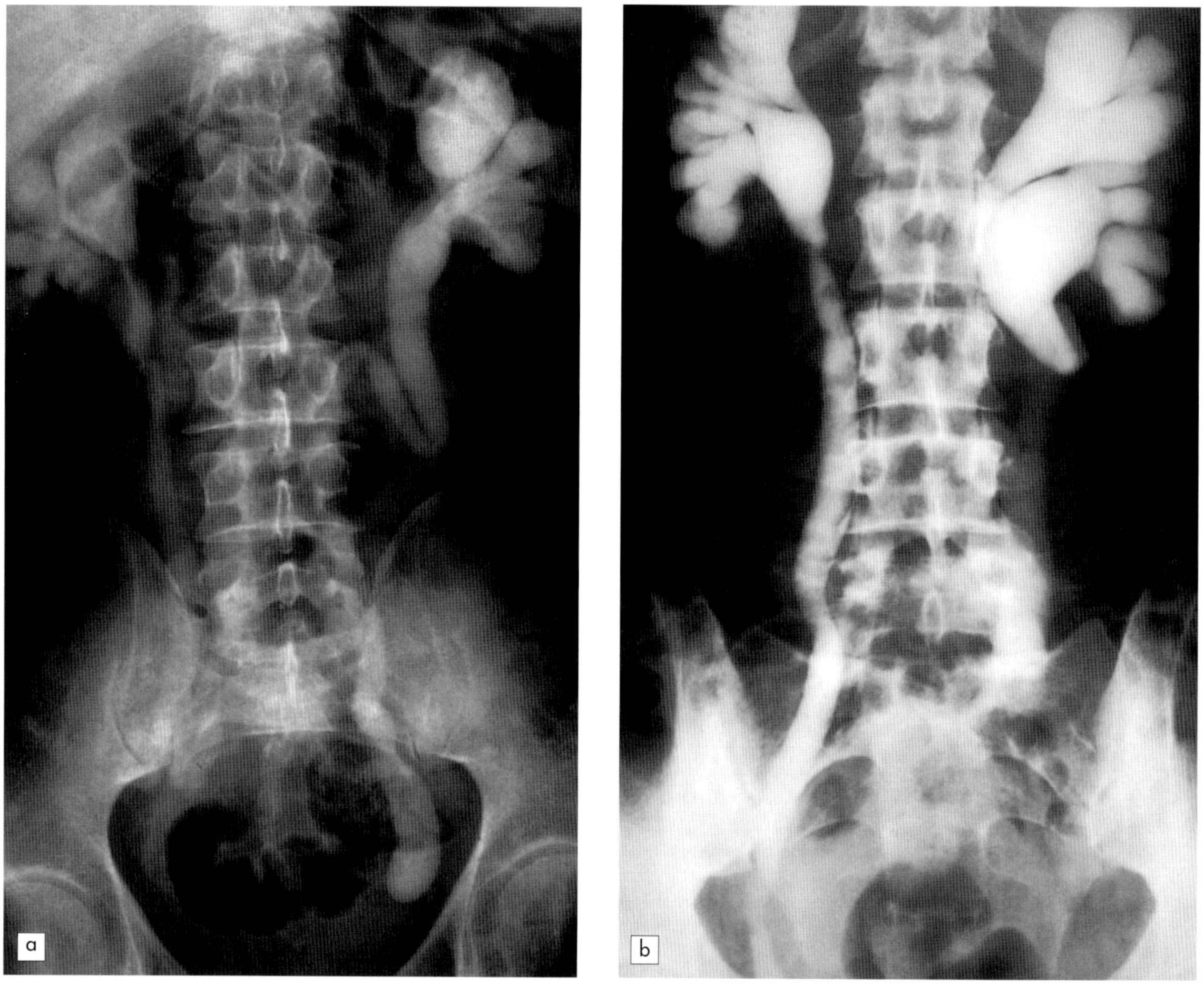

Figure 8.12 *(a, b) Radiological aspects of high-pressure retention.*

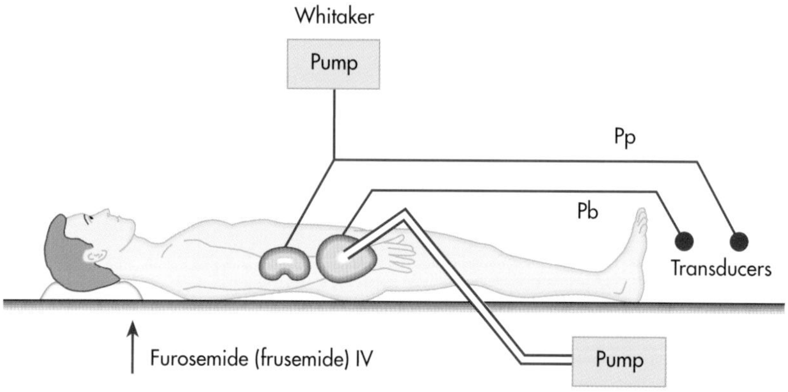

Figure 8.13 *Experimental protocol for bladder and renal pressure measurement.*

the renal substance to avoid leakage) and connected to standard Whitaker pump/measurement apparatus. A suprapubic pressure line was inserted, and finally a urethral catheter allowed bladder volume to be increased or decreased at will. The patient was made warm and comfortable on the investigation table, as the studies took an extended period of time. Patients rarely experienced any discomfort during the tests and commonly fell asleep during measurements.

States of hydration

Three differing states of hydration were identified. Baseline hydration determined that the patient was comfortable – enough water had been drunk to satisfy thirst. Water drinking determined that patients were asked to drink 1–1.5 litres of water fairly rapidly, a load well in excess of what they would normally ingest. A third level of fluid loading was attained by administration of furosemide (frusemide) 0.5 mg/kg IV. These three forms of hydration were used to 'front end load' the urinary tract – that is present differing diuretic loads to the drainage system of the renal mass.

In addition to fluid loads presented to the kidney, it was possible to vary the rate with which the fluid passed through the vesicoureteric junction. This was performed by filling and emptying the bladder through the urethral catheter, the resultant pressure being recorded by the suprapubic pressure line. As will be evident from Figure 8.9, such artificial filling and emptying of the bladder results in marked swings of intrinsic detrusor pressure, which may be expected to affect vesicoureteric transport.

Experimental observations

The results of these experiments are illustrated in Figures 8.14–8.20. During prolonged baseline recordings (Figure 8.14), in which the patient was resting comfortably and simply hydrated, there was no identifiable correlation or connection between bladder and pelvic pressure measurements. Occasional pelvic pressure waves were seen, as were occasional detrusor contractions (unstable waves), but these bore no temporal relationship to each other. Subsequently (Figure 8.15), the bladder was filled at a rate of 60 ml per minute and the effect on bladder and pelvic pressure noted. As expected from the pressure/volume characteristic of high-pressure bladders, the bladder pressure rose rapidly, but at the same time pelvic pressure was also seen to rise, albeit much more slowly. When 100 ml of water was removed from the bladder (Figure 8.16), bladder pressure dropped rapidly, as again would be expected, but pelvic pressure also dropped following the slow initial rise, demonstrating that the artificial 'cycling' of bladder pressure (see above) had induced a form of artificial 'cycling' of the upper tract pressure.

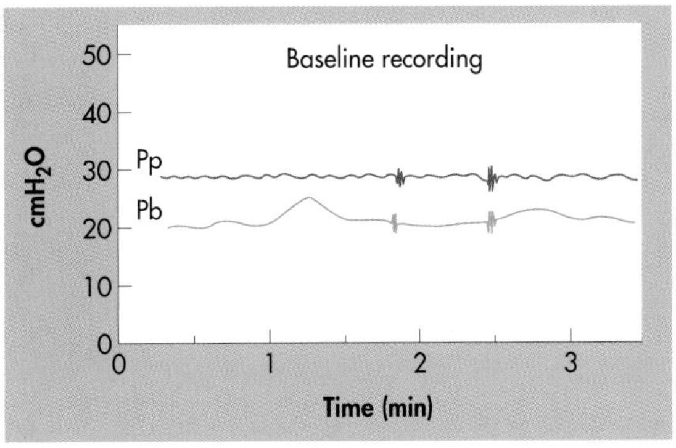

Figure 8.14 *Baseline recordings of renal pelvic (P_p) and bladder (P_b) pressures.*

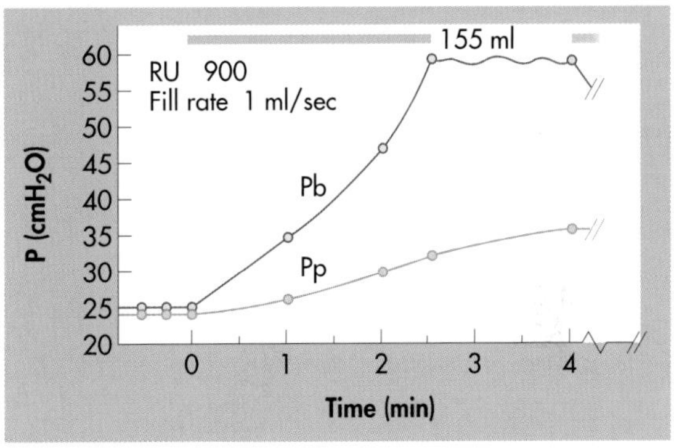

Figure 8.15 *Subsequent pressure variations.*

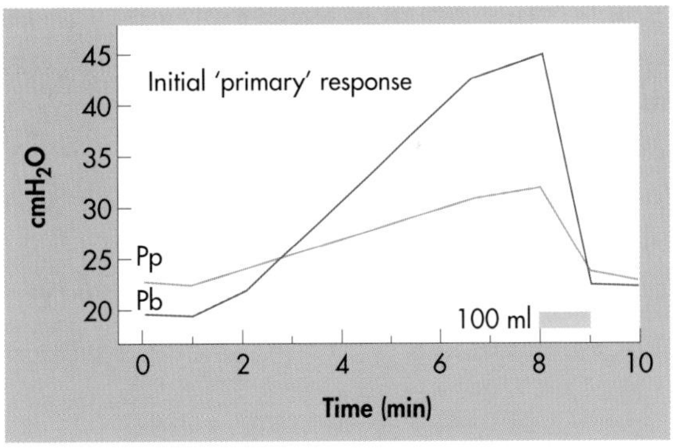

Figure 8.16 *Effect of bladder pressure variation.*

The cycling linkage continued but was more precisely interlinked when oral water loading increased the perfusion pressure at the proximal end of the urinary tract (Figure 8.17). Natural diuresis and subsequent bladder drainage produced sharp swings in bladder and pelvic pressure measurements,

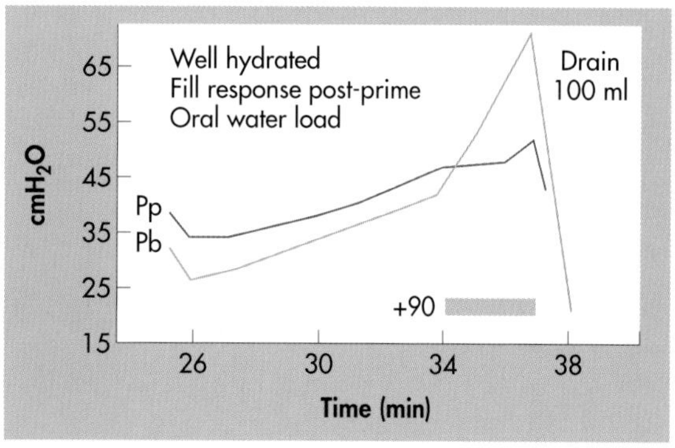

Figure 8.17 *Further pressure variations with water loading and an additional 90 ml in the bladder.*

although, as might be expected, bladder pressure swings were more acute than those seen in the renal pelvis.

Subsequently, under maximal 'front end loading' caused by furosemide (frusemide) IV, bladder pressure cycling via the urethral catheter led to similar sharp swings of pressure being recorded from the renal pelvis. Occasionally, small reductions in pelvic pressure were observed that were not related to any variation of bladder volume; these were thought to represent periods of ureteric 'creep', during which time smooth muscle of the upper urinary tract dilated marginally, thus reducing pressure and accommodating a greater volume. This is the mechanism thought experimentally to account for the development of hydroureter and hydronephrosis over the long term (Figure 8.19).

The interactive pressure experiments are summarized in Figure 8.20. During baseline periods, bladder and renal pressures are dissociated, and variation of bladder pressure in particular has no effect on upper tract distension. However, prolonged increase of bladder pressure (unlikely to be tolerated by the patient) or increased fluid loading/diuretic therapy (a reasonably common occurrence) might well 'prime' the upper tracts, and thereafter pressures within the pelvis may mimic precisely pressures within the bladder. It is very important to appreciate that this synchronous pressure state occurs in the *absence* of the vesicoureteric reflux. The pressure measured within the pelvis is not a reflection of bladder pressure 'passing backwards' up the ureter; it is a pressure required to be exerted by the upper tract if profusion through the vesicoureteric junction is to occur.

It is proposed therefore that these experiments give some insight into the development of hydronephrosis in the simple, uncomplicated (uninfected) case of high-pressure retention. It is now possible to consider what might be the consequences of such changes for renal function. By the same experimental model, it is possible to examine both renographic and biochemical aspects of renal function, and the technique and results of these studies will be briefly described.

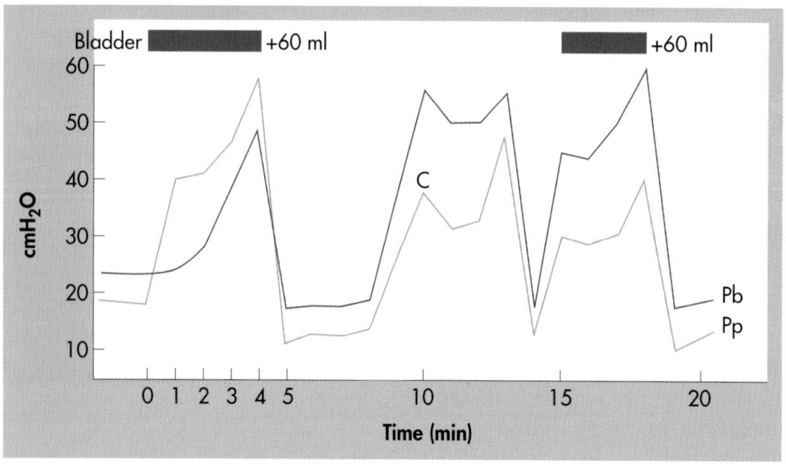

Figure 8.18 *Coordinated pressure movements within bladder and renal pelvis. Drainage volumes not shown. C: Possible time of ureteric 'creep'.*

EXCRETORY FUNCTION MEASURED BY GAMMA CAMERA RENOGRAPHY

It has already been noted that the lack of co-apting peristaltic waves would be likely fundamentally to affect drainage function from the upper urinary tract. The ureter, previously divided into segments, becomes an open column of fluid as hydronephrosis supervenes, and such an open column is capable of exerting forces very dissimilar to those acting in the normal state. It might be hypothesized, for example, that such an open hydroureter would, under certain critical circumstances, exert pressures on the vesicoureteric junction in the vertical position that would not be present in the horizontal position. Clearly, in this respect, the pressure on the other side of the vesicoureteric junction (that is, within the bladder) would be critical, but there might be defined circumstances where significant differences in drainage from the upper tracts would be seen when the patient was in the erect rather than the horizontal position.

Such patients can be identified, and one such is illustrated in Figures 8.21–23. The IVP of this 41-year-old man is not, at first glance, overtly hydronephrotic, but an open hydroureter can be seen on both sides, most marked on the left, and the typical 'snake's head' at the lower end of the ureter typical of high-pressure retention can be seen. The relatively small but high-pressure bladder fails to

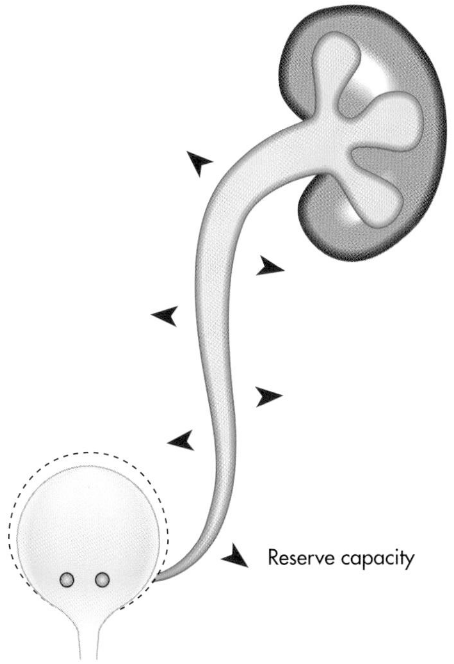

Figure 8.19 *Schematic diagram of ureteric 'creep' – gradual dilatation under stress.*

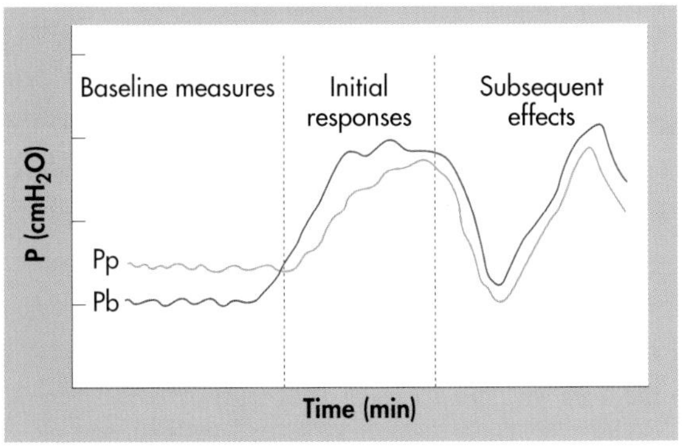

Figure 8.20 *Summary of interactive pressure–volume effects.*

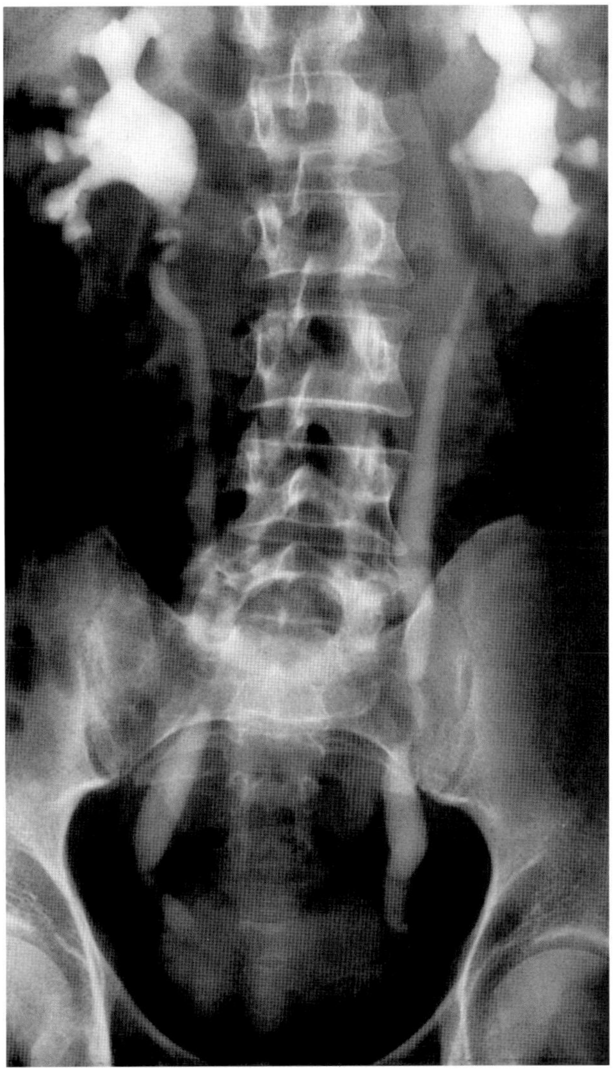

Figure 8.21 *Urographic changes in early high-pressure retention.*

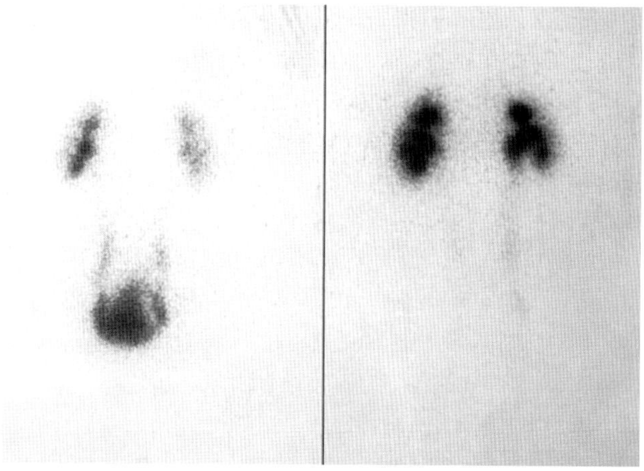

Figure 8.22 *Erect and supine renographic images.*

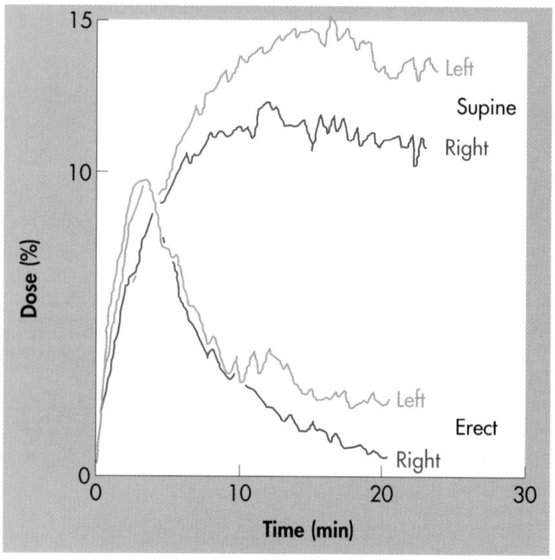

Figure 8.23 *Erect and supine renographic curves.*

opacify. ^{123}I gamma camera renography was performed in erect and supine positions under identical circumstances a few days apart. Figure 8.22 shows accumulated frames between 10 and 15 minutes. The panel showing the erect study clearly demonstrates upper tract drainage, particularly from the left, and bladder filling, while the panel relating to the supine study shows near total stasis within the renal pelvis and calyces and no image whatever of the bladder. Graphical analysis (Figure 8.23) shows equally good uptake for either test but little excretion in the supine position as compared to near normal excretion (renal area of interest demonstrated) in the erect position. This simple study in a young man with early high-pressure retention demonstrates conclusively that drainage through the vesicoureteric junction can be affected by postural conditions; loss of the normal co-apting mechanism might well be responsible for the observations.

GRAVITATIONAL THEORY OF DRAINAGE

This gravitational theory of the open hydroureter may be tested with the human high-pressure retention model (Figure 8.24). In these studies, men with sterile high-pressure retention have a suprapubic line and catheter inserted under local anaesthetic. Thus, the volume and hence pressure within the bladder may be varied at will while the patient is seated or lying in front of a gamma camera.

The results of various studies are depicted in Figures 8.25–8.28. In the first experiment, a man underwent ^{123}I gamma camera renography in the sitting position. He was comfortably hydrated but had been asked not to void prior to the examination. It was thus envisaged that his bladder pressure would be relatively advanced up the pressure–volume curve illustrated in Figure 8.9. Injection of the isotope was given, and the curves elaborated are shown. At 25 minutes, 120 ml of urine was withdrawn through the suprapubic catheter, and the effect on renal clearance of the isotope observed. The acute reduction in intravesical volume and thus pressure allowed vesicoureteric transport to take place, urine from the previously obstructed kidney passing rapidly onwards and down the hydroureter. In Figure 8.26, the same experiment is repeated, but the intravesical pressure is recorded on the same time base as the renogram curves. Under these conditions, little isotope escaped the renal substance until the reduction of the bladder volume once again caused a sharp drop of bladder pressure, following which rapid reduction in isotope counts from the kidney took place. These experiments demonstrate an important hydrodynamic aspect of high-pressure retention. A vertical line drawn at the moment isotope counts begin to reduce (urine leaving the kidney) bisects the intravesical pressure recording at approximately 25 cm of water. Thus, when the intravesical pressure is above this level, little or no drainage occurs from the

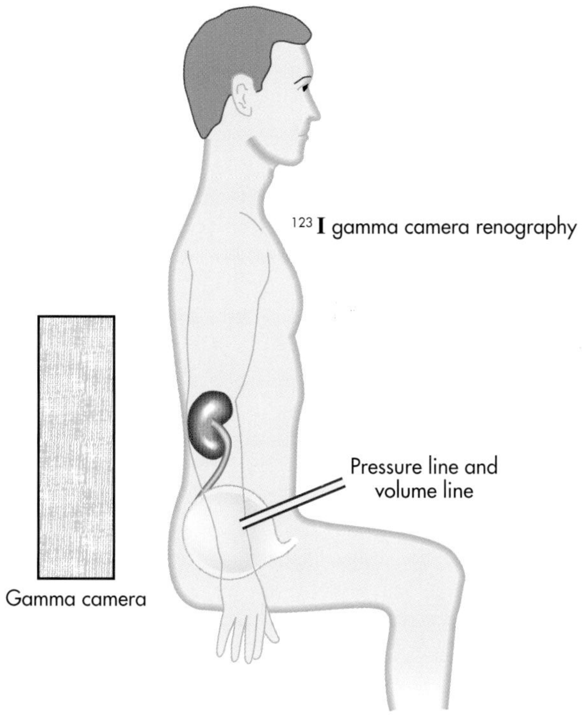

Figure 8.24 *Experimental protocol for drainage experiments.*

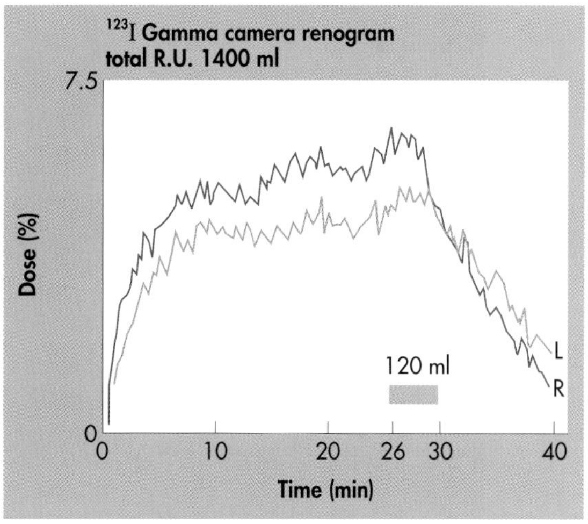

Figure 8.25 *Effect of bladder drainage.*

upper tract. As the pressure falls through 25 cm, rapid drainage starts to commence, suggesting that the figure of 25 cm, is particularly important for the maintenance of upper tract function.

The robust and resilient nature of the lower tract changes are illustrated in Figure 8.27. In these experiments, bladder pressure was recorded as before during gamma camera renography. However, to stimulate to the maximum the upper tract – and thus, if possible, to force perfusion into the bladder – an injection of furosemide (frusemide) was given 15 minutes after the isotope injection. As can be seen, despite this 'front end loading', the renographic counts do not diminish and the renographic curves do not deflect until, once again,

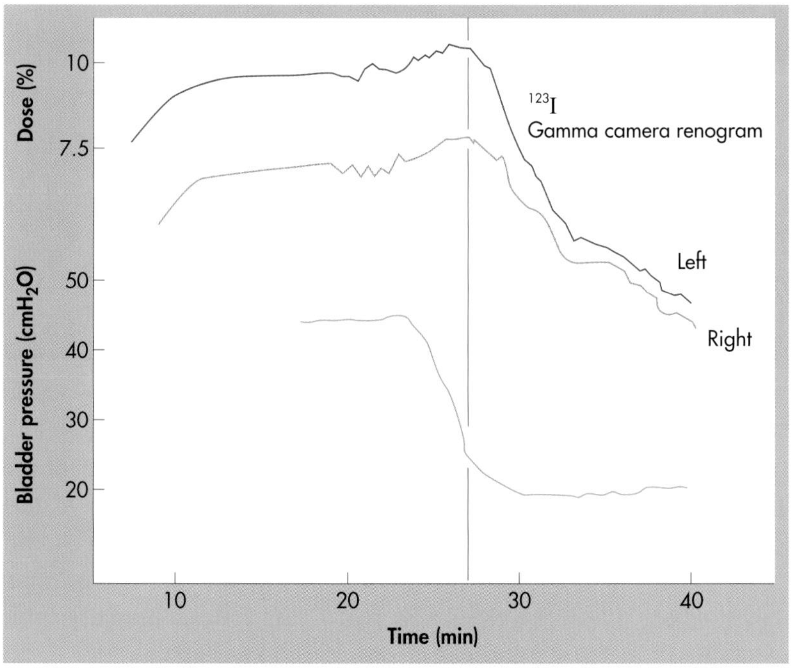

Figure 8.26 *Bladder pressure and renal drainage compared.*

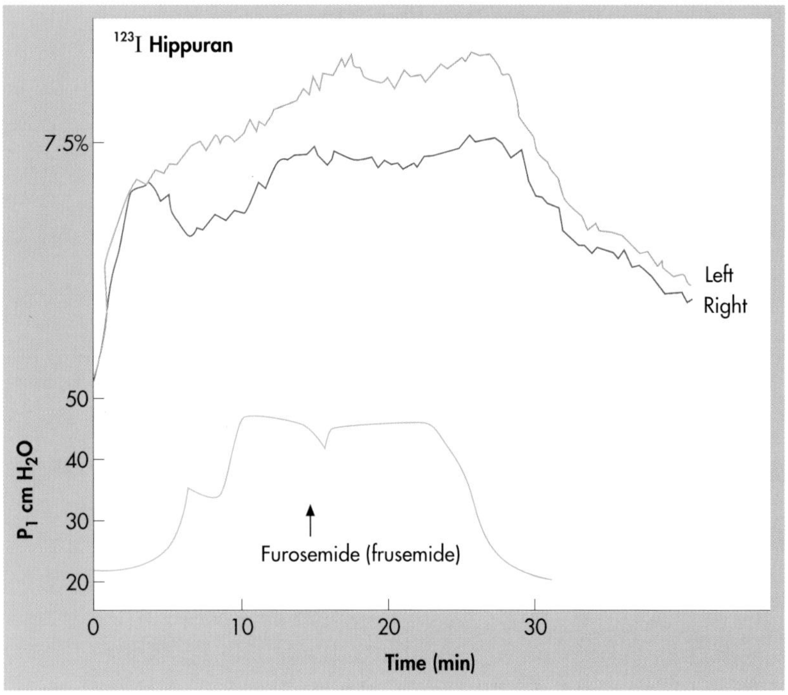

Figure 8.27 *Lack of furosemide (frusemide) effect until bladder drained. See text for details.*

bladder pressure has been significantly reduced by removing fluid from within. Lower tract intrinsic pressure and dynamics appear to dominate renal function, and such an effect may still be seen in relatively advanced obstructive renal failure (Figure 8.28). In this case, relatively poor uptake during gamma camera renography signifies relatively high serum creatinine, but, on draining the bladder, there is still an effect seen in the erect position that is not identified if the renography is carried out supine.

In conclusion, therefore, it is possible to advance an hypothesis on high-pressure chronic retention to account for the variation seen in upper and lower tract pressures. It is postulated that an open hydroureter (approximate length in the adult, 25 cm) (Figure 8.29) may maintain profusion through the vesicoureteric junction as long as the cyclic intrinsic detrusor pressure remains under 25 cm for the majority of the cycle. If the intrinsic detrusor pressure rises to >25 cm for the majority of the filling phase, ureteric stasis should supervene and obstructed renal failure would follow. This hypothesis was explored in the original paper describing high-pressure retention where a graph of intrinsic detrusor pressure against serum creatinine (Figure 8.30) appeared to show that above 25 cm of water

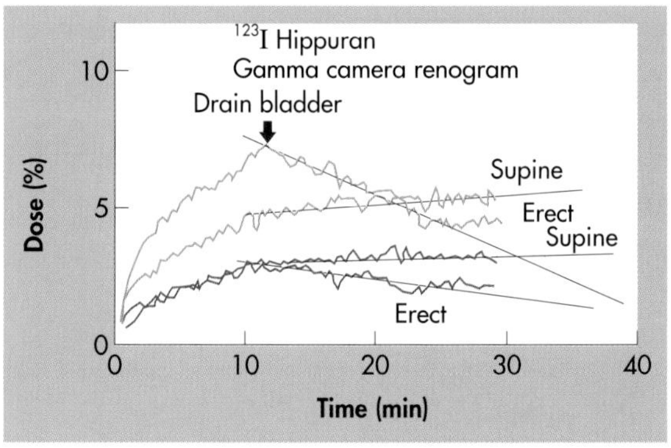

Figure 8.28 *Bladder effect in advanced renal failure.*

there was indeed a steep rise in creatinine, as would be expected from the experimental evidence. Although there were few patients with significantly raised creatinine levels in this series, other results from workers have tended to support the importance of the 25–30-cm water-pressure range with respect to maintenance of renal profusion and function. Similar figures also guide those who reconstruct the bladder, who should ensure that either tonic or phasic reservoir contraction waves do not reach this critical pressure limit for significant periods of the 24 hours.

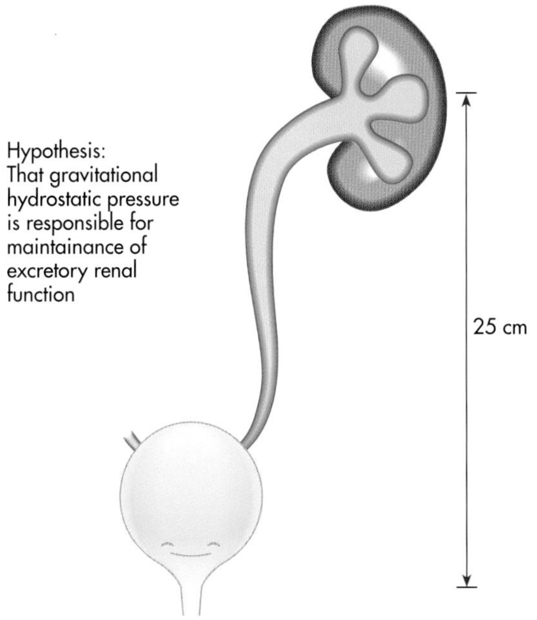

Figure 8.29 *Hypothesis for gravitational theory in open hydroureter.*

BIOCHEMICAL STUDIES BEFORE AND AFTER THE RELIEF OF OBSTRUCTION

This subject has been extensively studied in the literature and in our own department during the last few years by Jones and co-workers. An understanding of the abnormalities of tubular function that may occur under such circumstances is important for the practising urologist, who not infrequently has to manage a patient with post-obstructive diuresis on the urology ward. Absolute volumes (Figure 8.31) and electrolyte excretion (Figure 8.32) are maximal within 24 hours and usually stabilize by 14 days. Synchronous studies of glomerular filtration rate by various mechanisms (Figure 8.33) illustrate that most of the early improvement is related to tubular recovery, although a late glomerular recovery phase can be identified. Precisely similar urodynamic, renographic and biochemical changes may be seen in children as well as adults – infants and children with urethral valves

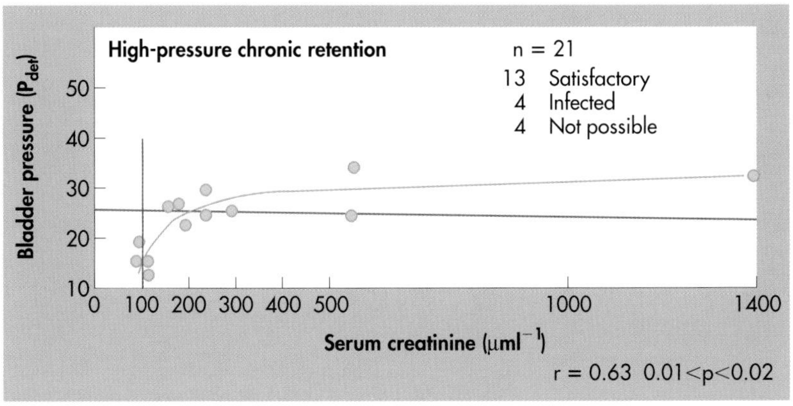

Figure 8.30 *Intrinsic detrusor pressure related to serum creatinine.*

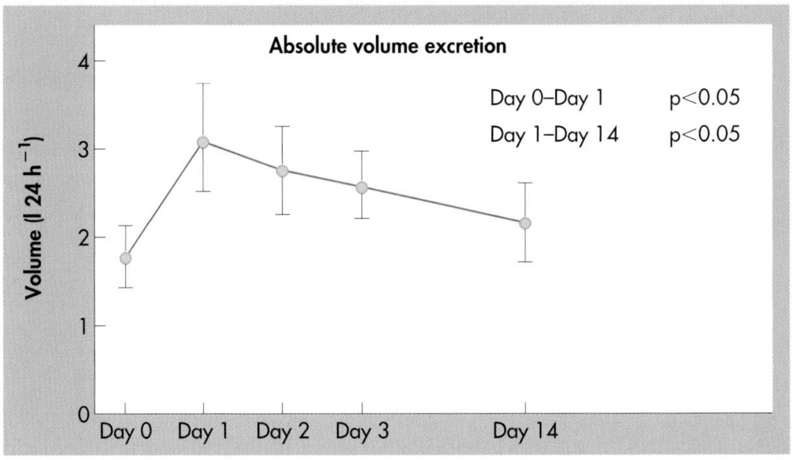

Figure 8.31 *Volume excretion before and after relief of obstruction. Day 0: prior to relief of obstruction by bladder catheterization.*

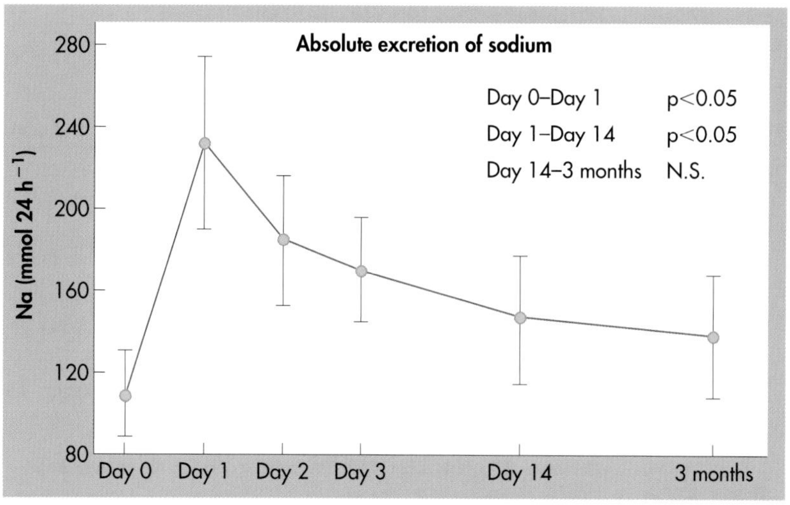

Figure 8.32 *Sodium excretion before and after release of obstruction. Day 0: as in Figure 7.31.*

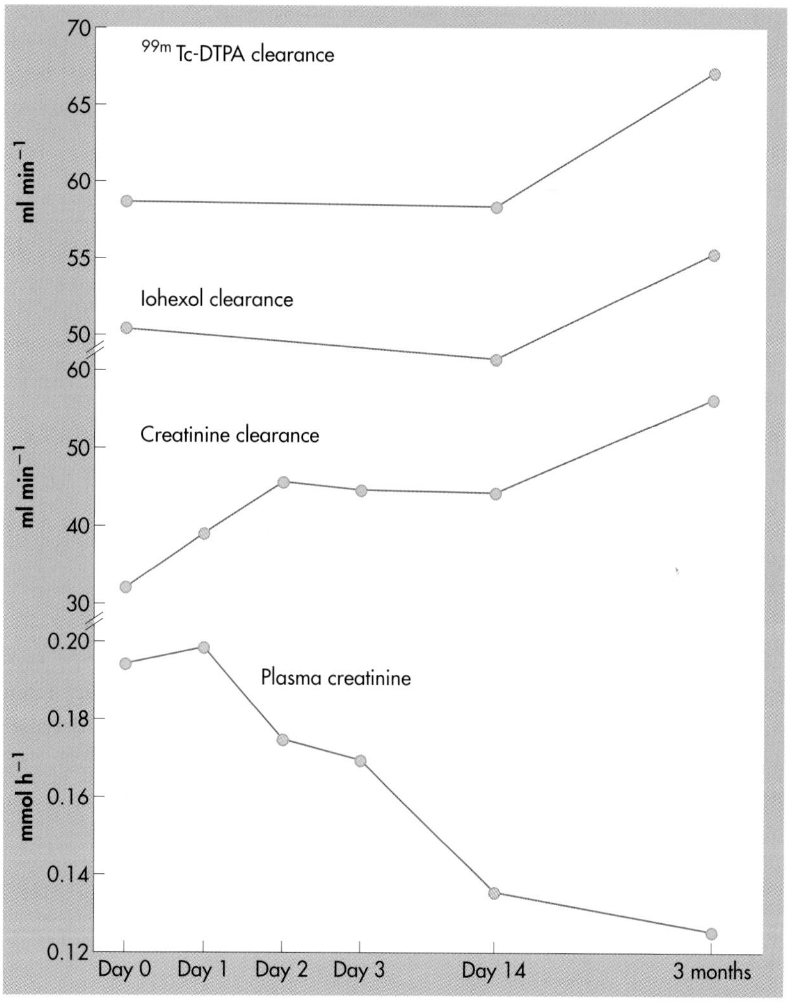

Figure 8.33 *Summary of glomerular and tubular changes in obstructive uropathy before and after the release of obstruction.*

have a near identical syndrome to high-pressure retention (the valve bladder), and in those cases that are not associated with reflux, similar patterns of obstructive renal failure take place. Unfortunately, the destructive nature of the severe obstruction on the detrusor muscle frequently leads to marked collagen infiltration and fibrotic damage, resulting in very poor compliance. By contrast, in the adult, long-term studies both from our own unit and others suggest that the majority of patients recover well, both as regards bladder and renal function.

The observations recorded above have, of course, been made in a particular group of patients studied with a particular form of bladder dysfunction. It might be argued that patients with neurogenic bladder dysfunction – acknowledged to be chiefly at risk because of obstructive renal problems – could not be linked urodynamically or therapeutically with the high-pressure retention group. There is no doubt that neurogenic bladders may demonstrate a profile of much more aggressive hyperreflexic contractions than that seen in high-pressure retention cases (although, in the latter, moderate instability may be seen on ambulatory studies), and it is possible that the hyperreflexic contractions themselves may be responsible for the obstructive renal failure. Nevertheless, there are enough signs in common (clinical, radiological, renographic and biochemical) to consider that the conditions may be associated at least in part; therapeutic and reconstructive lessons learned in one group may well be applicable to the other.

FURTHER READING

Badenoch AW. Congenital obstruction of the bladder neck. Ann RCS 1949; 4: 295–307

George NJR, O'Reilly PH, Barnard RJ et al. High pressure chronic retention. BMJ 1983; 286: 1780–1783

George NJR, O'Reilly PH, Barnard RJ et al. Practical management of patients with dilated upper tracts and chronic retention of urine. Br J Urol 1984; 56: 9–12

George NJR, Feneley RC, Roberts JBM. Identification of the poor risk patient with 'prostatism' and detrusor failure. Br J Urol 1986; 58: 290–295

Ghose RR. Prolonged recovery of renal function after prostatectomy for prostatic outflow obstruction. BMJ 1990; 300: 1376–1377

Holden D, George NJR, Rickards D et al. Renal pelvic pressures in human chronic obstructive uropathy. Br J Urol 1984; 56: 565–570

Jones DA, George NJR, O'Reilly PH et al. Reversible hypertension associated with unrecognised high pressure chronic retention of urine. Lancet 1987; 11: 1052–1054

Jones DA, George NJR, O'Reilly PH. Post-obstructive renal function. Semin Urol 1987; 5: 176–190

Jones DA, George NJR, O'Reilly PH et al. The biphasic nature of renal functional recovery following relief of chronic obstructive uropathy. Br J Urol 1988; 61: 192–197

Jones DA, Holden D, George NJR. Mechanism of upper tract dilatation in patients with thick walled bladders, chronic retention of urine and associated hydroureteronephrosis. J Urol 1988; 140: 326–329

Jones DA, Lupton EW, George NJR. Effect of bladder filling on upper tract urodynamics in man. Br J Urol 1990; 65: 492–496

Jones DA, Atherton JC, O'Reilly PH et al. Assessment of the nephron segments involved in post-obstructive diuresis in man, using lithium clearance. Br J Urol 1989; 64: 559–563

Jones DA, Gilpin SA, Holden D et al. Relationship between bladder morphology and long-term outcome of treatment in patients with high pressure chronic retention of urine. Br J Urol 1991; 67: 265–285

Sacks SH, Aparicio SAJR, Bevan A et al. Late renal failure due to prostatic outflow obstruction: a preventable disease. BMJ 1989; 298: 156–159

Styles RA, Neal DE, Ramsden PD. Chronic retention of urine. The relationship between upper tract dilatation and bladder pressure. Br J Urol 1986; 58: 647–651

Styles RA, Neal De, Griffiths CJ et al. Long term monitoring of bladder pressure in chronic retention of urine: the relationship between detrusor activity and upper tract dilatation. J Urol 1988; 140: 330–334

Wallace DM. The bladder neck in urinary obstruction. Proc R Soc Med 1951; 44: 434–437

9

Urinary tract infection

Nicholas J R George

INTRODUCTION

The infectious process encompasses a highly complex series of events which surround the relationship between the host attempting to defend itself against the offensive properties of the parasite. Virulence factors available to the micro-organism will be combated by a wide range of specific and non-specific defence mechanisms, and the result of this encounter, 'the microbiological battleground', will determine whether or not infectious disease is established.

Conventionally, accounts of infection of the urinary tract concentrate on the response of the urothelium to bacterial invasion. However, a continuing and perhaps increasing tendency to open surgery in certain groups of patients determines that a basic understanding of the broader concepts of the infectious process is likely to be advantageous for the practising urological surgeon. Therefore, in this account of urinary tract infection, before dealing with specific issues relating to organisms and the urothelium, a general description will be made of the host–parasite relationship as it applies to the urogenital system both in health and disease. Some important fundamental definitions are noted in Table 9.1. Such general microbiological points may be considered under the following headings.

1. colonizing micro-organisms in health
2. general defence mechanisms
3. general modifying factors
4. properties of commensal organisms.

Table 9.1 Essential definitions of basic microbiological terms.

Term	Definition
Pathogenicity	Ability to cause disease
Opportunistic infection	Weakened defences predispose to infection, often by non-pathogens
Virulence	Degree of pathogenicity

Colonizing micro-organisms in health

Table 9.2 lists common colonizing micro-organisms by site in healthy humans. The widespread presence of staphylococci and streptococci on the skin and surrounding the lower genitourinary tract will be appreciated, as will the occurence of *Candida* and lactobacilli within vaginal flora. The colon contains enormous numbers of bacteria – up to 10^{11} organisms per gram. The majority of these organisms are obligate anaerobes, although aerobic and facultative anaerobic organisms, such as Enterobacteriaceae and *Enterococcus* spp., are present in significant numbers (approximately 10^8/g of colonic contents), these species being the most common source of uropathogens.

The normally balanced environment of the bowel flora is significantly affected by antimicrobial agents. Antibiotic therapy results in normally sensitive *E. coli* strains as well as anaerobic species being replaced by more resistant strains and organisms such as *Pseudomonas aeruginosa*.[1] Cessation of broad-spectrum therapy allows recolonization by resident

Table 9.2 Organisms by site in health (normal flora). Commensal organisms which exist in symbiotic relationship with the host protecting against uropathogens.

Skin
Staphylococci (*Staph. aureus* and *Staph. epidermidis*)
Corynebacterium spp.
Candida spp.
Lower genitourinary tract
Staphylococci
Streptococci
Anaerobic cocci
Corynebacterium spp.
Lactobacilli (vagina)
Large intestine
Anaerobes
Bacteroides spp.
Clostridium spp.
Fusobacterium spp.
Aerobes/facultative anaerobes
Escherichia coli
Klebsiella spp.
Streptococci – Enterococci (*Strep. faecalis*)
Yeasts

flora, but slower-growing anaerobic organisms may initially be displaced by faster-growing Enterobacteriaceae. Hence, injudicious broad-spectrum therapy may increase the size of the colonic reservoir from which uropathogens are normally drawn[2] – as noted above, these organisms usually account for only 0.1% of total colonic flora. The presence of a large volume of potential uropathogens may clearly be an ascending threat to the lower urinary tract, particularly in the presence of any abnormality such as outflow tract obstruction or congenital anomalies.

General defence mechanisms

Non-specific host defence mechanisms are outlined in Table 9.3. General resistance to invasion may be described in terms of events at the surface of the host, events at a deeper level and mechanisms that depend on cellular function.

The role of commensal flora is further explored below. The mechanical integrity of skin and mucous membranes may clearly be breached in a number of ways. The breakdown of lipids into fatty acids (approximate pH 5–6) by skin flora constitutes a mildly hostile environment for pathogens. Lysozyme, found in every mucosal secretion, splits the muramic acid linkage in cell walls of Gram-positive organisms in particular. The iron-binding properties of lactoferrin disrupt the normal metabolism of the micro-organism. IgA secretion may prevent attachment of organisms to host cells.

Penetration of the initial line of defence leads to more substantial but non-specific reactions such as the acute-phase response and the inflammatory

Table 9.3 General non-specific (constitutive) host defence mechanisms. These are conveniently described in terms of the degree to which the organism penetrates the surface. General factors which may compromise these defences are noted.

Surface	Compromised	Subsurface	Compromised	Cellular	Compromised
Commensal flora	Antibiotics	Lysozyme	Drugs Corticosteroids Immunosuppression Infections (applies to all subsurface mechanisms)		Alcoholism Advanced cancer Renal disease Liver disease HIV (applies to all cellular mechanisms)
Mechanical integrity Acidity	Surgery Cannulae	Lactoferrin Acute phase response		Phagocytosis Polymorphonuclear Mononuclear	
Secretions Lysozyme Lactoferrin IgA		Inflammatory response			
Flow Peristalsis Irritation	Surgery Obstruction	Complement Fibronectin			

response. Humoral and cellular components, such as protease inhibitors and adherence proteins, are delivered to the site, and the classical inflammatory reaction supervenes. Activation of the complement cascade by the alternative pathway may lead to bacterial lysis as well as enhancement of phagocytosis. The antiadherence properties of the glycoprotein fibronectin may prevent attachment of pathogenic organisms. Increased phagocytosis by various cells, including neutrophil polymorphs, mononuclear phagocytes and natural-killer cells, is stimulated by a complex series of events which may vary according to the nature of the microbiological challenge.

General modifying factors

A number of generalized factors may affect the standard host defence mechanisms. Patients at the extremes of life are vulnerable to infections. Postmenopausal hormonal changes in the lower urinary tract are of particular interest to urologists.

Poor nutrition or overt malnutrition, particularly in the elderly, may weaken defences in a number of ways relating to protein synthesis and vitamin deficiency. Generalized disorders, such as diabetes mellitus, alcoholism and renal failure, may markedly increase susceptibility to disease, as may overwhelming infection and certain types of drug therapy as well as the general debility related to advanced malignancy. Pathological conditions which further expose the individual to risk of infection, such as stone disease or obstruction, will be considered below.

Properties of commensal organisms

Commensal organisms have an important role to play in the protection of the host by resisting the growth of more pathogenic organisms. The mechanisms by which they attain this objective are listed in Table 9.4. Competition for a limited supply of nutrients acts to restrict the growth of pathogens, while the ability of the commensal organisms to occupy certain cell-surface receptors (tropism) limits the adherence possibilities for the invader. Bacterial products known as bacteriocins may be toxic to other organisms, often of the same species. As noted above, fatty acid production by sebum and lipids results in a hostile microenvironment. Low-level but continued stimulation of the immune system, as well as the stimulation of cross-reacting 'natural' antibodies (such antibodies are raised against organisms which the host has not encountered because of antigenic cross-reaction with organisms that have been experienced), further enhances resistance to pathogenic bacteria. Apart from antibiotic therapy, the normal commensal flora may be significantly affected by general factors such as diet, hygienic habits and underlying disease.

Table 9.4 Mechanisms of protection by commensal flora. See text for details.

Competition for nutrients	(interference)
Competition for receptors	(tropism)
Bacteriocin production	
Fatty acid production	
Stimulation of immune system	
Stimulation of natural antibodies	

The described general mechanisms are, under the normal circumstances of health, remarkably effective at excluding pathogenic invasion. For a more complete account of the highly complex processes involved, the reader is referred to standard bacteriological texts. The remainder of this chapter will address, firstly, specific microbiological aspects of urinary tract infection in humans and, secondly, a clinical account of the more important forms of inflammatory disease.

HOST DEFENCE MECHANISMS – LOWER URINARY TRACT

Apart from the broad concepts outlined above, the lower urinary tract has a number of specific defence mechanisms which allow it to counter the threat posed by the reservoir of potential pathogens which is located chiefly in the lower bowel and on the perineal skin. Naturally, the anatomy of the male and in particular the length of the urethra determine that ascending infection is extremely uncommon when compared with the female. However, the lower urogenital tract, while clearly offering a bacteriological threat to the female urothelium, does offer some defence mechanisms against ascending infection by pathogenic bacteria.

Commensal organisms

An outline of the advantages of commensal flora has been described above. During the reproductive years, circulating oestrogens affect the vaginal epithelium, which stores increased amounts of glycogen within the cells (Figure 9.1). The glycogen is metabolized by *Lactobacillus acidophilus* into lactic acid, and the resultant drop in pH produces an unfavourable microenvironment for the majority of pathogenic bacteria attempting to ascend into the bladder (see also discussion of adhesion theory, below). Lactobacilli and other Gram-positive rods are collectively known as Döderlein's bacilli, and disruption of this vaginal flora by vaginitis or other infection leads to a rise in pH and loss of the natural defence barrier. Lactobacilli are one of the main causes of milk going sour and indeed are the active organisms in 'live' yoghurt, which for this reason is frequently advocated by health magazines as a topical application which can prevent recurrent lower urinary tract infection without the need for antibiotic therapy. Naturally, such protection is not available either before or after the menopause, one fact which possibly explains the increased incidence of ascending lower urinary tract infection in elderly women, whose introital skin is often thin and atrophic due to lack of circulating oestrogens.

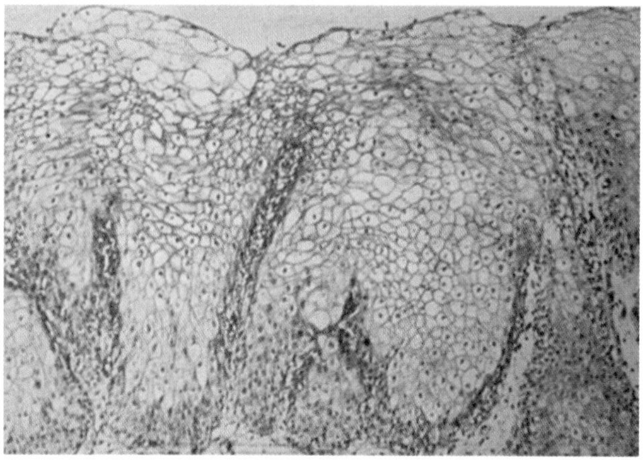

Figure 9.1 *Vaginal epithelial cells stuffed with glycogen. Produced in response to oestrogens, the glycogen is broken down by* Lactobacillus acidophilus, *thus increasing local vaginal acidity.*

Urine

Urine, normally a good culture medium, may under some circumstances be inhibitory or even bactericidal against some uropathogens. Low urinary pH levels in particular, as well as raised blood urea and high osmolarity, are inhibitory for some organisms.[3]

Genital skin

Although strictly unrelated to the urothelium, penetration of the natural barrier afforded by genital skin can have serious consequences for the patient (Figure 9.2a and b). Any perforation of penile skin may be followed by infection, but this is particularly the case when the patient is diabetic; such patients are commonly exposed to increased risk during self-administration of vasoactive substances for erectile dysfunction.

Urine flow

Urine flow from the kidney by ureteric peristalsis and from the bladder by periodic detrusor contraction constitutes the main defence mechanism of the urinary tract against ascending infection.[4] Loss of competence at the vesicoureteric junction for any reason may lead under certain circumstances to significant renal damage; additionally, reflux prevents efficient bladder emptying, thus compromising the flushing mechanism of micturition, which is similarly impeded by any form of lower urinary tract obstruction.

Bladder surface mucin

In a series of experiments on rabbit bladders, Parsons et al[5–7] proposed that a bladder surface mucin layer consisting of a glycosaminoglycan (GAG) was secreted by transitional cells and acted as an 'antiadherence factor' by inhibiting bacterial attachment to bladder mucosa, thereby facilitating removal of bacteria by the voiding process. These workers demonstrated that removal of the GAG layer by acid markedly increased adhesion to the urothelium (Figure 9.3) and, furthermore, that instillation of heparin (a synthetic GAG) into bladders previously

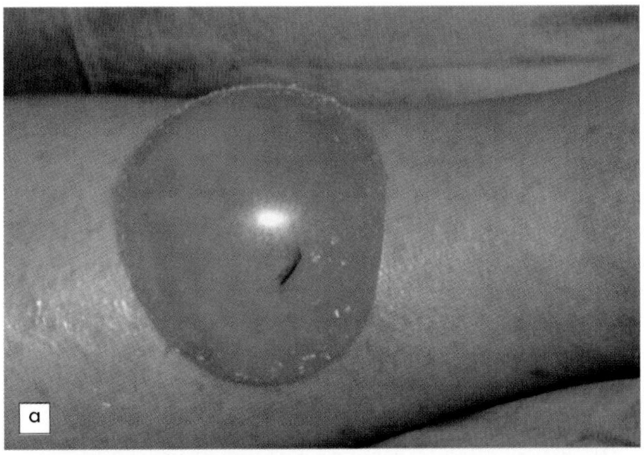

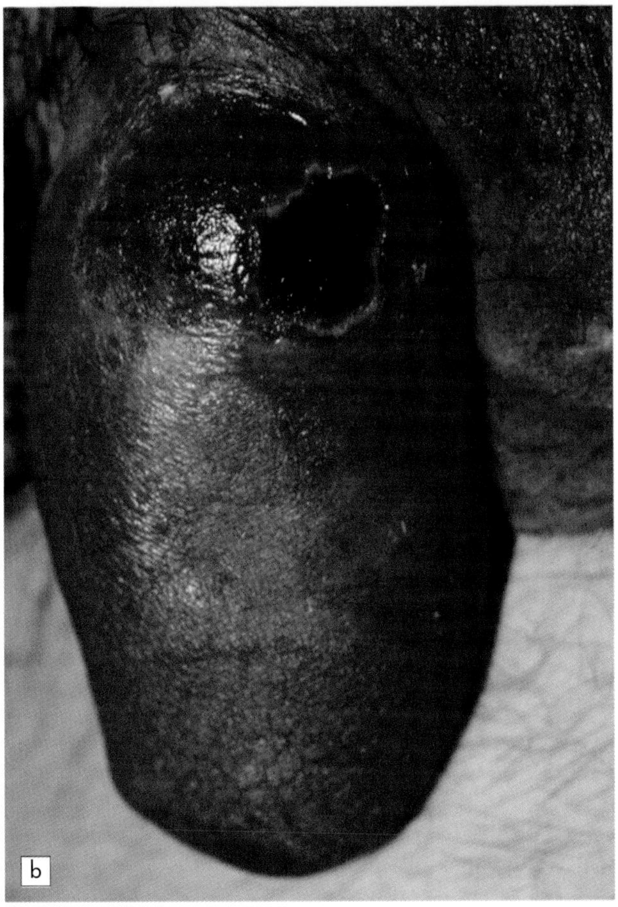

Figure 9.2 *The importance of skin epithelial integrity. (a) Large blister on forearm – no infection within perfect subblister culture medium due to integrity of ultra-thin residual epithelial covering. (b) Puncture site of intracavernosal therapy in diabetic – despite full precautions, serious widespread inflammation has taken place.*

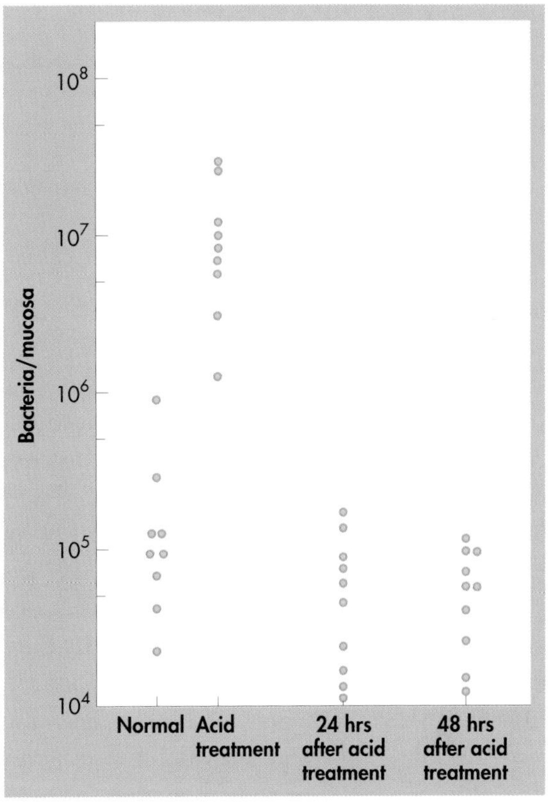

Figure 9.3 *Effect of bladder surface mucin. Binding of* ^{14}C*-labelled* E. coli *to normal bladder mucosa and acid-treated mucosa. Acid treatment removes the mucin layer, and bacterial adhesion to the bladder mucosa increases significantly. Twenty-four hours after acid treatment, the mucin layer has recovered sufficiently to prevent epithelial attachment. Rabbit bladder, (Reproduced with permission from Parsons CL, Greenspan C, Moore SW, Mulholland SG. Role of surface mucin in primary antibacterial defense of bladder.* Urology 1977; 9: 48–52.)

denuded of their GAG layer by acid resulted in restoration of the antimucosal adherence properties. Pretreatment of the bacteria with heparin had no effect on adherence, and the authors concluded that the surface mucin provided a protective barrier for the urothelium, thus preventing bacterial adherence to the uroepithelial cells. Subsequently, the bacteria trapped in the GAG layer are expelled by urination.[5–7]

Tamm-Horsfall protein

Tamm-Horsfall protein is secreted by the cells of the ascending loop of Henle and is the most common mucoprotein of renal origin in urine. Also known as uromucoid, Tamm-Horsfall protein was originally noted to react with influenza virus,[8] but, subsequently, it was established that the protein was capable of binding strongly to *E. coli* expressing type 1 manose-sensitive fimbriae,[9] probably because of manose-containing side chains within the mucoprotein. After entrapment, it is proposed that the uromucoid/

coliform complex is mechanically cleared from the urinary tract by urination. Recent studies confirm that in these circumstances the mannose-binding properties of type I pili are critically related to the Fim H tip adhesin (see below).[10]

Mucosal shedding

Attachment to uroepithelial cells by pathogenic bacteria offers both defence and attack possibilities for host and invading organism alike. Exfoliation rates for bladder mucosal cells under normal conditions of sterile urine are approximately 4 weeks;[11] following infection, greatly increased rates are observed within hours of inoculation, a process apparently linked to Fim H adhesion and the apoptotic pathway involving caspases and epithelial cell DNA fragmentation.[12,13]

Exfoliation of cells with adherent bacteria (Figure 9.4) by bulk flow of urine is likely to be of benefit to the host, although the consequent exposure of less mature epithelial cells may provide an opportunity for colonization and invasion by other uropathogenic organisms. It has been suggested that such sequestration of organisms within deeper layers of the bladder wall might explain problems related to persistent infection in some cases of cystitis.[14]

Local immune response

The role of immunity in the defence of the urinary tract remains poorly understood. Although considerable humoral and cellular response may be observed in upper urinary tract infection, serum production of urinary antibody in bladder infection is characteristically difficult to detect, perhaps reflecting the relative superficiality of the infection.

VIRULENCE MECHANISMS

Virulence mechanisms are those properties of the parasite which enable it first to colonize and then flourish within the host. Such mechanisms may be directed against external agents administered in order to eradicate the organism or against the host itself, including natural host defences which have developed over time to counter the invading microorganism. (Table 9.5).

Virulence against external agents – antimicrobial resistance

Before World War II there were few agents with reliable antimicrobial properties, and the virulence capability of organisms was almost entirely directed against the natural properties of the host. After the discovery and clinical usage of penicillin, organisms learnt rapidly to develop systems for evasion of the toxic effects of antibiotics, and the consequent

Table 9.5 General classification of virulence mechanisms.

Against external agents	Antimicrobial resistance
Against the host	Toxin production General mechanisms Adherence mechanisms

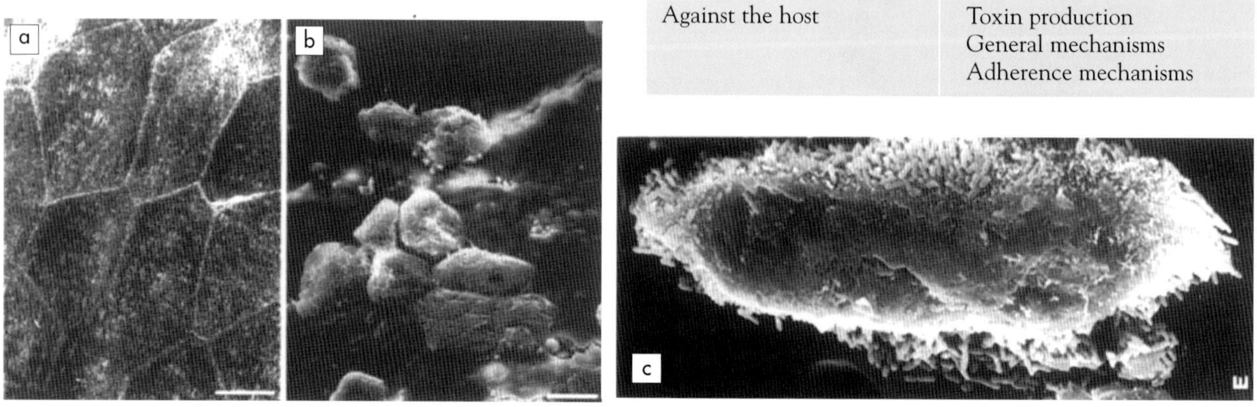

Figure 9.4 *Mucosal shedding of epithelial cells in response to* E. coli *infection. (a) Scanning electron micrograph of superficial epithelial cells of uninfected mouse bladder. (b) Following infection with type 1 pilated* E. coli, *superficial cells exfoliate, exposing deeper less mature cells. Scale bars 50 µm. (c) Magnified view of exfoliated mouse epithelial cell showing vesical surface coated with* E. coli *while the recently separated inferior surface is devoid of organisms (× 440). Illustrations courtesy of reference 15 (a, b) and reference 16 (c).*

emergence of resistant strains today constitutes a significant threat, particularly for certain groups of the population such as hospital inpatients. *Staphylococcus aureus*, once almost entirely penicillin sensitive, is now approximately 90% resistant to the agent. *Neisseria gonorrhoeae* remained penicillin sensitive for many years, but its acquisition of β-lactamase activity has resulted in high levels of penicillin resistance. Hospital-based doctors will be well aware of the extremely serious threat posed by methicillin-resistant *Staph. aureus* (MRSA) infections, which may spread rapidly throughout whole wards and effectively be untreatable. These examples underscore the extreme flexibility and adaptability of the invading micro-organism, which, through evolutionary processes, has managed to match and subsequently often overcome the best efforts of scientific antibiotic endeavour.

Types of resistance

Organisms may acquire antimicrobial resistance by two basic mechanisms. *Intrinsic resistance* means that the organism may naturally resist antibiotics by the production of natural enzymes, such as β-lactamases; or because the usual antibiotic target within the cell is lacking; or by the presence of an impenetrable cell wall. *Acquired resistance* develops as a result of the evolution of new or altered genetic material, which may occur through either mutations or gene transfer. Such mutations and transfers result in a number of well-described mechanisms by which the organism may evade the action of the antibiotic.

Enzyme inactivation

β-Lactamase production is the most important resistance mechanism of the penicillins and cephalosporins. The enzyme hydrolyzes the β-lactam bond in the antibiotic structure, rendering it inactive. β-Lactamase production is commonly found in *Staph. aureus*, *N. gonorrhoeae* and enterobacteria.

Altered permeability

Various alterations in receptor activity and transport mechanisms may prevent access of the antibiotic to the micro-organism. Aminoglycosides and tetracyclines are actively taken up into organisms, and resistance may occur either by inactivation of the transport mechanism or by development of additional systems allowing increased expulsion of the drug from the cell.

Alteration of binding site

Antibiotics may bind to specific targets within the cell. Genetic variation may alter or delete the antibiotic target, thus leading to resistance to the drug. The site of action of the more commonly used antibiotics is summarized in Table 9.6. The complex nature of antimicrobial resistance determines that a detailed account is beyond the scope of this text; for a comprehensive overview, the reader is referred to definitive studies of resistance mechanisms.[17]

Table 9.6 Target sites of common antimicrobial drugs. It is convenient to consider the action of the antibiotic as it relates to bacterial cell structure – cell wall, cytoplasmic membrane, ribosomal function and nucleic acid synthesis.

Drug	Target/mechanism
β-lactam (penicillin, cephalosporin)	Cell wall: disruption of peptidoglycan X-linkage
Aminoglycosides	Ribosomal interference: misreading mRNA
Erythromycin	Translocation interference
Tetracyclines	RNA-binding interference
Trimethoprim	Nucleic acid interference: dihydrofolate reductase inhibition
Fluoroquinolones (ciprofloxacin)	Inhibit DNA gyrase

VIRULENCE AGAINST THE HOST ITSELF

Toxin production

Toxins are proteins which are able to harm the cells or tissues of the host. Many organisms elaborate toxins which may either assist with the process of local invasion or be themselves responsible for the characteristics of disease. Important examples of such virulent toxins are those which produce the clinical manifestations of diphtheria, tetanus and botulism.

A number of organisms, including *E. coli*, exhibit *haemolysin* activity, which may damage erythrocytes in a variety of ways, including phospholipase C activity (cell-membrane damage) and osmotic lysis. *E. coli* strains commonly associated with urinary tract infection (01, 02, 04, 06, 07, 016, 018 and 075) frequently elaborate haemolysins, and such strains may be disproportionately promoted from the colonic reservoir.[18,19] Cytotoxic necrotizing factor 1 (cnf 1) is another toxin elaborated by pathogenic coliforms to facilitate colonization of the host.[20] Despite the strong association of such strains with the ability to cause ascending urinary tract infection, the precise mechanism of enhanced virulence remains unknown.

General mechanisms

Apart from toxin production, there are a number of general mechanisms which facilitate the organism's attempt to enter and multiply within the host.

1. penetration
2. antihumeral activity
3. evasion of phagocytosis
4. competition for nutrients.

Penetration

In general, organisms are unable to penetrate the intact epithelium of the host unless prior damage (Figure 9.2b) has taken place. However, certain parasites may do so, the best example in the urinary tract being the fork-tailed cercariae of *Schistosoma haematobium*, which are able to penetrate unbroken skin for a few hours after being shed by the intermediate snail host (Figure 9.5a).

Antihumeral activity

As noted above, antibodies such as secretory IgA may be active against organisms before mucosal invasion occurs. Organisms such as *N. gonorrhoeae* and *Proteus mirabilis* elaborate anti-IgA proteases that inactivate this defence mechanism. A further antihumeral virulence factor is exhibited by certain

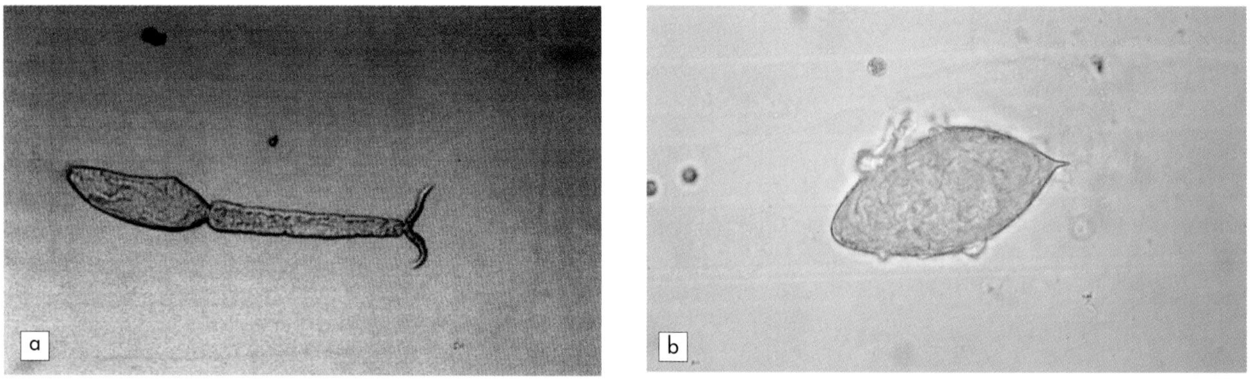

Figure 9.5 Schistosoma haematobium. *(a) The fork-tailed cercariae have a free-swimming existence of 24–28 hours. Intact skin or mucosa may be penetrated, the fork-tailed structure being lost in the process, allowing the organism (now known as a schistosomulum) to reach the subcutaneous tissues. (b) The spike-like projection at the end of the egg identifies the organism, in contrast to the projections of* Schistosoma mansoni, *which are located in the equatorial region. The eggs sequester within the wall of the urinary tract and are shed to the exterior in the urine. Typical egg dimensions of* S. haematobium: *112/170 × 40/70 μm. (Photomicrograph b courtesy of Dr Allan Curry, UHSM).*

isolates of *N. gonorrhoeae* that are able to resist the lytic effects of complement. Such strains are thus able to multiply and enter the host bloodstream, whereas those isolates which lack this virulence factor are unable to invade and so remain localized on the surface of the genital tract.[21] Resistance to the bactericidal effect of serum/complement has been linked to the integrity of the lipolysaccharide cell wall (O antigen). Additionally, loss of capsular polysaccharide (K antigen) has been associated with lack of resistance to compliment mediated lysis.[22]

Evasion of phagocytosis

A number of bacteria have developed mechanisms for resisting phagocytic attack by the host. Variation in surface antigens and the properties of some polysaccharide capsules may constitute a successful defence mechanism by preventing interaction between the phagocytic cell and the invading organism.[21]

Competition for nutrients

To be successful, any invading micro-organism will require an adequate supply of nutrients. In particular, free iron is required for metabolism and multiplication of *E. coli*, iron uptake being facilitated by the siderophore aerobactin and enterobactin.[20] The ability to produce these agents thus confirms an advantage on strains invading the urinary tract, and an association has been observed between aerobactin production and the expression of P fimbriae (see below) in patients with symptomatic urinary tract infection.[23]

Adherence mechanisms

The adherence of a cell to another structure is an extremely important biological characteristic that can be observed widely throughout nature. Early reports of this phenomenon[24] were slightly misleading, as the particular mechanisms of attachment were not fully understood at that time. General observations of bacteria and algae adhering to inert plastic or rocks in streams were brought together with other observations of various bacteria adhering in vivo to a number of epithelial surfaces. It is now possible to distinguish the individual mechanisms by which adhesion takes place in each of these specialized circumstances (Table 9.7). Although fimbriae are of overriding importance in urinary tract infection, it is helpful briefly to describe and contrast other methods of adhesion. Adherence is defined as the initial interaction of a micro-organism with the host. An adhesin is a microbiological molecule that leads to bacterial adhesion to cells or tissues. Adhesins predominantly react with specific receptors on the host cell surface, although non-specific adhesion (as by surface charge) may occur.[25]

Table 9.7 Recognized adhesion mechanisms. See text for details.
Afimbrial adhesins
Adherence pedestals
Fimbriae

Types of adhesins

Afimbrial adhesins consist of polymers, polysaccharides, lipoteichoic acid and other proteins associated with the cell wall of the organism. Collectively, these are known as a 'glycocalix', and together they serve to attach the organism to the target cell. The classical studies into glycocalix formation involved *Streptococcus mutans*, an organism that colonizes human teeth, leading to decay. Enzymatic activity at the cell surface degrades sucrose, providing fructose for ongoing nutrition, but it also polymerizes glucose into polysaccharide chains used to construct the glycocalix. Thus, the organism attaches itself to its target, at the same time protecting itself against attack and concentrating its nutrients by wrapping itself within the glycocalix – also known as a 'biofilm'.[26]

Helicobacter pylori provides a typical example of an organism which attaches itself via small cellular projections known as *adherence pedestals*. This organism, with its unmistakable flagella (approximately three times the size of fimbriae; see below), attaches itself to cells within the gastric epithelium, leading to ulceration and perhaps gastric carcinoma (Figure 9.6a). Presumably, the flagella drive the organism downwards into the mucosa, following which adhesion to the target cells take place (Figure 9.6b).

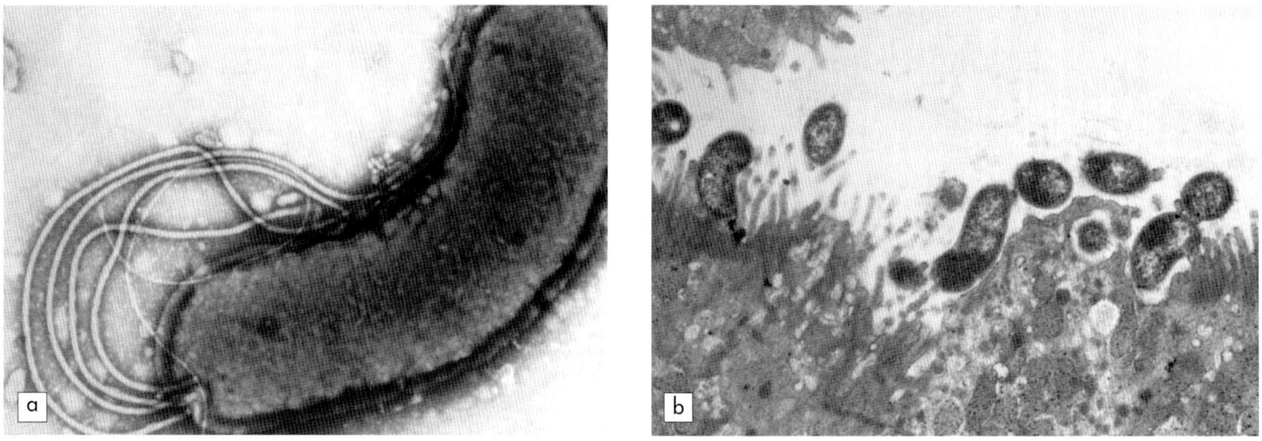

Figure 9.6 Helicobacter pylori. *(a) The flagella of the organism are easily identified (significantly larger than fimbriae). (b) Flagella used to propel organism into gastric mucosa where adhesins provide attachment. Photomicrographs courtesy of Dr Alan Curry, UHSM.*

Fimbriae

Fimbriae (also known as pili) are very important virulence structures that mediate attachment to host tissues and are particularly important in the pathogenesis of *E. coli* urinary tract infection. A typical organism may have 100–500 appendages, each approximately 5–10 nm in diameter and 2 μm in length (Figure 9.7). Isolates of *E. coli* may produce a number of antigenically distinct fimbriae, although some strains produce no fimbriae at all.

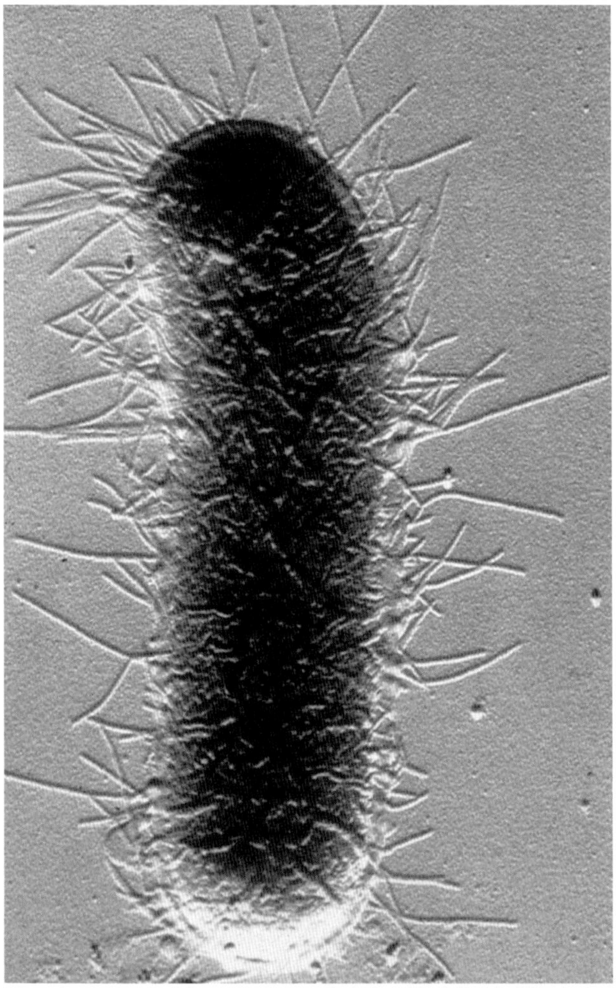

Figure 9.7 E. coli, *showing fimbriae. Photomicrograph courtesy of Dr Pauline Handley, University of Manchester.*

Supramolecular adhesins associated with pathogenic strains of *E. coli*

Early distinction between types of fimbriae was made by the ability of mannose, respectively, to inhibit (mannose-sensitive) or not to inhibit (mannose-resistant) the agglutination of guinea-pig erythrocytes. For some years, it had been known that type I pili were specifically bound to Tamm-Horsfall protein[9] and foreign bodies such as catheters and prosthetic implants.[27] More recently, a variety of techniques, including haemagglutination, electron microscopy, X-ray crystallography and molecular methodologies, have enabled a more precise identification of a number of specific adhesion organelles that are recognized as critically important virulence factors for uropathological *E. coli* (Table 9.8).

Table 9.8 Adhesin and receptor characteristics identified in pathogenic coliform infections. The description of the organelle, the characteristic of the tip adhesin and specific host receptor 'docking port' on particular host cells is tabulated. Data abstracted from references 15 and 20. The critical chemical structure of the PapG receptor has been emphasized by bold underlined text. For further details concerning the site of the disaccharide Gal-Gal core receptor, see reference 28. Globo A is similar but not identical to the Forsmann antigen and has been investigated as part of comparative receptor studies.[29,30]

Organelle	Guinea pig haemaglutination characteristic	Adhesin	Host receptors	Host cells	Clinical disease
Type I fimbriae	Inhibited by mannose (mannose sensitive)	Fim H	Uroplakin 1a (mannosylated glyco protein) Tamm-Horsfall protein (uromucoid) Collagen types I, IV Laminin Fibronectin	Bladder:kidney: Buccal epithelial cells Erythrocytes Neutrophils Foreign bodies (i.e. catheters)	Cystitis Sepsis
Type P fimbriae	Not inhibited by mannose (mannose-resistant)	PapG epitope class I	globo**<u>tria</u>**osylceramide		Not in human
		PapG epitope class II	globo**<u>tetra</u>**ceramide (globoside)	Kidney epithelial cells	Pyronephritis
		PapG epitope class III	globo**<u>penta</u>**ceramide (Forssmann antigen)	Human P blood group antigen	Cystitis
S/fic fimbriae		Sfas SfaA/FocH	Sialic acid Plasminogen	Bladder/kidney Epithelial cells Erythrocytes	Ascending UTI Sepsis Meningitis
Dr adhesins		Various	Type IV collagen $\propto 5\beta$, integrin	Bladder/kidney Epithelial cells	Cystitis Diarrhoea Sepsis

Type I fimbriae

These structures are the most common adhesion organelles found on pathogenic coliforms isolated from the urinary tract.[31] They are of variable length (1–2 μm) and approximately 7 nm thick, being of helical construction (Figure 9.8). The FimH terminal adhesin is a two-domain protein approximately 3 nm in width to which mannose-containing glycoprotein receptors can attach.[32,33] Uroplakin (UP1a) is a complex glycoprotein that covers the internal surface of the bladder in a form of membrane or plaque.[34] This and other related compounds (UP1b, UPII and UPIII) are the primary receptors (docking sites) for the type I pilus of pathogenic bacteria[33] (Table 9.8). The defensive role of Tamm-Horsfall protein, which preferentially binds type I pili, has been mentioned above.[10]

Initiation of the infective process

Traditionally, pathogenic coliforms were considered to exert their influence by epithelial adherence and subsequent metabolic disruption as a result of factors expressed from the epithelial locus. Recent work suggests that under certain circumstances coliform organisms may become opportunistic intracellular pathogens. Using human bladder epithelial cells, Martinez and co-workers observed cellular invasion by organisms expressing type I pili, but not by those with type G Pili.[35] The process required FimH-activated submembranous actin organization, phosphoinositide 3-kinase activation and tyrosine phosphorylation (Figure 9.9). Such internalization might allow (assuming no shedding) the organisms to replicate in the relative shelter (vacuole) of the uroepithelial cell, thus propagating the infective

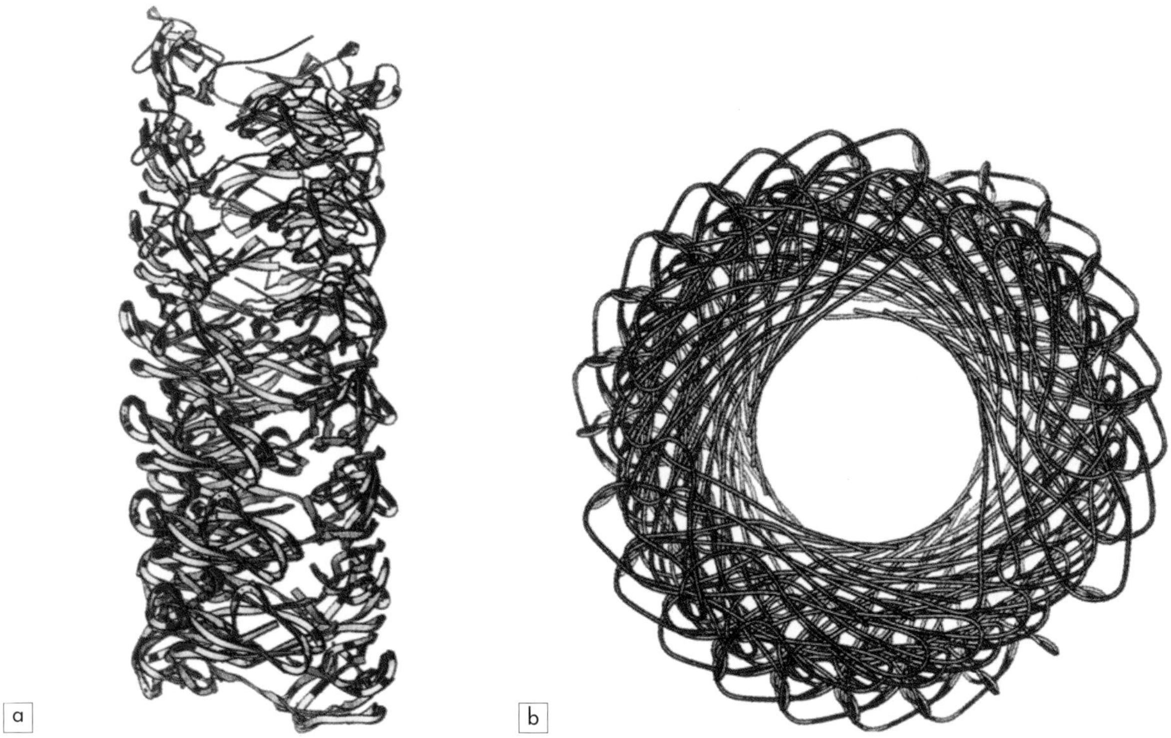

Figure 9.8 *Model of the type I pilus. (a) side view; (b) top view. External diameter approximately 70 Å. Tip adhesin – FimH; rod predominantly FimA subunits. Illustration courtesy of Choudhury D*[32].

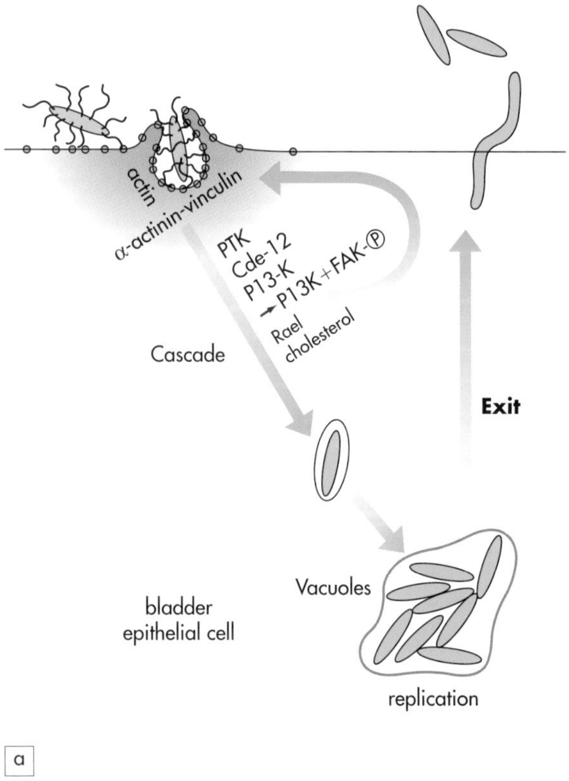

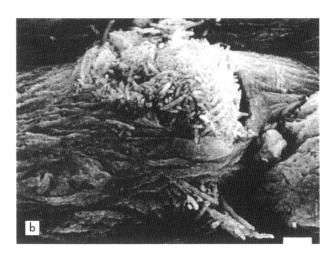

Figure 9.9 *(a) Possible mechanism of type I pilus-mediated invasion of bladder epithelial cells. FimH adhesion to cell surface triggers envelopment followed by activation of a cascade involving protein tyrosine kinases, PI-3 kinases and Cdc 42. The transduction cascade facilitates the internalization of the organism within membrane-bound vacuoles which protect it from host defence mechanisms. The organisms replicate within the intracellular environment, effectively converting the epithelial cell into a 'bacterial factory'. (b) Finally, the organisms burst out and are released from the surface of the epithelial cell. Note smaller rupture at base of cell with emerging rod-like organisms. Bar 5 μm.*
Cartoon courtesy of references 15, 35. Photomicrograph courtesy of reference 14.

process. Similar observations have been made relating to bacterial invasion of host macrophages.[36]

Expression of type I pili

Expression of adhesins can be markedly affected by a wide variety of factors, including environmental cues, adhesin 'cross talk' and the adherence environment in which the organism is placed; coliforms in liquid culture (no adherence required) may fail to develop any adhesion organelles at all.

Schwan and co-workers varied growth conditions and found that fewer type I pili were expressed in a low pH/high osmolarity environment.[37] Other cues include temperature change, oxygen tension and nutrient availability. Transcription of type I fimbrial genes is controlled by a promoter located on an invertible element; during urinary tract infection, the orientation of the element ('on') that allows the expression of type I pili was maximal at 24 hours, suggesting that the switch (phase variation) was a significant virulence mechanism in the early stages of an infection.[38] Expression of organelles is also significantly affected by other adhesins that may be present on the bacterium. Pap B, a regulator of type P pilus expression, may modulate type I expression, increasing the 'off' phase noted above.[39] Such interpilus variations may enable the organism to adapt and change targets; for example, such a mechanism would be advantageous for a Pap P pathogenic organism trying to reach the upper tracts via the bladder epithelial barrier of the bladder.

Type P fimbriae

P fimbriae are particularly important in disease of the upper urinary tract, and the clinical significance is discussed below. It has already been noted that some pathogenic organisms may variably express both type I and P pili,[40] a factor that may complicate attempts to identify virulence factors by in vitro bacterial studies.

Structure and ultrastructure of P fimbriae

Advances in molecular biology have enabled the structure of P fimbriae to be elucidated (Figure 9.10). The Pap pili (*p*ili *a*ssociated with *p*yelonephritis) essentially consist of four proteins, PapA, PapE, PapF and PapG, constructed and assembled on a platform of PapC protein, the fibre being 7 nm wide. PapG is chiefly responsible for binding to the receptor, while protein PapA constitutes the bulk of the 'stem' of the pilus, approximately 1000 subunits being arranged in a helical fashion between the surface of the organism and the active tip proteins.[20] Experimental observations suggest that the adhesion characteristics are maintained by the GFE tip proteins even in the absence of the helical structure of PapA stem subunits. It has been suggested that the reason for the seemingly dispensable fibre structure is that this length places the adhesin outside the lipopolysaccharide cell-surface structure of *E. coli* (see below), thus maintaining the integrity of the individual virulence mechanisms.[41]

Recent advances in the understanding of the receptor structure for the G tip protein are leading to significant advances in knowledge concerning the mechanisms of urinary tract infection. Table 9.8 annotates the globoseries glycolipid isoreceptor types, each of which contains the disaccharide α-GAL-1-4-β-GAL (known colloquially as GAL-GAL), and their association with disease. Different positioning of the disaccharide within the molecule in each of the isoreceptors determines the adherence capability

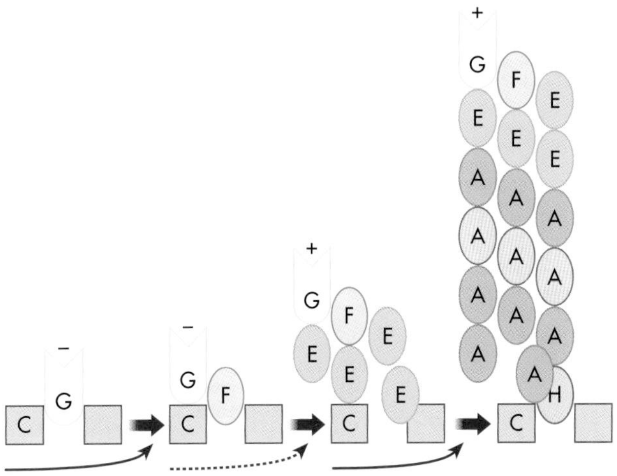

Figure 9.10 *Pilus assembly and structure. The PAP (pili associated with pyelonephritis) pilus is constructed and assembled on a platform of PAP C protein. The adhesion characteristics are chiefly determined by the terminal PAP G protein, which must be some distance from the platform before it is able to function (–, no adhesion; +, able to adhere). The PAP A subunits are formed in an helical fashion into the stem of the pilus, the entire structure being approximately 1000 subunits long. Data from Lindberg et al.*[41]

of the G tip proteins. Organisms with class I tip proteins do not adhere and do not cause disease in man due to the absence of the globo isoreceptor. Those with class II are strongly associated with pyelonephritis, while class III adhesins are commonly found in patients with cystitis.[28] Hence, the structure of the globo isoreceptor determines the outcome between invading organism and host – patients with infections from coliforms expressing class II adhesins are unlikely to suffer from cystitis, globoside being the major isoreceptor in the human kidney.[42] Similarly, the association of class III adhesion with cystitis suggests a predominance of Forssman receptors on the urothelium of the lower urinary tract. Further studies of receptor expression by means of differential blood group analysis[29] have demonstrated that minor differences in receptor core structure profoundly affect disease patterns, and emphasize the importance of precise 'fitness' if bacteria are to persist and multiply within the lower urinary tract.[30] Nevertheless, despite these studies of adhesin/receptor interactions, the importance played by non-specific mechanisms, such as electrostatic and hydrophobic attractive forces, should not be overlooked.[42]

Historical relevance of fimbrinated status

Long before the mechanisms of adherence were fully understood, observational studies had indicated a connection between the macroscopically observed bacterial adherence and severity of urinary tract infection. This phenomenon was first reported in *The Lancet* in 1976 by Catharina Svanborg Edén and colleagues from the Department of Immunology in Göteborg, Sweden, a department which has continued at the forefront of adherence research. Uroepithelial cells from freshly voided morning urine samples were added to bacterial cells, and the mixture was incubated during rotation for 60 minutes. Adherent bacteria (Figure 9.11) were counted under direct light microscopy. The results (Figure 9.12) demonstrated convincingly that pyelonephritic strains were more adherent than strains from other disorders of the lower urinary tract.[43] This effect was negated when the organisms were incubated with antibodies against the strain tested. These observations were extended by Fowler and Stamey, who studied adherence to vaginal cells from controls and from women susceptible to lower urinary tract infection (Figure 9.13). Significant adherence was demonstrated, suggesting the possibility that general cellular characteristics might be involved in the adherence process.[44] This concept was taken further by Schaeffer and co-workers, who confirmed the findings on vaginal cells and then showed that the same phenomenon could be observed on buccal cells (Figure 9.14). These observations clearly indicated

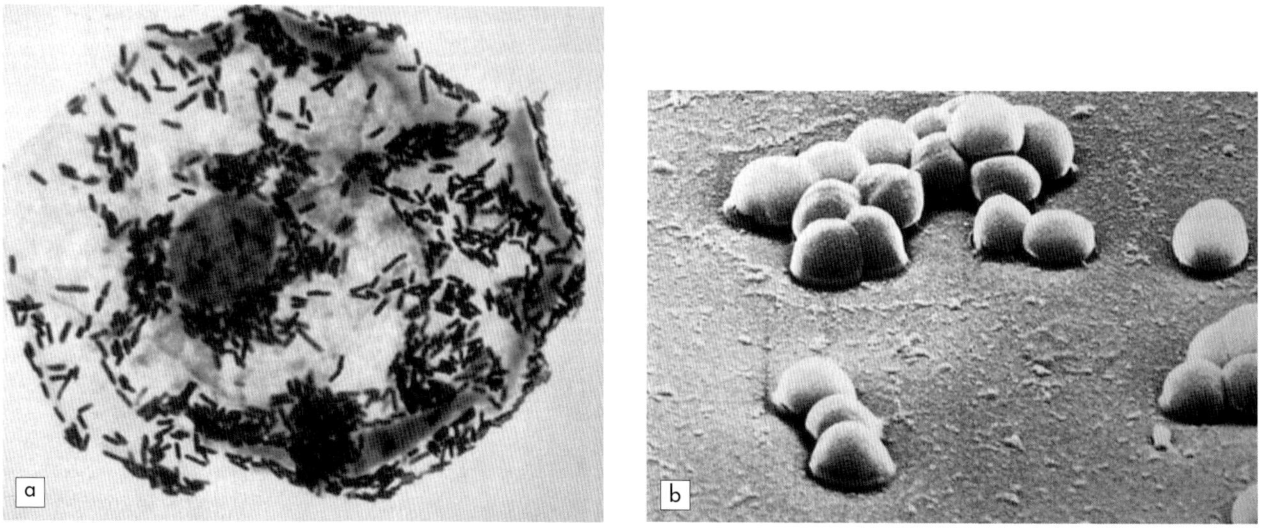

Figure 9.11 *Examples of bacterial adherence. (a) Adherence of* E. coli *to epithelial cell. (b) Adhesion of colonies to the surface of a urinary catheter. Such adhesion is thought to be mediated by type 1 fimbriae.*[27]

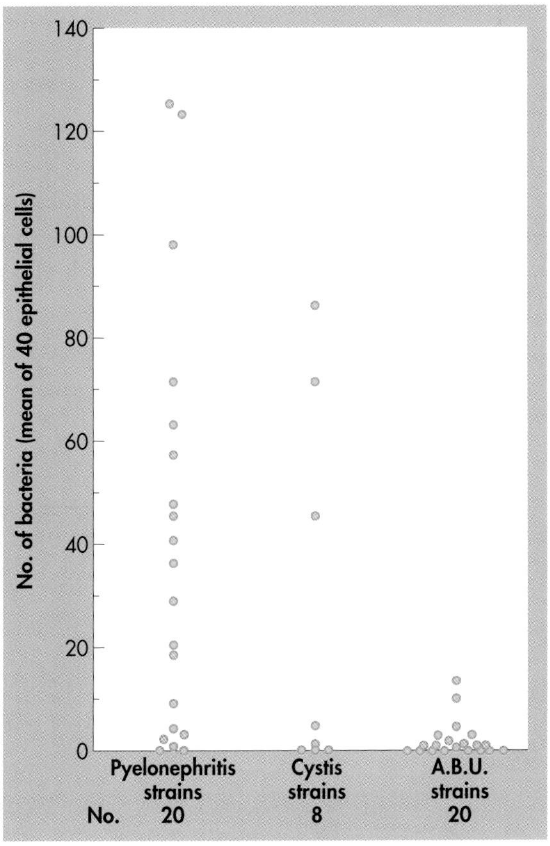

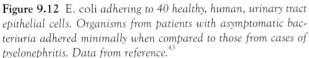

Figure 9.12 E. coli *adhering to 40 healthy, human, urinary tract epithelial cells. Organisms from patients with asymptomatic bacteriuria adhered minimally when compared to those from cases of pyelonephritis. Data from reference.*[43]

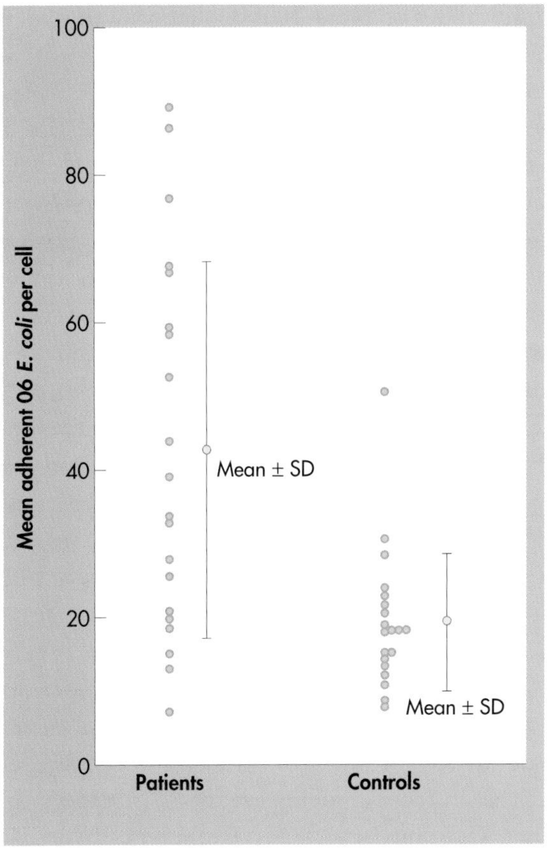

Figure 9.13 *In vitro adherence of* E. coli *to vaginal epithelial cells in patients susceptible to recurrent urinary tract infection compared to controls. Data from reference.*[44]

that there might be a widespread alteration in the surface characteristics of mucosal epithelial cells in particular susceptible individuals.[45]

Previously, Sellwood and co-workers at the Veterinary Agricultural Research Council had noted that *E. coli* strains expressing K-88 surface antigen caused neonatal diarrhoea when administered to some piglets, but not others. This phenomenon was observed to be due to K-88 adherence to intestinal cell brush borders in piglets that developed

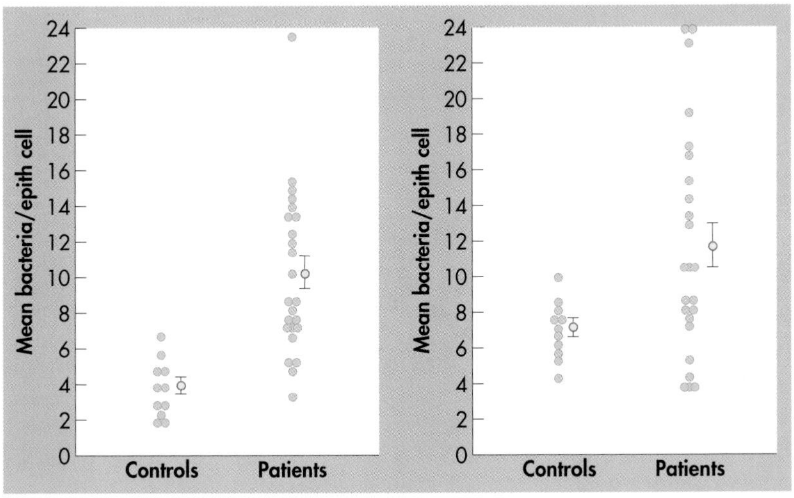

Figure 9.14 *In vitro adherence of* E. coli *to vaginal cells (left panel) and buccal cells (right panel) from patients with recurrent urinary tract infections as compared to controls. Data from reference.*[45]

diarrhoea, while those that remained well did not show this phenomenon.[46,47] Subsequently, it was found that 'adhesive' and 'non-adhesive' piglets inherited these intestinal cellular characteristics in a simple Mendelian manner, and these findings have since been acknowledged as the first report of a genetic basis for resistance to enteric disease.[48] Schaeffer, quoting this work, noted that it might explain in part why some patients' resistance to infectious disease could correlate with their blood groups.[49]

Subsequent ability to identify P fimbriated varieties of *E. coli* allowed further investigation into the mechanisms of urinary tract infection. Källenius et al[50] examined 97 children with urinary tract infection and compared them with 82 healthy controls. P fimbriated forms were found in 33/35 (91%) of urinary strains causing acute pyelonephritis, but in only 19% of patients with cystitis and 14% of cases with asymptomatic bacteriuria. By contrast, only 7% of faecal isolates from healthy controls carried such fimbriae. Further evidence of the importance of P fimbriation was observed by Johnson et al,[51] who investigated host conditions that might be associated with increased frequency of P fimbriae or other virulence factors. These studies clearly showed that, while P fimbriated forms remained *relatively* common in the presence of anatomical urinary tract abnormality or after instrumentation, the fimbriated form was absolutely essential if infection was to occur when none of these predisposing abnormalities were present. In summary, coliform strains with a variety of characteristics are capable of causing upper urinary tract infection in the presence of (that is, with the help of) obstruction or other abnormalities; however, for infection to supervene in a completely normal upper urinary tract, the presence of the P fimbriated form of *E. coli* is almost essential.

Recently, in an elegant experiment, Wullt and co-workers examined the ability of P fimbriae to induce inflammation in the human urinary tract, and at the same time they sought to satisfy Koch's 'molecular' postulates linking P pilus expression to the host inflammatory response. Koch's postulates state that, from diseased tissue, isolates should be recoverable, be reproducible in culture and, on reintroduction to a susceptible host, be the cause of further recognizable disease. At molecular level, the same postulates can be examined with respect to various factors such as the putative virulence mechanisms of the coliform bacillus.

It has already been noted that P fimbriation is associated with pyelonephritis in approximately 90% of cases, but in <20% of patients with asymptomatic bacteriuria (ABU).[50,52,53] Nevertheless, other adhesins – type I, type S and Dr adhesins – may also be isolated from patients with upper tract infection,

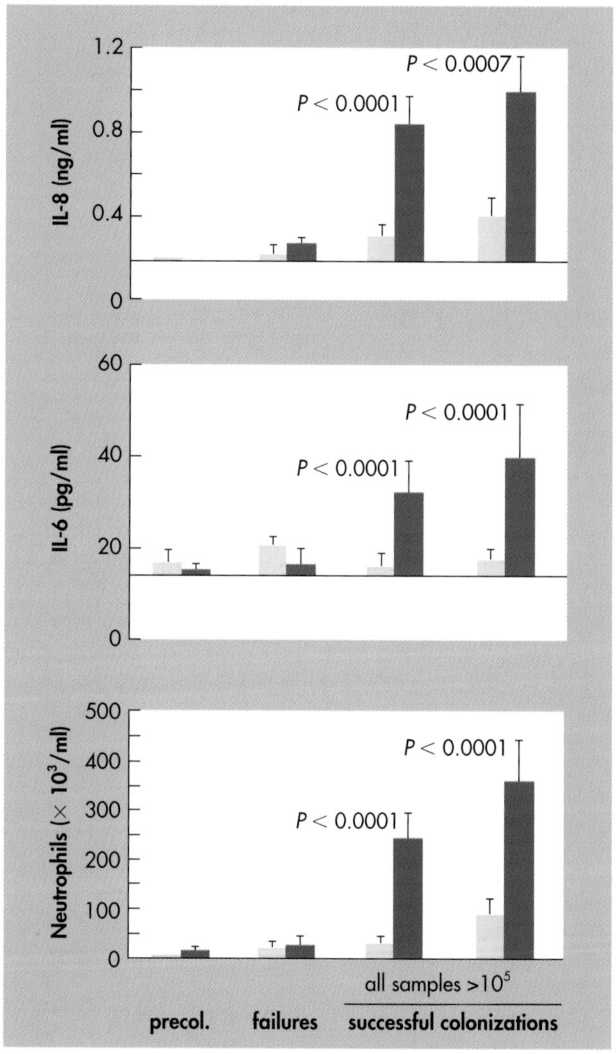

Figure 9.15 *Neutrophil, IL-6 and IL-8 responses to intravesical inoculation with ABU* E. coli *83972 non-fimbrinated strain (grey bars) and the same* E. coli *83972 strain transformed with recombinant plasmids encoding class II or class III P fimbriae (black bars). Responses identified in urine; see text for details. Precol.: Precolonization. Data from Wullt et al.*[54]

and the question arises as to which of these characteristics is the pre-eminent cause of disease. However, other lines of evidence (the ability to enter the bloodstream, to enhance experimental infection and to promote a cytokine response) suggest strongly that P fimbriae are indeed the significant independent virulence factors. To resolve this problem, 17 human volunteers received intravesical inoculation of either a non-fimbriated ABU coliform strain or Pap transformants of the same strain, the former acting as control to negate the possibility of non-specific adhesin formation linked to DNA sequences carried by the ABU strain. The result (Figure 9.15) demonstrated that the presence of the Pap transformants invariably caused higher neutrophil and cytokine responses; furthermore, loss of Pap expression was linked to a reduction in background inflammatory levels. Control strains did not cause a significant host response. Taken as a whole, the results provided convincing evidence that P fimbriation per se converted a low- into a high-virulence strain, suggesting in turn that Koch's 'molecular' postulates were indeed fulfilled.[54]

Type S pili

Less well defined than the preceding types of pili, S types nevertheless share a similar structure of Sfa A subunits, with the Sfa S subunit localized to the tip and interacting with sialic acid receptors on renal vascular and epithelial cells. The fimbriae may facilitate bacterial dissemination, and the type has been associated with pathogenic strains that are associated with sepsis and meningitis as well as ascending urinary tract infection.[55] FIC pili are homologous with type S and may be present on approximately 14% of pathogenic coliforms.

Dr adhesin family

The family includes both pilus-like adhesin Dr and non-fimbrial adhesion molecules. Their function remains open to question, but they can be isolated in a high proportion of children with urinary tract infection and one-third of pregnant women with pyelonephritis. They may be responsible for long-term bacterial persistence within the upper tract.[56]

Clinical aspects of adhesion theory

The ability to adhere and thus to persist within the host is an advantage to the micro-organism in a number of circumstances; it helps the pathogen to remain within its source (reservoir), to survive during the journey to the target tissue, and to establish and replicate on arrival within the lower urinary tract. Receptors for P fimbriae have been identified within the colon, and this attachment mechanism has been proposed to explain persistence of pathogenic organisms within the reservoir.[57] Such strains expressing Pap established themselves more rapidly in children susceptible to urinary tract infection than organisms without the adhesin.[53] Recent studies of cystitis in young schoolgirls,[58] chosen (by age) to exclude the effect of sexual intercourse, observed that the clones of organisms responsible for the infection were P fimbriated, whereas those forms were not usually found on the perineum – where clones exhibiting type I fimbriae and other virulence factors predominated. These observations, when summarized, indicate that both type I and type P fimbriae are commonly to be found in the faecal reservoir, as well as the periurethral zone, and may variously facilitate the initial move towards the lower urinary tract. Clearly, phase

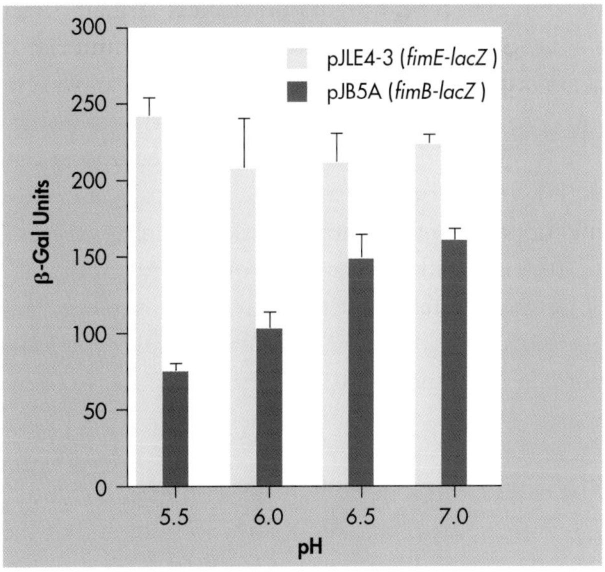

Figure 9.16 *Microenvironment and pathogenicity. Effect of altered pH in human urine on pilus expression. With a sodium phosphate buffer, the expression of FimB almost doubles at pH 7.0, whereas FimE levels remain constant throughout. Data from reference.*[37]

variation, 'cross-talk' and an altered microenvironment (the effect of *Bacillus acidophyllus* is noted above) may significantly alter fimbrial expression (Figure 9.16), both to evade host defences and to maintain optimal pathogenicity en route to the target cells. Needless to mention, this ability rapidly to vary expression makes the study of virulence factors particularly difficult for microbiological researchers. Hence, it is not entirely clear which virulence factors are responsible for colonization and for development of clinical disease in the lower urinary tract. Certainly, the variability mentioned above means that it is difficult at this time to predict infection on the basis of adhesin analysis of introital or periurethral organisms.[58]

Finally, it should be noted that the identification of certain forms of an organism associated with particular tissues does not per se prove a relationship with clinical disease – hence the need to test Koch's postulates. In particular, type I fimbriae are found in a majority of enterobacteria, on both non-pathogenic as well as pathogenic *E. coli*. In the experiments of Wullt and co-workers mentioned above, it was acknowledged that the inflammatory responses induced *in urine* were *not* observed systemically, where all patients remained well.[54] This, however, was an experiment on the bladder of humans, and not on the acknowledged target of Pap pili, the urothelium of the renal pelvis and calyces, a fact which might explain the observed lack of systemic response. Both type I and Pap III/Forsmann antigen mechanisms have been implicated in cystitis, but the interaction remains obscure, as do the various forms of inflammatory responses initiated during infection.[36,59] Transmission of the organism and subsequent establishment of clinical disease are clearly highly complex microbiological processes which remain minimally understood at the present time.

Therapeutic implications

The observations noted above might assist treatment of affected individuals in a number of ways. Variation in adhesion potential might identify at-risk groups. Fimbriae would appear to be a rational target for antimicrobial therapy and vaccine development. In the veterinary piglets experiment referred to above, effective vaccines based initially on the K-88 antigen were developed and successfully prevented neonatal diarrhoea in the susceptible groups. Immunization with purified P fimbriae has been attempted in a number of animal models, with variable success. In a primate setting, vaccination with a Fim H adhesin–chaperone complex protected three of four treated monkeys while all control animals developed cystitis, suggesting that such techniques might have application in humans with chronic lower urinary tract infection.[59a] As might be expected, phase variation and other types of antigen variability might be expected to cause problems in this type of therapeutic approach.

Virulence factors in other uropathogens

Not surprisingly, studies of other species involved in urinary tract infection have demonstrated the presence of adherence mechanisms. *Proteus mirabilis* and *Klebsiella* spp. have been found to express fimbriae in animal experiments.[60,61] *Staph. saprophyticus* is known to be able to adhere avidly to uroepithelial cells, probably by non-specific adherence mechanisms.

Summary of virulence factors in urinary tract infections

It is appropriate to bring together those factors which are thought to be important with respect to the virulence of Gram-negative bacteria in general and *E. coli* in particular (Table 9.9, Figure 9.17).

The antigenic structure of the bacterial surface is classically described in terms of three classes of antigens. O antigens represent the polysaccharide side chains of the lipopolysaccharide structure found in all Gram-negative bacteria. The polysaccharide is anchored to the outer membrane by lipid A (see also Figure 9.27), the agent thought to be responsible for endotoxic shock, as described below. O antigens are heat stable and classically certain serogroups (01, 02, 04, 06, 07, 016, 018 and 075) responsible for urinary infections, such strains being responsible for up to 80% of cases of pyelonephritis. Modern theory suggests that the O antigen is not itself specifically responsible for pathogenicity; rather, the identified serogroups represent clones of organisms with a selection or panel of various virulence properties that enable successful colonization of the urinary tract. Other serogroups and hence other combinations of virulence factors may enable successful colonization of other areas such as the gastrointestinal tract. *K* capsular antigen is partially heat stable and may, on occasion, partially obscure the O antigen (Figure 9.17). *K* capsular polysaccharide antigen has been strongly associated with pyelonephritis for many years, both in adults[62] and in children.[63] Some 70% of strains from children with pyelonephritis were associated with K1, K2, K3, K12 and K13 antigens, of which K1 is acknowledged to be the most frequently associated strain with pyelonephritic disease. Interestingly, K1 strains have also been associated with 80% of *E. coli* strains causing neonatal meningitis.[63]

Adherence mechanisms have been fully described above, and the relationship between type 1 fimbriae, P fimbriae and the ability to cause urinary tract infection has been noted. Typically, *E. coli* may be killed by serum bactericidal activity relating to both the classical and alternative pathway of complement. Cell-wall lipopolysaccharide (O antigen) is thought to provide a degree of resistance against complement-mediated digestion, and, recently, Leying and associates have suggested that the K1 polysaccharide antigen may also confer significant levels of serum resistance on the organism.[22] The advantages conferred on those organisms expressing haemolysin and aerobactin have been noted above. Colicin V is another virulence factor which has selectively been found to be present in isolates from urine, but not from isolates in the faecal reservoir. Colicin V is assumed to interfere with host defence mechanisms.[18,19]

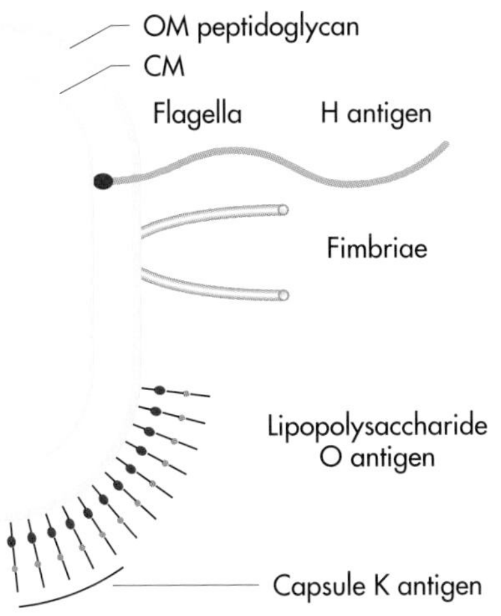

Figure 9.17 *Schematic diagram of cell-wall Gram-negative bacteria and associated structures. CM: cytoplasmic membrane; OM: outer membrane. Note differential size of flagella and fimbriae. Lipid A (see text) is on the innermost aspect of the lipopolysaccharide O antigen, next to the outer membrane (see also Figure 9.27).*

Table 9.9 Virulence factors associated with *E. coli.*
Specific O serotypes
K capsular antigen
Adherence mechanisms
Resistance to serum bactericidal activity
Haemolysin production
Aerobactin production
Colicin V

ORGANISMS RESPONSIBLE FOR URINARY TRACT INFECTION

The great majority of urinary tract infections are caused by single bacterial species; among these, *E. coli* is by far the most common, accounting for approximately 85% of general or community-based infections at the present time. Previous studies (Table 9.10) have emphasized the differences between general practice and hospital practice, where *E. coli* accounts for only approximately 50% of the isolates. *Proteus*, *Klebsiella*, enterococci and *Pseudomonas* are all more frequently isolated from hospital patients, especially if an in-dwelling catheter is present.[64,65] Remaining organisms include *Enterobacter*, *Citrobacter* and *Serratia*; fungal infections are rarely encountered outside hospital practice.

The presence of abnormalities in the urinary tract, as may be found in congenital abnormality or obstruction, often leads to infection by non-coliform organisms, such as *Proteus* and *Klebsiella*, and, under these circumstances, mixed infections are also frequently encountered. Naturally, obstruction related

Table 9.10 Organisms causing urinary tract infection in community and hospital practice. Although the proportions of organisms have remained relatively similar, it is accepted that in the 1990s approximately 80–85% of community urinary tract infection was related to *E. coli*. The comparable figure for hospital-based infections has remained steady at approximately 50%.

	General practice		Hospital practice	
	1976[1]	1971[2]	1971[2]	1978[2]
E. coli	72	78.5	55.4	50.7
Proteus mirabilis	9	9.2	11.4	10.6
Staphylococci	6	5.1	3..3	2.7
Strep. faecalis	3.3	2.3	4.0	4.3
Klebsiella spp.	2.7	2.3	16.8	21.6
Pseudomonas	–	–	2.7	2.8
Remainder	7.0	2.6	6.4	7.3

[1]Ref.64.
[2]Ref.65.

to stone formation is often associated with *Proteus mirabilis*. *Staph. saprophyticus* has been identified, particularly in the USA, as a cause of acute cystitis in young, sexually active females.[66] Anaerobic organisms are rarely pathogens in the urinary tract. Maskell et al supported the concept that slow-growing CO_2-dependent, Gram-positive bacteria might be responsible for the 'urethral syndrome',[67] although these suggestions that 'fastidious' organisms could be responsible for the symptom complex were strongly denied by other workers.[68] Apart from lactobacilli, *Gardinerella vaginalis* and *Ureaplasma urealyticum* are not infrequently isolated, but their role in infection of the lower urinary tract remains unproven.

Routes of infection

Organisms may enter the urinary tract via the ascending route, the haematogenous route or the lymphatic route.

Ascending route

The difference in the incidence of lower urinary tract infection between men and women strongly suggests that the ascending urethral route is the most common pathway for infection; in the female, organisms have been isolated from the bladder after both urethral massage[69] and sexual intercourse.[70] One insertion of a urinary catheter into the bladder has been observed to result in lower urinary tract infection in 1–2% of patients.[71] It is widely agreed that the presence of a urethral catheter for more than 36/48 hours almost invariably results in bladder bacteriuria. Recent studies suggest that spermicidal agents encourage the colonization of the introital region with uropathogenic bacteria.[72] The relationship between the introital flora and lower urinary tract infection is further considered below.

The question of ascent into the upper tract from the bladder in the absence of reflux appears problematical. Presumably, various virulence factors must aid progression through the vesicoureteric junction; perhaps mucosal oedema caused by local inflammation disrupts the valvular mechanisms and allows passage of organisms which then successfully colonize the upper tracts by means of the appropriate fimbrinated structures. Diuresis and loss of the usual co-apting ureteral mechanisms have also been suggested as a mechanism whereby organisms may gain entry into the upper tract.

Haematogenous route

Blood-borne infection of the kidney is a well-described though uncommon mechanism of renal infection in individuals who are otherwise normal. Staphylococcal spread from dental abscesses may occur, and these and other organisms may originate from sites such as diseased heart valves. Haematogenous spread of *Candida albicans* has been observed in experimental circumstances, although this fungus is not usually observed unless a chronic in-dwelling catheter is present. Interestingly, if one ureter is tied and bacteria are introduced into the bladder during experimentation on animals, infection supervenes in the non-obstructed kidney, but not on the hydronephrotic side.[73] This convincingly demonstrates the overriding importance of the ascending route and the relative resistance to haematological spread, even in the presence of severe obstruction – conditions under which it is acknowledged that haematogenous infection should easily supervene.

Lymphatic route

Theoretically, infection could spread via lymphatics into various parts of the urinary tract, but, in practice, there is little clinical evidence for such a mode of infection. Occasional experimental reports have failed to convince that the lymphatic route is other than of academic interest.

CLINICAL ASPECTS OF URINARY TRACT INFECTION

The significance of 'significance'

Historically, there have always been difficulties distinguishing between true bacteriuria, defined as actual residence of bacteria within the urinary tract, and contamination, defined as the adventitious entry of bacteria into the urine during the collection of the specimen. This problem was most notably tackled in the mid-1950s by Edward H Kass from Boston, who performed a number of studies on women with various disorders of the lower urinary tract in both the normal and pregnant state. In his most important study, the urine of female patients attending as outpatients was studied, specimens being obtained by catheterization and cultured promptly thereafter.[74] He found (Figure 9.18) that the patients could broadly be divided into two groups. In the first group were patients with bacterial counts between 0 and 100 000 per ml of urine; of these, only approximately 15% had a past history of urinary tract infection, instrumentation or catheterization of the urinary tract. He noted that the bacteria obtained in this group were usually the common saprophytes of the urinary tract, and his contention that these were contaminated specimens was further supported by the fact that second samples obtained from the same group usually demonstrated dissimilar organisms and counts.

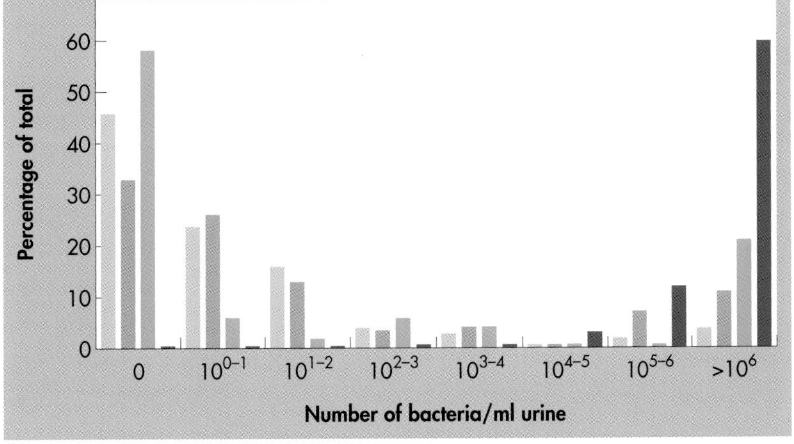

Figure 9.18 *Bacterial counts in urine of various population groups. Kass noted that most of the patients with low counts did not have a history of urinary tract infection, and in these cases reculture frequently demonstrated different organisms. However patients with $>10^5$ organisms, however, frequently had pure cultures associated with significant clinical infections (pyelonephritis). Data from reference.*[74]

By contrast, in the second group with more than 100 000 bacteria per ml, 55% had a past history of urinary tract infections, and repeat sampling in these patients revealed similarly high counts, both specimens yielding commonly accepted pathogens of the urinary tract. These simple yet ground-breaking observations define the level of 'bacterial significance' widely used to this day – 10^5 organisms or colony-forming units (CFU) per ml from midstream urine.

For a quarter of a century, the scientific distinction between patients with contaminants and patients with true infection was broadly welcomed. Gradually, however, it became clear that there were a significant number of women with dysuria and frequent urination whose midstream urines did not contain 'significant' bacteriuria, and to these women the label 'acute urethral syndrome' was applied. In an important study, Stamm et al investigated 59 women with 'acute urethral syndrome', from whom bladder urine was obtained either by suprapubic aspiration or clean urethral catheterization. Forty-two patients had abnormal pyuria, and 37 of these were infected with coliforms, *Staph. saprophyticus* or *Chlamydia trachomatis*. Patients without pyuria had little demonstrable infection. Stamm et al concluded that the classic Kass criteria of $>10^5$/ml was an insensitive diagnostic criterion when applied to symptomatic lower urinary tract infection in this group of relatively young, sexually active women.[75]

This and other similar studies[76] provoked a flurry of editorial comment.[77,78] Doubt was cast over the suggestion that 10^2 organisms per ml could reliably discriminate between patients with infected and uninfected lower urinary tracts. Additionally, it was noted that many midstream urine cultures were mixed – ignoring the conventional wisdom that true pathogens are usually found in pure culture. Nevertheless, it was acknowledged that most of Stamm's bacteriuric patients ($>10^2$, $<10^5$) had pyuria, suggesting that this was indeed a true infection.[52] Stamm himself made further comment and reviewed the situation in 1984.[78] He pointed out that the essence of Kass's original work (often forgotten) concerned patients with pyelonephritis, not women with acute frequency/dysuria lower tract symptoms. He made a plea for closer communication between clinicians and laboratory so as to obtain better information from the more flexible approach to quantitative bacteriological sampling. There is little doubt that urologists should be aware that 'no significant growth' may mean different things according to definitions in different bacteriological laboratories. It is the responsibility of each clinician to determine whether such a report refers to 10^5 CFU/ml or 10^2 CFU/ml – as usual, optimum results result only from close cooperation between clinical and laboratory service.

The introital question

Another major microbiological debate concerns the means whereby pathogenic organisms pass from the (presumed) faecal reservoir to the lower urinary tract. In particular, the importance of organisms that colonize the vaginal introitus and periurethral region has been discussed at great length, and the debate continues to the present day.

There seems little doubt that *E. coli* – pathogenic or otherwise – may obtain a foothold in the introital area, and, in this respect, it has been noted above that mannose-sensitive type 1 pili adhere powerfully to vaginal epithelial cells,[45] vaginal mucus[79] and uromucoid.[9] It has also been emphasized that type 1 fimbriae are to be found on non-pathogenic as well as pathogenic enterobacteria.

Three essential questions may be asked:

1. Do women at risk of urinary tract infections carry pathogenic organisms in the introital and periurethral area?
2. If so, are these organisms responsible for the symptomatic bladder or pyelonephritic infection?
3. In such cases, what is the state of the introital and periurethral area between overt symptomatic clinical infections?

A number of workers support the concept that abnormal periurethral flora are to be found in women with recurrent infections. Hinman's group[80] studied 43 patients and found that the flora contained a higher percentage of pathogenic microorganisms than that of female subjects without urological disease. In a general practice study from

London, Grüneberg observed that the infecting strain of *E. coli* was isolated from rectal, vaginal and periurethral flora in nearly all cases. Furthermore, he noted that chemotherapy eradicated the organism from the urine but not necessarily from the introital/urethral area.[81] Stamey studied cultures from 20 premenopausal controls compared to cultures from nine women with recurrent urinary infections.[82] He observed that not only was introital colonization significantly higher in the patients, but also enterobacteria persist after the infectious episode, and he postulated that the introital mucosa in women with infection was biologically different from the same area in women who never suffer from lower urinary tract infection. This postulate was supported some years later by Pfau and Sacks,[83] who had previously shown that the predominant bacterial flora of the introital and periurethral area consisted of lactobacilli and staphylococci, Gram-negative bacteria being infrequent and transitory. These workers found *E. coli* to be the predominant micro-organism recovered from 68% of introital, 60% of vaginal and 42% or urethral cultures.

Despite these apparently conclusive results by American researchers, a number of British workers failed to confirm the findings.[84–87] Nevertheless, although an absolute association between periurethral flora and lower urinary tract infection could not be demonstrated, it was acknowledged that the presence of *E. coli* in the introital area might constitute a 'permissive factor' for the subsequent development of overt infection.[84] Similarly, O'Grady et al could find no difference in the carriage rate between normal women and women with symptoms suggestive of urinary tract infection, although, again, these workers acknowledged that introital bacteria were more commonly recovered in patients when symptomatic (34%) than when symptom free (19%).[85] In a further development, Brumfitt observed that women with recurrent urinary infections were susceptible to perineal and periurethral colonization with Gram-negative bacteria, but they noted that the infection need not be with the colonizing enterobacteria.[86] Kunin, in an editorial comment, attempted to reconcile these positions[83] by suggesting that most workers could agree that infections were indeed preceded by colonization of the periurethral area with Gram-negative bacteria, but he considered that the evidence for colonization of this area between infections was less convincing. It may be argued that the presence or absence of organisms is not so critical as the ability of any organisms that may be present – that is, the virulence mechanism carried on those organisms – to ascend and invade the lower urinary tract. In summary, colonization is important, but the critical factor relates to the presence or absence of essential virulence mechanisms.

Urinary tract infection – variation by age and sex

It is appropriate at this point to review the changes that may occur in the urinary tract of either sex as a result of invasion by micro-organisms. Table 9.11 records the prevalence of bacteriuria by age in either sex as determined by studies in the literature. It is immediately apparent that bacteriuria is more common in females at all times of life, with the single exception of babies under 3 months old, among whom boys are more than twice as likely to have clinical infection than girls.

Infants

In the first month of life, there is a virtually identical incidence of urinary tract infection in girls and boys.[88] Interestingly, in infants under 3 months old, the infection rate in males depends on whether circumcision has been performed. For those who have had the operation, the incidence of infection is significantly less than that of girls of the same age. For uncircumcised infants, however, the risk is considerably greater, and it is clear that the presence of the foreskin is linked to an increased incidence of lower urinary tract infection. These observations were made in a remarkable study of 422 328 children born to members of the US services over a 10-year period. Precision military record keeping allowed the result of circumcision to be accurately documented (Figure 9.19). A surprising 80% of the male population underwent circumcision, but the 20% who did not suffered 70% of the male urinary tract infections.[88] The authors

Table 9.11 Prevalence of bacteriuria by age (%). The identified groups of patients are fully discussed in the text.

	Age years									
	<½	<³⁄₁₂	<5	School age	Young men	Non-pregnant females	Pregnant females	Pregnant females previous bacteriuria	65–70	>80
Male	0.075	Circumcised 0.07 Non-circumcised 0.77	0.5	0.03	<0.1	–	–	–	2–3	>20
Female	0.077	0.3	4.5	1.2	–	1.3	4–7	35	20	>20
Reference	63	63	67	68, 69, 70 70, 71, 72	–	73	72, 74, 75	70, 71	76	76

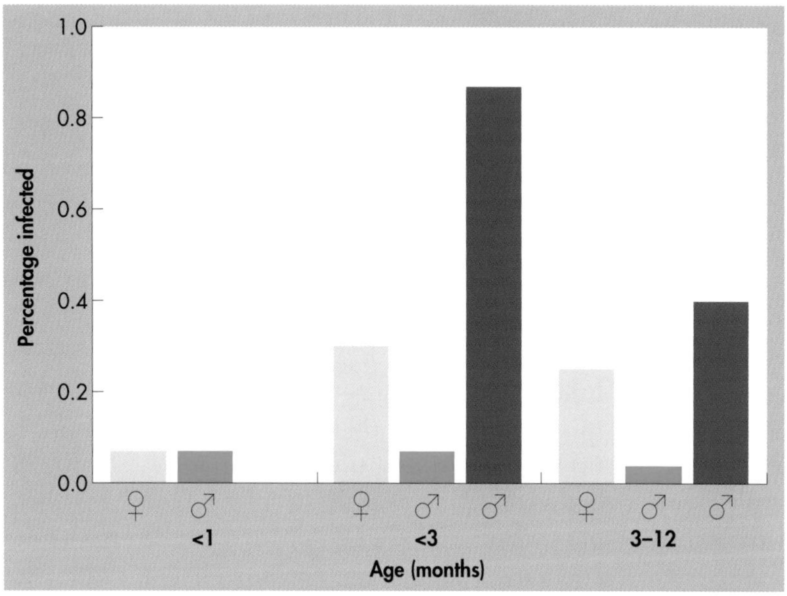

Figure 9.19 *Urinary tract infection in infants under 1 year. The incidence of infection between sexes is approximately similar under 1 month, but thereafter girls have more infections than boys unless the boys have not been circumcised. ■ Circumcised; ■ uncircumcised. Data from reference.*[88]

later proved their point by noting that a subsequent decline in the circumcision rate was associated with an increased incidence of male infant infection.[89]

Pre-school children

Urinary tract infection is important in children of this age group, as most paediatricians consider renal development to be most at risk at this time. Both symptomatic and asymptomatic infections are more common in girls, although the line between the two is difficult to draw – careful history taking in children with 'asymptomatic bacteriuria' often reveals symptoms strongly suggestive of urinary tract infection (UTI).[90] From the first year onward, infections become increasingly uncommon in male infants; indeed, the presence of such an infection may indicate significant disease or other abnormality of the urinary tract. Infections in girls may be troublesome and, as noted above, permanent damage relating to the reflux of infected urine may occur by mechanisms such as those described by Ransley.[91] It is difficult to avoid the conclusion that bacteriuria is a very important finding in this group of children.[92]

Bacteriuria in schoolchildren

As can be seen from Table 9.11, the problem of bacteriuria in schoolchildren relates almost entirely to girls. There is an impressive body of evidence concerning the nature and outcome of such infections. In Charlottesville, Virginia, an area with a stable local population, Kunin prospectively studied the characteristics and natural history of urinary tract infection in schoolgirls between 1959 and 1968. It was observed that bacteriuria was common in schoolgirls and symptoms were often absent; recurrence frequently occurred.[93] Approximately one-third of the girls had symptoms of the infection at the time of detection. In the UK, Meadow et al reported broadly similar findings in Birmingham schoolchildren. Infection in schoolboys was essentially undetectable, but 1% of girls had significant asymptomatic bacteriuria.[94] In another important prospective study, the Cardiff/ Oxford bacteriuria study group followed 208 girls from 5–12 years of age who had been identified as suffering from bacteriuria. The girls were followed for 4 years, and the authors noted that treatment had little effect on the emergence of symptoms, the clearance of vesicoureteric reflux, renal growth or the progression of renal scars. These observations seemed to suggest that renal damage had occurred before 5 years of age, as noted above.[95]

Effect of bacteriuria on subsequent pregnancy

Both Kunin's group and the Oxford/Cardiff group continued to follow their young women as they grew up and eventually became pregnant. These irreplaceable studies have emphasized the importance of vigilance with respect to young bacteriuric schoolgirls.

Gillenwater reported the US results in 1979. Sixty schoolgirls with bacteriuria and 38 matched controls had been followed for periods ranging up to 18 years. Renal scars and/or caliectasis were observed to occur only in the bacteriuric group, but renal function and blood pressure were not affected. The study group had 10 times as many bacteriuric episodes as did controls, and infections were particularly common during subsequent pregnancy. Most interestingly, seven children of the bacteriuric mothers, but none of the controls themselves, showed urinary tract infections.[96]

The Oxford/Cardiff group studied 52 pregnancies in 34 women who had been found to have bacteriuria in childhood. At the first antenatal visit, the prevalence of bacteriuria in the study group was significantly greater (35%) than that in the control group (5%). During pregnancy, pyelonephritis developed in 10% of the study group and in 4% of controls. The data suggested that previously bacteriuric women known to have renal scars were at increased risk of hypertension and pre-eclampsia of pregnancy, findings which have not been universally accepted. No comment was made about the children resulting from these pregnancies and their susceptibility or otherwise to urinary tract infection.[97]

In summary, therefore, these observations show that asymptomatic bacteriuria in schoolgirls persists over long periods of time. Subsequently, such young women are at greater risk of infection during pregnancy, and if renal damage has occurred in earlier life, the pregnancy may perhaps be complicated by hypertension or pre-eclampsia. The children of such women appear to inherit an ongoing susceptibility to bacteriuria and infection.

Young, non-pregnant females

It is generally accepted that the prevalence of bacteriuria in this group is approximately 1% per decade. To investigate the assumption that these cases were largely intercourse-related, Kunin's group compared the prevalence of significant bacteriuria in nuns and married women. As expected, they found that celibacy was associated with a lower frequency of infection, but young nuns still had a higher frequency of urinary infection than young males. He commented later that it was not clear from this study whether there was a subpopulation of women who were inherently susceptible to urinary infection that was not the result of sexual intercourse.[98]

Bacteriuria during pregnancy

There is general agreement that 4–7% of pregnant women have bacteriuria,[99,100] and of these 20–40% will develop symptomatic infection later in the pregnancy, usually in the third trimester. Bacteriuria in the lower urinary tract more commonly leads to pyelonephritis in pregnant than non-pregnant women, presumably because of the various changes that occur in the upper tracts as a result of the pregnancy. The prevalence of bacteriuria during pregnancy rises with parity, sexual activity, age, diabetes mellitus and sickle-cell trait. It has already been mentioned that pregnant women who were bacteriuric as schoolgirls carry a significantly greater risk of urinary tract infection during pregnancy.[95,96]

Urinary tract infection in young adult men

As previously emphasized, urinary tract infection in otherwise healthy adult men is very uncommon. Presumably, the large difference in prevalence between men and women is related to the length of the urethra and the difficulties which face uropathogens attempting to reach the urethral meatus from the faecal reservoir. The antibacterial nature of prostatic fluid is noted below. Presumably, most infections that occur arise due to sexual intercourse with an infected female partner, or, in the case of homosexuality, direct contamination from the faecal reservoir.

Older patients

The bias in favour of female patients which operates throughout most of life begins to reverse in old age. Presumably because of prostatic obstruction, residual urine and other problems in the lower urinary tract of older men, the incidence of bacteriuria rises steeply to significant levels, particularly after the age of 70 (Table 9.11). It has been observed that the place of residence has an important influence on the presence or otherwise of bacteriuria. Older men living at home have a lesser incidence of bacteriuria than those living in nursing homes, where the prevalence in both sexes is approximately 20%. Figures for those resident in hospital inpatient facilities are even higher.[101]

Uncomplicated cystitis in females

Approximately 20% of women experience an episode of simple cystitis during their lifetime. Most of these settle rapidly, but 2–3% suffer from repeat infections. In a Danish study, non-pregnant women 16–65 years of age were referred to the medical outpatient clinic, where a placebo study of patients with acute symptomatic lower urinary tract infection was undertaken. Fifty-three female patients were given placebo and were followed for longer than 12 months following the initial infection; 43 of these (81%) spontaneously cleared their urine within 5 months.[102] Unfortunately, nearly half these patients became reinfected within a year, and similar observations were found in the antibiotic-treated group. The author concluded that host defence and eradication mechanisms could be very effective, but to keep recurrence of bacteriuria to a minimum, it would be necessary to recheck urine samples for at least 6 months after the initial elimination of bacteriuria.

Typically, uncomplicated lower urinary tract infection is caused by *E. coli* in 80% of domicillary cases. *Staph. saprophyticus* may be implicated in up to 5% of cases, this organism being particularly noted in the literature from North America. The causes of the 'acute urethral syndrome', as reported by Stamm et al, have already been noted.[75] It seems reasonable that a pure growth of organism at concentrations between 10^2 and 10^5 accompanied by pyuria, should be accepted as a case of true cystitis. The case of bladder urine with mixed organisms and equivocal pyuria is much more debatable; these may perhaps be better described as equivocal cystitis, in contradistinction to the true urethral syndrome described below in which the symptoms of urethral irritation are accompanied neither by organisms nor by pyuria – the female equivalent of 'prostatodynia'.

The urethral syndrome

A critical definition of the female urethral syndrome refers to the symptoms of frequency and dysuria in the absence of bacteriuria and pyuria in both initial (VB1) and midstream (VB2) urine when analysis is made on several separate occasions. This definition assumes that such female patients have been thoroughly screened to exclude vesical motor dysfunction (bladder instability) as well as systemic and local (such as trauma, tumour and irradiation injury) disease.[103]

A number of workers have stressed the importance of pyuria in patients with such urethral symptomatology. O'Grady et al[104] proposed that pyuria was significant even when tests failed to identify bacteriuria. In their studies, if cultures were performed over extended periods of time, bacteria were eventually identified; thus, this patient group was designated as being 'between infections'.[104] *Chlamydia trochomatis* was identified in 10 of 16 patients with pyuria, but in only one of 16 patients without white cells in the urine.[50] The controversy surrounding more fastidious carbon dioxide-dependent organisms – chiefly lactobacilli – has also been noted.[67] In summary, although considerable effort may be required, the presence of pyuria may often give a clue as to the true bacteriological cause of the frequency dysuria syndrome. Those who have neither bacteriuria nor pyuria constitute the essential core of those who are said to suffer from the true 'urethral syndrome'.

Pyelonephritis

The clinical, radiographic and therapeutic aspects of acute and chronic pyelonephritis are beyond the remit of this work. The important virulence factors which enable colonization of the upper tract have been noted, as have those factors in childhood which later predispose to pyelonephritis of pregnancy. It is generally agreed that uncomplicated pyelonephritis in adults – as opposed to infants under 5 years – rarely leads to permanent and progressive renal damage with scarring. Renal function usually remains stable.

Stones and infection

Most urinary infections are caused by *E. coli*, but a substantial minority – around 10% – may be due to *Proteus mirabilis*, which is also found in the normal faecal flora. Most patients with simple proteus infections do not form stones, but stone formation is a risk, this being particularly high when stones are already present. Urease-producing bacteria, of which *Proteus* is the most notable genus, may split urea into ammonia and carbon dioxide, with alkalization of the urine and precipitation of crystals of magnesium, ammonia and calcium phosphate, 'triple phosphate', leading to stone formation. Such struvite stones may grow rapidly in infected urine, and a vicious circle ensues whereby the organisms themselves are trapped within the stone safe from the action of antibiotics and the natural host defence mechanisms. Urine cultures at these times may show pyuria but, misleadingly, no bacterial growth. Hence, removal of the stone is an essential part of the treatment of patients with *Proteus* and other urea-splitting urinary tract infections.

Infections of the male genital tract

Prostatitis

Until relatively recently, considerable confusion surrounded the symptom complex of men thought to have 'prostatitis'. In no small part, this was related to problems of terminology – various authorities were describing aspects of prostatitis in the literature but calling these symptom complexes by different names such as 'pelvic floor tension myalgia'. As a result, no one was sure exactly who was investigating which group of patients.

This situation was clarified by Drach et al, who suggested a classification in a letter to the *Journal of Urology*[105] which has since become accepted by most workers in the field. The categories are as follows:

1. acute bacterial prostatitis
2. chronic bacterial prostatitis
3. non-bacterial prostatitis
4. prostatodynia.

These four conditions have many symptoms in common, but they are also distinguished by specific clinical and microbiological features. Successful treatment in each group depends on meticulous attention to diagnostic detail, without which failure is inevitable.

Organisms responsible for acute bacterial and chronic bacterial prostatitis are generally similar and resemble those organisms responsible for lower urinary tract infection. The majority are grown in pure culture; most often, *E. coli* is isolated, while institutionalized patients may harbour more virulent organisms such as *Pseudomonas* or *Strep. faecalis*. It has been suggested that the (rare) episodes of cystitis that occur in young men are all secondary to infection of the prostatic ducts.

Aetiological factors thought to be important in acute or chronic bacterial prostatitis include ascending urethral infection and reflux of infected urine into ejaculatory and prostatic ducts. Blacklock[106] noted that patients with chronic bacterial prostatitis frequently had the same pathogens as identified in vaginal cultures of their sexual partners. Kirby et al injected carbon particles into the bladders of men about to undergo transurethral resection and found the particles within the prostate on later histological examination, thus proving that significant intraprostatic reflux had taken place.[107]

Localization of infection

It is evident that with a unified genitourinary tract emerging at the urethral meatus, specimens obtained there may relate to urethral, prostatic or bladder infections. To overcome this difficulty, specific techniques have been developed for localization of infection.[108] A possible scheme for carrying out such studies is illustrated in Figure 9.20. The localization tests are not difficult, but they do require attention to detail and a state of preparedness – failure to attend to such detail usually results in negative findings and a disappointed tertiary referral.

Following arrival in the clinic, the patient passes a VB1 specimen (10 ml – voided bladder 1). This is a 'washout' specimen and relates to urethral disease. After passage of a further 100–200 ml, the patient collects a standard specimen of midstream

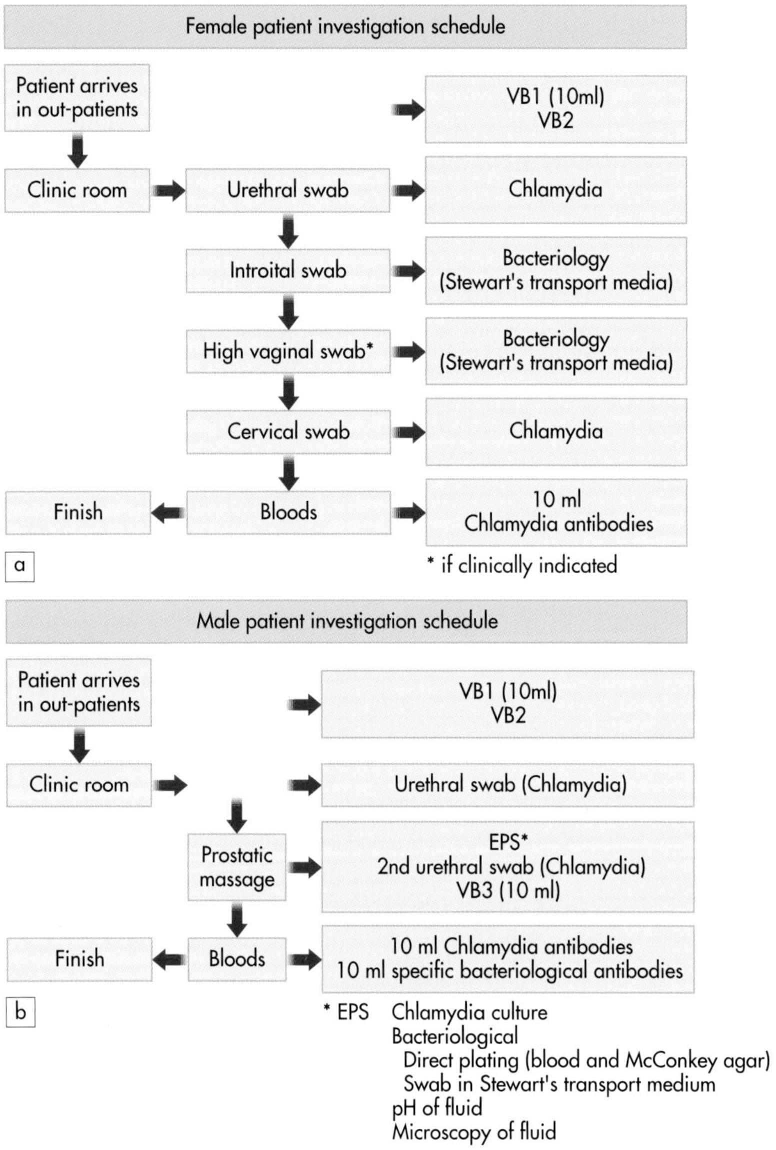

Figure 9.20 *Possible investigation schedule for female (a) and male (b) patients with possible urogenital infection. The tests are time intensive and require meticulous planning – see text for details.*

urine (VB2 [voided bladder 2]). Following this, the prostate is massaged in the usual fashion, and prostatic secretion is collected for analysis, as described below. Subsequently, the next voided 10 ml is collected for further examination (VB3 [voided bladder 3]), and, within this specimen, organisms of prostatic origin may be cultured. Hence, by comparison of specimens obtained from urethral urine, bladder urine and post-massage urine, it is generally possible to localize the source of the patient's infection.

Examination of prostatic fluid

Examination of material obtained after prostatic massage is an important step in the diagnosis of genital infection. In general, cases of prostatic inflammation are found to have more than 15 white cells per high-powered field when such microscopy is performed; as noted above, it is important to check that urethral and bladder specimens do not have similar levels of pyuria. A number of biochemical examinations may be made of expressed prostatic fluid (Figure 9.21). The pH of the fluid, normally around 6.5, becomes alkaline as a result of decreased levels of citric acid.[109] Zinc levels also reduce significantly,[110] this element having previously been known as prostatic antibacterial factor (PAF) due to its potent bactericidal action on most bacteria capable of causing urinary tract infection. It is not clear, however, whether these changes are the cause or the result of bacterial infection of the prostate gland.

Non-bacterial prostatitis

The cause of non-bacterial prostatitis is essentially unknown. Meticulous investigations may reveal pyuria, but no positive cultures may be obtained by the selective methodology described above. It is not clear whether the symptom complex – which is similar to chronic bacterial prostatitis – is related to infectious disease by an unidentified pathogen or is a non-infectious inflammatory process (Figure 9.22). A number of causes of non-bacterial prostatitis have been discussed in the literature, including previous antibiotic therapy, viral infection (herpes), *Ureaplasma urealyticum*, chemical inflammatory processes and autoimmune disease. The role of *Chlamydia trachomatis* is controversial. Mardh et al studied 53 patients with non-bacterial prostatitis and found only one positive chlamydial isolate,[111] and most other investigators have been similarly unsuccessful in identifying this organism in prostatic fluid or even in prostatic aspirates obtained by direct transrectal ultrasound-guided needle puncture of the gland.[112] Nevertheless, identification of this agent as the causative organism of epididymitis in younger men (Figure 9.25, see page 196) raises questions as to how the infection reaches the epididymis. In this study, a tender, swollen epididymis was associated with chlamydial infection in 19 of 23 patients (83%)

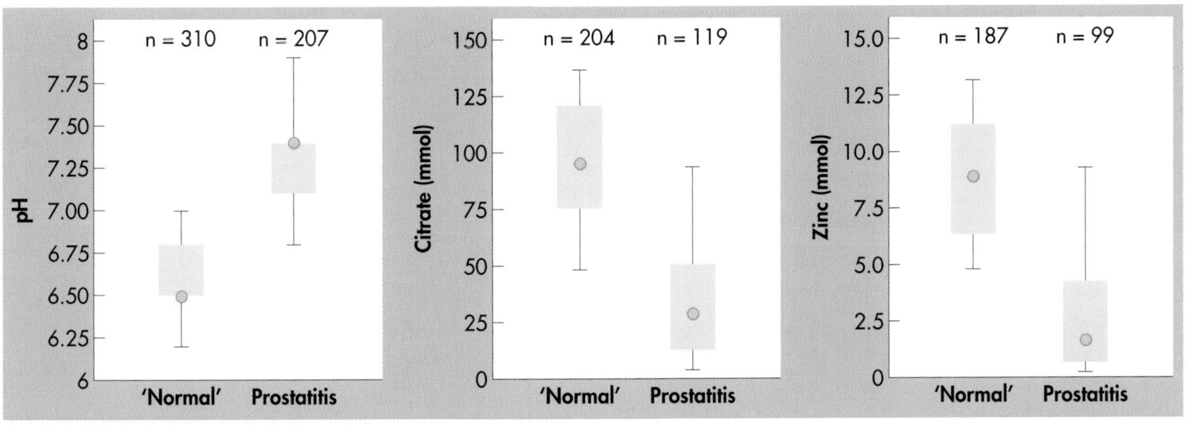

Figure 9.21 *Differences in expressed prostatic secretion composition (EPS) between 'normal' samples and men with prostatitis. Circles: median values; boxes: central 50% of samples. Error bars 10th/90th percentile. All differences significant (P < 0.001). Infection causes a rise in pH but a decrease in citrate and zinc concentration. See text for details. Data from reference.*[110]

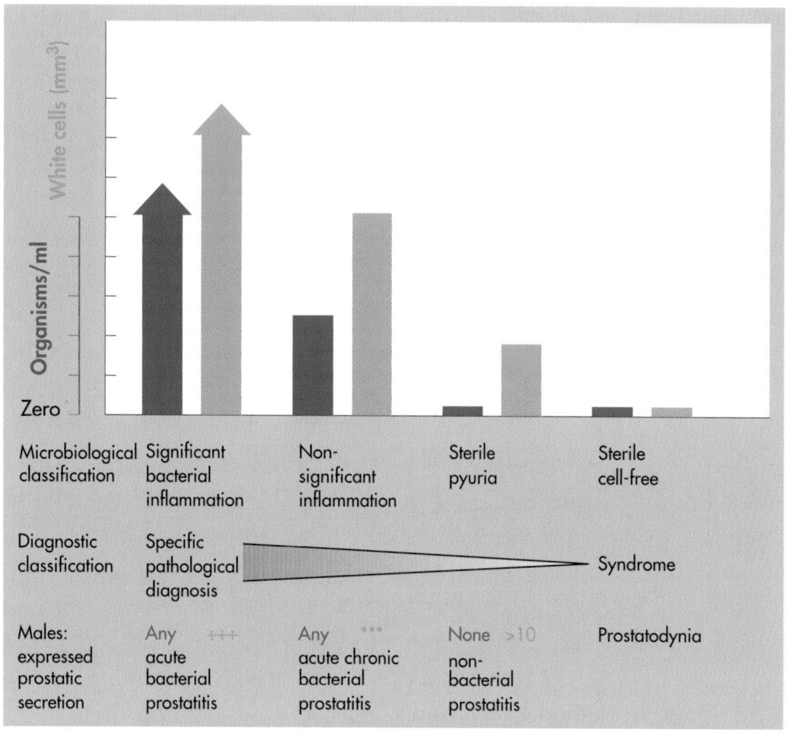

Figure 9.22 *The spectrum of microbiological activity in expressed prostatic secretion. Anticipated levels of both organisms and white cells in the four conditions classified by Drach et al*[105] *are illustrated. The major clinical problems relate to patients with non-bacterial prostatitis and prostatodynia.*

15–25 years of age, and these findings were consolidated by the observation that 9 of 12 consorts were also positive for this infection[127]. Presumably, these observations are reconciled by assuming that the organism may pass from urethra to epididymis, but the biological environment within the prostate ducts themselves is hostile to this agent.

Prevalence and diagnosis of *C. trachomatis*

Infection rates with *C. trachomatis* have markedly increased in recent years. Within the younger population, the infection rate is thought to be 3–12%.[113,114] The prevalence of the disease and its association with infertility has prompted a number of detection and screening schemes, which themselves are responsible in part for greatly increased reporting of the disease.[115]

Traditionally, the diagnosis of chlamydia has been made by the painstaking localization techniques described above. However, culture techniques for chlamydia are critical, and it is acknowledged that traditional diagnostic methods – usually based on the enzyme immunoassay (EIA) – lead to marked underestimation of the prevalence of the disease. For optimal detection, public health laboratories recommend that initial urine (VB1) should be analysed by polymerase chain reaction (PCR) techniques acknowledged as being extremely (90–95%) sensitive for the organism.[116] Within the UK, such molecular diagnostic techniques have not been widely taken up, usually because of financial implications as well as the logistics of managing large numbers of patients within urology clinics.

Antibiotic penetration in prostatitis

The specific physicochemical characteristics of the prostate and prostatic fluid govern the penetration of antibiotics into the organ. To penetrate the lipid membrane of the prostatic epithelium, a drug must be lipid soluble; furthermore, the acid–base characteristic of the drug will determine the concentration of the antibiotic in the fluid. Experiments on normal dog prostates (secretion pH 6.4) demonstrate that only bases are able to penetrate successfully into prostatic fluid. However, as noted above, during infection of the human prostate, pH becomes more alkaline and the dissociation gradient may reverse. Nevertheless, fat-soluble bases, such as erythromycin and trimethoprim, are effective in acute or chronic bacterial prostatitis despite experimental evidence which suggests that concentration of the drug should deteriorate as the pH of the expressed prostatic fluid becomes more alkaline.

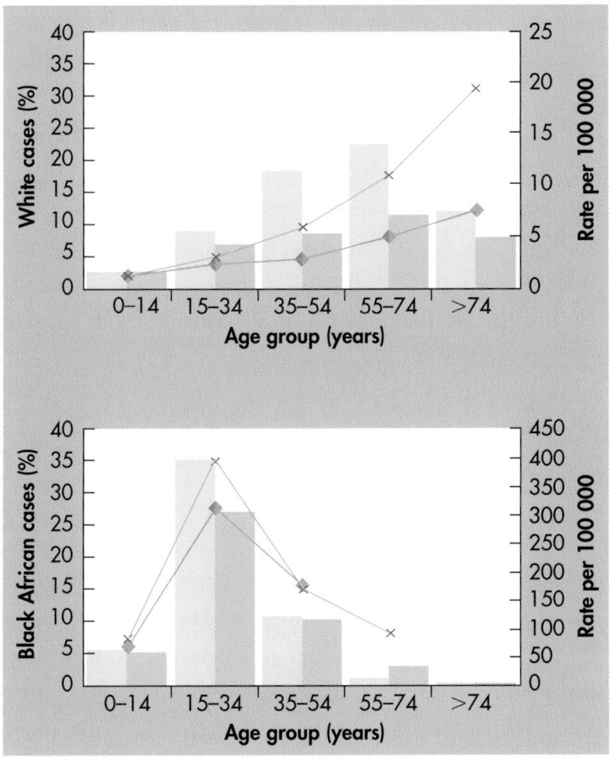

Figure 9.23 *Age and sex distribution of proportion of patients with tuberculosis, comparing (top) ethnic white population with (bottom) black African patients. Note very different age distribution and rate per 100 000 population. □: male; ■: female; ×: male rate; ◆: female rate. Data from reference.*[117]

Tuberculosis

Tuberculosis remains an important disease worldwide with an estimated 8–10 million new cases per annum. The incidence of the disease in its pulmonary form is increasing steadily, particularly in certain ethnic groups and geographical locations. A national survey in England and Wales in 1998 identified an annual rate of 10.9 per 100 000 population, representing increases of 11% and 21%, respectively, over similar surveys undertaken in 1993 and 1988.[117]

However, these figures mask a more complex picture; there has been relatively little change in most regions, but a 71% increase in London and other major urban areas with significant ethnic population. The per 100 000 rate among the whole population (4.4) was many times lower than that of immigrants from the Indian subcontinent (121), while significant increases were recorded for groups of black Africans (210) and Chinese (77.3) origin (Table 9.12). As expected, recent immigrants had a higher incidence of the disease than those who had arrived more than 5 years previously,[117] and the demographic profile of the disease shows wide variation between ethnic groups (Figure 9.23). Non-pulmonary disease in developed countries presents chiefly as lymphadenopthy or genitourinary disease,[118] the latter accounting for approximately 25% of cases surveyed in North America and the UK (Figure 9.24). Paradoxically, in these populations, genitourinary tuberculosis is less common in ethnic minority

Table 9.12 Annual number of patients with tuberculosis and rate of disease in England and Wales by ethnic group. Note the relatively stable data in whites and patients from the Indian subcontinent but marked increases within the Chinese and black African groups, especially those recently arrived from their native countries. Data from Rose et al.[117]

Ethnic group	Annual number cases/rate per 100, 000		
	1988	1993	1998
White	2504/5.36	2267/4.78	2108/4.38
Indian sub-continent	1784/132	2101/128	2141/121
Black African	77/64.4	355/151	743/210
Black Caribbean	137/29.4	104/21.6	125/26.4
Chinese	48/36.2	41/30.7	103/77.3

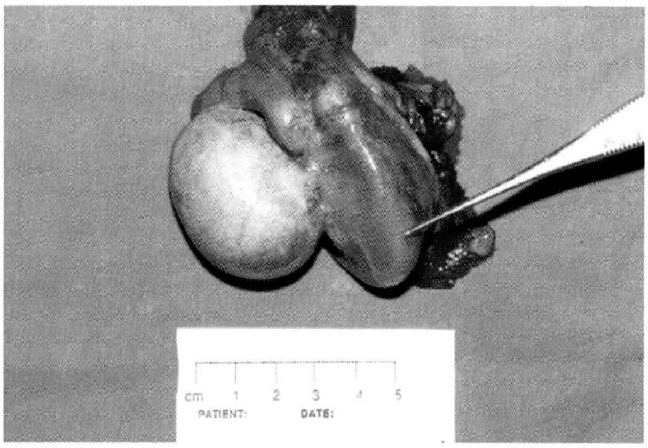

Figure 9.24 *Tuberculous epididymitis removed from 38-year-old white patient; histology revealed florid tuberculous changes within the descending genital tract.*

groups (approximately 5%) than in white Europeans (27%), although these observations might be related to age differences (Figure 9.25) at diagnosis.[119] Approximately 3% of all adults with pulmonary or non-pulmonary disease are co-infected with HIV.[120]

Clinical features

Descriptions of the classical presentation of genitourinary tuberculosis are to be found in clinical textbooks; some, however, are worthy of note to urologists. Disseminated disease may affect patients with renal or other types of organ transplantation, a situation further complicated by therapeutic immunosuppression.[121] Prophylactic chemotherapy (isoniazid) has been demonstrated to be of benefit in such high-risk renal transplant situations. In one study, 6 of 27 patients without prophylaxis developed disease while no treated patients became infected.[122] Length of treatment prophylaxis is probably best linked to the necessary duration of immunosuppression. Rarely, patients with chronic renal failure may develop genitourinary tuberculosis and hypercalcaemia.[123] Usually, raised calcitriol levels are more commonly found in patients with disseminated but non-genitourinary disease, probably due to active synthesis of vitamin D by activated macrophages within granulomas.

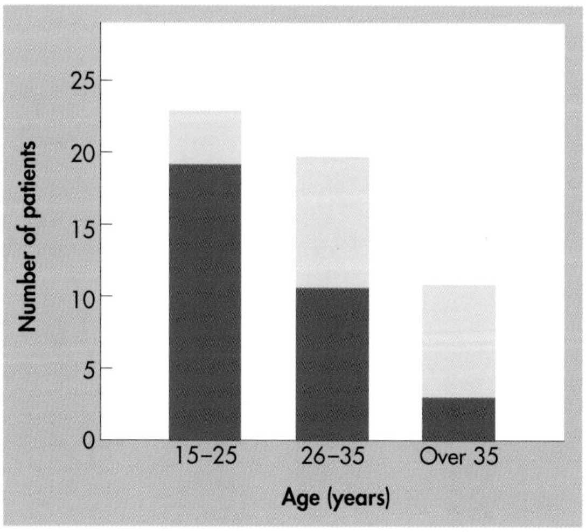

Figure 9.25 *Age distribution of patients with epididymitis according to recovered organism.* □ *negative for C. trachomatis,* ■ *positive for C. trachomatis. Data from reference.*[127]

Laboratory diagnosis

The great majority of cases are infected by the human tubercle bacillus, *Mycobacterium tuberculosis*. *M. bovis* is now rarely (1%) a cause of disease though it may be isolated in reactivated dormant disease or that associated with HIV infection. Bacille Calmette-Guérin vaccine strain-associated lesions are now regularly encountered by laboratories in those centres where intravesical immunotherapy of superficial bladder cancer is widely practised.

Classically, the diagnosis of genitourinary tuberculosis was made by culture on solid Lowenstein-Jensen median, the process taking up to 6 weeks. In cases with a high index of clinical suspicion, modern liquid-culture systems may deliver a diagnosis in half this time. In recent years, polymerase chain reaction (PCR) amplification techniques have been investigated for the diagnosis of both pulmonary and genitourinary tuberculosis and have been found to deliver good sensitivity and specificity.[124,125] Other workers have attempted to use the technique to diagnose active pulmonary tuberculosis in HIV patients by means of urine analysis.[124] It was concluded that PCR diagnostics may provide much faster confirmation of disease (24–48 hours), although the intermittent excretory nature of *M. tuberculosis* may lead to false-negative results, and urine concentration techniques may be required to reduce this error.[125]

To an extent, this diagnostic divide is a good example of the difference between an *efficacy* trial (what works in perfect conditions) and an *effectiveness* trial (what works in the real world).[126] It is well known that techniques that function satisfactorily with dedicated researchers and refined techniques perform poorly when applied to mass populations and routine laboratories. PCR diagnostics are suspect at organism concentrations of $<10^3$ per ml (roughly the lower detectable limit for light microscopy), and for most situations a high index of clinical suspicion, effective communication and modern culture systems lead to optimal outcomes in the search for M. *tuberculosis* in the genitourinary tract.

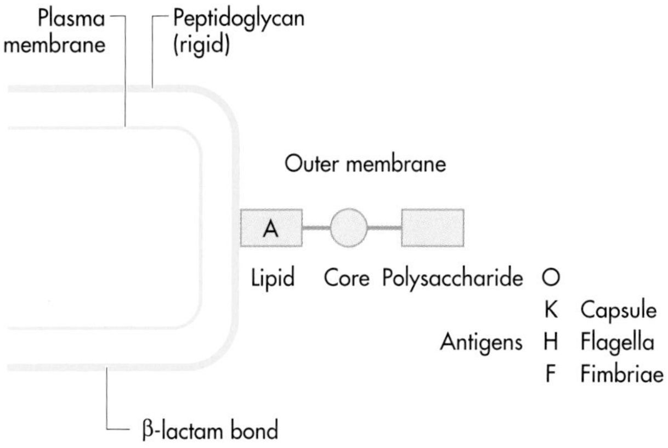

Figure 9.27 *Detailed structure of the O polysaccharide antigen associated with* E. coli. *Lipid adjacent to the outer membrane (lipid A) is thought to be responsible for the manifestations of endotoxic shock.*

Bacteraemia and septic shock

Septic shock is a relatively common and extremely serious complication of infection, usually of Gram-negative origin. In urological practice, the complication is most often encountered in the management of stones, usually complex in nature and located in the upper tract. Septicaemic shock, however, may occur after apparently simple and uncomplicated instrumentation of the urinary tract.

Figure 9.26 illustrates organisms isolated from blood cultures, and the surgical procedures involved are taken from a typically busy stone service. The endotoxin which is thought to trigger the septic cascade lies between the outer membrane and the core oligosaccharide that makes up the O serotype antigen common to Gram-negative bacteria (Figure 9.27, also see Figure 9.17). Known as lipid A, this lipopolysaccharide may trigger release of large amounts of cytokines, such as tumour necrosis factor and the interleukins, which participate in the classically described cascade illustrated

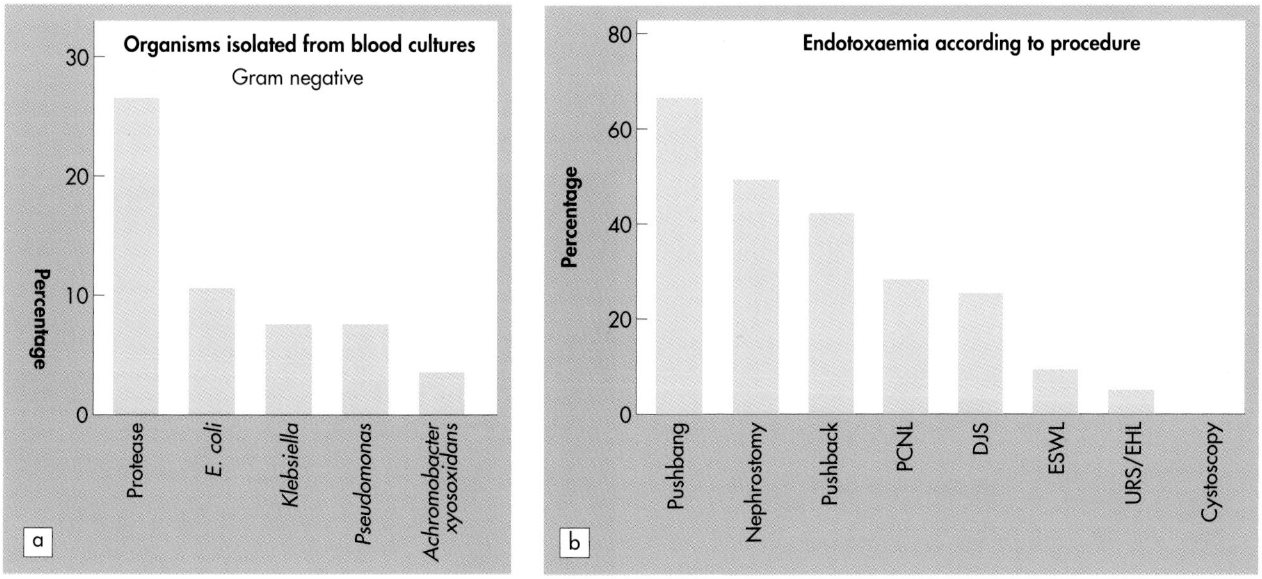

Figure 9.26 *Organisms (a) recovered from blood cultures following procedures (b) carried out in a busy interventional stone centre. Unfortunately, septic shock occurs in a significant number of these cases.*

in Figure 9.28. A full description of the sepsis syndrome is beyond the scope of this text, but urologists will be aware of the urgent need to maintain adequate tissue profusion by volume replacement at the same time as instituting appropriate antimicrobial therapy as judged by repeated blood cultures if necessary.

Papilloma viruses and cancer

Human papilloma viruses (HPV) are DNA-containing viruses which stimulate rapid cell division. External genital warts are most frequently caused by HPV types 6 and 11 (Figure 9.29). Other HPV types (mainly 16 and 18) are frequently present in the anogenital region and have been associated with the development of high-grade, premalignant cervical lesions (cervical intraepithelial neoplasia [CIN] III) as well as anogenital cancer, principally the anus and vulva. DNA sequences from such HPVs are detectable in the majority of cervical and anal tumours; PCR studies of apparently normal cervical smears showed increased levels of sequences from 'high-risk virus types', and subsequent colposcopy confirmed the presence of underlying high-grade CIN III.[128] Not all women infected with high-risk HPV types develop cancer, and the reason for this discrepancy remains unclear at the present time.

Localization studies in the urinary tract

It is pertinent to summarize the various localization studies that may be employed to identify the site of infection of any particular organism. When efficiently and accurately performed, such studies can be of great help to the urologist attempting to identify the source of organisms within the urinary tract.

Studies on prostatic fluid described by Meares and Stamey[108] have already been noted. Stamey has also refined localization studies designed to determine the source of bacteriuria emanating from the upper urinary tract. Essentially, this test involves ureteric catheterization of the appropriate unit in question after meticulous steps to eradicate bacteria from the bladder that would otherwise contaminate the ureteric sample. Such techniques have been equally useful when attempting to determine the source of cells with abnormal cytological features. Earlier methods for differentiating kidney from bladder infections (Fairley bladder washout test) have fallen into disuse, although such studies can, on occasion, be clinically helpful.

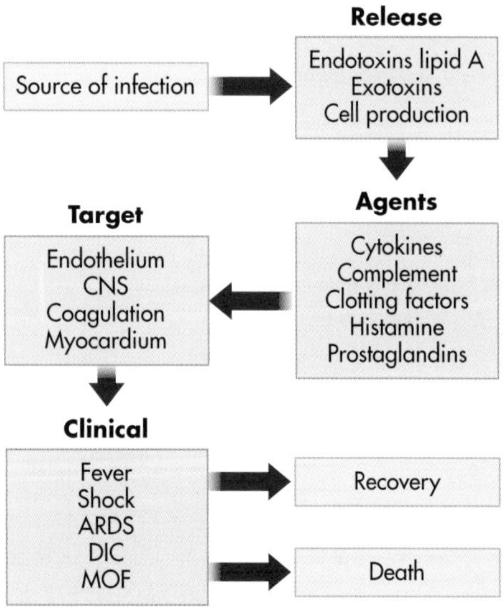

Figure 9.28 *The classical cascade described in endotoxic septicaemic shock. ARDS: adult respiratory distress syndrome; DIC: disseminated intravascular coagulation; MOF: multiple organ failure.*

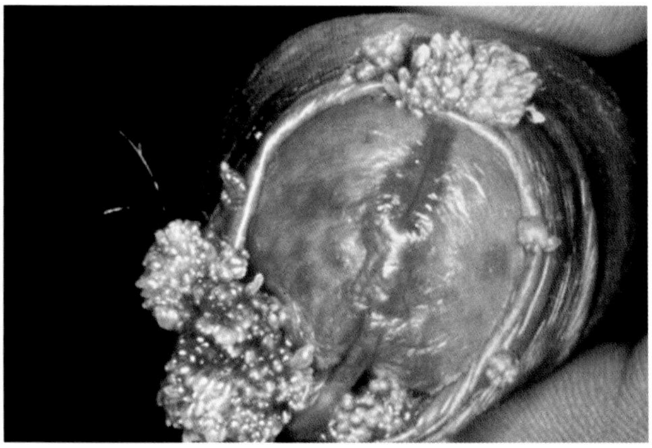

Figure 9.29 *Exophytic papilloma virus, usually caused by type 6 or type 11 infection*

Summary of definitions

Adherence	Initial interaction of micro-organism with host
Adhesin	Microbiological molecule that leads to adhesion to cells or tissues
Bacteriuria	The residence of bacteria within the urinary tract
Contamination	Adventitious entry of bacteria during urine collection
Fitness	The ability of bacteria to establish and maintain a population in a specific ecological habit
GAL-GAL	Essential core of disaccharide receptor for P fimbriae
Pathogenicity	The ability to cause disease
Phase variation	Variation of virulence antigens, often to protect organism
Tropism	The restriction of commercials and pathogens to certain host tissues and cell types
Virulence	The degree of pathogenicity

REFERENCES

1. Lincoln K, Lidin-Janson G, Winberg J. Resistant urinary infections resulting from changes in resistance pattern of faecal flora induced by sulphonamide and hospital environment. BMJ 1970; 3: 305–309
2. Finegold SM, Mathisen GE, George WL. Changes in human intestinal flora related to administration of antimicrobial agents. In: Hentges DJ, ed. Human Intestinal Microflora in Health and Disease. New York: Academic Press, 1983: 355–446
3. Kaye D. Antibacterial activity of human urine. J Clin Invest 1968; 47: 2374–2390
4. Cox CE, Hinman F Jr. Experiments with induced bacteriuria, vesical emptying and bacterial growth on a mechanism of bladder defence to infection. J Urol 1961; 86: 739–748
5. Parsons CL, Greenspan C, Mulholland SG. The primary antibacterial defence mechanism of the bladder. Investig Urol 1975; 13: 72–76
6. Parsons LC, Shrom SH, Hanno PM, Mulholland SG. Bladder surface mucin – examination of possible mechanisms for its antibacterial effect. Investig Urol 1978; 60: 196–200
7. Parsons CL, Mulholland SG, Anwar H. Antibacterial activity of bladder surface mucin duplication by exogenous glycosaminoglycan (heparin). Infect Immun 1979; 24: 552–557
8. Tamm I, Horsfall FL. A mucoprotein derived from human urine which reacts with influenza, mumps and Newcastle disease viruses. J Exp Med 1952; 95: 71–97
9. Ørskov I, Ferencz A, Ørskov F. Tamm-Horsfall protein or uro-mucoid is the normal urinary slime that traps type I fimbrinated *Escherichia coli*. Lancet 1980; 1: 887
10. Pak J, Pu Y, Xhang ZT et al. Tamm-Horsfall protein binds to type I fimbriated *E. coli* and prevents *E. coli* from binding to uroplakin 1a and 1b receptors. J Biol Chem 2001; 276: 9924–9930
11. Jost SP. Cell cycle of normal bladder urothelium in developing and adult mice. Virchows Arch B Cell Pathol Incl Mol Pathol 1989; 57: 27–36
12. Mulvey MA, Lopez-Boado YS, Wilson CL et al. Induction and evasion of host defences by type I pilated uro-pathological *E. coli*. Science 1998; 282: 1494–1497
13. Klump DJ, Weiser AC, Sangupta S et al. Uropathogenic *E. coli* potentiates type I pilus induced apoptosis by suppressing NF-kappaB. Infect Immun 2001; 69: 6689–6695
14. Mulvey MA, Schilling JD, Hultgren SJ. Establishment of a persistent *E. coli* reservoir during the acute phase of bladder infection. Infec Immun 2001; 69: 4572–4579
15. Mulvey MA. Adhesion and entry of uropathogenic *Escherichia coli*. Cell Microbiol 2002; 4: 257–271
16. Gunther NW, Lockatelle V, Johnson DE, Mobbley LT. In vivo dynamics of type I fimbria regulation in uropathogenic *Escherichia coli* during experimental urinary tract infection. Infect Immun 69: 2838–2853
17. Mayer KH, Opal SM, Mederios AA. Mechanisms of antibiotic resistance. In: Mandell GL, Douglas, Benett JE, Dolin R, eds. Principles and Practice of Infectious Diseases. Edinburgh: Churchill Livingstone, 1995: 212–224
18. Cooke EM, Ewins SP. Properties of strains of *Escherichia coli* isolated from a variety of sources. J Med Microbiol 1975; 8: 107–111
19. Minshew BH, Jorgenson J, Swanstrum M. Some characteristics of *E. coli* strains isolated from extra-intestinal infections of humans. J Infect Dis 1978; 137: 648–654
20. Johnson JR. Virulence factors in *E. coli* urinary tract infection. Clin Microbiol Rev 1991; 4: 80–128
21. Mayer TF. Pathogenic Neisseriae – a model of bacterial virulence and genetic flexibility. Int J Microbiol 1990; 274: 135–154
22. Leying H, Suerbaum S, Kroll H-P, Stahl D et al. The

capsular polysaccharide is a major determinant of serum resistance in K-1 positive blood culture isolates of *Escherichia coli*. Infect Immun 1990; 58: 222–227
23. Jacobson SH, Hammarlind M, Lidefeldt KJ, Österberg E et al. Incidence of aerobactin-positive *Escherichia coli* strains in patients with symptomatic urinary tract infection. Eur J Clin Microbiol Infect Dis 1988; 7: 630–634
24. Costerton JW, Geesey GG, Cheng K-J. How bacteria stick. Sci Am 1978; 238: 86–95
25. van Oss CJ, Good RJ, Chaudhury MK. The role of Van de Waals forces and hydrogen bonds in hydrophobic interactions between biopolymers and low energy surfaces. J Colloid Interface Sci 1986; 3: 378–384
26. Gibbons RJ, van-Houte J. Bacterial adherence in oral microbial ecology. Ann Rev Microbiol 1975; 29: 19–41
27. Mobley HLT, Chippendale GR, Tenney JH, Hull RA et al. Expression of type I fimbriae may be required for persistence of *Escherichia coli* in the catheterised urinary tract. J Clin Microbiol 1987; 25: 2253–2257
28. Roberts JA. Tropism in bacterial infections: urinary tract infections. J Urol 1996; 156: 1552–1559
29. Senior D, Baker N, Cedergren B, Falk P et al. Globo-A – a new receptor specificity for attaching *Escherichia coli*. FEBS Let 1988; 237: 123–127
30. Lindstedt R, Larson G, Falk P, Jodal U et al. The receptor repertoire defines the host range for attaching *Escherichia coli* strains that recognise Globo-A. Infect Immun 1991; 59: 1086–1092
31. Langermann S, Palaszynski S, Barnhart M et al. Prevention of mucosal *E. coli* infection by FimH adhesin based systemic vaccination. Science 1997; 276: 607–611
32. Choudhury D, Thompson A, Stojanoff V et al. X-ray structure of the FimC–FimH chaperone–adhesin complex from uropathogenic *E. coli*. Science 1999; 285: 1061–1066
33. Zhou G, Mo WJ, Sebbel P et al. Uroplakin is the urothelial receptor for uropathogenic *E. coli*: evidence from in vitro FimH binding. J Cell Sci 2001; 114: 4095–4103
34. Sunn TT, Zhao H, Provet J et al. Formation of asymmetric unit membrane during urothelial differentiation. Mol Biol Rep 1996; 23: 3–11
35. Martinez TS, Mulvey MA, Schilling JD. Type I pilus mediated bacterial invasion of bladder epithelial cells. EMBO J 2000; 19: 2803–2812
36. Baorto DM, Gao Z, Malaviya R et al. Survival of FimH expressing enterobacteria in macrophages relies on glycolipid traffic. Nature 1997; 389: 636–639
37. Schwan WR, Lee JL, Lenard FA et al. Osmolarity and pH growth conditions regulate *fim* gene transcription and type I pilus expression in uropathogenic *E. coli*. Infect Immun 2002; 70: 1391–1402
38. Gunther WW, Synder JA, Lockatell V et al. Assessment of virulence of uropathogenic *E. coli* type I fimbrial mutants in which the invertible element is phase locked on or off. Infect Immun 2002; 70: 3344–3354
39. Xia Y, Gally D, Forsman-Sembk et al. Regulatory cross talk between adhesin operant in *E. coli*: inhibition of fimbriae expression by the PapB protein. EMBO J 2000; 19: 1450–1457
40. Eisenstein BI. Phase variation of type I fimbriae in *Escherichia coli* is under transcriptional control. Science 1981; 214: 337–339
41. Lindberg F, Lund B, Johansson L, Normark S. Localisation of the receptor-binding protein adhesin at the tip of the bacterial pilus. Nature 1987; 328: 84–87
42. Roberts JA, Kaack MB, Baskin G, Marklund B-I et al. Epitotes of the P-fimbrial adhesin of *E. coli* cause different urinary tract infections. J Urol 1997; 158: 1610–1613
43. Svanborg Edén C, Hanson LÅ, Jodal U, Lindberg U et al. Variable adherence to normal human urinary tract epithelial cells of *Escherichia coli* strains associated with various forms of urinary tract infection. Lancet 1976; 2: 490–492
44. Fowler JE, Stamey TA. Studies of introital colonisation in women with recurrent urinary tract infections – role of bacterial adherence. J Urol 1977; 177: 472–476
45. Schaeffer AJ, Jones JM, Dunn JK. Association of in vitro *Escherichia coli* adherence to vaginal and buccal epithelial cells with susceptibility of women to recurrent urinary tract infections. N Engl J Med 1981; 304: 1062–1066
46. Sellwood R, Gibbons RA, Jones GW, Rutter JM. A possible basis for the breeding of pigs relatively resistant to neonatal diarrhoea. Vet Rec 95: 574
47. Sellwood R, Gibbons RA, Jones GW, Rutter JM. Adhesion of enteropathogenic *Escherichia coli* to pig intestinal brush borders: the existence of two pig phenotypes. J Med Microbiol 1975; 8: 405–411
48. Rutter JM, Burrows MR, Sellwood R, Gibbons RA. A genetic basis for resistance to enteric disease caused by *E. coli*. Nature 1975; 257: 135–136
49. Buckwalter JA, Naifeh GS, Auer JE. Rheumatic fever and the blood groups. BMJ 1962; 2: 1023–1027

50. Källenius G, Möllby R, Svenson SB, Helin I et al. Occurrence of P-fimbriated *Escherichia coli* in urinary tract infections. Lancet 1981; 2: 1369–1372
51. Johnson JR, Roberts PL, Stamm WE. P-fimbriae and other virulence factors in *Escherichia coli* urosepsis: association with patients' characteristics. J Infect Dis 1987; 156: 225–228
52. Leffler H, Svanborg-Éden C. Glycolipid receptors for uropathogenic *E. coli* on human erythrocytes and uroepithelial cells. Infect Immun 1981; 34: 920–929
53. Plos K, Carter T, Hull S et al. Intestinal carriage of P fimbriated *E. coli* and the susceptibility to urinary tract infection in young children. J Infect Dis 1995; 171: 625–631
54. Wullt B, Bergsten G, Connell H et al. P-fimbriae trigger mucosal responses to *E. coli* in the human urinary tract. Cell Microbiol 2001; 3: 255–264
55. Hacker J, Kestler H, Hoschntzky H et al. Cloning and characterisation of the S fimbrial adhesin II complex of *E. coli* 018 K1 meningitis isolate. Infect Immun 1993; 61: 544–550
56. Nowicki B, Selvarangan R, Nowick S. Family of *E. coli* Dr adhesins: delay-accelerating factor receptor recognition and invasiveness. J Infect Dis 2001; 183: S24–S27
57. Wold A, Thorssén M, Hull S, Svenborg-Éden C. Attachment of *E. coli* via mannose or Gal-Gal containing receptors to human colonic epithelial cells. Infect Immun 1988; 56: 2531–2537
58. Schlager TA, Whittam TS, Hendley JO, Hollis RJ et al. Comparison of expression of virulence factors by *Escherichia coli* causing cystitis and *E. coli* colonising the peri-urethra of healthy girls. J Infect Dis 1995; 172: 772–778
59. Hedlund M, Svensson M, Wilsson A et al. Role of the ceramide-signalling pathway in cytokine responses to P fimbriated *E. coli*. J Exp Med 1996; 183: 1037–1044
59a. Langermann S, Mollby R, Burlein JE et al. Vaccination with Fim H adhesin protects cynomolgus monkey from colonisation and infection by uropathogenic *E. coli*. J Infect Dis 2000; 181: 774–778
60. Silverblatt FS. Host–parasite interaction in the rat renal pelvis: a possible role of pili in the pathogenesis of pyelonephritis. J Exp Med 1974; 140: 1696–1699
61. Fader RC, Davis CP. Effect of pilation on *Klebsiella pneumoniae* infection in rat bladders. Infect Immun 1980; 30: 554–561
62. Glynn AA, Brumfitt W, Howard CJ. K antigens of *Escherichia coli* and renal involvement in urinary tract infections. Lancet 1971; 1: 514–516
63. Kaijser B, Hanson LA, Jodal U, Lidin-Janson G et al. Frequency of *E. coli* K antigens in urinary tract infections in children. Lancet 1977; 2: 663–664
64. Crump J, Pead L, Maskell R. Urinary infections in general practice. Lancet 1976; 1: 1184
65. Grüneberg RN. Antibiotic sensitivities of urinary pathogens, 1971–1978. J Clin Pathol 1980; 33: 853–856
66. Jordan PA, Iravani A, Richard GA. Urinary tract infection caused by *Staphylococcus saprophyticus*. J Infect Dis 1980; 142: 510–515
67. Maskell R, Pead L, Allen J. The puzzle of 'urethral syndrome': a possible answer? Lancet 1979; 1: 1058–1059
68. Brumfitt W, Hamilton-Miller JMT, Ludlam H, Gooding A. Lactobacilli do not cause frequency and dysuria syndrome. Lancet 1981; 2: 393–394
69. Bran JL, Levison ME, Kaye D. Entrance of bacteria into the female urinary bladder. N Engl J Med 1972; 286: 626–629
70. Buckley RM, McGuckin M, MacGregor RR. Urine bacterial counts following sexual intercourse. N Engl J Med 1978; 298: 321–324
71. Hinman F Jr. Mechanisms for the entry of bacteria and the establishment of urinary infection in female children. J Urol 1966; 96: 546–550
72. Hooton TM, Hillier S, Johnson C. *Escherichia coli* bacteriuria and contraceptive method. JAMA 1991; 265: 64–69
73. Vivaldi E, Cotran R, Zangwill DP. Ascending infection as a mechanism in pathogenesis of experimental non-obstructive pyelonephritis. Proc Soc Exp Biol Med 1959; 102: 242–247
74. Kass EH. Bacteriuria and the diagnosis of infections of the urinary tract. AMA Arch Intern Med 1957; 100: 709–714
75. Stamm WE, Wagner KF, Amsell R, Alexander ER et al. Causes of the acute urethral syndrome in women. N Engl J Med 1980; 303: 409–415
76. Stamm WE, Counts GW, Running KR, Fihn S et al. Diagnosis of coliform infection in acutely dysuric women. N Engl J Med 1982; 307: 463–468
77. Editorial. Can Kasstigation beat the truth out of the urethral syndrome? Lancet 1982; 2: 694–695
78. Stamm WE. Quantitative urine cultures revisited. Editorial. Eur J Clin Microbiol 1984; 3: 279–281
79. Venegas MF, Navas EL, Gaffney RA, Duncan JL et al. Binding of type I pilated *Escherichia coli* to vaginal mucous. Infect Immun 1995; 73: 416–421

80. Cox CE, Lacy SS, Hinman F Jr. The urethra and its relationship to urinary tract infection. II. The urethral flora of the female with recurrent urinary infection. J Urol 1968; 99: 632–638
81. Grüneberg RN. Relationship of infecting urinary organism to the faecal flora in patients with symptomatic urinary infection. Lancet 1969; 2: 766–768
82. Stamey TA, Sexton CC. The role of vaginal colonisation with Enterobacteriaceae in recurrent urinary infections. J Urol 1975; 113: 214–217
83. Pfau A, Sacks T. The bacterial flora of the vaginal vestibule, urethra and vagina in premenopausal women with recurrent urinary tract infections. J Urol 1981; 126: 630–634
84. Marsh FP, Murray M, Panchamia P. The relationship between bacterial cultures of the vaginal introitus and urinary infection. Br J Urol 1972; 44: 368–375
85. O'Grady FW, Richards B, McSherry MA, O'Farrell SM et al. Introital enterobacteria, urinary infection and the urethral syndrome. Lancet 1970; 2: 1208–1210
86. Brumfitt W, Grogan RA, Hamilton-Miller JMT. Periurethral enterobacterial carriage preceding urinary infection. Lancet 1987; 1: 824–826
87. Cattell WR, McSherry MA, Northeast A, Powell E et al. Periurethral enterobacterial carriage in the pathogenesis of recurrent urinary infection. BMJ 1974; 4: 136–139
88. Wiswell TE, Roscelli JD. Corroborative evidence for the decreased incidence of urinary tract infections in circumcised male infants. Paediatrics 1986; 78: 96–99
89. Wiswell TE, Enzenauer RW, Holton ME, Cornish JD et al. Declining frequency of circumcision: implications for changes in the absolute incidence and male to female sex ratio of urinary tract infections in early infancy. Paediatrics 1987; 79: 338–342
90. Feld L, Greenfield S, Ogra P. Urinary tract infections in infants and children. Paediatr Rev 1989; 11: 71–77
91. Ransley PG, Risdon RA. The pathogenesis of reflux nephropathy. Contrib Nephrol 1979; 16: 90–98
92. Siegel S, Siegel B, Sokoloff B. Urinary infection in infants and preschool children. Am J Dis Child 1980; 134: 369–372
93. Kunin CM. A ten year study of bacteriuria in schoolgirls: final report of bacteriologic, urologic, and epidemiologic findings. J Infect Dis 1970; 122: 382–393
94. Meadow RS, White RHR, Johnston NM. Prevalence of symptomless urinary tract disease in Birmingham schoolchildren. I. Pyuria and bacteriuria. BMJ 1969; 3: 81–84
95. Cardiff/Oxford Bacteriuria Study Group. Sequelae of covert bacteriuria in schoolgirls. A four-year follow-up study. Lancet 1978; 1: 889–894
96. Gillenwater JY, Harrison RB, Kunin CM. Natural history of bacteriuria in schoolgirls. N Engl J Med 1979; 301: 396–399
97. Sacks SH, Verrier Jones K, Roberts R, Asscher AW et al. The effect of symptomless bacteriuria in childhood on subsequent pregnancy. Lancet 1987; 2: 991–994
98. Kunin CM. Sexual intercourse and urinary infections. N Engl J Med 1978; 298: 336–337
99. Norden CW, Kass EH. Bacteriuria of pregnancy; a critical appraisal. Ann Rev Med 1968; 19: 431–437
100. Kass EH. Bacteriuria and pyelonephritis of pregnancy. AMA Arch Intern Med 1960; 105: 194–198
101. Brocklehurst JC, Dillane JB, Griffiths L. The prevalence and symptomatology of urinary infection in an aged population. Gerontol Clin 1968; 10: 242–253
102. Mabeck CE. Treatment of uncomplicated urinary tract infection in non-pregnant women. Postgrad Med J 1972; 48: 69–75
103. George NJR. Urethral syndrome – clinical features. In: George NJR, Gosling JA, eds. Sensory Disorders of the Bladder and Urethra. Springer-Verlag, 1986: 91–102
104. O'Grady FW, Charlton CAC, Fry IK, McSherry A et al. Natural history of intractable 'cystitis' in women referred to a special clinic. In: Brumfitt W, Ascher AW, eds. Urinary Tract Infection. Oxford: Oxford University Press, 1973: 81–91
105. Drach GW, Fair WR, Meares EM, Stamey TA. Classification of benign diseases associated with prostatic pain: prostatitis or prostatodynia? J Urol 1978; 120: 226
106. Blacklock NJ. Anatomical factors in prostatitis. Br J Urol 1974; 46: 47–50
107. Kirby RS, Lowe D, Bultitude MI. Intraprostatic urinary reflux: an aetiological factor in abacterial prostatitis. Br J Urol 1982; 54: 729–731
108. Meares EM Jr, Stamey TA. Bacteriologic localisation patterns in bacterial prostatitis and urethritis. Investig Urol 1968; 5: 492–518
109. Blacklock NJ, Beavis JP. Response of prostatic fluid pH in inflammation. Br J Urol 1974; 46: 537–542
110. Kavanagh JP, Darby C, Costello CB. Differences in expressed prostatic secretion composition (EPS) between 'normal' samples and from men with prostatitis. Int J Androl 1982; 5: 487–496

111. Mardh PH, Ripa KT, Colleen S, Treharne JD et al. Role of *Chlamydia trachomatis* in non-acute prostatitis. Br J Vener Dis 1978; 54: 330–334
112. Doble A, Thomas BJ, Walker MM. The role of *Chlamydia trachomatis* in chronic abacterial prostatitis: a study using ultrasound guided biopsy. J Urol 1989; 141: 332–335
113. Anderson B, Olesen F, Moller JK, et al. Population based strategies for outreach screening of urogenital *Chlamydia trachomatis* infections: a randomised controlled trial. J Infect Dis 2002; 185: 252–258
114. Fenton KA, Korovessis C, Johnson AM et al. Sexual behaviour in Britain: reported sexually transmitted infections and prevalent genital *Chlamydia trachomatis* infection. Lancet 2001; 358: 1851–1854
115. Pimenta J, Fenton KA. Recent trends in *Chlamydia trachomatis* in the United Kingdom and the potential for national screening. Euro Surveill 2001; 6: 81–84
116. Cheng H, Macaluso M, Vermund SH et al. Relative accuracy of nucleic acid amplification tests and culture in detecting *Chlamydia* in asymptomatic men. J Clin Microbiol 2001; 39: 3927–3937
117. Rose AMC, Watson JM, Graham C et al. Tuberculosis at the end of the 20th century in England and Wales: the results of a national survey in 1998. Thorax 2001; 56: 173–179
118. Garcia-Rodriguez JA, Garcia-Sanchez JE, Munoz Bellido JL et al. Genitourinary TB in Spain: a review of 81 cases. Clin Infect Dis 1994; 18: 557–561
119. Grange JM, Yates MD, Ormerod LP et al. Factors determining ethnic differences in the incidence of bacteriologically confirmed genitourinary tuberculosis in south east England. J Infect 1995; 30: 37–40
120. Churchill D, Hannan M, Miller R et al. HIV associated culture proved tuberculosis has increased in north central London from 1990–1996. Sex Transm Infect 2002; 76: 43–45
121. Gwoeltje KF, Matthew A, Rothstein M et al. Tuberculosis infection and anergy in haemodialysis patients. Am J Kidney Dis 1998; 31: 848–852
122. Higgins RM, Cahn AP, Porter D et al. Microbacterial infections after renal transplantation. Q J Med 1991; 78: 145–153
123. Paces R, de la Torre M, Alcazar F et al. Genitourinary tuberculosis as the cause of unexplained hypercalcaemia in a patient with pre-end stage renal failure. Nephrol Dial Transplant 1998; 13: 488–490
124. Romano L, Sanquinetti, Posteraro B et al. Early detection of negative BACTEC MCIT 960 cultures by PCR-reverse cross blot hybridization assay. J Clin Microbiol 2002; 40: 3499–3501
125. Van Vollenhoven P, Heynes CF, de Beer PM et al. PCR in the diagnosis of urinary tract tuberculosis. Urol Res 1996; 24: 107–111
126. When to act on evidence? Editorial. BMJ 2002; 325: 7371
127. Grant JBF, Costello CB, Sequeira PJL, Blacklock NJ. The role of *Chlamydia trachomatis* in epididymitis. Br J Urol 1987; 60: 355–359
128. Cuziack J, Szarewski A, Terry G. Human papilloma virus testing in primary cervical screening. Lancet 1995; 345: 1533–1536

10

The scientific basis of urinary stone formation

William G Robertson

INTRODUCTION

Urolithiasis is a disorder that has cut across all historical, geographical, demographic and social boundaries. From the days of the predynastic Egyptians until the present time, kidney stones have perplexed patients and physicians alike and, although during that time the methods for removing stones have advanced from the crudely barbaric to the highly sophisticated, the problem of how successfully to prevent their recurrence in a given patient continues to challenge urologists and nephrologists.

If patients are not provided with proper preventative management, the risk of recurrence is traditionally high – 40% within 3 years rising to 74% at 10 years and to 98% at 25 years in the days when open surgery and transurethral basket or loop extraction were the main techniques for removing stones.[1] Nowadays, in the era of extracorporeal shock-wave lithotripsy (ESWL) and percutaneous nephrolithotomy (PCNL), the recurrence rate is even higher (Figure 10.1), a fact which is not surprising since both techniques, particularly ESWL, often leave particles behind in the kidney that provide ideal nuclei for further stone formation.[2] Unfortunately, the relative success of ESWL, PCNL and ureteroscopy (URS) in the disintegration and removal of stones has lulled many into the belief that the problem can be managed solely by these means, a trend that has been increased by opportune cost-cutting by many Health Authorities, for although these minimally invasive techniques may be the procedures of choice for the removal of stones, *they do not treat the underlying cause(s) of stone formation*. Without biochemical screening and appropriate dietary and/or medical management, the patient will generally return for further stone removal in the future.

Not only is the failure to provide proper prophylactic treatment for the patient bad clinical management; in the long term, it is economically more expensive.[3] Financial analysis has shown that the projected cost of treating stone patients solely by removing their stones by minimally invasive technologies every time they form them is considerably more expensive than removing their initial stones and then screening the patients thoroughly to identify their risk factors in order to provide them with appropriate prophylactic management.[4]

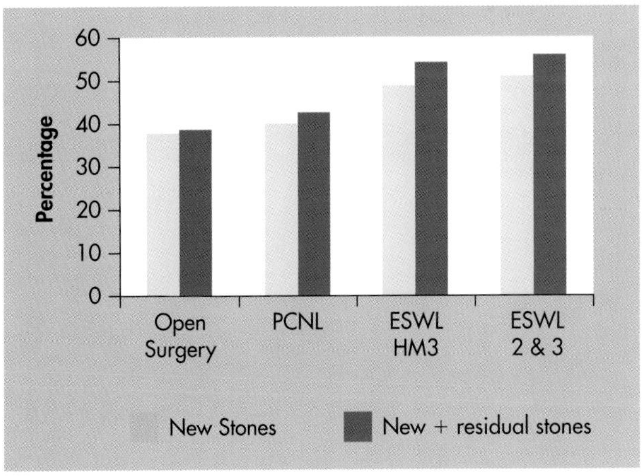

Figure 10.1 *The percentage of patients with new stones or with new plus residual stones within 3 years of the (a) open surgery, (b) percutaneous nephrolithotomy [PCNL], (c) extracorporeal shock wave lithotripsy using a Dornier HM3 lithotripter [ESWL HM3] or (d) extracorporeal shock wave lithotripsy using second- or third-generation lithotripters [ESWL 2 and 3].*

During the six millennia since the formation of the earliest recorded stones, the pattern of urolithiasis has changed in many respects, particularly within the past century. In Western countries before 1900, for example, stones occurred commonly in children, particularly boys, and were formed mainly in the bladder. These stones usually consisted of ammonium urate and/or calcium oxalate and were caused by poor nutrition. Although this form of the disorder is still found today in rural areas within the 'endemic stone belt' stretching from Jordan, through Iraq, Iran and the Indian subcontinent to the furthest extremities of South-East Asia, it is gradually disappearing with improving standards of nutrition, as it did in most developed countries about 100 years ago.[5]

As the incidence of bladder stones in children has decreased, however, the prevalence of upper urinary tract stones in adults has increased. Within this general increase in stone occurrence, there have been peaks and troughs in incidence that coincide with periods of economic prosperity and recession, respectively (Figure 10.2). Kidney stones occur more frequently in the more industrially developed nations and are less common in those countries whose economies are more dependent on agriculture. Overall, the incidence of upper tract stone disease increases in parallel with the level of affluence, presumably through the effect of the latter on diet and lifestyle.[6]

Other changes in the pattern of stone formation have also been noted during this time. Although stones generally occur more frequently in men than in women (male:female ratio about 2.5:1), recent studies have shown that, within the past 25 years, there has been a progressive decrease in the age at onset of stone formation in both males (Figure 10.3a) and females (Figure 10.3b), particularly females.[7] Within the population of stone-formers *as a whole*, the male:female ratio among patients who formed their first stone before the age of 20 is now 1.6:1 (cf. 3.0:1 in 1975). In those patients *currently* aged under 20, the ratio has fallen to 1.2:1 (cf 1.6:1 in 1975). The main changes have taken place in the teenage years and may be attributed to alterations in diet and lifestyle in that group during the past 25 years. The combination of an earlier age at onset and an increasing life expectancy means that more young first-time stone-formers will have a longer span of life over which they are likely to experience recurrence of the disorder. This will add to the burden on urological resources required to manage the stone problem in the future.

STONE COMPOSITION

The vast majority (75–80%) of urinary calculi consist predominantly of calcium oxalate (Figure 10.4), often on its own, but frequently mixed with calcium phosphate or, occasionally, uric acid.[8] In about 90%

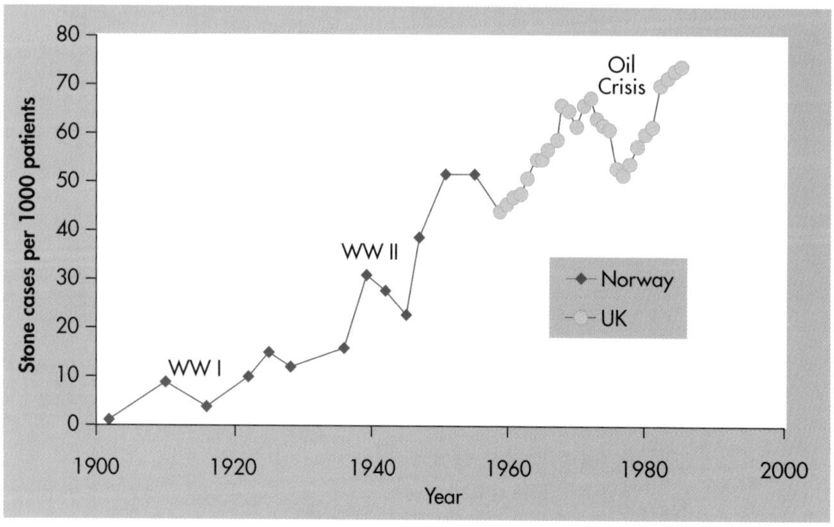

Figure 10.2 *The number of stone cases per 1000 patients attending hospital in Norway and in the UK during the past 100 years. (WWI and WWII refer to World War I and World War II, respectively, and Oil Crisis refers to the Middle East oil crisis in the early 1970s.)*

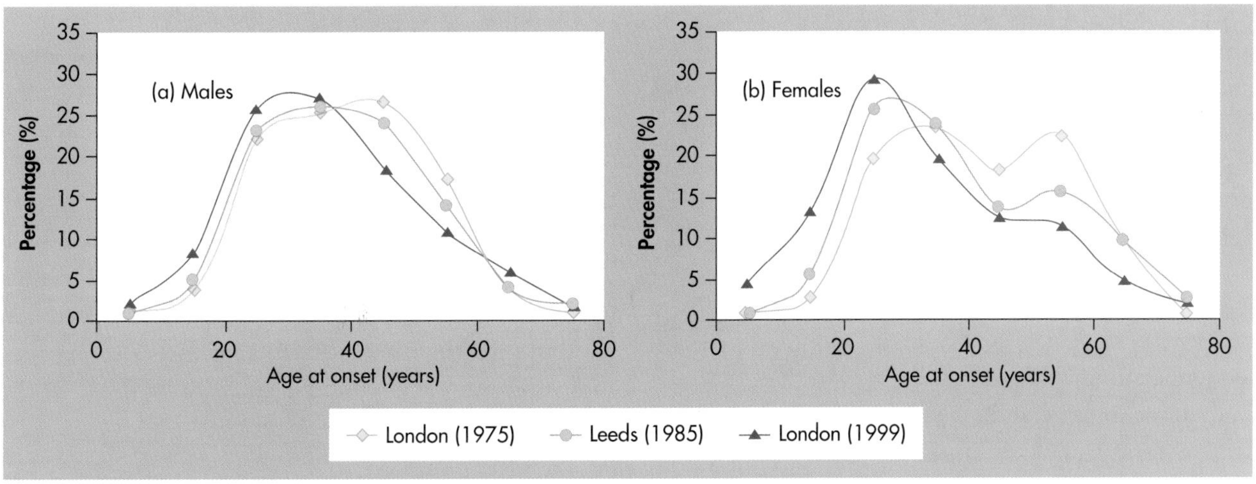

Figure 10.3 *The decrease in age at onset of stone formation in males and females in the UK during the past 25 years.*

of these cases, there is no obvious metabolic cause for their stones (idiopathic stone-formers). In the remainder, stones form secondarily to some disorder of calcium metabolism, oxalate metabolism or acid–base balance (see section on 'Calcium stone disease').

'Infection stones' composed of magnesium ammonium phosphate, usually in conjunction with calcium phosphate, constitute between 4% and 12% of all calculi. They are caused by urinary tract infections involving a urea-splitting organism and occur more commonly in women than in men.[9] They may also occur secondarily to the formation of most types of sterile stone. The relative incidence of infection stones has decreased over the past 25 years in most Western countries, presumably as a result of better clinical diagnosis and earlier treatment of urinary tract infections.

Uric acid calculi constitute between 4% and 15% of all stones depending on the relative consumption of animal and vegetable protein in the population concerned. 'Pure' uric acid stones are rare in developing countries and are most common in the oil-rich

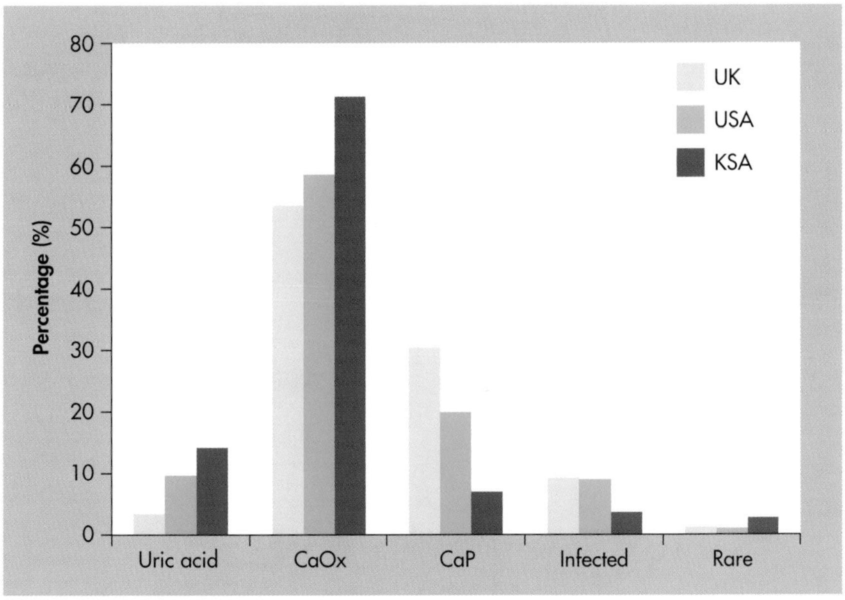

Figure 10.4 *The percentage of urinary stones classified according to the predominant mineral in the UK, USA and the Kingdom of Saudi Arabia (KSA). CaOx: calcium oxalate; CaP: calcium phosphate.*

states of the Arabian Gulf (Figure 10.4) and other affluent populations, or in countries where there is a cheap local source of animal protein.[8] Most uric acid stones are idiopathic in origin; a small number form secondarily to some disorder of purine metabolism or to some condition in which there is a high tissue turnover.

In all stone series, 1–3% of stones consist of one of a range of 'rare' constituents derived either from some hereditary or congenital inborn error of metabolism, such as cystinuria, xanthinuria or 2,8-dihydroxyadeninuria, or from a prescribed drug or one of its metabolites that is relatively insoluble in urine, such as silica, sulfonamides (such as sulfadiazine), indinavir or triamterene.

All stones contain a small percentage by weight of mucoproteinaceous matrix. A few consist almost entirely of mucoprotein ('matrix calculi') and usually result from inflammation of the urinary tract in patients whose urine is not sufficiently supersaturated to mineralize the organic matrix.[10] Apart from these rare entities, the role of the organic matrix in the formation of stones is unclear. By analogy with organized mineralized tissues such as bones and teeth, where the matrix plays a major role not only in the laying down of the mineral phase but also in defining the structure and architecture of the completed tissue, some researchers believe that the matrix of stones plays an equally important role in their initiation and growth.[11–13] Others, however, maintain that it is present merely as an adventitious inclusion, as a consequence of the calcium-binding properties of certain glycoproteins in the matrix material.[8]

THEORIES OF STONE FORMATION

The essential features of a complete theory of stone formation are that it should account for the formation and retention within the urinary system of some critical nucleus, which then enlarges by the processes of crystal growth and agglomeration until it produces the clinical symptoms associated with the disorder, namely, renal colic, dysuria and haematuria. In order to understand the current theories on how stones begin to form, it is necessary to appreciate some simple chemical principles involved in the stone-forming process.

CHEMICAL PRINCIPLES OF URINARY STONE FORMATION

Supersaturation

The overriding factor that is common to all types of stone is the relative insolubility of their respective mineral component(s) in urine. When a substance is allowed to dissolve in water, dissolution proceeds until the rate of return of the dissolved material to the solid phase equals the rate at which the solid phase goes into solution. The concentration of the substance in solution at this equilibrium point is known as the substance's solubility under the conditions of temperature and ionic strength concerned. Examples of the solubilities in water at 37° and at pH 6 of various salts and acids present in urine are shown in Table 10.1. Clearly, the substances that turn up in kidney stones have much lower solubilities than those that do not. For a sparingly soluble substance, it is usual to express this

Table 10.1 Solubilities of various possible urinary salts and acids in water at 37° and pH 6.

Salt	Solubility (g/l)	Properties
Calcium oxalate	0.0071	All occur in kidney stones
Calcium phosphate	0.08	
Uric acid	0.08	
Cystine	0.17	
Magnesium ammonium phosphate	0.36	
Calcium sulphate	2.1	Never occur in kidney stones
Calcium citrate	2.2	
Magnesium sulphate	293	
Calcium chloride	560	

equilibrium value as a product of the concentrations (or more correctly activities) of the constituent ions rather than as the absolute solubility of the substance in mass per unit volume. This equilibrium activity product is known as the thermodynamic solubility product of the substance concerned and is a constant at a given temperature.

In the absence of crystals of a particular substance, it is possible to add the ionic constituents of that substance to water and reach an activity product in the ensuing solution that is considerably above the solubility product of the substance without crystal nucleation occurring.[8] Such a solution is said to be in a state of metastable supersaturation, and it may survive in this state without de novo crystals forming for several hours. There is, however, an upper limit to this region of metastability, known as the 'formation product' of the substance. This is not a true thermodynamic constant, like the solubility product, but covers a band of supersaturation values within which de novo crystal nucleation may take place within a relatively short interval of time. Nucleation is dependent on the time of incubation and on the concentration of heterogeneous nuclei (that is, particles consisting of materials other than the substance under consideration) in the system. The upper limit of this band of formation products, beyond which the solution becomes completely unstable, corresponds to the level at which homogeneous nucleation takes place.[8]

From these general considerations of solubility, it is evident that urine may fall into one of three zones of relative supersaturation with respect to each of the stone-forming minerals (Figure 10.5). Urines lying below the solubility product of a given mineral are said to be undersaturated with respect to that mineral; in this region, no new crystals can form and any existing crystals will dissolve. *There is no risk of forming stones in undersaturated urine.* Urines lying between the solubility product and the 'formation product' band are in a state of metastable supersaturation; in this region, urines can exist for quite long time periods without new crystals forming, but any existing crystals of the mineral concerned would be expected to grow (subject to the presence of possible inhibitors of crystallization [see below]). Urines lying above the

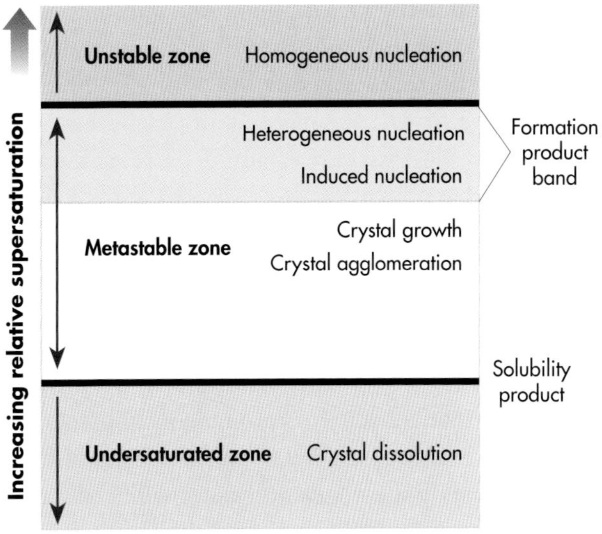

Figure 10.5 *Diagram showing the three main regions of relative supersaturation of urine with respect to a sparingly soluble mineral and the crystallization processes that may occur in each region.*

'formation product' band are said to be labile or unstable. Since urine is never a pure solution but usually contains particles of cell debris, polymerized glycoproteins, or even crystals of another salt, it is extremely unlikely that the point of homogeneous nucleation will ever be attained, since these particles will most likely have caused spontaneous heterogeneous nucleation to take place long before reaching this level of supersaturation.[8]

No simple method exists for measuring supersaturation directly in urine, and this has to be obtained indirectly by computational techniques. To calculate the relative supersaturation of urine with respect to every stone-forming salt and acid requires the measurement of the concentrations of 15 different urinary constituents.[14,15] These are fed into a computer that calculates the concentrations of all the soluble complexes formed between these constituents, the ionic strength of the urine and the activity coefficients of all the ions in solution. From this information, the activity products of each of the stone-forming substances are calculated and compared with the relevant solubility products. The ratio of activity product to solubility product is termed the relative supersaturation of urine with respect to the substance concerned. Values of 1 indicate that the urine is at the solubility product of the substance; values below 1 indicate that the urine is undersaturated with respect to the substance, and values greater than 1 indicate that the urine is supersaturated with that substance.[15]

Whether or not supersaturation is the only factor responsible for the formation of stones is still open to debate. Broadly, there are two main schools of thought regarding the initiation of stones. Proponents of the 'free-particle' model of urolithiasis believe that stones are initiated when urine becomes so excessively supersaturated with one of the salts or acids that turn up in kidney stones that crystals of that constituent spontaneously precipitate in urine.[16,17] If this happens frequently and if the crystals grow or aggregate sufficiently within the transit time of urine through the kidney, the risk increases that one of these particles will become trapped at some narrow point in the urinary tract and form the focus around which a stone may form.[18] Alternatively, blockage may occur through a 'log-jamming' mechanism in a urinary stream overcrowded with crystals (Figure 10.6).[8]

An alternative theory claims that the formation of a critical particle by such a 'free-particle' mechanism cannot take place within the transit time of urine through the kidney and that the only way that a stone can be initiated is through chemical 'fixation'

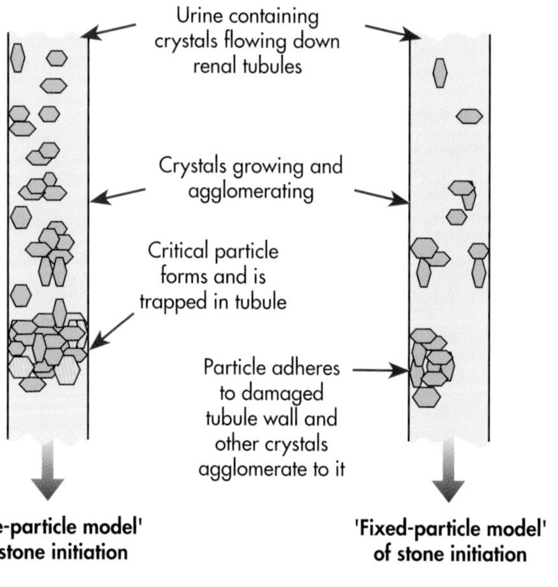

Figure 10.6 *Diagrammatic representation of how stones are initiated according to the 'free-particle' and 'fixed-particle' models of stone formation.*

of a crystal or aggregate of crystals to the renal epithelial lining (Figure 10.6). In this 'fixed-particle' theory, formation is postulated to occur either through damage to the cell walls (caused either by the crystals themselves or by viruses or bacteria) or through the participation of some 'gluing' material present in the urine of stone-formers (but absent from the urine of non-stone-formers) that causes crystals to adhere to these sites and there act as foci for stone-formation.[19–25] Both theories require urine to be supersaturated to some degree with respect to the stone-forming salt or acid concerned, sufficient to cause crystals to be formed by spontaneous or heterogeneous nucleation.

Processes of crystallization

Nucleation, as described above, is the first step in the process of crystallization. This causes a fall in the supersaturation of urine as new crystals are formed but does not usually reduce the level of supersaturation immediately down to the solubility product. There is then a period during which the initially formed nuclei grow in the remaining metastable urine, and in the moving stream of urine, the growing crystals may impact with each other and aggregate to form larger particles. *This process is called agglomeration and is the stage in the crystallization process during which the particle size increases most rapidly.*[17,18,26] In the 'free-particle' theory, crystal agglomeration is essential in order to create a particle that is large enough to be retained in the collecting tubule before the urine is expelled through the ducts of Bellini.[17,18,27] Crystal growth per se is normally too slow a process to allow this to happen within the transit time of urine through the renal tubule.

Agglomeration may be less important in the 'fixed-particle' model, since the initial particle that causes the stone to form round it is considered, by definition, to be 'glued' to the renal tubular epithelial wall. Once the initial entrapment ('free-particle' model) or fixation step ('fixed-particle' model) has taken place, both theories require the immobilized particle to increase in size through further crystal growth and agglomeration until it becomes a 'stone' that causes problems for the patient.[16–19,26,27]

Modifiers of crystallization

One factor that may affect the kinetics of the processes involved in both theories is the presence or absence in urine of so-called modifiers of crystallization.[8] These are claimed to be of particular importance in the formation of calcium-containing stones. Indeed, no specific, naturally occurring modifier has been reported to have any effect on the crystallization of cystine, uric acid or magnesium ammonium phosphate. One group of crystallization modifiers is claimed to *retard* the rate of growth and/or aggregation of crystals of calcium salts and/or the binding of calcium-containing crystals to cell walls. These are known as *inhibitors* of crystallization and include magnesium,[28] citrate,[29] pyrophosphate,[30,31] adenosine diphosphate,[32] adenosine triphosphate,[32] at least two phosphopeptides,[33] various glycosaminoglycans,[34,35] non-polymerized Tamm-Horsfall protein (also known as uromodulin),[36–38] nephrocalcin,[38–41] calgranulin,[42] various plasma proteins,[11] osteopontin (also known as uropontin),[43] α-1-microglobulin,[12] β-2-microglobulin,[44] urinary prothrombin fragment 1[45,46] and inter-α-trypsin inhibitor (bikunin light chain).[47]

The second group of modifiers is claimed to *stimulate* one or more of the processes involved in the crystallization of calcium salts. These are known as *promoters* of stone formation and include matrix substance A,[12] various uncharacterized urinary proteins and glycoproteins,[48–50] and the polymerized form of Tamm-Horsfall protein (uromucoid).[51–53]

Unquestionably, urine does possess a certain ability to modify the rate of crystal growth and/or agglomeration of calcium oxalate crystals and may also contain factors that influence the binding of these crystals to renal epithelial cells. Currently, it would seem, however, that the 'crystallization-modifying activity' is unlikely to be attributable to one single magic factor X but is probably due to the net effect of all the above promoters and inhibitors (and probably others not yet identified). None of the above factors appears to dominate the kinetics of crystal nucleation, growth, aggregation and binding to cells, and none has yet been accepted as being uniquely different, either quantitatively or qualitatively, between stone-formers and normal subjects. Therefore, the assertion that a deficiency in one particular inhibitor or an excess of one particular promoter is *the* cause of stone formation is open to question.[54]

In the final analysis, stone formation is probably due to an abnormal combination of factors that affect both the thermodynamic driving force (supersaturation) and the kinetic (rate-controlling) processes involved in the crystallization of the various stone-forming minerals. For some types of stone formation (cystine, xanthine, 2,8-dihydroxyadenine, uric acid and probably magnesium ammonium phosphate), the thermodynamic factors appear to predominate; in others (calcium-containing stones), both sets of factors may be involved.[8]

Crystalluria

Whatever the detailed mechanism of stone initiation, an individual's propensity to produce crystals of one of the stone-forming constituents is an important prerequisite for stone formation, either because the crystals lead directly to the initiation of stones (as postulated in the 'free-particle' model) or because their production is a signal that urine is so supersaturated with respect to that constituent that heterogeneous nucleation and crystal growth are likely to occur at one of the critical sites postulated in the 'fixed-particle' model. Crystalluria occurs more frequently and more abundantly in the urine of stone-formers than in that of controls, and, in patients with calcium-stone disease, the crystals are larger and more agglomerated.[17,18] The severity of the disorder, as defined by the stone episode rate in a given patient is proportional to the percentage of large crystals and aggregates in the patient's urine (Figure 10.7). It would appear that particle size is a vital factor in the stone-forming process.

CYSTINE STONE FORMATION

Cystinuria is a congenital disorder characterized by a defect in the renal tubular reabsorption of cystine, lysine, ornithine and arginine, but the lesion also affects the intestine.[55,56] As a consequence, the urinary excretion of these amino acids is greatly increased. Lysine, ornithine and arginine are all fairly

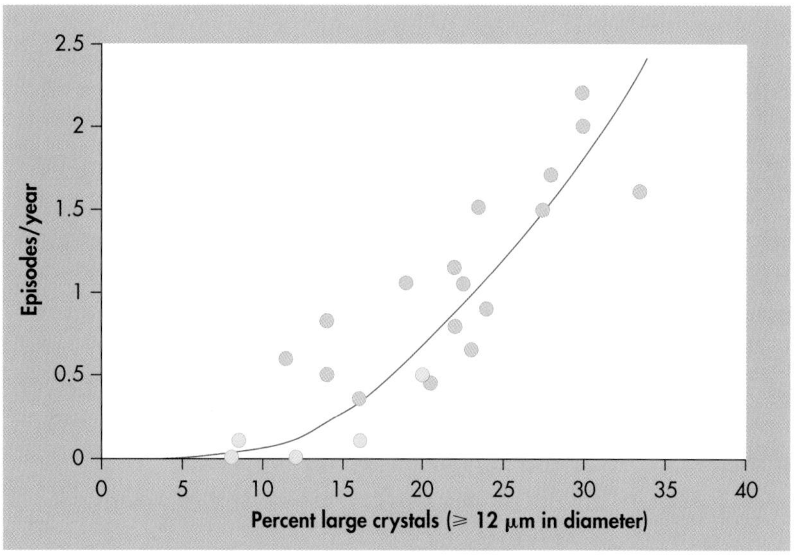

Figure 10.7 *The relationship between the severity of stone formation (as defined by the stone episode rate) in recurrent calcium oxalate stone-formers and the proportion of large calcium oxalate crystals and aggregates in their freshly voided urine; (●): untreated patients; (○): patients on orthophosphate supplements.*

soluble in urine, but cystine is relatively insoluble and, as a result, these patients tend to have cystine crystalluria and to form cystine stones.[57,58]

The sole risk factor for cystine stone formation is the supersaturation of urine with respect to cystine, as defined by the urinary concentration of cystine and urine pH (Figure 10.8). Within the normal pH range of urine (5–7), the supersaturation is defined by the concentration of cystine. In normal urine, this is generally low (10–100 μmol/l), at which concentrations urine is well undersaturated with respect to cystine; therefore, cystine crystalluria is never found in normal urine. In heterozygous cystinurics, whose urinary cystine concentrations are in the range 20–1000 μmol/l, the supersaturation values are higher but still below the solubility of cystine in urine. As a rule, these patients do not have cystine crystalluria in fresh urine and do not form cystine stones.[59] Homozygous cystinurics, however, have much higher urinary concentrations of cystine (1400–4200 μmol/l), above the solubility of cystine in saline at 37° (1250 μmol/l), and so their urines are considerably supersaturated with respect to cystine (Figure 10.8). These patients often pass large cystine

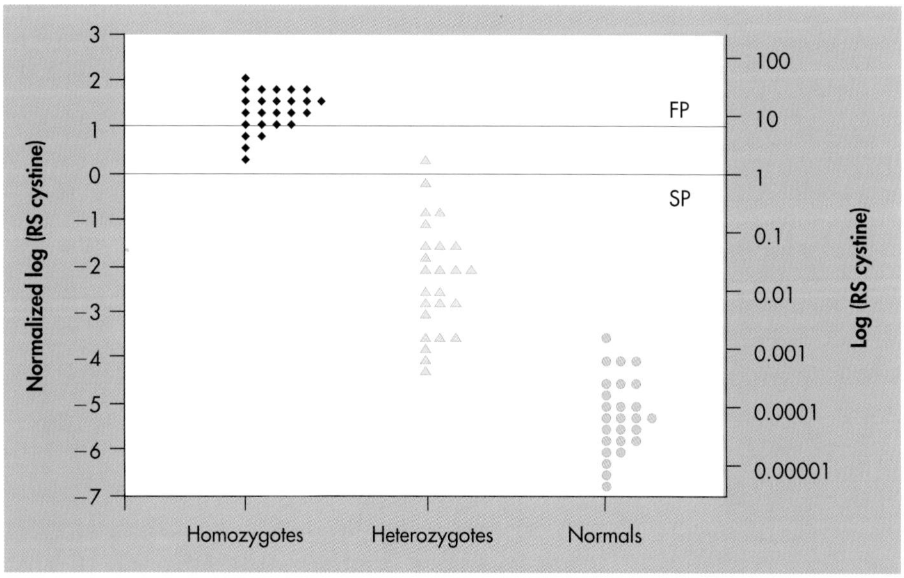

Figure 10.8 *The relative supersaturation (RS) of urine with respect to cystine in homozygous cystinurics, heterozygous cystinurics and normal subjects. The data are plotted on a log scale, where the solubility product (SP) has a value of 1, and on a normalized log scale such that the SP has a value of 0 and the upper limit of the formation product band (FP) has a value of 1.*

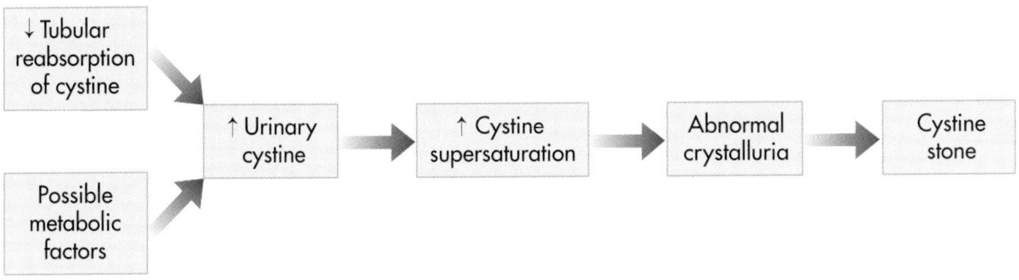

Figure 10.9 *A risk factor model of cystine stone formation.*

crystals in their urine and form cystine stones.[57,58] This form of stone formation is therefore readily explained in terms of excessive excretion → excessive supersaturation → abnormal crystalluria → stones. The complete risk factor model of cystine stone formation is outlined in Figure 10.9.

Prevention of cystine stones requires the supersaturation of urine to be substantially reduced in order to prevent continued crystalluria (Figure 10.10). Although cystine is more soluble in alkaline urine than under acidic or neutral conditions, alkali therapy is not always practicable, as large doses of sodium bicarbonate are required to maintain urinary pH above 7.6.[60] Less alkali may be required if the patient is also put on a high fluid intake (>3 l/day).[61] Alternatively, reduction in cystine concentration may be achieved by administration of 2–4 g/day of D-penicillamine, which forms an S–S link with the cysteine subunits of cystine to form a disulphide that is more soluble than cystine (Figure 10.11).[62] However, this form of therapy has a high risk of side-effects, including rashes, neutropenia, thrombopenia, nephrotic syndrome and fever. Severe proteinuria is experienced in about 10–15% of patients.[58] A number of analogues, such as *N*-acetyl-D-penicillamine and α-mercaptopropionyl-glycine, have been tried with some degree of success as less toxic alternatives. If the above forms of therapy are pursued tenaciously, the supersaturation of urine with respect to cystine can be reduced (Figure 10.10) and with it the risk of stone recurrence.[58,66,67]

It is also possible to explain the formation of the other 'rare' stones (such as 2,8-dihydroxyadenine, xanthine and silica) simply on the basis of their insolubility in urine. These stones form purely from the excessive excretion in urine of the particular substance concerned, either as a result of some metabolic defect or from the administration of a drug that is itself insoluble (or one of its metabolites is insoluble) in urine. Urine becomes excessively supersaturated with the substance concerned, resulting in abnormal crystalluria and stone formation.[8]

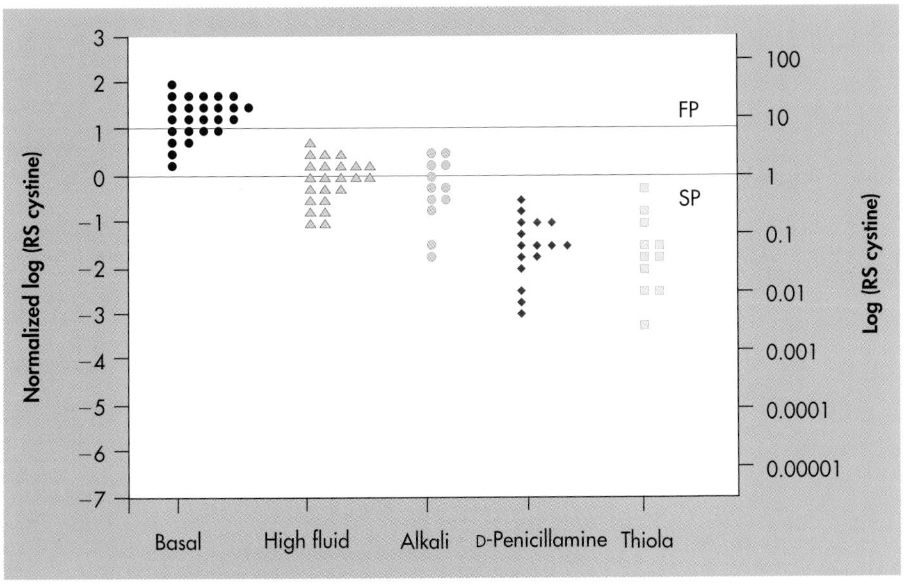

Figure 10.10 *The effect of various treatments on the relative supersaturation (RS) of urine with respect to cystine in cystinuric stone-formers. The data are plotted on a log scale, where the solubility product (SP) has a value of 1, and on a normalized log scale such that the SP has a value of 0 and the upper limit of the formation product band (FP) has a value of 1.*

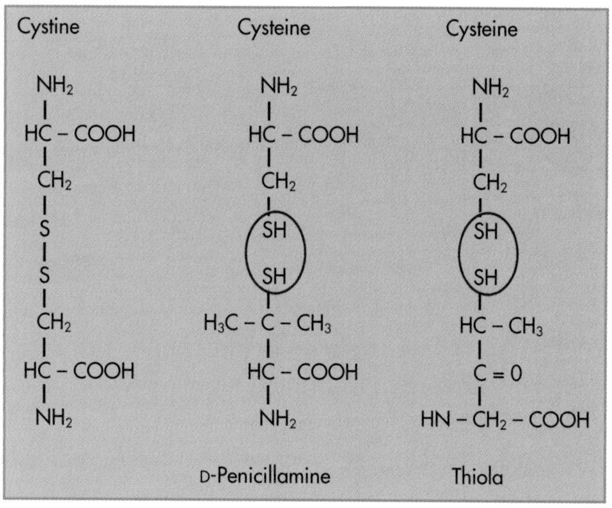

Figure 10.11 *The structures of cystine, cysteine and various analogues which form S–S complexes with cysteine that are soluble in urine.*

URIC ACID STONE FORMATION

Uric acid is the end-product of purine metabolism and is normally excreted in urine in the range 2–5 mmol/day.[68,69] Patients with urinary excretions above this range are prone to form uric acid stones, but hyperuricosuria per se is not the sole cause or even the most important factor in uric acid lithiasis.[70] Dehydration is almost as important as hyperuricosuria, and a low urine pH is more critical than both of these factors.[71,72] The main causes of hyperuricosuria are listed in Table 10.2.

Table 10.2 Causes of hyperuricosuria.
Primary gout
Increased purine intake
Glycogen storage disease – glucose-6-phosphatase deficiency
Increased phosphoribosyl pyrophosphate synthetase activity
Hypoxanthine – guanine phosphoribosyltransferase deficiency (Lesch-Nyhan syndrome)
Neoplastic disease
Secondary polycythaemia
Anaemia and haemoglobinopathy
Psoriasis
Cystinuria

As with the formation of 'rare' stones, uric acid stone formation can be completely explained in terms of excessive supersaturation of urine with respect to uric acid.[8] Chemically, the two factors that determine the risk of uric acid crystalluria are the concentration of uric acid and the pH of urine. The pKa of uric acid is 5.46, so that any urine with a pH of less than this figure will contain more of the relatively insoluble, undissociated form of the acid. Uric acid crystalluria becomes increasingly more likely as urine pH drops below 5.3.[73] Normal urine, on the other hand, generally lies in the metastable or undersaturated region with respect to uric acid[8] with little or no risk of forming uric acid crystals (Figure 10.12).

The causes of an acid urine are listed in Table 10.3. These include a high acid-ash diet containing large amounts of meat, fish and poultry.[74] As this type of diet is also high in purines, these patients usually have hyperuricosuria in conjunction with their acid urine, and so the risk of uric acid stone formation is compounded.[8] In the idiopathic uric acid stone-formers, the tendency to pass an acid urine has been attributed to a low rate of ammonia synthesis;[71,75] ammonia is normally synthesized in the kidney to buffer hydrogen ions. Ileostomy patients also pass urine that is highly supersaturated with respect to uric acid.[76] Their urine is highly concentrated and very acidic as a result of losing water and bicarbonate through their ileostomy. The risk factor model of uric acid stone formation is shown in Figure 10.13.

Table 10.3 Possible causes of acid urine.
Dehydration
Oliguria
Diarrhoea
Permanent ileostomy
Colostomy
Low rate of renal production of ammonia
Increased titratable acidity
High acid-ash diet (as in a high intake of animal protein)

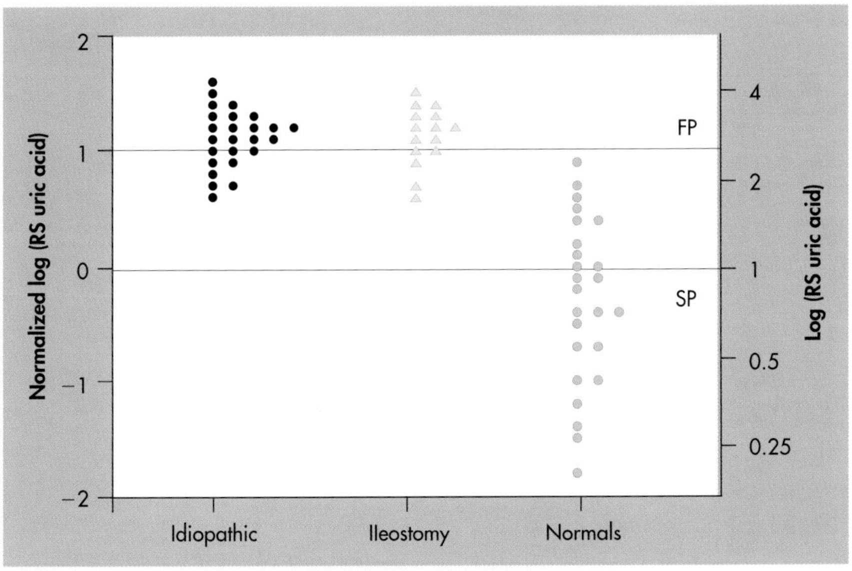

Figure 10.12 *The relative supersaturation (RS) of urine with respect to uric acid in idiopathic uric acid stone-formers, patients with an ileostomy and uric acid stones and normal subjects. The data are plotted on a log scale, where the solubility product (SP) has a value of 1, and on a normalized log scale such that the SP has a value of 0 and the upper limit of the formation product band (FP) has a value of 1.*

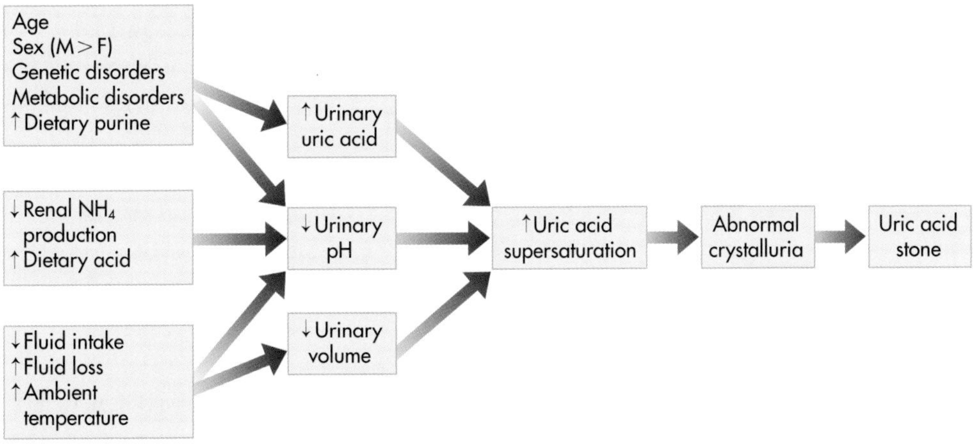

Figure 10.13 *A risk factor model for uric acid stone formation.*

Treatment is designed to lower the supersaturation of urine with respect to uric acid (Figure 10.14). This can be achieved relatively cheaply by increasing urinary pH to above 6.2 (but not higher than 6.5 in order to avoid formation of calcium phosphate stones) with oral sodium bicarbonate or potassium citrate and maintaining the urine volume above 2 l/day with a high fluid intake.[71,72,77] Allopurinol, which inhibits the metabolic production of uric acid from xanthine by blocking the enzyme xanthine oxidase, may be necessary for patients who cannot tolerate alkali.[78,79] Allopurinol has few side-effects, but care has to be taken with patients with enzyme defects that lead to a very high production of uric acid (such as Lesch-Nyhan syndrome or neoplastic disease), since allopurinol administration may result in xanthinuria and xanthine stones.[80,81]

INFECTED STONE FORMATION

Urinary tract infections involving urea-splitting organisms often lead to the formation of stones that consist of calcium phosphate often mixed with magnesium ammonium phosphate.[82] Chemically, the process involves the breakdown of urea by the enzyme urease to form ammonium, bicarbonate and hydroxyl ions (Figure 10.15) with an accompanying marked alkalinization of urine (pH > 7.2). Under these conditions, the supersaturation of urine with

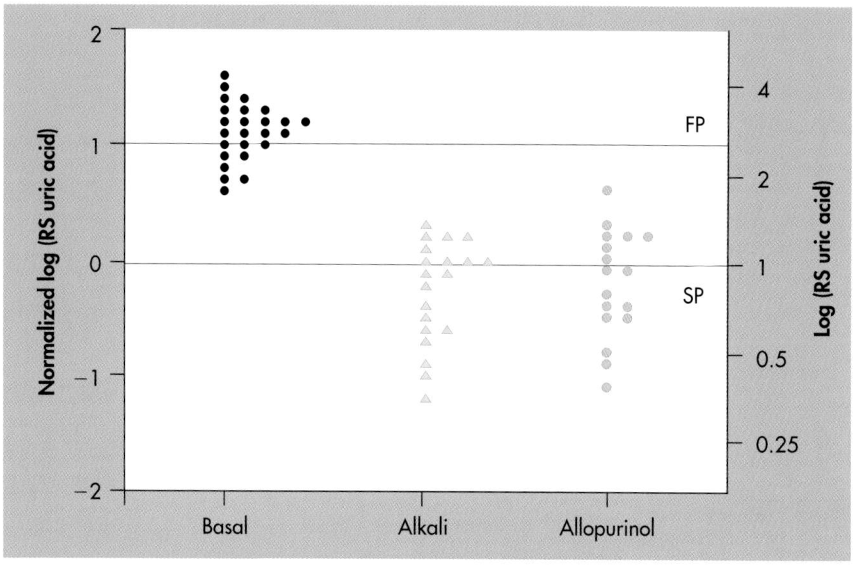

Figure 10.14 *The effect of various treatments on the relative supersaturation (RS) of urine with respect to uric acid in uric acid stone-formers. The data are plotted on a log scale, where the solubility product (SP) has a value of 1, and on a normalized log scale such that the SP has a value of 0 and the upper limit of the formation product band (FP) has a value of 1.*

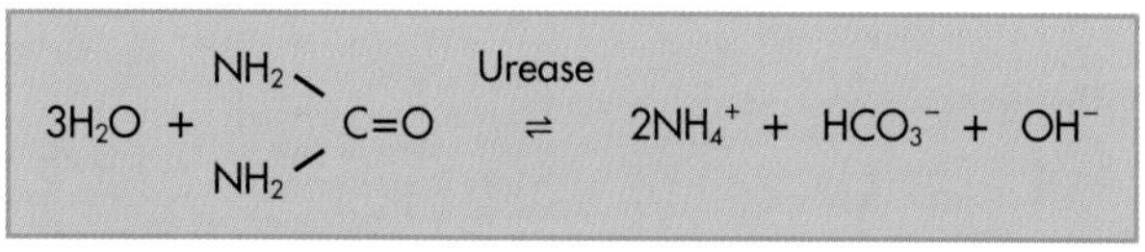

Figure 10.15 *The breakdown of urea by urease to form ammonium ions and alkali.*

respect to both calcium phosphate and magnesium ammonium phosphate reaches values that cause spontaneous precipitation of these salts and massive crystalluria (Figure 10.16).[82,83] In addition, two of the known inhibitors of calcium phosphate crystal growth, pyrophosphate and citrate, are often low in the urines of patients with urinary tract infections, and this may allow the formation of larger than normal

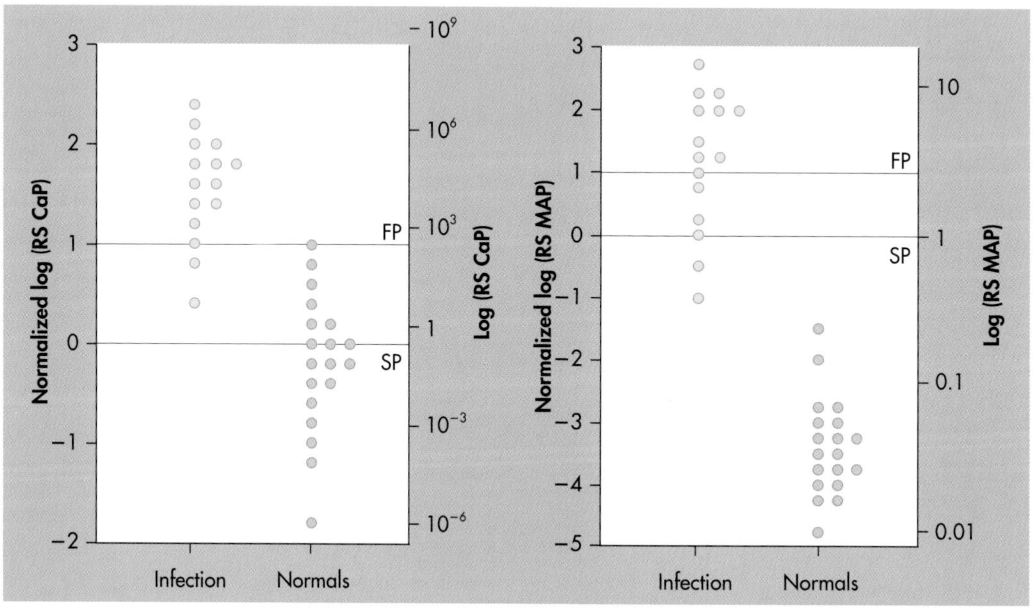

Figure 10.16 *The relative supersaturation (RS) of urine with respect to calcium phosphate (CaP) [left panel] and magnesium ammonium phosphate (MAP) [right panel] in infected stone-formers and normal subjects. The data are plotted on a log scale, where the solubility product (SP) has a value of 1, and on a normalized log scale such that the SP has a value of 0 and the upper limit of the formation product band (FP) has a value of 1.*

crystals and aggregates of calcium phosphate, thereby increasing the risk of stone formation.[8] A list of the organisms causing urinary tract infection and their ability to produce urease is contained in Table 10.4. The risk-factor model of infected stone formation is shown in Figure 10.17.

Treatment of infected stone patients usually involves the combined efforts of the surgeon and the physician. The first stage is to remove the stone completely and, if possible, to correct any anatomical obstruction that might have caused the underlying infection. Medical management is necessary before and after stone removal in order to sterilize the urine.[84] This may not always be easy to achieve since the infecting organism may be resistant to several antibiotics.[85,86] In this situation, urease-inhibiting drugs, such as acetohydroxamic acid, may be helpful,[87–89] although there may be side-effects (Figure 10.18).[87] A high fluid intake is necessary in all patients, and some acidification may be required to lower the urine pH to around 6. Drinking cranberry juice may be beneficial in this respect.[90]

CALCIUM STONE DISEASE

Stones consisting of calcium oxalate, often mixed with calcium phosphate, are the most common types of calculi in most series.[8] 'Pure' calcium phosphate stones are quite rare, suggesting that calcium oxalate is the main problem behind the formation of calcium-containing stones. The reason for this is the very poor solubility of calcium oxalate in aqueous media (Table 10.1). Whereas urine can often be undersaturated with respect to all other constituents of urinary calculi, particularly in non-stone-formers, in the case of calcium oxalate urine is always supersaturated to

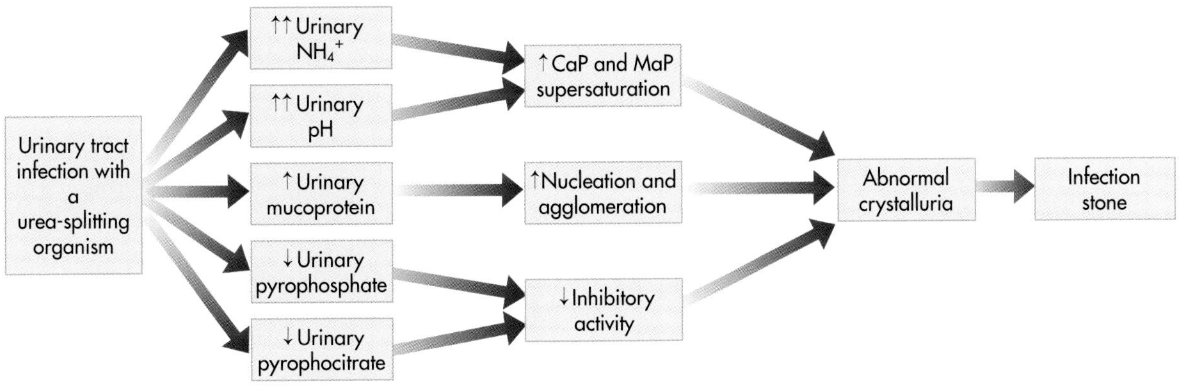

Figure 10.17 *A risk factor model of infected stone-formation.*

Table 10.4 The relative prevalence of organisms causing urinary tract infection and their ability to produce urease.

Organisms causing urinary tract infection	Patients with infection (%)		Ability to produce urease	
	In hospital	At home	Frequently	Occasionally
Escherichia	5	0	0	+
Proteus	16	5	+	0
Klebsiella	9	2	0	+
Streptococcus	7	0	0	0
Staphylococcus	5	3	+	0
Pseudomonas	3	0	0	+
Ureaplasma urealyticum	1	0	+	0

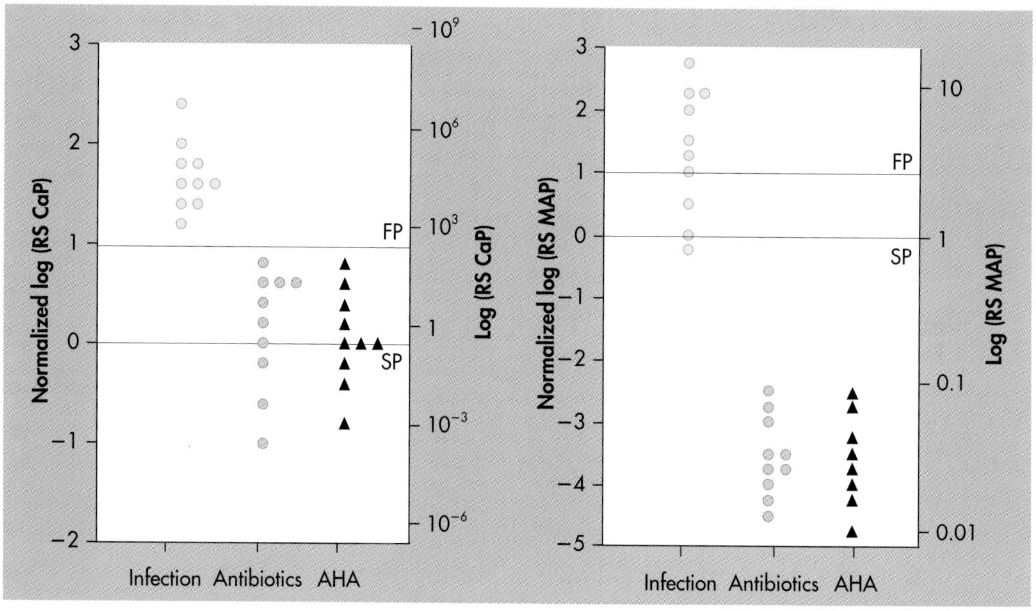

Figure 10.18 *The effect of various treatments on the relative supersaturation (RS) of urine with respect to calcium phosphate (CaP) [left panel] and magnesium ammonium phosphate (MAP) [right panel] in infected stone-formers (AHA: acetohydroxamic acid). The data are plotted on a log scale, where the solubility product (SP) has a value of 1, and on a normalized log scale such that the SP has a value of 0 and the upper limit of the formation product band (FP) has a value of 1.*

some degree with the salt, *even in normal subjects* (Figure 10.19). This means, firstly, that urine is relatively close to the formation product of calcium oxalate in most individuals and, secondly, that once calcium oxalate deposits form and become lodged in the kidney, they can never dissolve spontaneously. Stones containing calcium oxalate can be disintegrated by ESWL and other methods and the fragments (probably) passed, but they cannot be easily redissolved, even with aggressive irrigation techniques.

The vast majority of calcium stone-formers are said to be idiopathic, since they exhibit no obvious metabolic cause for their stones. About 10–12% of patients are found to have a metabolic cause, such as primary hyperparathyroidism, distal renal tubular acidosis or primary or enteric hyperoxaluria.[8] The complete list of conditions that lead to secondary calcium stones is contained in Table 10.5.

Unlike most other types of stone formation, calcium lithiasis does not appear to be attributable to a single urinary abnormality or even to a simple combination of abnormalities. It is a truly multifactorial disorder in which various combinations of (often) small increases or decreases in certain urinary factors may compound the risk of forming stones.[8] These include a low urine volume (<1.3 l/day),[91,92] a raised urinary pH (>6.3),[8,93] hypercalciuria (>6 mmol/day)[94–98], mild hyperoxaluria (>0.45 mmol/day),[26,99,100] hypocitraturia (<2 mmol/day),[101–103] hyperuricosuria (> 4.5 mmol/day)[74]

Table 10.5 List of conditions that may lead to secondary calcium stone formation.

Primary hyperparathyroidism
Distal renal tubular acidosis (type I)
Hereditary hyperoxaluria
Enteric hyperoxaluria
Medullary sponge kidney
Cushing's disease and steroid treatment
Sarcoidosis
Immobilization
Milk-alkali syndrome
Vitamin D intoxication
Betel-nut chewing

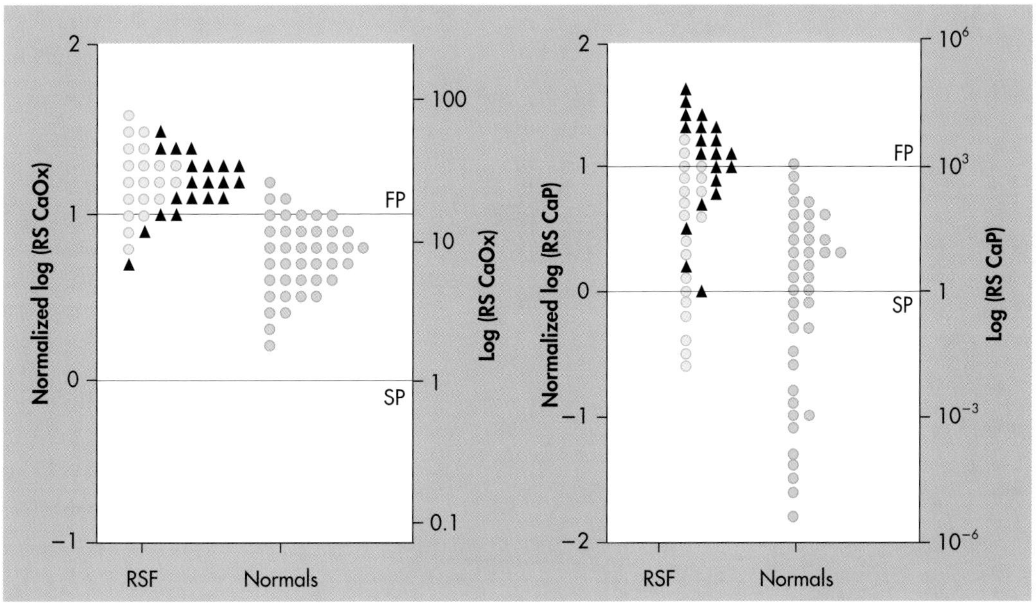

Figure 10.19 *The relative supersaturation (RS) of urine with respect to calcium oxalate (CaOx) [left panel] and calcium phosphate (CaP) [right panel] in recurrent idiopathic calcium stone-formers (RSF) and normal subjects. The RSF are divided into those with 'pure' CaOx stones (●) and those with 'mixed' CaOx/CaP stones (▲). The data are plotted on a log scale, where the solubility product (SP) has a value of 1, and on a normalized log scale such that the SP has a value of 0 and the upper limit of the formation product band (FP) has a value of 1.*

and a low urinary magnesium excretion (<3.2 mmol/day).[104] All of these factors have been found to be different between stone-formers and normals, although in each case there is a considerable overlap between the data in the two groups.[105,106] All the abnormalities described are known to increase the supersaturation of urine with respect to calcium oxalate and/or calcium phosphate, although they are not all equally important in this respect. In addition to their ability to influence supersaturation, citrate and magnesium are mild inhibitors of crystallization of calcium salts,[28,29] and uric acid is a mild promoter of calcium stone formation.[107,108] Risk factor analysis has shown that, taking all their properties into account, the overall order of importance of the above seven factors in determining the risk of forming calcium-containing stones is as follows: low urine volume > mild hyperoxaluria > raised urinary pH > hypercalciuria > hypocitraturia > hyperuricosuria > hypomagnesiuria.[106]

The risk-factor model of calcium stone formation makes use of these seven measurements to generate a number of algorithms that represent an estimate (P_{SF}) of the overall biochemical risk of forming various types of calcium-containing stones.[105,106] The model has recently been extended to include uric acid-containing stones so that predictions can be made from an analysis of two 24-hr urines on the likelihood of forming all combinations of stone types involving uric acid, calcium oxalate and calcium phosphate.[106] The values of P_{SF}, which are calculated on a probability scale from 0 to 1, are higher in stone-formers than in non-stone-formers. In recurrent stone-formers, the values are generally over 0.5 whereas in normal subjects they are usually under 0.5. This function therefore provides quite a good discriminator between the two groups (Figure 10.20). Furthermore, within the group of recurrent stone-formers, the severity of the disorder (as defined by the stone-recurrence rate of the patient) is related to the patient's average P_{SF} value. This method of combining risk factors is a useful means of assessing the risk of forming stones in a given individual and for following the efficacy of the particular form of prophylaxis prescribed for the patient. A summary of the urinary risk factors involved in all types of stone formation is given in Table 10.6.

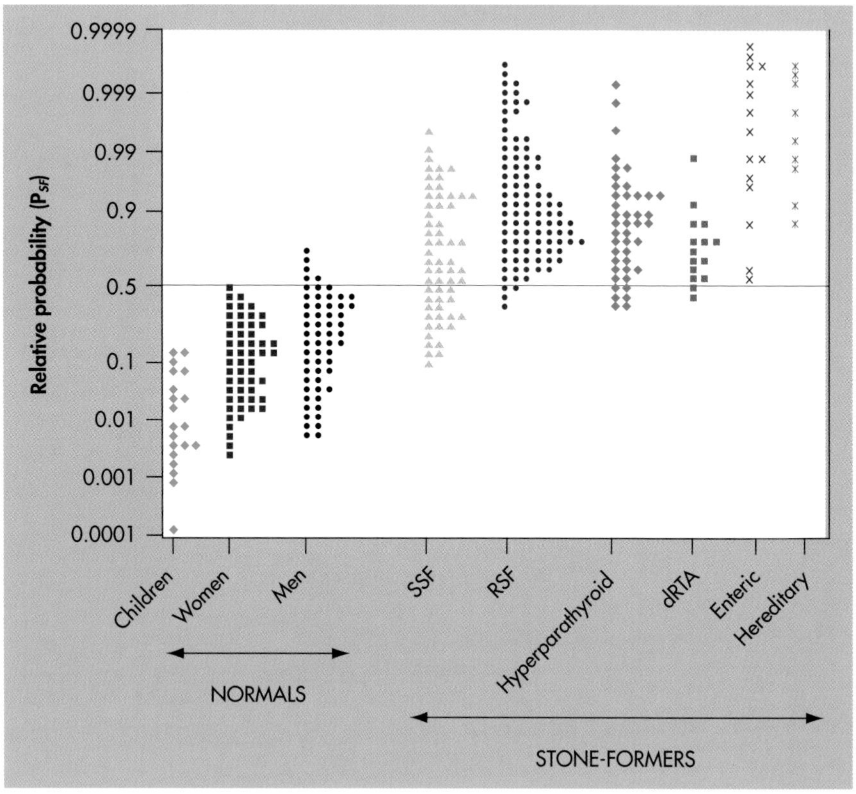

Figure 10.20 *The overall relative probability of forming calcium-containing stones (P_{SF}) in normal children and adults and in single episode (SSF) and recurrent (RSF) idiopathic calcium stone-formers. Also shown are the P_{SF} values in various groups of patients at risk of forming secondary calcium stones. Hyperparathyroid: patients with primary hyperparathyroidism; dRTA: distal renal tubular acidosis; enteric: patients with enteric hyperoxaluria; hereditary: patients with hereditary hyperoxaluria.*

Table 10.6 Summary of the urinary risk factors for the various types of stone formation and their effects on the parameters of crystallization.

Stone type	Urinary risk factor	Chemical effect
Rare stones	↑ Xanthine, ↑ 2,8-dihydroxyadenine, ↑ silica, ↑ indinavir, etc.	↑ Supersaturation of relevant stone constituent
Cystine stones	↑ Cystine	↑ Cystine supersaturation
Uric acid stones	↓ pH ↑ Uric acid ↓ Volume	↑ Uric acid supersaturation
Infection stones	↑↑ pH ↑ Ammonium ions ↑ Mucosubstances	↑ Magnesium ammonium phosphate and calcium phosphate supersaturation ↑ Agglomeration of crystals
Calcium stones	↓ Volume ↑ Oxalate ↑ Calcium ↑ pH ↓ Citrate ↓ Magnesium ↓ Macromolecular inhibitors ↑ Uric acid ↑ Macromolecular promoters	↑ Calcium oxalate and/or calcium phosphate supersaturation ↓ Crystallization inhibitory activity ↑ Crystallization promotive activity

Epidemiological factors in the formation of urinary stones

There are three groups of epidemiological factors that have been found to be of importance in the formation of urinary stones – demographic, environmental and pathophysiological. Each of these groups contains a number of categories. These are summarized in Table 10.7. Each has been shown to increase the risk of stone formation through its effect on the balance between supersaturation, inhibitors and promoters of crystallization in urine.[8] For calcium stone formation, the most common form of the disorder, the main epidemiological factors are age,[8] gender,[8] season,[109,110] climate,[111,112] stress,[113] occupation,[112,114,115] affluence,[116–118] diet (including fluid intake)[8,119–123] and genetic/metabolic factors.[124–126]

The role of diet, in particular, has been studied in detail, and it appears to explain much of the changing pattern of stone incidence over the past 100 years.[8,121,127] As the composition of the diet becomes 'richer' in a given population (owing to an increased consumption of protein, particularly animal protein, refined sugars and salt), the incidence of stones increases.[121,127] This often follows periods of economic expansion (Figure 10.2). During periods of recession, on the other hand, the incidence of stones has been noted to decrease in parallel with a return to a more healthy form of diet containing more fibre and fewer energy-rich foods.[8,127] The risk factor model for calcium stone formation, incorporating all of these factors, is shown in Figure 10.21.

Prevention of stone recurrence

The main aim in the prevention of stone recurrence is to decrease the likelihood of crystals forming in the urinary tract by reducing the supersaturation of urine with respect to the particular constituent(s)

Table 10.7 The epidemiological factors involved in uric-acid and calcium stone formation and their effects on urinary risk factors.

Epidemiological factor	Urinary risk factors
Age and sex	↑ Calcium, ↑ oxalate, ↑ uric acid, ↑ pH, ↓ volume, ↓ citrate, ↓ magnesium, ↓ macromolecular inhibitors, ↑ promoters
Climate and season	↓ Volume, ↑ calcium, ↑ oxalate, ↓ pH
Stress	↑ Calcium, ↑ oxalate, ↑ uric acid, ↓ magnesium
Low fluid intake or exercise	↓ Volume, ↓ pH
Affluence and diet	↑ Calcium, ↑ oxalate, ↑ uric acid, ↓ citrate, ↓ pH
Metabolic disorders	
Gout	↑ Uric acid
Glycogen storage disease	↑ Uric acid
Lesch-Nyhan syndrome	↑ Uric acid
Neoplastic disease	↑ Uric acid
Ileostomy	↓ Volume, ↓ pH
Primary hyperparathyroidism	↑↑ Calcium, ↑ pH
Distal renal tubular acidosis	↑ pH, ↑ calcium, citrate
Hereditary hyperoxaluria	↑↑ oxalate
Enteric hyperoxaluria	↑ Oxalate, ↓ pH, ↓ citrate, ↓ magnesium
Medullary sponge kidney	↑ Calcium
Cushing's disease	↑ Calcium, ↑ pH
Vitamin D intoxication	↑↑ Calcium
Milk-alkali syndrome	↑ Calcium, ↑ pH
Sarcoidosis	↑↑ Calcium
Betel-nut chewing	↑↑ Calcium, ↑ pH
Immobilization	↑ Calcium, ↑ pH (from urinary tract infection)

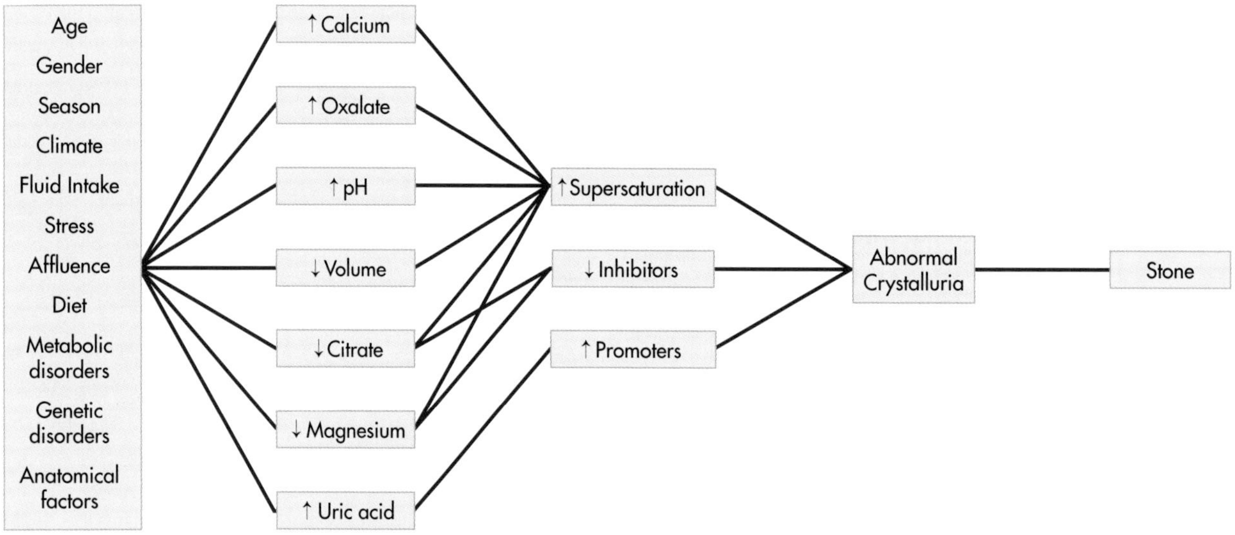

Figure 10.21 *A risk-factor model for calcium stone formation.*

Table 10.8 Medical methods for prevention of urinary stone disease.

Stone type	Treatment
2,8-Dihydroxyadenine	Very high fluid intake (>3 l/day) + allopurinol (300 mg/day)
Silica	Discontinue magnesium trisilicate antacids
Xanthine	Hereditary form: high fluid intake + oral alkali (urine pH >7.4) Iatrogenic form: withdraw allopurinol
Cystine	Very high fluid intake (>3 l/day) + oral alkali (urine pH >7.5) or D-penicillamine (2–4 g/day) or α-mercaptopropionylglycine
Uric acid	High fluid intake (>2.5 l/day) + oral alkali (urine pH >6.2) or reduce purine intake or allopurinol (300 mg/day)
Infected	High fluid intake + antibiotics + oral acid (pH < 6.2)
Calcium	
Idiopathic	High fluid intake + dietary advice or thiazide diuretics (bendrofluazide 10 mg/day) or phosphate supplements (1–1.5 g P/day) or magnesium supplements (500 mg Mg/day) or potassium citrate (20 mequiv t.d.s)
Hyperparathyroid	Parathyroidectomy or, if contraindicated, high fluids + oral acid
Hereditary hyperoxaluric	High fluid intake (>3 l/day) + pyridoxine (400 mg/day)
Enteric hyperoxaluric	High fluid intake + low oxalate/high calcium diet or potassium citrate
Renal tubular acidotic	High fluid intake + thiazides or potassium citrate
Medullary sponge kidney	Treat as for idiopathic
Corticosteroid-induced	Discontinue corticosteroids: treat as for idiopathic
Sarcoidosis	High fluid intake
Milk-alkali syndrome	Discontinue alkali and moderate calcium intake + high fluid intake
Vitamin D intoxication	Discontinue high vitamin D intake + high fluid intake
Betel-nut chewing	Discontinue practice
Immobilization	High fluid intake; remobilize as far as possible; treat any urinary tract infection with antibiotics
Iatrogenic	Discontinue drug concerned as far as possible and replace with alternative therapy + high fluid intake

that occur in the patients' stones.[128–130] A summary of the available dietary and medical treatments for the various types of urinary calculi is shown in Table 10.8. Although most of these are effective in reducing the risk of stone recurrence, the main problem in the long-term management of stone patients is compliance.[131] Generally, stone-formers feel well for most of the time, except when they are experiencing an attack of renal colic. It is often difficult, therefore, to maintain their cooperation and motivation to adhere to their preventative treatment over a long period after their stone episode. If they do not have a recurrence of their problem within a few months of their episode, most stone-formers will regress to their original abnormal pattern of urine biochemistry within 3–6 months and will eventually produce another stone.[132] Once they have had several episodes of renal colic, it is usually easier to motivate them on a more continuous basis. It is important to review the patient regularly as an outpatient and to repeat the 24-hr urine analysis, preferably annually but at least biennially, to ensure that they are adhering to the prophylaxis prescribed and to check that their biochemical risk of stones remains low.[106,131]

REFERENCES

1. Williams RE. Long-term survey of 538 patients with upper urinary tract stone. B J Urol 1963; 35: 416–437
2. Pearl MS, Clayman RV. Outcomes and selection of surgical therapies of stones in the kidney and ureter. In: Coe FL, Favus MJ, Pak CYC, Parks JH et al, eds. Kidney Stones – Medical and Surgical Management. Philadelphia: Lippincott-Raven, 1996: 709–755
3. Robertson WG. The economic case for the biochemical screening of stone patients. In: Rodgers AL, Hibbert BE, Hess B, Khan S et al, eds. Urolithiasis 2000. Cape Town: University of Cape Town, 2000: 403–405
4. Parks JH, Coe FL. The financial effects of kidney stone prevention. Kidney Int 1996; 50: 1706–1712
5. Andersen DA. Environmental factors in the aetiology of urolithiasis. In: Cifuentes Delatte L, Rapado A, Hodgkinson A, eds. Urinary Calculi. Basel: Karger, 1973: 130–144
6. Robertson WG, Peacock M, Heyburn PJ, Hanes FA et al. The risk of calcium stone-formation in relation to affluence and dietary animal protein. In: Brockis JG, Finlayson B, eds. Urinary Calculus. Littleton, MA: PSG Publishing, 1981: 3–12
7. Robertson WG, Whitfield HN, Unwin RJ, Mansell MA et al. Possible causes of the changing pattern of the age of onset of urinary stone disease in the UK. In: Rodgers AL, Hibbert BE, Hess B, Khan S et al, eds. Urolithiasis 2000. Cape Town: University of Cape Town, 2000: 366–368
8. Robertson WG. Urinary tract calculi. In: Nordin BEC, Need AG, Morris HA, eds. Metabolic Bone and Stone Disease. 3rd edn. Edinburgh: Churchill Livingstone, 1993: 249–311
9. Griffith DP, Osborne CA. Infection (urease) stones. Miner Electrolyte Metab 1987; 13: 278–285
10. Wickham JEA. Matrix and the infective renal calculus. Br J Urol 1976; 47: 727–732
11. Boyce WH, King JS. Present concepts concerning the origin of matrix and stones. Ann N Y Acad Sci 1963; 104: 563–578
12. Morse RM, Resnick MI. A new approach to the study of urinary macromolecules as a participant in calcium oxalate crystallization. J Urol 1988; 139: 869–873
13. Morse RM, Resnick MI. A study of the incorporation of urinary macromolecules onto crystals of different mineral compositions. J Urol 1989; 141: 641–644
14. Robertson WG. Measurement of ionized calcium in biological fluids. Clin Chim Acta 1969; 24: 149–157
15. Werness P, Brown C, Smith LH, Finlayson B. EQUIL2: a BASIC computer program for the calculation of urinary saturation. J Urol 1985; 134: 1242–1244
16. Vermeulen CW, Ellis JE, Hsu TC. Experimental observations on the pathogenesis of urinary calculi. J Urol 1966; 95: 681–690
17. Robertson WG, Peacock M, Nordin BEC. Calcium crystalluria in recurrent renal stone-formers. Lancet 1969; 2: 21–24
18. Kok DJ, Papapoulos SE, Bijvoet OLM. Crystal agglomeration is a major element in calcium oxalate urinary stone-formation. Kidney Int 1990; 37: 51–56
19. Finlayson B, Reid F. The expectation of free and fixed particles in urinary stone disease. Investig Urol 1978; 15: 442–448
20. Kumar S, Sigmon D, Miller T, Carpenter B et al. A new model of nephrolithiasis involving tubular dysfunction/injury. J Urol 1991; 146: 1384–1389
21. Bigelow MW, Wiessner JH, Kleinman JG, Mandel NS. Calcium oxalate crystal attachment to cultured kidney epithelial cell lines. J Urol 1998; 160: 1528–1532

22. Verkoelen CF, van der Boom BG, Houtsmuller AB, Schröder FH et al. Increased calcium oxalate monohydrate crystal binding to injured tubular epithelial cells in culture. Am J Physiol 1998; 274: F958–F965
23. Scheid C, Koul H, Hill WA, Luber-Narod J et al. Oxalate toxicity in LLC-PK_1 cells: role of free radicals. Kidney Int 1996; 49: 413–419
24. Lieske JC, Leonard R, Swift HS, Toback FG. Adhesion of calcium oxalate monohydrate crystals to anionic sites of renal epithelial cells. Am J Physiol 1996; 270: F192–F199
25. Koul H, Menon M, Koul S, Santosham V, Snow M. Effect of oxalate on calcium oxalate crystal adherence to renal epithelial cells in culture. In: Rodgers AL, Hibbert BE, Hess B, Khan S et al, eds. Urolithiasis 2000. Cape Town: University of Cape Town, 2000: 267–269
26. Robertson WG, Peacock M, Nordin BEC. Calcium oxalate crystalluria and urine saturation in recurrent renal stone-formers. Clin Sci 1971; 40: 365–374
27. Kok DJ, Khan SR. Calcium oxalate nephrolithiasis, a free or fixed particle disease? J Urol 1994; 46: 847–854
28. Borden TA, Lyon ES. The effects of magnesium and pH on experimental calcium oxalate stone disease. Investig Urol 1969; 6: 412–422
29. Meyer JL, Smith LH. Growth of calcium oxalate crystals. II. Inhibition by natural urinary crystal growth inhibitors. Investig Urol 1975; 13: 36–39
30. Fleisch H, Bisaz S. Isolation from urine of pyrophosphate, a calcification inhibitor. Am J Physiol 1962; 203: 671–675
31. Fleisch H, Bisaz S. The inhibitory effect of pyrophosphate on calcium oxalate precipitation and its relation to urolithiasis. Experientia 1964; 20: 276–277
32. Meyer JL, McCall JT, Smith LH. Inhibition of calcium phosphate crystallization by nucleoside phosphates. Calcif Tissue Res 1974; 15: 289–293
33. Howard JE, Thomas WC, Barker LM, Smith LH et al. The recognition and isolation from urine and serum of a peptide inhibitor to calcification. Johns Hopkins Med J 1967; 120: 119–136
34. Robertson WG, Peacock M, Nordin BEC. Inhibitors of the growth and aggregation of calcium oxalate crystals in vitro. Clin Chim Acta 1973; 43: 31–37
35. Ryall RL, Harnett RM, Marshall VR. The effect of urine, pyrophosphate, citrate, magnesium and glycosaminoglycans on the growth and aggregation of calcium oxalate crystals in vitro. Clin Chim Acta 1981; 112: 349–356
36. Robertson WG, Scurr DS, Bridge CM. Factors influencing the crystallization of calcium oxalate in urine – a critique. J Crystal Growth 1981; 53: 182–194
37. Worcester EM, Nakagawa Y, Coe FL. Glycoprotein calcium oxalate crystal growth inhibitor in urine. Miner Electrolyte Metab 1987; 13: 267–272
38. Worcester EM, Nakagawa Y, Wabner CL, Kumar S et al. Crystal adsorption and growth slowing by nephrocalcin, albumin and Tamm-Horsfall protein. Am J Physiol 1988; 255: F1197–F1205
39. Nakagawa Y, Ahmed MA, Hall SL, Deganello S et al. Isolation from human calcium oxalate stones of nephrocalcin, a glycoprotein inhibitor of calcium oxalate crystal growth. Evidence that nephrocalcin from patients with calcium oxalate nephrolithiasis is deficient in gamma-carboxyglutamic acid. J Clin Invest 1987; 79: 1782–1787
40. Hess B, Nakagawa Y, Coe FL. Inhibition of calcium oxalate monohydrate crystal aggregation by urine proteins. Am J Physiol 1989; 257: F99–F106
41. Coe FL, Parks JH. Defenses of an unstable compromise: crystallization inhibitors and the kidney's role in mineral regulation. Kidney Int 1990; 38: 625–631
42. Pillay SN, Asplin JR, Coe FL. Evidence that calgranulin is produced by kidney cells and is an inhibitor of calcium oxalate crystallization. Am J Physiol 1998; 275: F255–F261
43. Shiraga H, Min W, Van Dusen WJ, Clayman MD et al. Inhibition of calcium oxalate crystal growth in vitro by uropontin: another member of the aspartic acid-rich protein superfamily. Proc Natl Acad Sci USA 1992; 89: 426–430
44. Dussol B, Geider S, Lilova A, Leonetti F et al. Analysis of the soluble matrix of five morphologically different kidney stones. Urol Res 1995; 23: 45–51
45. Stapleton AMF, Dawson CJ, Grover PK, Hohmann A et al. Further evidence linking urolithiasis and blood coagulation: urinary prothrombin fragment 1 is present in stone matrix. Kidney Int 1996; 49: 880–888
46. Grover PK, Ryall RL. Inhibition of calcium oxalate crystal growth and aggregation by prothrombin and its fragments in vitro: relationship between protein structure and inhibitory activity. Eur J Biochem 1999; 263: 50–56
47. Dawson CJ, Grover PK, Ryall RL. Inter-alpha-inhibitor in urine and calcium oxalate urinary crystals. Br J Urol 1998; 81: 20–26
48. Spector AR, Gray A, Prien EL. Kidney stone matrix. Differences in acidic protein composition. Investig Urol 1976; 13: 387–389

49. Lian JB, Prien EL, Glimcher MJ, Gallop PM. The presence of protein-bound γ-carboxyglutamic acid in calcium-containing renal calculi. J Clin Invest 1977; 59: 1151–1157
50. Jones WT, Resnick MI. The characterization of soluble matrix proteins in selected human renal calculi using two-dimensional polyacrylamide gel electrophoresis. J Urol 1990; 144: 1010–1014
51. Rose GA, Sulaiman S. Tamm-Horsfall mucoproteins promote calcium oxalate crystal formation in urine: quantitative studies. J Urol 1982; 127: 177–179
52. Scurr DS, Robertson WG. Modifiers of calcium oxalate crystallization found in urine. III. Studies on the role of Tamm-Horsfall mucoprotein and of ionic strength. J Urol 1986; 136: 505–507
53. Grover PK, Ryall RL, Marshall VR. Does Tamm-Horsfall mucoprotein inhibit or promote calcium oxalate crystallization in human urine? Clin Chim Acta 1990; 190: 223–238
54. Robertson WG. 'Take-home message' on the epidemiology and basic science of stone-formation. In: Rodgers AL, Hibbert BE, Hess B, Khan S et al, eds. Urolithiasis 2000. Cape Town: University of Cape Town, 2000: 841–849
55. Dent CE, Senior B, Walshe JM. The pathogenesis of cystinuria. II. Polarographic studies of the metabolism of sulphur-containing amino acids. J Clin Invest 1954; 33: 1216–1226
56. Milne MD, Asatoor AM, Edwards KDG, Loughridge LW. The intestinal absorption defect in cystinuria. Gut 1961; 2: 323–337
57. Ettinger B, Kolb FO. Factors involved in crystal formation in cystinuria. In vivo and in vitro crystallization dynamics and a simple colorimetric assay for cystine. J Urol 1971; 106: 106–110
58. Dahlberg PJ, Van den Berg CJ, Kurtz SB, Wilson DM et al. Clinical features and management of cystinuria. Mayo Clin Proc 1977; 52: 533–542
59. Crawhall JC, Purkiss P, Watts RWE, Young EP. The excretion of amino acids by cystinuric patients and their relatives. Ann Hum Genet 1969; 33: 149–169
60. Dent CE, Friedman M, Green H, Watson LCA. Treatment of cystinuria. Br Med J 1965; 1: 403–407
61. Dent CE, Senior B. Studies on the treatment of cystinuria. Br J Urol 1955; 27: 317–332
62. Crawhall JC, Scowen EF, Watts RWE. Effect of penicillamine on cystinuria. Br Med J 1963; 1: 588–590
63. Stokes GS, Potts JT, Lotz M, Bartter FC. New agent in the treatment of cystinuria: *N*-acetyl-D-penicillamine. BMJ 1968; 1: 284–288
64. Remien A, Kallistratos G, Burchardt P. Treatment of cystinuria with thiola (α-mercapto-propionyl glycine). Eur Urol 1975; 1: 227–228
65. Pak CYC, Fuller C, Sakhaee K, Zerwekh JE et al. Management of cystine nephrolithiasis with mercaptopropionylglycine. J Urol 1986; 136: 1003–1008
66. Frimpter GW. Medical management of cystinuria. Am J Med Sci 1968; 255: 348–357
67. Koide Y, Kinoshita K, Takemoto M, Yachiku S et al. Conservative treatment of cystine calculi: effect of oral alpha-mercaptopropionylglycine on cystine stone dissolution and on prevention of stone recurrence. J Urol 1982; 128: 513–516
68. Gutman AB, Yü TF. Uric acid nephrolithiasis. Am J Med 1968; 45: 657–779
69. Seegmiller JE, Grayzel AI, Laster L, Liddle L. Uric acid production in gout. J Clin Invest 1961; 40: 1304–1314
70. Atsmon A, De Vries A, Frank M. Uric Acid Lithiasis. Amsterdam: Elsevier, 1963
71. Metcalfe-Gibson A, MacCallum FM, Morrison RBI, Wrong O. Urinary excretion of hydrogen ion in patients with uric acid calculi. Clin Sci 1965; 28: 325–345
72. Kursh ED, Resnick MI. Dissolution of uric acid calculi with system alkalinization. J Urol 1984; 132: 286–287
73. Cifuentes Delatte L, Rapado A, Abehsera A, Traba ML et al. Uric acid lithiasis and gout. In: Cifuentes Delatte L, Rapado A, Hodgkinson A, eds. Urinary Calculi. Basel: Karger, 1973: 115–118
74. Coe FL, Moran E, Kavalich AG. The contribution of dietary purine over-consumption to hyperuricosuria on calcium oxalate stone-formers. J Chron Dis 1976; 29: 793–800
75. Henneman PH, Wallach S, Dempsey EF. The metabolic defect responsible for uric acid stone-formation. J Clin Invest 1962; 41: 537–542
76. Bambach CP, Robertson WG, Peacock M, Hill GL. Effect of intestinal surgery on the risk of urinary stone formation. Gut 1981; 22: 257–263
77. Pak CYC, Sakhaee K, Fuller C. Successful management of uric acid nephrolithiasis with potassium citrate. Kidney Int 1986; 30: 422–428
78. Rundles WR, Wyngaarden JB, Hitchings GH, Elion GB et al. Effect of xanthine oxidase inhibitor on thiopurine metabolism, hyperuricaemia and gout. Trans Assoc Am Physicians 1963; 76: 126–140
79. Godfrey RG, Rankin TJ. Uric acid renal lithiasis: management by allopurinol. J Urol 1969; 101: 643–647

80. Greene ML, Fujimoto WY, Seegmiller JE. Urinary xanthine stones – a rare complication of allopurinol therapy. N Engl J Med 1969; 280: 426–427
81. Band PR, Silverberg DS, Henderson JF, Ulan RA et al. Xanthine nephropathy in a patient with lymphosarcoma treated with allopurinol. N Engl J Med 1970; 283: 354–357
82. Griffith DP, Musher DM, Itin C. Urease. The primary cause of infection-induced urinary stones. Investig Urol 1976; 13: 346–350
83. Robertson WG, Peacock M, Nordin BEC. Activity products in stone-forming and non-stone-forming urine. Clin Sci 1968; 32: 579–594
84. Lerner SP, Gleeson MJ, Griffith DP. Infection stones. J Urol 1989; 141: 753–758
85. Cox CE. Urinary tract infection and renal lithiasis. Urol Clin N Am 1974; 1: 279–297
86. Chinn RH, Maskell R, Mead JE, Polak A. Renal stone and urinary infection: a study of antibiotic treatment. BMJ 1976; 2: 1411–1413
87. Griffith DP, Gibson JR, Clinton CW, Musher DM. Acetohydroxamic acid: clinical studies of a urease inhibitor in patients with staghorn renal calculi. J Urol 1978; 119: 9–15
88. Martelli A, Buli P, Cortecchia V. Urease inhibitor therapy in infected renal stones. Eur Urol 1981; 7: 291–293
89. Griffith DP, Gleeson MJ, Lee H, Longuet R et al. Randomized, double-blind trial of Lithostat (acetohydroxamic acid) in the palliative treatment of infection-induced urinary calculi. Euro Urol 1991; 20: 243–247
90. Kinney AB, Blount M. Effect of cranberry juice on urinary pH. Nurs Res 1979; 28: 287–290
91. Pak CYC, Sakhaee K, Crowther C, Brinkley L. Evidence justifying a high fluid intake in treatment of nephrolithiasis. Ann Intern Med 1980; 93: 36–39
92. Jaeger P, Portmann L, Jacquet AF, Burckhardt P. Drinking water for stone-formers: is the calcium content relevant? Eur Urol 1984; 10: 53–54
93. Marshall RW, Cochran M, Robertson WG, Hodgkinson A et al. The relation between urine saturation and stone composition in patients with calcium-containing renal stones. Clin Sci 1972; 43: 433–441
94. Albright F, Henneman P, Benedict PH, Forbes AP. Idiopathic hypercalciuria. Proc R Soc Med 1953; 46: 1077–1081
95. Hodgkinson A, Pyrah LN. The urinary excretion of calcium and inorganic phosphate in 344 patients with calcium stone of renal origin. Br J Surg 1958; 46: 10–18
96. Pak CYC, Kaplan RA, Bone H, Townsend J et al. A simple test for the diagnosis of absorptive, resorptive and renal hypercalciurias. N Engl J Med 1975; 292: 497–500
97. Coe FL, Favus MJ. Idiopathic hypercalciuria in calcium nephrolithiasis. Disease-a-Month 1980; 26: 1–36
98. Halabé A, Sutton RAL. Primary hyperparathyroidism and idiopathic hypercalciuria. Miner Electrolyte Metab 1987; 13: 235–241
99. Robertson WG, Peacock M. The cause of idiopathic calcium stone disease: hypercalciuria or hyperoxaluria? Nephron 1980; 26: 105–110
100. Rose GA. Current trends in urolithiasis research. In: Rous SN, ed. Stone Disease: Diagnosis and Management. Orlando, FL: Grune & Stratton, 1987: 383–416
101. Rudman D, Kutner MH, Redd SC, Waters WC et al. Hypocitraturia in calcium nephrolithiasis. J Clin Endocrinol Metab 1982; 1052–1057
102. Nicar MJ, Skurla C, Sakhaee K, Pak CYC. Low urinary citrate excretion in nephrolithiasis. Urology 1983; 21: 8–14
103. Hosking DH, Wilson JW, Liedtke RR, Smith LH et al. Urinary citrate excretion in normal persons and patients with idiopathic calcium urolithiasis. J Lab Clin Med 1985; 106: 682–689
104. Tiselius H-G, Almgård LE, Larsson L, Sörbo B. A biochemical basis for grouping of patients with urolithiasis. Eur Urol 1978; 4: 241–249
105. Robertson WG, Peacock M, Heyburn PJ, Marshall DH et al. Risk factors in calcium stone disease of the urinary tract. Br J Urol 1978; 50: 449–454
106. Robertson WG. A simplified procedure for assessing the biochemical risk of forming stones in patients with uric acid or calcium-containing urinary calculi. In: Borghi L, Meschi T, Briganti A, Schianci T et al, eds. Kidney Stones. Cosenza: Editoriale Bios, 1999: 403–406
107. Coe FL, Kavalich AG. Hypercalciuria and hyperuricosuria in patients with calcium nephrolithiasis. N Engl J Med 1974; 291: 1344–1350
108. Grover PK, Ryall RL. Urate and calcium oxalate stones: from repute to rhetoric to reality. Miner Electrolyte Metab 1994; 20: 361–370
109. Prince CL, Scardino PL, Wolan CT. The effect of temperature, humidity and dehydration on the formation of renal calculi. J Urol 1956; 75: 209–215

110. Robertson WG, Peacock M, Marshall RW, Speed R et al. Seasonal variations in the composition of urine in relation to calcium stone-formation. Clin Sci Mol Med 1975; 49: 597–602
111. Pierce LW, Bloom B. Observations on urolithiasis among American troops in a desert area. J Urol 1945; 54: 466–470
112. Blacklock NJ. The pattern of urolithiasis in the Royal Navy. In: Hodgkinson A, Nordin BEC, eds. Proceedings of the Renal Stone Research Symposium. London: Churchill, 1969: 33–47
113. Brundig P, Berg W, Schneider HJ. Stress und Harnsteinbildungsrisiko. I. Einfluss von Stress auf lithogene Harnsubstanz. Urol Int 1981; 36: 199–207
114. Larsen JF, Phillip J. Studies on the incidence of urolithiasis. Urol Int 1962; 13: 53–54
115. Clark JY. Renal calculi in army aviators. Aviat Space Environ Med 1990; 61: 744–747
116. Robertson WG, Peacock M, Hodgkinson A. Dietary changes and the incidence of urinary calculi in the UK between 1958 and 1976. J Chron Dis 1979; 32: 469–476
117. Robertson WG, Peacock M, Baker M, Marshall DH et al. Studies on the prevalence and epidemiology of urinary stone disease in men in Leeds. Br J Urol 1983; 55: 595–598
118. Power C, Barker DJP, Blacklock NJ. Incidence of renal stones in 18 British towns. Br J Urol 1987; 59: 105–110
119. Robertson WG, Peacock M, Heyburn PJ, Hanes FA et al. Should recurrent calcium oxalate stone-formers become vegetarians? Br J Urol 1979; 51: 427–443
120. Robertson WG, Peacock M, Marshall DH. Prevalence of urinary stone disease in vegetarians. Eur Urol 1982; 8: 334–339
121. Robertson WG. Diet and calcium stones. Miner Electrolyte Metab 1987; 13: 228–234
122. Iguchi M, Umekawa IT, Ishikawa T, Katayama Y et al. Dietary intake and habits of Japanese renal stone patients. J Urol 1990; 143: 1093–1095
123. Curhan GC, Willett WC, Rimm EB, Stampfer MJ. A prospective study of dietary calcium and other nutrients and the risk of symptomatic kidney stones. N Engl J Med 1993; 328: 833–838
124. Resnick MI, Pridgen DB, Goodman HO. Genetic predisposition to formation of calcium oxalate renal calculi. N Engl J Med 1968; 278: 1313–1318
125. Coe FL, Parks JH, Moore ES. Familial idiopathic hypercalciuria. N Engl J Med 1979; 300: 337–340
126. Aladjem M, Modan M, Lusky A, Georgi R et al. Idiopathic hypercalciuria: a familial generalized renal hyperexcretory state. Kidney Int 1983; 24: 549–554
127. Blacklock NJ. Epidemiology of renal lithiasis. In: Wickham JEA, ed. Urinary Calculous Disease. Edinburgh: Churchill Livingstone,1979: 21–39
128. Coe FL, Parks JH, Asplin JR. The pathogenesis and treatment of kidney stones – medical progress. N Engl J Med 1992; 327: 1142–1152
129. Fine JK, Pak CYC, Preminger GM. Effect of medical management and residual fragments on recurrent stone formation following shock wave lithotripsy. J Urol 1995; 153: 27–33
130. Pak CYC. Kidney stones. Lancet 1998; 351: 1797–1801
131. Robertson WG. Is it possible to motivate patients with recurrent stones to adhere to their treatment regimen? In: Rodgers AL, Hibbert BE, Hess B, Khan S et al, eds. Urolithiasis 2000. Cape Town: University of Cape Town, 2000: 624–627
132. Norman RW, Bath SS, Robertson WG, Peacock M. When should patients with symptomatic stone disease be evaluated metabolically? J Urol 1984; 132: 1137–1139

11

Shock

David A Brealey and Andrew R Webb

NORMAL PHYSIOLOGY

In health, 90% of the total body oxygen utilization is by aerobic respiration for the generation of ATP. Oxygen delivery (DO_2), the product of cardiac output, haemoglobin and oxygen saturation, is about 1000 ml/min in the normal resting adult. About 250 ml of this is utilized for aerobic respiration and other oxygen-consuming processes (VO_2); that is, DO_2 is well in excess of the body's VO_2. In response to increased demand, as in exercise, oxygen delivery is enhanced by both an increase in cardiac output and an increased extraction of oxygen from haemoglobin. The increase in extraction is mainly a result of nutrient capillary recruitment but also of a reduced haemoglobin affinity for oxygen in the presence of hypoxaemia (right shift of the oxyhaemoglobin dissociation curve). Once the oxygen supply falls below demand (DO_2crit) (Figure 11.1), oxygen consumption becomes dependent on delivery (physiological supply dependency), and it is believed the tissues switch to anaerobic respiration to make up any energy shortfall.[1] Lactic acid accumulates and the tissues build up an 'oxygen debt'.

PATHOPHYSIOLOGY OF SHOCK

Shock is the inability of the circulation to supply adequate oxygen and nutrients to metabolizing tissues. Oxygen delivery can be impaired by decreasing any of its components. For example, a loss of cardiac output may occur as a result of a large myocardial infarction, pulmonary embolism or severe haemorrhage. In addition, haemorrhage will also decrease the haemoglobin, and a significant pulmonary embolism is associated with a decrease in arterial oxygen saturation. Certain disease states such as sepsis may have direct toxic effects on the cell, preventing the utilization of oxygen, although this is often compounded by hypovolaemia and myocardial depression. Although often conveniently boxed into various categories, shock states often have a number of components. It is important to understand and recognize these to manage shock appropriately.

Without the appropriate supply, or the ability to use oxygen, the cellular ATP levels start to fall, with a resultant decrease in cell function. Energy production becomes increasingly dependent on accelerated glycolysis, with a resulting accumulation of lactate. There is a failure[2] of DNA and protein synthesis and

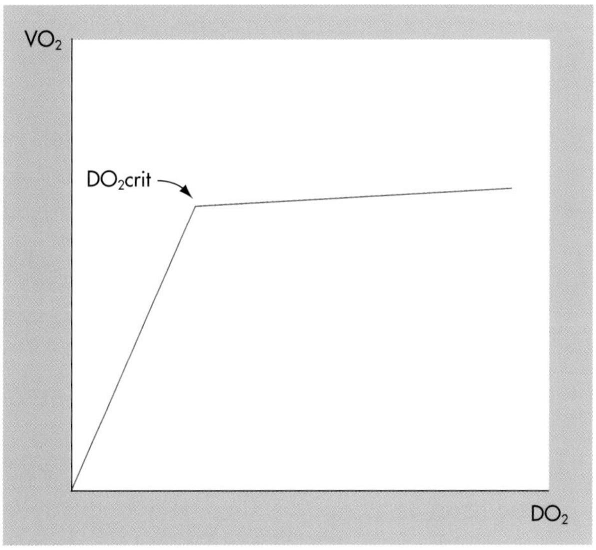

Figure 11.1 *Relationship between VO_2 and DO_2.*

an eventual failure of transmembrane ion pumps, leading to an intracellular accumulation of sodium and calcium. If the ATP concentration falls to a certain level, the cell undergoes apoptosis,[3] an energy-requiring process where cell death follows a predetermined sequence of events, culminating in phagocytosis by macrophages. Apoptosis prevents the spillage of cell contents and so does not initiate an inflammatory reaction, allowing the macrophage to recycle the cellular building blocks. If the insult is very severe, ATP levels fall markedly and cell death occurs by necrosis; the cells lyse in an uncontrolled fashion, releasing their contents and initiating an inflammatory response. Certain cells, such as neurons, are more sensitive to alteration in oxygen availability than others, and acute alteration is more devastating than gradual deterioration.

Inflammation

Shock and hypoxia are often associated with a stimulation of proinflammatory pathways, including activation of macrophages, neutrophils, platelets, endothelium, complement, coagulation and fibrinolytic pathways. A multitude of inflammatory mediators is produced, including cytokines, arachidonic acid metabolites, nitric oxide and endothelins, with consumption of endogenous defence mechanisms such as antithrombin-III and activated protein C. The expression, affinity and activity of numerous receptors (such as soluble tumour necrosis factor (TNF) receptors, adrenoreceptors and glucocorticoid receptors) are also affected. There is an associated vasodilatation, and the capillary endothelial cells become damaged and 'leaky' during the inflammatory response. This results in oedema formation, further compromising tissue oxygenation by increasing diffusion distance and by exerting pressure on the surrounding capillaries.

Occasionally, this response is inappropriate and excessive, and, through a number of ill-understood mechanisms, there is resultant damage to many of the body's vital organs, leading to the syndrome of multiorgan dysfunction (MODS).[4] This is the leading cause of mortality in the surgical ICU[5] (with an average mortality of 50%), and it has no specific treatment.

Ischaemia-reperfusion injury

The inflammatory process is well documented in ischaemia-reperfusion injury. During the ischaemic, shock phase, cells generate a number of reactive oxidant species through the action of xanthine oxidase and other enzymes released into the general circulation on reperfusion. These oxidants have numerous actions, including inhibiting enzymes, damaging lipid bilayers and cleaving DNA. They activate a number of genes involved in the inflammatory cascade, such as nuclear factor (NF)-κβ, which are capable of upregulating cytokines, such as TNF, and modifying the expression of adhesion molecules on leucocytes and endothelial cells. Clinically, this can manifest itself as vasodilatation, cardiac dysrhythmia, and myocardial stunning after coronary reperfusion.

The sphlanchnic circulation and shock

During the shock phase, blood flow is redistributed away from areas such as the sphlanchnic bed to maintain perfusion of more 'vital' organs, such as the brain and the heart. However, it has long been recognized that the gut mucosa, ischaemic as a result of redistribution of its already precarious blood supply (and loss of luminal derived substrates), is no longer able to act as a barrier to resident, intestinal flora.[6,7] This is believed to lead them to translocate the mucosa, entering portal blood and lymph, disseminating to distant sites and potentiating the inflammatory response. Though disruption of bowel mucosa and translocation have been demonstrated in critically ill humans,[8,9] it is not clear whether it is pathological or physiological.

CLASSIFICATION OF SHOCK

Classically, shock states are classified as cardiogenic, hypovolaemic, distributive or obstructive. It is important to remember there is often a great deal of cross-over between them.

Cardiogenic shock

Cardiogenic shock is the inability of the heart to perfuse the tissues adequately. There is usually associated hypotension, low cardiac output and high pulmonary artery occlusion pressure. The most common cause is acute myocardial infarction, though other causes include myocarditis, cardiomyopathy, valvular heart disease and pericardial tamponade. Cardiogenic shock is associated with both systolic and diastolic cardiac dysfunction.[10,11]

The body can recognize a decrease in left ventricular function only as low blood pressure and a loss of circulating volume. There is a resultant increase in sympathetic tone and, later, activation of salt- and water-retaining mechanisms (such as renin-angiotensin-aldosterone and vasopressin). These 'compensatory' mechanisms increase the work of the heart thereby compounding any dysfunction. As a result of sympathetic stimulation, myocardial compliance decreases, heart rate increases and myocardial oxygen demand increases. Since cardiogenic shock is often the result of limited coronary perfusion, the myocardial ischaemia increases. The peripheral effects of sympathetic stimulation include vasoconstriction, forcing the heart to pump against an increasing peripheral resistance and increasing left ventricular work.

Reversible myocardial dysfunction – hibernation and stunning

Originally, contractile dysfunction following myocardial ischaemia was thought to be irreversible. Contractile dysfunction occurs within seconds of a severe reduction in coronary blood flow. If this persists for 20–40 min there is widespread cardiomyocyte necrosis, and the dysfunction becomes irreversible – myocardial infarction. However, there are two forms of reversible myocardial dysfunction, hibernation and stunning. If ischaemia is less profound, the degree of contractile function becomes matched to perfusion, but cardiomyocytes remain viable and recover fully on reperfusion. This is known as short-term myocardial hibernation.[12] The reason for the contractile dysfunction is unclear. Though there is a rapid decrease in myocardial ATP, the contractile dysfunction occurs before this. Decrease in intracellular pH,[13] increased lactate production and disturbed calcium handling[14] have all been implicated. However, a rise in inorganic phosphate (the result of ATP hydrolysis) may uncouple myofibrillar ATPase activity.[15] Thus, there is a decrease in myocardial activity but a preservation of the energy supply and demand relationship. The hibernating myocardium maintains its sensitivity to inotropes, such as adrenaline (epinephrine), but the increased energy requirements upset the supply–demand balance and precipitate infarction. Downregulation of β-receptors and alteration of ion-channel activity may also promote the development of hibernation. In long-term hibernating myocardium (weeks to months), there is a dedifferentiation of cardiomyocytes to a more embryonic form.

Myocardial stunning occurs after short episodes of ischaemia followed by reperfusion and is associated with histological integrity.[16,17] Stunning is associated with a decrease in the myofilament's sensitivity to calcium, possibly effected by the release of oxygen radicals. The contractile dysfunction is entirely reversible, though recovery may take several weeks. The myocardium retains a sensitivity to inotropes, but, unlike hibernation, there is no accompanying metabolic deterioration. Table 11.1 illustrates some of the cellular characteristics of both stunned and hibernating myocardium which can coexist and are difficult to distinguish clinically.

Hypovolaemic shock

Hypovolaemic shock occurs when there is insufficient intravascular volume to maintain an adequate cardiac output. This can occur as a direct loss of fluid from the body (as in haemorrhage, diarrhoea and burns) or as a redistribution of fluid from the

Table 11.1 Cellular characteristics of myocardial stunning and hibernation.

	Timing	[ATP]	Histology	Duration
Stunning	After reperfusion	Low ATP	No necrosis	Slowly reversible
Hibernation	During low coronary flow	Normal ATP	No necrosis	Rapidly reversible

intra- to the extravascular spaces (as in sepsis, trauma and pancreatitis). Young, fit adults are able to maintain a normal blood pressure and pulse despite blood losses of up to 25% of predicted blood volume, making clinical assessment of blood loss difficult. However, a postural increase in pulse rate of >30 bpm or severe postural dizziness (inability to stand) are sensitive and specific (97% and 98%, respectively) indicators of hypovolaemia due to large blood losses (>630 ml).[18] The sensitivity of these signs may be reduced in the elderly and those on medications such as β-blockers.

A loss of intravascular volume decreases cardiac filling pressures and end diastolic volume. This leads to a decrease in the length of cardiac muscle fibres and, through the Starling mechanism, a fall in stroke volume and mean arterial pressure. This fall in pressure is sensed by the baroreceptors, with resulting sympathetic stimulation of the myocardium and an increase in myocardial contractility and heart rate. Occasionally, hypovolaemia is associated with a normal heart rate or even bradycardia. Sympathetic stimulation also mediates vasoconstriction of the capacitance vessels and precapillary arterioles; this reduces the transcapillary hydrostatic pressure and encourages movement of extravascular fluid into the intravascular space – autotransfusion. Venoconstriction and autotransfusion increase preload, and autotransfusion decreases the haematocrit (and hence viscosity), thus improving flow through the microvasculature. With mild blood loss (around 10%) there is little redistribution of blood supply, but more severe haemorrhage (20–30%) will see a preservation of blood flow to vital organs, such as heart, brain and kidneys, at the expense of flow to other organs, such as bowel and pancreas. Should haemorrhage continue (>30%), cardiac output and mean arterial pressure decrease in a linear fashion. The compensatory mechanisms are unable to cope with the loss of volume, and flow to vital organs starts to decrease, manifesting as confusion or a decreased level of consciousness, oliguria and an increasing lactic acidosis. As diastolic pressure falls and heart rate increases, myocardial blood flow will also decrease, and at a critical point myocardial ischaemia occurs, further impairing cardiac output. This point occurs earlier in those with coronary artery disease.

The hypovolaemia associated with burns and trauma is compounded by the diffuse capillary leak that occurs in these conditions. Thus, unlike haemorrhage, water, salts and protein leak from the microvasculature into the interstitium, reducing preload and increasing haematocrit. These conditions may be associated with paradoxical vasodilatation, a disruption of the microvasculature with shunting of blood away from the capillary bed and a depression in cardiac output as a result of circulating 'myocardial depressant factors'.

Activation of the salt- and water-conserving mechanisms, with release of aldosterone and antidiuretic hormone, acts as a slower, more long-term measure to improve intravascular volume and hence preload.

Distributive shock

Distributive shock results from a redistribution of blood supply between and within organs, often associated with a decrease in the tone arterioles and the venous capacitance vessels. Causes include systemic inflammation, anaphylaxis, spinal cord injury and spinal anaesthesia, and the result is a loss of sympathetic tone.

The shock resulting from the systemic inflammatory response syndrome (SIRS)[19] has classically been included under the category of distributive shock. However, more recent evidence suggests this may be incorrect. SIRS is a state of generalized inflammation (Table 11.2). Sepsis is the most common cause, but other aetiologies include pancreatitis, burns, trauma, cardiac arrest, drug overdose and drowning. It is thought to result from an inappropriate and generalized activation of proinflammatory pathways, including activation of macrophages, neutrophils, platelets, endothelium, complement, coagulation and fibrinolytic pathways.

The pathophysiology of this form of shock is far more complex than other forms. There is an associated vascular dilatation leading to a relative hypovolaemia. Diffuse vascular endothelial damage leads to a leakage of plasma components into the extravascular space, further compounding the hypovolaemia. Global myocardial depression is common in septic shock,[20] but is often masked by tachycardia and low systemic vascular resistance.

Table 11.2 Clinical definitions of SIRS and sepsis.[50]

Systemic inflammatory response syndrome (SIRS)	The systemic inflammatory response to a variety of severe clinical insults. Requires two or more of: – core temperature >38°C or <36°C – heart rate > 90 bpm – respiratory rate >20 breaths/min or $PaCO_2$ <4.3kPa – white blood count >12000/mm^3 or <4000/mm^3 or >10% immature neutrophils
Sepsis	The systemic response to infection Requires SIRS criteria in the presence of proved or suspected infection
Severe sepsis	Sepsis associated with organ dysfunction, hypoperfusion or hypotension
Septic shock	Sepsis associated with hypotension (despite adequate fluid resuscitation) and perfusion abnormalities

Despite the myocardial depression, patients often have a raised tissue-oxygen delivery but exhibit an inability to extract this oxygen. These patients also have evidence of lactic acidosis, a decrease in the arteriovenous oxygen saturation gap and a DO_2crit shifted to the left, suggesting that anaerobic respiration occurs at higher levels of DO_2 than normal – this is termed 'pathological supply dependency'. These findings led investigators to believe that sepsis and the associated organ dysfunction resulted from shunting of blood away from the nutrient capillary bed, leaving the tissues relatively ischaemic; hence, the term 'distributive shock'. This may arise from a loss of microvascular control (nitric oxide, prostaglandins, altered adrenoreceptor densities)[21,22] or by capillaries becoming blocked by plugs of activated white cells, platelets or fibrin deposits.

Further work has suggested that the cells in sepsis are not hypoxic but *dysoxic*; in other words, oxygen is present but is not being utilized. Some have demonstrated an absence of hypoxia in septic organs,[23] while others have demonstrated a raised tissue-oxygen tension in both septic animals[24,25] and patients[26] despite evidence of organ dysfunction and metabolic acidosis. In contrast, patients with cardiogenic shock and haemorrhage show falls in tissue P_{O_2} in line with the severity of the insult.[27] Resolution of the septic process and eventual survival were associated with normalization of the muscle P_{O_2} in septic patients, though non-survivors had persistently raised values.[28]

As ATP generation by oxidative phosphorylation utilizes over 90% of total body VO_2, the changes seen in critical illness suggest failure of bioenergetic pathways as a possible mechanism of organ dysfunction and failure. Disruption of key enzymes within the pathway leading from glycolysis, via the tricarboxylic acid (Krebs) cycle, to the electron transport chain, has been demonstrated in in vitro models of sepsis. Nitric oxide and its metabolites (such as peroxynitrite), which are produced in significant excess in sepsis, inhibit complexes I and IV (cytochrome oxidase) of the electron transport chain (Figure 11.2).[29]

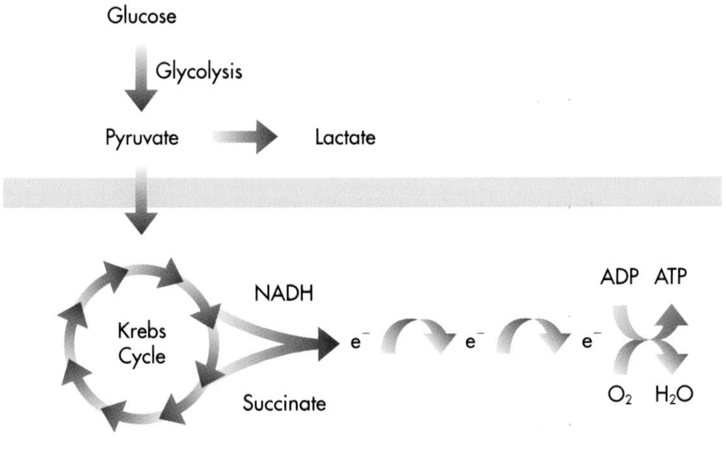

Figure 11.2 *The electron transport chain. For explanation, see text.*

Human data are scanty, although there is anecdotal evidence of decreased ATP levels in sepsis.[30,31] We have also found altered activity of mitochondrial enzymes in muscle biopsies taken from patients in septic shock.[32]

Anaphylaxis

This is an immediate immune reaction of a sensitized individual being exposed to the causative antigen. It is an extreme example of a type 1 hypersensitivity reaction. Other, less dramatic examples include eczema, hay fever and asthma.[33]

The individual becomes sensitized when a B cell recognizes an antigen as foreign and produces IgE antibodies against it. These antibodies then bind to specific, high-affinity receptors on the surface of blood basophils and tissue mast cells. On re-exposure, the antigen causes cross-linking of these antibodies. This results in the activation of a number of intracellular signalling mechanisms, causing degranulation of preformed histamine and various eosinophil chemotactic factors and de novo synthesis of leucotrienes, prostaglandins and platelet-activating factor. These compounds lead to vasodilatation, increased vascular permeability and the recruitment of eosinophils. Occasionally, an anaphylactoid response occurs without prior exposure to the antigen; though rare it can happen with morphine, pethidine or a number of anaesthetic drugs such as atracurium, thiopental and propofol. Other antigens capable of eliciting an anaphylactoid response include drugs (penicillin), antiserum, low-molecular-weight radiological dyes, snake and bee venom, pollen and certain foods.[34] Signs develop within minutes of re-exposure, with the eruption of discrete, cutaneous wheals. Laryngeal oedema presents as a hoarse voice or stridor. Lower airway involvement includes bronchospasm, submucosal oedema and eosinophilic infiltration, presenting as wheeze and hyperinflated lungs. There may be generalized non-pitting oedema. Patients complain of nausea and abdominal cramps. Cardiovascular collapse may occur secondary to the acute respiratory failure but also as a result of a generalized vasodilatation, a loss of plasma volume. There may be myocardial depression as a result of coronary vasoconstriction and possible myocardial infarction.

Obstructive shock

Obstructive shock occurs after an acute obstruction to flow in the central circulation and can be broadly divided into intrinsic (as in pulmonary embolism and acute pulmonary hypertension) and extrinsic (as in tension pneumothorax and pericardial tamponade) causes. Pulmonary embolism is the most common cause. Immobilization, surgery, trauma, carcinomatosis and heart failure predispose to venous thromboembolic disease. Pulmonary emboli usually originate from the deep veins of the legs or pelvis. However, up to 12% of emboli arise from other areas such as the right heart, deep veins of the arm and the internal jugular.[35,36] Occlusion of the major pulmonary arteries leads to profound right ventricular failure and pulmonary insufficiency, resulting in rapid cardiovascular collapse and death. Less severe occlusion results in varying degrees of right ventricular strain and ventilation/perfusion mismatching. Release of local vasoactive substances, such as bradykinins, may lead to pulmonary arteriolar constriction, compounding the strain on the right ventricle.

Acute pulmonary hypertension often occurs in the setting of acute respiratory failure. Hypoxia leads to pulmonary vasoconstriction. There is often an influx of white cells to the pulmonary circulation, resulting in microvascular congestion and endothelial damage.[37] There are associated fluid shifts into the extravascular spaces and capillary compression. Microemboli have been seen in patients with acute respiratory distress syndrome, further compounding the problem.[38] The sudden rise in pulmonary pressure leads to strain and failure of the right ventricle and a consequent reduction in left ventricular filling and cardiac output.[39]

Tension pneumothorax occurs when gas accumulates in the intrapleural space, resulting in a localized rise of intrathoracic pressure and displacement of lung and the mediastinum. This causes 'kinking' of the inferior vena cava and a decrease in venous return and hence cardiac output; this decrease in venous return is exacerbated if the patient is ventilated with positive pressure. Intrapulmonary shunting may worsen the effects.

MANAGEMENT OF SHOCK

To manage shock, we follow the basic principles of resuscitation and then devote attention to the cause. The latter is beyond the scope of this chapter. Successful management of shock requires a functional approach to shock, after ensuring adequate oxygenation and appropriate haemodynamic monitoring. Blind therapy adrenaline [epinephrine] 0.2 mg IV titrated to blood pressure only) is excusable only in the pulseless or dangerously hypotensive patient. No matter what the cause of shock, resuscitation must target the four main components of the circulation individually, that is, the blood volume and constituents, the heart, the blood vessels and the tissues. Figure 11.3 shows the functional components of the circulation and a step-by-step approach to correction of circulatory failure.

Correction of blood volume

Usually, the blood volume will be targeted first. The reference standard for the diagnosis of hypovolaemia is the measurement of blood volume. The techniques available rely on the principles of indicator dilution, usually involving radioisotopes as the indicators. Most techniques do not lend themselves to rapid, bedside estimation and, therefore, preclude rapid intervention. Furthermore, patients with acute shock may require a higher than normal blood volume to maintain an adequate circulation. We therefore rely on surrogate markers of volume status.

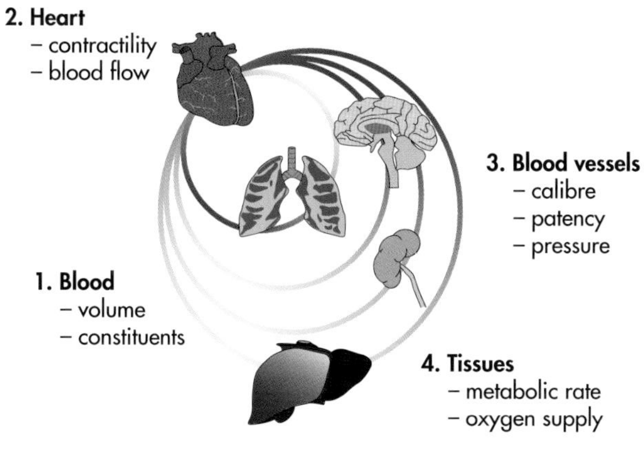

Figure 11.3 *The functional components of the circulation. Management of circulatory failure should follow a step-by-step approach with attention to the volume and constituents of the blood first. After correction of hypovolaemia, the cardiac output should be corrected, followed by attention to the calibre of blood vessels to maintain perfusion pressure. Finally, the metabolic rate of the tissues should be controlled to cope with a limited circulation.*

Clinical signs of hypovolaemia

Clinical signs of hypovolaemia (reduced skin turgor, oliguria, tachycardia and postural hypotension) are late indicators. The presence of these signs signifies hypovolaemia of a degree that requires urgent intervention. The absence of these signs does not exclude hypovolaemia. More difficult is the diagnosis of lesser degrees of hypovolaemia which require treatment for maintenance of tissue perfusion and avoidance of organ dysfunction. Clinical assessment is dependent on patient position, there being an increase in plasma volume, and therefore a minimization of clinical signs, associated with supine positioning.[40] Where hypovolaemia is suspected in a supine patient, lifting the legs and watching for an improvement in the circulation is a useful indicator.

The central venous pressure (CVP)

The central venous pressure (CVP) is the most popular surrogate marker of volume status. Its popularity is based on ease of measurement, but there are a number of pitfalls. CVP is dependent on venous return to the heart, right ventricular compliance, peripheral venous tone[41] and posture.[42] A normal CVP does not exclude hypovolaemia,[43] and CVP is particularly unreliable in pulmonary vascular disease, right ventricular disease, isolated left ventricular failure and valvular heart disease. In patients with an intact sympathetic response to hypovolaemia, the CVP may fall in response to fluid.[44]

Pulmonary artery wedge pressure (PAWP)

The PAWP provides similar information regarding fluid status to the CVP. As with the CVP, the absolute level of PAWP does not confirm or exclude hypovolaemia. Left ventricular disease may increase the level of PAWP required for an adequate circulating volume, and interpretation of PAWP requires caution in ventilated patients.[45] PAWP is a useful indicator of relative hypovolaemia where CVP is high and PAWP is significantly lower; for example, in selective right ventricular dysfunction or chronic airflow limitation where the CVP is unreliable.

The fluid challenge

The fluid challenge is a method of safely restoring circulating volume.[46] Rather than using fixed haemodynamic end points, fluid is given in small aliquots to produce a known increment in circulating volume with assessment of the dynamic haemodynamic response to each aliquot. No fixed haemodynamic end point is assumed, and the technique provides a diagnostic test of hypovolaemia (via an appropriate positive response of the circulation to fluid) and a method of titrating the optimal dose of fluid to the individual's requirement.

The change in CVP or PAWP after a 200-ml increment in circulating volume depends on the starting circulating volume (Figure 11.4).

A 3-mmHg rise in CVP or PAWP represents a significant increase and is probably indicative of an adequate circulating volume. It is important to assess the clinical response and the adequacy of tissue perfusion in addition; if inadequate, it is necessary to monitor stroke volume before further fluid challenges or considering further circulatory support.

Choice of fluid

In the bleeding or anaemic patient, correction of the circulating red cell mass will be necessary. However, resuscitation of the circulating volume can be done with any available fluid. For the purposes of the fluid challenge approach, it is more appropriate to use colloid fluids than crystalloid fluids, and it should be remembered that packed red cells have a high haematocrit and therefore high viscosity. An immediate transudation to the interstitial space of three-quarters of the volume of saline[47–49] infused implies that oedema is a necessary side effect of any increase in intravascular volume and therefore any correction of the shock state with crystalloid resuscitation. Although colloid will undoubtedly contribute to oedema in states of capillary leak,[49] the argument that the transfer of colloid to the interstitial space in capillary leak may contribute to further oedema formation has been refuted consistently by experimental evidence.[50–53] There is no difference in the process of oedema formation whether the cause is an increase in capillary hydrostatic pressure or a capillary leak. In the lung, this process follows the sequence of interstitial fluid accumulation, followed by distension of the alveolar capillary barrier and finally alveolar flooding.[54] Thus, it is the intravascular Starling forces that are most relevant, and any increase in capillary hydrostatic pressure through resuscitation will contribute to an increase in interstitial volume.[55]

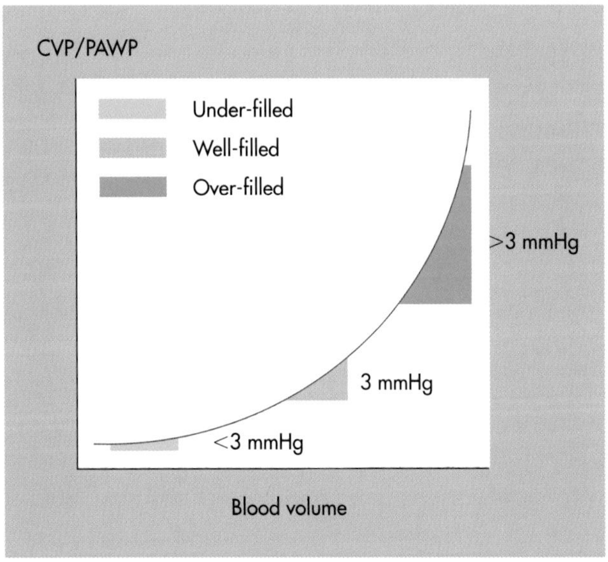

Figure 11.4 *The response of CVP or PAWP to a 200-ml increment of blood volume. In the hypovolaemic patient, no significant rise in CVP or PAWP would be expected. In the optimally filled patient, a rise in CVP or PAWP would be expected.*

Recently, the crystalloid–colloid controversy has been fuelled by several meta-analyses demonstrating no benefit to mortality with colloid resuscitation.[56–58] It is of importance to note that the research on which these meta-analyses were based did not titrate fluid requirements by the dynamic fluid-challenge method; in many cases, titration was not to a haemodynamic end point at all.[59] The aim of a fluid challenge is to produce a small but significant (200 ml) and rapid increase in circulating volume. Colloid fluids are ideal in that they give a reliable increase in plasma volume; crystalloids are rapidly lost from the circulation, and larger volumes would be required to achieve an increase of 200 ml in circulating volume.[47,48] Furthermore, fluid administration would have to be repeated more frequently to maintain microcirculatory blood flow.[60]

Correction of blood constituents

For the purposes of shock management the most important constituent is the red cell because of its oxygen carriage. Over-aggressive resuscitation with non-red-cell fluids will inevitably lead to reduced oxygen-carrying capacity. This may be compensated for by an increased cardiac output, and tissue oxygen supply may be improved by a reduced whole-blood viscosity associated with the reduced haematocrit. Standard practice is to maintain a haemoglobin level of 8–10 g/dl, although the practice is not evidence-based. A recent study[61] has suggested better outcomes for some critically ill patients when the trigger to blood transfusion is 7.5 g/dl rather than liberal transfusion to the 10 g/dl target. Part of the problem of correction of red-cell mass is that we mostly use stored blood cells, as these may not be effective in guaranteeing tissue oxygen supply.[62]

In the absence of good evidence, it would seem sensible to avoid excessive anaemia by red-cell transfusion but concentrate on the provision of an adequate circulating volume as the most critical aspect of managing the blood component of the circulation. Where haemorrhage is obvious, the use of blood as a volume agent, as well as a method of correcting red-cell mass deficit, is, of course, reasonable.

Assessment and correction of cardiac output and stroke volume

Although filling pressures are useful in assessing the response to fluid challenges, a failure to correct the shock state requires further investigation of cardiac function. There are a variety of methods available to measure the cardiac output and stroke volume. Thermodilution techniques via a pulmonary artery catheter were the standard method for many years. More recently, these techniques have been modified to allow continuous monitoring or intermittent monitoring with central venous and arterial catheters. Minimally or non-invasive methods include oesophageal Doppler,[63] bioimpedence[64] and lithium dilution.[65] Once the stroke volume can be monitored, the responsiveness of the heart to fluid should be assessed once again by fluid challenge. In the inadequately filled left ventricle, a fluid challenge will increase the stroke volume (Figure 11.5).

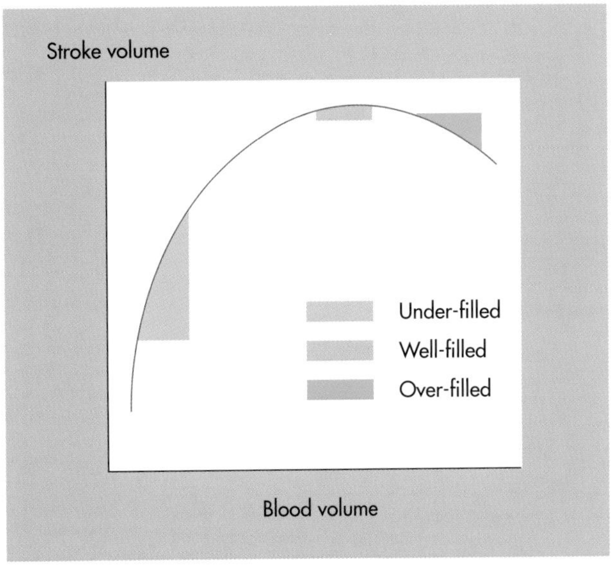

Figure 11.5 *The response of stroke volume to small-volume fluid challenges. In the hypovolaemic patient, an increase in stroke volume would be expected. In the optimally filled patient, no significant rise in stroke volume would be expected.*

Failure to increase the stroke volume with a fluid challenge may represent an inadequate challenge, particularly if the PAWP or CVP fails to rise significantly (by at least 3 mmHg). This indicates that cardiac filling was inadequate, as the increment in circulating volume fills the depleted peripheral vascular space. In this case, the fluid challenge should be repeated. It is important to monitor stroke volume rather than cardiac output during a fluid challenge. If the heart rate falls appropriately in response to a fluid challenge, the cardiac output may not increase despite an increase in stroke volume.

A low stroke volume that is not increasing with fluid support may require inotropic support or, in cardiogenic shock, vasodilator therapy with or without inotropic therapy.

Correction of a low stroke volume in cardiogenic shock

If an acute ischaemic cardiac event is the cause of the shock, the increase in myocardial oxygen demand as a result of inotropes may worsen the ischaemia. The use of vasodilators may improve stroke volume by reducing peripheral resistance, the main limitation to their use being hypotension.

Figure 11.6 shows that reducing peripheral resistance increases stroke volume and reduces filling pressures. Associated hypotension should be treated with further fluid challenges to ensure maintenance

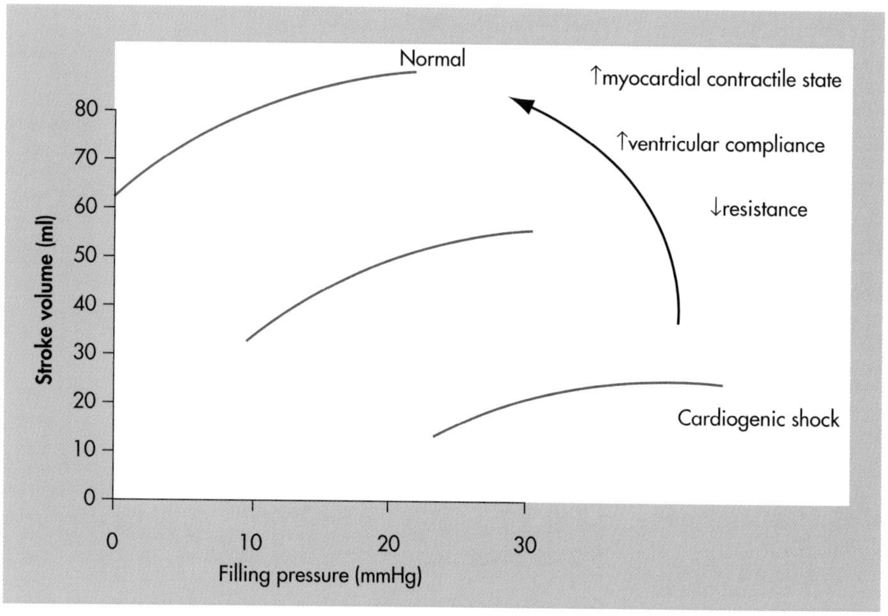

Figure 11.6 *The Frank–Starling mechanism relates cardiac contractility to preload. In clinical practice, the stroke volume is related to filling pressures and depends on myocardial contractile state, ventricular compliance and peripheral resistance. Improvements in stroke volume in cardiogenic shock can be achieved by increasing filling pressures, reducing peripheral resistance or increasing myocardial contractility.*

of the circulating volume before resorting to other methods of circulatory support. Glycerltrinitrate (GTN) is the mainstay of vasodilator therapy in cardiogenic shock. A dose of 1–20 mg/hr IV is titrated to the goal of a normal stroke volume while accepting a reduction in mean arterial pressure to 60–70 mmHg (higher in the patient with premorbid hypertension).

In severe cardiogenic shock, it may not be possible to normalize the stroke volume. In these cases, it is appropriate to consider early mechanical ventilation to reduce tissue oxygen demand (see later) or the use of inotropes to increase myocardial contractility. The severest cases do not respond to drug therapy and require mechanical circulatory support (intra-aortic balloon counterpulsation or left ventricle (LV) assist devices).

Correction of a low stroke volume in non-cardiogenic shock

In other forms of shock, a low stroke volume that is not responsive to fluid therapy should be corrected with inotropic drugs. At present, none of the inotropic drugs are pure, all having various effects on the peripheral circulation, and some possessing both vasoconstrictor and vasodilator properties, depending on the dose (Table 11.3). The most popular inotropic drugs are dobutamine and adrenaline (epinephrine). Both exert their inotropic effects by stimulation of cardiac β-receptors. Dobutamine is used in a dose of 1–20 μg/kg per min IV, and it has mainly vasodilator effects on the peripheral circulation (which may exacerbate any hypotension). Adrenaline (epinephrine), titrated from low doses of 0.05 μg/min IV, vasodilates mainly the muscle vasculature at low doses, this giving way to vasoconstriction at higher doses. No ceiling is placed on the dose of adrenaline (epinephrine), and, in cases where the ceiling dose of dobutamine is reached, it is usual to use adrenaline (epinephrine). With either drug, or any other inotropic agent, it is essential to titrate the dose against the stroke volume, a normal stroke volume being the target. Small, incremental doses with continuous monitoring of response are essential.

Correction of blood pressure

One of the hallmarks of shock and often the first clinical indicator of circulatory failure is low blood pressure. It should be remembered that the body monitors its own circulation primarily through the baroreceptors, and homeostatic mechanisms to maintain blood pressure are well developed. Low blood pressure, although often the first clinical indicator, is a late feature of failing circulation. A healthy adult can lose 25% of predicted normal blood volume without hypotension.[66] Because of the late failure of homeostasis to maintain blood pressure, the management of shock attempts to correct other components

Table 11.3 Classification of expected effects of inotropic agents. The main receptor affected is shown in bold.

	Receptors	SV	HR	BP	Renal	Splanchnic	Lung	Limb
Dobutamine	**β1**, β2, α1	↑↑	↑↑	↑	↑	↓	↑	↑↑
Dopamine (low)	**DA**	↑			↑↑	↑↑		↑
Dopamine (med)	**β1, DA**	↑↑	↑	↑	↑↑		↓	↑
Dopamine (high)	**α1, β1, DA**	↑	↑↑	↑↑	↑	↓	↓↓	
Adrenaline (epinephrine) (low)	**β1**, α1, α2	↑↑	↑↑	↑		↑	↓	↑
Adrenaline (epinephrine) (high)	**α1, β1**, α2	↑↑	↑	↑↑	↓↓	↓↓	↓↓	↓↓
Noradrenaline (norepinephrine)	**α1**, β1	↑		↑↑	↓↓	↓↓	↓↓	↓↓
Isoproterenol	**β1, β2**	↑	↑↑				↑↑	↑↑
Dopexamine	**DA, β1, β2**	↑↑	↑↑		↑↑	↑↑	↑	↑

of the circulation before attending to the blood pressure, except in the situation of a dangerously low (that is, incompatible with sustaining life) blood pressure. If the blood pressure remains low despite correction of volume status and cardiac function, vasoconstrictor drugs are titrated to maintain a safe perfusion pressure. The most common vasoconstrictor used is noradrenaline (norepinephrine) with a starting dose of 0.05 μg/min IV. Correcting blood pressure to normal levels is rarely necessary, so long as blood flow to all tissues has been restored. As a rule of thumb, a mean arterial pressure of 60 mmHg and above is adequate for perfusion if blood volume and blood flow are adequate. Raising the blood pressure to higher levels is necessary only if there is continuing evidence of poor tissue perfusion (for example, persisting oliguria or lactic acidosis) and is more commonly required in those with premorbid hypertension.

Patients who fail to respond to the vasoconstrictor effects of noradrenaline (norepinephrine) may show a beneficial response to other vasoconstrictor drugs. Antagonizing the vasodilator effects of peripheral nitric oxide with methylthioninium chloride, in a dose of 2 mg/kg IV, has proved beneficial in these resistant cases.[67]

Correction of tissue perfusion

Irrespective of the circulatory status, adequate tissue perfusion does not require treatment. Global assessment of tissue perfusion is based on demonstration of the absence of anaerobic metabolism, that is, no lactic or metabolic acidosis. The presence of lactic acidosis does not necessarily indicate an inadequate circulation, as in liver dysfunction, and the absence of lactic acidosis does not guarantee adequate perfusion of all tissues.[68] However, in the absence of clinically useful tools to monitor regional perfusion, the demonstration of no lactic acidosis is the most useful goal in assessing tissue perfusion. If a pulmonary artery catheter is in situ, the demonstration of a mixed venous oxygen saturation of >60% suggests adequate arterial oxygen delivery. However, inability of tissues to utilize available oxygen, as in sepsis, often leads to a high mixed venous saturation (>75%) with co-existing lactic acidosis. There are, at present, no treatments to improve oxygen uptake in this situation.

Reducing metabolic demand

Finally, in the resuscitative process, attention must be focused on the metabolic demand of the tissues. Practical methods of reducing metabolic rate include control of pyrexia, pain and anxiety. Avoiding physical activity includes the reduction of respiratory work; mechanical ventilation is a useful adjunct to successful management of shock and should not be delayed until blood gases are deteriorating. This is particularly true in patients with cardiogenic shock where the reduction in respiratory work reduces the cardiac output required to perfuse other tissues.

Preventing shock

High-risk surgical patients who have low levels of oxygen delivery in the perioperative period fare worse than those with high levels. It has been proposed that these patients develop a higher 'oxygen debt' and a greater inflammatory response during and after the operation. Trials investigating whether driving the circulation (using fluid and vasoactive drugs) to the higher values seen in survivors demonstrated a consistent 4–5-fold decrease in mortality and a reduction in the number of organ failures in the immediate post-operative period.[69–71]

Unfortunately, driving the circulation of patients who are already critically ill neither improves outcome nor decreases mortality.[72,73] The reason for this difference is poorly understood but may be a result of more profound microcirculatory and metabolic derangement in the critically ill, or of the limited physiological reserve of elderly patients. In most studies, those that responded to fluid resuscitation alone fared better than those requiring vasoactive drug support.

Table 11.4 Therapeutic goals in shock.

Fluid challenge	• Maximum SV • > 3 mmHg rise in CVP • > 3 mmHg rise in PAWP but maintained < 20 mmHg
Inotropic therapy	• SV at least normal • Mixed venous saturation > 60% • Arterial lactate < 1.5 mmol/l • Correction of metabolic acidosis
Adjunctive therapy	• Vasodilators to accommodate volume therapy • Vasodilators to counteract α1 effects • Vasoconstrictors if MAP < 60 mmHg or higher in those with premorbid hypertension • Decrease metabolic rate

CONCLUSION

Shock remains a challenge to the clinician. Clinical methods must be supplemented with appropriate haemodynamic monitoring and frequent reassessment to ensure the variety of treatments commonly used are of benefit to the patient. It is not possible to achieve this goal with clinical methods alone. Suitable goals of therapy are shown in Table 11.4.

REFERENCES

1. Vallet B. Vascular reactivity and tissue oxygenation. Intensive Care Med 1998; 24: 3–11
2. Buttgereit F, Brand MD. A hierarchy of ATP-consuming processes in mammalian cells. Biochem J 1995; 312: 163–167
3. Richter C, Schweizer M, Cossarizza A, Franceshi C. Control of apoptosis by the cellular ATP. FEBS Lett 1996; 378: 107–110
4. Pinsky MR, Vincent JL, Deviere J, Algere M et al. Serum cytokine levels in human septic shock. Relation to multiple organ failure and mortality. Chest 1993; 103: 565–575
5. Deitch EA. Multiple organ failure. Pathophysiology and potential future therapy. Ann Surg 1992; 216: 117–134
6. Harris CE, Griffiths RD, Freestone N, Billington D et al. Intestinal permeability in the critically ill. Intensive Care Med 1992; 18: 38–41
7. O'Dwyer ST, Michie HR, Zeigler TR, Revhaug A et al. A single dose of endotoxin increases intestinal permeability in healthy humans. Arch Surg 1988; 123: 1459–1464
8. O'Boyle C, MacFie J, Mitchell CJ, Johnstone D et al. Microbiology of bacterial translocation in humans. Gut 1998; 42: 29–35
9. MacFie J, O'Boyle C, Mitchell CJ, Buckley PM et al. Gut origin of sepsis: a prospective study investigating associations between bacterial translocation, gastric microflora, and septic morbidity. Gut 1999; 45: 223–228
10. Califf RM, Bengtson JR. Cardiogenic shock. N Engl J Med 1994; 330: 1724–1730
11. Hollenberg SM, Kavinsky CJ, Parillo JE. Cardiogenic shock. Ann Intern Med 1999; 131: 47–59
12. Heusch G, Schulz R. Hibernating myocardium: a review. J Mol Cell Cardiol 1996; 28: 2359–2372
13. Flaherty JT Weisfeldt ML, Bulkley BH, Gardner TJ et al. Mechanisms of ischemic myocardial cell damage assessed by phosphorus-31 nuclear magnetic resonance. Circulation 1982; 65: 561–570

14. Kusuoka H, Weisfeldt ML, Zweier JL, Jacobus WE et al. Mechanism of early contractile failure during hypoxia in intact ferret heart: evidence for modulation of maximal Ca^{2+}-activated force by inorganic phosphate. Circ Res 1986; 59: 270–282
15. Kusuoka H, Weisfeldt ML, Zweier JL, Jacobus WE et al. Mechanism of contractile failure during hypoxia in intact ferret heart: evidence for modulation of maximal Ca-activated force by inorganic phosphate. Circ Res 1996; 59: 270–282
16. Jeroudi MO, Hartley CJ, Bolli R. Myocardial reperfusion injury: role of oxygen radicals and potential therapy with antioxidants. Am J Cardiol 1994; 73: 2B–7B
17. Marban E. Myocardial tunning and hibernation. The physiology behind the colloquialisms. Circulation 1991; 83: 681–688
18. McGee S, Abernethy WB, Simel DL. Is this patient hypovolemic? JAMA 1999; 281: 1022–1029
19. American College of Chest Physicians/Society of Critical Care Medicine Consensus Conference. Definitions for sepsis and organ failure and guidelines for the use of innovative therapies in sepsis. Crit Care Med 1992; 20: 864–874
20. Parker MM, Shelhamer JH, Bacharach SL, Green MV et al. Profound but reversible myocardial depression in patients with septic shock. Ann Intern Med 1984; 100: 483–490
21. Lehrs HA, Bittinger F, Kirkpatrick CJ. Microcirculatory dysfunction in sepsis: a pathogenetic basis for therapy? J Pathol 2000; 190: 373–386
22. Ince C, Sinaasappel M. Microcirculatory oxygenation and shunting in sepsis and shock. Crit Care Med 1999; 27: 1369–1377
23. Hotchkiss RS, Rust RS, Dence CS, Wasserman TH et al. Evaluation of the role of cellular hypoxia in sepsis by the hypoxic marker [^{18}F] fluoromisonidazole. Am J Physiol 1991; 261: R965–972
24. Rosser DM, Stidwill RP, Jacobson D, Singer M. Oxygen tension in the bladder epithelium increases in both high and low output endotoxemic sepsis. J Appl Physiol 1995; 79: 1878–1882
25. VanderMeer TJ, Wang H, Fink MP. Endotoxemia causes ileal mucosal acidosis in the absence of mucosal hypoxia in a normodynamic porcine model of septic shock. Crit Care Med 1995; 23: 1217–1226
26. Boekstegers P, Weidenhofer S, Pilz G, Werdan K. Peripheral oxygen availability within skeletal muscle in sepsis and septic shock: comparison to limited infection and cardiogenic shock. Infection 1991; 19: 317–323
27. Gosain A, Rabkin J, Reymond JP, Jensen JA et al. Tissue oxygen tension and other indicators of blood loss or organ perfusion during graded hemorrhage. Surgery 1991; 109: 523–532
28. Boekstegers P, Weidenhofer S, Kapsner T, Werdan K. Skeletal muscle partial pressure of oxygen in patients with sepsis. Crit Care Med 1994; 22: 640–650
29. Singer M, Brealey D. Mitochondrial dysfunction in sepsis. Biochem Soc Symp 1999; 66: 149–166
30. Bergstrom J, Bostrom H, Furst P, Hultman E et al. Preliminary studies of energy-rich phosphagens in muscle from severely ill patients. Crit Care Med 1976; 4: 197–204
31. Liaw K, Askanazi J, Michelson C, Kantrowitz L et al. Effect of injury and sepsis on high-energy phosphates in muscle and red cells. J Trauma 1980; 20: 755–759
32. Brealey D, Hargreaves I, Heales S, Land J et al. Mitochondrial dysfunction in human septic shock. Intensive Care Med 1999; 25: S58
33. Brostoff J, Hall T. Hypersensitivity – type I. In: Roitt I, Brostoff J, Male D, eds. Immunology. 5th edn. Mosby International, 1998: 302–317
34. Kemp SF, Lockey RF, Wolf BL, Lieberman P. Anaphylaxis. A review of 266 cases. Arch Intern Med 1995; 155: 1749–1754
35. Kisel DJ. Pulmonary embolism from axillosubclavian thrombosis on a rehabilitation unit: case report. Arch Phys Med Rehabil 1997; 78: 319–323
36. Hingorani A, Ascher E, Lorenson E, DePippo P et al. Upper extremity deep venous thrombosis and its impact on mortality rates in a hospital based population. J Vasc Surg 1997; 26: 853–860
37. Weiland JE, Davis WB, Holter JF, Mohammed JR et al. Lung neutrophils in the adult respiratory distress syndrome. Clinical and pathophysiologic significance. Am Rev Respir Dis 1996; 133: 218–225
38. Vesconi S, Rossi GP, Pesenti A, Fumagalli et al. Pulmonary microthrombosis in severe adult respiratory distress syndrome. Crit Care Med 1988; 16: 111–113
39. Marshall RE, Hanson CW, Frasch F, Marshall C. The role of hypoxic pulmonary vasoconstriction in pulmonary gas exchange and blood flow distribution. Intensive Care Med 1994; 20: 379–389
40. Hagan RD, Diaz FJ, Horvath SM. Plasma volume changes with movement to supine and standing positions. J Appl Physiol 1978; 45: 414–417
41. Widgren B, Berglund G, Wikstrand J, et al. Reduced venous compliance in normotensive men with

positive family histories of hypertension. J Hypertens 1992; 10: 459–465
42. Amoroso P, Greenwood R. Posture and central venous pressure measurement in circulatory volume depletion. Lancet 1989; 2: 258–260
43. Weil M, Shubin H, Rosoff L. Fluid repletion in circulatory shock – central venous pressure and other practical guides. JAMA 1965; 192: 668–674
44. Baek SM, Makabali GG, Byran-Brown CW, Kusek JM, Shoemaker WC. Plasma expansion in surgical patients with high central venous pressure; the relationship of blood volume to hematocrit, CVP, pulmonary wedge pressure, and cardiorespiratory changes. Surgery 1975; 78: 304–315
45. Shasby D, Dauber I, Pfister S et al. Swan-Ganz catheter location and left atrial pressure determine the accuracy of the wedge pressure when positive end-expiratory pressure is used. Chest 1981; 80: 666–670
46. Webb A. The fluid challenge. In: Webb A, Shapiro M, Singer M, Suter P, eds. Oxford Textbook of Critical Care. Oxford: Oxford University Press, 1999: 32–34
47. Falk J, Rackow E, Weil M. Colloid and crystalloid fluid resuscitation. Acute Care 1983; 10: 59–94
48. Shoemaker W, Schluchter M, Hopkins JA, et al. Comparison of the relative effectiveness of colloids and crystalloids in emergency resuscitation. Am J Surg 1981; 142: 73–84
49. Shoemaker W. Comparisons of the relative effectiveness of whole blood transfusions and various types of fluid therapy in resuscitation. Crit Care Med 1976; 4: 71–78
50. Metildi LA, Shackford SR, Virgilio RW, et al. Crystalloid versus colloid in fluid resuscitation of patients with severe pulmonary insufficiency. Surg Gynecol Obstet 1984; 158: 207–212
51. Rackow E, Falk J, Fein I. Fluid resuscitation in shock: a comparison of cardiorespiratory effects of albumin, hetastarch and saline solutions in patients with hypovolaemic shock. Crit Care Med 1983; 11: 839–850
52. Nylander W, Hammon J, Roselli R, et al. Comparison of the effects of saline and homologous plasma infusion on lung fluid balance during endotoxemia in unanesthetized sheep. Surgery 1981; 90: 221–228
53. Appel P, Shoemaker W. Evaluation of fluid therapy in adult respiratory failure. Crit Care Med 1981; 9: 862–869
54. Staub N, Nagano H, Pearce M. Pulmonary edema in dogs, especially the sequence of fluid accumulation in the lung. J Appl Physiol 1967; 2: 227–240
55. Rackow EC, Astiz ME, Janz TG, Weil MW. Absence of pulmonary edema during peritonitis and shock in rats. J Lab Clin Med 1989; 112: 264–269
56. Schierhout G, Roberts I. Fluid resuscitation with colloids or crystalloids in critically ill patients: a systematic review of randomised trials. BMJ 1998; 316: 961–964
57. Cochrane Injuries Group Albumin Reviewers. Human albumin administration in critically ill patients: a systematic review of randomised controlled trials. BMJ 1998; 317: 235–239
58. Choi PT, Yip G, Quinonez LG, Cook DJ. Crystalloids versus colloids in fluid resuscitation: a systematic review. Crit Care Med 1999; 27: 200–210
59. Webb A. Crystalloid or colloid resuscitation. Are we any the wiser? Crit Care Forum 1999; 3: R25–R28
60. Funk W, Baldinger V. Microcirculatory perfusion during volume therapy. Anesthesiology 1995; 82: 975–982
61. Hebert PC, Wells G, Tweeddale M, Martin C. Does transfusion practice affect mortality in critically ill patients? Transfusion Requirements in Critical Care (TRICC) Investigators and the Canadian Critical Care Trials Group. Am J Respir Cri Care Med 1997; 155: 1618–1623
62. Fitzgerald RD, Martin CM, Dietz GE, Doig GS, Potter RF, Sibbald WJ. Transfusing red blood cells stored in citrate phosphate dextrose adenine-1 for 28 days fails to improve tissue oxygenation in rats. Crit Care Med 1997; 25: 726–732
63. Singer M, Allen MJ, Webb AR, Bennett ED. Effects of alterations in left ventricular filling, contractility, and systemic vascular resistance on the ascending aortic blood velocity waveform of normal subjects. Crit Care Med 1991; 19: 1138–1145
64. Kubicek WG, Karnegis JN, Patterson RP, Witsoe DA, Mattson RH. Development and evaluation of an impedance cardiac output system. Aerosp Med 1966; 37: 1208–1212
65. Kurita T, Morita K, Kato S et al. Comparison of the accuracy of the lithium dilution technique with the thermodilution technique for measurement of cardiac output. Br J Anaesth 1997; 79: 770–775
66. Hamilton-Davies C, Mythen MG, Salmon JB, Jacobson D, Shukla A, Webb AR. Comparison of commonly used clinical indicators of hypovolaemia with gastrointestinal tonometry. Intensive Care Med 1997; 23: 276–281
67. Schneider F, Lutun P, Hasselmann M, Stoclet JC, Temple JD. Methylene blue increases systemic vascular resistance in human septic shock. Preliminary observations. Intensive Care Med 1992; 18: 309–311

68. Gutierrez G, Clark C, Brown SD, Price K, Ortiz L, Nelson C. Effect of dobutamine on oxygen consumption and gastric mucosal pH in septic patients. Am J Respir Crit Care Med 1994; 150: 324–329
69. Shoemaker W, Appel P, Kram H, Waxman K et al. Prospective trial of supranormal values of survivors as therapeutic goals in high-risk surgical patients. Chest 1988; 94: 1176–1186
70. Boyd O, Grounds R, Bennett E. A randomized clinical trial of the effect of deliberate perioperative increase of oxygen delivery on mortality in high-risk surgical patients. JAMA 1993; 270: 2699–2707
71. Wilson J, Woods I, Fawcett J, Whall R et al. Reducing the risk of major elective surgery: randomised controlled trial of preoperative optimisation of oxygen delivery. BMJ 1999; 318: 1099–1103
72. Hayes MA, Timmins AC, Yau EH, Palazzo M, Hinds CJ, Watson D. Elevation of systemic oxygen delivery in the treatment of critically ill patients. N Engl J Med 1994; 330: 1717–1722
73. Gattinoni L, Brazzi L, Pelosi P, Latini R et al. A trial of goal oriented hemodynamic therapy in critically ill patients. N Engl J Med 1995; 333: 1025–1032

12

Acute renal failure

Guy H Neild

CLINICAL OVERVIEW

Epidemiology

Acute renal insufficiency is a sudden decline in renal function. There are no standard definitions. This chapter discusses life-threatening acute renal failure when the renal function falls towards zero. In the UK, about 50 people per million population develop acute renal failure requiring dialysis each year. Acute renal failure complicates about 5% of admissions to hospital and 30% of admissions to intensive care.

Aetiology

By far the most common causes of acute renal failure today are seen on the intensive care unit and are related to sepsis, trauma and surgery. The kidney fails, often with one or more other organs. In this setting, the kidney switches off, but if a kidney biopsy is taken, the tissue appears to be virtually normal and the kidney failure is (potentially) reversible; this is referred to as acute tubular necrosis. In such cases, there is usually little or no doubt about the antecedent factors – although the actual cause of acute tubular necrosis is usually multifactorial, such as a combination of hypotension, sepsis and nephrotoxic drugs.

Differential diagnosis of acute renal failure
There are three levels or categories at which kidney failure may occur (see Table 12.1):

1. There is interruption of adequate blood flow or perfusion of the kidney (pre-renal failure).
2. There is something wrong with the kidney itself (parenchymal injury).
3. There is obstruction of the ouflow of urine from the kidneys.

Table 12.1 Differential diagnosis of acute renal failure.

1.	Pre-renal failure: inadequate perfusion of blood through kidney
2.	Renal (parenchymal): intrinsic injury to the diseased kidney
3.	Post-renal failure: obstruction of the urine outflow

It is sensible to divide the first group into (a) physiological pre-renal failure, in which correction of the underlying hypovolaemia restores adequate perfusion to the kidney and (b) pathological pre-renal failure, in which there is anatomical disruption of the blood supply (such as aortic dissection). The different causes of acute renal failure are shown in Table 12.2.

Presentation

The clinical symptoms are usually dominated by those of the underlying pathology (Table 12.2). The symptoms of severe renal failure (uraemia) are not specific (see Chapter 13). The classical (but not obligatory) feature of acute renal failure is reduction of the urine volume (oliguria), defined as a urine volume of less than 400 ml per day. This will often be associated with fluid retention leading to oedema. Clinical situations in which acute tubular necrosis occurs are shown in Table 12.3.

Table 12.2 Aetiology of acute renal failure.

Pre-renal
Physiological
- Shock (hypovolaemia)
  - Primary underfilling of circulating blood volume due to loss of blood, colloid or crystalloid
  - Primary dilatation of peripheral circulation (loss of peripheral resistance) due to septicaemia, anaphylaxis
- Heart failure (cardiogenic shock)
- Changes in glomerulo-haemodynamics
  - Hepatorenal syndrome
  - Septicaemia
  - Angiotensin-converting enzyme inhibitors, non-steroidal anti-inflammatory drugs

Pathological
- Renal artery thrombosis or embolus
- Dissection of aorta
- Renal artery trauma
- Cholesterol emboli

Renal
- Acute tubular necrosis
- Acute glomerulonephritis
- Acute interstitial nephritis
- Acute tubular obstruction
  - Pigments (myoglobin, haemoglobin)
  - Crystals
  - Myeloma
- Acute infection (pyelonephritis)
- Occlusion of renal microcirculation (haemolytic uraemic syndrome)

Post-renal
- Involvement of both ureters
  - Stones, papillae (intrinsic)
  - Retroperitoneal fibrosis (extrinsic)
  - Glands, aorta
- Bladder
  - Tumour
  - Prostate
  - Bladder neck obstruction

Investigations

When sick patients are admitted, there is a range of routine tests that is done (Table 12.4). This range will be extended depending on the known diagnosis or the likely differential diagnoses.

Biochemistry

The fact that somebody has renal failure is established by blood tests showing high values of urea and creatinine. With renal failure, whether it is acute

Table 12.3 Clinical situations in which acute tubular necrosis occurs.

Pre-renal leading to ischaemic renal failure	Hypovolaemia Cardiac failure Neural (sympathetic overactivity), such as aortic dissection Septicaemia Cyclosporin toxicity Vasoactive drugs, such as non-steroidal anti-inflammatory drugs, angiotensin-converting enzyme inhibitors Renal artery occlusion, as in aortic surgery
Renal	Nephrotoxins, such as gentamicin, amphotericin, cisplatinum Toxin, such as paraquat or radiocontrast agents Toxicity, as in pancreatitis, multiple organ failure Sepsis, including pneumonia Idiopathic/unknown Myeloma Haemoglobinuria, myoglobinuria
Outflow obstruction	Renal colic (neural reflex)

Table 12.4 Investigations for acute renal failure.

Blood tests
Biochemistry
  Blood
  Urine
Haematology
  Full blood count
  Coagulation screen
Serology (antibody tests)

Urine tests
Dipstick urine
Microscope urine
Quantify urine Na^+, urea, creatinine and protein
Culture urine (midstream urine, MSU)

Bacteriology
Culture urine (MSU)
Culture blood (blood cultures)

Imaging
Radiology
Nuclear medicine

Renal biopsy

or chronic, a number of other biochemical tests are abnormal, but these do not usually help distinguish between acute and chronic renal failure. Generally, with renal failure, the plasma levels of potassium, phosphate and urate are raised and that of calcium is reduced.

Haematology

With any patient, a full blood count (FBC) would be done and the blood-clotting times checked (the prothrombin time, the activated partial thromboplastin time (APTT) or kaolin clotting time (KCT), and the thrombin time). The presence of prolonged clotting times and thrombocytopenia indicates disseminated intravascular coagulation, which is usually secondary to septicaemia.

Serology

The presence of antibodies may help to establish the cause of an autoimmune disease (such as antinuclear, or antineutrophil cytoplasm) or may be necessary in diagnosing an infectious disease.

Urine test

It is mandatory that urine is tested on admission for blood and protein. A urine sample must also be sent to the laboratory to be placed under the microscope (to look for red cells, white cells and protein casts, and bacteria) and cultured. With pre-renal failure, as there is no renal injury, the urine should not contain blood or protein; with established acute tubular necrosis, or outflow obstruction, again there is no expectation of blood or protein of glomerular origin, and no more than trace amounts should be found. With acute glomerular disease, the urine will be loaded with blood, protein and casts of these products.

Often, in acute renal failure, a spot sample of urine will be sent to the laboratory to measure the sodium, potassium and urea concentration in the urine. Pre-renal failure is characterized by urine sodium of <20 mmol/l and a urine/plasma urea ratio of >8. This is because the tubules are working normally and reabsorbing salt and water maximally. Once ischaemic damage occurs to the tubules and there is acute tubular necrosis, the tubules can no longer reabsorb sodium or concentrate the urine, and so urine sodium is typically >40 mmol/l and urine/plasma urea ratio <3.

Radiology and nuclear medicine

The essential information required concerning the cause of renal failure is anatomical information regarding the shape and size of the kidneys and their texture. This can all be obtained with ultrasound. The minimum information reported should be the size and shape of each kidney and whether its texture shows evidence of increased fibrosis, reported as increased echogenicity. In acute renal failure, the kidneys will be normal sized or larger than normal. In contrast, in chronic renal failure, the kidneys are not only smaller than expected but show increased echogenicity.

In certain circumstances, specialist X-rays or isotope scans will be performed. Dynamic renal isotope scanning is helpful to confirm equal blood flow to both kidneys and to demonstrate the pattern of uptake that is typical of acute tubular necrosis, and therefore predictive of recovery.

Renal biopsy

In many instances, it is clear that the injury is to the kidney itself, but the different tests will not, for example, discriminate between different types of glomerular disease. Only a renal biopsy can determine the precise diagnosis. Renal biopsies are important not only for the diagnosis but for establishing which treatment would be best and the prognosis, that is, the likely response to the treatment.

Differential diagnosis

In summary, the first step is to take a history and examine the patient and treat any underlying hypovolaemia or outflow obstruction. With new patients, one must determine whether the problem is acute, chronic or, sometimes, acute-on-chronic. Renal ultrasound is the key investigation. It will demonstrate obstruction when present, and in acute renal failure confirm that kidneys are of normal or increased size. Urine dipstick and urine microscopy are also necessary to categorize the type of renal injury.

Complications of acute renal failure

Fluid overload

This can commonly occur either before the patient is seen by the doctor or after the patient is treated with intravenous fluids. The patient will often complain of increasing breathlessness, and physical examination will show signs of fluid overload (peripheral oedema, raised jugular venous pressure or central venous pressure, and gallop rhythm) and pulmonary oedema. A chest X-ray is often necessary to confirm that there is pulmonary oedema. If the kidneys are still working, they may be able to pass more urine after treatment with diuretics; otherwise, dialysis may be necessary to remove the fluid.

Hyperkalaemia

This is a recognized medical emergency. The patient will generally not have any specific symptoms, but an electrocardiogram will show a typical appearance of hyperkalaemia. If the potassium is not lowered, the patient may have a cardiac arrest. There are a number of strategies involving intravenous drugs to lower the potassium in the short term, but once renal failure is established, the potassium will only be controlled by dialysis.

Hypertension

The hypertension may be due to general fluid retention and/or it may be generated by the kidney. The high blood pressure may improve when fluid is removed. In addition to this, blood pressure-lowering drugs are often given. It is very important that the blood pressure should not be lowered too quickly from very high levels, particularly for patients presenting with very severe hypertension (malignant hypertension), who may suffer serious consequences. It is well known for vessels to thrombose, resulting in strokes; thrombosis of arteries to the spinal cord can result in paraplegia.

Bleeding tendency

Patients with severe renal failure have an increased likelihood of bleeding, which may occur even though their platelet count and clotting are normal. This is because the platelets, for reasons that are not clearly understood, do not adhere normally to the endothelium and arrest bleeding. In addition, sick patients may have either a low platelet count or abnormal clotting, which may be other causes of an increased bleeding tendency. Patients are at increased risk of gastrointestinal haemorrhage, particularly from the stomach, which can be prevented by a number of therapeutic measures to reduce the acidity inside the stomach.

Infection

Patients may present with infection. Moreover, uraemic patients have a slightly suppressed immune system, rendering them more susceptible to infection and to severe infection.

Treatment

General conservative measures

A patient must first be resuscitated in the appropriate way. This may mean giving, or sometimes removing, fluid. All efforts should be made to re-establish a good circulatory state in the patient, which means a good cardiac output and a warm and well-perfused periphery. Patients who are anaemic may need a blood transfusion; others may be managed with intravenous saline or dextrose solutions. Attention should be paid to the blood potassium and to establishing the urine output. It is often much easier to catheterize a sick patient so that the urine output can be monitored on an hourly basis.

Specific treatment of underlying disease

This refers to the aetiology of the renal failure. If it is established, for example, that the patient has obstruction to the ureters, it is usually appropriate to drain the kidneys with a percutaneous nephrostomy. If the obstruction is at the level of the bladder neck or below, simple bladder catheterization may be sufficient.

Clearly, if the underlying problem is an infection, this should be appropriately diagnosed and treated. In some cases, the intrinsic disease of the kidney will become clear only after the biopsy, and it may require specific treatment with immunosuppressive drugs. Rapidly progressive glomerulonephritis is a medical emergency, as delay in treatment can result in irreversible renal failure.

Dialysis

There are three absolute indications for dialysis:

1. fluid overload that is resistant to diuretic therapy
2. increasing hyperkalaemia
3. severe uraemia and acidosis.

Generally, patients with acute renal failure will be treated with haemodialysis rather than peritoneal dialysis. However, there are times when peritoneal dialysis may be indicated or haemodialysis may be unavailable.

Prognosis

In acute renal failure, the prognosis depends on the number of organs, in addition to the kidneys, that are failing. If the kidney is the single affected organ and the patient is otherwise well, survival is in excess of 80%. Patients with more than one organ failing are likely to be managed on the intensive care unit. For such patients, the outlook is very poor. With one other organ failing (such as the lungs requiring ventilation), there is a 45% chance of survival. With two other organs failing (for example, needing ventilation and cardiac support), the mortality rate is in excess of 80%. With three or more other organs failing, the mortality rate is in excess of 90%. There is no indication that outcome has improved in the past decade.

Those who have just renal involvement and ischaemic damage to their kidney resulting in acute tubular necrosis can expect to make an almost complete recovery, with renal function returning eventually to normal. At follow-up, they may have mild evidence of residual injury, such as small amounts of protein in the urine, but do not develop chronic renal failure.

PATHOGENESIS OF ACUTE TUBULAR NECROSIS

Introduction

The pathogenesis of acute tubular necrosis is complex. The normal kidney filters 120 ml of ultrafiltrate from plasma per minute, or 173 litres per day. This is equivalent to processing the entire blood volume 36 times a day. Clearly, the kidney has to have not only the normal ability to reabsorb 99% of this tubular fluid, but also multiple and complex mechanisms to protect the circulation if tubular function is compromised. Not only are there often multiple insults causing acute tubular necrosis, but there are also multiple mechanisms contributing to the final result of no urine. In attempting to unravel these mechanisms, there are three factors to consider:

1. The kidney does not function (glomerular filtration rate <5 ml/min).
2. The injury is potentially reversible.
3. The renal histology shows only (minor) tubular changes.

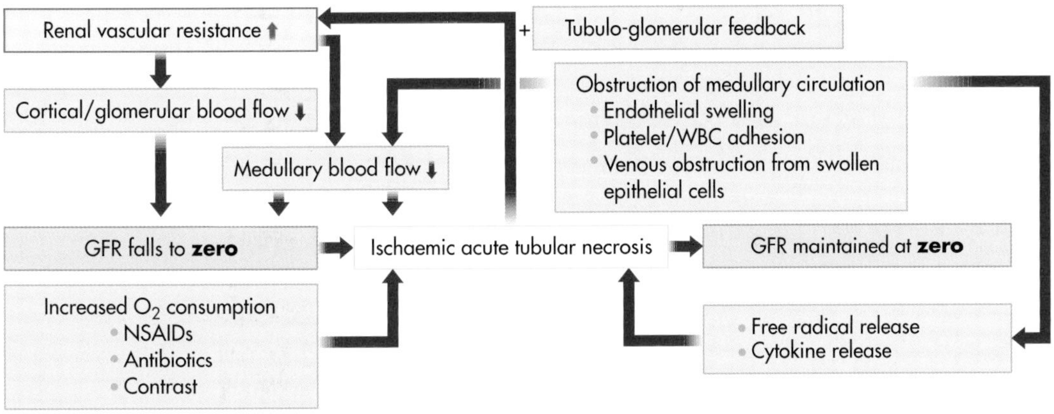

Figure 12.1 *Pathogenesis of acute tubular necrosis.*

Two considerations underlie research into the pathogenesis of acute tubular necrosis:

1. Can strategies be developed to prevent it?
2. Can strategies be developed to accelerate its recovery?

Pathogenesis is best considered with reference to these two considerations. Firstly, what mechanisms lead to the glomerular filtration rate falling to zero? Secondly, what mechanisms maintain the glomerular filtration rate at zero even after the blood supply is returned to near normal?

There are a number of clinical situations in which acute tubular necrosis occurs (see Table 12.3). This section discusses the mechanisms initiated by these clinical insults. The key components in the pathogenesis are shown in Figure 12.1. In reality, there is rarely a single cause, but a number of events that summate, and this is typified by the patient on the intensive care unit. This review only attempts to summarize the facts and present the current consensus views.

One major clue to the pathogenesis is provided by our clinical experience: in almost all experimental models of acute renal failure and in humans, volume loading with saline and the establishment of a natriuresis will prevent or minimize acute tubular necrosis. Conversely, volume contraction will increase the risk of acute tubular necrosis. If we could understand the mechanisms activated by this simple manoeuvre, we would have real insight into the pathogenesis.

Renal anatomy and physiology relevant to acute tubular necrosis

Anatomy

The kidneys (less than 0.5% of the body mass) have one of the highest blood flow rates per unit tissue mass in the body and receive approximately 20% of the cardiac output. This is to filter the blood – only a small percentage is required to supply oxygen for metabolism. Renal blood flow, per gram of tissue, declines progressively from the outer to the inner cortex. Glomerular density shows a similar gradient and this ensures that the outer cortical glomeruli contribute most to total glomerular filtration rate.

The medullary blood supply is derived from the efferent arterioles of the inner cortical glomeruli. These arterioles branch and descend into the descending vasa rectae, which themselves descend in vascular bundles and at intervals leave to supply the adjacent peritubular capillary plexus. In the region of the thick ascending limb, the plexus is very dense.

The loops of Henle have two origins. There are short loops that descend from glomeruli in the outer cortex and they are located furthest from the vascular bundles and are most susceptible to ischaemia. Long loops, from inner cortical glomeruli, are located close to the bundles.

The capillary plexus drains upwards via the ascending vasa rectae, which empty into the arcuate veins at the corticomedullary junction. Both descending and ascending vasa rectae are resistance vessels, which regulate medullary blood flow. Ascending vessels have very thin walls and are potentially susceptible to compression by swollen tubules.

Flow in the outer cortex is approximately sixfold greater than in the outer medulla and 20-fold greater than in the inner medulla. Autoregulation also occurs in the medulla. The limited blood supply to the medulla prevents washout of the gradients of solute formed by the loops of Henle, which are important for normal urine concentration.

Oxygen tension

In the kidney there are gradients of oxygen availability.[1] Medullary partial pressure of oxygen (p_{O_2}) is 10–20 mmHg and much lower than cortical p_{O_2} (about 50 mmHg). The corticomedullary gradient of p_{O_2} is maintained by the countercurrent diffusion of oxygen between arterial and venous branches of the vasa rectae, thus reducing the oxygen supply to the deeper medulla. The ambient p_{O_2} in the renal medulla is low, but demand for oxygen is also low because medullary tubular metabolism is mainly by anaerobic glycolysis.

Glomerular filtration

The rate of glomerular ultrafiltration depends not only on the hydrostatic pressure within the capillary but also on the total capillary surface area available for filtration. Reduction in glomerular capillary surface area due to mesangial contraction is an attractive theoretical concept and might play a role in the maintenance of reduced glomerular filtration rate. Although vasoconstrictors, such as angiotensin and endothelin, do cause mesangial cell contraction in vitro, there is no direct evidence that this does happen in vivo.[2]

Vasomotor tone in the kidney is regulated by a complex series of dilator and constrictor mediators. Some are likely to be more important than others, but we no longer have the naivety to believe that one (such as endothelin) is the principal mediator. What is clear, and verified in experimental models, is that if there is afferent constriction and reciprocal efferent dilatation, then glomerular plasma flow may be normal, and yet the net hydrostatic pressure is too low to permit ultrafiltration and urine is therefore not formed.

Events that lead to a fall in glomerular filtration rate to zero

The renal tubules of healthy kidneys reabsorb over 7 litres of ultrafiltrate per hour. Failure, even partial, of tubular reabsorption would be disastrous, and so highly effective feedback mechanisms have developed to reduce or switch off glomerular filtration.

Shutdown in cortical blood flow (pre-renal failure)

When the circulation is threatened, as in hypovolaemia, the kidney reduces glomerular filtration ('pre-renal failure'). There is a great reduction in cortical blood flow, but, at all costs, medullary flow is maintained. This is partly achieved by the two circulations being independently regulated.

Heterogeneity

The immediate increase in renal vascular resistance in response to hypoperfusion, whether due to hypovolaemia or heart failure, is partly the result of massive sympathetic activity with secondary activation of the renin-angiotensin system. Although renal blood flow is decreased, glomerular filtration rate is initially preserved by a disproportionate rise in efferent tone, which is mediated in particular by angiotensin. Moreover, the increased tone in the afferent vessels is offset by vasodilatory prostaglandins and nitric oxide; for these reasons, the use of angiotensin-converting enzyme inhibitors or inhibitors of cyclooxgenase (such as non-steroidal anti-inflammatory drugs) can cause a precipitous decline in glomerular filtration rate.

A very attractive hypothesis proposes that the independent regulation of the cortical and medullary blood supplies is in part achieved by the differential action of adenosine, itself a product of ischaemia. In conditions of ischaemia in other organs, adenosine is a vasodilator and is cytoprotective. In the kidney, it is a potent vasoconstrictor of the cortical circulation (via A1 receptors), but a vasodilator in the medulla (via A2 receptors).[3]

Loss of autoregulation

Following the induction of acute tubular necrosis, there is loss of endothelium-dependent vasodilatation within the kidney, which contributes to the loss of autoregulation. This may have two consequences: firstly, there will be loss of the compensatory vasodilatation following ischaemic injury; secondly, the kidney will not be protected from any subsequent falls in perfusion pressure.

Tubuloglomerular feedback

Glomerular haemodynamics are locally regulated by the tubuloglomerular feedback mechanism. Early in the course of ischaemic injury to the thick ascending limb, there is loss of chloride reabsorption and activation of this feedback mechanism at the macula densa, which in turn leads to afferent arteriolar constriction and a decrease in glomerular filtration rate.[4] Adenosine is a potent enhancer of tubuloglomerular feedback and acts in synergism with other vasoactive agents, such as angiotensin, to produce renal vasoconstriction. This effect is more pronounced in salt-restricted than in salt-loaded rats.

Vasoactive mediators

In addition to adenosine, there are many potent vasoactive mediators, both endogenous and exogenous, that are important. Moreover, loss of vasodilators (such as nitric oxide) will exacerbate vasoconstriction. It would be premature to single out a principal mediator, but endothelin would seem an obvious candidate as a key factor.[5]

What is intriguing, and still unexplained, is the reduction in glomerular filtration rate seen in the hepatorenal syndrome (and some other situations). Although the glomerular filtration rate can be virtually zero, the kidney mimics pre-renal failure; that is, the urine is concentrated and there is avid retention of sodium, implying that the tubular (medullary) blood supply is still intact. The kidney is resistant to volume expansion. This glomerular haemodynamic state can be achieved only by afferent constriction with reciprocal efferent dilatation. No pharmaceutical intervention is yet capable of reversing this situation. Similarly, no pharmaceutical intervention will reverse cyclosporin nephrotoxicity.

Shutdown in medullary blood flow (leading to acute tubular necrosis)

Hypovolaemia

When the renal circulation is initially compromised, medullary blood flow is maintained, but beyond a certain point the medullary flow becomes inadequate to maintain oxygenation of the medullary tubules.

Sepsis and cytokine activation

In the past decade, there has been an enormous increase in our understanding of the physiology of septicaemia.[6] Endotoxin (lipopolysaccharide) triggers the release of a series of cytokines and vasoactive mediators. Septic shock is associated with a fall in peripheral vascular resistance and mean arterial blood pressure. This is initially associated with a rise in cardiac output. However, venous pooling occurs, causing a fall in cardiac preload and cardiac output. This reduction in cardiac output is exacerbated by myocardial depressant factors that are generated. In the kidney, independently of these systemic effects, there is a rise in renal vascular resistance, and a fall in renal blood flow and glomerular filtration rate. These changes are due to the mediators released, which include tumour necrosis factor, interleukin-1, platelet-activating factor, thromboxane, leukotriene and endothelin. Lipopolysaccharide itself has no direct effect on the renal circulation.[6]

In septicaemia, renal haemodynamics can be altered so that, as in the hepatorenal syndrome, the glomerular filtration rate may be reduced with volume-resistant oliguria, and yet there is still avid retention of sodium. More commonly, critically ill patients with septicaemia or multiple organ failure have a progressive fall in glomerular filtration rate with gradually increasing oliguria, although they may initially have non-oliguric renal failure. No pharmacological intervention significantly alters this course of events (except treatment and resolution of the underlying problem). The final sequence of events that leads to tubular ischaemia and acute tubular necrosis is still unknown.

Vascular obstruction

In experimental models of acute tubular necrosis, focal and segmental necrosis of the media in resistance arterioles is found. This is probably a consequence of the initial severe vasospasm, but may contribute to the continuing reduction in blood flow. Endothelial swelling is patchy and transient,[7] except in the corticomedullary area, where it is consistent and persists.

The lumens of capillaries are occluded not only by swollen endothelial cells but also by platelets and leucocytes adhering to sites of endothelial injury and thus contributing to the mechanical obstruction. Following ischaemic injury, free radical production by damaged endothelium and activated adherent neutrophils will inactivate endothelium-derived nitric oxide, thus further promoting the cycle of vasoconstriction and leucocyte adhesion. Endothelial injury will also lead to loss of endothelial tight junctions, an increase in vascular permeability and interstitial oedema. Nevertheless, there is a rationale for giving drugs (such as prostacyclin and nitric oxide donors) that may dilate the microcirculation and prevent leucocyte adhesion and platelet aggregation.

Although endothelial cell injury is likely to trigger thrombosis and the generation of fibrin, it is very difficult to find morphological evidence of this due to the great fibrinolytic capacity of endothelium, and fibrin may be found only when the fibrinolytic pathways are overwhelmed.

Venous obstruction

In post-mortem specimens, the dark zone at the outer medulla seen in acute tubular necrosis is due to intense vascular congestion of the ascending vasa rectae. Obstruction of the venous return from the medulla is thought to be an important factor contributing to tubular ischaemia.[8] The medullary circulation is drained by the very thin-walled ascending vasa rectae. After ischaemic injury to medullary tubules, there is cell swelling and interstitial oedema, and these swollen tubules obstruct the ascending vessels. Sufficient cell swelling to contribute to 'no reflow' does not occur until anoxia has persisted for 30–40 minutes. Thus, a vicious circle is set up, with increasing venous obstruction increasing tubular ischaemia.

Tubular obstruction

The role of tubular obstruction in the maintenance of oliguria has provoked much debate for many years. Tubular obstruction plays a major role in some experimental models, but there is less evidence in humans. However, as described in the previous section, cell swelling is thought to play an important role in venous obstruction of the medullary circulation.

There are secondary causes of acute renal failure in which tubular obstruction is relevant. These include myeloma, crystalluria, haemoglobinuria and myoglobinuria. Although the pathogenesis of acute renal failure in, for example, myoglobinuria is complex and multifactorial, it seems sensible from a clinical point of view to minimize the risk of cast obstruction. Thus, establishing a diuresis and alkalinizing the urine are logical strategies.[9]

Reperfusion injury and no reflow phenomenon

In acute tubular necrosis following ischaemia and reperfusion, the mechanism of continued reduction in renal blood flow that occurs after correction of systemic pressure and volume – the 'no-reflow' phenomenon – is poorly understood. There are a number of factors that contribute to it. Both the interruption and subsequent restoration of blood flow (reperfusion) cause tissue injury in any organ, although the consequences vary greatly. The impact is greatest in the heart, and cardiological science has been increasingly successful at developing interventions to protect the myocardium. Ischaemia and reperfusion in the kidney contribute not only to the renal dysfunction after periods of hypoperfusion, but also to the non-immunological damage that complicates cadaveric renal transplantation and revascularization surgery. One must be cautious about overextrapolating from the heart and central nervous system to the kidney because, in the former, interruption of flow is often complete and associated with infarction.

Leucocytes and activation of adhesion molecules

Trapping and adhesion of leucocytes in the microcirculation play a key role in ischaemic injury, and activated neutrophils can release reactive oxygen species and a variety of enzymes, including proteases, elastase and myeloperoxidase. Neutrophils will adhere to endothelium when adhesion molecules on endothelial cells (such as ICAM-1) are activated, as by reperfusion injury or sepsis.

In models of myocardial and intestinal ischaemia, depletion of neutrophils, blockade of neutrophil adhesion and inhibition of complement all reduce tissue injury.[10,11] Recent powerful support for their relevance to acute renal failure comes from blocking adhesion molecules. Monoclonal antibodies against ICAM-1 protect against experimental ischaemia, even when given 2 hours after the insult,[12] and mice deficient in ICAM-1 are protected against acute renal failure.[10] It is therefore of potential relevance that both adenosine and nitric oxide can downregulate adhesion molecules.

Free radicals

Reperfusion with oxygenated blood is associated with free-radical generation, leading to lipid peroxidation, polysaccharide depolymerization and deoxyribonucleotide degradation. Damaged endothelial cells not only now fail to generate vasodilators, but also release vasoconstrictors and swell, which leads to an increase in vascular permeability. These local events will also lead to progressive trapping of leucocytes, which in turn contribute to the no-reflow phenomenon. Reactive oxygen species contribute to tissue injury in models of myocardial and renal ischaemia. Although, in renal ischaemia, the use of different combinations of xanthine oxidase inhibitors, superoxide dismutase, catalase and glutathione can, in general, protect, the results have been disappointing. This probably reflects the difficulty in delivering exogenous antioxidants to target tissues.

Events that maintain glomerular filtration rate at zero

Ischaemic injury to tubules

Extensive research in rodent models of acute tubular necrosis has identified the thick ascending limb as the most vulnerable site for ischaemic injury. In humans, it is not certain whether this part of the tubule is necessarily the most vulnerable. Histological and microdissection studies of tubules suggest a more diffuse injury (although, even by electron microscopy, changes are often inconspicuous, with little evidence of tubular necrosis).

The discussion that follows relates to work on rodent models. For the reasons given above, one must be cautious about over-extrapolating the potential of protective strategies defined in these models.

Structural changes

Following ischaemic injury, a consequence of morphological changes occurs in the proximal tubule. First, 'blebs' appear on the apical surface and the brush-border is lost. Cells lose their polarity (with relocation of Na^+/K^+-ATPase from the basolateral to the apical membrane) and the integrity of their tight junctions, with integrins redistributed to the apical membrane. These changes are a consequence of alteration in the cytoskeleton and microtubule assembly. Cells (both dead and alive) exfoliate into the lumen, an effect which may lead to an increase in intratubular pressure and exacerbate any back leak of ultrafiltrate that is occurring through the destructive tubules into the interstitium.[13]

Tubular energetics

The principal determinant of medullary oxygen consumption is the rate of active reabsorption in the thick ascending limb. Morphological injury to the thick ascending limb (in rats) can be greatly reduced by inhibiting active transport by these cells. Furosemide (frusemide), which blocks chloride reabsorption, reduces the injury, and ouabain, which eliminates active transport (by inhibiting Na^+/K^+-ATPase), prevents the lesion entirely. The lesion can also be prevented by abolishing glomerular filtration (achieved by raising glomerular oncotic pressure with albumin).[1] In contrast, increasing the work load makes the injury worse. This can be achieved acutely by fluid depletion or adding amphotericin, an ionophore that increases sodium reabsorption and thus the activity of the sodium/potassium pump and oxygen demand.

Another important way in which hypovolaemia, by causing oliguria, may predispose to acute tubular necrosis is by permitting high concentrations of potential toxins (such as radiocontrast and gentamicin) to be present in the ascending tubule.[1] To cope with this potentially unstable, and hypoxic, environment in the medulla, a number of cytoprotective systems have evolved. Vasodilatory prostaglandins, nitric oxide and adenosine are all cytoprotective by inhibiting transport mechanisms (principally for sodium and chloride) and reducing tubular work. Cytochrome P-450-dependent arachidonate metabolites and platelet-activating factor also inhibit transport, and intracellular acidosis is another powerful cytoprotective force.

Biochemical events during acute ischaemic cell injury

Cortical renal tubular epithelia are strictly aerobic and are particularly susceptible to damage during periods of respiratory arrest. There have been few attempts to study biochemical events in models of acute tubular necrosis. In a study of cellular hypoxia, the ability of the rat kidney to recover and continue to pass urine after 30 minutes of ischaemia from haemorrhage was related to the magnitude and duration of the renal adenosine triphosphate (ATP) deficit (as measured in vivo by ^{32}P-NMR).[14]

There is currently much interest in in vitro models of the cell biology of acute tubular necrosis, as there are some surprising and exciting ways in which injury may be prevented. The most remarkable is glycine cytoprotection. In models of 60-minute hypoxia, reoxygenation results in 80% cell death, which is prevented by coincubation of cells with glycine.[15] Glycine is also cytoprotective against cell ischaemia induced by inhibitors of oxidative phosphorylation and glycolysis. The cells maintain structure and recover full metabolic function and ATP content after the removal of the inhibitors.[15,16] The protective effect of glycine occurs at a stage beyond calcium dysregulation and ATP preservation.[16]

Cellular injury is associated with an increase in intracellular calcium. The influx of calcium exacerbates the medullary hypoxia and the injury, and thus the therapeutic potential for calcium channel antagonists to protect against acute tubular necrosis.[17]

SUMMARY AND THERAPEUTIC IMPLICATIONS

Until recently, most experimental models of acute tubular necrosis involved a single massive insult, which bore little relation to the onset of acute tubular necrosis in humans. More recently, models have been developed that combine multiple insults, although individually they have no effect. These are based on inhibiting the multiplicity of homeostatic mechanisms that protect the medulla. For instance, rats can be salt depleted and then given a non-steroidal anti-inflammatory drug and radiocontrast medium. The combination produces acute tubular necrosis, whereas two of the three do not.[18]

Can acute tubular necrosis be prevented? Volume expansion and salt loading, which reduce the work of urine concentration and stimulate medullary vasodilatation, are vital in preventing critical medullary ischaemia. Synergy between hypovolaemia and toxic insults (such as gentamicin) results from the increased renal concentration of toxins in medullary tubules at a time when tubular reabsorption is increased and oxygen supply is reduced.[1] Establishing a diuresis, and thus reducing the tubular concentration of toxins, will protect against the onset of acute tubular necrosis. Although experimental work provides a rationale for the clinical use of furosemide (frusemide), recent data suggest that it confers no benefit over saline infused alone. Similarly, mannitol may prevent cell swelling, promote urine flow, release vasodilatory mediators and even act as an antioxidant, but clinical studies have not shown any reproducible benefit, either for it or for dopamine, in the prevention or amelioration of acute tubular necrosis.[13]

Nevertheless, there are encouraging developments that focus on repair and regeneration. The work cited on the role of ICAM-1 inhibition is very exciting, and studies on tubular cell recovery and regeneration are promising. A number of growth factors (epidermal growth factor, hepatocyte growth factor and insulin-like growth factor-1), when given to animals with renal ischaemia, reduce the extent of injury and accelerate recovery.[19] Clinical trials of insulin-like growth factor-1 are in progress.

REFERENCES

1. Brezis M, Rosen S. Hypoxia of the renal medulla – its implications for disease. N Engl J Med 1995; 332: 647–655
2. Neild GH. Endothelial and mesangial cell dysfunction in acute renal failure. In: Bihari D, Neild GH, eds. Acute Renal Failure in the Intensive Therapy Unit. London: Springer-Verlag, 1990: 77–89
3. Dinour D, Agmon Y, Brezis M. Adenosine: an emerging role in the control of renal medullary oxygenation? Exp Nephrol 1993; 1: 152–157
4. Thurau K, Boylan JW. Acute renal success. The unexpected logic of oliguria in acute renal failure. Am J Med 1976; 61: 308–315
5. Woolfson RG, Millar CGM, Neild GH. Ischaemia and reperfusion injury in the kidney: current status and future direction. Nephrol Dial Transplant 1994; 9: 1529–1533
6. Zager RA. Sepsis-associated acute renal failure: some potential pathogenetic and therapeutic insights. Nephrol Dial Transplant 1994; 9(Suppl. 4): 164–167
7. Kashgarian M, Siegel NJ, Ries AL, DiMeola HJ et al. Hemodynamic aspects in development and recovery phases of experimental postischemic acute renal failure. Kidney Int 1976; 10: 5160–5168
8. Mason J, Welsch J, Torhorst J. The contribution of vascular obstruction to the functional defect that follows renal ischaemia. Kidney Int 1987; 31: 65–71
9. Better OS, Stein JH. Early management of shock and prophylaxis of acute renal failure in traumatic rhabdomyolysis. N Engl J Med 1990; 322: 825–829
10. Kelly KJ, Williams WW Jr, Colvin RB, Meehan SM et al. Intercellular adhesion molecule-1-deficient mice are protected against ischemic renal injury. J Clin Invest 1996; 97: 1056–1063
11. Granger DN, Korthuis RJ. Physiologic mechanisms of postischaemic tissue injury. Ann Rev Physiol 1995; 57: 311–332
12. Kelly KJ, Williams WW, Colvin RB, Bonventre JV. Antibody to intercellular adhesion molecule 1 protects the kidney against ischemic injury. Proc Natl Acad Sci USA 1994; 91: 812–816

13. Thadhani R, Pascual M, Bonventre JV. Acute renal failure. N Engl J Med 1996; 334: 1148–1160
14. Ratcliffe PJ, Moonen CTW, Holloway PAH, Ledingham JGG et al. Acute renal failure in hemorrhagic hypotension: cellular energetics and renal function. Kidney Int 1986; 30: 355–360
15. Weinberg JM, Buchanan DN, Davis JA, Abarzua M. Metabolic aspects of protection by glycine against hypoxic injury to isolated proximal tubules. J Am Soc Nephrol 1991; 1: 949–958
16. Weinberg JM, Davis JA, Roeser NF, Venkatachalam, MA. Role of increased cytosolic free calcium in the pathogenesis of rabbit proximal tubule cell injury and protection by glycine or acidosis. J Clin Invest 1991; 87: 581–590
17. Schrier RW, Arnold PE, van Putten VJ, Burke TJ. Cellular calcium in ischaemic acute renal failure: role of calcium entry blockers. Kidney Int 1987; 32: 313–321
18. Heyman SN, Brezis M, Reubinoff CA, Greenfield Z et al. Acute renal failure with selective medullary injury in the rat. J Clin Invest 1988; 82: 401–412
19. Hammerman MR, Miller SB. Therapeutic use of growth factors in renal failure. J Am Soc Nephrol 1994; 5: 1–11

13

Chronic renal failure

Guy H Neild

INTRODUCTION

Definition

Chronic renal failure is recognized by consistently high plasma urea and creatinine concentrations. The degree of renal failure can be arbitrarily divided into mild, moderate or severe, based on the plasma creatinine (Table 13.1). It is convenient (and accurate) to consider the value of glomerular filtration rate or creatinine clearance as a percentage of normal (for example, 20 ml/min is equivalent to 20% of normal function).

Aetiology

There are many causes of renal failure. The cause will vary depending on age and to some extent on ethnic origin and geographical location. For instance, a paediatric population waiting for a renal transplant will be dominated by those with nephrourological malformations. An elderly population will be dominated by renovascular disease and diabetes. In developing countries, glomerulonephritis remains a major cause of renal failure.

Table 13.2 shows a typical range of the diseases causing renal failure in an adult population in the UK. As an increasingly elderly population is accepted for dialysis, the percentages change, and hypertension and diabetes become more prevalent. In the USA, these two diagnoses alone account for more than 50% of all new dialysis patients.[1]

Table 13.2 Aetiology of chronic renal failure.

Cause	Percentage
Glomerulonephritis	28
Scarred kidneys (reflux nephropathy) and malformations of the urinary tract	17
Diabetes mellitus	16
Uncertain	13
Polycystic kidney disease	10
Hypertension and renovascular disease	8
Hereditary nephritis	1
Others	7

Table 13.1 Degrees of renal failure.

Renal failure	Glomerular filtration rate (ml/min per 1.73 m^2)	Creatinine (μmol/l)
Mild	30–50	150–300
Moderate	10–30	300–700
Severe	<10	>700

Incidence and epidemiology

In the UK, around 80 per 1 million population are accepted on to dialysis programmes each year. This is an increase from the recommended target of 60 per million in 1991. The target was increased after an audit in five different parts of the UK showed that many patients were not being considered for dialysis, and that 80 per million was a consistent figure in all parts of the UK for those generally considered as suitable for dialysis.[2] This figure underestimates the need in inner cities, where there are large ethnic populations. For reasons that are still not clear, renal failure is four to six times more common in Asians and Afro-Caribbeans, than in the white (Caucasian) population. This increased disease burden is true for hypertension, diabetes and non-diabetic forms of chronic renal failure.[3]

In the USA, the figure is more than 200 new patients per 1 million population each year and reflects the larger percentage of the non-white population. In all countries, the incidence rises exponentially with age, and by 80 years of age, end-stage renal failure will occur in approximately 800 per million population.[1]

Presentation/symptoms

Progressive renal failure due to disease of the kidney is often insidious and asymptomatic. Symptoms attributable to the kidney failure per se are not specific (Table 13.3) and do not usually occur until 80–90% of kidney function is lost.

The predominant early symptoms of severe renal failure or 'uraemia', such as fatigue, lethargy and tiredness, are attributable to the anaemia of renal failure and improve when the anaemia is corrected by blood transfusion or the recombinant hormone erythropoietin.

Intrinsic kidney disease is most commonly due to progressive glomerular disease, which is invariably associated with proteinuria, and usually some haematuria, hypertension and a tendency to retain salt and water. In contrast, some progressive disease is predominantly due to tubulointerstitial disease, and this is typically seen when there is a primary urological disease or dysplasia. Tubular disease is characterized by minimal proteinuria, early loss of renal concentrating ability, a tendency to salt wasting (therefore no peripheral oedema), early onset of acidosis and normal blood pressure.

Table 13.3 Uraemic symptoms.

Early (due to anaemia)
Malaise, lethargy, tiredness
Shortness of breath on exertion
Late (due to uraemic toxins)
Itching (pruritis)
Loss of appetite (anorexia)
Nausea and vomiting
Variable (related to abnormal calcium, phosphate)
Muscle weakness
Bone and joint pain
Severe (after dialysis should have been started)
Pericarditis
Impaired mental performance, drowsiness, stupor, coma
Rapid respiration (tachypnoea) due to acidosis

Signs

There are few specific signs of uraemia:

1. Patients may be pale because of anaemia and, if both anaemia and renal failure are severe, often have a yellow tinge to their skin.
2. Patients tan easily in the sun, and the pigmentation fades more slowly than normal.
3. If the renal failure is long-standing since childhood, the patient may be of small stature (in relation to other family members).
4. There may be excoriation of the skin from scratching.

PATHOPHYSIOLOGY

This section first discusses the universal mechanisms that lead to progressive, inexorable renal failure. Secondly, the consequences of loss of kidney tissue are reviewed.

Mechanisms of progressive renal failure

Not all kidney disease is progressive, but once the kidney is sufficiently damaged, for any reason, progressive loss of the remaining nephrons is almost inevitable and is associated with a progressive glomerular disease which leads to glomerulosclerosis.[4] This is invariably associated with proteinuria and hypertension. Thus, there is a final common pathway even when, for example, the original cause of scarred kidneys was urological. This process is the consequence of glomerular capillary hypertension and the concomitant 'glomerular hyperfiltration'.

Different diseases progress at different rates. The prognostic factors are predominantly:

1. hypertension
2. magnitude of proteinuria.

It is now established that careful control of blood pressure slows the rate of loss of renal function.[5,6]

Glomerular capillary hypertension and glomerular hyperfiltration injury

Our understanding of these important mechanisms is based almost exclusively on a reproducible experimental model in which rats have five-sixths or more of their renal mass ablated. Following nephrectomy, the 'remnant kidney' initially hypertrophies and hyperfiltrates in an attempt to improve the glomerular filtration rate. Subsequently, over a number of months, the animals develop increasing proteinuria, hypertension and progressive renal failure with a glomerular lesion that is characterized histologically by focal and segmental glomerulosclerosis.[7]

Following the initial nephrectomy, a predictable sequence of glomerular haemodynamic events occurs. Renal blood flow per glomerulus increases, and the glomerular capillary hydrostatic pressure increases, leading to a great increase in single nephron glomerular filtration rate, or 'hyperfiltration'. This glomerular capillary hypertension appears to be the central event in the mechanism of progressive glomerular injury. The mechanism by which this capillary hypertension causes injury and focal and segmental glomerulosclerosis is less certain. Nevertheless, there is good evidence that the hypertension leads to endothelial damage, which in turn causes platelet adhesion, fibrin formation and subsequent sclerosis. In favour of this mechanism is the ability of various anticoagulant and antiplatelet regimens to reduce the injury and protect the kidney. Secondly, there is increasing evidence that glomerular epithelial cell injury occurs and contributes to the sclerosis.[7]

In these animals, a low-protein diet is effective at reducing this injury and is associated with a fall in single nephron glomerular filtration rate, capillary flow and pressure.[4] More importantly, it has also been shown that treatment of this model with an angiotensin-converting enzyme inhibitor is able to prevent the development of the proteinuria, focal and segmental glomerulosclerosis, and renal failure. In contrast, conventional hypotensive drugs, which are equally effective at reducing systemic blood pressure, have no beneficial effect on the disease process.[8,9] The explanation for this is that while all hypotensive agents will tend to lower glomerular capillary pressure through a reduction in afferent arterial pressure, only angiotensin-converting enzyme inhibitors are able to lower the glomerular pressure, independently of systemic pressure, by their ability to reduce efferent arteriolar tone. Subsequently, it has been shown that angiotensin II receptor antagonists are equally effective, and there is no additional benefit from combining the two drugs. There is now conclusive evidence in progressive renal disease that reducing systemic blood pressure slows the rate of loss of glomerular filtration rate.[5] Moreover, angiotensin-converting enzyme inhibitors are more effective than other hypotensive agents at reducing the loss of glomerular filtration rate and reducing proteinuria.[10–12] Angiotensin II receptor antagonists appear to be equally effective as angiotensin-converting enzyme inhibitors in short-term studies.

Consequences of progressive renal failure

The kidney not only excretes toxins and regulates salt and water balance (Table 13.4), but is also an important source of hormones and enzymes that regulate:

1. the normal production of red cells by the bone marrow (erythropoiesis)
2. calcium and phosphate homeostasis and normal bone mineralization
3. blood pressure.

Table 13.4 Roles of the kidney.

Excretion of toxic metabolites
Regulation of salt and water balance
Regulation of acid–base balance
Hormonal role promoting:
erythropoietin – which stimulates red cell production
renin – which regulates blood pressure
enzymes to activate vitamin D
uncharacterized factor – which lowers blood pressure

Failure of these systems leads to the endocrine problems associated with renal failure (Table 13.5).

Uraemic toxins

The principal role of the kidney is to excrete the metabolic products of nitrogen catabolism. The two conventional markers that are routinely measured as indices of renal function are urea and creatinine. Urea and creatinine are not themselves toxic. The toxins that give rise to the symptoms and complications of chronic renal failure are poorly characterized, and there are very many of them. They are clearly related to protein catabolism, as symptoms will improve on a low-protein diet and are made worse by a high-protein diet. The majority of toxins are filtered by the glomerulus and are therefore removed by dialysis, but some are protein bound, depend normally for excretion on tubular secretion, and are therefore not readily removed by dialysis.

Compounds increased in uraemia include guanidines (methylguanidine and guanidinosuccinic acid), products of nucleic acid catabolism, amines from gut bacteria, phenoles, carbohydrate derivatives (myoinositol, mannitol and sorbitol) and large numbers of unknown molecules of sizes 500–5000 Da known as 'middle molecules'.[13]

Table 13.5 Complications of uraemia.

Endocrine
Hypertension
Accelerated atherosclerosis
Anaemia
Renal bone disease (osteodystrophy)
Acidosis
Toxic
Skin: pruritis
Gastrointestinal system: anorexia, nausea, vomiting
Cardiovascular system: pericarditis
Peripheral nervous system: neuropathy
Central nervous system: convulsions, coma

The regulation of salt and water balance

The kidney's principal role is to filter the plasma. In a healthy young adult kidney, approximately 120 ml of this plasma is filtered per minute; that is, 120 ml of ultrafiltrate is produced per minute. This means that in 1 hour 7200 ml (120 × 60) of ultrafiltrate are produced; in 24 hours, 173 litres (7.2 × 24) are produced. Because we produce only 1–2 litres of urine a day, there is obviously a very efficient system of recovery, or tubular fluid reabsorption.

A normal daily urine volume of, say, 1.7 litres would mean that only 1% of the ultrafiltrate was excreted, while 99% was reabsorbed. The 99% is all the 'good things' that need to be recovered; that is, water, salts, sugar and amino acids. The toxic metabolites remain in the tubules and are excreted in the urine.

Water

The medullary component of the tubules is responsible for the ability to concentrate the urine by reabsorbing water, as well as diluting the urine in response to a water load. Both these abilities are progressively lost until urine of a fixed concentration is produced in end-stage renal failure. The ability to concentrate urine requires several mechanisms to be intact, including the following conditions:

1. the countercurrent system normally generates a very high interstitial osmolality in the medulla.
2. the descending tubule and collecting ducts are impermeable to water in the presence of vasopressin (antidiuretic hormone).

It is now known that water crosses cell membranes via specific water channels called aquaporins. The most important one is aquaporin 2, which is the vasopressin-regulated water channel found exclusively in the renal collecting ducts. Mutations in aquaporin 2 result in severe nephrogenic diabetes insipidus, with the kidney unable to respond to vasopressin.[14] In experimental models of lithium toxicity, expression of this receptor is very greatly reduced, presumably accounting for the inability to concentrate urine.

In chronic renal failure, several factors disrupt the ability to concentrate urine. Damage to the medulla causes a progressive loss of the hypertonic interstitium, damage to tubules causes resistance to antidiuretic hormone ('nephrogenic diabetic insipidus'), and an increasing solute load per remaining nephron causes an obligatory solute diuresis. The inability to concentrate urine in the presence of dehydration is one of the earliest symptoms in tubular disease, leading to symptoms of nocturia and polyuria.

Sodium

As renal function decreases, hormonal mechanisms increase the fraction of filtered sodium excreted from less than 1% in normals up to 30% in end-stage renal failure. Thus, sodium balance and extracellular fluid volume are maintained until the glomerular filtration rate is <10 ml/min.[15,16] Eventually, the kidney cannot maintain the homeostasis, and the extracellular fluid increases, leading to hypertension and dependent oedema, or, in severe cases, pulmonary oedema. When we discuss extracellular fluid homeostasis, sodium is a shorthand for sodium and chloride. It is the retention of chloride anions that leads to volume overload and hypertension.

In renal (tubulointerstitial) disease in which medullary damage predominates, there can be an inability to conserve sodium chloride. Such patients are usually normotensive, do not develop oedema and may require salt supplementation.

Potassium

Potassium is excreted into the urine by tubular secretion. This occurs principally in the distal tubule, where sodium is exchanged for potassium in the presence of aldosterone. Most patients can maintain potassium homeostasis down to a glomerular filtration rate of 5 ml/min, but capacity to increase excretion is limited, and severe hyperkalaemia can occur with a sudden reduction of glomerular filtration rate.[16,17]

Acidosis raises plasma potassium by potassium ion transfer out of cells (in exchange for hydrogen ions), and prevents tubular secretion of potassium (as hydrogen will be exchanged preferentially for sodium in the distal tubule). Conversely, correction of acidosis can lead to a rapid fall in plasma potassium.

In some forms of renal disease (particularly diabetes and amyloid), there may be inappropriately raised potassium for the degree of renal impairment. This is usually due to relative deficiency of aldosterone ('hyporeninaemic hypoaldosteronism'), and this disorder responds to supplementation with fludrocortisone.

The regulation of acid–base balance

The kidney is responsible for acid–base homeostasis, a key role of which is the excretion of non-volatile acids (Table 13.6).[16,18] Non-volatile acids are principally derived from the metabolism of sulphur-containing amino acids (methionine and cystine). The kidney maintains acid–base balance by:

1. the reabsorption of filtered bicarbonate
2. hydrogen ion excretion and acidification of urinary buffers (mainly filtered monobasic phosphate salts, HPO_4^{2-})
3. the generation and secretion of ammonia from the proximal tubule (which traps urinary H^+ as NH_4^+).

In this way, homeostasis is generally maintained down to glomerular filtration rates of 20 ml/min. When renal disease is principally due to tubular damage, acidosis can occur early in renal insufficiency. Although it has been recognized for many years that chronic acidosis may cause osteomalacia and particularly rickets in children, a number of other sequelae are now recognized (Table 13.7).

Anaemia

One of the earliest features of chronic renal failure is anaemia,[19] which is multifactorial but predominantly due to a failure of renal erythropoietin synthesis. The renal cells responsible for erythropoietin synthesis have been identified as interstitial cells present

Table 13.6 Uraemic acidosis I.
Failure to excrete non-volatile acids
Failure of bicarbonate ion reabsorption (proximal renal tubular acidosis)
Failure of hydrogen ion secretion (distal renal tubular acidosis)
Failure of ammonia synthesis (distal renal tubular acidosis)

Table 13.7 Uraemic acidosis II.

Reduced cardiac output
Increased muscle catabolism
Reduced bone mineralization and growth
Osteomalacia
Increased urinary and faecal calcium ion excretion
Inhibition of 1-α-hydroxylase

in the renal cortex. Anaemia in severe chronic renal failure is also due to reduced red cell survival, increased blood loss from the gastrointestinal tract associated with an increased bleeding tendency, and uraemic suppression of erythropoiesis. Typically, there is a normochromic normocytic anaemia.

The effects of the anaemia are partly compensated for by a shift in the oxygen-dissociation curve to the right due to increased concentration of 2,3-diphosphoglycerate and phosphates in red cells.

Hypertension

Two principal mechanisms lead to hypertension in renal disease:

1. salt and water retention leading to an expansion of extracellular fluid
2. renal damage leading to activation of the renin-angiotensin system.

In addition, there is evidence that the kidney produces a lipid mediator that lowers blood pressure. It is certainly remarkable that hypertension can regress following a successful renal transplant. There is also increasing interest in the role of endothelium-derived vasorelaxant factors that counteract the resting sympathetic tone of blood vessels. The most potent and significant of these is nitric oxide, and there is evidence that in uraemia this ability of the normal vessel to produce nitric oxide is reduced or the action of nitric oxide is antagonized, leading to an increase in resting tone and hypertension.

Renal bone disease

Renal bone disease is a mixture of hyperparathyroidism, osteomalacia and osteoporosis. Typically, hyperparathyroidism predominates. A fourth but rare component is the radiological appearance of osteosclerosis. In dialysis patients, or patients who have received aluminium hydroxide as phosphate binders, aluminium toxicity can play a role and cause a severe form of osteomalacia.[20]

Hyperparathyroidism

Three separate forces activate the parathyroid glands to cause secondary hyperparathyroidism. Firstly, the earliest metabolic derangement in chronic renal failure is phosphate retention due to a reduction in glomerular filtration of PO_4^{2-}. The rise in plasma PO_4^{2-} causes a reciprocal fall in plasma calcium, and directly activates the parathyroids to release more parathyroid hormone. The increase in parathyroid hormone acts on the tubules to increase urinary phosphate excretion and correct the rise in plasma phosphate.

Secondly, as the kidney fails, there is simultaneous loss of the renal tubular enzyme 1-α-hydroxylase and thus falling plasma levels of 1,25-dihydroxycholecalciferol (calcitriol), and therefore plasma calcium. If untreated, this leads to the state of 'vitamin D-resistant rickets' (osteomalacia). Reduction in 1,25-dihydroxycholecalciferol is a powerful stimulus to parathyroid hormone release, which in turn activates the failing enzyme. Hyperphosphataemia also inhibits calcitriol synthesis.

Finally, hypocalcaemia directly activates the parathyroids to produce more parathyroid hormone. Parathyroid hormone also has a direct effect on the enzyme 1-α-hydroxylase, which is responsible for the final activation of vitamin D to calcitriol. This activation will act to correct the hypocalcaemia.

The ability to maintain extracellular concentrations of calcium in a narrow physiological range is mediated by a G protein-coupled cell surface receptor called the calcium-sensing receptor. The receptor is expressed predominantly in the parathyroid gland, but also along the kidney tubule, and it regulates renal tubular calcium reabsorption.[21] Via this calcium-sensing receptor, increased plasma concentration of calcium inhibits parathyroid hormone synthesis. In contrast, phosphate activates parathyroid hormone synthesis.

Thus, there is a complex interplay of kidney, parathyroid gland and gut attempting to maintain calcium homeostasis. The parathyroid glands also have vitamin D receptors to which calcitriol binds, and the latter is a potent inhibitor of parathyroid hormone synthesis. This inhibition is itself antagonized by hyperphosphataemia. The situation becomes more complex in renal failure, as the sensitivity and density of these parathyroid receptors change in response to the prevailing milieu.

The management of secondary hyperparathyroidism has been made much easier by the availability of sensitive and specific assays for the intact hormone (as opposed to previous assays for metabolites, which are retained in chronic renal failure). A rise in parathyroid hormone is the earliest detectable metabolic derangement in chronic renal failure and starts to occur even with glomerular filtration rates of 50–60 ml/min.

Osteomalacia

The natural history of progressive renal failure is of progressive vitamin D resistance (see above). Restriction of dietary calcium, or a diet or lifestyle that promotes vitamin D deficiency, will exacerbate the problem. Thus, in Asian patients, osteomalacia may be the predominant form of renal bone disease. Osteomalacia is also caused by chronic metabolic acidosis, when the bones take on a major role as a buffer for the acid.

Osteoporosis

Osteoporosis is a natural part of the ageing process, but it may be exacerbated in renal patients by premature ovarian failure, long-term use of glucocorticosteroids, chronic ill-health associated with immobility, hypercatabolism or injudicious protein/calcium dietary restriction. Today, based on our understanding of all these processes, we have a very effective treatment to prevent bone disease, according to the following steps:

1. early restriction of dietary phosphate
2. the use of phosphate binders (calcium carbonate, aluminium hydroxide) to reduce the gut adsorption of phosphate
3. the use of analogues of calcitriol that will increase plasma calcium and inhibit parathyroid hormone secretion
4. when appropriate, the correction of acidosis with oral sodium bicarbonate.

Hyperlipidaemia

The uraemic state itself causes hypertriglyceridaemia and hypercholesterolaemia. Moreover, many patients have other risk factors for hyperlipidaemia, including hypertension and hyperinsulinaemia (particularly common in non-white ethnic groups), diabetes, drugs used to treat hypertension (diuretics), other drugs (steroids) and unfitness.

Bleeding tendency

In severe uraemia, there is an increased bleeding tendency, although this is not apparent until the creatinine is usually in excess of 600 μmol/l. The defect is due to the impairment of normal platelet adhesion to damaged endothelium. In addition, platelet function is abnormal and, ex vivo, platelets are hyperaggregable in response to aggregating agents.

In uraemia, it is becoming increasingly acknowledged that there is a generalized defect in normal endothelial function, with evidence of impaired activity of endothelium-derived nitric oxide.

Atherosclerosis

The commonest cause of death in dialysis and transplant patients is cardiovascular disease as a consequence of premature and accelerated atherosclerosis. There are many factors, some well defined, others less clear. They can be divided into two groups (Table 13.8).

On the one hand, there are the usual factors, which are overrepresented in renal failure patients and are very similar to those associated with hyperlipidaemia and hypertension. On the other hand, there are factors that are uniquely uraemic and ill-defined. It is still not clear whether haemodialysis or

Table 13.8 Uraemia and atherosclerosis.

Burden of risk factors
Hypertension
Hyperlipidaemia
Unfit
Therapy (including steroids)
Uraemic factors
Endothelial injury
Increased oxidative stress
Platelet dysfunction

continuous ambulatory peritoneal dialysis imposes a greater burden and risk of atheroma. The uraemic factors probably relate to the abnormal endothelial function that is present plus the increased oxidative stress that occurs. The latter will cause, in particular, an increase in oxidatively modified low-density lipoproteins.

REFERENCES

1. USRDS 1994 Annual Data Report. IV. Incidence and causes of treatment ESRD. Am J Kidney Dis 1994; 4(Suppl. 2): S48–56
2. Roderick PJ, Ferris G, Feest TG. The provision of renal replacement therapy in England 1993–5 and Wales 1995. I. Report to the Renal Assoc Executive. 1997: 1–13
3. Roderick PJ, Raleigh VS, Hallam L, Mallick NP. The need and demand for renal replacement therapy in ethnic minorities in England. J Epidemiol Community Health 1996; 50: 334–339
4. Brenner BM, Meyer TW, Hostetter TH. Dietary protein intake and the progressive nature of kidney disease: the role of hemodynamically mediated glomerular injury in the pathogenesis of progressive glomerular sclerosis in aging, renal ablation, and intrinsic renal disease. N Engl J Med 1982; 307: 652–659
5. Klahr S, Levey AS, Beck GJ, Caggiula AW et al. The effects of dietary protein restriction and blood-pressure control on the progression of chronic renal disease. N Engl J Med 1994; 330: 877–884
6. Lazarus JM, Bourgoignie JJ, Buckalew VM, Greene T et al. Achievement and safety of a low blood pressure goal in chronic renal disease. Modification of Diet in Renal Disease Study Group. Hypertension 1997; 29: 641–650
7. El Nahas AM. Mechanisms of experimental and clinical renal scarring. In: Davison AM, Cameron JS, Grunfeld J-P, Kerr DN et al, eds. Oxford Textbook of Clinical Nephrology. 2nd edn. Oxford: Oxford University Press, 1998: 1749–1788
8. Zatz R, Dunn BR, Meyer TW, Anderson S, Rennke HG, Brenner BM et al. Prevention of diabetic glomerulopathy by pharmacological amelioration of glomerular capillary hypertension. J Clin Invest 1986; 77: 1925–1930
9. Anderson S, Rennke HG, Brenner BM. Therapeutic advantage of converting enzyme inhibitors in arresting progressive renal disease associated with systemic hypertension in the rat. J Clin Invest 1986; 77: 1993–2000
10. Bjorck S, Mulec H, Johnsen SA, Norden G et al. Renal protective effect of enalapril in diabetic nephropathy. BMJ 1992; 304: 339–343
11. Lewis EJ, Hunsicker LG, Bain RP, Rohde RD. The effect of angiotensin-converting enzyme inhibition on diabetic nephropathy. The Collaborative Study Group. N Engl J Med 1993; 329: 1456–1462
12. The GISEN Group (Gruppo Italiano di Studi Epidemiologici in Nefrologia). Randomised placebo-controlled trial of effect of ramipril on decline in glomerular filtration rate and risk of terminal renal failure in proteinuric, non-diabetic nephropathy. Lancet 1997; 349: 1857–1863
13. Hoerl WH. Genesis of the uraemic syndrome. In: Davison AM, Cameron JS, Grunfeld J-P, et al, eds. Oxford Textbook of Clinical Nephrology. 2nd edn. Oxford: Oxford University Press, 1998: 1821–1836
14. Deen PM, Verdijk MA, Knoers NV, Wieringa B et al. Requirement of human renal water channel aquaporin-2 for vasopressin-dependent concentration of urine. Science 1994; 264: 92–95
15. Kumar S, Berl T. Sodium. Lancet 1998; 352: 220–228
16. Rose BD, Rennke HG. Renal pathophysiology – the essentials. Baltimore, MD: Williams and Wilkins, 1994
17. Halperin ML, Kamel KS. Potassium. Lancet 1998; 352: 135–140
18. Gluck SL. Acid-base. Lancet 1998; 352: 474–479
19. Macdougall IC, Eckardt K-U. Haematological disorders. In: Davison AM, Cameron JS, Grunfeld J-P, et al, eds. Oxford Textbook of Clinical Nephrology. 2nd edn. Oxford: Oxford University Press, 1998: 1935–1954
20. Reichel H, Druecke TB, Ritz E. Skeletal disorders. In: Davison AM, Cameron JS, Grunfeld J-P, et al, eds. Oxford Textbook of Clinical Nephrology. 2nd edn. Oxford: Oxford University Press, 1998: 1954–1981
21. Brown EM. Physiology and pathophysiology of the extracellular calcium-sensing receptor. Am J Med 1999; 106: 238–253

14

Structure and function of the lower urinary tract

Anthony R Mundy

INTRODUCTION

Before starting, the reader should be aware of certain problems in discussing the subject.

First of all, a great deal is known (relatively speaking) about the microscopic structure of the bladder, urethra and pelvic floor, but as one works back proximally through the innervation of the lower urinary tract to the spinal cord and up to the brain, and as one turns more from structure to function, so knowledge of the subject becomes exponentially less.

Secondly, much of the published research on the lower urinary tract has been done on animals other than humans and there are considerable species differences that make interpretation of such work very difficult.

Thirdly, in the same vein, many of the experimental studies have been done after neuronal ablation or otherwise in circumstances that are very far from physiological. Extrapolation from ablative pathophysiology in experimental animals to normal physiology in humans is also problematic.

Fourthly, many experimental studies have been based on the identification of receptors for neurotransmitters, or on the demonstration by radioimmunoassay of the presence of neurotransmitters themselves or have attempted to infer the presence of a physiologically significant mechanism from the presence of one component of a presumed 'reflex arc'. One or two examples will show the fallacy of such an extrapolation. Firstly, one of the most significant medical advances in recent years has been in the development of beta adrenergic receptor-active drugs for the treatment of bronchospasm, but there is no significant beta sympathetic innervation to the human lung. Receptors are present that may be therapeutically manipulated, but they have no apparent physiological significance. Secondly, and more obviously, 'receptors' can be identified in human platelets but no one imagines that platelets have an innervation.

Finally, it should be appreciated that just because a reflex mechanism exists does not mean that that mechanism is active, let alone important in normal circumstances. Thus, a reflex may be present or elicitable or evident in disease, but it does not necessarily mean that it is active or important in health.

These various points should be borne in mind when reading about studies of the structure and function of the lower urinary tract. Equally, it is hoped that the reader will forgive the author for the speculation that will creep in to provide a reasonably smooth narrative when substance is lacking.

The discussion begins distally in the bladder and urethra and then moves proximally, considering structure first and function second but integrating both as far as possible.

THE STRUCTURE OF THE BLADDER AND URETHRA

The bladder consists of three layers: an epithelial layer, a muscular layer and an adventitial layer, which on its posterior aspect is covered with peritoneum. The adventitial layer is circumscribed by two fascial layers – the first on the anterior and lateral aspect of the bladder and the second on the dome and posterior aspect of the bladder – the two fusing together anteriorly and laterally to form what Uhlenhuth[1] described as the superior hypogastric wing (Figure 14.1), which runs laterally to the external iliac vessels and anteriorly on to the anterior abdominal wall, ensheathing the medial umbilical ligaments and the urachus. The same two layers form the anterior layer of the sheath around the ureters and the superior and inferior vesical vessels posterolaterally in what Uhlenhuth described as the inferior hypogastric wing (Figure 14.2). Posteriorly, the sheet of fascia that covers the dome and posterolateral aspect of the bladder sweeps back onto the posterolateral pelvic side wall and to ensheath the rectum as Uhlenhuth's presacral fascia (Figure 14.3). These fascial layers and the neurovascular structures that they ensheath hold the bladder in place, as does the

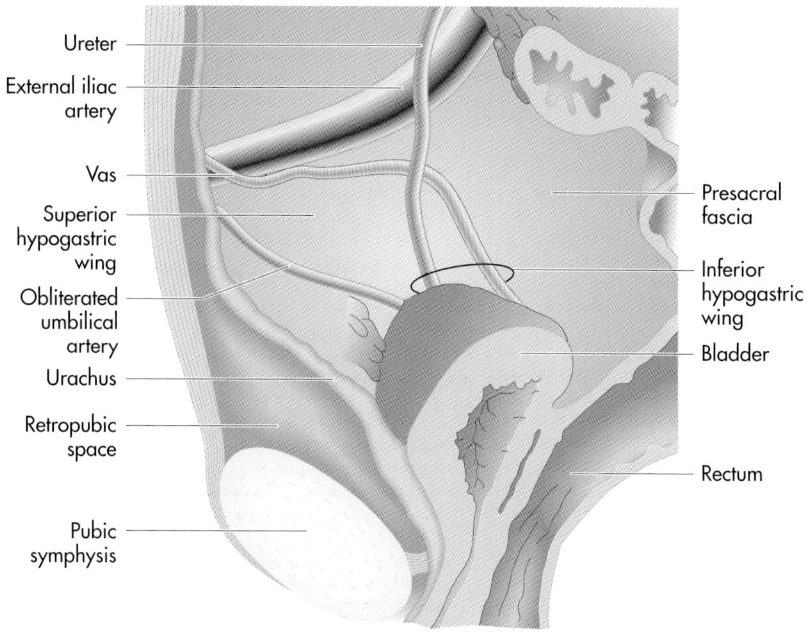

Figure 14.1 *Diagram of the distribution of pelvic fascia to show the superior hypogastric wing. (Reproduced with permission from Mundy AR. Urodynamic and Reconstructive Surgery of the Lower Urinary Tract. Edinburgh: Churchill Livingstone, 1993.)*

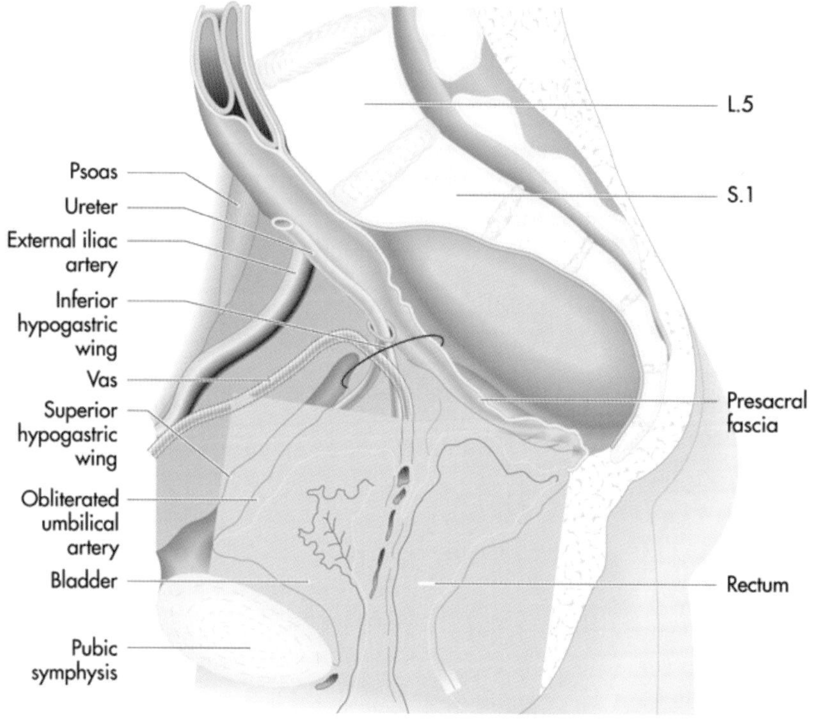

Figure 14.2a *Diagram of the pelvic fascia to show the inferior hypogastric wing. (Reproduced with permission from Mundy AR. Urodynamic and Reconstructive Surgery of the Lower Urinary Tract. Edinburgh: Churchill Livingstone, 1993.)*

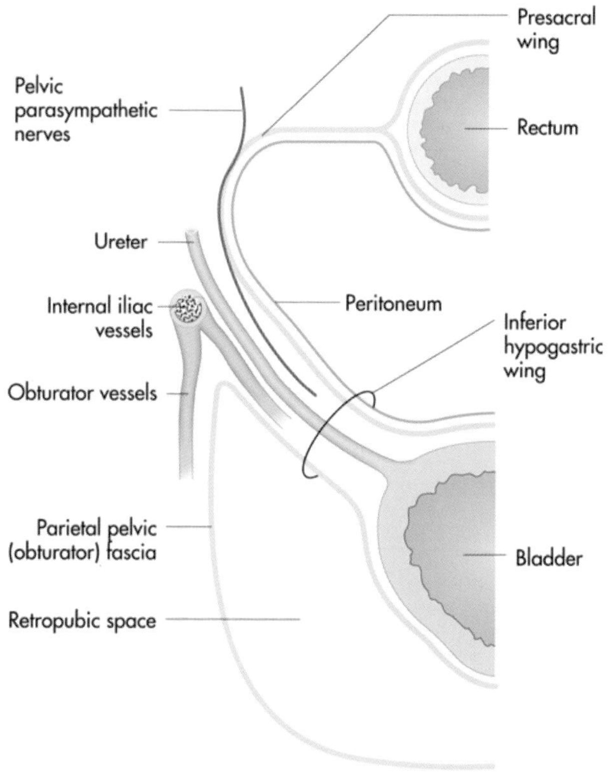

Figure 14.2b *Cross-section of the inferior hypogastric wing to show its structure, origin, disposition and contents. (Reproduced with permission from Mundy AR. Urodynamic and Reconstructive Surgery of the Lower Urinary Tract. Edinburgh: Churchill Livingstone, 1993.)*

urethra, and the prostate in males, with which the bladder is continuous. The urethra and prostate have their attachments too, notably the endopelvic fascia, which tethers them to the pelvic side wall and the periurethral component of the levator ani muscle in males (it is vestigial in females) and the posterior vaginal wall in females, to which the female urethra is intimately related (Figure 14.4).

There are other supporting structures that are thought to be important in lower urinary tract function, particularly in the female.

First and foremost, in the female, are the pubo-urethral ligaments, which sling the full length of the urethra but particularly the proximal urethra from the inferior pubic area (Figure 14.5). These have been particularly studied by Zacharin[2] and his findings have since been confirmed by others, and all of these authors have sought somehow to link a deficiency in these ligaments to the genesis of stress incontinence.

The homologous structures in the male are the puboprostatic ligaments, which have become of particular interest since the development by Walsh[3] of his technique of radical retropubic prostatectomy.

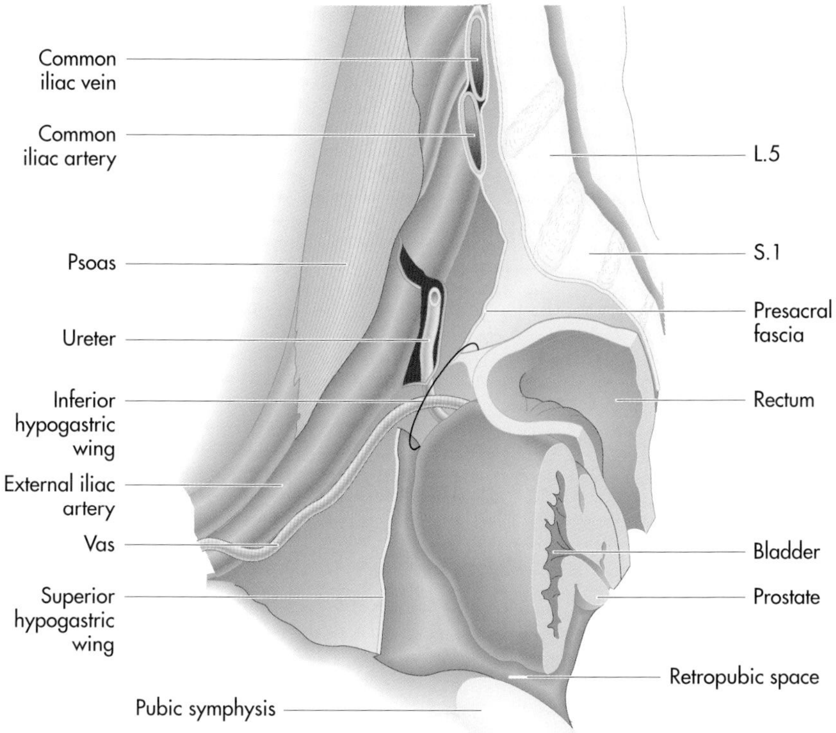

Figure 14.3 *Diagram of the pelvic fascia to show the distribution of the presacral fascia. (Reproduced with permission from Mundy AR. Urodynamic and Reconstructive Surgery of the Lower Urinary Tract. Edinburgh: Churchill Livingstone, 1993.)*

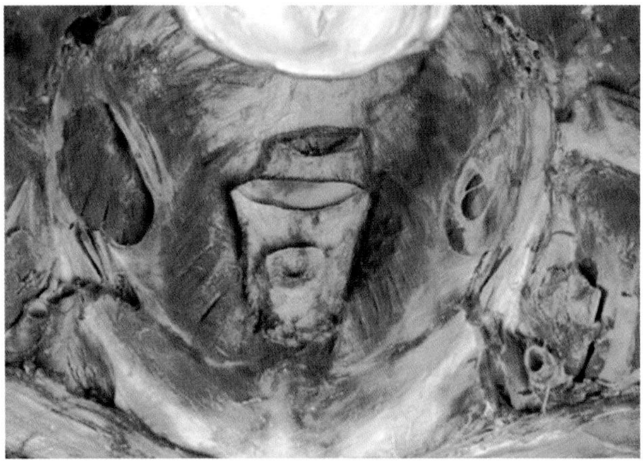

Figure 14.4a *The relationship of the urethra to the anterior vaginal wall. (Reproduced with permission from Gosling JA, Dixon JS, Humpherson JR. The Functional Anatomy of the Urinary Tract. Edinburgh: Churchill Livingstone, 1983.)*

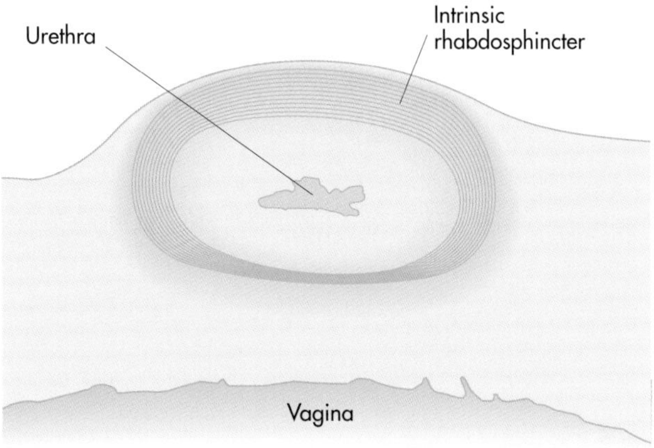

Figure 14.4b *Cross-section to show the integration of the urethra, below the bladder neck within the anterior vaginal wall. (Reproduced with permission from Mundy AR. Urodynamic and Reconstructive Surgery of the Lower Urinary Tract. Edinburgh: Churchill Livingstone, 1993.)*

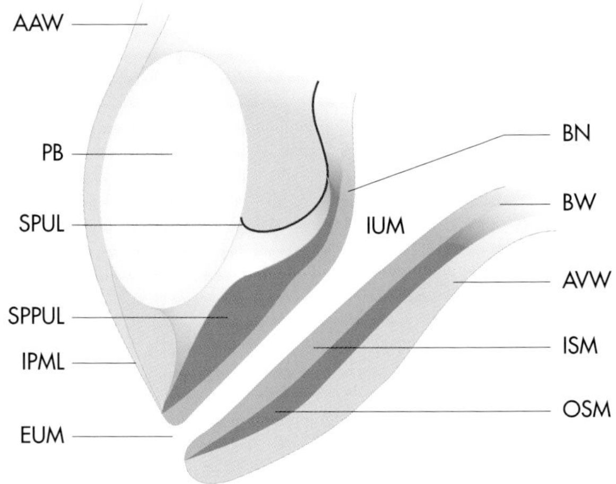

Figure 14.5 *The orientation of the pubourethral ligaments. AAW = anterior abdominal wall; PB = pubic bone; BN = bladder neck; BW = bladder wall; AVW = anterior vaginal wall; ISM = inner smooth muscle; OSM = outer striated muscle; IUM = internal urinary meatus; EUM = external urinary meatus; SPUL = superior pubourethral ligament; SPPUL = subpubic pubourethral ligament; IPML = inferior pubomeatal ligament. (Reproduced with permission from Chilton CP. The urethra. In: Webster G, Kirby R, Goldwasser B, King L, eds. Reconstructive Urology. Cambridge, MA: Blackwell Scientific Publications, 1993.)*

One supporting structure identified in the anatomical and more traditional urological literature, the existence of which is now disputed, is the so-called urogenital diaphragm. Described as the layer upon which the prostate sits,[4] it has proved elusive to others[5] and probably does not exist as a separate entity.

The urothelial layer is a multilayered transitional epithelium that is continuous with the ureters above and the prostatic urethra below. Under the light microscope, the urothelium is similar in the bladder and the prostatic urethra, but there are differences on scanning electron microscopy that become more marked the further one proceeds down the urethra towards the bulbar segment where it changes to a columnar epithelium. The urothelium has numerous so-called tight junctions (see Chapter 1), which make it impermeable to fluids and solutes. This relative impermability should not be taken to mean that the urothelium is inert. Indeed, various drugs can be absorbed from the bladder and instilled intravesically. In addition, the urothelium may have a sensory role. Various sensory nerves have been recognized in the subepithelium which have been presumed to act as touch receptors and chemoreceptors. There may also be cells in the epithelium sensitive to hydrostatic pressure which may have an important role in continence and voiding.

The smooth muscle of the bladder, which accounts for most of the thickness of the bladder wall, is called the detrusor layer. There have been various attempts to identify specific bundles of muscle within the bladder wall,[6] largely in order to substantiate a hypothetical mechanism to account for the opening of the bladder neck at the initiation of voiding, but there is no good evidence that such layering exists.[7] The bladder should be considered as a single homogeneous layer of relatively large muscle bundles in a relatively small amount of connective tissue. These muscle bundles have no particular orientation (Figure 14.6). As one approaches the bladder base from above down, there is the triangular region of the trigone between the two ureters and the internal urinary meatus, where there is a flimsy additional superficial layer of smooth muscle quite separate from the underlying smooth muscle, which is typical detrusor. This additional trigonal layer is derived from the ureters and shows several distinct characteristics. The muscle fibres form bundles that are much smaller with a higher connective tissue component and a fairly dense adrenergic innervation[8] (Figure 14.7). The trigonal muscle was once thought also to have a role in opening the bladder neck, but this too has not been substantiated. As one approaches closer to the bladder neck, the disposition and orientation of the detrusor change uniformly around it. The muscle bundles get smaller, there is a relatively greater amount of connective tissue, and the orientation of the muscle bundles becomes more uniform, to loop obliquely around the bladder neck (Figure 14.8).

Below the bladder neck in both sexes, the muscle bundles continue to be relatively small in size and interspersed with a relatively larger connective tissue component and they continue to show an oblique looping arrangement around the urethra. The vascular component of the wall increases by comparison with the bladder, particularly in females.[9] In the male, the prostate forms an additional component at this level, and at the upper part, where the prostate and the bladder neck merge, there is the pre-prostatic sphincter in which adrenergically innervated smooth muscle bundles form a distinct sphincter around the urethra to prevent retrograde ejaculation (Figure 14.9).[8] It should be emphasized that this adrenergically innervated smooth muscle component – the pre-prostatic sphincter – which is present in males

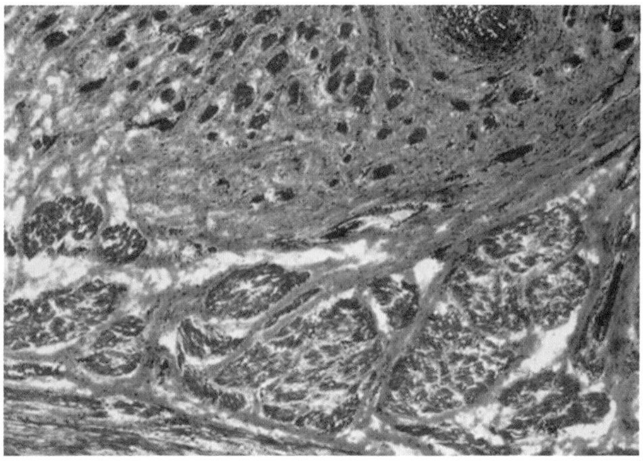

Figure 14.7a *Low-power microscopy of the detrusor stained with Masson's trichrome to show the distribution of the smooth muscle bundles in relation to the trigone superficially, compared with the detrusor proper, more deeply. (Reproduced with permission from Gosling JA, Dixon JS, Humpherson JR. The Functional Anatomy of the Urinary Tract. Edinburgh: Churchill Livingstone, 1983.)*

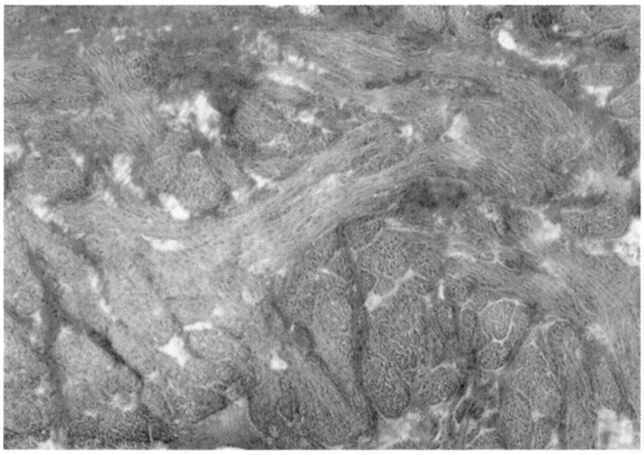

Figure 14.6 *Low-power microscopy of the detrusor stained with Masson's trichrome to show the orientation of the smooth muscle bundles. (Reproduced with permission from Gosling JA, Dixon JS, Humpherson JR. The Functional Anatomy of the Urinary Tract. Edinburgh: Churchill Livingstone, 1983.)*

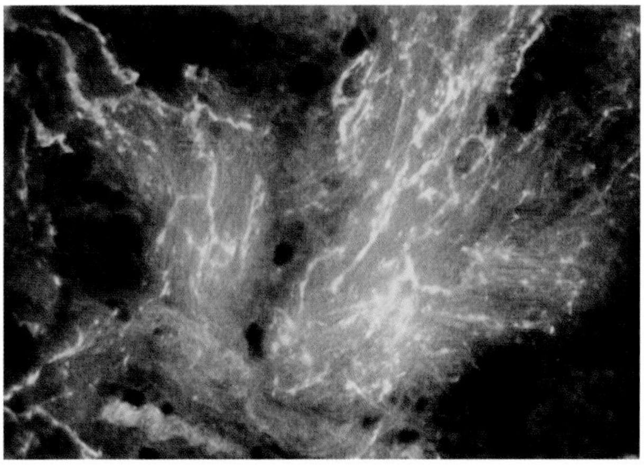

Figure 14.7b *Immunofluorescent microscopy study to show the presence of adrenergic nerves in the trigone. (Reproduced with permission from Gosling JA, Dixon JS, Humpherson JR. The Functional Anatomy of the Urinary Tract. Edinburgh: Churchill Livingstone, 1983.)*

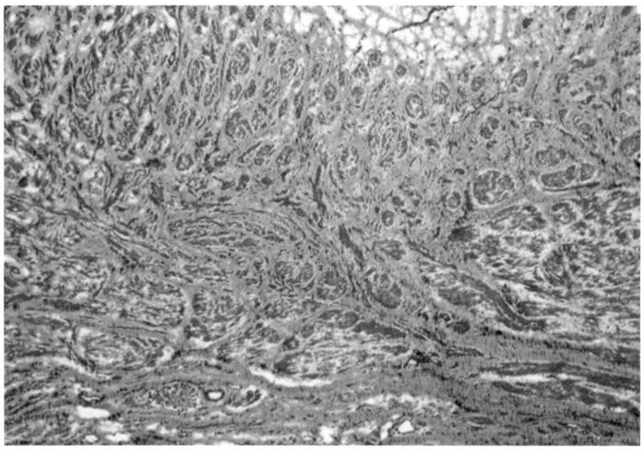

Figure 14.8a *Low-power microscopy of the detrusor stained with Masson's trichrome to show the distribution of the smooth muscle bundles at the bladder neck. (Reproduced with permission from Gosling JA, Dixon JS, Humpherson JR. The Functional Anatomy of the Urinary Tract. Edinburgh: Churchill Livingstone, 1983.)*

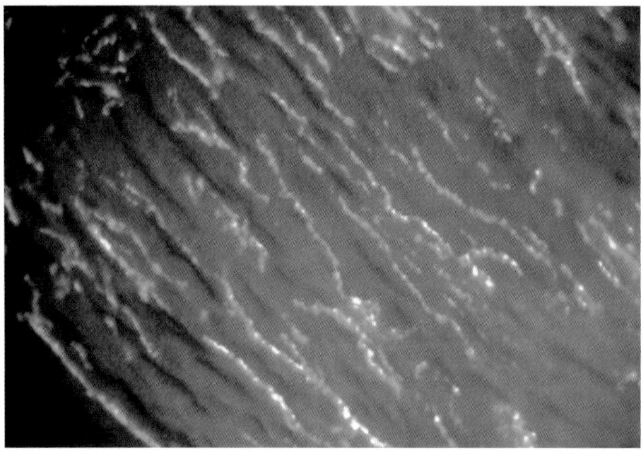

Figure 14.8b *Immunofluorescent microscopy to show the presence of adrenergic nerve fibres in the bladder neck. (Reproduced with permission from Gosling JA, Dixon JS, Humpherson JR. The Functional Anatomy of the Urinary Tract. Edinburgh: Churchill Livingstone, 1983.)*

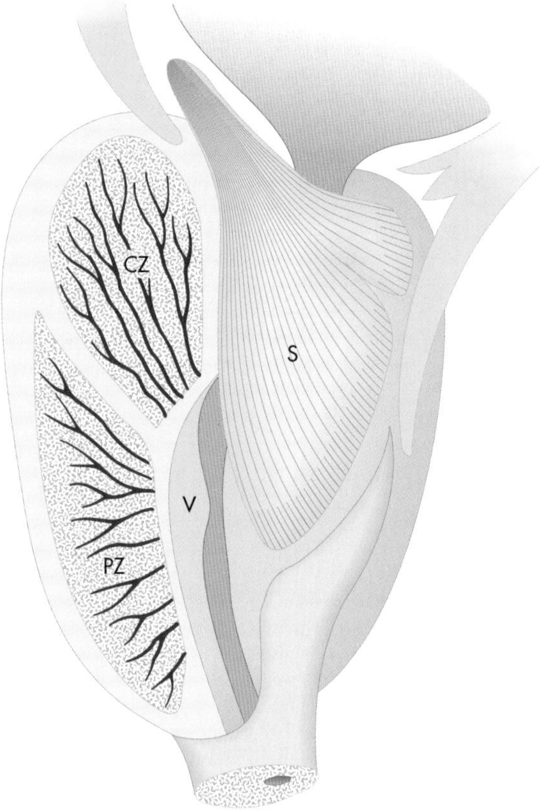

Figure 14.9 *A diagram to show the pre-prostatic sphincter. CZ = central zone; PZ = peripheral zone; S = pre-prostatic sphincter; V = verumontanum.*

but not in females, is a genital sphincter and not the bladder neck urinary sphincter mechanism in the strict sense, which is presumably the same in both sexes.

The pre-prostatic sphincter and the trigone are the only areas to show a distinct adrenergic innervation; otherwise the only adrenergic neurons in the bladder are those that supply the blood vessels.[8] This is not to say that there are not adrenergic receptors present; indeed, there are alpha receptors in the bladder base and beta receptors elsewhere in the bladder dome,[10] but there is no evidence that there is a functionally important innervation to these receptors in the normal individual. Further down the urethra at the apex of the prostate in males and in the mid-urethra in females, there is the urethral sphincter mechanism, sometimes called the 'distal sphincter mechanism' to distinguish it from the proximal sphincter mechanism, which is the other name for the bladder neck. Whereas there is a readily identifiable sphincter mechanism in the 'sphincter active' area of the urethra in both sexes, there is no anatomically identifiable sphincter mechanism at the bladder neck in either sex (using the term 'bladder neck' in its strictest sense – as distinct from the pre-prostatic sphincter). The urethral sphincter mechanism has three components (Figure 14.10). The innermost is the urethral smooth muscle and the middle layer is the striated muscle component within the urethral wall. These two components within the urethral wall itself are separated from the third component, which is the periurethral component of

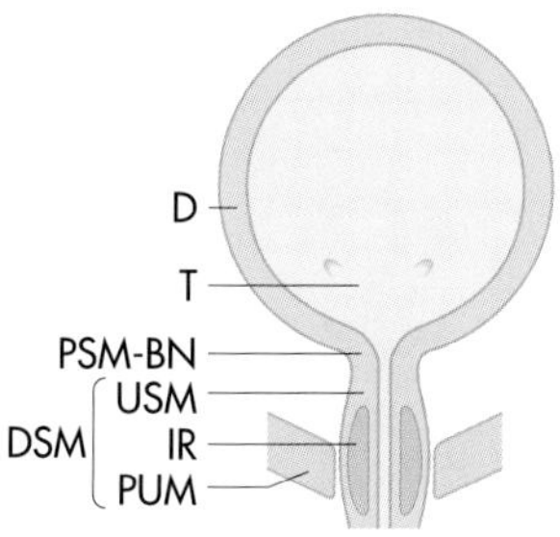

Figure 14.10 *Diagrammatic representation of the components of the urethral sphincter mechanism. D = detrusor; T = trigone; PSM-BN = proximal sphincter mechanism-bladder neck; DSM = distal sphincter mechanism; USM = urethral smooth muscle; IR = intrinsic rhabdosphincter; PUM = peri-urethral musculature.*

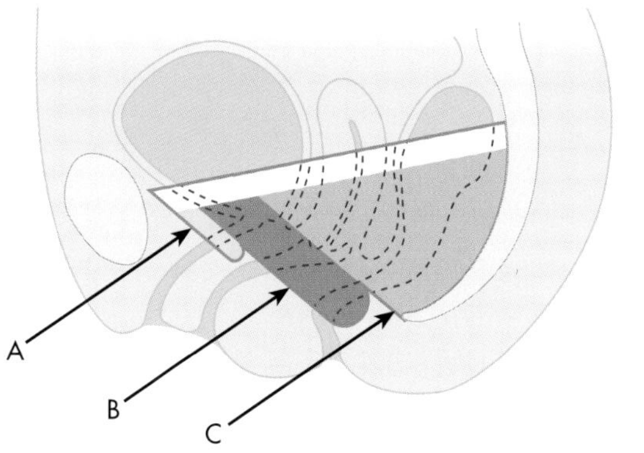

Figure 14.11 *Illustration of the various components of levator ani showing separate sling and diaphragmatic components. A = pubo-urethral sling; B = pubo-rectal sling; C = levator diaphragm.*

the levator ani, or pubouretheral sling, which is slung around the urethra in much the same way as the puborectal sling is disposed round the rectum.[11] These two sling components, the pubourethral and the puborectal slings, are distinct from and below the diaphragmatic layer of the levator ani (Figure 14.11).[12] They both form substantial components of their respective sphincter mechanisms and they share several common features.

THE URETHRAL SPHINCTER MECHANISM

Of the three layers of the urethral sphincter mechanism, two are relatively quickly dealt with. The outermost layer – the pubourethral sling – is the levator ani component most closely related to the urethra;[11] it is typical striated muscle; it has typical striated muscle innervation; it is relatively insignificant in the female compared to the male because of the presence of the vagina; and it is activated along with the rest of the levator ani under 'stress conditions', acting specifically on the urethra at such times to augment urethral occlusion pressure.

The urethral smooth muscle is dealt with relatively quickly for an entirely different reason: we know very little about its function. The innervation is more complicated than the detrusor with both excitatory and inhibitory innervation. Small ganglia, smaller than in and around the bladder, are present, and both acetylcholine and noradrenaline (norepinephrine) mediate contraction. The sympathetic innervation involves a distinct subtype of the alpha 1 adrenoceptor in the male, particularly in the prostatic urethra, which has particular implications for the treatment of bladder outflow obstruction due to benign prostatic hyperplasia as described in Chapter 15.

When the striated muscle of the urethral sphincter mechanism is paralysed, the urethral smooth muscle continues to produce a high-pressure zone, which suggests that it is tonically active[12] – whereas the bladder smooth muscle is phasically active – and recent experimental studies suggest that this tonic smooth muscle contraction may be relaxed by nitric oxide.[13,14] Indeed, there are both ganglia and nerves innervating the urethral smooth muscle which contain nitric oxide synthase. The current opinion is that this nitric oxide-related relaxant mechanism in this area of the urethra and bladder neck opening, and urethral relaxation that occurs when the bladder contracts at the onset of voiding.

It appears that it is the striated muscle component within the urethral wall that is the most important component for continence. It is sometimes called the intrinsic rhabdosphincter.[8] This striated muscle is unusual in a number of ways.[8] It is orientated predominantly anteriorly in both the vertical and horizontal planes and is relatively deficient posteriorly, giving it, overall, a signet ring distribution (Figure 14.12). This is clearly seen microscopically in both sexes (Figure 14.13). The reason for this is not clear, but it is common experience that the easiest way of stopping water flowing through a hosepipe is to kink it rather than to squeeze it circumferentially. It may

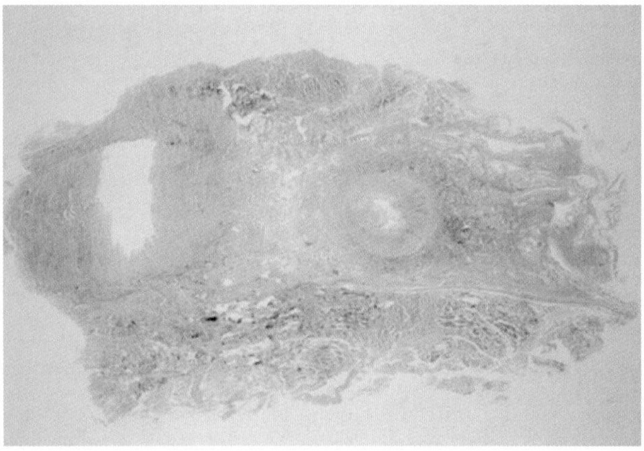

Figure 14.12 *Low-power microscopy of a transverse section of the male sphincter-active urethra to show the 'signet ring' distribution of the intrinsic rhabdosphincter. (Anterior to the right of the figure.)*

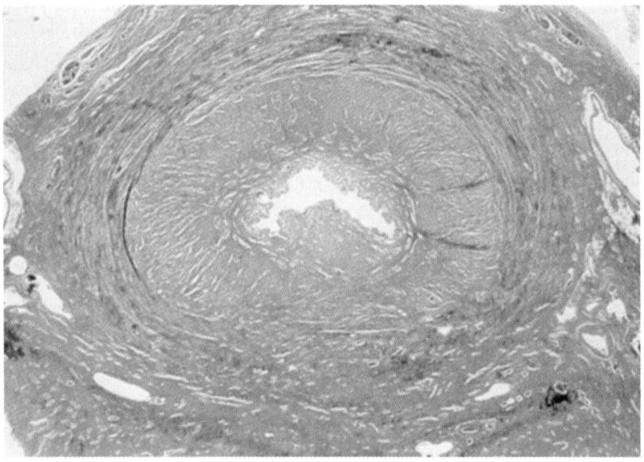

Figure 14.13 *Low-power microscopy of a transverse section of the female sphincter-active urethra to show the 'signet ring' distribution of the intrinsic rhabdosphincter. (Anterior to the top of the figure.)*

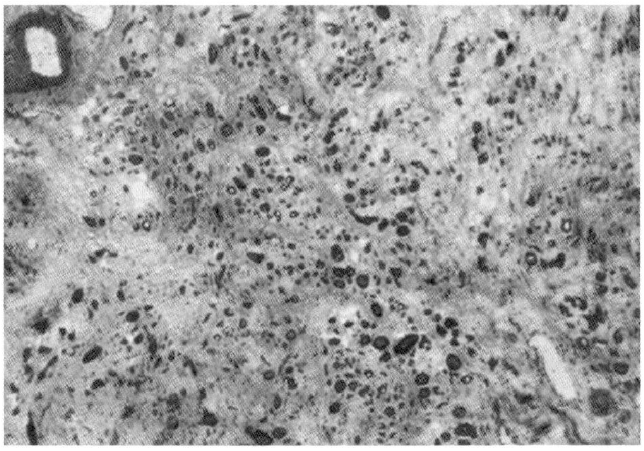

Figure 14.14 *Low-power microscopy of the intrinsic rhabdosphincter to show the relative distribution of muscle bundles and connective tissue. (Reproduced with permission from Gosling JA, Dixon JS, Humpherson JR. The Functional Anatomy of the Urinary Tract. Edinburgh: Churchill Livingstone, 1983.)*

be that the distribution of the fibres of the intrinsic striated muscle of the urethra produces a kinking rather than a circumferential compression when it contracts, for this sort of reason, but this is entirely conjectural. This intrinsic striated muscle sphincter is composed of relatively very small muscle fibres when compared with typical striated muscle; the fibres themselves are disposed in small muscle bundles within a very much greater connective tissue component than is seen in typical striated muscle (Figure 14.14); the muscle fibres themselves are stuffed with mitochondria; there are no muscle spindles; and there are several distinct histochemical staining characteristics of these muscle fibres, most notably a uniform staining with acid-stable myosin adenosine triphosphatase (ATPase) (Figure 14.15).[15] By contrast, the typical striated muscle of the pubourethral sling that is immediately adjacent to the intrinsic rhabdosphincter shows larger muscle fibres in larger muscle bundles, with little connective tissue, fewer mitochondria, muscle spindles present and a mixed pattern of staining for acid-stable myosin ATPase (Figure 14.16). Furthermore, whereas the nerve supply to the levator ani originates in typical cell bodies in the motor cell nuclei of the anterior horn of the sacral spinal cord, the cell bodies of the fibres that innervate the intrinsic rhabdosphincter appear to arise in a nucleus more medially situated in the sacral anterior horn, as do the fibres innervating the anal sphincter mechanism, and this spinal cord nucleus is known as spinal nucleus X, sometimes called Onuf's nucleus (Figure 14.17).[16] The fibres from Onuf's nucleus to the intrinsic rhabdosphincter run out of the anterior primary rami and the nerve fibres run initially with the nervi erigentes, which are the preganglionic parasympathetic neurons. They run with these fibres through the pelvic plexuses and down with the postganglionic parasympathetic neurons into the urethra.[8]

Whether this is the sole innervation of the intrinsic rhabdosphincter or whether there is a separate component arising from the pudendal nerve is not clear,[17] but after pudendal neurectomy or pudendal

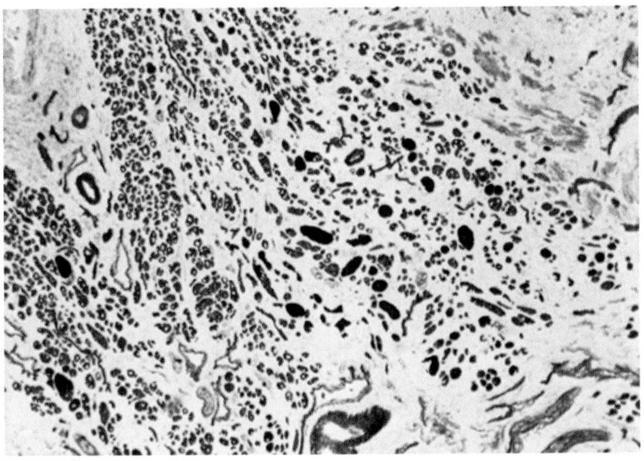

Figure 14.15 *Low-power histochemistry of the intrinsic rhabdosphincter to show the distribution of acid-stable myosin ATPase. (Reproduced with permission from Gosling JA, Dixon JS, Humpherson JR. The Functional Anatomy of the Urinary Tract. Edinburgh: Churchill Livingstone, 1983.)*

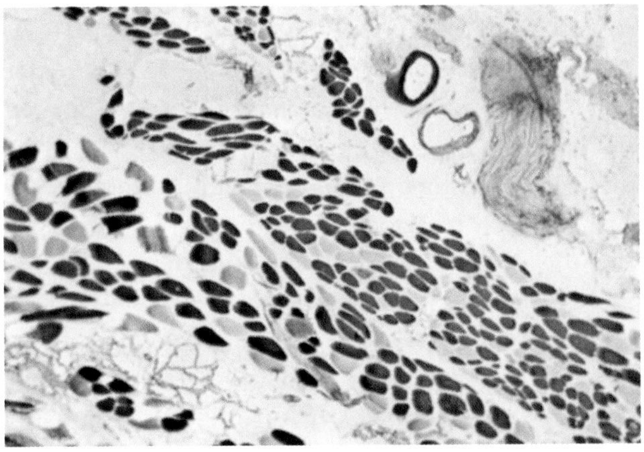

Figure 14.16 *Low-power histochemistry of the typical striated muscle, in this case the pubourethral sling, to show the distribution of acid-stable myosin ATPase. (Reproduced with permission from Gosling JA, Dixon JS, Humpherson JR. The Functional Anatomy of the Urinary Tract. Edinburgh: Churchill Livingstone, 1983.)*

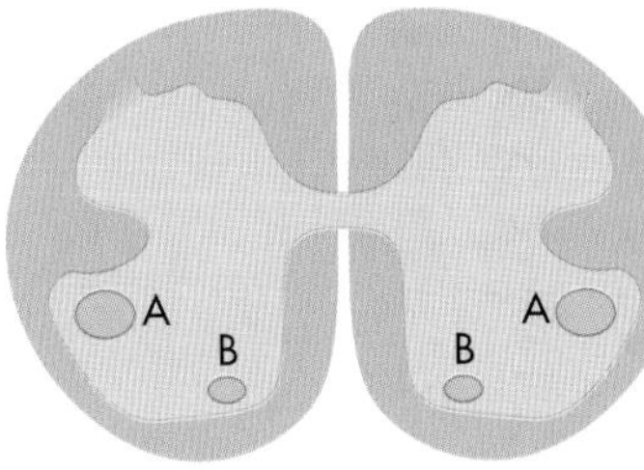

Figure 14.17 *Diagram to show the separate origin of the innervation of the intrinsic rhabdosphincter from Onuf's nucleus as distinct from the site of origin of typical striated msucle from anterior horn cells. A = α motorneuron group; B = Onuf's nucleus.*

nerve blockade, the urethral sphincter mechanism is intact so there is clearly a source other than the pudendal nerve.

These characteristics of the intrinsic rhabdosphincter are very unusual but not unique; the intrinsic laryngeal muscles are very similar in structure and in the nature of their innervation.

THE INNERVATION OF THE BLADDER AND URETHRA

Four separate neuronal pathways to the lower urinary tract have been alluded to (Figure 14.18). The principal one is derived from cell bodies in the intermediolateral column of the second, third and fourth sacral segments of the spinal cord. These are preganglionic parasympathetic fibres that run out of the anterior primary rami of S2, S3 and S4 and then separate out from the somatic component which runs to the sacral plexus, to run as the nervi erigentes to the pelvic plexuses. These preganglionic parasympathetic neurons end by synapsing in ganglia on the cell bodies of

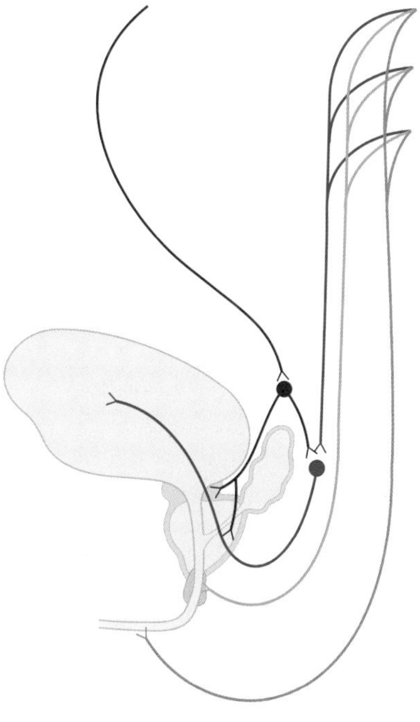

Figure 14.18 *Diagram to show the four components of innervation of the lower urinary tract. (—) Sympathetic; (—) parasympathetic; (—) somatic innervation of intrinsic rhabdosphincter; (—) pudendal nerve. (Reproduced with permission from Gosling JA, Dixon JS, Humpherson JR. The Functional Anatomy of the Urinary Tract. Edinburgh: Churchill Livingstone, 1983.)*

the postganglionic parasympathetic nerves, which then run to the bladder and to the urethra (and more proximally to the rectum and the genital structures). In humans, 50% of the ganglia of the pelvic plexus are in the adventitial tissue around the base and posterolateral aspects of the bladder and 50% are within the bladder wall itself.[8] For this reason it is, strictly speaking, technically impossible to denervate the bladder because the 50% within the bladder wall itself will still remain and there will therefore still be reflex activity, even if this is not physiologically significant. A more semantically correct term would therefore be 'decentralization' rather than 'denervation' when discussing the stripping of the nerves from around the outside of the bladder.

The somatic nerve fibres that arise from Onuf's nucleus and that travel with the otherwise autonomic parasympathetic nerve fibres of the nervi erigentes and pass ultimately to the intrinsic rhabdosphincter have already been mentioned.

The third component is the sympathetic nerve component that arises from the intermediatolateral column of the 10th, 11th and 12th thoracic and the 1st and 2nd lumbar segments of the spinal cord. These preganglionic sympathetic fibres and their postganglionic sympathetic derivatives travel as the hypogastric nerves, which innervate the trigone, the blood vessels of the bladder and the smooth muscle of the prostate in males, including the pre-prostatic sphincter. They also have postganglionic branches that end in the parasympathetic ganglia,[8] where they exert an inhibitory effect that is described in detail below.

Finally, there is the pudendal nerve component, also arising from S2, S3 and S4, in this instance from typical anterior horn motor neuron cell bodies, which innervates the urethra and the pelvic floor musculature and provides afferent innervation to the urethra.

By comparison with typical anatomical 'nerves' such as the obturator nerve, the femoral nerve and even the sciatic nerve, the total mass of the autonomic nerves in the pelvis is large. The autonomic nerves are not as discrete and easily identifiable as the somatic nerves referred to, disposed as they are as a sheet within the fascial layers that invest the rectum, the genital structures and the lower urinary tract, but if the nerve fibres are dissected out and considered as a whole, their volume is considerable. It is this sheer mass that protects pelvic autonomic function from extensive damage during pelvic surgery such as hysterectomy or rectal resection, but they are nonetheless vulnerable to traction injuries during such procedures,[18] as of course they are in females during childbirth.

Functional aspects of the innervation of the bladder and urethra

Cholinergic nerves cannot be stained directly for microscopical study – only indirectly by staining for acetylcholinesterase, the enzyme that breaks down acetylcholine at the neuromuscular junction. Staining for acetylcholinesterase shows a dense 'presumptive-cholinergic' innervation of the detrusor smooth muscle (Figure 14.19) with a nerve to muscle cell ratio of about 1:1, and a less dense cholinergic innervation of the urethral smooth muscle.[8] Under the electron microscope, the terminal branches of the parasympathetic neurons within the bladder wall are seen to contain varicosities (Figure 14.20). These varicosities are there because of the presence of numerous vesicles within the terminal neuron at that point and these vesicles contain neurotransmitter substances. Alongside the varicosity is the

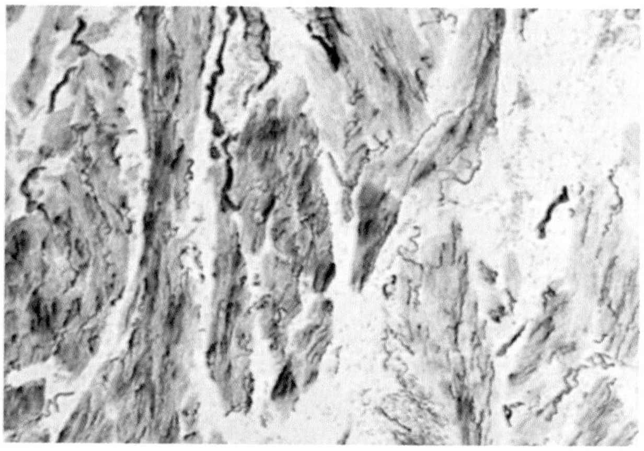

Figure 14.19 *Low-power microscopy of the muscle wall after staining with acetylcholinesterase to show the distribution of presumptive cholinergic nerves in the bladder wall. (Reproduced with permission from Gosling JA, Dixon JS, Humpherson JR. The Functional Anatomy of the Urinary Tract. Edinburgh: Churchill Livingstone, 1983.)*

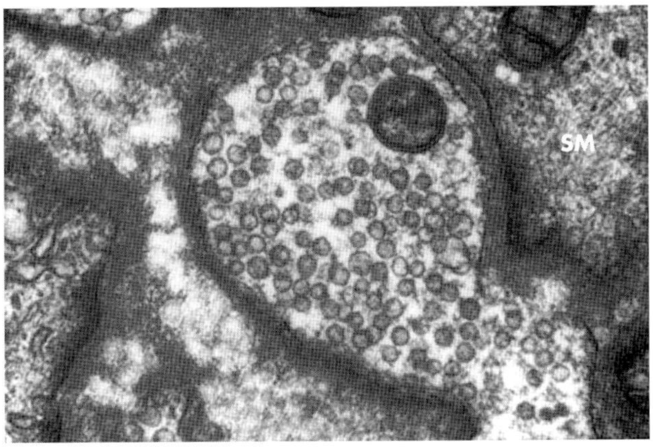

Figure 14.20 *Electron microscopy of a terminal neuron within the detrusor smooth muscle layer to show a varicosity containing small clear vesicles containing acetylcholine. (Reproduced with permission from Gosling JA, Dixon JS. Anatomy of the bladder, urethra and pelvic floor. In: Mundy AR, Stephenson TP, Wein AJ, eds. Urodynamics – Principles, Practice and Application. Edinburgh: Churchill Livingstone, 1984.)*

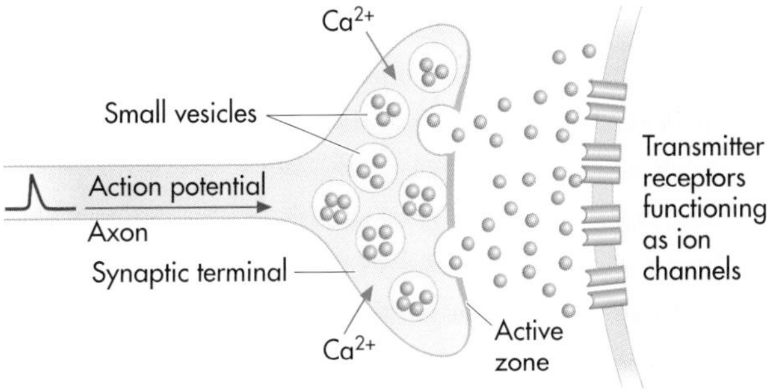

Figure 14.21 *Diagram of a nerve ending and neuromuscular junction to show the release of 'fast' neurotransmitters into the neuromuscular junction. (Reproduced with permission from Goodman SR. Medical Cell Biology. Philadelphia: JB Lippincott, 1994.)*

specialized area of the smooth muscle that constitutes the receptor site, although this is not very specialized by comparison with the receptor site – the neuromuscular junction – in striated muscle. Adjacent smooth muscle cells are connected by so-called 'regions of close approach', like gap junctions in effect, which could, at least theoretically, allow electrotonic spread of activity from one smooth muscle cell to the next and which thereby confer so-called 'cable properties' on the smooth muscle fibres. This would supplement the spreading neuronal stimulus as a sort of 'parallel pathway', and help to ensure a uniform simultaneous contraction of all the bladder smooth muscle cells at the time of voiding.

Vesicles are of two main types:[19] small clear vesicles and larger vesicles with a dense core. The small clear vesicles are thought to contain so-called 'fast' neurotransmitter substances, which are released directly into the area between the neuron and the adjacent neuron across a synapse, or the adjacent smooth muscle cell across a neuromuscular junction (Figure 14.21) to open ligand-gated ion channels on the receptor site that will initiate an action potential. Outside the central nervous system, the commonest neurotransmitter to be found in these small clear vesicles is acetylcholine and the commonest receptor is the nicotinic acetylcholine receptor, although acetylcholine does not exclusively act as a fast neurotransmitter to open ligand-gated ion channels in this way. In the central nervous system, gamma-aminobutyric acid (GABA) is also found in small clear vesicles.[20]

Large, dense-cored vesicles contain so-called 'slow' neurotransmitters,[20] which are called 'slow' because they are released non-specifically from around the area of the varicosity (Figure 14.22) rather than specifically into the receptor site; and because they generally act by binding to G-protein-linked receptors (see Chapter 1) and initiating smooth muscle contraction through second messengers systems. This is so-called 'pharmacomechanical' coupling of the neuronal stimulus to smooth muscle contraction, as distinct from the 'electromechanical' coupling initiated by the binding of ligand-gated ion channels by fast neurotransmitters.

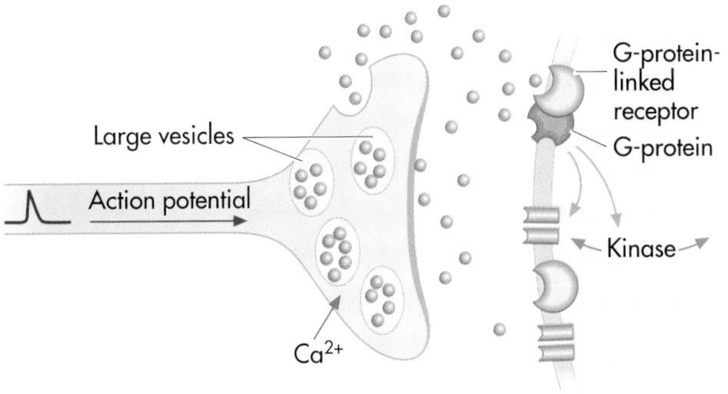

Figure 14.22 *Diagram of a nerve ending and neuromuscular junction to show the release of 'slow' neurotransmitters from around the neuromuscular junction. (Reproduced with permission from Goodman SR. Medical Cell Biology. Philadelphia: JB Lippincott, 1994.)*

A single nerve impulse will empty about half the vesicles in a varicosity, each of which will release about 5000 molecules of acetylcholine as a quantum. These vesicles empty their contents in response to a rise in cytosolic calcium within the varicosity as a result of the opening of membrane calcium channels induced by the neuronal electrical impulse (voltage-gated calcium channels), causing an influx of extracellular calcium.[21]

There are other ways of demonstrating the primacy of parasympathetic cholinergic activity in the excitatory innervation of the bladder other than by showing its density on light microscopy and electron microscopy. The most convincing way is by the physiological study of strips of detrusor smooth muscle in an organ bath (Figure 14.23). The organ bath keeps the muscle strip at the right temperature, sufficiently oxygenated and in the right fluid medium to keep it viable sufficiently long for adequate study. The excitatory nerve supply to the muscle fibres within the muscle strip is stimulated by using an electrical impulse. If the strength and amplitude are optimized and the frequency of the electrical stimulus is then varied, a frequency–response curve is produced between about 0.5 Hz and 20 Hz, above which the response rate plateaus until the electrical impulse is of sufficiently high frequency to cause damage (Figure 14.24). This response can be abolished by the application of tetrodotoxin, which is a sodium channel blocker which therefore blocks nerve conduction.[21] (Tetrodotoxin is extracted from the liver of the puffer fish – called fugu in Japan – and will be known as such to James Bond aficionados.) If a frequency–response curve is plotted after the application of tetrodotoxin, there will be a very small response at higher frequencies that is not nerve mediated but due to direct stimulation of the smooth muscle cell membrane itself. If the frequency–response curve is performed after the application of atropine at a sufficient dose to give complete cholinergic blockade, then the only response left will be the same as that after tetrodotoxin (Figure 14.25). In other words, in the normal human specimen (stressing both adjectives), there is no excitatory component left after atropine blockade and there is no 'atropine-resistant' component to excitatory neurotransmission. Normal excitatory neurotransmission in the human bladder is exclusively muscarinic cholinergic.[22–24] In other mammals, it is a completely different story. In some small mammals, there may be as much as 30% of the frequency–response curve that is atropine resistant. This is thought to be due to the presence of an alternative excitatory neurotransmitter that, in most animal species showing this type of excitatory neurotransmission, is thought to be adenosine triphosphate (ATP).[20] This is

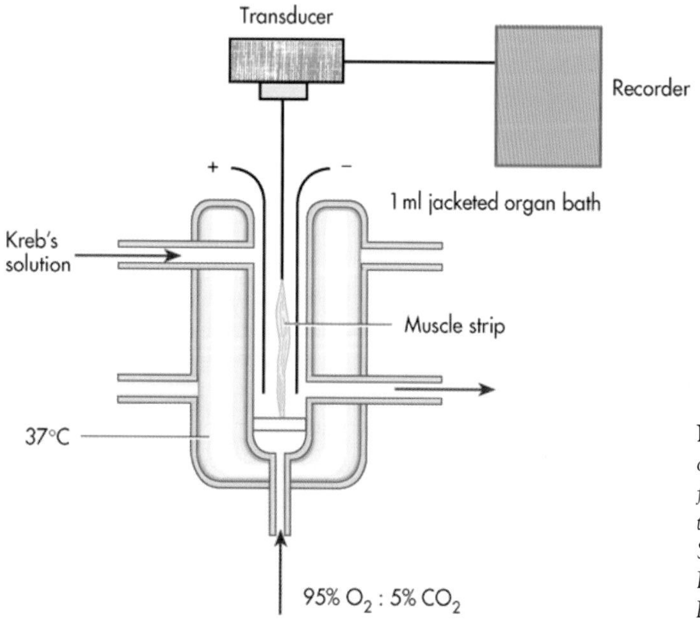

Figure 14.23 *Diagrammatic representation of an organ bath experiment. (Reproduced with permission from Mundy AR, Thomas PJ. Clinical physiology of the bladder, urethra and pelvic floor. In: Mundy AR, Stephenson TP, Wein AJ, eds. Urodynamics – Principles, Practice and Application. 2nd edn. Edinburgh: Churchill Livingstone, 1994.)*

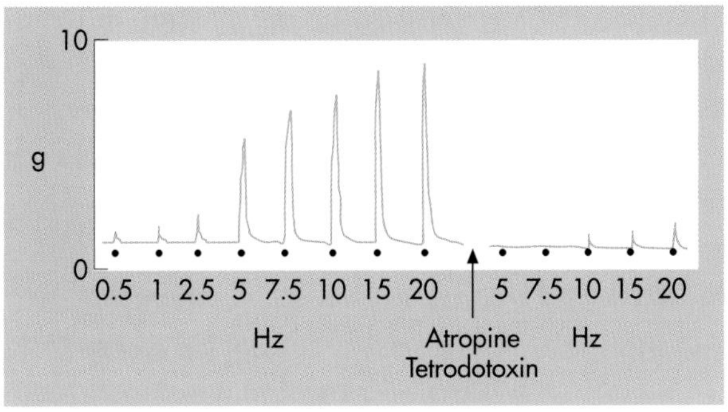

Figure 14.24 *A frequency–response curve before and after tetrodotoxin showing a very small residual contraction that is not nerve mediated and due to direct smooth muscle stimulation. (Reproduced with permission from Mundy AR, Thomas PJ. Clinical physiology of the bladder, urethra and pelvic floor. In: Mundy AR, Stephenson TP, Wein AJ, eds. Urodynamics – Principles, Practice and Application. 2nd edn. Edinburgh: Churchill Livingstone, 1994.)*

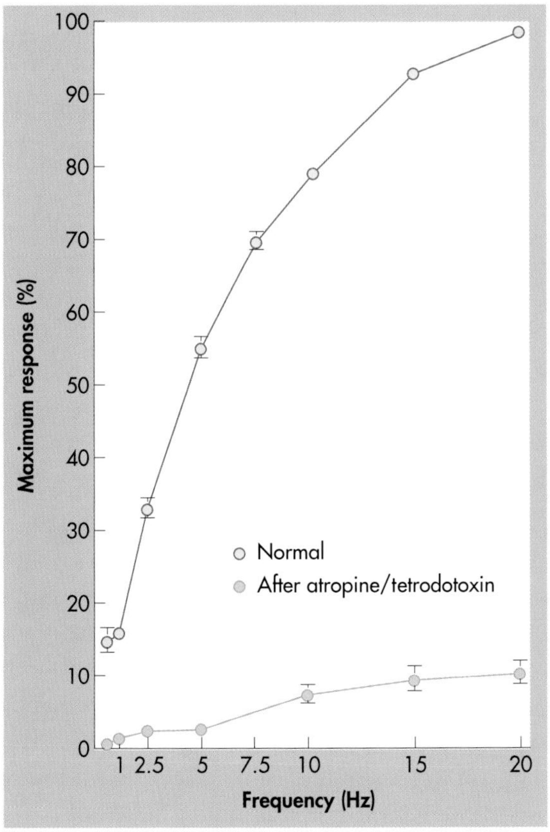

Figure 14.25 *A frequency–response curve before and after atropine in a human showing a very small residual response. In this case it is a graphical representation of the percentage response. (Modified from Mundy AR, Thomas PJ. Clinical physiology of the bladder, urethra and pelvic floor. In: Mundy AR, Stephenson TP, Wein AJ eds. Urodynamics – Principles, Practice and Application. 2nd edition. Edinburgh: Churchill Livingstone, 1994.)*

thought to give rise to the type of bladder contraction responsible for the excretion of a small amount of urine for the purposes of territorial marking. In those animals that exhibit territorial marking, it seems likely that a normal voiding detrusor contraction is cholinergic in origin, whereas the small-volume 'squirt' of urine excreted for territorial marking is under so-called purinergic (ATP-mediated) innervation.

This is not to say that ATP cannot be made to cause contraction of human detrusor smooth muscle. It has indeed been shown to do so,[21] but it does not appear to be a component of normal human voiding. It may, however, be a cause of abnormal detrusor function in detrusor instability.

Mechanisms of contraction and relaxation of the bladder and urethral smooth muscle in health and disease

This is described in detail in the next chapter.

OTHER NEUROTRANSMITTERS

To qualify as a neurotransmitter, a potential candidate must satisfy certain stringent criteria. In the last 15 years or so, numerous compounds have been identified as potential neurotransmitters, many of which fail to satisfy these criteria but nonetheless appear to be involved in the process of neurotransmission, either as neurotransmitters or as neuromodulators.[20]

A further observation is that many of these compounds seem to be related to nerves that show the characteristics of cholinergic or adrenergic neurons. In other words, the putative neurotransmitter or neuromodulator appears to be 'co-localized' with a known 'classical' transmitter or with another putative neurotransmitter.[20]

Several of these putative neurotransmitters are peptides, which have been grouped together as neuropeptides. This group includes substance P[25,26] vasoactive intestinal polypeptide[27,28] and neuropeptide Y, to name but a few. Substance P is thought to be involved in afferent neurotransmission.[26] Vasoactive intestinal polypeptide relaxes detrusor smooth muscle[27] and has been shown in some studies to be co-released with acetylcholine. Similarly, neuropeptide

Y has been co-localized in adrenergic neurons. This concept of co-localization, co-release and co-transmission is interesting as it provides a means of modifying the effects of neural activity either temporally or spatially. Thus, the same nerves could produce two transmitters with different effects, both being simultaneously released but with one predominating in one area and the other in the other area. For example, an excitatory and an inhibitory transmitter, if co-released, might cause bladder contraction if the former predominated in the bladder and relaxation of the bladder neck if the latter predominated at that site. This neuromodulatory activity could have other effects which would less dramatically act to 'fine tune' the actions of the lower urinary tract.

THE AFFERENT INNERVATION OF THE BLADDER

So far, we have mainly concentrated on the efferent innervation of the bladder. The afferent innervation is equally important, but is less well understood. Afferent impulses arise from the nerve plexus in the lamina propria immediately deep to the urothelium, from within the muscle layer itself, and, presumably, from the adventitia. Afferent nerve endings have been identified, but their nature is poorly understood.[29] Substance P and ATP are thought to be sensory neurotransmitters and there is good evidence to support this view, but again the mechanism is not well understood. Other presumptive sensory nerves have been shown to contain calcitonin gene-related peptide (CGRP) and other transmitters, including neurokinan A.[30]

Pelvic nerve afferents consist of myelinated A-delta and unmyelinated C axons. The A-delta myelinated axons arise from tension receptors in the smooth muscle of the bladder and respond to increasing muscle wall tension during bladder filling. These are the afferent neurons responsible for eliciting the so-called micturition reflex in normal healthy individuals. Most of the C-fibre unmyelinated axons arise from receptors in the sub-urothelial layer, although some nociceptors sensitive to overdistension may also be found in the muscle and adventitia. Some of the sub-urothelial receptors respond to stretching of the mucosa and thus act as bladder volume sensors. The remainder are insensitive to normal bladder distension and are referred to as 'silent afferents'.[31] These afferents are thought to become mechanosensitive when irritated or inflamed, thereby lowering the threshold of bladder contraction in such situations. It is thought that this may be due to the release of neurokinin A, which then acts on its own specialist receptor binding sites and sensory nerve endings in the sub-urothelial layer.[32]

What is clear, from the work of Nathan,[33] is that there are three types of sensation arising from the bladder (Figure 14.26). The first and most general sensation of bladder filling arises from receptors throughout the bladder. The afferent fibres run with the parasympathetic nerves back to the sacral cord, where there is some local synapsing on preganglionic parasympathetic cell bodies in the intermediolateral column of the sacral cord, but the majority of afferent neurons run in the ascending tracts of the spinal cord and up to the pons, where they synapse with preganglionic neurons in the nucleus locus coeruleus in the rostral pons. Other fibres pass up to the cerebral cortex to give rise to sensory awareness. This type of afferent stimulus gives rise to a volume-related awareness of bladder filling that is easily suppressed.

Less easily suppressed is the next type of bladder sensation, which is stimulated by definite fullness of the bladder. This is a stimulus that arises in the trigonal area and the afferent impulses are transmitted in neurons that run with the sympathetic nerves up to the thoracolumbar cord. Once again, there are local relays in the cord, but most fibres run up in the ascending tracts to the pons and to the cerebral cortex to give awareness.

Finally, there is the feeling of severe urgency and the sense that voiding is imminent. This sensation cannot be overlooked. It arises in the urethra and the afferent fibres run with the pudendal nerve, again giving rise to local relays in the sacral cord, but with most fibres running in the ascending tracts to the pons and to the cerebral cortex.

Within the spinal cord, the ascending and descending fibres all run in an equatorial plane through the spinal canal, as also shown by Nathan[34] (Figure 14.27). The medial tracts are visceral efferent, the intermediate tracts are somatic efferent to the

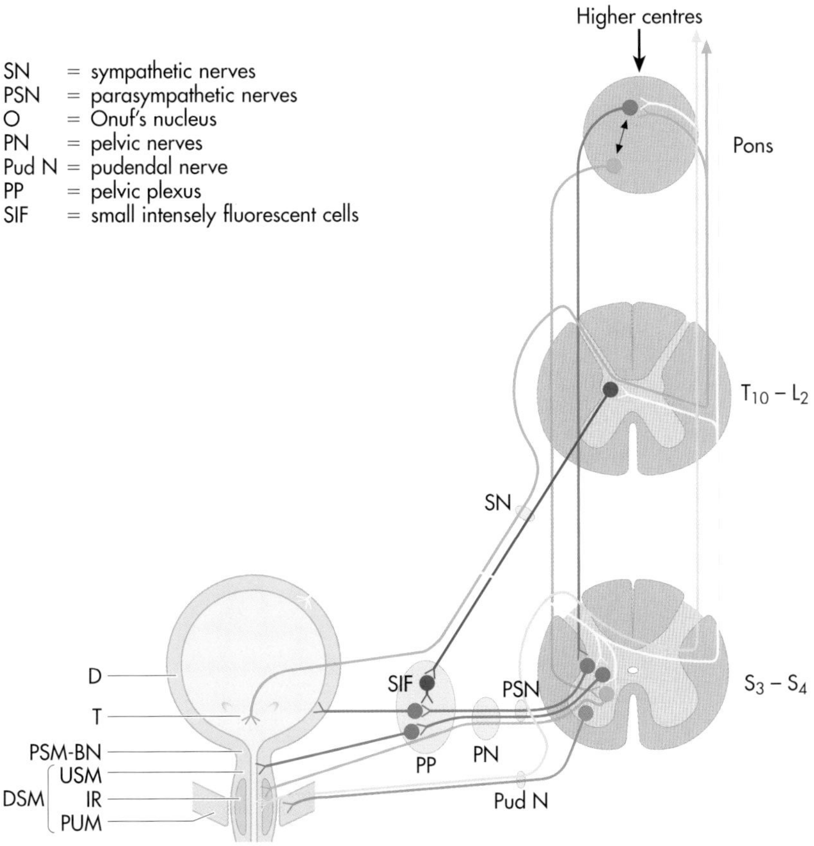

Figure 14.26 *The nervous pathways concerned with the three different types of sensation from the lower urinary tract; ( ) from the bladder, (—) from the trigone, ( ) from the urethra and pelvic floor. (Reproduced with permission from Mundy AR, Thomas PJ. Clinical physiology of the bladder, urethra and pelvic floor. In: Mundy AR, Stephenson TP, Wein AJ, eds. Urodynamics – Principles, Practice and Application. 2nd edn. Edinburgh: Churchill Livingstone, 1994.)*

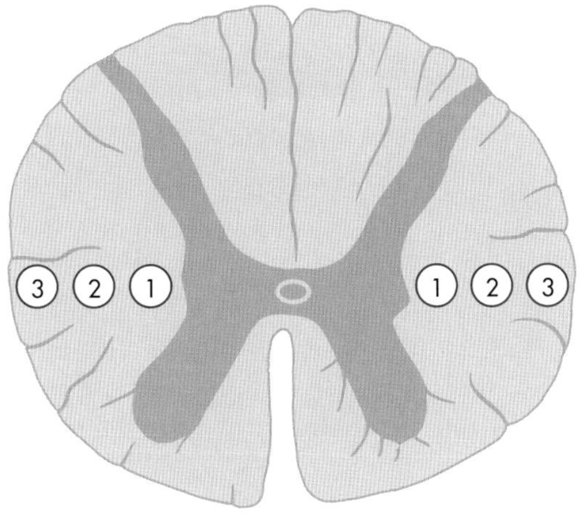

Figure 14.27 *The orientation within the spinal cord of the pathways related to lower urinary tract function. 1 = autonomic efferent; 2 = somatic efferent; 3 = afferent. (Reproduced with permission from Mundy AR, Thomas PJ. Clinical physiology of the bladder, urethra and pelvic floor. In: Mundy AR, Stephenson TP, Wein AJ, eds. Urodynamics – Principles, Practice and Application. 2nd edn. Edinburgh: Churchill Livingstone, 1994.)*

intrinsic rhabdosphincter and the pelvic floor, and the most lateral fibres lying at the periphery of the cord between the corticospinal and the spinothalamic tracts are visceral afferent. The location of these tracts in relation to the urinary tract was found by post-mortem studies of patients who had undergone the neurosurgical procedure of percutaneous cordotomy during life for relief for severe visceral pain, usually malignant in origin.

The nature of the neurotransmitters in both the afferent and efferent pathways of the spinal cord[35] is still largely unknown.[36] Glutamic acid is thought to be the principal excitatory transmitter of both the ascending and descending limbs of the micurition reflex pathway as well as in the reflex pathway controlling sphincter function at both the spinal and supra-spinal levels. Likewise, gamma amino butyric acid (GABA) is the most important inhibitory modulator. It is clear that several other substances may exert significant modulatory influences, including supraspinal cholinergic and dopaminergic influences at the supra-spinal level and adrenergic influences at the spinal level.

CEREBRAL CONTROL OF VOIDING

Within the brain, there are five areas that are concerned with continence and voiding (Figure 14.28). The first has already been alluded to – the nucleus locus coeruleus in the rostral pons where afferent nerves synapse on the cell bodies of efferent nerve fibres. There are two connections of importance at this site. The first is the synapse, by which means an adequate afferent impulse gives rise to an efferent impulse that will generate a detrusor contraction that is sufficient in amplitude and duration to cause complete bladder emptying. The second connection that occurs at this site co-ordinates this contraction with relaxation of the bladder outflow in order to given unobstructed voiding. The details of these two mechanisms and their co-ordination are unclear; it is, however, quite clear that this is the site where both these actions – generation of a normal voiding contraction and reciprocal relaxation of the sphincter mechanism – occur and are co-ordinated. If there is such a thing as a 'micturition centre', then this is it.[37]

This view of a unitary 'pontine micturition centre' has been revised in recent years largely by the work of Blok and Holstege.[38] They have shown experimentally that micturition and continence are independently organized in the brain, and this has since been confirmed by PET scanning in humans.[39] Their experimental studies in the cat have shown that the pontine micturition centre is exactly where Barrington said it was in the medial part of the dorso-lateral pons. This they call the M-region. Neurons from the M-region project downwards to

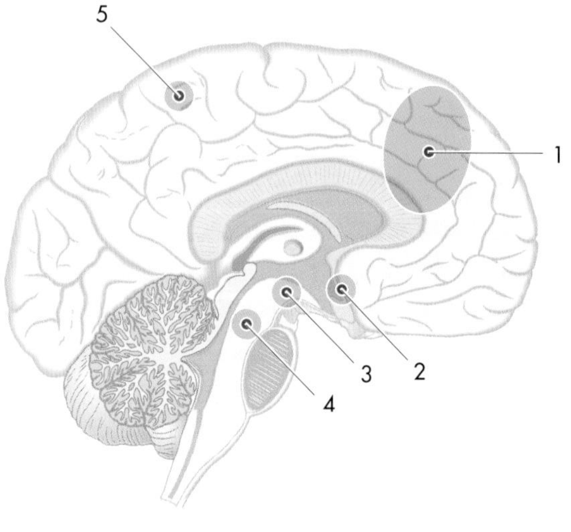

Figure 14.28 *Five areas of the brain concerned with lower urinary tract function. 1 = medial aspect of frontal lobe; 2 = septal and pre-optic nuclei; 3 = hypothalamus; 4 = nucleus locus coeruleus (Barrington's Pontine Micturition Centre); 5 = paracentral lobule. (Reproduced with permission from Mundy AR, Thomas PJ. Clinical physiology of the bladder, urethra and pelvic floor. In: Mundy AR, Stephenson TP, Wein AJ, eds. Urodynamics – Principles, Practice and Application. 2nd edn. Edinburgh: Churchill Livingstone, 1994.)*

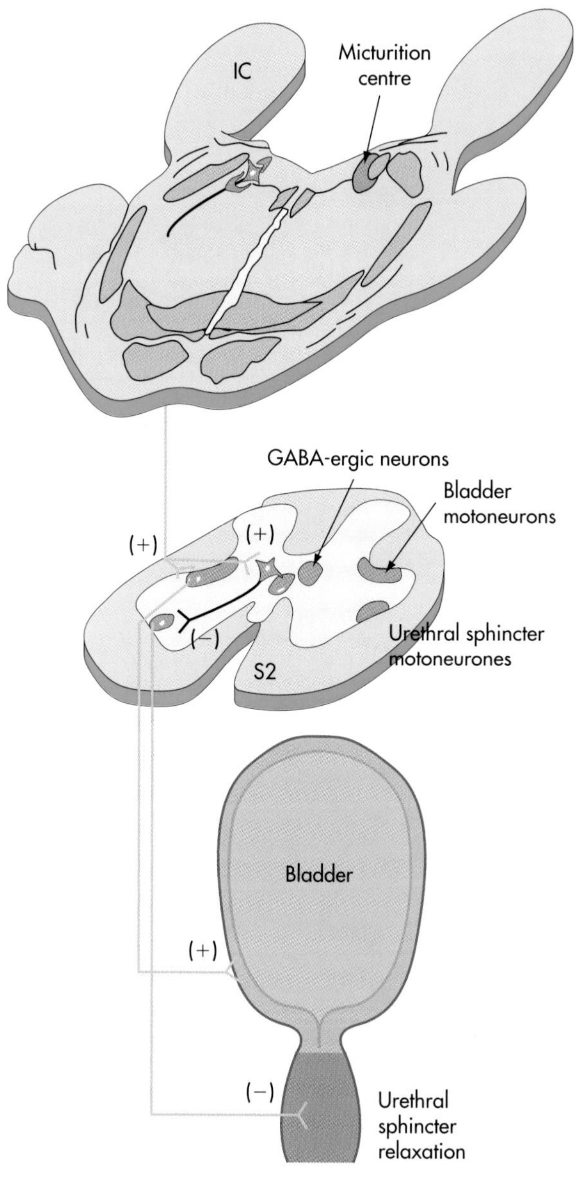

Figure 14.29 *Schematic diagram of the spinal and supraspinal structures and their pathways involved in micturition. Pathways are indicated on one side only. IC = inferior cellulus; S2 = second sacral segment.*

the sacral intermedio-lateral grey column. There are also projections to the sacral intermedio-medial cell column, which is also known as the dorsal grey commissure (DGC). Thus, impulses from the M-region simultaneously excite the preganglionic parasympathetic neurons in the sacral intermedio-lateral grey column to cause bladder contraction and excite GABA-ergic interneurons in the DGC in the same area of the spinal cord which inhibit the urethral sphincter motor neurons and thereby cause relaxation of the sphincter. The presence of the M-region has been shown in exactly the same area in humans by PET.

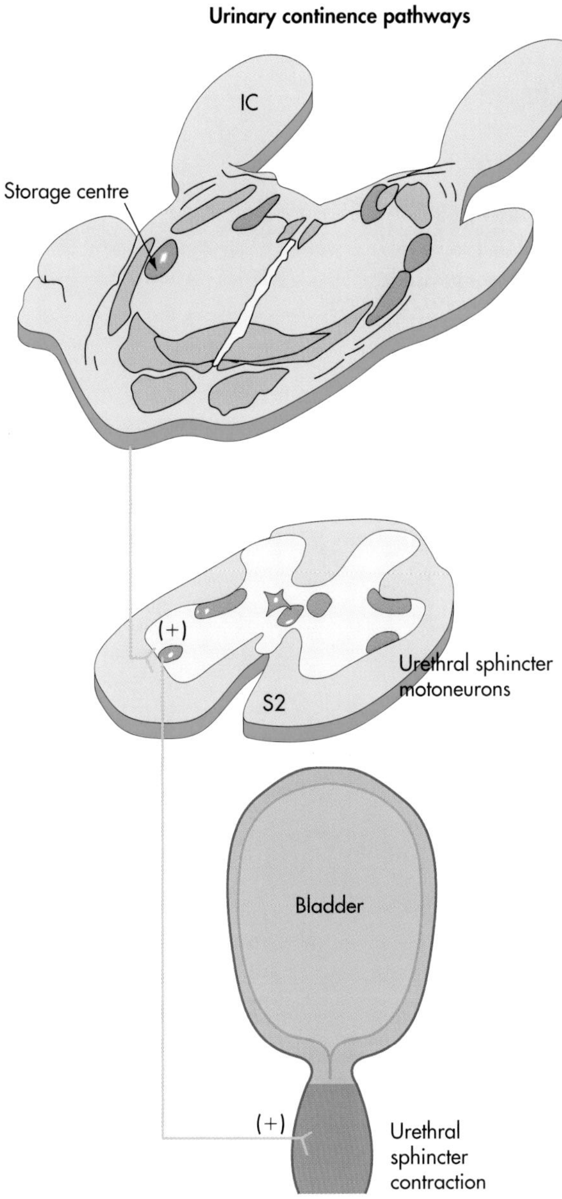

Figure 14.30 *Schematic diagram of the spinal and supraspinal structure and their pathways involved in bladder control problems.*

It has also been shown that afferent impulses do not project directly to the pontine micturition centre (M-region) but to a relay centre in the mesencephalic periaqueductal grey matter (PAG).

Ventral and lateral to the pontine micturition centre of M-region is another group of neurons responsible for the storage of urine during continence. This is known as the pontine storage centre (PSC) or L-region (Figure 14.30). Neurons project from the L-region to the urethral sphincter motor neurons in Onuf's nucleus, reducing tonic urethral sphincter contraction. The presence of this centre in humans has also been confirmed on PET scanning.

Clearly, as this is largely an autonomic event, parasympathetically mediated, the hypothalamus is important, and this is the second of the five centres. The third is the paracentral lobule of the cerebral cortex, which is responsible for the control of the pelvic floor musculature. The importance of this centre becomes manifest in spastic conditions such as congenital cerebral palsy, in which failure of relaxation can cause quite severe voiding difficulties. The normal physiological role of other related areas of the brain, such as the basal ganglia, is not clear, although diseases that affect these areas, such as Parkinson's disease and multiple system atrophy, have obvious adverse effects.

At the junction of the diencephalon and telencephalon are the septal and pre-optic nuclei where the 'associated acts' of both micturition and defecation (and, for that matter, coition) are coordinated.[40] In some animals, such as the cat, these associated acts of voiding are quite elaborate, but in the human being they are restricted to fixation of the diaphragm and anterior abdominal wall musculature.

Finally, there is the area in the medial aspect of the frontal lobe that, although described initially as an inhibitory area,[41] seems to facilitate or inhibit voiding according to circumstances. Thus, it would appear, this area of the frontal lobe can facilitate the nucleus locus coeruleus to cause voiding when the bladder is only partially full and afferent activity is therefore subthreshold. This is the way in which the bladder can be emptied before going to bed or before undertaking a long journey to avoid, perhaps, the need to void during the night or the journey. Equally, if afferent activity has reached a threshold level but there is a good programme on the television, then this area of the frontal lobe can suppress the need to void until a more appropriate time.

The details of our understanding of the spinal cord mechanisms involved in voiding are sparse – in the brain, our knowledge of the mechanisms involved in continence and voiding is scant indeed.

THE NORMAL BLADDER FILLING–VOIDING CYCLE

So far, a summary has been given of our anatomical and physiological knowledge peripherally in the bladder and urethra themselves and then centrally within the nervous system. It has been seen that the most important 'reflex arcs' are mediated through the nucleus locus coeruleus in the rostral pons; that excitatory neurotransmission in the human is exclusively cholinergic, and specifically muscarinic in origin; that relaxation of the bladder neck and urethral smooth muscle is probably mediated through the action of nitric oxide; and that the intrinsic rhabdosphincter is the most important component of the sphincter mechanism for continence and must be reciprocally relaxed through a coordinating mechanism in the rostral pons for normal voiding to occur. However, these issues and the other matters discussed do not explain all that we need to know about normal continence and voiding.

It is apparent during the normal filling and voiding cycle of a cystometrogram, with synchronous measurement of pressure within the sphincter-active urethra (Figure 14.31), that bladder pressure stays almost completely unchanged throughout filling to a

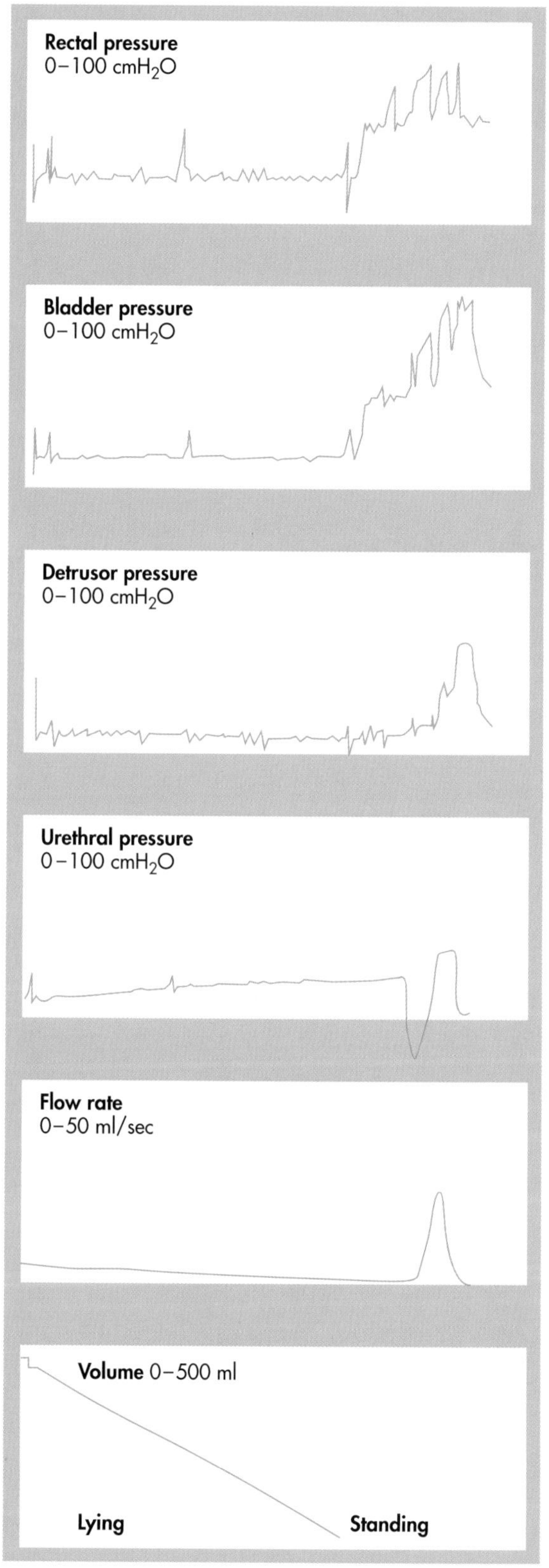

Figure 14.31 *Synchronous urethral and bladder pressure studies to show the urethra pressurized during bladder filling and pressure fall before the onset of detrusor contraction. (Reproduced with permission from Mundy AR, Thomas PJ. Clinical physiology of the bladder, urethra and pelvic floor. In: Mundy AR, Stephenson TP, Wein AJ, eds. Urodynamics – Principles, Practice and Application. 2nd edn. Edinburgh: Churchill Livingstone, 1994.)*

normal capacity despite an increasing afferent stimulus. There is, however, a small but definite rise in intraurethral pressure that is volume related. Then, just before or synchronous with the onset of voiding, there is a drop in intraurethral pressure, matched by a cessation of the electromyographic activity of the intrinsic rhabdosphincter, after which or synchronous with which detrusor pressure starts to rise.[12] This rise in pressure is then sustained until the bladder is empty, by which time detrusor pressure has returned to normal and urethral resistance has risen back to normal. The cycle then starts over again.

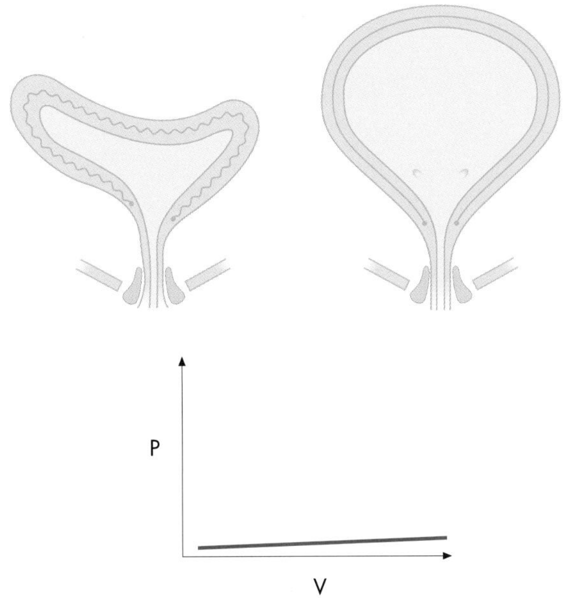

Figure 14.32 *The contribution of passive properties of the bladder wall to normal bladder compliance. (Reproduced with permission from Mundy AR, Thomas PJ. Clinical physiology of the bladder, urethra and pelvic floor. In: Mundy AR, Stephenson TP, Wein AJ eds. Urodynamics – Principles, Practice and Application. 2nd edn. Edinburgh: Churchill Livingstone, 1994.)*

WHAT KEEPS THE BLADDER PRESSURE LOW DURING FILLING?

This ability of the bladder to keep its pressure almost unchanging irrespective of bladder volume and afferent stimulation is known as compliance. The bladder is highly compliant: it shows very little change in pressure for a substantial change in volume. A steady rise in pressure during filling, which is sometimes seen when the bladder wall is 'stiff' due to disease, is known as low compliance or poor compliance.

The exact nature of normal bladder compliance is not clear, but it can be observed to be present in the bladder post-mortem, at least up to a certain filling volume.[42] This has been explained on the basis of the physical characteristics of the protein fibres that constitute the cellular and connective tissue structures of the bladder wall. They can be imagined as being coiled in the collapsed bladder and filling simply uncoils them, at least until 100–200 ml of filling has occurred (Figure 14.32). Detrusor smooth muscle cells have a striking ability to change their length without any change in tension. They may lengthen as much as fourfold during bladder filling, in a linear relationship with increasing bladder radius.

Our understanding of what happens over and beyond this elastic component and a certain 'viscoelastic' property of the bladder is due to the work of de Groat and his co-workers, who have studied this mechanism in great detail in the cat.[43] In a series of elegant experiments, de Groat has shown that there is a 'gating' mechanism in the parasympathetic ganglia of the pelvic plexuses, which means that subthreshold activity in the preganglionic neurons is not transmitted to postganglionic efferent neurons (Figure 14.33). There is also an inhibitory interneuron mechanism within the spinal cord that helps to keep afferent impulses from being transmitted onwards until they reach a critical level. At low levels of afferent activity, the inhibitory interneurons prevent the transmission of impulses from the afferent nerves to the preganglionic efferent nerves. As

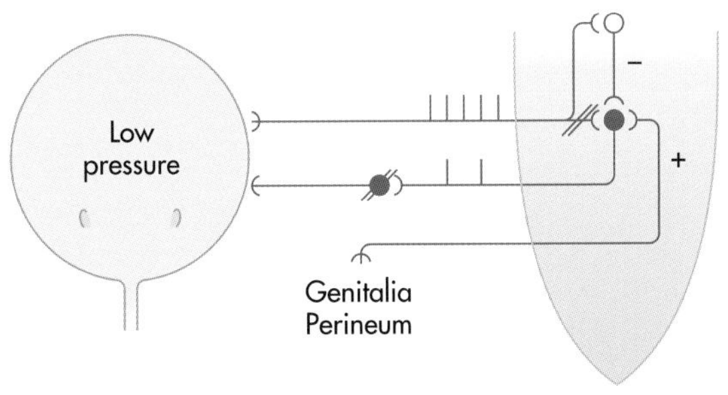

Figure 14.33 *The 'gating' mechanism by which, with minor degrees of activity in the afferent and preganglionic efferent nerves, there is no transmission to postganglionic efferent nerves.*

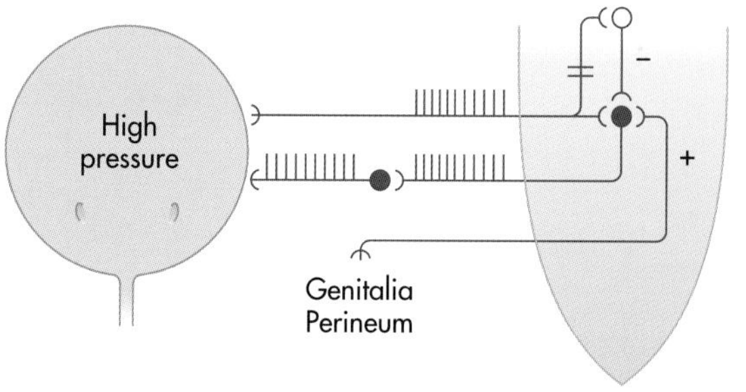

Figure 14.34 *The 'gating' mechanism showing that, with threshold afferent and preganglionic efferent activity, efferent activity is transmitted to postganglionic neurons.*

afferent activity builds up, the inhibitory interneurons are progressively inhibited and impulses start to appear in the preganglionic efferent neurons, but the gating mechanism prevents these from being transmitted to the postganglionic efferent neurons until preganglionic efferent activity has reached a critical 'threshold' level. When this level is reached, a barrage of impulses is then transmitted down the postganglionic efferent neuron to the bladder, which therefore contracts (Figure 14.34).

In addition, there are the inhibitory effects of the sympathetic neurons that have postganglionic branches ending on parasympathetic ganglion cells, as mentioned earlier in the chapter. The afferent fibres are presumably those that arise in the trigone, conveying fullness of the bladder and running up to the thoracolumbar cord, where the local relay gives rise to efferent sympathetic activity that tends to inhibit neurotransmission across the parasympathetic ganglia of the pelvic plexuses, thereby enhancing de Groat's gating mechanism (Figure 14.35).

WHAT CAUSES THE RISE IN URETHRAL PRESSURE DURING BLADDER FILLING?

This appears to be due to local reflex activity within the sacral cord by which afferent impulses from the bladder cause a local reflex rise in efferent activity to

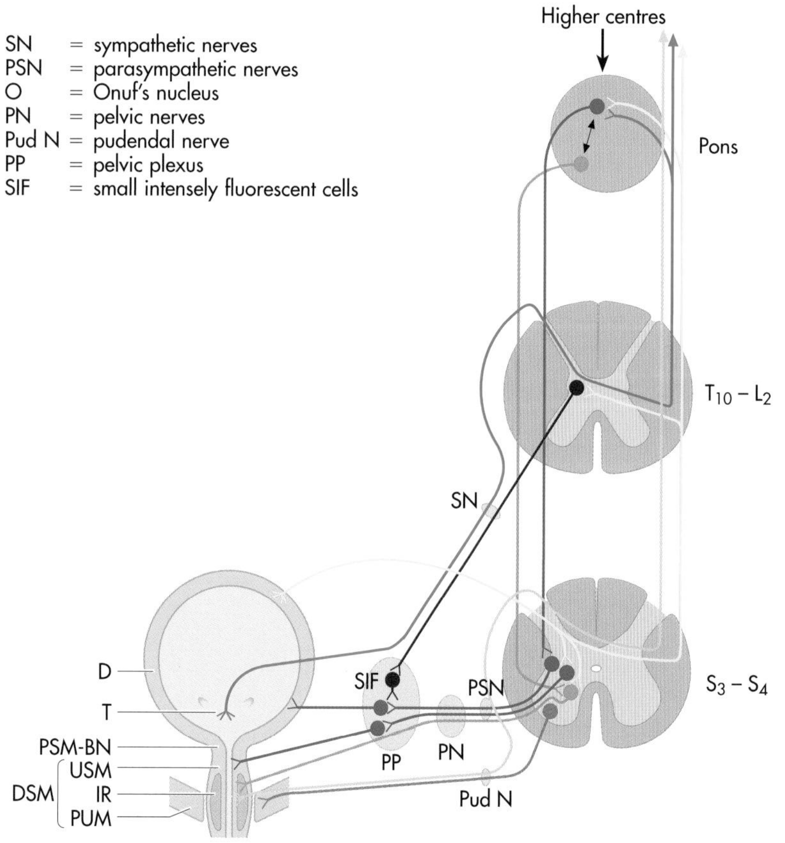

Figure 14.35 *The action of sympathetic fibres (—) on parasympathetic ganglia. (Reproduced with permission from Mundy AR, Thomas PJ. Clinical physiology of the bladder, urethra and pelvic floor. In: Mundy AR, Stephenson TP, Wein AJ, eds. Urodynamics – Principles, Practice and Application. 2nd edn. Edinburgh: Churchill Livingstone, 1994.)*

the urethral smooth muscle. It is thought to be spinal because it persists after complete spinal cord transection above the level of the sacral segments. Other than that, the mechanism is unclear.

WHAT CAUSES THE FALL IN URETHRAL PRESSURE AT THE ONSET OF VOIDING?

The mechanism of this is not clear either, but it has regularly been observed that intraurethral pressure drops to a degree that indicates that both the smooth and the striated components of the urethral sphincter mechanism are relaxed.[12] Cessation of rhabdosphincter electromyogram activity synchronous with the fall in urethral pressure has also been observed to support this conclusion. This possibly explains why the most urgent sense of a very full bladder is more a urethral than a bladder sensation, transmitted through the pudendal nerve. It seems, in fact, that the urethral sphincter mechanism is reflexly opening, and only voluntary contraction of the pelvic floor and suppression of the micturition reflex can stop it occurring. It seems, therefore, that at this point there has been threshold activation of the efferent cell bodies in the nucleus locus coeruleus and only positive intervention by higher centres to suppress the process can prevent the urethra from relaxing and stop reflex detrusor contraction from following.

HOW DOES THE BLADDER NECK OPEN?

There have been several theories to account for this. It used to be thought that there was a reciprocal innervation of the bladder by the parasympathetic system and of the bladder neck by the sympathetic system and that when the one caused contraction the other caused relaxation (Figure 14.36),[44] but that was discounted when the role of the sympathetic system in the lower urinary tract was effectively ruled out, as discussed above. With the recent discovery of the role of nitric oxide, however, this reciprocal innervation theory might well be resuscitated. Nitric oxide may be co-transmitted with acetylcholine and it may be that the acetylcholine component causes contraction of the detrusor smooth muscle, whereas at the bladder neck and in the urethra there is a more dominant nitric oxide effect released from the same type of neurons, which causes bladder neck and urethral relaxation. This does not explain the relaxation of the intrinsic rhabdosphincter, but if one presupposes that relaxation of the rhabdosphincter is a necessary precondition for detrusor contraction to occur, then bladder neck and urethral smooth muscle relaxation at the onset of detrusor contraction is all that is left to explain.

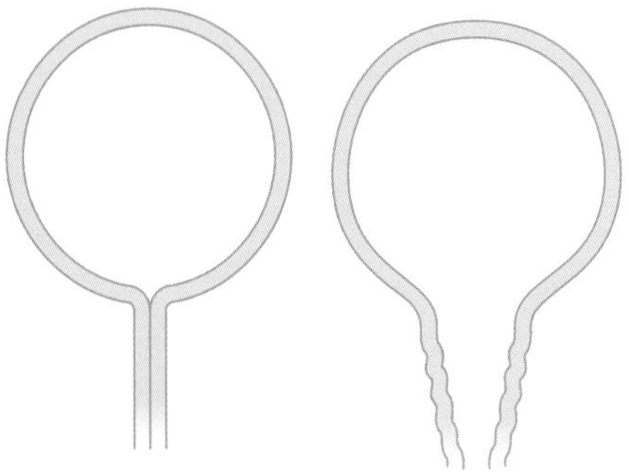

Figure 14.36 *Diagrammatic representation of the theory of 'reciprocal innervation'.*

Another explanation popularized by Lapides[45] (Figure 14.37) was that the bladder neck and the urethral musculature were continuous and fixed like a system of guy ropes at the urogenital diaphragm. Contraction therefore caused shortening, which therefore caused opening of the bladder neck. This theory was never widely held and was eventually discounted by the demonstration that the urogenital diaphragm did not exist.

The next theory to explain bladder neck opening was Hutch's 'base plate' theory (Figure 14.38).[46] This

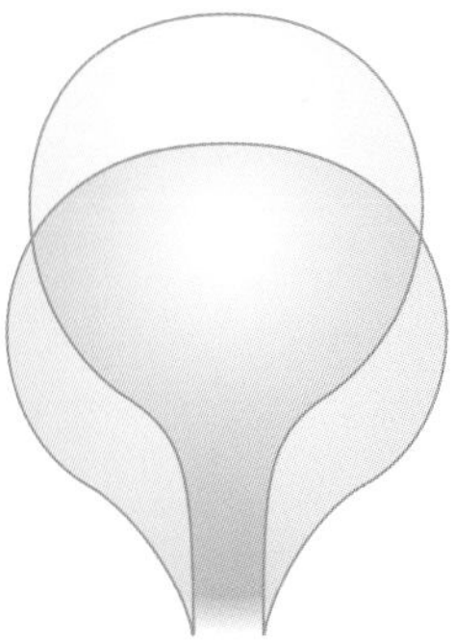

Figure 14.37 *Diagrammatic representation of Lapides' theory of bladder neck opening.*

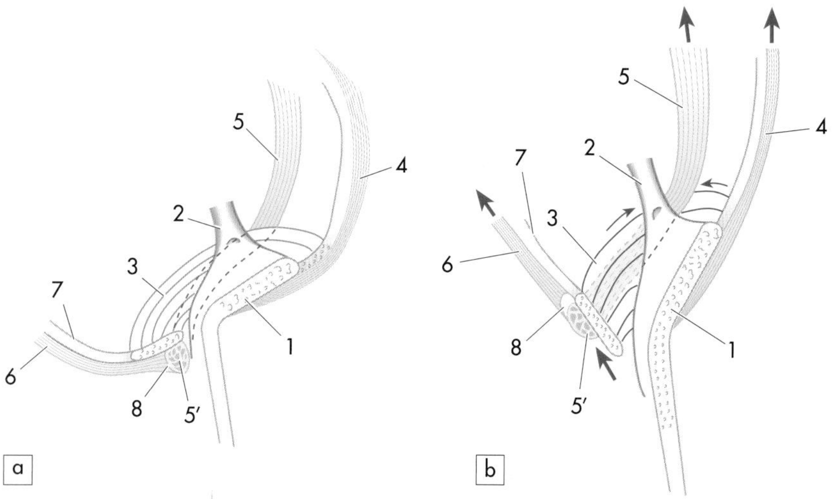

Figure 14.38 *(a, b) Diagrammatic representation of Hutch's theory of bladder neck opening. Figures refer to hypothetical muscle bundles identified by Hutch. (Reproduced with permission from Hutch JA. Anatomy and Physiology of the Bladder, Trigone and Urethra. London: Butterworths, 1972.)*

was based on the importance of the trigonal musculature and of certain bands of detrusor smooth muscle that acted to trip open the base plate of the bladder neck, but the presence of such layers and bands has never been demonstrated convincingly by anybody else and so this theory, too, has been discounted.

There is the simple hydrokinetic observation that there is only actually one way out of the bladder and that is through the bladder neck, so that when the detrusor contracts, the force is likely to be transmitted in that direction (Figure 14.39). It may well be that this simplistic point of view is at least in part correct, perhaps in conjunction with the reciprocal relaxation theory modified to incorporate the action of nitric oxide rather than the sympathetic nervous system. In addition, it should be noted that it has been observed in spinal cord-injured patients fitted with a sacral anterior root stimulator that the bladder neck can be made to open and close separately from events in the main body of the detrusor, indicating that there may be a separate innervation to the bladder neck (Giles Brindley, personal communication). Clearly, as it can only be demonstrated in this way and then only under certain circumstances and in some patients, this innervation cannot readily be dissected out from innervation of the bladder as a whole, but again it would tend to support the reciprocal innervation theory, with the co-release of nitric oxide in the sphincter-active area to explain opening coincident with cholinergic-mediated detrusor contraction.

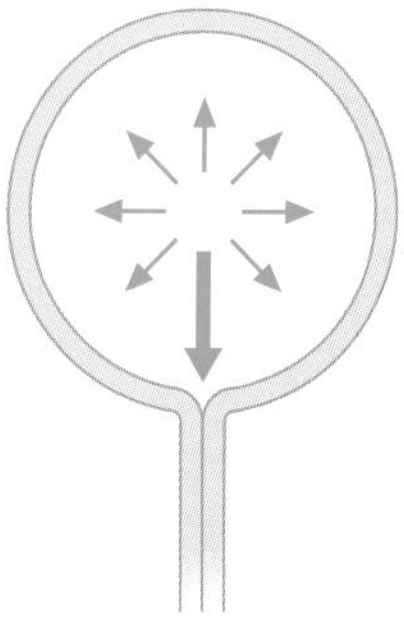

Figure 14.39 *A simple hydrokinetic explanation of bladder neck opening.*

VESICO-URETHRAL REFLEXES

As many as 12 'micturition reflexes' have been described, largely following the descriptions by Barrington earlier this century[37] and by Kuru more recently.[47] Some of these are only active in experimental animals subject to various neural ablation procedures and at least one of them is the genital reflex of closing off the bladder neck to ensure antegrade ejaculation. Some have been observed in animals but not in humans. So far in this chapter, reference has been made to four reflexes (Figure 14.40). The first is the afferent impulse routed up to the pons to cause the parasympathetic efferent contraction of the bladder of sufficient amplitude and duration to give complete bladder emptying; and the second is that which causes reciprocal relaxation of the

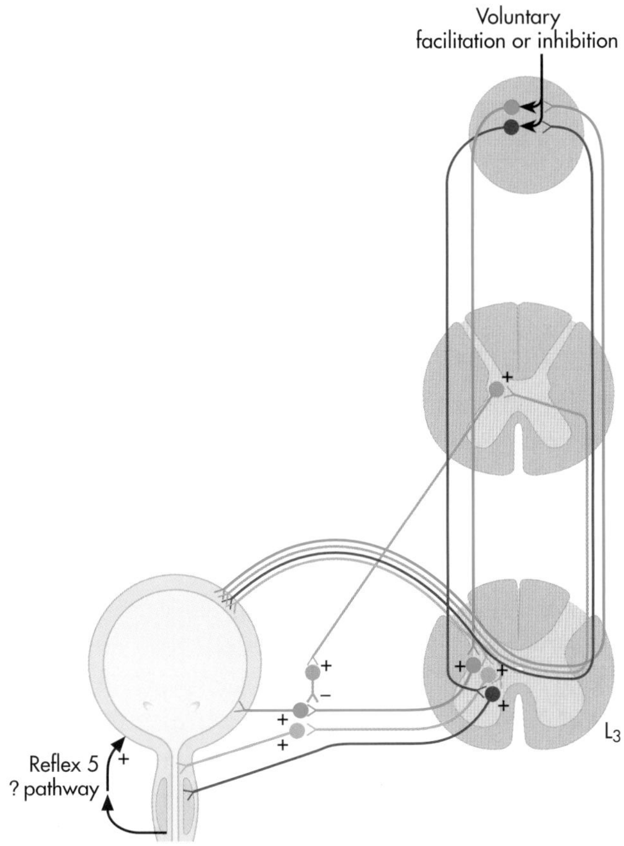

Figure 14.40 *Diagram to show the bladder reflexes described in this chapter. Reflex 1 (—); Reflex 2 (—); Reflex 3 (—); Reflex 4 (—). (Reproduced with permission from Mundy AR, Thomas PJ. Clinical physiology of the bladder, urethra and pelvic floor. In: Mundy AR, Stephenson TP, Wein AJ eds. Urodynamics – Principles, Practice and Application. 2nd edn. Edinburgh: Churchill Livingstone, 1994.)*

intrinsic rhabdosphincter to allow unobstructed voiding. The third is the local spinal reflex increase in urethral pressure during bladder filling. The fourth reflex is the one that causes sympathetic inhibition of parasympathetic ganglionic transmission in the pelvic plexuses with more advanced degrees of bladder filling.

There is, therefore, one local sacral reflex causing a rise in urethral pressure during filling, and one thoracolumbar reflex causing sympathetic inhibition of ganglionic transmission in the parasympathetic innervation to the bladder, thereby supporting de Groat's gating mechanism that keeps the bladder quiescent during filling. Then, there are the two pontine reflexes, the one to cause a bladder contraction of adequate amplitude and duration and the second to co-ordinate this with reciprocal relaxation of the intrinsic rhabdosphincter.

In addition, there is a reflex facilitation that occurs during a detrusor contraction that is mediated by afference in the pudendal nerve. The mechanism for this is unclear, but Brindley has noted that after pudendal blockade, the force of detrusor contraction is considerably reduced;[48] hence, the afferent pathway can be identified as pudendal but the rest of the reflex is unclear.

This is not to say that other reflexes do not exist and particularly that other reflexes do not exist in disease, but these are the only ones that can be positively identified as being important in health.

SUMMARY

It will be apparent to the reader that there is a great deal to be learnt about the structure and even more about the function of the lower urinary tract, particularly about the spinal and supraspinal mechanisms that control it.

The fundamental features are that during bladder filling, intravesical pressure changes very little despite the bladder filling by 400 ml or more, and this 'compliance' is achieved by a 'gating' mechanism that prevents afferent neuronal activity being transmitted to postganglionic efferent activity until that afferent activity reaches a critical level. Critical afferent activity is transmitted by ascending spinal pathways that synapse on cell bodies in the nucleus locus coeruleus in the rostral pons in addition to providing conscious awareness of bladder filling. When afferent activity to the nucleus locus coeruleus, subject to suprapontine facilitation or inhibition, reaches a threshold level, efferent activity is initiated, mediated through the pelvic parasympathetic nerves and muscarinic receptors. This causes a detrusor contraction of sufficient amplitude and duration to give complete bladder emptying and a synchronous coordinated reciprocal relaxation of the urethral sphincter mechanism to allow unobstructed voiding until the bladder is empty. It seems clear that excitatory neurotransmission in the normal human detrusor is exclusively cholinergic, and it is becoming increasingly clear that reciprocal relaxation of the urethral sphincter is a prerequisite for detrusor contraction, and that the synchronous relaxation of the bladder neck and urethral smooth muscle is probably mediated by nitric oxide, which is co-transmitted with acetylcholine from postganglionic parasympathetic neurons. Unfortunately, although this fundamental mechanism appears reasonably clear, a lot of the details are lacking at present.

REFERENCES

1. Uhlenhuth E, Hunter DT, Loechel WE. Problems in the Anatomy of the Pelvis. Philadelphia: Lippincott, 1953
2. Zacharin RF. The anatomical supports of the female urethra. Obstet Gynaecol 1968; 32: 754–759
3. Walsh PC. Radical retropubic prostatectomy. In: Walsh PC, Gittes RF, Perlmutter AD, Stamey TA, eds. Campbell's Urology. 5th edn. Philadelphia: WB Saunders, 1986: 2769–2771
4. Redman JF. Anatomy of the genitourinary system. In: Gillenwater JR, Grayhack JT, Howards SS, Duckett JN, eds. Adult and Pediatric Urology. 3rd edn. Philadelphia: Mosby, 1996: 3–61
5. Kaye KW, Milne N, Creed K, Van-der-Werf B. The urogenital diaphragm external urethral sphincter and radical prostatectomy. Aust N Z J Surg 1997; 67: 40–44
6. Hutch JA. Anatomy and physiology of the bladder, trigone and urethra. London: Butterworths, 1972
7. Gosling J. The structure of the bladder and urethra in relation to function. Urol Clin North Am 1979; 6: 31–38
8. Dixon J, Gosling J. Structure and innervation in the human. In: Torrens M, Morrison FB, eds. The Physiology of the Lower Urinary Tract. London: Springer Verlag, 1987: 3–22
9. Raz S, Caine M, Zeigler M. The vascular component in the production of intraurethral pressure. J Urol 1972; 108: 93–96
10. Sundin T, Dahlstrom A, Norlen L, Svedmyr N. The sympathetic innervation and adrenoreceptor function of the human lower urinary tract in the normal state and after parasympathetic denervation. Investig Urol 1977; 14: 322–328
11. Chilton CP. The urethra. In: Webster G, Kirby R, King L, Goldwasser B, eds. Reconstructive Urology. Cambridge, MA: Blackwell Scientific, 1993: 59–73
12. Tanagho EA. The anatomy and physiology of micturition. Clin Obstet Gynaecol 1978; 5: 3–26
13. James MJ. Relaxation of the human detrusor. University of Nottingham, MD Thesis, 1993
14. Bridgewater M, MacNeil HF, Brading AF. Regulation of tone in pig urethral smooth muscle. J Urol 1993; 150: 223–228
15. Gosling JA, Dixon JS, Critchely HOD, Thompson SA. A comparative study of the human external sphincter and periurethral levator ani muscles. Br J Urol 1981; 53: 35–41
16. Schroder HD. Onuf's nucleus X: a morphological study of a human spinal nucleus. Anat Embryol 1981; 162: 443–453
17. Zrara P, Carrier S, Kour NW, Tanagho EA. The detailed neuroanatomy of the human striated urethral sphincter. Br J Urol 1994; 74: 182–187
18. Mundy AR. An anatomical explanation for bladder dysfunction following rectal and uterine surgery. Br J Urol 1982; 54: 501–504
19. Burnstock G. Autonomic innervation and transmission. Br Med Bull 1979; 35: 255–262
20. Burnstock G. The changing face of autonomic transmission. Acta Physiol Scand 1986; 126: 67–91
21. Brading AF. Physiology of the urinary tract smooth muscle. In: Webster G, Kirby R, King L, Goldwasser B, eds. Reconstructive Urology. Cambridge, MA: Blackwell Scientific, 1993: 15–26
22. Brindley GS, Craggs MD. The effect of atropine in the urinary bladder of the baboon and of man. J Physiol 1975; 255: 55P
23. Kinder RB, Mundy AR. Atropine blockade of nerve-mediated stimulation of the human detrusor. Br J Urol 1985; 57: 418–421
24. Sibley GA. An experimental model of detrusor instability in the obstructed pig. Br J Urol 1985; 57: 292–298
25. Alm P, Alumets J, Brodin E, Hakanson R et al. Peptidergic (substance P) nerves in the genito-urinary tract. Neuroscience 1978; 3: 419–425
26. Maggi CA, Barbanti G, Santicioli P, Beneforti P et al. Cystometric evidence that capsaicin-sensitive nerves modulate the afferent branch of the micturition reflex in humans. J Urol 1989; 142: 150–154
27. Gu J, Restorick J, Blank MA, Huang WM et al. Vasoactive intestinal polypeptide in the normal and unstable bladder. Br J Urol 1983; 55: 645–647
28. Alm P, Alumets J, Hakenson R, Sundler F. Peptidergic (vasoactive intestinal peptide) nerves in the genito-urinary tract. Neuroscience 1977; 2: 751–754

29. Fergusson DR, Kennedy I, Burton TJ. ATP release from rabbit urinary bladder epithelial cells by hydrostatic pressure change – a possible sensory mechanism. J Physiol 1997; 505: 503
30. De Groat WC. Spinal cord projections and neuropeptides in visceral afferent neurons. Prog Brain Res 1986; 67: 165–188
31. Habler HJ, Janig W, Koltzenburg M. Activation of unmyelinated afferent fibres by mechanical stimuli and inflammation of the urinary bladder in the cat. J Physiol 1990; 425: 545
32. Wen J, Morrison JFB. Sensitisation of pelvic afferent neurones from the rat bladder. J Auton Nerv Sys 1996; 58: 187
33. Nathan PW. Sensations associated with micturition. Br J Urol 1956; 28: 126–131
34. Nathan PW. The central nervous connections of bladder. In: Chisholm GD, Williams DI, eds. Scientific Foundation of Urology. London: Heinemann, 1976
35. MacMahon SB, Morrison JFB. Spinal neurones with long projections activated from the abdominal viscera of the cat. J Physiol 1982; 332: 1–20
36. Sillen U. Central neurotransmitter mechanisms involved in the control of urinary bladder function. Scand J Urol Nephrol 1980; Suppl. 58
37. Barrington FJF. The effect of lesions on the hind and midbrain on micturition in the cat. Q J Exp Physiol 1915; 15: 181–202
38. Blok BFM, Holstege G. The central control of micturition and continence: implications for urology. BJU Intl 1999; 83 (Suppl. 2): 1–6
39. Blok BFM, Williamsen ATM, Holstege G. A PET study on brain control of micturition in humans. Brain 1997; 120: 111–121
40. Hess WR. The Functional Organisation of the Diencephalon. London: Grune & Stratton, 1957
41. Andrew J, Nathan PW. Lesions of the anterior frontal lobes and disturbances of micturition and defecation. Brain 1964; 87: 233–261
42. Tang PC, Ruch TC. Non-neurogenic basis of bladder tonus. Am J Physiol 1955; 181: 249–257
43. De Groat WC. Physiology of the urinary bladder and urethra. Ann Int Med 1980; 92: 312–315
44. Denny-Brown D, Robertson EG. On the physiology of micturition. J Physiol 1933; 56: 149–190
45. Lapides J. Structure and function of the internal vesical sphincter. J Urol 1958; 80: 341–353
46. Hutch J. A new theory of the anatomy of the internal urinary sphincter and the physiology of micturition. Invest Urol 1965; 3: 36–58
47. Kuru M. Nervous control of micturition. Physiol Rev 1965; 45: 425–494
48. Brindley GS, Craggs MD. The pressure exerted by the external sphincter of the urethra when its motor nerve fibres are stimulated electrically. Br J Urol 1974; 46: 453–462

15

Detrusor smooth muscle physiology

Christopher H Fry

PHYSICAL PROPERTIES OF THE BLADDER INFLUENCE WHAT IS RECORDED

Bladder intravesical pressure and detrusor wall tension

The bladder is a hollow organ that works to expel urine by raising intravesical pressure. This is achieved by increasing the wall stress (tension) of the bladder, which in turn is brought about by contracting the detrusor smooth muscle in the wall. However, the relationship between the force of detrusor contraction and a rise in bladder luminal pressure is not a proportional one but requires that bladder geometry is also taken into account. Failure to recognize this complicating factor can lead to the erroneous conclusion that different intraluminal pressures are dependent solely on the contractile state of detrusor smooth muscle.

The relationship between vesical pressure (P) and wall stress (T) is given by Laplace's law where r is the radius of the vessel, as shown in Figure 15.1:

$$P = \frac{2T}{r}$$

Contraction of a muscular element in bladder wall will generate a force that acts tangentially to the wall. This force will be counteracted by a distending force (Newton's laws), thus acting perpendicularly to the wall, which can be called a pressure P; the magnitude of the force is shown to be equivalent to P^*r. More details can be found in any textbook of physics. The model is slightly complicated in the case when the wall is a finite thickness, d, when Laplace's law becomes $P = (2Td / r)$. Figure 15.2 shows model calculations that calculate P for two initial volumes, 400 and 200 ml – in all cases, the increase of wall stress, T, is the same. Two situations are shown: when volume is constant (Figure 15.2a) and when volume declines (Figure 15.2b). These situations can be analogized to when the bladder contracts when the sphincter is closed, and during voiding. A number of points can be made:

- The relationship between wall stress and pressure is linear only when volume is constant. Thus, extrapolation to the contractile properties of the muscle wall from the rise of pressure is not always straightforward.
- The rise of pressure is greater for a smaller volume.
- The rise of pressure is greater when the volume decreases compared to the constant volume case.

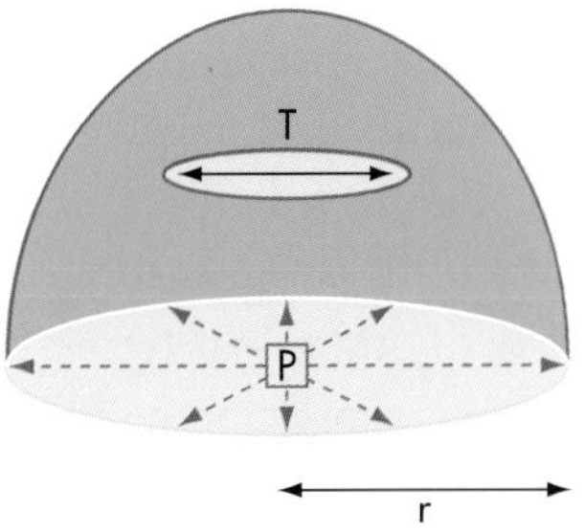

Figure 15.1 *The relation between pressure, (P), wall tension, (T) and radius, (r) of a hollow spherical organ. P acts on the wall of the sphere; T is a force per unit length acting tangentially to the wall. The wall tension is shown acting perpendicularly to a theoretical slit in the wall.*

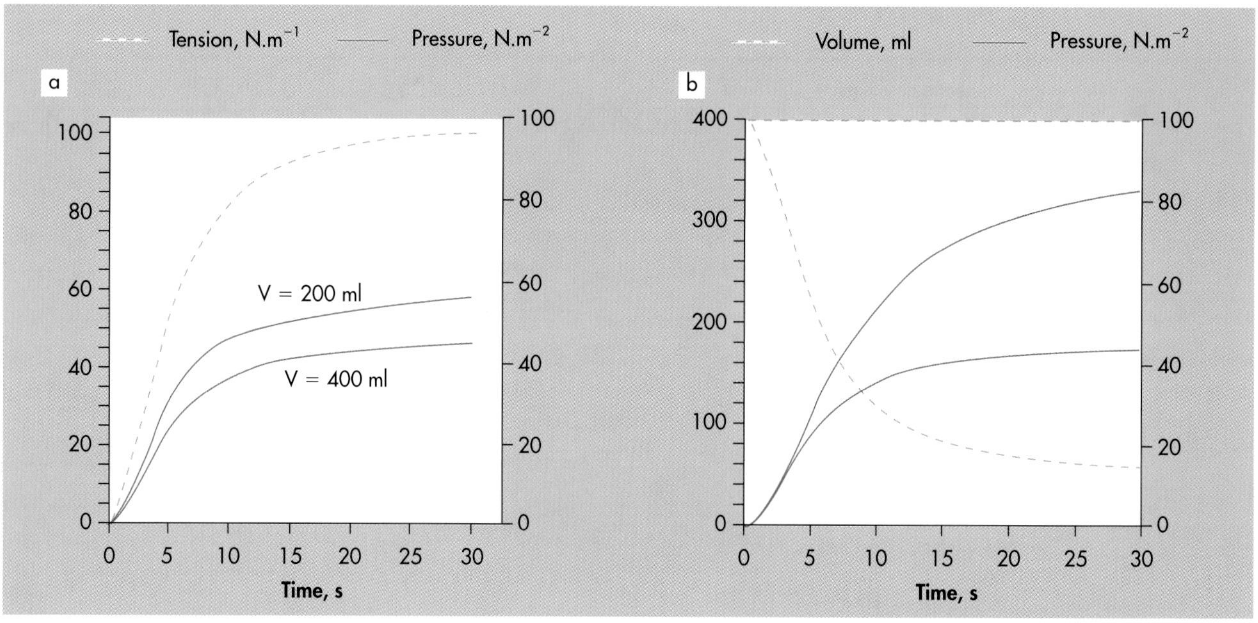

Figure 15.2 *Calculations from Laplace's law. (a) The rise of intraluminal pressure for an increase of wall tension (dotted line). The pressure change is shown for two constant volumes: 400 and 200 ml. (b) The change of intraluminal pressure for the same change of wall tension as in (b). In this case, the volume again either remains constant at 400 ml (brown traces) or changes from 400 to 50 ml (green traces) during tension development.*

Models of the bladder and stress-relaxation

Early models of whole muscle recognized that muscle cells exist within a complex tissue arrangement of extracellular material such as collagen and other non-contractile cellular components. Recorded tension in a muscle is transmitted from the contractile regions through these other elements, and this may contribute significantly to the overall mechanical properties of the tissue.[1,2] If these other elements were truly rigid, they would transmit such forces faithfully, and an accurate estimate of contractile force could be made. If a muscle shortens, ?*l*, in response to a developed force, *F*, the relation between the two (*F*/?*l*) is a measure of muscle stiffness – the inverse of stiffness is termed 'compliance'. In three dimensions, that is, in the bladder, the terms *F* and *l* are replaced by pressure, *P*, and volume, *V*. Thus, bladder compliance is given by the ratio (?*P*/?*V*) when a known volume of fluid is injected into the bladder (the change of wall stress can also be found from ?*P* by Laplace's law, assuming the bladder remains spherical in shape).

However, viscous forces will tend to dissipate some of this force as heat, both attenuating and slowing the force change.[3] Estimation of compliance is now more difficult – it could be measured when viscoelastic forces have dissipated, or before they have had a chance to dissipate. Figure 15.3 shows a model situation, and in either case the value of

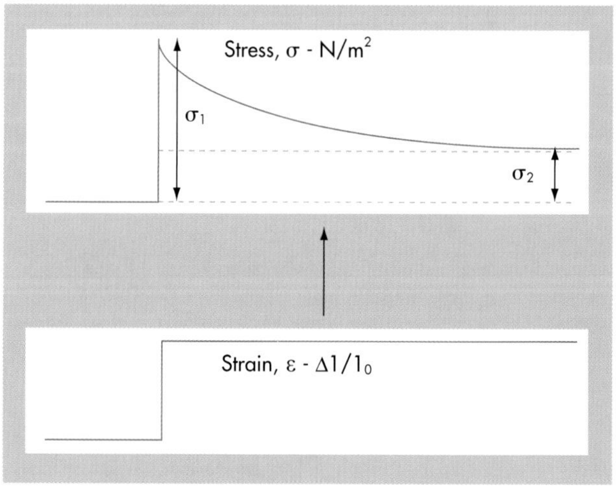

Figure 15.3 *Schematic representation of changes to muscle stress, σ, after a rapid stretch or change of strain, ε. Muscle compliance can be measured before or after stress relaxation.*

compliance will be very different. Estimation of bladder compliance ($\Delta V/\Delta P$) deserves equal consideration.[4] Injection of a known volume of fluid will raise intravesical pressure and subsequently decay towards the initial value. This pressure decay (stress relaxation) will be due to viscoelastic relaxation, and possibly (and controversially) some component of active relaxation of the detrusor muscle. The initial rise of pressure and the subsequent decay will be greater if the volume is injected quickly compared to the stress-relaxation time, rather than more slowly.

Glossary

Several physical terms have been used in this Chapter, and will be used, which perhaps require definition, as their misuse can sometimes cause confusion. Some have already been defined, such as **compliance**.

Force and tension. **Force**, a general term in physics, is a measure of interaction between bodies; the unit is the newton (N). When a body such as a muscle contracts, or is artificially stretched, it is under **tension**, which is equal to the force exerted at that point.

Weight and mass. **Mass** (m) characterizes the inertial properties of a body; that is, the force needed to produce a given acceleration. **Weight** (w) is a force exerted on a body by the earth. A mass of 1 kg has a weight of 9.8 N; that is, $w = m.g$ ($g = 9.8$ m.s^{-2}). Many authors quote muscle contraction in units of grams, but this is erroneous; the units should be those of force (N).

Stress and strain. A bar (or muscle) that is pulled or compressed by a force F is in tension. **Stress** is F per unit cross-sectional area (units N.m^{-2}). Muscle contractile performance is often quoted in these units to normalize different muscle dimensions. The change of length ($\Delta l/l_0$) occurring from stress development is **strain** and is dimensionless.

Pressure and wall tension. **Pressure** is a force per unit area acting perpendicularly on a surface; its unit is N.m^{-2} (or pascal, [Pa]). **Wall tension** (like surface tension) is a force acting along a length; its unit is N.m^{-1}.

Speed and velocity. **Speed** is a scalar quantity; that is it has a magnitude. **Velocity** is a vector quantity; that is, it has magnitude and direction. When we talk about the velocity of muscle contraction, it is assumed that this is occurring along the longitudinal axis of the muscle.

SMOOTH MUSCLE MECHANICS AND ENERGETICS

All muscles, striated and smooth muscles, share a number of contractile characteristics by virtue of the molecular apparatus which generates force. For example, the magnitude of a contraction is dependent on the resting length of the muscle, and the rate at which a muscle shortens is a function of the load it has to move. The exact length- and load-dependence of these variables is governed by particular features of the muscle cell, but, in general, smooth muscles from various sources have similar characteristics. Because muscle mechanics has not been extensively investigated in the detrusor, this section will be more general.

Isometric contractions

In this state, a muscle develops force but does not change its length – the cellular processes are discussed below. Stretch of the muscle in an unstimulated (passive) state increases its tension, and Figure 15.4 shows that this rises steeply at larger stretches. If the muscle is stimulated, an active tension is additionally developed. A plot of the active component shows a bell-shaped dependence on length, known as the length–tension relationship. In striated muscle, this is explained by variation in the overlap of the actin and myosin filaments, embodied in the sliding-filament hypothesis,[5] and a similar explanation may hold true for smooth muscle. Smooth muscle differs from striated muscle in the relative wide range of resting lengths over which active force can be developed. This is a useful feature of smooth muscle as it ensures that active force can be developed despite a wide variation in stretch; that is, detrusor smooth muscle can still generate a contraction despite large variations in bladder volume.

Isotonic contractions

Figure 15.5 shows the arrangement for an isotonic contraction whereby a muscle shortens while lifting a load. The speed, v, of shortening is reduced as the tension (T) on the muscle imposed by a load is increased. The precise relationship is embodied in the force–velocity relation, described by A.V. Hill[6] and shown in Figure 15.5, which has played a fundamental role in our understanding of muscle energetics:

$$v = b\,(T_0 - T)/(T + a)$$

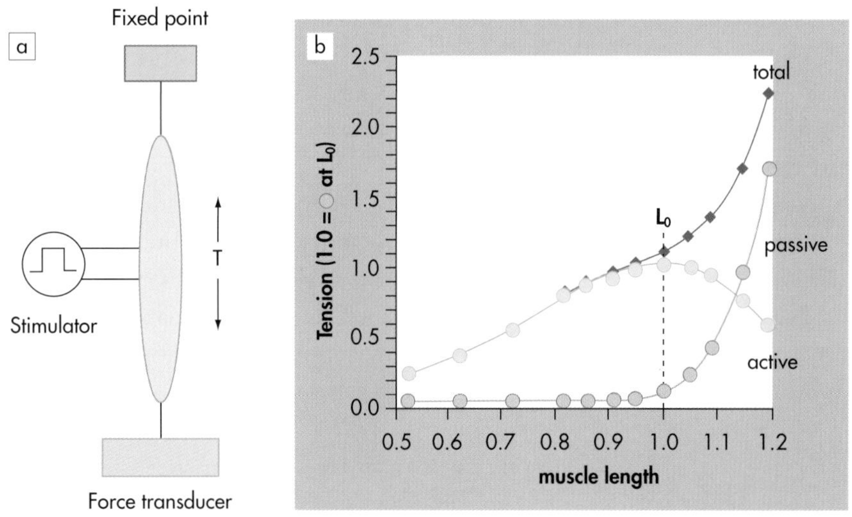

Figure 15.4 *Isometric contraction of muscle. (a) The experimental arrangement; a muscle is artificially stimulated and the active tension, (T), developed is measured by a force transducer. A force transducer is an instrument that ideally does not move when placed under stress, but measures the change in stress. The fixed point can be varied to alter the resting length of the muscle. (b) The relationship between the resting length of a detrusor strip and the passive, active and total tension. The axes are expressed as a proportion of each variable at L_0 – the muscle length generating optimum active force.*

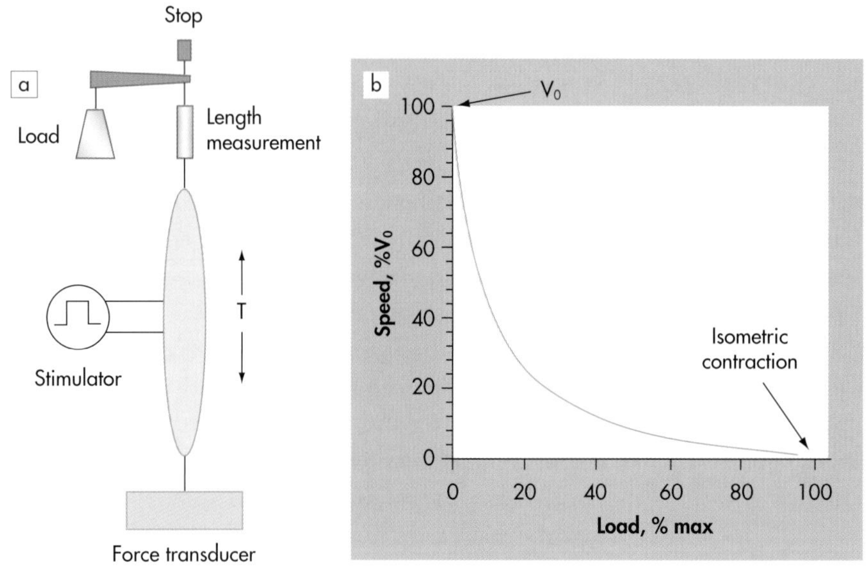

Figure 15.5 *Isotonic contraction of muscle. (a) The experimental arrangement; a muscle is allowed to shorten when stimulated and lifts the load via a fulcrum. The Stop prevents the muscle from being extended too greatly. (b) The relationship between the initial shortening speed of a contraction and the load – the force–velocity (f–v) relationship. The speed is expressed as a percentage of a maximum value, V_0, when lifting no load and is obtained by extrapolation of the experimental curve with the Hill equation. By definition, the isometric contraction occurs when the load is too great to lift and no shortening occurs.*

where *a* and *b* are constants and T_0 is the maximum (isometric) tension at zero speed. A useful feature of this curve is the extrapolation to a maximum velocity of shortening at zero load, V_0, as this is related to the maximum frequency of cross-bridge cycling (see below). The curve bears a superficial resemblance to the derived pressure flow plots obtained in urodynamics,[7] which have been analysed by the same formulation to estimate the contractile state of the bladder.[8]

A feature of smooth muscle is that it is capable of maintaining tension for considerable periods of time with relatively little consumption of metabolic energy; this has been termed the 'latch state'.[9] Again, this is an advantageous feature of smooth muscle, which frequently has to maintain an active state for longer periods than smooth or cardiac muscle. An explanation is that unphosphorylated myosin can also maintain cross-bridges but that the cycling rate is slow, accounting for the low ATP consumption. The low cross-bridge cycling rate is mirrored in a reduction of the V_0 during the development of a contraction (Figure 15.6). Thus, in the latch state, smooth muscle can maintain tension for a relatively long period with little expenditure of energy, but its ability to respond rapidly is diminished. The relationship between tension development, ATP consumption, V_0 and myosin

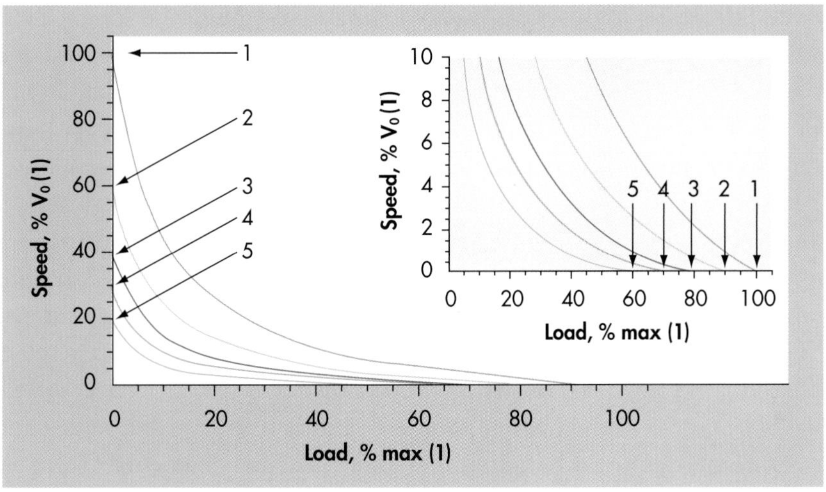

Figure 15.6 *Variation of the f–v relationship during the time course of an active contraction in a smooth muscle. The curves from 1 to 5 would be obtained at successive intervals during the contraction, when V_0 and the isometric tension decline. Note that V_0 declines more than isometric tension. The axes are expressed as a percentage of the V_0 and isometric contraction for curve 1. The inset shows at higher resolution the intercepts with the abscissa.*

light-chain phosphorylation is shown schematically in Figure 15.7.

The term 'muscle contractility'

It is of considerable interest for the scientist and clinician to be able to quantify the contractile state of a muscle. However, for hollow organs such as the bladder, the measured output is a change of vesical (detrusor) pressure. It would be desirable to know whether pathological changes to pressure result from a primary dysfunction of the muscular component or have other explanations; otherwise, the choice of treatment will have no rational basis. To the muscle physiologist, the term contractility, has a precise and specific meaning; namely, an alteration to isometric

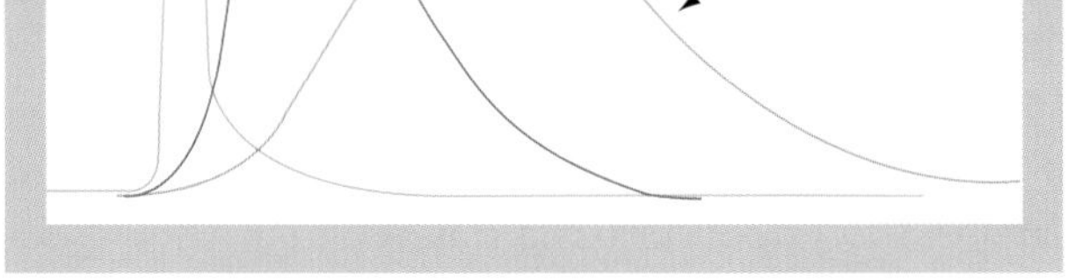

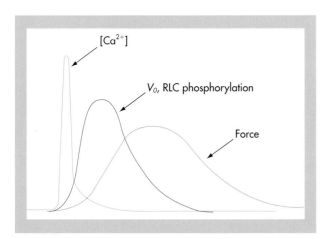

Figure 15.7 *A diagrammatic representation of the time course of changes to intracellular [Ca^{2+}], the maximum velocity of shortening (V_0), light-chain phosphorylation and muscle tension in a tonic smooth muscle as detrusor.*

tension or V_0, independent of resting muscle length – that is, an inotropic effect. The term 'contractility' is used by the urologist rather loosely to describe any factor that may change detrusor pressure; be it a change of muscle contractility, the amount of muscle tissue in the detrusor mass, the resting length of the muscle or even the shape and volume of the bladder. Confused communication between the physiologist and the clinician can arise from the use of a term which has different meanings.

Smooth muscle energetics

Compared to striated muscle, smooth muscle has a high economy, as contractions can be maintained for a relatively long period of time with a lower ATP consumption than in the initial stages of force development. However, when external work is being generated (remember: work = force × distance), smooth muscle has a lower *efficiency* than striated muscle. Efficiency may be defined as the work produced per unit free energy change of the driving chemical reaction, that is, ATP hydrolysis, and is about 20 and 5 $kJ.mol^{-1}$ in striated and smooth muscle, respectively.[10,11] The reason for this decreased efficiency is unclear, but one hypothesis is that the ATP required to phosphorylate the myosin light chain (see below) in addition to that needed for cross-bridge cycling contributes to the overall metabolic load.[9,12] However, contraction speeds are rarely as high in smooth muscle as those in striated muscles, so that the requirement for a phosphocreatine (PCr) pool is much less. Even in more phasic muscles such as detrusor, although PCr levels decrease slightly, the total high-energy phosphate pool remains constant in well-oxygenated tissue.[13]

A particular feature of smooth muscle metabolism is that oxidative metabolism and lactate production occur together and that their respective rates are not correlated. In some vascular smooth muscles, it has been shown that force development and O_2 consumption are closely correlated, whereas lactate production is associated with other ATP-consuming processes such as the Na pump.[14] This has led to the suggestion that metabolism is functionally compartmentalized, with O_2 consumption above basal levels directed towards meeting the needs for actomyosin ATP consumption. However, the proponents of this hypothesis emphasize that this is not a rigid compartmentalization and that cross-talk between the aerobic and anaerobic pathways is possible. The relevance of this metabolic division to detrusor muscle has not been tested.

THE CONTRACTILE MACHINERY

The process of muscle contraction, or generation of tension within a muscle cell, involves the interaction of actin and myosin filaments to form a cross-bridge. In detrusor smooth muscle, as in most other smooth muscles, these protein filaments are dispersed irregularly throughout the cell, unlike striated muscle, where they form regular arrays. This disorganized arrangement results in a less rapid contraction and one not oriented necessarily along the longitudinal axis of the myocyte. However, this suits the function of smooth muscle, which compared to striated muscle, requires a more prolonged active state, and reduced orientation of tension development along a particular axis.

Figure 15.8 is a schematic picture of two adjacent smooth muscle cells, showing contractile proteins anchored to dense bodies within the cell and dense plaques on the cell membrane. These proteins consist of actin and myosin filaments, as well as several regulatory proteins, such as tropomyosin, caldesmon and calponin. Intermediate filaments form a cytoskeletal array and are believed to maintain the spacing of the dense bodies and plaques, as well as distribute force generated by the contractile components throughout the cell. Dense plaques from adjacent cells can be opposed to form mechanical junctions which distribute tension development evenly throughout the muscle mass. Shown also are gap junctions which can form electrical junctions between cells.

Cross-bridge cycling is powered by ATP hydrolysis but regulated by a transient rise of the sarcoplasmic [Ca^{2+}]. Ca^{2+} in the sarcoplasm binds to a soluble protein calmodulin (Cm), to form a complex, Ca_4Cm, which activates the contractile machinery. In smooth muscle, Ca_4Cm activates the myosin molecule via activation of a myosin light-chain kinase (MLCK), culminating in phosphorylation of the so-called regulatory myosin light chain (RLC):[15] the

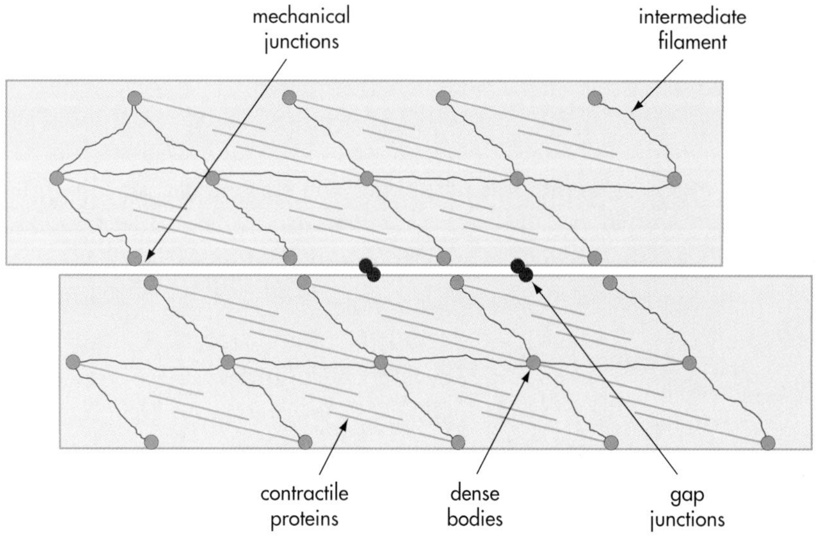

Figure 15.8 *A diagram of two opposing smooth muscle cells showing the relationship between the contractile elements and their attachments.*

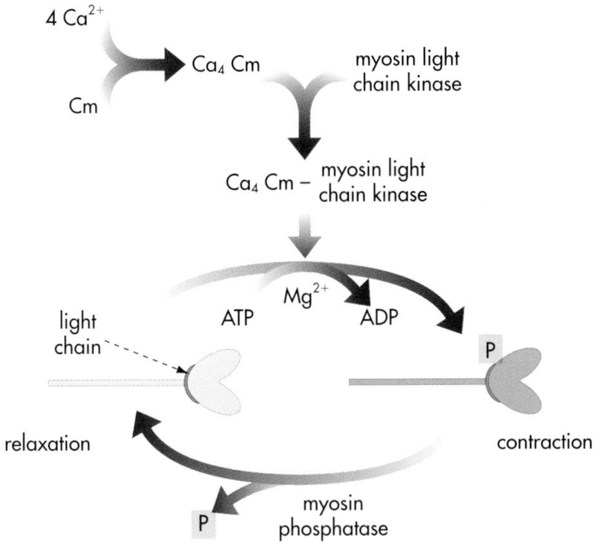

Figure 15.9 *The cellular cascade of reactions showing the activation (phosphorylation) of the myosin regulatory light chain – shown as a dark collar around the myosin heads. Cm: calmodulin.*

process illustrated in Figure 15.9. RLC phosphorylation greatly increases actin-activated myosin MgATPase activity, which results in the heavy chain of the myosin molecule forming a cross-bridge with an actin filament which generates force. Cross-bridge cycling – the continuous process of making and breaking of cross-bridges with the consumption of ATP – can proceed as long as myosin is activated by Ca_4Cm, thus generating a contraction. Relaxation occurs when the RLC is dephosphorylated by a myosin phosphatase.[16] This generally occurs when the Ca_4Cm concentration falls due to a reduction of the sarcoplasmic [Ca^{2+}], but other Ca^{2+}-independent mechanisms may also stimulate RLC dephosphorylation and also cause relaxation – an example is considered below.

Experiments with isolated contractile proteins[17] show that the Ca^{2+}-dependent regulation of the contractile apparatus in detrusor smooth muscle occurs over a range of ionized [Ca^{2+}] between 0.1 μM and 10 μM (Figure 15.10). This is precisely the range of [Ca^{2+}] that is measured in the sarcoplasm of intact detrusor myocytes when they are relaxed, or activated by contractile agonists such as acetylcholine or its analogue, carbachol.[18] Quantitative measurements such as these are important as they reinforce the importance of modulation of the sarcoplasmic [Ca^{2+}] as the key determinant of contractile regulation.

Although modulation of the sarcoplasmic [Ca^{2+}] is the most important regulator of contraction in smooth muscle such as detrusor, other factors may modulate this process. Their significance is not fully understood, but they offer additional routes to fine-tune the contractile state of the muscle, both physiologically and pharmacologically. Such control points include phosphorylation of MLCK itself[19] and activation of myosin phosphatase,[20] both of which depress myosin ATPase activity and hence contraction. Phosphorylation of MLCK suppresses its own activation by Ca_4Cm, and activation of myosin phosphatase would reduce RLC phosphorylation.

An example of such modulation is given by the cyclic nucleotides, cAMP and cGMP, both of which relax smooth muscle. The role played by cGMP will be considered later (see 'Regional differences in

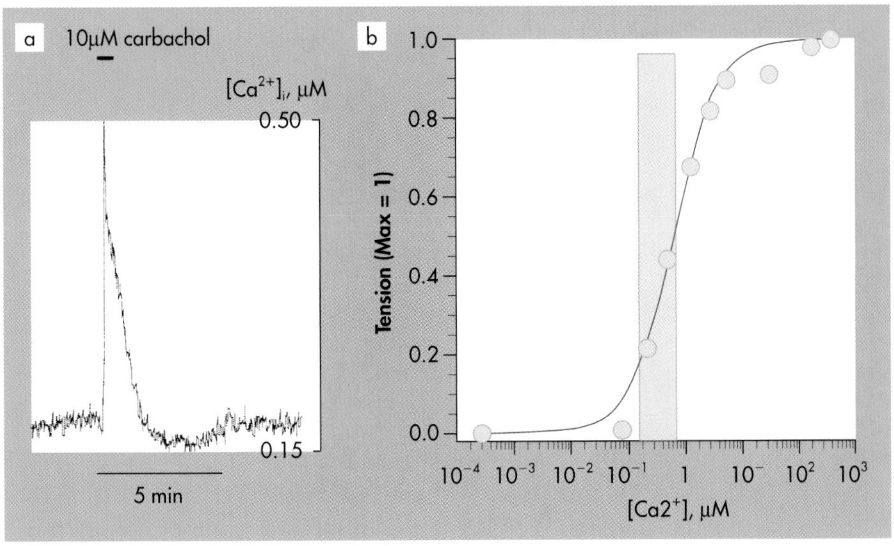

Figure 15.10 *(a) The change of the intracellular [Ca^{2+}] in an isolated detrusor myocyte on application of the acetylcholine analogue, carbachol. (b) The relationship between the [Ca^{2+}] and the tension developed by contractile filaments in a guinea-pig detrusor strip. The shaded bar shows the range of [Ca^{2+}] encompassed by the Ca^{2+}-transient on the left. Methods from references 17 and 18.*

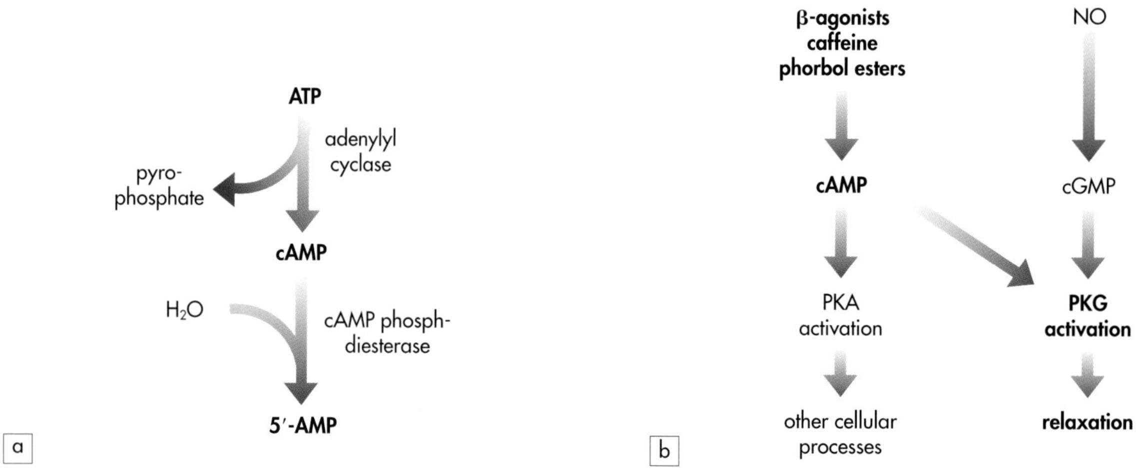

Figure 15.11 *(a) the reactions leading to the formation of cyclic-AMP (cAMP) from ATP and its breakdown to 5′-adenosine monophosphate (5′-AMP). (b) the postulated pathways leading to the activation of protein kinase A (PKA) and protein kinase G (PKG) by the cyclic nucleotides cAMP and cGMP: NO, nitric oxide.*

bladder smooth muscle'). Cellular cAMP levels are increased (Figure 15.11a), either by increasing the activity of adenylyl cyclase (as by β-receptor activation) or by phosphodiesterase inhibition (as in application of caffeine). Addition of caffeine to a detrusor cell is a good example of the relevance of the cyclic nucleotide-dependent mechanisms. Caffeine evokes a substantial rise of the $[Ca^{2+}]_i$, as it can evoke near maximal release of Ca^{2+} from intracellular stores; but, paradoxically, it generates little contractile activity,[21] presumably by increasing cellular cAMP (Figure 15.12). cAMP activates a kinase (protein kinase A [PKA]), and it was believed that PKA would mediate relaxation by, for example, phosphorylating MLCK,[22] or myosin phosphatase. More recently, it has been proposed that cAMP can also activate protein kinase G (PKG – the kinase activated by cGMP),[23] and it is by this route that relaxation is mediated (Figure 15.11b). The precise details remain to be elucidated in lower urinary tract smooth muscles.

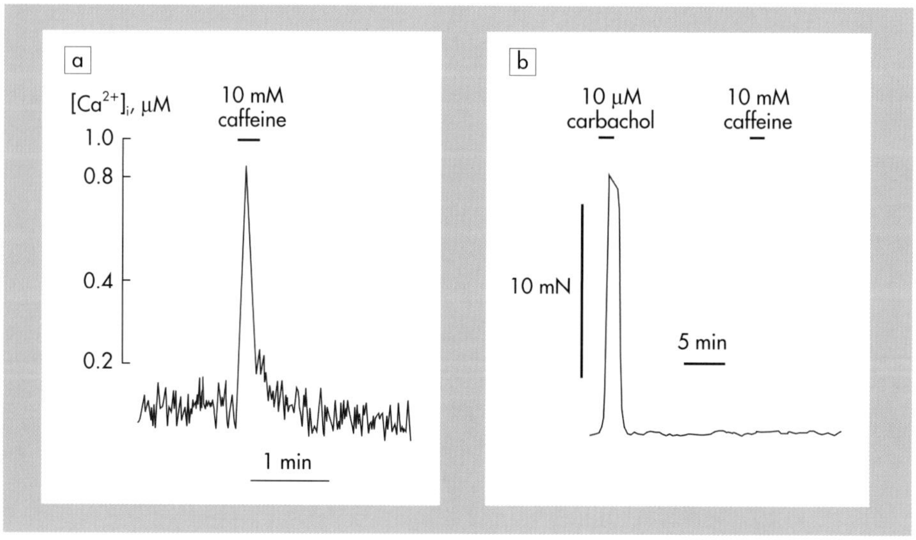

Figure 15.12 *(a) The increase of the intracellular $[Ca^{2+}]$ evoked by caffeine in an isolated human detrusor myocyte (methods[18]). (b) The effect of carbachol and caffeine on isometric tension in an in vitro strip of human detrusor. The agents were added to the superfusate during the times indicated by the horizontal bars.*

MOTOR INNERVATION OF THE DETRUSOR

Role of motor nerves

A phasic detrusor smooth muscle contraction is controlled by a dense network of parasympathetic motor nerves that ramify through the detrusor mass. The nerve fibres expand, along their length, into varicosities that contain small vesicles of neurotransmitters, such that virtually every detrusor myocyte is in functional contact with a motor nerve (Figure 15.13). These nerves can be stained for acetylcholinesterase (Figure 15.14), an extracellular enzyme that degrades acetylcholine, and are therefore designated as cholinergic fibres.

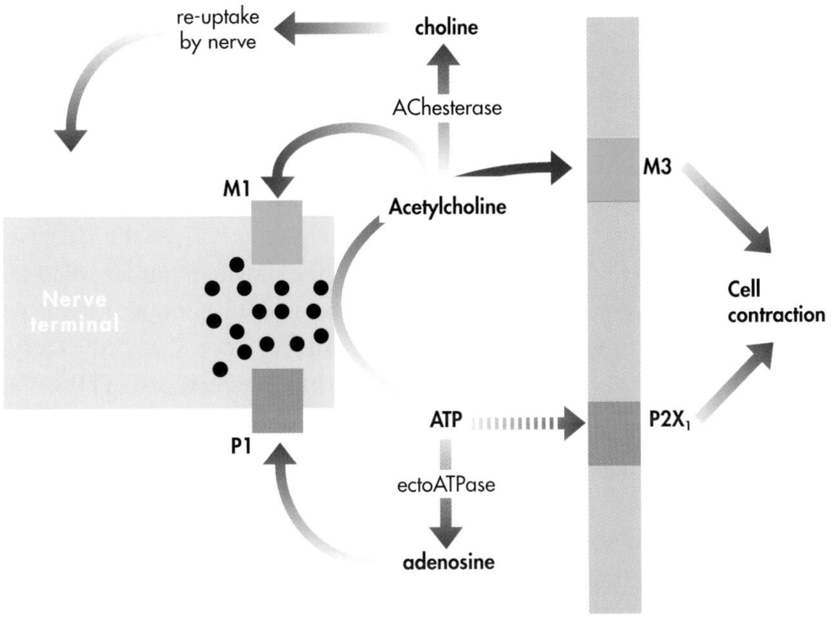

Figure 15.13 *A schematic representation of the neuromuscular junction at a detrusor cell. The nerve terminal releases acetylcholine and ATP. The transmitters bind to receptors on the muscle membrane to evoke contraction. Their lifetime is limited by enzymes in the junctional cleft. The transmitter acetylcholine or the ATP breakdown product adenosine can also exert prejunctional effects modifying further transmitter release. Choline is taken up the nerve terminal to resynthesize acetylcholine.*

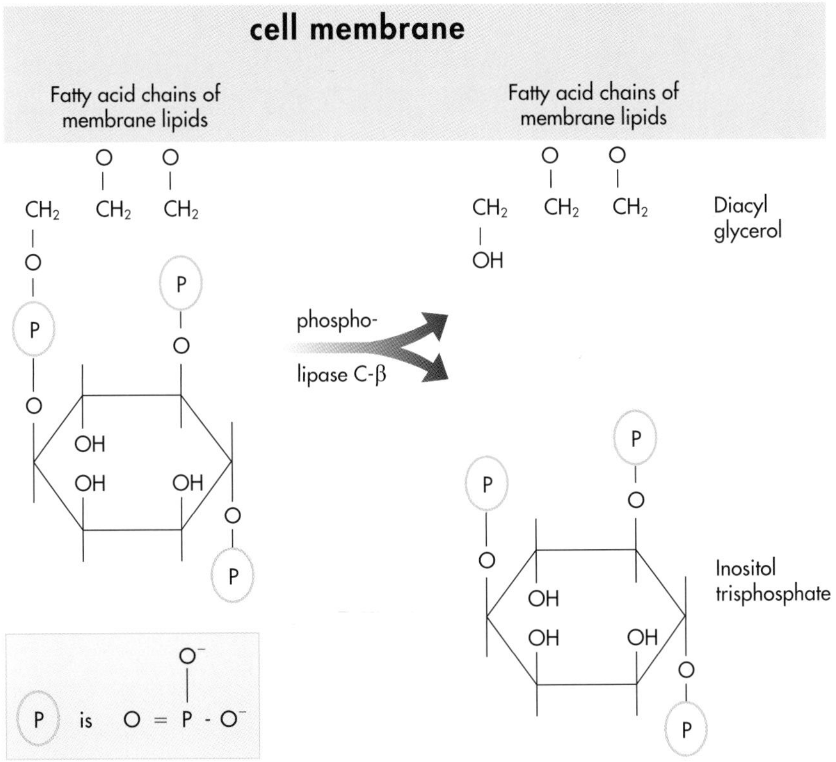

Figure 15.14 *Biochemical reaction leading to the production of inositol trisphosphate and diacylglycerol from membrane phosphoinositides.*

The functional neurotransmitters can be identified by in vitro experiments using detrusor strips. Tetanic stimulation of a strip with short pulses (50–100 μs) evokes a contraction which can be blocked completely by the neurotoxin, tetrodotoxin.[24] Tetrodotoxin blocks Na^+ channels responsible for the depolarizing phase of the nerve (and also skeletal muscle and working myocardium) action potential but has no direct action on detrusor smooth muscle, as it lacks such Na^+ channels. It may therefore be inferred that the contraction arises after stimulation of the motor nerves and their release of transmitters which diffuse to the muscle membrane. In the case of detrusor from stable human bladders, this contraction can also be blocked virtually completely by atropine, implying that the functional transmitter is exclusively acetylcholine (Figure 15.15).[25]

Detrusor from non-primate bladders and from some unstable human bladders, exhibit a degree of atropine resistance, whereby a residual contraction is obtained in the presence of atropine.[24] This additional component of contraction is believed to be mediated by a second neurotransmitter ATP, as this fraction can be abolished by prior desensitization of purinergic receptors on the smooth muscle membrane.[25]

Breakdown of neurotransmitters in the synaptic cleft

The lifetime of transmitters in the synaptic cleft is limited due to their removal by extracellular enzymes, acetylcholinesterase and ectoATPases.[26] Choline is one product of acetylcholine breakdown which is taken up by the nerve terminal by a Na^+-linked secondary active transport; ATP is hydrolysed ultimately to adenosine. Transmitter breakdown ensures that receptor occupation on the muscle membrane is transient. Any factor which alters the activity of these enzymes will therefore change the effectiveness of these neurotransmitters. For example, physostigmine, which inhibits acetylcholinesterase, enhances the detrusor contraction.[24] Even in the normal human bladder, it is believed that both acetylcholine and ATP are released by the motor nerve,[27] but that only acetylcholine has any functional effect, as ATP is so effectively hydrolysed in the synaptic space. The pathophysiological aspects of this system will be considered in Chapter 16.

The neurotransmitter breakdown products and the neurotransmitters themselves can exert further modulatory roles on transmitter release by having

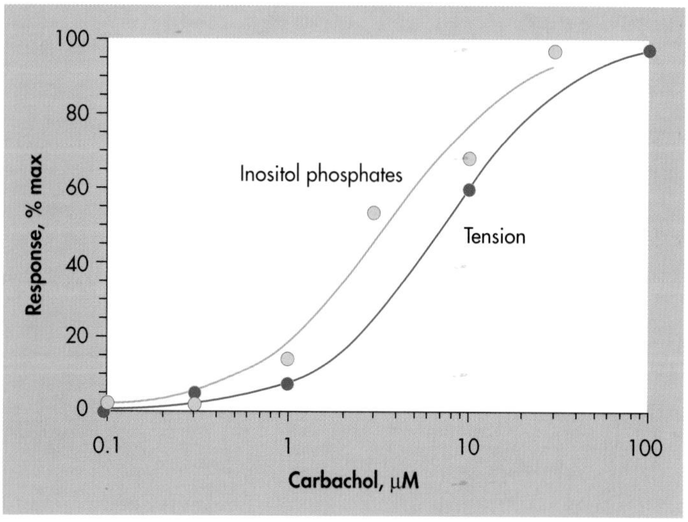

Figure 15.15 *The dependence of inositol phosphate production and tension generation on the extracellular carbachol concentration in detrusor preparations. Adapted from reference 40.*

effects via the pre-synaptic membrane. Acetylcholine can bind to M1 receptors[28] and adenosine (from ATP) to P1 receptors on the nerve terminal[29] and modulate further release of transmitter. Moreover, there may be considerable functional cross-talk of this feedback, as adenosine binding to the motor nerve terminal has also been demonstrated to inhibit acetylcholine release in ileal smooth muscle.[30] This autoinhibition will ensure that the quantity and time-course of transmitter release is modulated, so as not to deplete excessively the store of transmitter and risk desensitization of the muscle receptors. A scheme of transmitter release is shown in Figure 15.13.

THE CELLULAR ACTION OF TRANSMITTERS AND THE REGULATION OF INTRACELLULAR Ca^{2+}

Mode of action of transmitters

Acetylcholine binds to muscarinic receptors on the smooth muscle membrane. Pharmacologically, three different types of muscarinic receptors have been identified (M1, M2 and M3) with respect to their differential antagonism to different ligands: that is, pirenzipine (M1), methoctramine (M2), 4-diphenylacetoxy-N-piperidine or 4-DAMP (M3).[31] Recently an M4 subtype has also been identified.[32] Molecular approaches have yielded five subtypes (m1–m5), of which the first three correspond to those identified by pharmacological methods,[33,34] although only the m2 and m3 subtypes may be abundant in human bladder. In the bladder, most quantitative binding studies demonstrate that the dominant receptor is the m2 subtype,[34,35] but the M3 subtype is believed to mediate contraction.[31,35] The role that M2 receptors play is unclear, but they could assist in contraction development,[36] possibly by their G-protein-dependent inhibition of adenylyl cyclase.

Extracellular ATP also binds to specific purinergic receptors. On the detrusor smooth muscle membrane, this is predominantly of the $P2X_1$ subtype, based on the binding of specific probes.[37] In each case, agonist binding to the receptor initiates a series of cellular events that initiate the process of contraction.

Muscarinic receptors and contractile activation

M3 receptors are coupled to membrane-bound G-proteins (Chapter 1), in this instance the Gq subtype, which activates a phospholipase (phospholipase C-β) to break down membrane-bound phosphatidylinositol ultimately to inositol trisphosphate (IP_3) and diacylglycerol (DAG) – Figure 15.14 (see also Figure 15.18). DAG remains associated with the cell membrane and is fairly rapidly metabolized. However, it has two important functions in many cells: (1) it can be further cleaved to arachidonic acid, which in turn acts as a precursor for eicosanoid production; (2) it activates several of the isoforms of protein kinase C, which in turn can modulate ion channel function. The significance of this pathway remains to be fully explored in detrusor.

IP_3 is soluble within the sarcoplasm and diffuses to the sarcoplasmic reticulum (s.r.), an intracellular organelle which can store Ca^{2+} to high concentrations by pumping the ion into its lumen via a Ca^{2+}-activated ATPase. IP_3 receptors on the s.r. membrane are linked to Ca^{2+} release channels such that production of the second messenger leads to a rapid rise of the sarcoplasmic $[Ca^{2+}]$.[38] Several subtypes of the IP_3 receptor have been identified,[39] but the functional significance of these has yet to be defined. The importance of inositol phosphates in mediating cholinergic-dependent contraction has been well illustrated in detrusor. Figure 15.15 shows that the generation of tension and production of inositol phosphates in detrusor samples is stimulated by similar concentrations of the acetylcholine analogue, carbachol.[40]

An important sequela of this scheme is that initiation of tension by muscarinic agonists, and mediated by soluble second messengers, is independent of electrical membrane events, such as action potentials. This is well illustrated by an experiment in which the membrane potential is measured simultaneously with the rise of intracellular Ca^{2+} in response to carbachol exposure (Figure 15.16). Addition of carbachol to an isolated detrusor cell

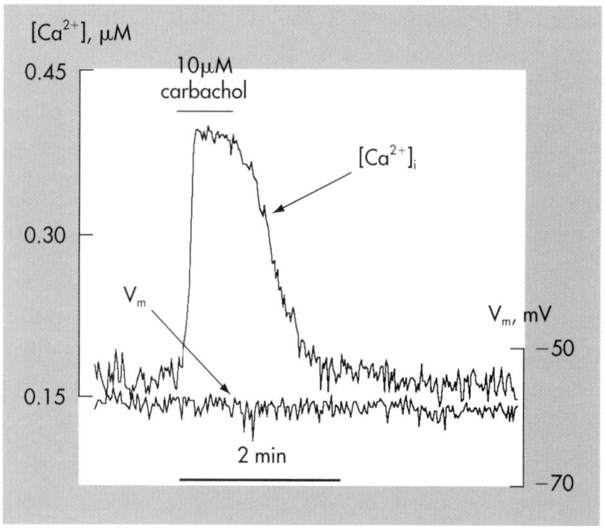

Figure 15.16 *The effect of 10 µM extracellular carbachol on the intracellular [Ca^{2+}] and membrane potential, V_m, in an isolated detrusor myocyte.*

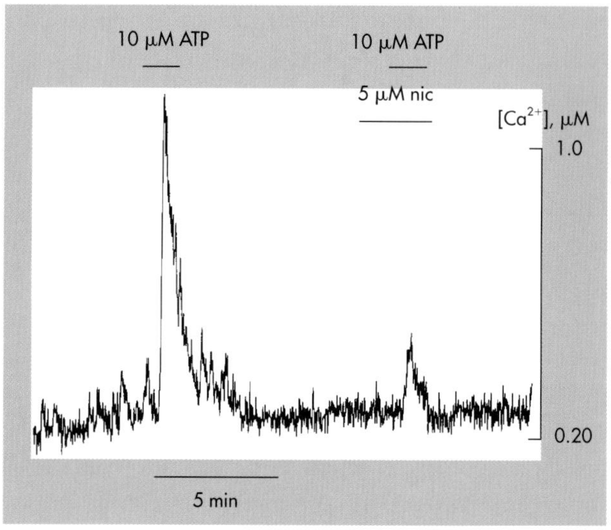

Figure 15.17 *The effect of 10 µM ATP on the intracellular [Ca^{2+}] in an isolated detrusor myocyte. Two applications are shown. Preceding and during the second ATP exposure, the myocyte was also exposed to 5 µM nicardipine.*

generates a transient rise of intracellular Ca^{2+} but no alteration to the membrane potential.

Purinergic receptors and contractile activation

The $P2X_1$ receptor is a ligand-gated ion channel which is activated when ATP binds. The channel is relatively non-selective to cations, so that Na^+ carries most charge, although some direct Ca^{2+} entry can occur by this route.[41] However, the depolarization mediated by the inward movement of cations is sufficient to open L-type Ca^{2+} channels, which initiate a secondary, more substantial Ca^{2+} influx. Figure 15.17 shows that ATP, when added to a detrusor myocyte, generates a transient rise of the intracellular [Ca^{2+}], which can be largely abolished by L-type channel antagonists such as nicardipine. The substantial rise of the intracellular [Ca^{2+}] mediated by this influx is again partially supplemented by release from the sarcoplasmic reticulum through a process of Ca^{2+}-induced Ca^{2+} release.[42,43] This phenomenon occurs when a rapid rise of intracellular [Ca^{2+}] opens Ca^{2+} channels in the s.r. membrane – the so-called ryanodine receptor – which are structurally similar to the IP_3-gated s.r. Ca^{2+} channels. Figure 15.18 summarizes the relationship between extracellular agonists and intracellular Ca^{2+} release.

IP_3 is rapidly degraded by specific phosphatases, and this limits the phase of Ca^{2+} release from the s.r. However, termination of contraction is importantly brought about by a reduction of the sarcoplasmic [Ca^{2+}] to resting levels. The most potent way the cell achieves this is by an uptake of Ca^{2+} back into the s.r., via a CaATPase.[44] This ATPase can be blocked by agents such as cyclopiazonic acid or thapsigargin, and in the presence of these inhibitors, subsequent addition of agents such as caffeine evoke little Ca^{2+} release.

However, other mechanisms may also be active, but their relative roles need to be established in detrusor. By analogy with other smooth muscles,[45] Ca^{2+} may be removed from the cell by two possible routes: (1) a separate CaATPase in the cell membrane;[46] (2) a Na^+/Ca^{2+} countertransporter which ejects one Ca^{2+} for the influx of three Na^+ (these Na^+ can then be removed by the Na pump).[47] Finally, the mitochondria may participate in Ca^{2+} removal from the sarcoplasm via a so-called uniporter, using the energy in the mitochondrial membrane potential created by the generation of a proton gradient.[48,49] Although this route has been ignored in recent years, due to its relatively slow uptake rate, it is regaining favour by those who study intracellular Ca^{2+} regulation. It is also a sensible mechanism, as several

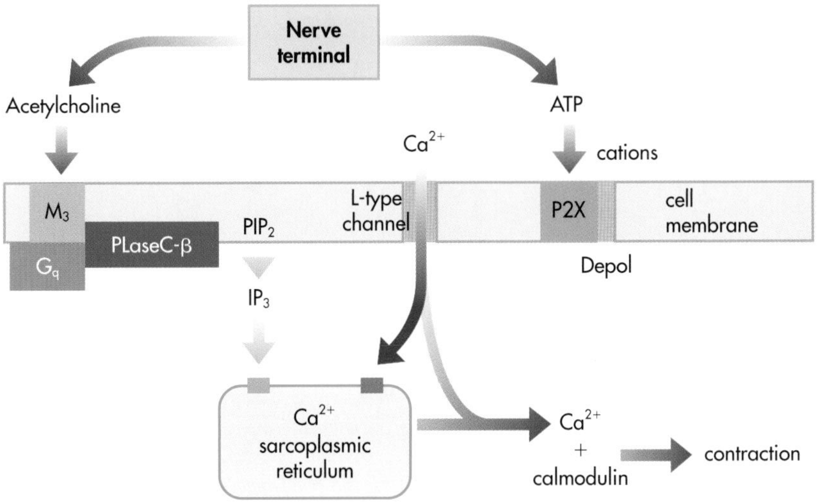

Figure 15.18 *The membrane and intracellular events leading to the rise of the intracellular [Ca^{2+}] in response to the release of acetylcholine and ATP in a detrusor myocyte. Ca^{2+} release from the sarcoplasmic reticulum is evoked by IP_3 binding to a receptor on the organelle surface or a transient Ca^{2+} influx through ion channels (Ca^{2+}-induced Ca^{2+} release). G_q: G-protein subtype G_q; PLaseC-β: phospholipase C-β.*

mitochondrial enzymes involved in aerobic ATP production are Ca^{2+} sensitive. Contraction is an ATP-consuming process and is mediated by a rise of sarcoplasmic Ca^{2+}; therefore, any mitochondrial Ca^{2+} influx would be an ideal sensor to match ATP consumption and production.[50] Figure 15.19 summarizes the possible routes for removing Ca^{2+} from the sarcoplasm to terminate the contraction.

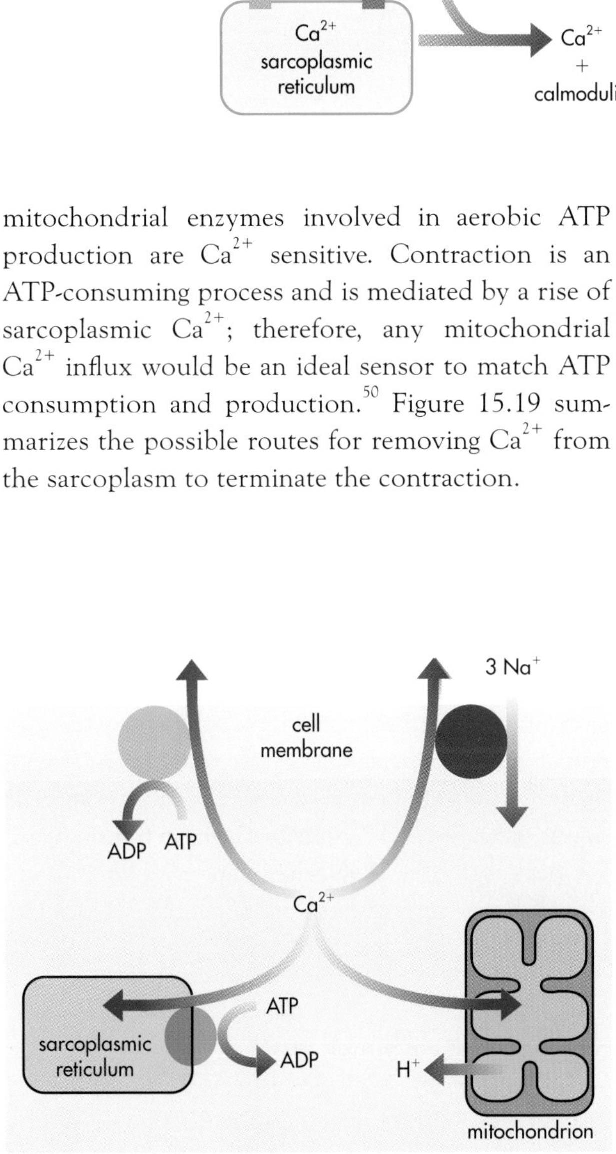

Figure 15.19 *Possible routes for Ca^{2+} clearance from the sarcoplasm in a detrusor myocyte. Intracellular routes are via a CaATPase into the sarcoplasmic reticulum or into the mitochondria by utilization of the energy in the proton gradient across the inner membrane. Efflux routes are via a separate ATPase or a Na^+/Ca^{2+} exchange. See text for details.*

ELECTROPHYSIOLOGICAL PROPERTIES OF DETRUSOR SMOOTH MUSCLE

The transfer of ions across the cell membrane is generally mediated either via ion transporters or through ion channels. A net flux of cations or anions will also change the membrane potential – a flux of cations into the cell will depolarize it and an efflux cause hyperpolarization. Ion transporters move ions relatively slowly (about 10^3 ions per second) and serve important functions to regulate the intracellular concentrations of, for example Na^+ (via the Na pump) or H^+ (via Na^+/H^+ counterexchange). They generally produce minor effects on the membrane potential, as the net flux of ions is relatively small. Net flux through an ion channel is much greater (about 10^6 ions per second), so that more profound effects on membrane potential will generally ensue. Thus, the electrophysiological properties of detrusor will be determined largely by ion channel properties.

Ion channels and membrane events

Transmembrane ion fluxes are often measured as the current they carry, by the voltage-clamp method shown in Figure 15.20a. The membrane potential, V_m, is measured with an intracellular electrode (often a 'patch' electrode which forms a tight seal with the surface membrane and ruptures a hole in it, thus gaining access to the intracellular space).[51,52] An

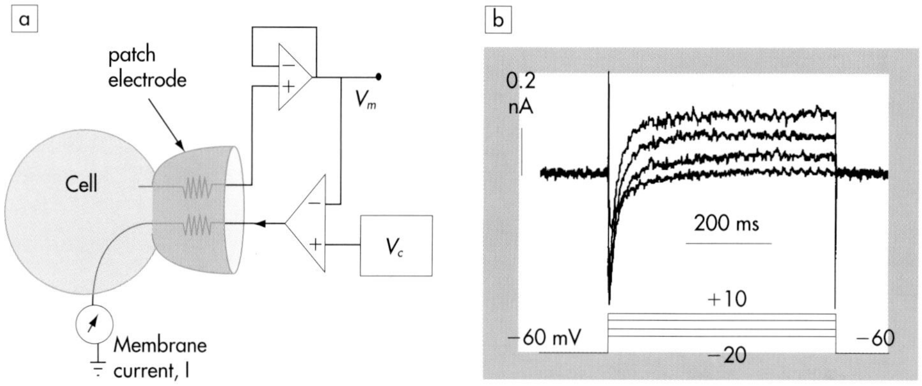

Figure 15.20 *(a) Schematic representation of the voltage-clamp of an isolated cell with a patch electrode. The membrane potential (V_m), of the cell is recorded by a unity-gain amplifier (represented by the upper triangle in the figure) for one fraction of a duty cycle, usually at about 4 kHz. The value serves as the negative (inverting) input of a second amplifier of which the non-inverting input is a second command potential (V_c). A current proportional to the difference V_c–V_m is fed back into the cell for the remainder of the duty cycle, and is equivalent to the membrane current flowing when the membrane potential is switched from V_m to V_c. (b) Sample current traces when the membrane potential is clamped for 500 ms to different potentials (–20, –10, 0, +10 mV), from a resting (or holding) potential of –60 mV. An inward current transiently flows before an steady-state outward current is established. The calibration bar represents a current of 200 pA (2.10^{-10} A).*

advantage of using a patch electrode is that the composition of the cell interior can be controlled as the solution in the patch electrode displaces the sarcoplasm of the cell. Thus, the effect of changing the extracellular and intracellular environment on ionic currents can be measured.

The value of V_m is compared to a command potential, V_c, and a current which is proportional to the difference between V_c and V_m is then passed into the cell, usually by the same patch electrode, by electronic switching systems. This current is equivalent to the ionic current that would flow across the cell membrane if V_m was suddenly changed to V_c. The type of experimental traces are shown in Figure 15.20b. Cation influx (or anion efflux, but this will not be considered here) is represented as a current trace below the baseline, and is called an inward current: an outward current results from cation efflux. The particular ion carrying a current can be determined by changing the extracellular or intracellular concentrations of different ions and measuring the effect on the magnitude of the resultant ionic current.

Ionic channels mediating depolarization

Two major classes of ion channels have been identified: (1) voltage-activated Ca^{2+} channels; (2) non-specific cation channels.[53]

Voltage-activated Ca^{2+} channels

In human and animal detrusor, two Ca^{2+} channels have been identified; an L-type[54–56] and a T-type channel.[57] L-type channels are opened at membrane potentials more positive than –40 mV, and the magnitude of the current is large – sufficient to support the depolarizing phase of the action potential.[54] Therefore, activation of these channels can generate a significant rise of the intracellular [Ca^{2+}] (Figure 15.21a). The channels are blocked by agents such as verapamil and nicardipine, and they have biophysical characteristics similar to L-type channels in other cell types. T-type channels are opened at more negative potentials (about –65 mV), and the current is more transient and the peak value smaller. They can be distinguished from L-type currents by their selective block by 100 μM $NiCl_2$ (Figure 15.21b).[57]

Non-specific cation channels

Receptors which bind extracellular ATP are rapidly deactivating cation channels,[58,59] causing depolarization (Figure 15.22) of a magnitude sufficient to activate L-type Ca^{2+} channels. Activation of these purinergic receptors thus causes a transient rise of intracellular Ca^{2+}, which can be almost completely blocked by L-type channel antagonists (Figure 15.17).

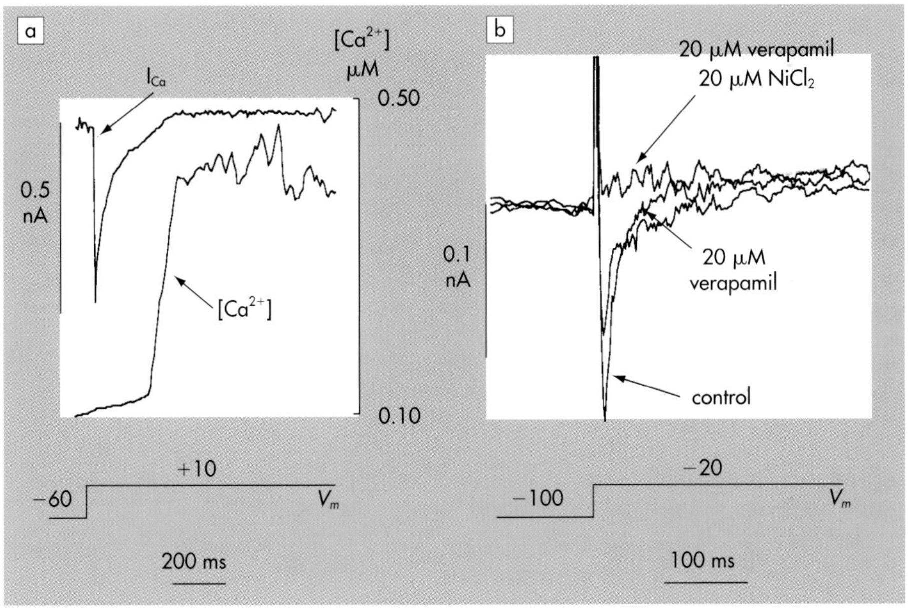

Figure 15.21 *(a) Simultaneous recording of L-type Ca^{2+} current and intracellular $[Ca^{2+}]$ in an isolated detrusor myocyte on a change of membrane potential (V_m), from −60 to +10 mV. (b) Inward currents recorded on changing V_m, from −100 to −20 mV, under control conditions, in the presence of 20 μM verapamil and 20 μM verapamil + 100 μM NiCl2. The patch pipette contained Cs^+ to block outward K^+ currents.*

Recent work has identified a large number of purinoreceptors, but the available evidence shows that the $P2X_1$ subtype predominates in human detrusor smooth muscle.[37]

Stretch-activated channels have also been described in detrusor cells,[60,61] whereby physical stretch of the membrane opens a cation channel, depolarizing the cell. It has been proposed that this channel could mediate a rise in muscle tone in the bladder wall during filling, although this remains to be proved.

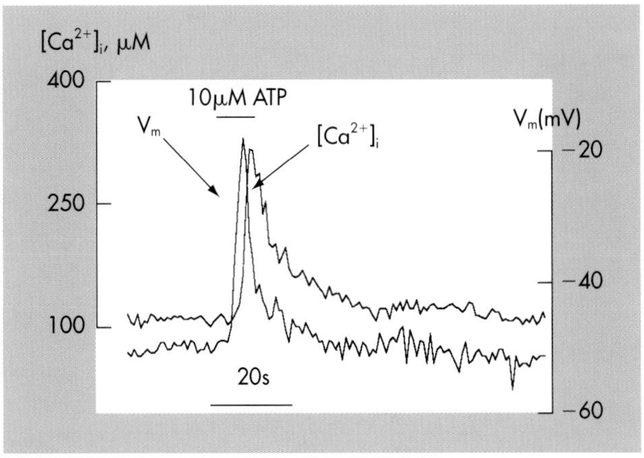

Figure 15.22 *The effect of 10 μM extracellular carbachol on the intracellular $[Ca^{2+}]$ and membrane potential (V_m), in an isolated detrusor myocyte.*

Ionic channels mediating repolarization

A number of K^+ channels have been identified in detrusor smooth muscle, but two types are likely to predominate; namely, K^+ channels activated by a rise of intracellular Ca^{2+} and channels opened by a reduction of intracellular ATP. Both channels exhibit a property called outward-going rectification; that is, they pass a larger current at positive membrane potentials. Thus, the more depolarized V_m becomes, the greater is the tendency for repolarization, and this results in brief rather than prolonged changes to membrane potential.

Ca^{2+}-activated K^+ channels

Several different such channels have been identified, distinguished by the amount of current that individual channels can carry. In detrusor, the so-called large conductance (BK) channel is predominant, based on the observation that the current is greatly attenuated by toxins such as iberiotoxin and charybdotoxin.[61,62] The channel is opened by a rise of $[Ca^{2+}]$ on the intracellular face of the membrane, in particular when Ca^{2+} is released from intracellular stores.[63,64] A rise of intracellular $[Ca^{2+}]$ will therefore open a K^+ channel, an effect which causes membrane hyperpolarization and may limit further Ca^{2+} influx

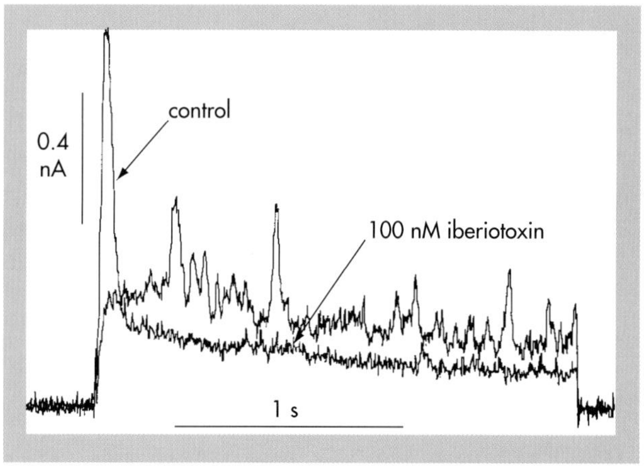

Figure 15.23 *Spontaneous transient outward currents (STOCs) superimposed on a background outward current in an isolated detrusor myocyte. 100 nM iberiotoxin abolished the STOCs. Currents evoked by a change of* V_m *from –60 to +40 mV.*

by reducing the likelihood of Ca^{2+} channel activation. This feedback process can lead to oscillations of membrane current, called STOCs[65] (spontaneous transient outward currents, Figure 15.23), which would in turn lead to oscillations of membrane potential.

ATP-dependent K^+, K_{ATP}, channels

These represent another important class of K^+ channels whose role in detrusor smooth muscle regulation is unclear. A reduction of the intracellular [ATP] opens such channels, which again may serve as a feedback protective device.[66,67] Figure 15.24 shows an experiment when the channel is artificially opened with the drug levcromakalim, despite a high intracellular [ATP]. Reduced cellular ATP levels will occur during metabolic stress, when further ATP consumption by contracting the muscle cell would be undesirable. Hyperpolarization of the membrane would tend to limit Ca^{2+} influx and thereby reduce tension development, and ATP consumption, by the cell.

The functions of ion channels in detrusor smooth muscle

Several functions have already been alluded to. Greater opening of K^+ channels will hyperpolarize the membrane, providing a negative feedback over Ca^{2+} influx and ATP consumption. In addition, K^+ channels will be the main determinant of the resting potential, as these will be the class of ion channels mainly open at such potentials.

Ca^{2+} channels have been proposed to play a role in refilling intracellular stores in other smooth muscles,[68] and in detrusor contractions mediated by muscarinic agonists can be attenuated by L-type Ca^{2+} channel antagonists.[69] Because of the interplay between intracellular Ca^{2+} levels and BK channel activation, the membrane potential is likely to oscillate between levels that will span the range of potentials at which T-type and even L-type channels will open. Recordings from isolated detrusor cells show that V_m may indeed show significant oscillations, which can occasionally even trigger

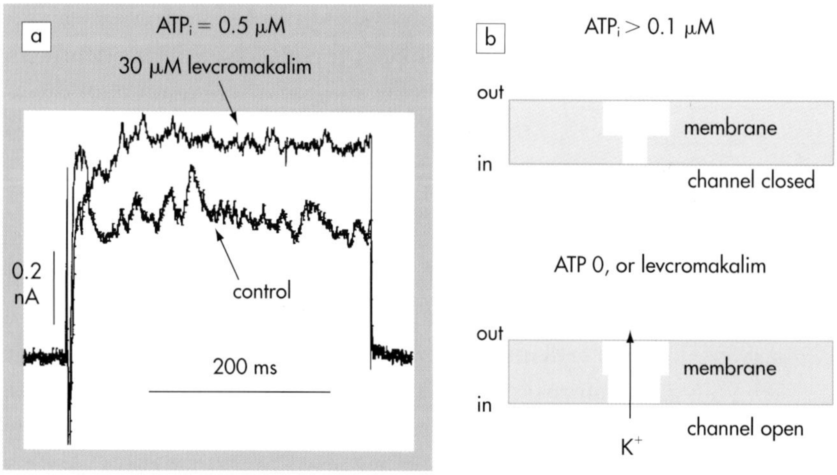

Figure 15.24 *(a) Ionic currents recorded in an isolated detrusor myocyte in the absence (green) and presence (brown) of levcromakalim. The patch electrode contained 1 mM ATP. (b) Diagram of* K_{ATP} *channels; in the presence of intracellular [ATP] of >0.5 mM, the channel is closed. In the presence of levcromakalim or when the intracellular [ATP] is reduced, the channel opens, allowing* K^+ *efflux.*

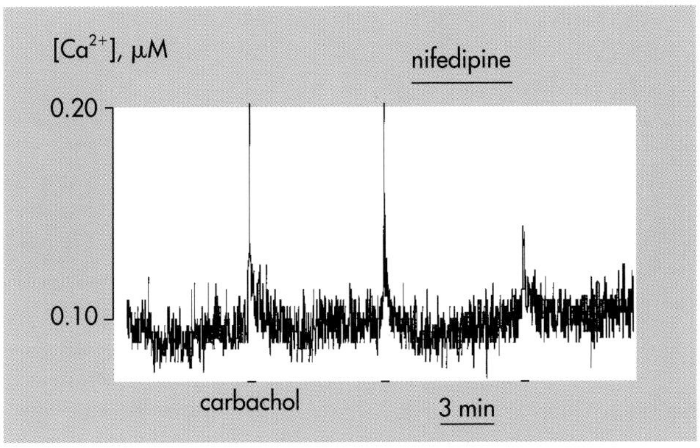

Figure 15.25 *Recording of the intracellular [Ca^{2+}] in an isolated guinea-pig detrusor myocyte. The myocyte was briefly exposed to 10 μM carbachol on three separate occasions. Between the second and third exposure, the cell was also exposed to 10 μM nicardipine.*

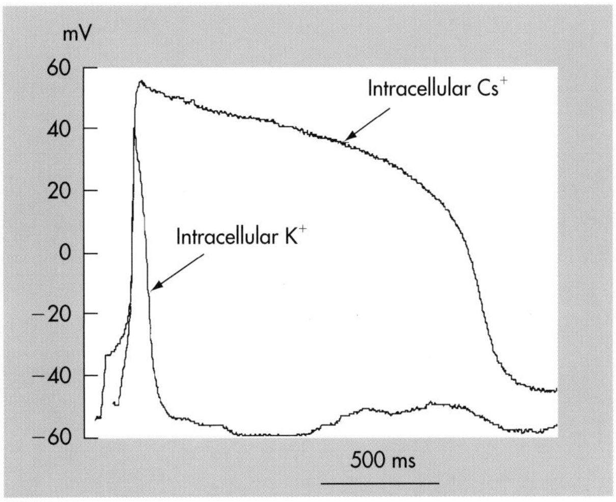

Figure 15.26 *Action potentials recorded in an isolated human detrusor myocyte in response to passage of a current (0.04 nA) into the cell via a patch electrode. The patch electrode contained either a K^+-based or a Cs^+-based solution.*

action potentials. The role of Ca^{2+} channels in refilling intracellular stores is illustrated in Figure 15.25. A myocyte is exposed twice to caffeine, which releases stored Ca^{2+}. In the interval between the second and third exposures, a Ca^{2+} channel antagonist is added, attenuating the third carbachol-induced Ca-transient. Such an experiment is consistent with Ca^{2+} channels providing an influx route in the interval between successive exposures, to fill intracellular Ca^{2+} stores. T-type channels may aid this process, as they open at more negative membrane potentials and thus will provide an additional influx route.

Action potentials

Detrusor smooth muscle can generate action potentials (APs),[70] which are capable of propagating considerable distances. Figure 15.26 shows an example from human detrusor. The depolarizing phase (upstroke) is attenuated in zero-Ca solutions, and quantitative measurements show that the magnitude of the L-type Ca^{2+} current is sufficient to support this phase. Repolarization is slowed by intracellular Cs^+, which is known to block K^+ channels.[71,72] However, the fact that muscarinic agonists can generate contraction independently of membrane potential changes shows that APs are not a *requirement* for the initiation of contraction. However, their study is warranted, as AP generation may modulate force production under the following circumstances:

- Purinergic transmitters (ATP) will depolarize the cell sufficiently to open L-type Ca^{2+} channels and initiate an AP. This is relevant to detrusor from some unstable human bladders and from non-primate bladders, which have both functional cholinergic and purinergic neurotransmission.
- Membrane potential oscillations may generate localized APs, as may occur, for example, during transient intracellular Ca depletion after a large release of Ca^{2+} from intracellular stores.

Propagation of electrical signals?

An area of current controversy is whether an electrical signal (APs or membrane oscillations) can propagate between adjacent cells. In tissues such as cardiac muscle, cell-to-cell propagation is easy, and the myocardial mass constitutes the functional syncytium of cells.[73] Therefore, an action potential generated in one part of the myocardium will activate a much larger region. Connectivity is ensured by gap junctions; they contain a family of proteins, connexins, which form a large pore connecting the sarcoplasm of adjacent cells.[74]

Gap junctions can be visualized under the electron microscope and in myocardium are concentrated at the intercalated disks. In detrusor, many investigators have been unable to observe gap junctions, or see

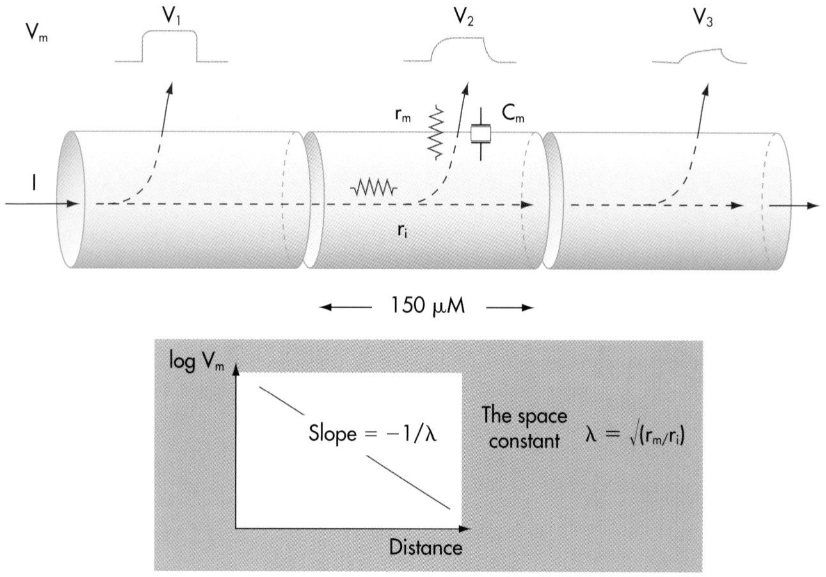

Figure 15.27 *Diagram of several detrusor myocytes to illustrate the experimental arrangement designed to demonstrate electrical coupling between adjacent cells. A current is injected into one cell (left). The current can leave the cell across the surface membrane (represented by a resistance [R_m], and capacitance [C_m]) and, if possible, crossing to the next cell, where the current again has these two possible pathways. When current leaves the cell, it generates a change to membrane potential represented by the transients, V_1, V_2 and V_3. The more extensive is electrical coupling, the greater the distance voltage transients can be recorded.*

them only very occasionally,[75] a fact which has led to the conclusion that detrusor smooth muscle cells are not electrically coupled. However, electrophysiological studies have suggested that adjacent cells may be coupled.[76,77] Experiments with muscle strips have demonstrated electric current flow over considerable distances between cells. Figure 15.27 shows the experimental system: current, *I*, is injected into a set of cells and the change of membrane potential, V_m, measured at various distances from the injection site. The further away voltage changes can be recorded, the greater the distances current will travel, and thus the better, cells will be connected. With such experiments, currents can be shown to flow several cell lengths, implying significant coupling. The quantification of such data is carried out by cable analysis, so-called because the mathematical background was originally formulated by William Thompson (Lord Kelvin) when investigating the feasibility of transmitting telegraphic signals via an insulated trans-Atlantic cable. In practice, the magnitude of the voltage responses (illustrated in Figure 15.27) is used to generate a parameter called the space constant, λ. A large value of λ implies good electrical coupling, and, in detrusor, values of several millimetres are recorded.[76] This suggests that currents can flow over many cell lengths, which are about 150 µm at their greatest dimension. The interested reader is referred to more mathematical treatments of the subject.[78–81] To corroborate these observations, connexin subtypes have recently been demonstrated in human detrusor by using specific antibodies (GP Sui and NJ Severs, unpublished data). The sparsity of antibody binding and the relatively high electrical resistance measured means that detrusor is not electrically coupled as well as the myocardium; nevertheless, signals can pass between adjacent cells.

The consequences of intercellular coupling are important and not yet fully explored. Firstly, the *speed* at which electrical signals travel depends upon the actual magnitude of the coupling resistance: a relatively high resistance results in a slow speed.[82] It remains to be determined how effectively and how rapidly electrical signals can propagate through detrusor tissue and whether they may be responsible for coordinating any mechanical activity in the muscle mass. Secondly, small molecules can also pass through gap junctions, thus ensuring chemical coupling of cells also.[83] The importance of such cell-to-cell transference in harmonizing the biochemical behaviour of the tissue is an unexplored subject.

REGIONAL DIFFERENCES IN BLADDER SMOOTH MUSCLE

Most work on detrusor smooth muscle has used muscle from the dome of the bladder, and the physiology of bladder neck and trigone has been less intensively studied. However, a number of differences in smooth muscle have emerged. These regions have a sympathetic innervation, as well as a cholinergic supply,[84,85] which is mediated via α_1, and possibly also α_2, receptors.[86] The sympathetic supply may well enhance the more profound spontaneous contractile behaviour found in these regions of the bladder.

Upon blockade of cholinergic and adrenergic (both α- and β-dependent) receptors, the tetrodotoxin-dependent contractile response can still be observed; it has been termed a NANC (non-adrenergic, non-cholinergic) response. At higher stimulation frequencies or in muscle that has been precontracted, this NANC response evokes a relaxation[87,88] and has been postulated to contribute to the relaxation of the bladder neck during micturition. Histochemical studies have identified a nerve population which contains NADPH-diaphorase activity,[89,90] a feature of nitric oxide synthase (NOS). NOS catalyses the conversion of arginine to citrulline with the consequent production of the signalling molecule, nitric oxide (NO). This system has been proposed to contribute to the NANC-induced relaxation.[91] NO is an extremely diffusible substance and, in spite of a short lifetime, can diffuse to adjacent cells, including smooth muscle cells. The only certain receptor for NO is soluble guanylate cyclase, which in turn catalyses the conversion of guanosine triphosphate (GTP) to cyclic GMP, a nucleotide which relaxes smooth muscle.[92] The whole process is shown in Figure 15.28.

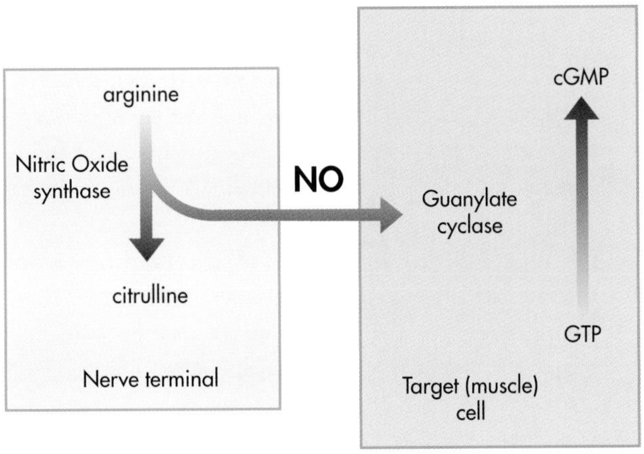

Figure 15.28 *A scheme to show the relationship between nitrergic nerves, which generate nitric oxide (NO), and the target cells which utilize the messenger to increase their production of cyclic GMP.*

DRUGS AND DETRUSOR FUNCTION

One of the purposes of studying detrusor smooth muscle is to identify particular features that would offer attractive drug targets. Two ideals are of relevance in this case: (1) to identify unique features of detrusor smooth muscle to minimize the effect of agents on other tissue, and (2) to characterize changes to detrusor function associated with bladder dysfunction to avoid compromising the normal function of the bladder. Reviews concerning the pharmacological control of the bladder frequently appear.[93–96] The purpose of this section is to provide, where possible, an outline of the action on smooth muscle of different types of bladder-active agents.

Muscarinic agents

The M3 muscarinic receptor is the functional subtype in the human bladder and M3-selective agents such as darifenacin are available for the treatment of bladder overactivity.[97] However, M3 receptors are also important for regulating intestinal motility and saliva production, so that tissue specificity is difficult to attain.[98] Moreover, the role that M2 receptors play in regulating muscle function is unclear. Some muscarinic antagonists, such as tolterodine, have less subtype selectivity and may influence other uncharacterized aspects of muscarinic activation in detrusor.[99]

Adrenergic agents

The sympathetic nervous system appears to play little direct role in bladder function, although it may modulate parasympathetic activity,[100] possibly by decreasing acetylcholine release by stimulating α_2 receptors.[101] In detrusor from the bladder dome, β-adrenoreceptors are more abundant than α-receptors,[102] and adrenergic agents exert β-mediated relaxation, possibly by activation of adenylyl cyclase. An unusual β_3 subtype has been described, which, along with the β_2-receptor, may provide promising drug targets.[103] α_1 (possibly α_{1A}) receptors are the physiologically important adrenergic receptor in the bladder neck and trigone as well as the prostate stroma, and selective antagonists, such as tamsulosin, are effective in relaxing noradrenaline (norepinephrine)-evoked contractions in these tissues.[104]

Nitrergic modulators

Regulation of bladder neck opening by modulation of the nitrergic system has not been investigated. In principle, there are several points of regulation.[91] Much current work is directed towards inhibition of the system; nonetheless, this provides fundamental information for its potential upregulation for the hyperactive bladder.

- inhibition of NO synthesis by N^G-substituted L-arginines such as L-NMMA and L-NAME
- inhibition of release – muscarinic, α_2 and opioid receptors on the nerve terminal preventing release
- removal of NO by some superoxide generators such as hydroquinone and pyrogallol
- modulation of soluble guanylate cyclase activity.

Cyclic nucleotide modulators

In principle, phosphodiesterase (PDE) inhibitors, such as the methylxanthines, and stimulators of adenylyl cyclase, such as phorbol esters, should promote relaxation. For example, rolipram, a PDE-4 inhibitor, reduces detrusor contractility, but the PDE-5 inhibitor zaprinast had no effect.[105]

Ion channel modulators

Ca^{2+} channel antagonists, by reducing Ca^{2+} influx, should depress detrusor contractility. The problem with such agents is that their similar potency on myocardium and vascular smooth muscle generates significant cardiovascular side effects.[106,107] The K_{ATP} channel has also been the object of scrutiny in trying to achieve bladder relaxation. K_{ATP}-channel openers such as pinacidil and cromakalim, although effective, also had cardiovascular side effects. More bladder-selective agents, such as ZD6169, have recently been described.[108] The BK channel has received less pharmaceutical attention, but, as it is the major K^+ conductance channel, when intracellular Ca^{2+} is raised, it offers potential as a possible target.[109]

Prostanoids

Prostanoids contract human detrusor and are produced during bladder distension.[110] However, it is uncertain, in vivo, whether they have a direct effect on the muscle or activate sensory capsaicin-sensitive afferent nerves.[111]

ACKNOWLEDGEMENTS

The work quoted from the Institute of Urology was carried out with grants from the MRC, the Wellcome Trust and St Peter's Research Trust. I am particularly indebted to Dr C Wu and Dr G-P Sui, with whom I have had the pleasure to collaborate in collecting many of the illustrated data.

REFERENCES

1. Alexander RS. Series elasticity of urinary bladder smooth muscle. Am J Physiol 1976; 231: 1337–1342
2. Glerum JJ, Van Mastrigt R, Van Koeveringe AJ. Mechanical properties of mammalian single smooth muscle cells. III. Passive properties of pig detrusor and human *a terme* uterus cells. J Muscle Res Cell Motil 1990; 11: 453–462
3. Wagg A, Fry CH. Visco-elastic properties of isolated detrusor smooth muscle. Scand J Urol Nephrol Suppl 1999; 201: 12–18
4. Finkbeiner A, Lapides J. Effect of distension on blood flow in dog's urinary bladder. Investig Urol 1974; 12: 210–212
5. Huxley AF. The origin of force in skeletal muscle. Ciba Foundation Symposium 1975; 31: 271–290
6. Hill AV. The force–velocity relation in shortening muscle. In First and Last Experiments in Muscle Mechanics. Cambridge: Cambridge University Press, 1970: 23–41
7. Griffiths DJ. The mechanics of the urethra and of micturition. Br J Urol 1973; 45: 497–507
8. Malone-Lee J, Wahedna I. Characterisation of detrusor contractile function in relation to old age. Br J Urol 1993; 72: 873–880
9. Hai CM, Murphy RA. Ca^{2+}, crossbridge phosphorylation, and contraction. Ann Rev Physiol 1989; 51: 285–298
10. Paul RJ. Smooth muscle energetics. Ann Rev Physiol 1989; 51: 331–349

11. Paul RJ, Strauss JD, Krisanda J. The effects of calcium on smooth muscle mechanics and energetics. In: Siegman MJ, Somlyo AP, Stephens NL, eds. Regulation and Contraction of Smooth Muscle. New York: Liss, 1987: 319–332
12. Murphy RA. The muscle cells of hollow organs. News Physiol Sci 1988; 3: 124–128
13. Hellstrand P, Paul RJ. Phosphagen content, breakdown during contraction and oxygen consumption in rat portal vein. Am J Physiol 1983; 244: C250–C258
14. Paul RJ, Bauer M, Pease W. Vascular smooth muscle: aerobic glycolysis linked to Na-K transport processes. Science 1979; 206: 1414
15. Stull JT, Krueger JK, Kamm KE et al. Myosin light chain kinase. In: Bárány M, ed. Biochemistry of Smooth Muscle Contraction. San Diego, CA: Academic Press, 1996: 119–130
16. Erdödi F, Ito M, Hartshorne DJ. Myosin light chain phosphatase. In: Bárány M, ed. Biochemistry of Smooth Muscle Contraction. San Diego, CA: Academic Press, 1996: 131–142
17. Wu C, Kentish JC, Fry CH. Effect of pH on myofilament Ca^{2+}-sensitivity in alpha-toxin permeabilized guinea pig detrusor muscle. J Urol 1995; 154: 1921–1924
18. Wu C, Fry CH. The effects of extracellular and intracellular pH on intracellular Ca^{2+} regulation in guinea-pig detrusor smooth muscle. J Physiol 1998; 508: 131–143
19. Stull JT, Hsu LC, Tansey MG, Kamm KE. Myosin light chain kinase phosphorylation in tracheal smooth muscle. J Biol Chem 1990; 265: 16683–16690
20. Rembold CM. Modulation of the $[Ca^{2+}]$ sensitivity of myosin phosphorylation in intact swine arterial smooth muscle. J Physiol 1990; 429: 77–94
21. Hockey JS, Wu C, Fry CH. The actions of metabolic inhibition on human detrusor smooth muscle contractility from stable and unstable bladders. BJU 2000; 86: 531–537
22. Conti MA, Adelstein RS. The relationship between calmodulin binding and phosphorylation of smooth muscle myosin kinase by the catalytic subunit of 3′:5′ cAMP-dependent protein kinase. J Biol Chem 1981; 256: 3178–3181
23. Lincoln TM, Cornwell TL, Taylor AE. cGMP-dependent protein kinase mediates the reduction of Ca^{2+} by cAMP in vascular smooth muscle cells. Am J Physiol 1990; 258: C399–C407
24. Sibley GN. A comparison of spontaneous and nerve-mediated activity in bladder muscle from man, pig and rabbit. J Physiol 1984; 354: 431–443
25. Bayliss M, Wu C, Newgreen D, Mundy AR et al. A quantitative study of atropine-resistant contractile responses in human detrusor smooth muscle, from stable, unstable and obstructed bladders. J Urol 1999; 162: 1833–1839
26. Westfall TD, Kennedy C, Sneddon P. The ecto-ATPase inhibitor ARL 67156 enhances para-sympathetic neurotransmission in the guinea-pig urinary bladder. Eur J Pharmacol 1997; 329: 169–173
27. Hoyle CH. Non-adrenergic, non-cholinergic control of the urinary bladder. World J Urol 1994; 12: 233–244
28. Somogyi GT, de Groat WC. Function, signal transduction mechanisms and plasticity of presynaptic muscarinic receptors in the urinary bladder. Life Sci 1999; 64: 411–418
29. King JA, Huddart H, Staff WG. Purinergic modulation of rat urinary bladder detrusor smooth muscle. Gen Pharmacol 1997; 29: 597–604
30. Gusraffson LE, Wiklund NP, Lundin J, Hedqvist P. Characterization of the pre- and post-junctional adenosine receptors in guinea-pig ileum. Acta Physiol Scand 1985; 123: 195–203
31. Hegde SS, Eglen RM. Muscarinic receptor subtypes modulating smooth muscle contractility in the urinary bladder. Life Sci 1999; 64: 419–428
32. D'Agostino G, Bolognesi ML, Lucchelli A, Vicini D et al. Prejunctional muscarinic inhibitory control of acetylcholine release in the human detrusor: involvement of the M4 receptor subtype. Br J Pharmacol 2000; 129: 493–500
33. Nilvebrant L, Andersson KE, Gillberg PG, Stahl M et al. Tolterodine – a new bladder-selective antimuscarinic agent. Eur J Pharmacol 1997; 327: 195–207
34. Yamaguchi O, Shishido K, Tamura K, Ogawa T et al. Evaluation of mRNAs encoding muscarinic receptor subtypes in human detrusor muscle. J Urol 1996; 156: 1208–1213
35. Wang P, Luthin GR, Ruggieri MR. Muscarinic acetylcholine receptor subtypes mediating urinary bladder contractility and coupling to GTP binding proteins. J Pharmacol Exp Ther 1995; 273: 959–966
36. Hegde SS, Choppin A, Bonhaus D, Briand S et al. Functional role of M2 and M3 muscarinic receptors in the urinary bladder of rats in vitro and in vivo. Br J Pharmacol 1997; 120: 1409–1418

37. Longhurst PA, Schwegel T, Folander K, Swanson R. The human P2X1 receptor: molecular cloning, tissue distribution, and localisation to chromosome 17. Biochim Biophys Acta 1996; 1308: 185–188
38. Berridge MJ. Inositol trisphosphate and calcium signalling. Nature 1993; 361: 315–325
39. Cardy TJ, Traynor D, Taylor CW. Differential regulation of types-1 and -3 inositol trisphosphate receptors by cytosolic Ca^{2+}. Biochem J 1997; 328: 785–793
40. Iacovou JW, Hill SJ, Birmingham AT. Agonist-induced contraction and accumulation of inositol phosphates in the guinea-pig detrusor: evidence that muscarinic and purinergic receptors raise intracellular calcium by different mechanisms. J Urol 1990; 144: 775–779
41. MacKenzie AB, Surprenant A, North RA. Functional and molecular diversity of purinergic ion channel receptors. Ann N Y Acad Sci 1999; 868: 716–729
42. Bolton TB, Prestwich SA, Zholos AV, Gordienko DV. Excitation-contraction coupling in gastrointestinal and other smooth muscles. Ann Rev Physiol 1999; 61: 85–115
43. Taggart MJ, Wray S. Contribution of sarcoplasmic reticular calcium to smooth muscle contractile activation: gestational dependence in isolated rat uterus. J Physiol 1998; 511: 133–144
44. Rohrmann D, Zderic SA, Wein AJ, Levin RM. Effect of thapsigargin on the contractile response of the normal and obstructed rabbit urinary bladder. Pharmacology 1996; 52: 119–124
45. Himpens B, Missiaen L, Casteels R. Ca^{2+} homeostasis in vascular smooth muscle. J Vascular Res 1995; 32: 207–219
46. Shmigol A, Eisner DA, Wray S. Carboxyeosin decreases the rate of decay of the $[Ca^{2+}]_i$ transient in uterine smooth muscle cells isolated from pregnant rats. Pflugers Arch 1998; 437: 158–160
47. Hryshko LV, Philipson KD. Sodium–calcium exchange: recent advances. Basic Res Cardiol 1997; 92 (Suppl 1): 45–51
48. Fry CH, Powell T, Twist VW, Ward JP. Net calcium exchange in adult rat ventricular myocytes: an assessment of mitochondrial calcium accumulating capacity. Proc R Soc Lond, Series B 1984; 223: 223–238
49. Ganitkevich VYA. Clearance of large Ca^{2+} loads in a single smooth muscle cell: examination of the role of mitochondrial Ca^{2+} uptake and intracellular pH. Cell Calcium 1999; 25: 29–42
50. Robb-Gaspers LD, Burnett P, Rutter GA, Denton RM et al. Integrating cytosolic calcium signals into mitochondrial metabolic responses. EMBO J 1998; 17: 4987–5000
51. Hamill OP, Marty A, Neher E, Sakmann B et al. Improved patch-clamp techniques for high-resolution current recording from cells and cell-free membrane patches. Pflugers Arch 1981; 391: 85–100
52. Neher E, Sakmann B. The patch clamp technique. Sci Am 1992; 266: 28–35
53. Fry CH, Wu C, Sui GP. Electrophysiological properties of the bladder. Int Urogynecol J 1998; 9: 291–298
54. Montgomery BS, Fry CH. The action potential and net membrane currents in isolated human detrusor smooth muscle cells. J Urol 1992; 147: 176–184
55. Nakayama S, Brading AF. Evidence for multiple open states of the Ca^{2+} channels in smooth muscle cells isolated from the guinea-pig detrusor. J Physiol 1993; 471: 87–105
56. Nakayama S, Brading AF. Inactivation of the voltage-dependent Ca^{2+} channel current in smooth muscle cells isolated from the guinea-pig detrusor. J Physiol 1993; 471: 107–127
57. Sui GP, Wu C, Fry CH. Inward Ca^{2+} currents in cultured and freshly isolated detrusor smooth muscle cells – evidence of a T-type Ca^{2+} current. J Urol 2001; 165: 621–626
58. Inoue R, Brading AF. The properties of the ATP-induced depolarization and current in single cells isolated from the guinea-pig urinary bladder. Br J Pharmacol 1990; 100: 619–625
59. Inoue R, Brading AF. Human, pig and guinea-pig bladder smooth muscle cells generate similar inward currents in response to purinoceptor activation. Br J Pharmacol 1991; 103: 1840–1841
60. Wellner MC, Isenberg G. Properties of stretch-activated channels in myocytes from the guinea-pig urinary bladder. J Physiol 1993; 466: 213–227
61. Wellner MC, Isenberg G. cAMP accelerates the decay of stretch-activated inward currents in guinea-pig urinary bladder myocytes. J Physiol 1995; 482: 141–156
62. Hollywood MA, Cotton KD, McHale NG, Thornbury KD. Enhancement of Ca^{2+}-dependent outward current in sheep bladder myocytes by Evan's blue dye. Pflugers Arch 1998; 435: 631–636
63. Ganitkevich VY, Isenberg G. Dissociation of subsarcolemmal from global cytosolic $[Ca^{2+}]$ in myocytes from guinea-pig coronary artery. J Physiol 1996; 490: 305–318
64. ZhuGe R, Tuft RA, Fogarty KE, Bellve K, Fay FS, Walsh JV Jr. The influence of sarcoplasmic reticulum Ca^{2+} concentration on Ca^{2+} sparks and spontaneous

transient outward currents in single smooth muscle cells. J Gen Physiol 1999; 113: 215–228
65. Bolton TB, Imaizumi Y. Spontaneous transient outward currents in smooth muscle cells. Cell Calcium 1996; 20: 141–152
66. Wammack R, Jahnel U, Nawrath H, Hohenfellner R. Mechanical and electrophysiological effects of cromakalim on the human urinary bladder. Eur Urol 1994; 26: 176–181
67. Gopalakrishnan M, Whiteaker KL, Molinari EJ, Davies-Taber R et al. Characterization of the ATP-sensitive potassium channels (KATP) expressed in guinea pig bladder smooth muscle cells. J Pharmacol Exp Ther 1999; 289: 551–558
68. Qian Y, Bourreau JP. Two distinct pathways for refilling Ca^{2+} stores in permeabilized bovine trachealis muscle. Life Sci 1999; 64: 2049–2059
69. Kishii K, Hisayama T, Takayanagi I. Comparison of contractile mechanisms by carbachol and ATP in detrusor strips of rabbit urinary bladder. Jpn J Pharmacol 1992; 58: 219–229
70. Sui GP, Wu C, Fry CH. The electrophysiological properties of cultured and freshly isolated detrusor smooth muscle cells. J Urol 2001; 165: 627–632
71. Mostwin JL. The action potential of guinea pig bladder smooth muscle. J Urol 1986; 135: 1299–1303
72. Heppner TJ, Bonev AD, Nelson MT. Ca^{2+}-activated K^+ channels regulate action potential repolarization in urinary bladder smooth muscle. Am J Physiol 1997; 273: C110–C117
73. Weidmann S. The diffusion of radiopotassium across intercalated disks of mammalian cardiac muscle. J Physiol 1966; 187: 323–342
74. Severs NJ. Cardiac muscle cell interaction: from microanatomy to the molecular make-up of the gap junction. Histol Histopathol 1995; 10: 481–501
75. Gabella G. Cells and cell junctions in the muscle coat of the bladder. Scand J Urol Nephrol 1997; Suppl 184: 3–6
76. Seki N, Karim OM, Mostwin JL. Changes in electrical properties of guinea pig smooth muscle membrane by experimental bladder outflow obstruction. Am J Physiol 1992; 262: F885–F891
77. Fry CH, Cooklin M, Birns J, Mundy AR. Measurement of intercellular electrical coupling in guinea-pig detrusor smooth muscle. J Urol 1999; 161: 660–664
78. Hodgkin AL, Rushton WAH. The electrical constants of a crustacean nerve fibre. Proc R Soc Lond, Series B 1946; 133: 444–479
79. Chapman RA, Fry CH. An analysis of the cable properties of frog ventricular myocardium. J Physiol 1978; 283: 262–282
80. Weidmann S. Electrical constants of trabecular muscle from mammalian heart. J Physiol 1970; 210: 1041–1054
81. Jack JJB, Noble T, Tsien RW. Electric Current Flow in Excitable Cells. Oxford: Clarendon Press, 1976
82. Delmar M, Michaels DC, Johnson T, Jalife J. Effects of increasing intercellular resistance on transverse and longitudinal propagation in sheep epicardial muscle. Circ Res 1987; 60: 780–785
83. Beye EC. Gap junctions. Int Rev Cytol 1993; 137C: 1–37
84. Ek A, Alm P, Andersson KE, Persson CG. Adrenergic and cholinergic nerves of the human urethra and urinary bladder. A histochemical study. Acta Physiol Scand 1977; 99: 345–352
85. Gosling JA, Dixon JS, Jen PY. The distribution of noradrenergic nerves in the human lower urinary tract. A review. Eur Urol 1999; 36 (Suppl 1): 23–30
86. Ueda S, Satake N, Shibata S. Alpha 1- and alpha 2-adrenoceptors in the smooth muscle of isolated rabbit urinary bladder and urethra. Eur J Pharmacol 1984; 103: 249–254
87. Klarskov P, Gerstenberg TC, Ramirez D, Hald T. Non-cholinergic, non-adrenergic nerve mediated relaxation of trigone, bladder neck and urethral smooth muscle in vitro. J Urol 1983; 129: 848–850
88. Klarskov P. Non-cholinergic, non-adrenergic inhibitory nerve responses of bladder outlet smooth muscle in vitro. Br J Urol 1987; 60: 337–342
89. Triguero D, Prieto D, Garcia-Pascual A. NADPH-diaphorase and NANC relaxations are correlated in the sheep urinary tract. Neurosci Lett 1993; 163: 93–96
90. Smet PJ, Edyvane KA, Jonavicius J, Marshall VR. Distribution of NADPH-diaphorase-positive nerves supplying the human urinary bladder. J Auton Nerv Sys 1994; 47: 109–113
91. Rand MJ, Li CG. Nitric oxide as a neurotransmitter in peripheral nerves: nature of transmitter and mechanism of transmission. Ann Rev Physiol 1995; 57: 659–682
92. Denninger JW, Marletta MA. Guanylate cyclase and the NO/cGMP signalling pathway. Biochim Biophys Acta 1999; 1411: 334–350
93. Wein AJ. Pharmacologic options for the overactive bladder. Urology 1998; 51(Suppl 2A): 43–47
94. Andersson KE. Advances in the pharmacological control of the bladder. Exp Physiol 1999; 84: 195–213

95. Andersson KE, Appell R, Cardozo LD, Chapple C et al. The pharmacological treatment of urinary incontinence. Br J Urol 1999; 84: 923–947
96. Andersson KE. Treatment of overactive bladder: other drug mechanisms. Urology 2000; 55 (Suppl 5A): 51–57
97. Alabaster VA. Discovery and development of selective M3 antagonists for clinical use. Life Sci 1997; 60: 1053–1060
98. Chapple CR. Muscarinic receptor antagonists in the treatment of overactive bladder. Urology 2000; 55 (Suppl 5A): 33–46
99. Yono M, Yoshida M, Wada Y, Kikukawa H et al. Pharmacological effects of tolterodine on human isolated urinary bladder. Eur J Pharmacol 1999; 368: 223–230
100. Chai TC, Steers WD. Neurophysiology of micturition and continence. Urol Clin North Am 1996; 23: 221–236
101. Andersson KE. The pharmacology of lower urinary tract smooth muscles and penile erect tissues. Pharmacol Rev 1993; 45: 253–308
102. Goepel M, Wittmann A, Rubben H, Michel MC. Comparison of adrenoceptor subtype expression in porcine and human bladder and prostate. Urol Res 1997; 25: 199–206
103. Igawa Y, Nishizawa O, Yamazaki Y et al. Functional and molecular biological evidence of β_3-adrenoreceptors in the human detrusor. J Urol 1997; 157: 175 (Abstract 677)
104. Williams TJ, Blue DR, Daniels DV, et al. In vitro alpha1-adrenoceptor pharmacology of Ro 70-0004 and RS-100329, novel alpha1A-adrenoceptor selective antagonists. Br J Pharmacol 1999; 127: 252–258
105. Longhurst PA, Briscoe JA, Rosenberg DJ, Leggett RE. The role of cyclic nucleotides in guinea-pig bladder contractility. Br J Pharmacol 1997; 121: 1665–1672
106. Shapiro E, Tang R, Rosenthal E, Lepor H. The binding and functional properties of voltage dependent calcium channel receptors in pediatric normal and myelodysplastic bladders. J Urol 1991; 146: 520–523
107. Brixius K, Mohr V, Muller-Ehmsen J, Hoischen S et al. Potent vasodilatory with minor cardiodepressant actions of mibefradil in human cardiac tissue. Br J Pharmacol 1998; 125: 41–48
108. Wojdan A, Freeden C, Woods M, Oshiro G et al. Comparison of the potassium channel openers, WAY-133537, ZD6169, and celikalim on isolated bladder tissue and in vivo bladder instability in rat. J Pharmacol Exp Ther 1999; 289: 1410–1418
109. Hu S, Kim HS. Modulation of ATP-sensitive and large-conductance Ca^{2+}-activated K^+ channels by Zeneca ZD6169 in guinea pig bladder smooth muscle cells. J Pharmacol Exp Ther 1997; 280: 38–45
110. Morita T, Ando M, Kihara K, Kitahara S et al. Effects of prostaglandins E_1, E_2 and F_2 alpha on contractility and cAMP and cGMP contents in lower urinary tract smooth muscle. Urol Int 1994; 52: 200–203
111. Maggi CA. Prostanoids as local modulators of reflex micturition. Pharmacol Res 1992; 25: 13–20

16

The cellular pathophysiology of bladder dysfunction

Christopher H Fry

MYOGENIC BASIS OF BLADDER DYSFUNCTION

Definition of the problem

From the point of view of detrusor muscle physiology, the bladder presents two problems: (1) the overactive bladder, whereby large, uncontrolled changes of detrusor pressure occur; and (2) the underactive bladder, whereby an insufficient increase of intravesical pressure occurs for complete expulsion of the contents. When there are no obvious neurological defects in patients, the presumption is that changes to the cellular characteristics of tissue in the bladder wall, including detrusor smooth muscle, are the primary cause of the conditions, and the problem may be classified as myogenic. It is important to emphasize that from a clinical aspect a syndrome such as bladder instability is *associated* with a number of conditions (such as outflow tract obstruction) or symptoms (such as frequency and/or urge). However, these give no indication to the researcher as to what is the basic *cause* of the problem. Outflow tract obstruction, for example, may precipitate a chain of events which eventually causes bladder instability, but it is essential to identify the fundamental changes which manifest themselves as instability.

Moreover, a simple division of bladder dysfunction into either a neurogenic or myogenic cause is too simplistic. There is no doubt that primary neurological defects result also in changes to the function of smooth muscle, and, in addition, factors that have a direct impact on smooth muscle activity (such as bladder wall hypoxia) also affect the nervous supply to the detrusor. Therefore, it is more appropriate to characterize those changes which occur to smooth muscle function, whatever the cause, and determine whether they result in changes to bladder function.

Further philosophical issues confront the experimenter. It cannot always be proven that the changes that occur to cell, tissue and organ function are the primary cause of bladder dysfunction, or occur as a secondary consequence of a pre-existing condition. Furthermore, although changes can be documented in muscle from dysfunctioning bladders, it is by no means certain whether they are responsible for abnormal function, or are mere epiphenomena. However, the identification of any derangements to the cell physiology of bladder wall tissues has a number of motivations:

- It may assist in identifying those conditions that might initiate changes to the cell physiology.
- It will determine which particular characteristics of the cell are changed.
- It could identify useful drug targets, that is, targets which are specific to abnormally functioning tissue, while leaving normal tissue relatively unaffected.

Bladder overactivity

Bladder overactivity is the predominant condition, and therefore most research has gone in this direction: this section of the chapter will consequently have the same emphasis. The key unanswered question that remains is, what is an unstable contraction: an increase in the existing contractile activity of detrusor muscle, generation of additional contractions, or greater coordination of pre-existing activity? This chapter will document changes to detrusor function which occur in dysfunctioning bladders, but only working hypotheses can be presented as to what causes bladder overactivity. In keeping with the general trend, data will be drawn from three sources: (1) obstructed bladders (with or without documented instability); (2) bladders that are idiopathically unstable; and (3) neurogenic or hyperreflexic bladders, that is, those with documented neurological deficits. The reader will also be struck by often inconsistent observations in the literature. These will be pointed out when they occur, and this emphasizes the fact that bladder dysfunction is a multifaceted problem, and that important and unknown differences exist between different experimental models.

Experimental models and approaches

Two general approaches are used: (1) bladder instability and/or obstruction induced in animal models, and the consequent study of the whole bladder and tissue in vivo and in vitro;[1–3] (2) studies of human tissue taken from patients with and without bladder dysfunction.[4–7] Each approach has advantages, so that they are complementary: animal models are well defined, as specific lesions can be induced to generate the condition, it is easier to make more controlled in vivo measurements and tissue samples come from more homogeneous populations. On the other hand, human tissue may have fundamental differences from animal tissue so that extrapolation from the animal to the human condition is not always possible. It is also important to add a caveat that much research has used human and animal detrusor obtained from obstructed bladders. In such cases, bladder dysfunction may not always be observed, or even tested for, especially in samples from patients, and this may account for some variability of the data in the literature.

BLADDER INSTABILITY AND INCREASED MYOGENIC ACTIVITY – OUTLINE

If an increase of bladder activity results from an augmentation of detrusor function, there are several stages in excitation–contraction coupling that may be altered (Figure 16.1). The reader may care to refer back to this scheme, as they will not always be considered in turn.

- augmentation of action potential generation or an increase of transmitter release
- increased lifetime of transmitters

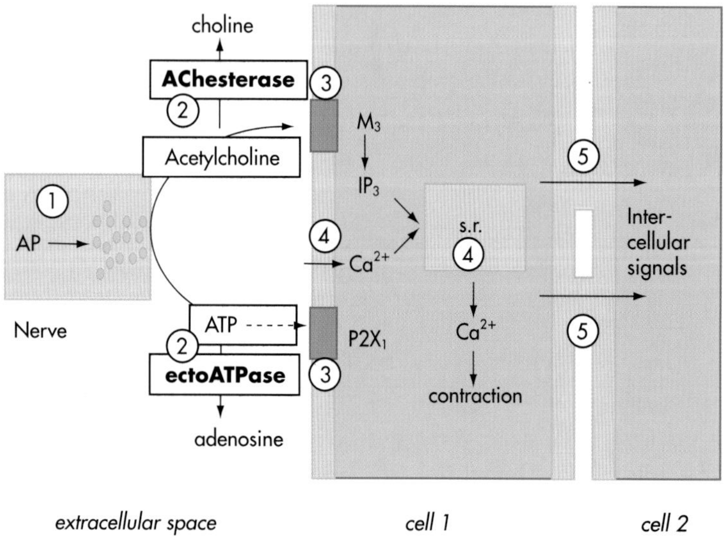

Figure 16.1 *A schematic diagram of tension generation in a multicellular portion of detrusor smooth muscle. The numbers circled 1–5 refer to the particular stages discussed in the text, which are altered in tissues from patients with detrusor instability.*

- increase of receptor response to transmitters
- sensitization of the detrusor cell mechanisms, leading to contraction
- increased coupling of detrusor cells to form a more effective syncytium.

RESPONSE OF TISSUE TO NERVE-MEDIATED AND RECEPTOR-ACTIVATED STIMULATION

Response to electrical stimulation

Stimulation of the motor nerves embedded in a detrusor sample with a tetanic train of impulses results in a muscle contraction which is blocked by the neurotoxin, tetrodotoxin. The contraction is increased as the impulse frequency in the tetanic train is raised, presumably as action potential frequency is also raised, generating a frequency–response relationship. Figure 16.2 shows a frequency–response curve for human detrusor muscle obtained from a normal bladder: the contraction is normalized to that which is obtained at high frequencies. A leftward shift indicates that a greater proportion of tension is generated with a lower stimulation frequency; a shift to the right would indicate reduced sensitivity to stimulation.

Several studies have shown a shift to the right with samples from patients[4,8] or animals[9,10] with obstructed bladders, or patients with idiopathic instability.[7] However, other studies have recorded opposite shift[6] or no shift[3] in samples from idiopathically unstable bladders. Detrusor biopsies from patients with a neurogenic basis to their instability generally demonstrate a leftward shift.[6,11,12] In view of the variability of the shift of the frequency–response relationship in pathological bladders, it is unlikely that an increase of the sensitivity of the motor nerves to external stimulation is the sole reason for bladder instability, but it may contribute to the condition in neurogenic bladders.

It has also been suggested that the detrusor muscle cell itself is electrically more excitable, so that a given stimulus would be more likely to evoke a depolarizing response and even an action potential. However, the response of human detrusor muscle to direct electrical stimulation is not different in samples from stable, unstable and obstructed bladders.[7] Moreover, the magnitude of the membrane potential and resting membrane resistance, both important determinants of electrical excitability, are not different in detrusor cells from stable and unstable bladders (GP Sui and CH Fry, unpublished data).

Response to muscarinic agonists

An alternative possibility is that the post-junctional receptors on the detrusor cell membrane – in

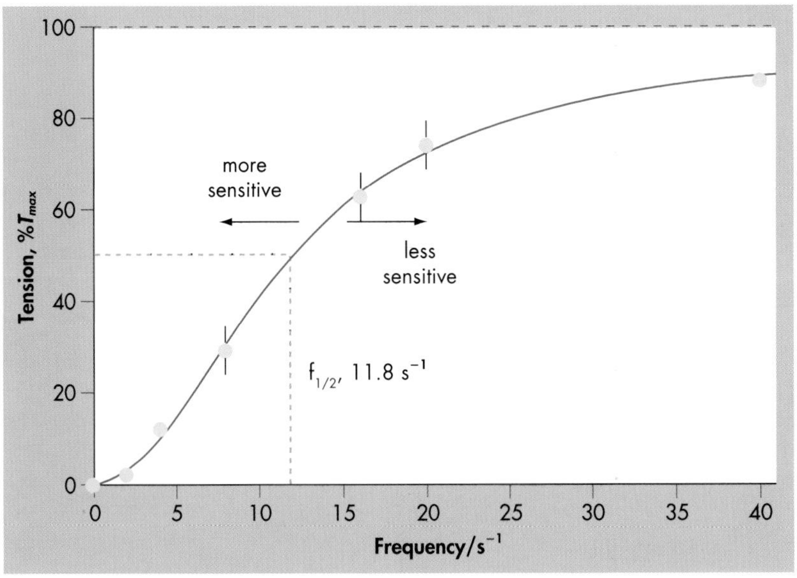

Figure 16.2 *A frequency–response curve for an isolated strip of detrusor muscle. The abscissa shows the frequency of pulses in a tetanic stimulating train, and the ordinate the magnitude of the peak contractile response, normalized to a maximum, T_{max}, obtained from a curve-fit to the data. The data (mean ± s.e., n = 12) are from experiments on normal detrusor muscle.[42] A least-squares curve-fit to the data was used:*

$$T = \frac{T_{max} \cdot f^n}{f_{1/2}{}^n \cdot f^n},$$

where T is tension; f, stimulating frequency; $f_{1/2}$, the frequency at which $T = 0.5T_{max}$ and n, a constant: the value of $f_{1/2}$, is shown on the plot. A right- or left-hand shift to the plot is also indicated – see text for details.

particular, the muscarinic receptors – show an enhanced sensitivity to transmitters. Thus, a given release from the nerve terminal would evoke a greater response, especially at low concentrations. Such a phenomenon is known as post-junctional supersensitivity and has been described in many tissues, especially in combination with relative denervation of the tissue. Microscopical studies of detrusor samples from obstructed bladders and idiopathically unstable bladders do indeed show denervation, which may not be homogeneous but distributed unevenly throughout the sample.[8,13,14] However, denervation is also not a ubiquitous observation in the unstable bladder. In a pig model of instability induced by circumferential supratrigonal bladder transection,[3] there was no loss in the density of cholinergic fibres.

A large number of studies has demonstrated supersensitivity to acetylcholine or its analogue carbachol, in multicellular samples from obstructed and/or unstable human and animal bladders.[3,8–10,15–18] In many studies, experimental denervation was induced or was observed concomitantly. However, supersensitivity is not a ubiquitous finding,[4,6,7,13] and in one model of instability associated with outflow obstruction,[19] supersensitivity to muscarinic agonists developed only when the obstruction was removed and instability had disappeared.

Several explanations may be given for the supersensitivity observed in some studies. The most straightforward is an increase in the affinity of M3 receptors to muscarinic agonists. However, an increase in the sensitivity to carbachol cannot be demonstrated in isolated human detrusor smooth muscle cells obtained from stable, unstable and obstructed bladders.[20] In these experiments, the transient rise of the intracellular [Ca^{2+}] on addition of carbachol was used as the experimental variable. Figure 16.3 shows the response of single cells to carbachol in biopsies obtained from stable and unstable bladders from an individual study[7,20] – responses were identical in the two groups. This was corroborated in a study with obstructed rat bladders, which showed that the affinity of the M3 antagonist 4-DAMP was not different from that in control samples.[21] Alternatively, an increase in the number of M2 receptors has also been proposed to sensitize the muscle[22] to muscarinic agonists. Finally, a decrease in the breakdown of acetylcholine in the synaptic cleft could produce the phenomenon (see below, Synaptic breakdown).

Response to purinergic agonists

A feature of detrusor from normal human bladders is that nerve-mediated contractions are abolished completely by atropine, whereas in most other animals an atropine-resistant,[23] purinergic component remains – see Chapter 15. However, several studies have shown that tissue from human bladders with a variety of pathologies also shows atropine-resistant,

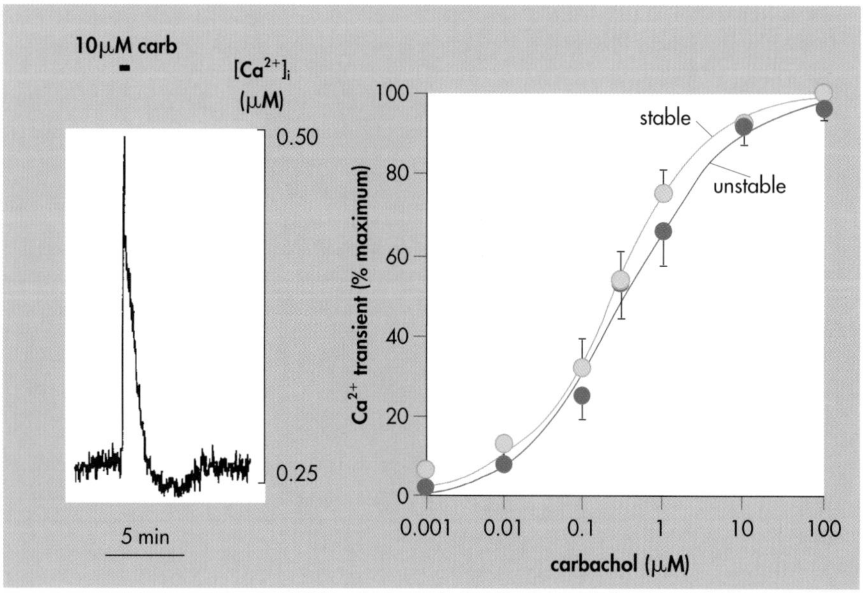

Figure 16.3 *The action of carbachol on the intracellular [Ca^{2+}] in isolated detrusor myocytes. The left-hand trace illustrates a Ca^{2+}-transient in response to 10 μM carbachol. Intracellular Ca^{2+} was measured by the Ca^{2+}-sensitive fluorochrome Fura-2. The left-hand plots show dose–response curves to carbachol, using the magnitude of the Ca^{2+}-transient as the dependent variable. Data were obtained from cells isolated from stable or unstable bladders.*[20] *The curve-fits were identical in form to that used in Figure 16.2.*

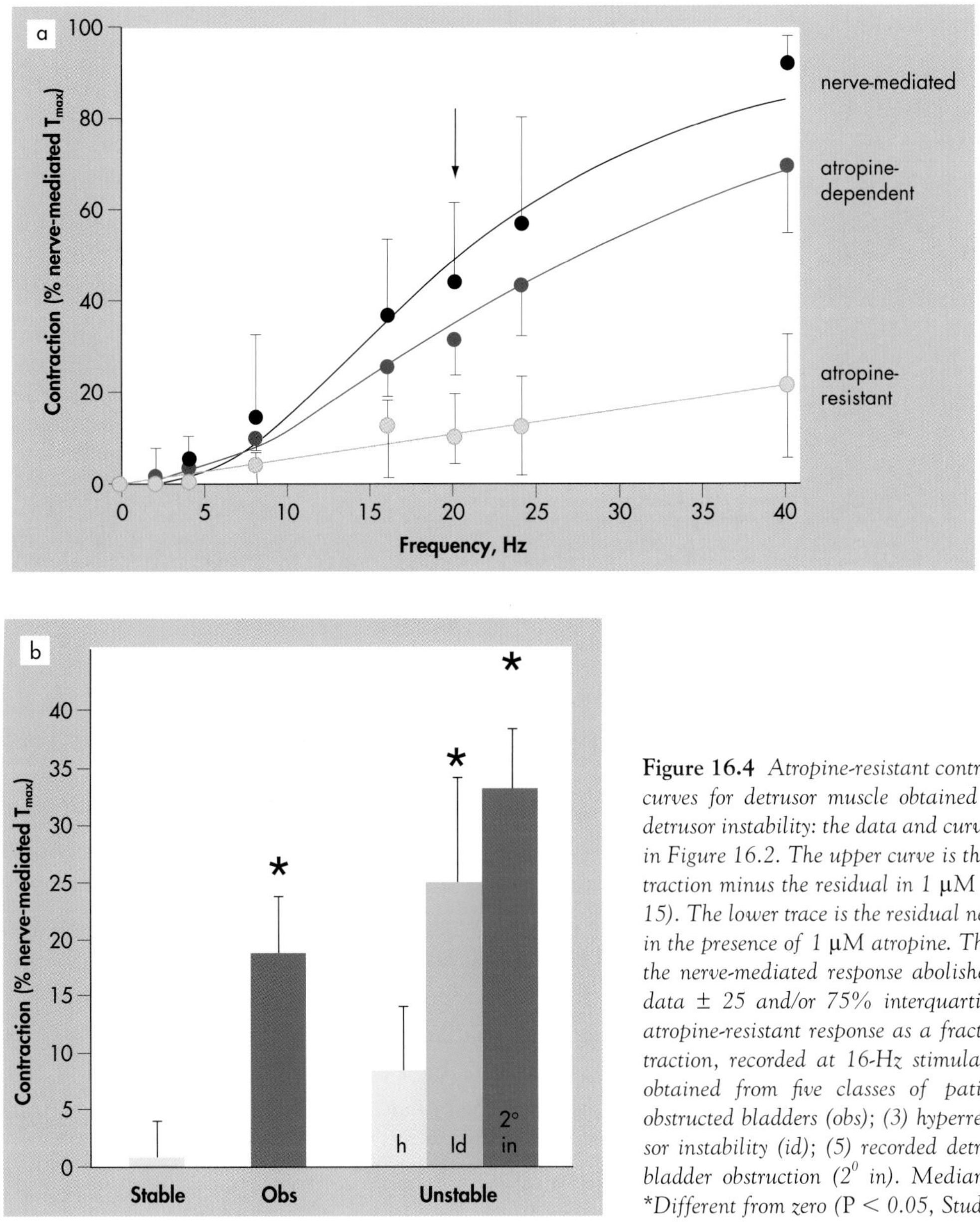

Figure 16.4 *Atropine-resistant contractions. (a) Frequency–response curves for detrusor muscle obtained from patients with idiopathic detrusor instability: the data and curve-fits were obtained as described in Figure 16.2. The upper curve is the nerve-mediated response (contraction minus the residual in 1 μM tetrodotoxin – see also Chapter 15). The lower trace is the residual nerve-mediated response recorded in the presence of 1 μM atropine. The middle trace is the fraction of the nerve-mediated response abolished by 1 μM atropine. Median data ± 25 and/or 75% interquartiles. (b) The proportion of the atropine-resistant response as a fraction of the nerve-mediated contraction, recorded at 16-Hz stimulation frequency. The data were obtained from five classes of patients: (1) stable bladders; (2) obstructed bladders (obs); (3) hyperreflexia (h); (4) idiopathic detrusor instability (id); (5) recorded detrusor instability associated with bladder obstruction (2⁰ in). Median values + 75% interquartile. *Different from zero (P < 0.05, Student's t-test).*

purinergic contractions.[7,24–26] Figure 16.4 shows nerve-mediated force–frequency curves of human detrusor from stable and unstable bladders – unstable bladder samples exhibit an atropine-resistant component, itself abolished by prior treatment with α,β-methylene ATP, an agent which desensitizes purinergic (specifically P2X1) receptors. It is proposed therefore that such an additional excitatory mechanism would increase the likelihood of contractile activation in such bladders. However, this purinergic component is not ubiquitous in tissue from unstable bladders; it is present in those with idiopathic instability, but absent in those with hyperreflexia[7] emphasizing that instability has a heterogeneous aetiology.

Figure 16.5 shows that an additional, purinergic component of contraction is not a result of the detrusor cell itself showing an increased affinity to ATP.[20] ATP also induces a transient rise of the intracellular [Ca^{2+}] (see Chapter 15), and the figure shows that the Ca^{2+}-transients are evoked over a similar range of ATP concentrations in cells from stable and idiopathically unstable bladders.

Much of the above data indicate that the contractile responses to cholinergic and purinergic transmitters may be enhanced in certain instabilities and

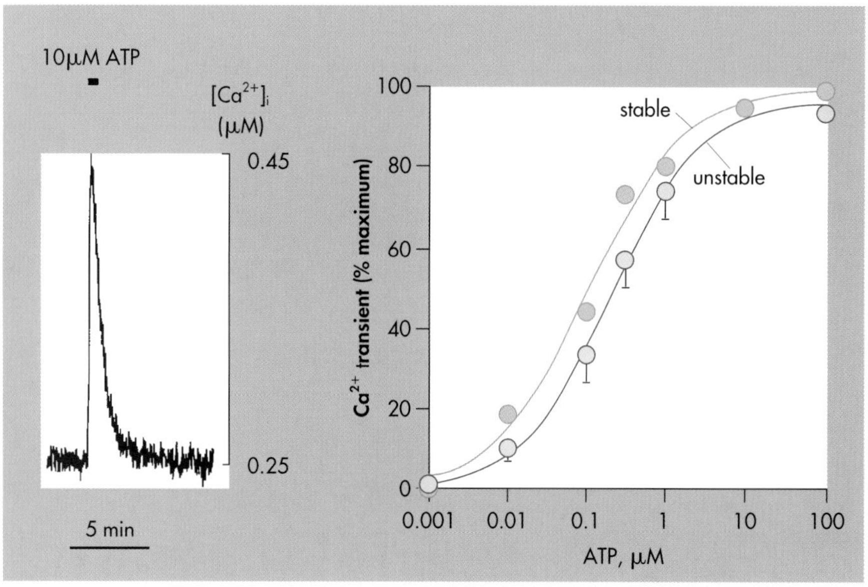

Figure 16.5 *The action of ATP on the intracellular [Ca^{2+}] in isolated detrusor myocytes. The left-hand trace illustrates a Ca^{2+}-transient in response to 10 μM ATP. The left-hand plots show dose–response curves to carbachol, using the magnitude of the Ca^{2+}-transient as the dependent variable. Data were obtained from cells isolated from stable or unstable bladders.[20] The curve-fits were identical in form to that used in Figure 16.2.*

could represent an important mechanism underlying bladder overactivity in disease. It is unlikely that it is due solely to a change in detrusor smooth muscle sensitivity to transmitters, so that other explanations must also be sought – these will be considered below.

RELEASE AND BREAKDOWN OF TRANSMITTERS

Synaptic breakdown

Acetylcholine and ATP are hydrolysed in the synaptic cleft by acetylcholine esterase (AChE) and ectoATPase, respectively. In principle, a decrease in the activity of either enzyme would prolong the lifetime of the transmitter and thus enhance the magnitude of the response and increase the potency of the agonist. For example, application of the AChE inhibitor physostigmine enhances nerve-mediated contractions.[23] Furthermore, one study has indicated that AChE activity may indeed be decreased in neurogenic bladders, which are often associated with unstable activity, although these measurements were not accompanied by an evaluation of the sensitivity of the tissue to acetylcholine itself.[27]

The ectoATPase present in detrusor may be inhibited by the agent ARL 67156.[28] Application of ARL 67156 to guinea-pig bladder strips has also been shown to increase the magnitude of nerve-mediated contractions,[29] indicating that the action of ATP on the muscle cell is attenuated by its extracellular hydrolysis.

Therefore, one explanation for atropine-resistant contractions in detrusor from unstable and obstructed bladders may be that ectoATPase activity is reduced, so that a proportion of released ATP would reach the detrusor cell membrane. Figure 16.6 shows the dose–response curves of ATP and its non-hydrolysable analogue, α,β-methylene ATP (ABMA), on human detrusor contractions. The potency of ABMA is much greater than ATP, although comparable measurements on isolated cells show similar potencies. Therefore, the lower potency of ATP on the strip could be due to its hydrolysis outside the cell. Preliminary data (D Skennerton, R Harvey, CH Fry; unpublished data) show that the potency of ATP is increased in detrusor strips from obstructed and unstable bladders. This suggests that ectoATPase activity is indeed reduced in these samples and could account for the atropine-resistant contractions.

Transmitter release

Pre-synaptic muscarinic (M1) receptors exert an autofacilitatory effect on acetylcholine release, mediated

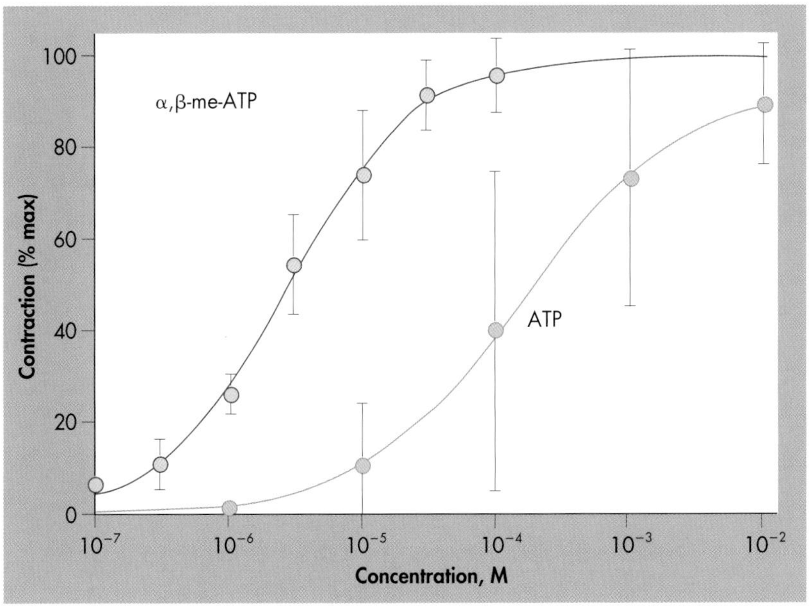

Figure 16.6 *The contraction of detrusor smooth muscle strips to ATP and the non-hydrolysable analogue α,β-methylene ATP (ABMA). Mean data ± s.d. The data were fitted to a function of the form shown in Figure 16.2.*

by protein kinase C[30,31] with a possible concomitant downregulation by M2 and M4 receptors.[32,33] There is evidence that the facilitatory mechanism at least is upregulated in animals with spinal cord transection[34,35] and represents a further site which may enhance the overall contractile state of detrusor.

Less is known about the control of ATP release in detrusor nerve terminals. One study in mouse bladder has suggested that different presynaptic Ca^{2+} channels may regulate release of acetylcholine (predominantly N-type channels) and ATP (predominantly P- and Q-type channels).[36]

PROPERTIES OF DETRUSOR SMOOTH MUSCLE – ELECTROMECHANICAL FUNCTIONS

The previous discussion has indicated that important changes take place outside the detrusor cell in tissue from dysfunctioning bladders. There is also evidence that the detrusor cell itself is altered. Two main areas have been studied: contractile activation and intercellular communication, and some of the changes have been recently summarized.[37] Chapter 15 summarizes the process in normal detrusor whereby receptor activation leads to a contraction.

Contractile activation

The basic presumption is that bladder overactivity results from a raised sarcoplasmic $[Ca^{2+}]$. A raised extracellular [K] will depolarize the cell, enhance Ca^{2+} influx and generate a contraction. Studies using human samples from idiopathically unstable or hyperreflexic bladders show an enhanced contractile sensitivity to a raised [K][13,16] (although others show no difference[38,39]) via an as yet undefined process. However, this may be offset by a reduction in the absolute contractility of muscle, whether induced by a raised [K][21,40,41] or electrical field stimulation[13,15,16] (but see other reports.[6,42]). Reduction of contractility may result from reduced cholinergic innervation[13,15,16] and replacement of muscle tissue by extracellular matrix or other components.[14,43,44]

Membrane Ca^{2+} channels, particularly L-type channels, play an important role in filling intracellular Ca-stores (Chapter 15) and changes to the biophysical properties of these channels have been reported in cells obtained from unstable and obstructed bladders.[45] The net result would be to enhance, over the long term, Ca^{2+} influx. These changes are indicative of changes to the molecular subunit structure of the Ca^{2+} channel.

The sarcoplasmic reticulum (s.r.) plays a predominant role in regulating the sarcoplasmic [Ca^{2+}]. In experimental models of obstruction, the s.r. shows a diminished ability to regulate intracellular Ca^{2+},[46] and may be correlated with a reduction of mitochondrial oxidative function[47,48] (but see Damaser et al[49]). The inability to regulate intracellular Ca^{2+} in tissues such as myocardium results in spontaneous intracellular Ca^{2+} transients and contractions[50,51] and, in particular, is induced by excessive Ca^{2+} influx into the cell and reduction of s.r. uptake. Spontaneous Ca^{2+} oscillations have been observed in detrusor myocytes after exposure to ATO or carbachol, and are significantly more likely in myocytes isolated from unstable than normal bladders.[52]

Spontaneous contractions are a feature of isolated detrusor smooth muscle, although it occurs more readily in samples from rodents and mustelids than man. However, the incidence of spontaneous activity is increased in samples from experimentally obstructed animal bladders[53–55] and from patients with instability.[6] These contractions are insensitive to tetrodotoxin[55] but abolished by raised extracellular Mg,[56] and are presumed to be myogenic in origin. A recent study has shown that human detrusor is also characterized by spontaneous fluctuations of membrane potential,[57] which, although they are not large enough to be classified as action potentials, would be sufficient to open Ca^{2+} channels. It remains to be ascertained whether they are correlated with spontaneous intracellular Ca^{2+} oscillations and provide the link to equivalent contractile phenomena. However, if spontaneous contractions are significant phenomena, they may contribute to the decrease in bladder compliance that is associated with the obstructed bladder.[58,59]

Electrophysiological changes

There has been less emphasis on electrophysiological changes associated with bladder obstruction and instability. Experimental and modelling studies have demonstrated a prolongation of the action potential[45,60] with no change to the membrane potential and a similar responsiveness to alteration of extracellular K.[60,61] The latter observation is in contrast to the increased contractile sensitivity to raised [K] observed by some groups.[13,16] In smooth muscles with a high membrane resistance, such as detrusor, the Na pump may influence the actual level of the action potential. Na-pump blockade generated a larger depolarization in tissue from obstructed bladders.[61] There are two implications of this observation: (1) other ion conductances, such as to K^+, may be of less importance as the membrane potential itself is unchanged; (2) Na-pump blockade, as may occur during severe hypoxia, may have a greater depolarizing influence.

PROPERTIES OF DETRUSOR SMOOTH MUSCLE – INTERCELLULAR COMMUNICATION

Conventional wisdom holds that detrusor cells are poorly coupled, as evidenced by the sparsity or absence of gap junctions between adjacent cells[62,63] and the difficulty by which electrical currents pass from cell to cell.[64] Although other studies have demonstrated some electrical coupling,[61,65] it remains much less than in well-coupled tissues such as myocardium. It has been proposed that unstable activity in the bladder may be facilitated by enhanced coupling in this tissue.[13] In a subset of patients with detrusor overactivity, a microscopical study showed that samples from their bladders had a greater number of so-called protrusion junctions, indicative of intercellular coupling.[66] Equivalent electrical recordings are sparse in detrusor from dysfunctional bladders. One study[61] in a model of guinea-pig obstruction has shown a decrease in the space constant, λ (see Chapter 15). λ is a measure of the ratio of membrane resistance (r_m), to the intercellular resistance (r_i), such that $\lambda^2 = r_m/r_i$. r_i includes the sarcoplasm resistance (which can be assumed to be constant) and the gap junction resistance. If all else remains unchanged, a reduction of λ would imply reduced intercellular coupling (that is, increased r_i) – opposite to what has been suggested above for the overactive bladder.

This subject therefore deserves study and comparison with tissues such as myocardium, where electrical current spread has been more extensively investigated. The value of *quantitative* investigation is of considerable importance, as it has been shown in myocardium that a 10–20-fold increase of gap junction resistance can create the conditions for conduction block, and smaller increases create conditions for re-entry circuits as a basis for arrhythmias. The interested reader is referred to numerous chapters in Zipes and Jalifé.[67]

BLOOD FLOW, ACIDOSIS AND DETRUSOR FUNCTION

Bladder filling is associated with a decrease of blood flow to the bladder wall, tissue hypoxia[68,69] and acidosis.[70] These changes are presumed to occur by stretching of the bladder wall and deformation of the blood vessels. In the hypertrophied bladder, which can occur, for example, as a compensation for an increase of bladder outflow resistance,[71] angiogenesis does not keep pace with the increase of muscle growth, so that such ischaemic conditions would be exacerbated. Tissue hypoxia has complex effects on detrusor function which may contribute to unstable contractions. In the short term (that is, over several minutes), there is an increase of detrusor contractility before a longer-term reduction.[72] The increased contractility may be ascribed to an intracellular acidosis which, in contrast to striated muscle, augments the force of contraction.[73] In the long term, the reduction of aerobic metabolism will limit the ability of the cell to regulate the intracellular [Ca^{2+}] and thus facilitate the conditions for spontaneous oscillations of [Ca^{2+}], as described above. It remains to be determined whether an unstable bladder contraction is accompanied during filling by a local ischaemic-acidotic response.

CONCLUSIONS

It is not possible at the time of writing to determine the cellular basis of detrusor instability. Although most forms of instability are associated with changes to the cell physiology of detrusor smooth muscle, these changes are not always the same. Most likely, detrusor instability is a multifaceted symptomatic condition with a number of aetiologies, many of which manifest themselves as uncontrolled contractions of the bladder wall. However, the following strands emerge:

- The motor innervation to the detrusor alters – the density and local distribution of nerve fibres changes – an effect which may disrupt the coordinated excitation of the bladder mass.
- The nerve–muscle interface is receiving increasing attention – *in vitro*, different functional changes occur in multicellular strips of detrusor from unstable bladders when compared to isolated cells from the same sources. One explanation is that the quantity and type of neurotransmitters, as well as their fate in the synaptic cleft, are altered.
- Biochemical changes take place in the detrusor in many models of bladder obstruction and instability, disrupting the intracellular regulation of Ca^{2+}. The particular alterations that occur have been recently summarized.[74]
- Hypoxia, caused by a reduced blood flow per unit amount of tissue, may be a key instigator of the biochemical and physiological processes.

REFERENCES

1. Sethia KK, Brading AF, Smith JC. An animal model of non-obstructive bladder instability. J Urol 1990; 143: 1243–1246
2. Mostwin JL, Karim OM, van Koeveringe G, Brooks EL. The guinea pig as a model of gradual urethral obstruction. J Urol 1991; 145: 854–858
3. Buttyan R, Chen MW, Levin RM. Animal models of bladder outlet obstruction and molecular insights into the basis for the development of bladder dysfunction. Eur Urol 1997; 32 (Suppl 1): 32–39
4. Eaton AC, Bates CP. An in vitro physiological study of normal and unstable human detrusor muscle. Br J Urol 1982; 54: 653–657
5. Palfrey ELH, Fry CH, Shuttleworth KED. A new in vitro perfusion method for the investigation of human detrusor muscle. Br J Urol 1984; 56: 635–640
6. Kinder RB, Mundy AR. Pathophysiology of idiopathic detrusor instability and detrusor hyperreflexia. An in vitro study of human detrusor muscle. Br J Urol 1987; 60: 509–515

7. Bayliss M, Wu C, Newgreen D, Mundy AR et al. A quantitative study of atropine-resistant contractile responses in human detrusor smooth muscle, from stable, unstable and obstructed bladders. J Urol 1999; 162: 1833–1839
8. Harrison SC, Hunnam GR, Farman P, Ferguson DR et al. Bladder instability and de-nervation in patients with bladder outflow obstruction. Br J Urol 1987; 60: 519–522
9. Speakman MJ, Brading AF, Gilpin CJ, Dixon JS et al. Bladder outflow obstruction – a cause of denervation supersensitivity. J Urol 1987; 138: 1461–1466
10. Harrison SC, Ferguson DR, Doyle PT. Effect of bladder outflow obstruction on the innervation of the rabbit urinary bladder. Br J Urol 1990; 66: 372–379
11. Nurse DE, Restorick JM, Mundy AR. The effect of cromakalim on the normal and hyper-reflexic human detrusor muscle. Br J Urol 1991; 68: 27–31
12. Saito M, Kondo A, Kato T, Levin RM. Response of isolated human neurogenic detrusor smooth muscle to intramural nerve stimulation. Br J Urol 1993; 72: 723–727
13. Mills IW, Greenland JE, McMurray G, McCoy R et al. Studies of the pathophysiology of idiopathic detrusor instability: the physiological properties of the detrusor smooth muscle and its pattern of innervation. J Urol 2000; 163: 646–651
14. Charlton RG, Morley AR, Chambers P, Gillespie JI. Focal changes in nerve, muscle and connective tissue in normal and unstable human bladder. Br J Urol 1999; 84: 953–960
15. Sibley GN. The physiological response of the detrusor muscle to experimental bladder outflow obstruction in the pig. Br J Urol 1987; 60: 332–336
16. German K, Bedwani J, Davies J, Brading AF et al. Physiological and morphometric studies into the pathophysiology of detrusor hyperreflexia in neuropathic patients. J Urol 1995; 153: 1678–1683
17. Yokoyama O, Nagano K, Kawaguchi K, Komatsu K et al. The influence of pelvic nerve transection on the neuromuscular system of the canine urinary bladder. Urol Res 1992; 20: 45–48
18. Persson K, Alm P, Uvelius B, Andersson KE. Nitrergic and cholinergic innervation of the rat lower urinary tract after pelvic ganglionectomy. Am J Physiol 1998; 274: R389–397
19. Malmgren A, Uvelius B, Andersson KE, Andersson PO. On the reversibility of functional bladder changes induced by infravesical outflow obstruction in the rat. J Urol 1990; 143: 1026–1031
20. Wu C, Bayliss M, Newgreen D, Mundy AR et al. A comparison of the mode of action of ATP and carbachol on isolated human detrusor smooth muscle. J Urol 1999; 162: 1840–1847
21. Krichevsky VP, Pagala MK, Vaydovsky I, Damer V et al. Function of M3 muscarinic receptors in the rat urinary bladder following partial outlet obstruction. J Urol 1999; 161: 1644–1650
22. Braverman AS, Luthin GR, Ruggieri MR. M2 muscarinic receptor contributes to contraction of the denervated rat urinary bladder. Am J Physiol 1998; 275: R1654–1660
23. Sibley GN. A comparison of spontaneous and nerve-mediated activity in bladder muscle from man, pig and rabbit. J Physiol 1984; 354: 431–443
24. King JA, Huddart H, Staff WG. Effect of choline ester analogues, noradrenaline and nifedipine on normal and hypertrophied human urinary bladder detrusor muscle. Gen Pharmacol 1998; 30: 131–136
25. Sjogren C, Andersson K-E, Husted S, Mattiasson A et al. Atropine resistance of transmurally stimulated isolated human bladder muscle. J Urol 1982; 128: 1368–1371
26. Palea S, Artibani W, Ostardo E, Trist DG et al. Evidence for purinergic neurotransmission in human urinary bladder affected by interstitial cystitis. J Urol 1993; 150: 2007–2012
27. Yoshida Y, Akimoto Y, Tatsumi H, Koda A. Experimental neurogenic bladder in rats and effect of Robaveron, a biological prepared from swine prostate, on it. Jpn J Pharmacol 1986; 40: 149–159
28. Westfall TD, Kennedy C, Sneddon P. Enhancement of sympathetic purinergic neurotransmission in the guinea-pig isolated vas deferens by the novel ecto-ATPase inhibitor ARL 67156. Br J Pharmacol 1996; 117: 867–872
29. Westfall TD, Kennedy C, Sneddon P. The ecto-ATPase inhibitor ARL 67156 enhances parasympathetic neurotransmission in the guinea-pig urinary bladder. Eur J Pharmacol 1997; 329: 169–173
30. Somogyi GT, Tanowitz M, de Groat WC. M1 muscarinic receptor-mediated facilitation of acetylcholine release in the rat urinary bladder. J Physiol 1994; 480: 81–89
31. Somogyi GT, Tanowitz M, Zernova G, de Groat WC. M1 muscarinic receptor-induced facilitation of ACh and noradrenaline release in the rat bladder is mediated by protein kinase C. J Physiol 1996; 496: 245–254
32. D'Agostino G, Bolognesi ML, Lucchelli A, Vicini D

et al. Prejunctional muscarinic inhibitory control of acetylcholine release in the human isolated detrusor: involvement of the M4 receptor subtype. Br J Pharmacol 2000; 129: 493–500
33. Inadome A, Yoshida M, Takahashi W, Yono M et al. Prejunctional muscarinic receptors modulating acetylcholine release in rabbit detrusor smooth muscles. Urol Int 1998; 61: 135–141
34. Somogyi GT, Zernova GV, Yoshiyama M, Yamamoto T et al. Frequency dependence of muscarinic facilitation of transmitter release in urinary bladder strips from neurally intact or chronic spinal cord transected rats. Br J Pharmacol 1998; 125: 241–246
35. Somogyi GT, de Groat WC. Function, signal transduction mechanisms and plasticity of presynaptic muscarinic receptors in the urinary bladder. Life Sci 1999; 64: 411–418
36. Waterman SA. Multiple subtypes of voltage-gated calcium channel mediate transmitter release from parasympathetic neurons in the mouse bladder. J Neurosci 1996; 16: 4155–4161
37. Brading AF, Turner WH. The unstable bladder: towards a common mechanism. Br J Urol 1994; 73: 3–8
38. Saito M, Kondo A, Kato T, Hasegawa S et al. Response of the human neurogenic bladder to KCl, carbachol, ATP and $CaCl_2$. Br J Urol 1993; 72: 298–302
39. Saito M, Kondo A, Kato T, Levin RM. Response of isolated human neurogenic detrusor smooth muscle to intramural nerve stimulation. Br J Urol 1993; 72: 723–727
40. Yu HJ, Levin RM, Longhurst PA, Damaser MS. Ability of obstructed bladders to empty is dependent on method of stimulation. Urol Res 1997; 25: 291–298
41. Saito M, Wein AJ, Levin RM. Effect of partial outlet obstruction on contractility: comparison between severe and mild obstruction. Neurourol Urodyn 1993; 12: 573–583
42. Hockey JS, Wu C, Fry CH. The actions of metabolic inhibition on human detrusor smooth muscle contractility from stable and unstable bladders. BJU 2000; 86: 531–537
43. Gosling JA. Modification of bladder structure in response to outflow obstruction and ageing. Eur Urol 1997; 32 (Suppl 1): 9–14
44. Elbadawi A, Yalla SV, Resnick NM. Structural basis of geriatric voiding dysfunction. IV. Bladder outlet obstruction. J Urol 1993; 150: 1681–1695
45. Gallegos CR, Fry CH. Alterations to the electrophysiology of isolated human detrusor smooth muscle cells in bladder disease. J Urol 1994; 151: 754–758
46. Rohrmann D, Levin RM, Duckett JW, Zderic SA. The decompensated detrusor I. The effects of bladder outlet obstruction on the use of intracellular calcium stores. J Urol 1996; 156: 578–581
47. Bilgen A, Wein AJ, Haugaard N, Packard D et al. Effect of outlet obstruction on pyruvate metabolism of the rabbit urinary bladder. Mol Cell Biochem 1992; 117: 159–163
48. Gosling JA, Kung LS, Dixon JS, Horan P et al. Correlation between the structure and function of the rabbit urinary bladder following partial outlet obstruction. J Urol 2000; 163: 1349–1356
49. Damaser MS, Haugaard N, Uvelius B. Partial obstruction of the rat urinary bladder: effects on mitochondria and mitochondrial glucose metabolism in detrusor smooth muscle cells. Neurourol Urodyn 1997; 16: 601–607
50. Kort AA, Lakatta EG. Calcium-dependent mechanical oscillations occur spontaneously in unstimulated mammalian cardiac tissues. Circ Res 1984; 54: 396–404
51. Eisner DA, Valdeolmillos M. A study of intracellular calcium oscillations in sheep cardiac Purkinje fibres measured at the single cell level. J Physiol 1986; 372: 539–556
52. Wu C, Fry CH. Spontaneous action potentials and intracellular Ca^{2+} transients in human detrusor smooth muscle cells isolated from stable and unstable bladders. Br J Urol 1997;
53. Kato K, Wein AJ, Radzinski C, Longhurst PA et al. Short term functional effects of bladder outlet obstruction in the cat. J Urol 1990; 143: 1020–1025
54. Malmgren A, Andersson KE, Sjögren C, Andersson PO. Effects of pinacidil and cromakalim (BRL 34915) on bladder function in rats with detrusor instability. J Urol 1989; 142: 1134–1138
55. Ekstrom J, Uvelius B. Length-tension relations of smooth muscle from normal and denervated rat urinary bladders. Acta Physiol Scand 1981; 112: 443–447
56. Montgomery BS, Thomas PJ, Fry CH. The actions of extracellular magnesium on isolated human detrusor muscle function. Br J Urol 1992; 70: 262–268
57. Visser AJ, van Mastrigt R. Intracellular recording of spontaneous electrical activity in human urinary bladder smooth muscle strips. Arch Physiol Biochem 1999; 107: 257–270

58. Rohrmann D, Zderic SA, Duckett JW, Levin RM et al. Compliance of the obstructed fetal rabbit bladder. Neurourol Urodyn 1997; 16: 179–189
59. Damaser MS, Arner A, Uvelius B. Partial outlet obstruction induces chronic distension and increased stiffness of rat urinary bladder. Neurourol Urodyn 1996; 15: 650–665
60. Seki N, Karim OM, Mostwin JL. Changes in action potential kinetics following experimental bladder outflow obstruction in the guinea pig. Urol Res 1992; 20: 387–392
61. Seki N, Karim OM, Mostwin JL. Changes in electrical properties of guinea pig smooth muscle membrane by experimental bladder outflow obstruction. Am J Physiol 1992; 262: F885–891
62. Gabella G, Uvelius B. Urinary bladder of rat: fine structure of normal and hypertrophic musculature. Cell Tissue Res 1990; 262: 67–79
63. Elbadawi A, Yalla SV, Resnick NM. Structural basis of geriatric voiding dysfunction. II. Aging detrusor: normal versus impaired contractility. J Urol 1993; 150: 1657–1667
64. Bramich NJ, Brading AF. Electrical properties of smooth muscle in the guinea-pig urinary bladder. J Physiol 1996; 492: 185–198
65. Fry CH, Cooklin M, Birns J, Mundy AR. Measurement of intercellular electrical coupling in guinea-pig detrusor smooth muscle. J Urol 1999; 161: 660–664
66. Elbadawi A, Yalla SV, Resnick NM. Structural basis of geriatric voiding dysfunction. III. Detrusor overactivity. J Urol 1993; 150: 1668–1680
67. Zipes DP, Jalifé J, eds. Cardiac Electrophysiology: From Cell to Bedside. Philadelphia: WB Saunders.
68. Batista JE, Wagner JR, Azadzoi KM, Krane RJ et al. Direct measurement of blood flow in the human bladder. J Urol 1996; 155: 630–633
69. Azadzoi KM, Pontari M, Vlachiotis J, Siroky MB. Canine bladder blood flow and oxygenation: changes induced by filling, contraction and outlet obstruction. J Urol 1996; 155: 1459–1465
70. Bellringer JF, Ward J, Fry CH. Intramural pH changes in the anaesthetised rabbit bladder during filling. J Physiol 1994; 480: 82–83P
71. Williams JH, Turner WH, Sainsbury GM, Brading AF. Experimental model of bladder outflow tract obstruction in the guinea pig. Br J Urol 1993; 71: 543–554
72. Thomas PJ, Fry CH. The effects of cellular hypoxia on contraction and extracellular ion accumulation in isolated human detrusor smooth muscle. J Urol 1996; 155: 726–731
73. Liston TG, Palfrey EL, Raimbach SJ, Fry CH. The effects of pH changes on human and ferret detrusor muscle function. J Physiol 1991; 432: 1–21
74. Levin RM, Haugaard N, Hypolite JA, Wein AJ et al. Metabolic factors influencing lower urinary tract function. Exp Physiol 1999; 84: 171–194

17

Scientific basis of urodynamics

Michael Craggs and Sarah Knight

INTRODUCTION

The lower urinary tract comprises the bladder, urethra and striated sphincter, which act as a single functional unit under nervous control. The bladder has two principal functions; first, to be a secure low-pressure storage reservoir for the entire urine output from the kidneys and, second, to contract efficiently and empty at socially convenient times. The normal person voids on average about 300 ml completely in about 40 seconds six times a day with no leakage and little sensation of bladder filling in between. However, if these functions are ever compromised, as, for example, in patients presenting with symptoms such as incontinence, urgency, frequency or obstructed voiding, it is important that we are able to assess the operation of the lower urinary tract objectively during both the storage and voiding phases.

Such investigations form the basis of urodynamics, a study which attempts to measure and determine the relationship between bladder volume, bladder pressure (cystometry) and urine flow (flowmetry) under the best physiological conditions possible. The physiological basis and coordination of normal bladder and sphincter function are described fully elsewhere (see Chapter 15).

Much is said about the lack of correlation between symptoms and urodynamic measures in some patients; for example, it is not always possible to observe unstable contractions of the detrusor in the untreated patient complaining of urge incontinence. This sort of finding has made some urologists sceptical of the value of invasive urodynamics (pressure monitoring by catheter per urethra) to the extent that they believe the method is unnatural, offers little to the diagnosis of a patient's problems and introduces infection to the bladder. On the other hand, there are many clinicians who do accept urodynamics as a useful investigative tool but only as a practised art requiring years of experience and careful evaluation.

However, there is an important scientific basis of urodynamics which, if properly standardized and interpreted, can lead to significant findings for making a proper diagnosis of a patient's problems. An example of this is in the derived measure of 'urethral resistance', where an analysis relating detrusor pressure to flow can objectively define obstructed voiding, a condition not always accurately diagnosed from flow measurement alone.[1] Therefore, to transform urodynamics from an art form to a science, we must have a full understanding of the principles of the technique, the underlying physics and mechanics, the derivation of parameters and an appreciation of the extent and limitations of urodynamics as a diagnostic tool.

PHYSICS AND MECHANICS OF THE LOWER URINARY TRACT

From an engineering point of view, the bladder and urethra act as a single functional unit, which can be modelled as a system comprising reservoir, valves and connecting tubes, with pressure, flow and volume as measured variables. To understand the working of this unit during the normal micturition cycle, it is easiest to consider storage and voiding separately, but before that we should be clear about the definition of the measures, specifically, pressure.

Pressure is defined as the force acting per unit area, and force is a vector quantity which has a direction; however, pressure is scalar and has no direction. In urodynamics, pressure is usually quoted in the units of cmH_2O. The standard international (SI) unit is the kilopascal (kPa), which is approximately equal to 10 cmH_2O.

Storage phase

Bladder filling is an essentially passive process during which the normal functional capacity of 300–500 ml should be reached with only a small increase in pressure and before sensations of bladder fullness are perceived. It is possible to account for the bladder as a low-pressure, high-capacity reservoir in purely physical terms.

The small pressure rise within the bladder as it fills is mainly the result of elastic forces generated within the bladder wall. If the bladder is assumed to behave as a thin-walled sphere, its pressure volume characteristics can be described by Laplace's law ($P = 2T/R$) where P = pressure, R = radius and T = tension per unit width of bladder wall (Figure 17.1). As the bladder fills and the volume increases (R↑), the wall tension increases (T↑), but the ratio T/R remains constant, resulting in little change in intravesical pressure until the bladder is almost full.

The use of Laplace's law to determine wall tension and pressure is based on the assumption that the bladder is a thin-walled sphere during the whole of the filling phase. However, the bladder actually progresses from a relatively thick-walled irregular shape when empty to a thin-walled multicurved vessel when full, but the model is a sufficient approximation for a relatively full bladder.

The property of the bladder wall that allows a large increase in volume with only a small associated pressure rise is known as compliance, which is defined as the change in volume divided by the corresponding change in pressure ($\Delta V/\Delta P$). The wall also exhibits the property of elasticity, as it can return to its normal size after voiding with no permanent deformation (plastic) changes. The bladder wall is composed of three layers: an outer covering of connective tissue (serosa), a smooth muscle layer (detrusor) and a mucous membrane (urothelium) which lines the interior of the bladder. These layers comprise collagen and elastin fibres as well as muscle. The layers in combination make the bladder very compliant until the structural capacity of the bladder is reached, and further increases in volume cause increased wall stiffness as the properties of the collagen fibres in the wall dominate and reduce compliance (Figure 17.2).

In addition to compliance and elasticity, the bladder exhibits the time-dependent property of viscoelasticity in which the bladder wall tension and extension are dependent upon rate of filling. When the bladder wall is stretched rapidly, as during fast filling, it appears stiffer than when filled more slowly;

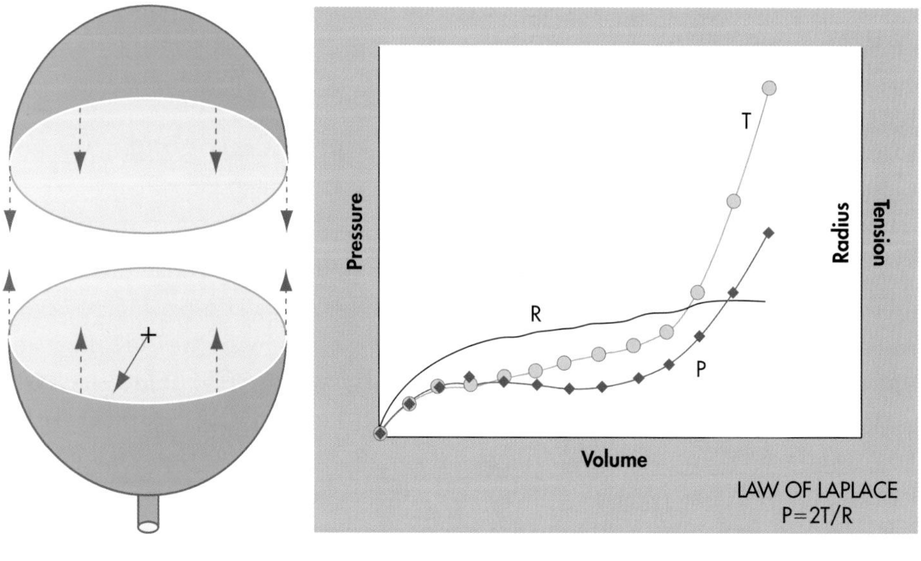

Figure 17.1 *The physics of the bladder as a low-pressure reservoir. The bladder modelled as a thin-walled sphere obeying the law of Laplace. Relationships between volume, pressure, radius and tension in a thin-walled sphere.*

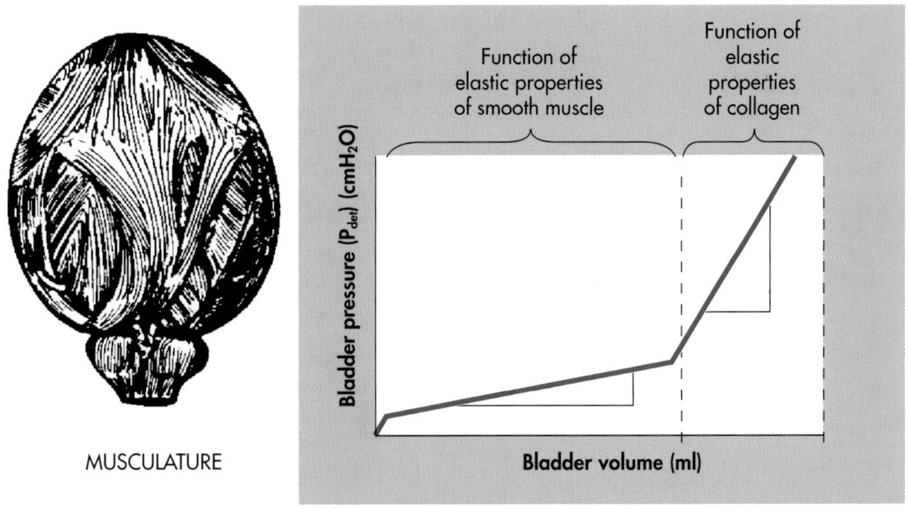

Figure 17.2 *Structure, compliance and capacity of the bladder. Bladder musculature and graph showing relationship between bladder volume and pressure with respect to structural properties.*

however, when the filling is stopped, the wall exhibits relaxation in an exponential manner. Viscoelasticity is often modelled as a combination of spring (purely elastic) and dash-pot (purely viscous) elements[2] (Figure 17.3).

These properties of the bladder wall during storage are likely to be purely passive physical mechanisms attributable to the properties of the tissues, although there may be some active neuromodulatory effects brought about by reflex contractions of the detrusor muscle.

Throughout the storage phase, the urethra must remain closed with a pressure (P_{ura}) which exceeds that of the bladder pressure (P_{ves}) to ensure no leakage of urine ($P_{ura} > P_{ves}$). The urethral closure pressure may be divided into passive and active forces.[3] Passive forces are maintained by the mucosal seal which occurs when the urethral walls oppose each other. Active forces are exerted by the contraction of the urethral and periurethral muscles.

The urethral pressure increases as the bladder fills and during periods when the intraabdominal pressure increases – for example, as a result of postural change or coughing and sneezing – thus maintaining continence.

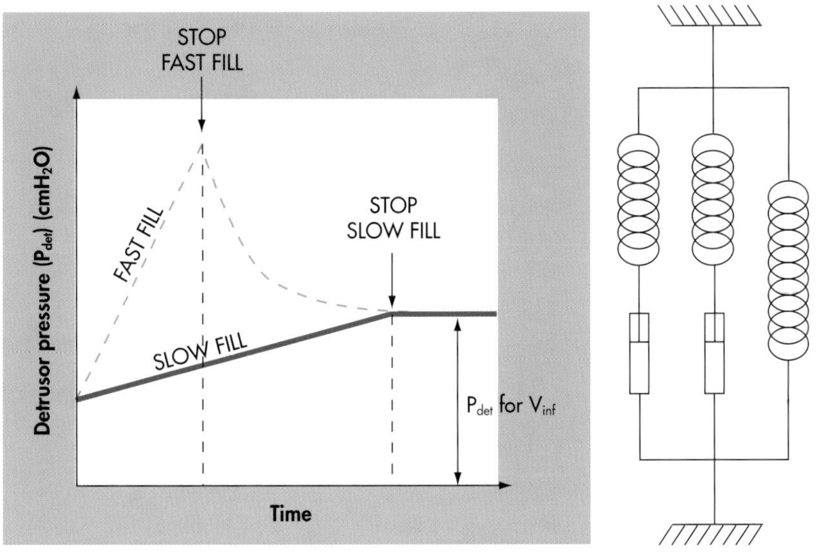

Figure 17.3 *Viscoelastic properties of the bladder wall. The effect of bladder fill rate on measured detrusor pressure. A typical spring and dashpot model of the viscoelastic behaviour of the bladder wall.*

Voiding phase

Voiding is initiated voluntarily following sensation of bladder fullness and is preceded by relaxation of the urethral sphincter. The detrusor muscle contracts in response to uninhibited parasympathetic stimulation, but urine does not flow until the bladder pressure exceeds the urethral pressure ($P_{ves} > P_{ura}$). This initial detrusor contraction is isometric since there is no significant change in bladder volume and no external work done in passing urine.

As soon as the bladder pressure exceeds the urethral closure pressure, the detrusor contraction becomes isotonic, and there is shortening of the detrusor muscle, producing increased external work as the flow reaches a maximum. The isotonic contraction is sustained by reflex activation mediated by increased tension in the receptors in series with the contracting muscle fibres until it falls below a threshold as the detrusor begins to relax at the end of voiding (Figure 17.4).

As with any fluid flow, the rate of urine output (Q_{ura}) is dependent upon both the driving force (P_{ves}), and the resistance to flow (R_{ura}) ($Q_{ura} \propto P_{ves}/R_{ura}$). Other fluid properties, such as viscosity, are normally constant and relatively unimportant, but the use of radio-opaque substances, which can be quite viscous, for X-ray imaging of the urinary tract during urodynamics may have small effects on flow. Physiologically, the isometric part of the detrusor contraction should follow the standard force–length (or volume) and force–velocity curves that can be demonstrated for other muscles[4] (Figure 17.5).

If the bladder is overstretched or not sufficiently full, a submaximal isometric contraction will be produced and reduced flow rate will be achieved. The optimal contraction of the detrusor will be at bladder volumes within the normal functional capacity. The isotonic contraction of the detrusor, that is, when the bladder is emptying, is related to the velocity of shortening of the detrusor muscle. As the force changes from isometric to isotonic, the maximum speed of shortening increases with decreasing load until, in the theoretical limit, no force is required when the muscle becomes unloaded. The resistance to flow is dependent upon both active and passive factors in the urethra, including urethral lumen shape and length, active contraction of the sphincter, and intrinsic muscle and anatomical features. These factors may change throughout the voiding phase; therefore, a simple interpretation of urethral resistance may be difficult to evaluate, and it may be more useful to describe these changes in terms of impedance that includes a time-dependent element. Although the viscosity of urine can be approximated as a constant, the type of urine flow is likely to alternate between laminar and turbulent, depending on changes in the urethral impedance.

Understanding these basic principles of physics and mechanics is important if we are to develop good scientific methodology for urodynamic investigations, the measurement of and relationship between pressure, flow and volume during the storage and voiding phases of bladder function.

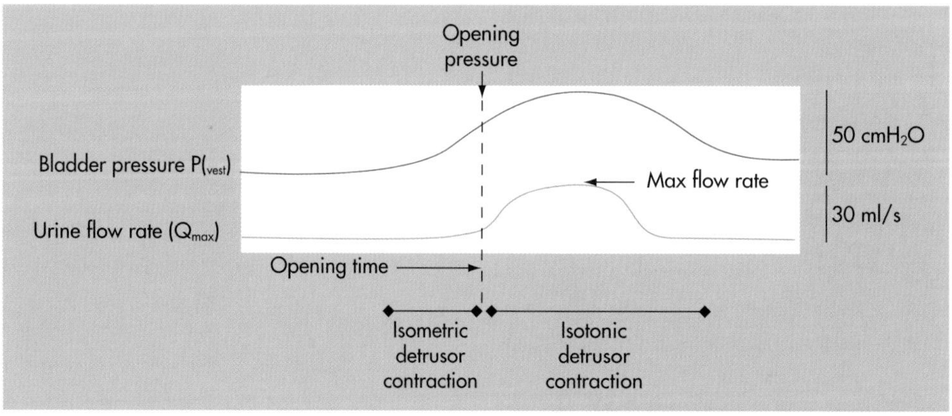

Figure 17.4 *Pressure relationships from storage to voiding, indicating the transition from isometric to isotonic detrusor contraction.*

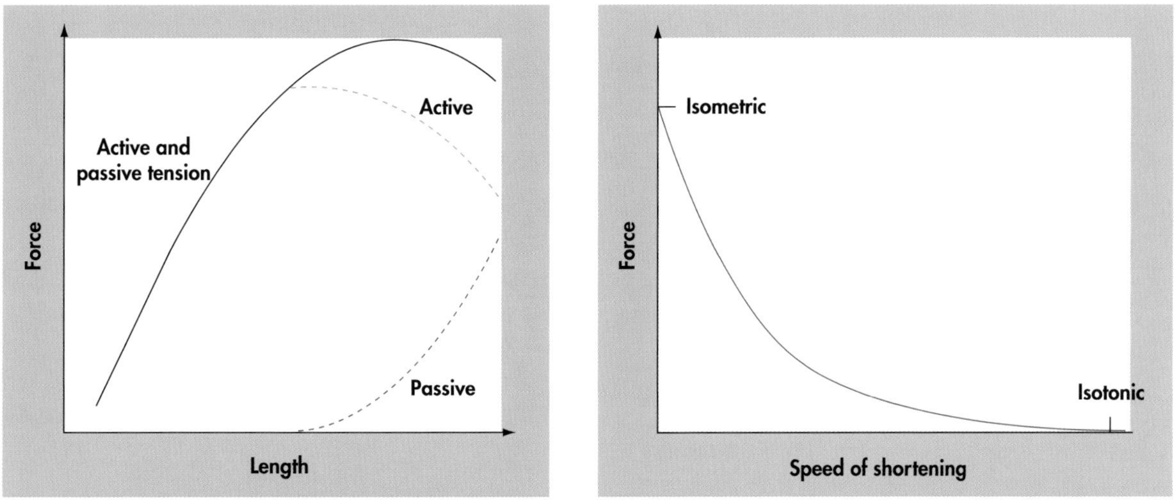

Figure 17.5 *Force–length curve and force–velocity curve for detrusor muscle contraction.*

METHODOLOGY, PRACTICE AND PROBLEMS

The basic aim of urodynamics is to provoke the lower urinary tract in the relatively controlled environment of a clinical laboratory so as to provide an objective basis for a patient's symptoms, lead to a clear diagnosis of the dysfunction and, hopefully, give a guide to rational treatment. Perhaps the greatest failure in this endeavour is poor practice and the misinterpretation of urodynamic tests. There are a number of techniques available for the practice of urodynamics depending on whether the individual patient has a voiding or storage problem, or a combination of both, these are summarised in Table 17.2. In standard urodynamic testing, we usually measure only pressure, flow and volume and leave other physiological measures, such as the electromyography of sphincters, to more specialized investigations. In order to interpret accurately the results of urodynamic tests and carry them out in a scientific and reproducible manner, free from technical artefact, it is important to have a full understanding of the physical principles of these measurements, as described in the previous section.

Pressure can be measured in a number of ways; simple manometry is based on the height of a fluid column, with the pressure proportional to the height of the column. Alternatively, the fluid column can be connected (for example, via a fluid-filled catheter) to an external strain gauge pressure transducer in which the pressure is proportional to the electrical signal output from the transducer. This is the most commonly used pressure measurement technique in urodynamics. Microtip catheter transducers utilize a miniature pressure sensor mounted in the tip (or along the side) of a catheter which can be inserted into the bladder.

Bladder pressure is usually expressed with reference to atmospheric pressure; therefore, the correct zeroing of transducers to atmospheric pressures is very important. In addition, the position of the catheter tip transducer within the bladder can affect the pressure recording, as the pressure measured at the top of the bladder is approximately 10 cmH_2O lower than that at the base due to the height of the water within the bladder itself, and the fluid-filled catheters are very dependent upon relative height of external transducer and tip of catheter (Figure 17.6). The standard zero reference is the level of the symphisis pubis (International Continence Society).

Cystometry

The aim of cystometry is to investigate the pressure–volume relationship of the bladder during the filling and storage phases. In order to measure pressure, a catheter is introduced into the bladder either per urethra or, if access is available, suprapubically. In addition to measuring bladder pressure, it is important to measure intra-abdominal pressure, usually

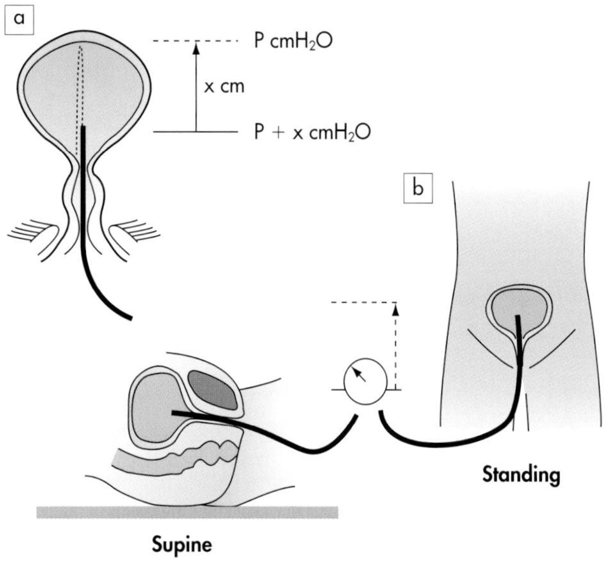

Figure 17.6 *Effect of catheter position in bladder on recorded pressure. (a) Effect of intravesical catheter position of microtip pressure transducer. (b) Effect of relative position of external pressure transducer.*

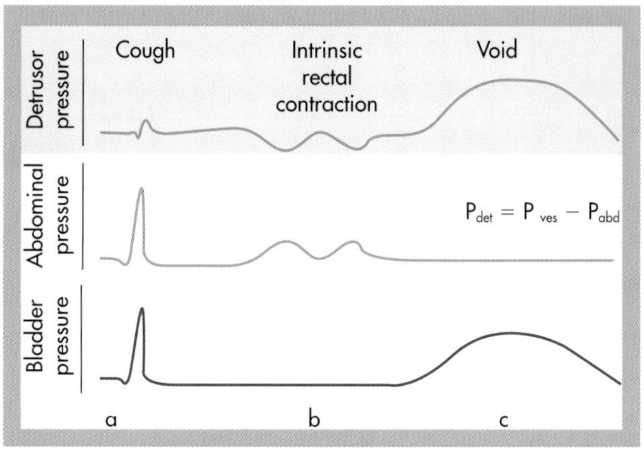

Figure 17.7 *Subtraction cystometry with detrusor pressure calculated from difference between vesical and rectal pressure measurement. (a) Cough appears in both P_{ves} and P_{abd} and therefore no P_{det}. (b) Intrinsic bowel contraction appears in P_{abd} only; therefore, P_{det} shows inverse trace. (c) Bladder contraction activity appears in P_{ves} alone and therefore in P_{det}.*

through a catheter placed in the rectum. In this way, the intra-abdominal pressure (P_{abd}) can be subtracted from the intravesical pressure (P_{ves}) to give a true detrusor pressure (P_{det}) free from artefacts caused by extravesical pressure increases, such as coughing or straining. However, it must be noted that in addition to abdominal pressure changes, P_{abd} will also reflect intrinsic bowel activity (Figure 17.7).

During a filling cystometrogram, fluid is retrogradely instilled into the bladder in a physiological manner. In the ideal situation, this means using isotonic saline at body temperature, at a rate close to that of natural diuresis from the kidneys (< 10 ml/min). However, due to constraints of time and convenience, filling rates are normally much faster (10–100 ml/min), though these rates may be too provocative for some overactive bladders, and may lead to overfilling in others that are hypoactive. As described earlier, a normal bladder shows very little change in pressure during filling (high compliance – see earlier section), but because of possible decreases in the viscoelastic nature of the bladder wall (for example, in the neuropathic bladder), it may be necessary to fill much more slowly in some patients. A further matter is the position of the patient during cystometry – lying down, sitting or standing may be important if we are to replicate the conditions in which patients' symptoms are revealed, but this cannot always be practical. Most filling cystometry is performed with the patients lying either supine or semirecumbent and then raised to sitting or standing position for voiding cystometry (see later in this section).

Urethral pressure profilometry (UPP)

This technique is used to determine the intraluminal pressure along the length of the urethra, during the storage phase. This investigation has lost favour among some clinicians, probably as a result of its relative complexity and inaccuracy if not performed correctly. However, knowledge of urethral resistance can be useful in identifying urethral incompetence (as in anatomical obstruction by stricture, benign prostatic hyperplasia (BPN), or active dyssynergic sphincters). There are two principal techniques for measuring UPP: fluid perfusion profilometry[5] and solid-state microtip pressure transducers.

The perfusion technique is based on the pressure required to perfuse fluid through a catheter at a constant rate; this is best achieved with a syringe driver rather than a peristaltic pump. A catheter with side holes is introduced into the urethra and zeroed in the standard way, and the catheter is attached via a three-way tap to a pressure transducer and an infusion pump. The pressure recorded is defined as the resistance the urethral wall produces to the perfusing fluid. The catheter is then withdrawn slowly along the length of the urethra, thus giving a pressure profile. A profile can also be obtained by withdrawing a solid-state pressure tip transducer at a constant rate (Figure 17.8).

There are a number of factors that must be taken into account when performing UPP to ensure accuracy. As described earlier, pressure has no direction, and therefore measuring in a particular orientation along the urethral wall may introduce errors due to position of side holes or transducer sensors. In addition, bladder volume, patient position and artefacts caused by movement or abdominal straining can also introduce errors.

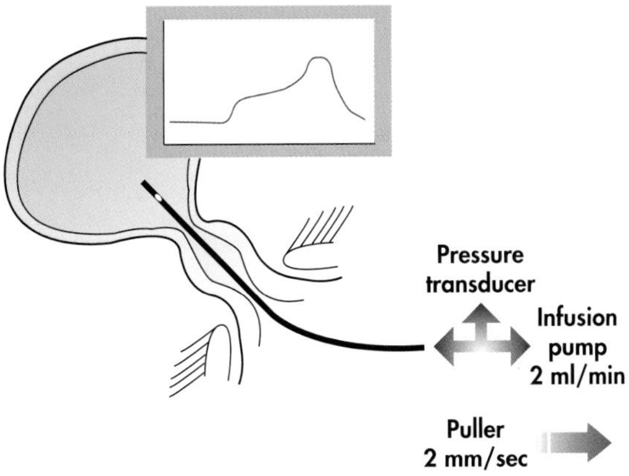

Figure 17.8 *Brown–Wickham perfusion technique for measurement of urethral pressure profile.*

Urethral pressure profiles can be measured in steady-state or static conditions, or, alternatively, under conditions of stress such as coughing or straining.

Flowmetry

Of all urodynamic tests, this is the least invasive and easiest to perform with modern flow-rate recorders and should certainly be the first line of investigation for suspected voiding problems. As described in the previous section, the flow rate of urine from the bladder is dependent upon both the driving force of the pressure generated in the bladder and the resistance of the urethra. A simple flow-rate measurement cannot accurately distinguish the relative importance of these two factors; therefore, accurate diagnosis is often not possible without measuring both bladder pressure and flow rate simultaneously. Even then, the effect of urethral resistance may be an important additional factor.

There are a number of techniques available for measuring urine flow, based on the different principles described in Table 17.1.

Modern electronic devices can output a number of parameters based on the voiding characteristics. However, a single flow rate on a single occasion is unlikely to be of much diagnostic value, and a number of factors should be taken into account when performing meaningful flowmetry. The bladder volume at which the flow rate was measured is extremely important, especially with respect to the

Table 17.1 Methods of measuring urine flow.

Type of flowmeter	Principle	Comments
Weight transducer	Weight of urine voided measured and differentiated with respect to time to calculate flow rate	
Rotating disc	A servomotor rotates the disc at a constant rate, but rate of urine flow tends to slow the disc, requiring greater power to keep at a constant speed. Power consumption of servomotor is proportional to flow rate and can be integrated for voided volume	'Cruising' (moving urine stream over disc and sides of collecting container) can cause artefact
Capacitance	A capacitor comprised of a metal strip is placed vertically in the collecting vessel. As volume of urine increases, the level of urine on the strip changes and capacitance decreases. The signal is proportional to voided volume and can be differentiated for flow rate	Urinating on to capacitance strip may cause artefact

force–length curve of the detrusor muscle. An over- or understretched bladder will not be capable of generating the maximal force to expel urine and thus may give a lower than optimal flow rate (Figure 17.9). The urethral resistance may also change with bladder volumes and also give rise to different flow rates.

It is important to estimate the total bladder volume not only from the voided volume but also taking into account any residual volume in the bladder. This can be calculated by ultrasound or by catheter. In unfamiliar surroundings, a patient may feel uncomfortable, be inhibited or strain during voiding, and this may lead to an unnatural flow pattern and incomplete voiding. Technical artefacts can occur if the stream of flow is not aimed directly into the flow meter, and 'cruising' or moving the stream across the flow meter can lead to abnormal traces. Flowmetry can also now be carried out with portable devices at home. This can lead to more accurate results, as the patient is more comfortable and multiple measurements can be recorded.

The ideal situation in which to carry out flowmetry is in conjunction with cystometry, so that voiding pressure and flow rate can be measured simultaneously, although the delay in urine flow exiting the bladder and reaching the flow meter must be taken into account. Pressure flow studies can, for example, help to identify whether a low flow rate is due to a urethral obstruction or a hypocontractile bladder; this information could not be inferred from a flow rate alone.

INTERPRETATION: ART OR SCIENCE?

Interpretation of urodynamic investigations is very much dependent on both a proper understanding of the physiological factors controlling and affecting the lower urinary tract and the technical aspects of urodynamic technique. This is particularly important if the interpreters did not undertake the investigations themselves, Table 17.3 summarises some important factors which may influence urodynamic findings.

The diagnostic potential of urodynamic studies relies on a number of measures which should be quantified and standardized to minimize subjective interpretation. The International Continence Society (ICS) Standardization Committee has been pivotal in introducing procedures and guidelines for the standardization of terminology of lower urinary tract function, dysfunction and rehabilitation, including derived parameters and indices of function.[5a] However, it should be appreciated that rather little of this standardization has been based on comparative control data from healthy volunteers. Therefore, interpretation of urodynamic data on patients, in the hope of providing definitive diagnosis, can still remain unclear.

Filling cystometry

From the filling cystometrogram, we can determine information about bladder compliance, the incidence of 'unstable' detrusor activity, and the sensa-

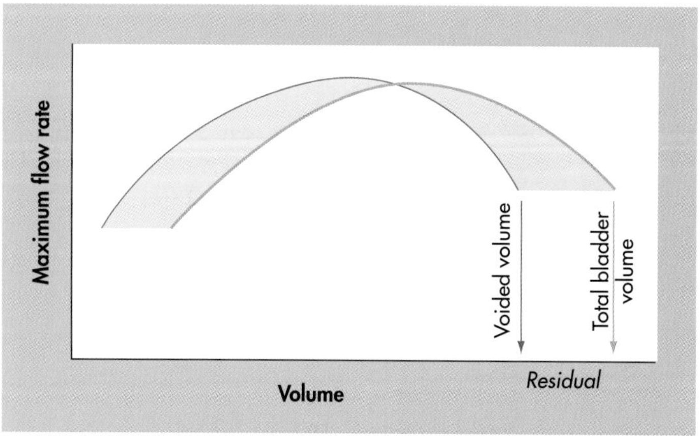

Figure 17.9 *The relationship between maximum flow rate out of the bladder and bladder volume, demonstrating the reduction in flow rate at bladder volumes significantly larger or smaller than the functional volume.*

tions perceived by subjects as the bladder volume increases to capacity.

As described in the previous section, bladder compliance is defined as the ratio of volume change to pressure change – ΔV/ΔP. For a normal healthy bladder, the maximum capacity should be reached with only a small change in bladder pressure, to give a high value for compliance (about 40 ml/cmH_2O). As the bladder becomes stiffer, particularly towards maximum capacity, the pressure per unit volume can increase, and the compliance becomes smaller in a non-linear fashion. It is important to recognize the effect that the rate that bladder filling can have on compliance, and in some cases it may be necessary to stop the fill and wait until the bladder pressure has returned to its stress-relaxed state before calculating a value for compliance. This might be particularly important in the pathologically small bladder where fibrosis, a reduction in elasticity and other factors might be expected to reduce compliance severely. Indeed, in the neurogenic bladder of spinal cord injury, the rate of filling cystometry is usually kept low at 10–20 ml/min.

During filling, the normal bladder should remain stable up to full bladder capacity, showing little or no activity. Unlike the slow rises in detrusor pressure associated with lowered bladder compliance, detrusor overactivity is characterized by phasic events which rise relatively and then fall again within a few tens of seconds. Bladder activity can also be provoked by rapid filling (for example, 10 ml/s) or ice water, and these may be more useful provocative tests than the standard filling cystometrogram in some patients, such as those with a neurological cause for their overactive detrusor, as in spinal cord injury. Although it is not common practice in routine urodynamic laboratories, quantifying detrusor overactivity is important if a proper assessment of interventions is to be made. Various approaches have been adopted, including measuring the peak pressure, calculating the area under the unstable contraction and recording the frequency of events. For many urodynamic tests, overactivity presents itself as a single 'end-fill' event which occurs when the bladder reaches its maximum cystometric volume (Figure 17.10).

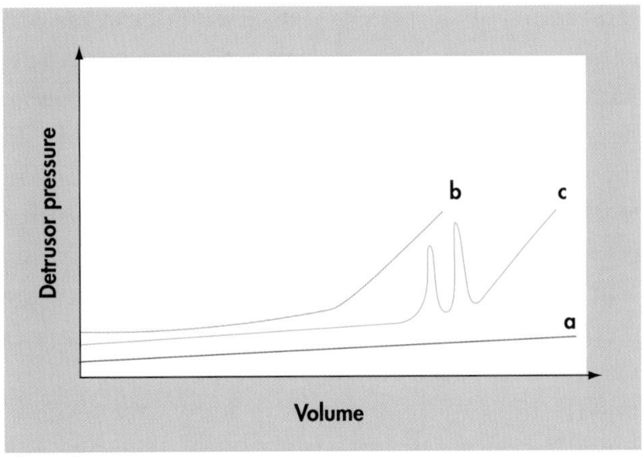

Figure 17.10 *Typical filling cystometrogram traces illustrating (a) normal bladder, (b) bladder with loss of compliance at end fill and (c) instability and end-fill loss of compliance.*

The sensations recorded by subjects during a filling cystometrogram usually receive much less attention than the occurrence of abnormal pressure changes. The standard technique for monitoring bladder sensations is the use of markers for the first sensation (FS), first desire to void (FDV), and strong desire to void (SDV), which is sometimes described as strong urge and occasionally associated with severe discomfort and pain, though it is not always associated with changes in detrusor pressure. However, these markers may be very subjective, variable and susceptible to prompting by the investigator. Bladder sensations may also be confused due to interference from catheterization, non-physiological fill rates and embarrassment.

With the development of a new technique for investigating bladder sensations during cystometry, it may now become possible to determine the relevance of urodynamics and symptomatology more objectively. This will be especially useful in conditions such as urgency, frequency and urge incontinence where overactivity cannot always be reliably demonstrated even at full capacity.[6]

The maximum capacity of the bladder is described as the volume at which patients feel they can no longer delay micturition. This measure can be very different in the same individual in everyday life and probably depends on many factors. Of course, functional bladder capacity, rather than maximum capacity, may be more accurately reflected in frequency–volume diaries. However, in the relatively controlled environment of the urodynamics laboratory, repeated cystometries can give a reasonable indication of a person's maximum capacity. Of course this is more difficult to determine in patients with poor or absent sensation such as those with a neurological cause for their bladder problems. In these patients, it is possible to get a reasonable estimate of maximum capacity by filling until detrusor overactivity occurs. Interestingly, patients who present with intractably small bladder capacities are sometimes found to have relatively normal capacities when tested under general anaesthesia.

Urethral pressure profiles

A number of parameters can be derived from the static urethral pressure profile, including maximum urethral pressure (MUP), maximum urethral closure pressure (MUCP) and functional profile length (FPL) (Figure 17.11). Although the functional profile length may not be diagnostically useful in itself, it can be used to calculate a further index by multiplying it with maximum urethral pressure. This index has been used to diagnose stress incontinence.

The stress UPP can be used to determine the decrease in transfer of abdominal pressures to the urethra during manoeuvres such as the Valsalva and cough to determine degree of stress incontinence (Figure 17.12).

However, it has been shown that the position of the patient during these studies can dramatically alter the results. Diagnostic interpretations of urethral function can also be made from the characteristic shape of the UPP. However, it should be noted that there are a number of differences caused by both age and sex that may lead to inaccuracies in these interpretations. For example, the MUP often decreases with age, and, in women, it often decreases, especially after the menopause. The MUP is often lower in patients with stress incontinence, though the findings are not always consistent with symptoms reported by the patient, and there is a significant overlap in the values found in incontinent and continent subjects.

Flowmetry and voiding cystometry

As described in the earlier section, the most useful voiding study involves the simultaneous measurement of voiding pressure and flow rate. This allows the derivation of a number of factors that may be useful in the diagnosis of lower urinary tract dysfunction, particularly obstructive disorders. However, if flowmetry alone is undertaken, there are a number of factors that are measured, including maximum flow rate, average flow rate, flow time, voiding time, voided volume and time to maximum flow. Several nomograms have been developed for determining the degree of obstruction from flow rate alone. These include the Liverpool nomogram, which was constructed after analysing flow rates and bladder volumes collected from many hundreds of patients.[7] The shape of the normal flow curve is near Gaussian and deviations from this shape may suggest pathology; for example, a low flat curve may be indicative of a stricture, while an intermittent flow with low flow rate may indicate obstruction. It is also important during uroflowmetry to determine the residual volume; this can be calculated most accurately by catheterizing the patient, or by ultrasonography.

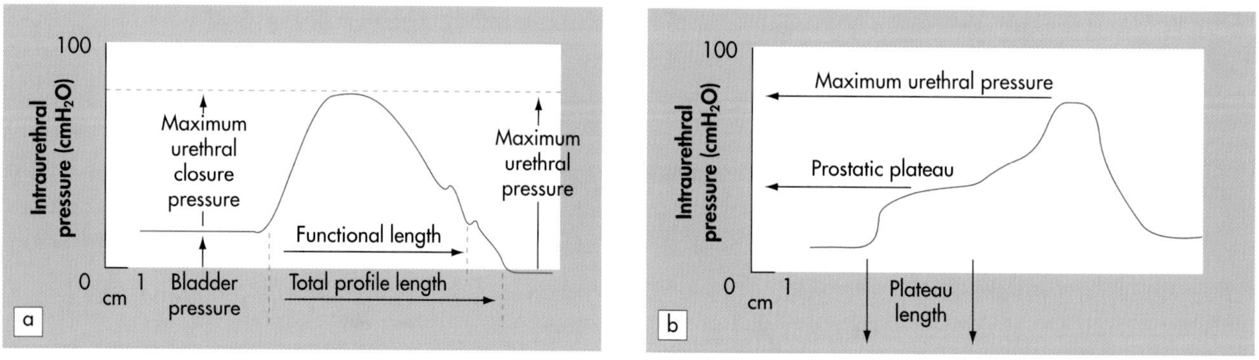

Figure 17.11 *Typical urethral pressure profiles in (a) female and (b) male subjects.*

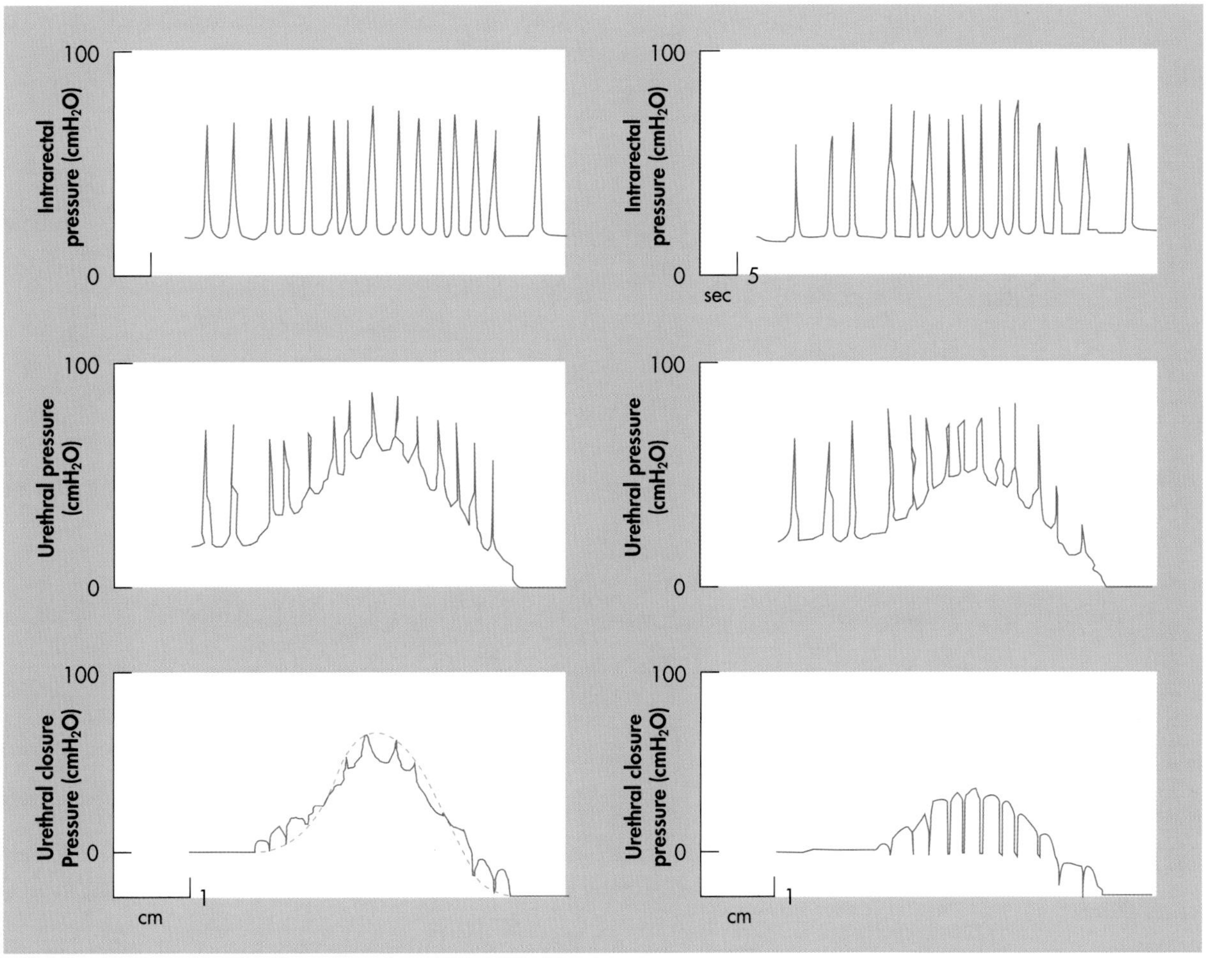

Figure 17.12 *The stress urethral pressure profile in a healthy volunteer and a female with stress urinary incontinence.*

Pressure–flow studies are carried out to determine whether the low flow rate recorded during flowmetry is attributable to a high urethral resistance or a low bladder pressure. The interrelationship between these variables means that accurate diagnosis of dysfunction requires simultaneous measurement of flow rate and detrusor pressure. The most common variables measured are the maximum flow rate (Q_{max}) and the detrusor pressure at this flow rate ($P_{det}Q_{max}$). As for simple flowmetry, a number of nomograms have been derived for these variables to identify patients with obstructive disorders (Figure 17.13).[8,9]

It is important to note that nearly all of these nomograms have a large equivocal region, which makes a definitive diagnosis impossible.

If a low flow rate is also associated with a low detrusor pressure, it is may be necessary to determine the contractility of the detrusor muscle. Detrusor contractility is an important parameter that is relatively complicated to measure and understand. An isometric detrusor contraction can be produced by asking a patient to stop voiding as soon as the maximum flow rate is reached. As the detrusor muscle continues to contract against a closed outlet, the contraction is assumed to be isometric, the resulting pressure is defined as $P_{det.iso}$. A single stop test is often used, and a single value for $P_{det.iso}$ is derived from this. However, the definition of contractility includes a dependence upon the muscle length. The serial stop test has therefore been suggested as a more accurate method for determining a true contractility curve.[10,11]

In this way, the detrusor force at each given volume can be determined for each stop test. It should be noted that patients with severe stress incontinence

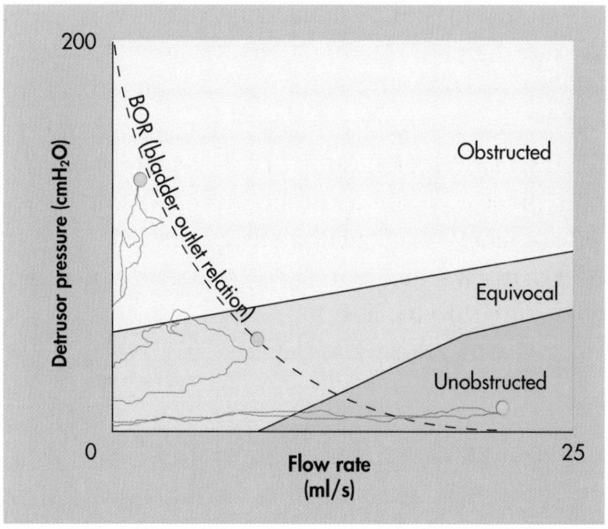

Figure 17.13 *Nomogram for determining bladder outlet obstruction.*

may not be able to stop urine flow sufficiently, and there is the theoretical possibility that repeated cessation may cause an inhibition of detrusor contraction.

The Watts factor (WF) developed by Griffiths[12] is an alternative method for deriving a continuous calculation of detrusor contractility. The WF is defined as the power per unit area of bladder and is numerically equal to isometric detrusor pressure throughout voiding (Figure 17.15).

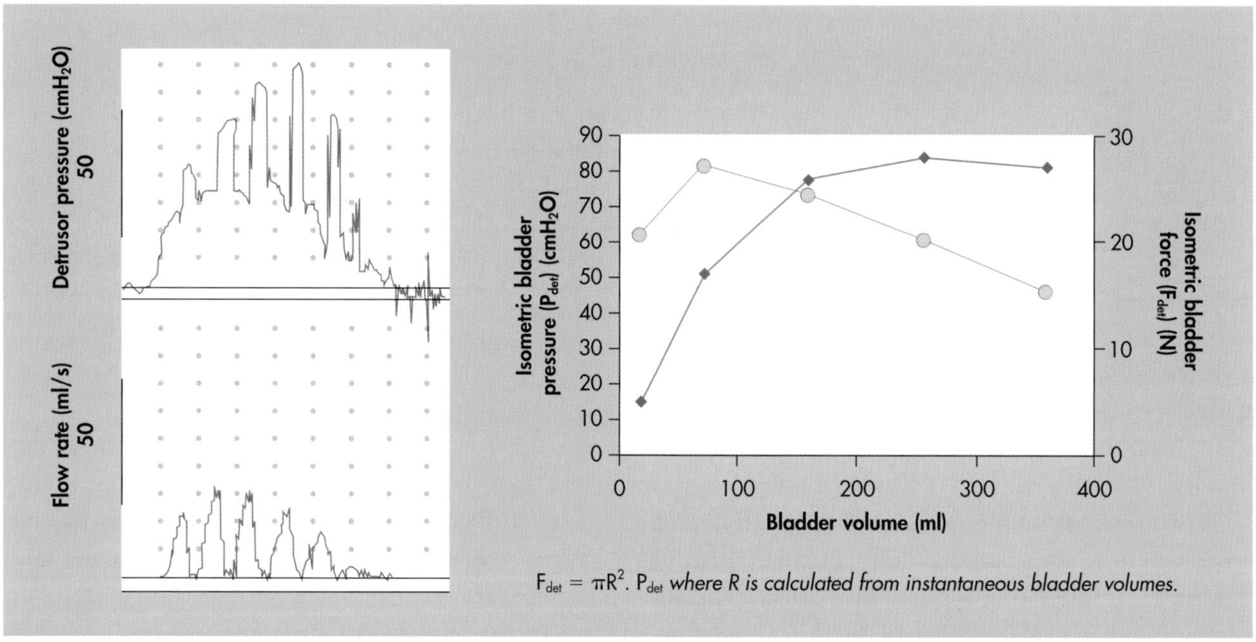

Figure 17.14 *A graph showing typical serial stop test during voiding.*

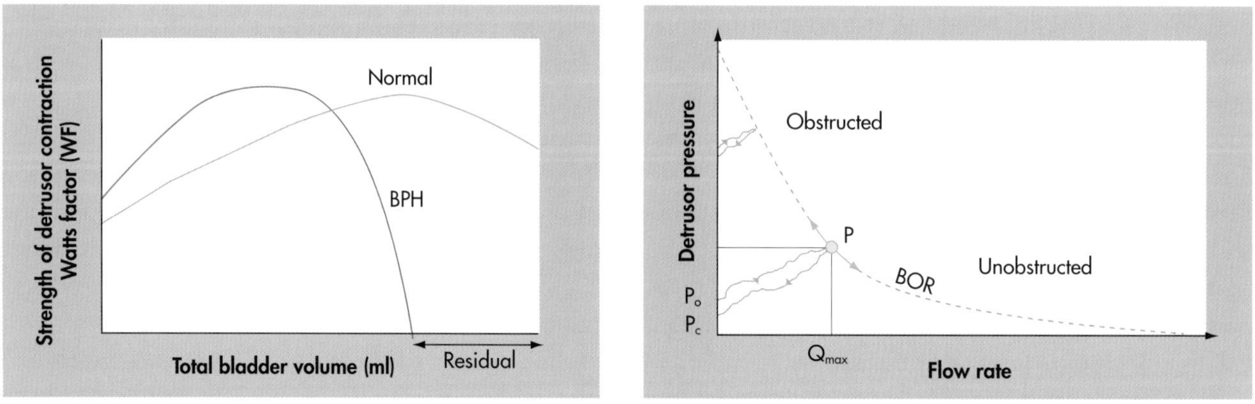

Figure 17.15 *Graphs illustrating derived bladder parameters Watts factor (WF) and bladder output relationship (BOR).*

ADVANCED TECHNIQUES AND NEW DEVELOPMENTS

In recent times, more specialized techniques to assist diagnosis have been introduced into the practice of urodynamics. Of these, the videocystometrogram (VCMG), in which X-ray imaging of the urinary tract with a contrast medium is combined with urodynamic measurements, is the most common. Although it can yield valuable information about bladder morphology, urethral dysfunction (for example, in assessing dyssynergic sphincters or bladder neck obstruction) and ureteral reflux (important to identify and eliminate for the preservation of renal function), which cannot be obtained with urodynamics alone, it has the danger of overexposure to X-rays and is relatively expensive, thus precluding frequent use.

Another technique gaining much favour is ambulatory urodynamics, where bladder pressure, rectal pressure and leakage can be monitored continuously over a long period on a portable data-logger to assess the effects of 'normal' activities on lower urinary tract function. Considerable technical back-up is required for this type of study, and much time and care are needed in data analysis, especially for the identification and elimination of artefacts. Although expensive, it is said to be a valuable aid in diagnosing conditions such as idiopathic instability where standard urodynamics has been unsuccessful.

Newer methods are now being investigated which may overcome some of the other problems associated with conventional urodynamics. As we have seen, bladder pressure is conventionally measured by catheterization with the attendant risk of traumatizing the urethra and introducing infection into the bladder (estimated to occur in about 1–5% of urodynamic investigations), so by eliminating the need for catheters in the bladder, this morbidity could be reduced. One such technique is non-invasive urodynamics. For a proper diagnosis of bladder outlet obstruction, such as that associated with benign prostatic hyperplasia, it is necessary to study the relationship between urinary flow rate and bladder pressure. A new and novel technique for measuring bladder pressure non-invasively is currently being developed into a practical device which does not require catheters in the bladder.[13] Essentially, the technique is simple; it uses an inflatable cuff placed around the penis to apply compressive obstruction sufficient to stop urine flow. At the point where flow just stops, the cuff pressure is a reasonably good approximation of bladder pressure. A successful non-invasive bladder pressure technique could provide a more cost-beneficial diagnostic method for selecting patients for surgery as well as lowering morbidity through infection.

Future developments include the use of functional magnetic resonance imaging (fMRI) to produce high-quality anatomical characterization of the function of the bladder, urethra and pelvic floor. However, the use of MRI combined with urodynamics is still in an experimental phase,[14] but it has the potential for giving three-dimensional views of the bladder and urethra during filling and voiding. More recently, PET (positron-emission tomography) studies have been used to determine which areas of the brain are responsible for sensations of bladder filling.[15] Although this technique is likely to remain purely a research tool, the results may increase our knowledge and understanding of the micturition cycle.

SYMPTOMS AND URODYNAMICS

Although we may now have a good scientific understanding of the basis of urodynamics, the question still remains, 'What exactly is the relationship between urinary symptomatology and urodynamics?' There have been many studies and papers written about this topic but without a firm conclusion as to whether they do correlate in any urological problem.

In a recent study of women questioned about their complaints of urinary incontinence, it was found that not only were the subjective answers by patients not helpful in differentiating the aetiology of incontinence but also that almost no questions were helpful in predicting which patients would have normal video urodynamics.[16] Interestingly, questions about nocturia, frequency, urgency and urge incontinence, among others, were not statistically significant for any group. If there is so little correlation between symptoms and urodynamics, what is the purpose of urodynamics? If it is the symptoms that drive patients to seek help in the first place, what additional information is urodynamics providing? Are the rather non-physiological techniques used in urodynamics part of the problem?

Perhaps for some urological problems, such as urge incontinence, the difficulty in urodynamics has to do with measuring the sensations of bladder filling and urge itself rather than looking just for instability as a cause for their symptoms. Diaries show that these patients void frequently, suggesting that they may be having strong sensations of urge and the desire to void at relatively low bladder volumes.

During urodynamics, patients are asked through dialogue to report on any sensations; for example, the standard measures are 'first sensation of filling', 'first desire to void' and, finally, 'strong desire to void'. Prompting the patient for answers probably helps to undermine the value of these measures of sensation, and this may be very important if we are trying to get an accurate picture of the bladder volume at the time. Perhaps we should pay more attention to the sensations experienced by patients during urodynamics and get accurate measures of bladder volumes for each level of reported sensation. So, in urge incontinence at least, there may be a more positive correlation between symptoms and urodynamics.[17]

CONCLUSION: URODYNAMICS – ART OR SCIENCE?

This chapter has outlined the scientific basis of urodynamics and how simple physical principles can be applied to explain the functions of the bladder during filling and voiding cystometry. The techniques for measuring and recording pressure changes and flow accurately are described together with how we can relate these measurements to some functions of the lower urinary tract. For the urologist, it is important to know when and in what ways the lower urinary is dysfunctional, so comparisons with 'normal function' are crucial. There are some tabulated examples of normal versus patient data in the form of nomograms or charts, such as flow versus voided volume[18] or detrusor pressure.[19] From these charts, clinicians can relate their findings on urodynamics to the variation of the 'normal population' and draw conclusions about departure of their patients from normality. Even more sophisticated graphs have evolved which describe the contractility and urethral resistance[20] calculated as derivations from pressure, volume and flow measured during urodynamics. Applying these graphs 'blindly' and without full appreciation of urodynamic techniques, their errors and their artefacts is very likely to lead to false information about a patient's true lower urinary tract function.

Table 17.2 Techniques used in urodynamics for measurement of lower urinary tract function.

Technique	Function	Indication
Cystometry	Measurement of bladder storage and voiding function, including sensation	Incontinence and dysfunction of detrusor
Flowmetry	Measurement of voiding function	Incontinence and voiding dysfunction
Urethral pressure profilometry	Measurement of urethral closure pressures	Incontinence due to sphincter incompetence
Ambulatory urodynamics	Behaviour of bladder and urethra during activities of daily living	Incontinence
Video-urodynamics	Measurement of bladder storage and voiding in conjunction with imaging of bladder morphology	Multifactorial incontinence or suspected abnomalities in lower urinary tract
Neurophysiological	Neurophysiological assessment of urethral sphincter and pelvic floor function	Incontinence or dyssynergic voiding

Table 17.3 Potential factors which may lead to inaccuracies in urodynamic findings.

Problem	Artefact and possible effects
Transducer zeroing and position	Incorrect pressure with respect to reference and poor subtraction of P_{ves} and P_{abd}
Poor subtraction	Incorrect P_{det} recording, best checked by continuous coughing which should show equal pressure changes on P_{ves} and P_{abd}
Patient position	May not reproduce patients' symptoms and give false pressure
Filling medium, temperature, viscosity, pH	May cause irritation, increasing sensations and possibly provoking overactivity
Filling rate	Filling too fast may provoke unstable contractions and underestimate compliance
Catheter size	A large catheter may cause irritation and partial obstruction
Air bubbles in water-filled lines	This will cause a damped pressure recording and incorrect pressure values
Misplaced catheter	Will not represent true P_{ves} or P_{det}; that is, catheter being expelled during voiding or coughing
Overfilling of bladder	May reduce ability to void, especially in patients with reduced sensation or outflow obstruction
Presence of infection	May increase urgency symptoms
Concomitant medication	May affect symptoms

Finally, if we are to relate some types of urinary symptoms with urodynamics, we must include more objective ways of recording the sensations of filling and urge in our studies. Reading urodynamic records in an intelligent way is both an art form and a science requiring considerable experience in order to reach a high standard of interpretation.

FURTHER READING

Abrams P. Urodynamics. 2nd edn. London: Springer-Verlag, 1997

Chapple C, Christmas TJ, Fallows J, Turner-Warwick RT, eds. Urodynamics Made Easy. Churchill Livingstone, 1999

Jonas U. Evolutions in Urodynamics. Karger, 1991

The Mechanics and Hydrodynamics of the Lower Urinary Tract. Medical Physics Handbooks 4. Bristol: Adam Hilger Limited, 1980

Mundy AR, Stephenson TP, Wein AJ, eds. Urodynamics: Principles, Practice and Application. 2nd edn. Churchill Livingstone, 1994

Sand PK, Ostergard DR. Urodynamics and the Evaluation of Female Incontinence. London: Springer-Verlag, 1995

REFERENCES

1. Schafer W. Urethral resistance? Urodynamic concepts of physiological and pathological bladder outlet function during voiding. Neurourol Urodyn 1985; 4: 161–201
2. van Mastrigt R, Coolsaet BL, van Duyl WA. Passive properties of the urinary bladder in the collection phase. Med Biol Eng Comput 1978; 16: 471–482
3. Zinner NR, Sterling AM, Ritter RC. Role of inner urethral softness in urinary continence. Urology 1980; 16: 115–117
4. Hill AV. The heat of shortening and the dynamic constants of muscle. Proc R Soc Lond B Biol Sci 1938; 126: 136–195
5. Brown M, Wickham JE. The urethral pressure profile. Br J Urol 1969; 41: 211–217

5a. Abrams P, Cardozo L, Fall M et al. The standardisation of terminology in lower urinary tract function: report from the standardisation sub-committee of the International Continence Society. Urology 2003; 61: 37–49

6. Oliver SE, Fowler CJ, Mundy AR, Craggs MD. Measuring the sensations of urge and bladder filling during cystometry in urge incontinence and the effects of neuromodulation. Neurourol Urodyn 2003; 22: 7–16

7. Haylen BT, Parys BT, Anyaegbunam WI, Ashby D, West CR. Urine flow rates in male and female urodynamic patients compared with the Liverpool nomograms. Br J Urol 1990; 65: 483–487
8. Griffiths D, Hofner K, van Mastrigt R et al. Standardisation of terminology of lower urinary tract function: pressure-flow studies of voiding, urethral resistance, and urethral obstruction. International Continence Society Sub-Committee on Standardisation of Terminology of Pressure-Flow Studies. Neurourol Urodyn 1997; 16: 1
9. Schafer W. Analysis of bladder outlet function with the linearized passive urethral resistance relation, linPURR and a disease specific approach for grading obstruction: from complex to simple. World J Urol 1995; 13: 47
10. Susset JG, Brissot RB, Regnier RB. The stop-flow technique: a way to measure detrusor strength. J Urol 1982; 127: 489–494
11. Craggs MD, Knight SL, McFarlane JA. Detrusor force measured by serial stop-tests in healthy volunteers. Neurourology Urodyn 1998; 17: 1–2
12. Griffiths DJ. Mechanics of micturition. In: Yalla SV, McGuire EJ, Elbadawi E, Blaivas G, eds. Neurology and Urodynamics: Principles and Practice. New York: Macmillan, 1988
13. Griffiths CJ, Rix D, MacDonald AM, Drinnan MJ et al. Noninvasive measurement of bladder pressure by controlled inflation of a penile cuff. J Urol 2002; 167: 1344–1347
14. Simmons A, Williams SC, Craggs M, Andrew C et al. Dynamic multi-planar EPI of the urinary bladder during voiding with simultaneous detrusor pressure measurement. Magn Reson Imaging 1997; 15: 295–300
15. Athwal BS, Berkley KJ, Hussain I, Brennan A et al. Brain responses to changes in bladder volume and urge to void in healthy men. Brain 2001; 124(Pt 2): 369–377
16. Amundsen C, Lau M, English SF, McGuire EJ. Do urinary symptoms correlate with urodynamic findings? J Urol 1999; 161: 1871–1874
17. Oliver S, Fowler C, Mundy A, Craggs M. Measuring the sensations of urge and bladder filling during cystometry in urge incontinence and the effects of neuromodulation Neurourol Urodyn 2003; 22(1): 7–16
18. Haylen BT, Ashby D, Sutherst JR, Frazer MI, West CR. Maximum and average urine flow rates in normal male and female populations – the Liverpool nonograms. Br J Urol 1989; 64(1): 30–8
19. Abrams PH, Griffiths DJ. The assessment of prostatic obstruction from urodynamic measurements and from residual urine. Br J Urol 1979; 51: 129–134
20. Schäfer W. Basic principles and clinical application of advance analysis of bladder voiding function. Urol. Clin N Am 1990; 17: 553–566

18

Male sexual function

Suks Minhas, John P Pryor and David J Ralph

INTRODUCTION

Normal male sexual function is considered to be essential for good health and it is important to remember that psychological factors impinge upon all elements of it. This chapter concentrates on erectile function and fertility but commences with discussion of the hormone testosterone, which is of paramount importance to male sexual function.

TESTOSTERONE METABOLISM

The Y chromosome (Figure 18.1) determines that an embryo will develop into a male and is essential for normal sexual function. It contains fewer genes than other chromosomes but does contain the sex (or testis)-determining gene (SRY), which controls gender by triggering the formation of a testis in the male embryo (see Chapter 28). The azoospermic factor (AZF) and DAZ group of genes are also associated with spermatogenesis. Deletions of the Y chromosome in these regions can be associated with abnormal spermatogenesis.

The cells in the primitive genital ridge differentiate in the presence of the SRY gene during the seventh week of fetal life into Leydig and Sertoli cells (Figure 18.2). The Leydig cells produce testosterone, initially under the influence of maternal chorionic gonadotrophin and then pituitary gonadotrophins. This causes mesonephric (Wolffian) duct differentiation to become the seminal vesicles, vasa deferentia and the body and tail of the epididymis. Testosterone, in the presence of intracellular 5a-reductase, is converted into dihydrotestosterone in the genital sinus and accounts for external virilization of the penis and scrotum. The Sertoli cells produce a glycoprotein, Müllerian inhibitory factor, which causes

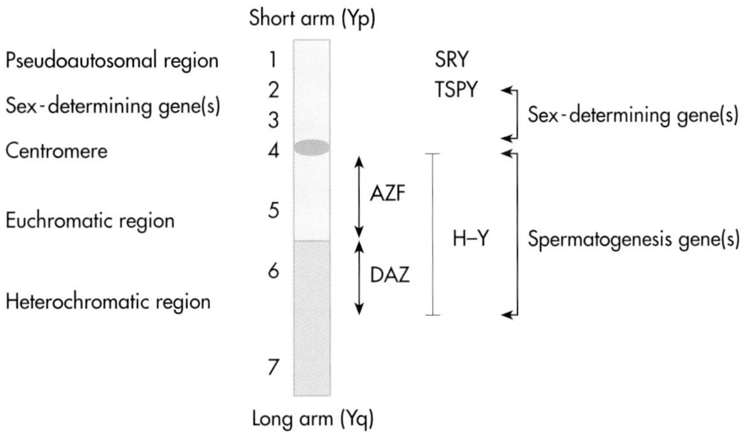

Figure 18.1 *The Y chromosome is critical for normal male sexual determination.*

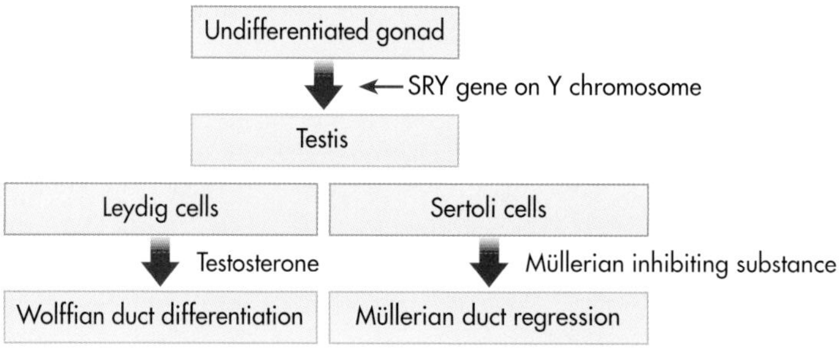

Figure 18.2 *Male genital development in the fetus.*

regression of the paramesonephric (Müllerian) ducts and also stimulates the first phase of testicular descent. Müllerian inhibiting factor may now be measured and has clinical implications. The second stage is androgen dependent, and additional roles are played by the genitofemoral nerve and calcitonin-related peptide. An understanding of these factors helps to explain abnormalities of gender and testicular maldescent. Testosterone is the most important circulating androgen in man and is bound to sex hormone-binding globulin and albumin. The latter binds to all steroids with low affinity, whereas the former is a glycoprotein, synthesized in the liver, and with a high affinity but low capacity for testosterone. In man, 60% of the circulating testosterone is bound to sex hormone-binding globulin, 38% is bound to albumin and the remaining 2% is free. Free and albumin-bound testosterone constitute the bioavailable functions of circulating testosterone, but some sex hormone-binding globulin-bound testosterone may be found in the prostate and testes.

The biosynthesis of testosterone (Figure 18.3) takes place in the Leydig cells. Steroidogenesis is stimulated through a cyclic adenosine monophosphate (cAMP)/protein kinase C-dependent mechanism, which mobilizes cholesterol substrate and promotes the conversion of cholesterol through pregnanilone, dihydroepiandrosterone, androstenedione to testosterone. Testosterone is converted to dihydrotestosterone by 5α-reductase within the target organ. Enzyme defects may lead to intersex states.

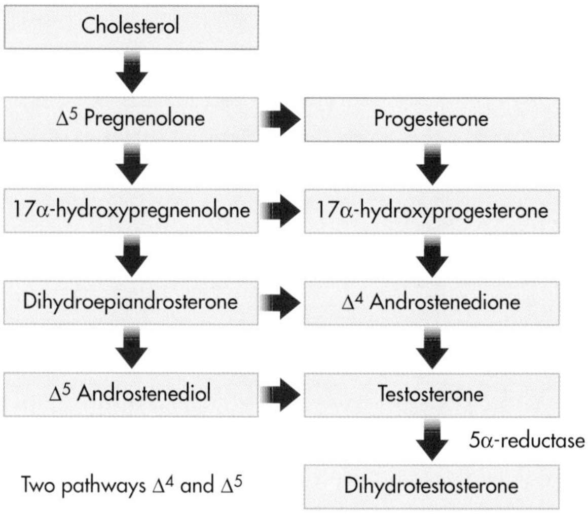

Figure 18.3 *The metabolic pathway for androgen production.*

HYPOTHALAMIC-PITUITARY-TESTICULAR AXIS

Anterior pituitary gonadotrophin secretion is controlled by hypothalamic gonadotrophin-releasing hormone (GnRH) released into the pituitary portal circulation by axon terminals in the median eminence of the hypothalamus. These neurosecretory neurons are responsive to a wide variety of sensory inputs as well as to gonadal negative feedback. GnRH stimulates both luteinizing hormone and follicle-stimulating hormone secretion from the anterior pituitary gland. These hormones are glycoproteins of 115 amino acids and have a molecular mass of about 30 000 daltons. They are produced by the gonadotrophic cells of the adenohypophysis and differ only in the structure of their beta-subunit. The GnRH precursor gene has been identified and mapped to chromosome 8p. In the adult male, GnRH (a decapeptide), is released episodically into the pituitary portal circulation every 90–140 minutes; each volley of GnRH elicits an immediate release of luteinizing hormone, producing the typical pulsatile pattern of luteinizing hormone in the systemic circulation. Though also secreted episodically, follicle-stimulating hormone and testosterone pulses are not apparent in normal men because of the slower secretion of newly synthesized rather than stored hormone, and the longer circulating half-lives. The intermittent mode of GnRH stimulation within a narrow physiological range of frequency is obligatory for sustaining the normal pattern of gonadotrophin secretion. Continuous or high-frequency GnRH stimulation paradoxically desensitizes the pituitary gonadotrophin response because of the depletion of receptors and the refractoriness of post-receptor response mechanisms.

Testosterone exerts the major negative feedback action on gonadotrophin secretion. Its effect is predominantly to restrict the frequency of GnRH pulses from the hypothalamus to within the physiological range. Testosterone also acts on the pituitary to reduce the amplitude of luteinizing hormone response to GnRH; this may require the local conversion of testosterone to oestradiol in the pituitary. These inhibitory actions are best seen in agonadal or castrated males, in whom high-frequency and high-amplitude luteinizing hormone pulsatile secretion prevails. Feedback inhibition of pituitary follicle-stimulating hormone synthesis is also affected by testosterone, particularly at high concentrations, as well as the glycoprotein Sertoli cell product inhibin. Inhibin exists in two forms that have a common alpha-subunit but distinct beta-subunits. Low levels of inhibin B may indicate absence of spermatogenesis.

Testosterone levels vary throughout life. There is a relatively high level in late fetal life, which falls to a very low level throughout childhood. Puberty is associated with a surge in testosterone production that remains high until late adult life. The fall in testosterone levels after the age of 55 is not sudden, but the mean plasma testosterone level in healthy men falls by about 0.17 nmol/annum.

THE ACTION OF ANDROGENS

Androgens are essential for normal male sexual differentiation and function, and a deficiency results in a failure of sexual development, delayed or absent puberty, and other clinical syndromes (Table 18.1). In men, there is no sudden fall in androgen secretion to cause a male menopause. The decline in testosterone levels may be associated with partial androgen deficiency in the ageing man, but the mental changes occurring in the mid-fifties are likely to be the result of social stresses rather than of hormonal deficiency. Declining androgen levels appear to be more important with regard to the onset of osteoporosis than to erectile dysfunction (ED). Androgen replacement may be done with testosterone patches applied to the skin daily; oral medication, a 2-weekly to 3-weekly injection of testosterone esters (Sustanon); or the implantation of a testosterone pellet (6-monthly).

THE PHYSIOLOGY AND PHARMACOLOGY OF PENILE ERECTION

Penile erection is a complex neurovascular process, which is dependent upon the relaxation of the cavernous smooth muscle. This requires integration

Table 18.1 Testosterone deficiency.

Primary (hypergonadotrophic hypogonadism)
Congenital testicular agenesis
Klinefelter's syndrome
Sterogenic enzyme defects
Testicular maldescent
Acquired
Bilateral orchidectomy
Bilateral torsion testis
Bilateral orchitis
Radiotherapy/chemotherapy
Secondary (hypogonadotrophic hypogonadism)
Congenital
Idiopathic (e.g. Kallmann's syndrome)
Fertile eunuch
Acquired
Pituitary lesions:
trauma
surgery
tumour (N.B.: hyperprolactinaemia)
haemochromatosis

of both somatic and autonomic peripheral neural pathways, as well as central coordination of these pathways in the brain.

Recently, there have been rapid advances in our knowledge and understanding of the physiology and molecular biology of this process. This has led to the emergence of novel pharmacotherapies for the treatment of male erectile dysfunction.

Functional anatomy of the penis

The human penis should be considered as a vascular organ; as such, it shares many common physiological properties with other vascular smooth muscles. The penis consists of a pair of corpora cavernosa and a ventrally placed corpus spongiosum (Figure 18.4). The cavernosal bodies are invested by the tunica albuginea, which is fused to form a midline septum. The corpus spongiosum is ventral to the corpus cavernosa and surrounds the urethra. Distally, the corpus spongiosum expands to form the glans penis.

In essence, each corpus cavernosum consists of a meshwork of vascular smooth muscle, which surrounds a complex series of spaces called the sinusoids (Figure 18.5). The sinusoidal spaces are themselves lined by an endothelium, which plays an important functional role in regulating corporal smooth muscle tone. Each sinusoidal space is supplied by a helicine artery, which is derived from the cavernosal artery. The cavernosal artery is a branch of the common penile artery, which is a branch of the internal pudendal artery (Figure 18.6).

During penile erection, both the smooth muscle of the arterioles supplying the sinusoidal spaces and the trabecular muscle relax, resulting in an increase in blood flow into the cavernous bodies. Arteriolar and cavernosal smooth muscle relaxation leads to engorgement of the sinusoidal spaces with blood, leading to compression of a series of subtunical veins. During penile erection, these veins become compressed, with the result that there is a reduction in venous return and the penis becomes erect. This process is known as the veno-occlusive mechanism (Figure 18.7).

Haemodynamic phases of erection

During erection, the penis enlarges and becomes hard. The vascular changes that occur have been divided into five different phases (Figure 18.8).

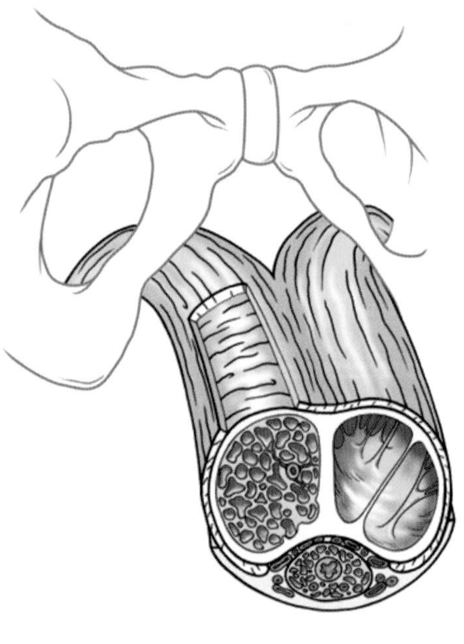

Figure 18.4 *The structure of the penis.*

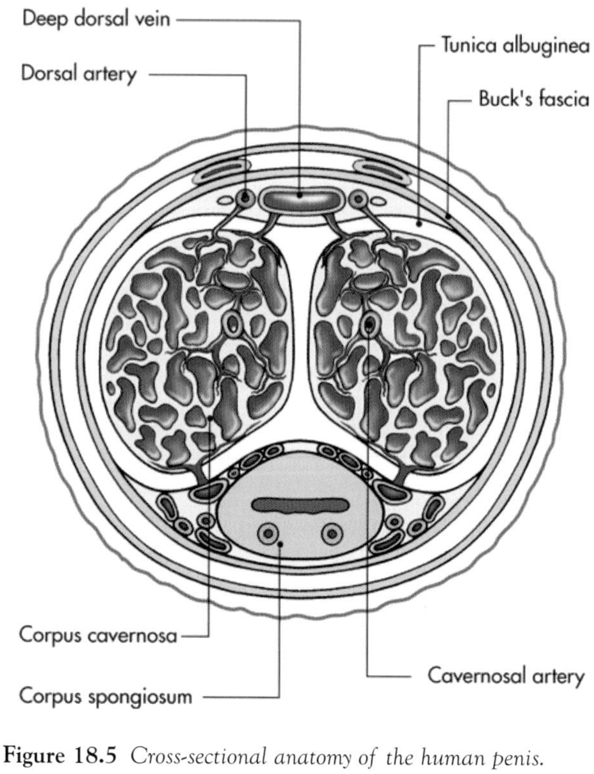

Figure 18.5 *Cross-sectional anatomy of the human penis.*

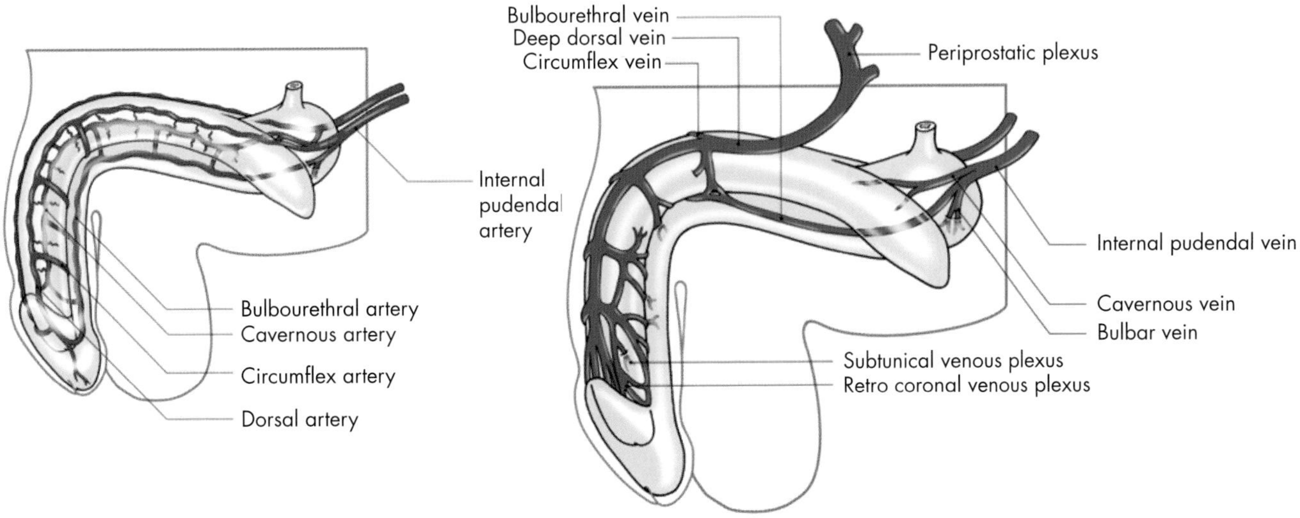

Figure 18.6 *Arterial supply and venous drainage of the human penis.*

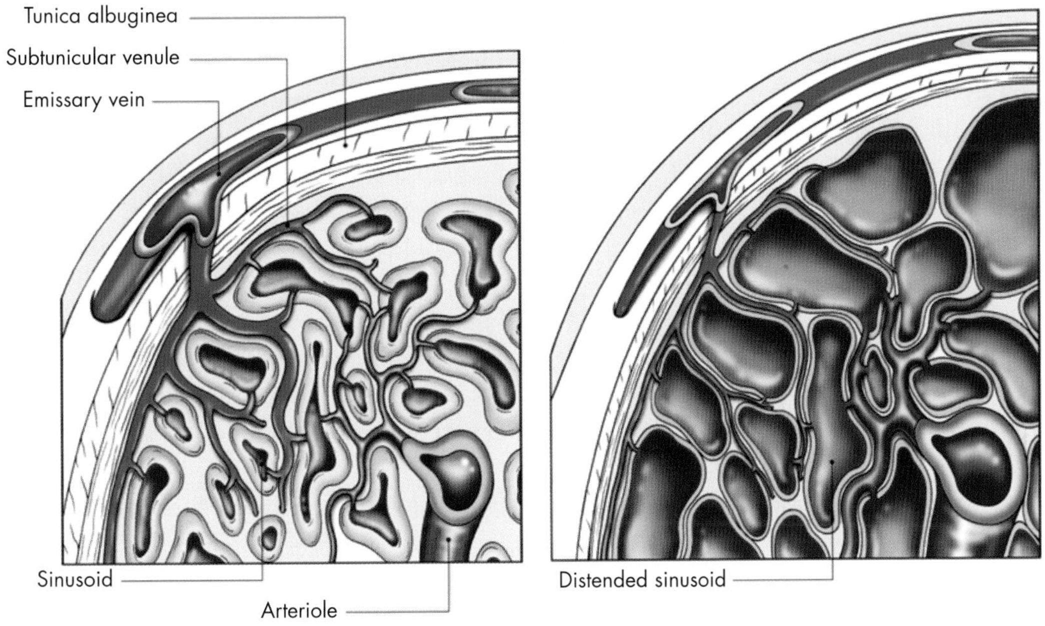

Figure 18.7 *Veno-occlusive mechanism. During sexual stimulation, the smooth muscle surrounding the sinusoidal spaces relaxes leading to engorgement of the spaces with blood. This leads to compression of subtunical venules and emissary veins, causing penile erection.*

Latent phase

The start of an erection is preceded by relaxation of arterial and cavernous smooth muscle. This leads to a fall in vascular resistance, with a resulting rapid inflow of blood into the cavernous spaces. For a short period, there is no increase, or even a slight fall, in the intracorporeal pressure. This period of isometric filling of the sinusoidal spaces is associated with the highest flow rate of the whole erectile process and may be more than double the resting value. During this phase, there is only slight elongation and fullness of the penis.

Tumescence phase

As the inflow of blood continues, it becomes associated with increasing cavernous pressure. When the intracavernous pressure rises above diastolic pressure, flow occurs only during systole. This phase is

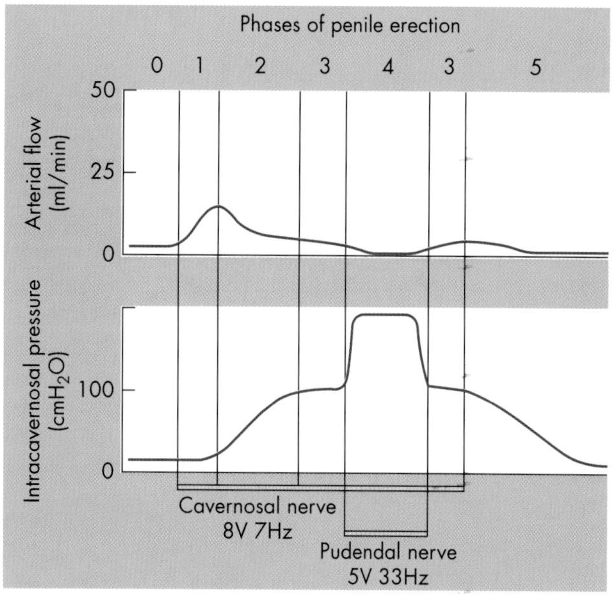

Figure 18.8 *The haemodynamic phases of penile erection.*

characterized by rapid expansion and elongation of the penis to its full size. The duration of this phase is age dependent and is influenced by the strength of stimulation.

Full-erection phase

The continued inflow of blood and the distension of the sinusoidal spaces compress the subtunical venous plexus against the non-compliant tunica albuginea. This impedes the outflow of blood through the emissary veins, and the intracavernous pressure rises further. The stage of full erection is reached when the intracorporeal pressure equals mean systolic pressure. The pressure remains steady during this phase, indicating that the rate of arterial inflow is lower than during the tumescence phase and equals the venous outflow.

Rigid-erection phase

Penile rigidity is achieved by contraction of the ischiocavernosus muscles, and this raises the intracavernous pressure to well above systolic blood pressure. There is no flow in the cavernosal artery at this stage, and, at the same time, there is further obstruction of the venous channels and flow in them also approaches zero. Consequently, for a short period of a few minutes, the corpora cavernosa become functionally dead spaces with hardly any inflow or outflow. This phase occurs naturally during sexual intercourse or masturbation, and its duration is limited by muscle fatigue, an effect which obviates the risk of tissue ischaemia.

Detumescence phase

This commences with the relaxation of the ischiocavernosus muscles, but detumescence is also an active process due to the contraction of the cavernosal smooth muscle under sympathetic nervous stimulation. This contraction expels blood from the sinusoidal spaces, and it is accompanied by arterial vasoconstriction to reduce the inflow to the resting level. The penis becomes smaller and shorter and eventually flaccid.

The changes described above all take place in the corpora cavernosa, but similar changes take place in the corpus spongiosum, including the glans penis. However, the pressure rise is not so great, as there is no limiting investing layer of tunica albuginea. Furthermore, the venous outflow into the deep dorsal vein is unimpeded. There is some compression of the deep dorsal vein between the overlying stretched skin and the expanded corpora during full erection. This raises pressure in the glans and increases its engorgement and fullness. There is a further increase in venous resistance with contraction of the ischiocavernosus and bulbocavernosus muscles during the rigid phase of erection.

Neurological control of erection

Central control of penile erection

The central pathways for controlling penile erection are complex and not completely understood. Much of our knowledge of these pathways is derived from experimental animal models, particularly the rat. The main coordinating centre for erectile activity appears to be the medial pre-optic area, which is contiguous with the hypothalamus. There is strong evidence to support the involvement of regions within the hypothalamus, and activation of dopamine receptors in animals is associated with the induction of penile erection. Central dopaminergic neurons have been found in the hypothalamus with projections to the medial pre-optic area (MPOA) and paraventricular nucleus (PVN). Further pathways are found projecting from the caudal hypothalamus to the lumbosacral spinal cord. When the dopamine receptor agonist apomorphine is administered systemically in male rats it can induce penile erection. The major families of dopamine receptors, D1-like (D1 and D5) and D2-like (D2, D3 and D4), have been implicated in the erectile process, although the D2 receptor appears to predominate functionally. Interestingly, injection of apomorphine into the PVN of rats can also induce seminal emission.

In contrast to the peripheral neural pathways, central noradrenergic neurons appear to facilitate penile erection. Central alpha-2 receptors appear to exist in the MPOA, which may suppress sexual activity. Interestingly, antagonists of these receptors appear to reverse these effects.

The importance of oxytocin neurons in penile erection is unclear, although oxytocinergic neurons derived from the PVN project to the spinal autonomic nuclei. Stimulation of these neurons may provoke erections. Table 18.2 summarizes the effects of other centrally acting agents on penile erection.

Peripheral neural pathways

The penis is innervated by the autonomic nervous system, which consists of cholinergic (parasympathetic) and adrenergic (sympathetic) nervous systems. The parasympathetic and sympathetic pathways are intimately involved in the process of penile erection (Figure 18.9). The penis also receives a somatic innervation via the pudendal nerves.

Table 18.2 Central neurotransmitters involved in penile erection.

Neurotransmitter	Action on erectile pathways
Dopamine	Excitatory
5 Hydroxytryptamine	Mainly inhibitory
Noradrenaline (norepinephrine)	Excitatory
GABA	Inhibitory
Oxytocin	Excitatory
Nitric oxide	Excitatory

Sympathetic pathways

Noradrenergic fibres originate from pre-ganglionic cell bodies within the intermediolateral grey matter of the spinal cord between the levels of T10 and L2. These then pass to the paravertebral chain and hypogastric plexi, from where post-ganglionic fibres pass to the pelvic, cavernous and pudendal nerves to reach the penis. Sympathetic stimulation leads to the release of noradrenaline (norepinephrine) from post-ganglionic nerve terminals, resulting in smooth muscle contraction, via alpha-adrenoreceptor stimulation.

Parasympathetic pathways

Parasympathetic nerve fibres originate from the intermediolateral grey matter of the spinal cord segments S2 to S4 and pass to the pelvic plexus via the nervi erigentes. The cavernous nerves arise here and carry the autonomic nerve supply to the penis. Parasympathetic stimulation leads to arterial dilatation and penile smooth muscle relaxation.

Sensory pathways

Afferent impulses from the genitalia pass via the dorsal penile nerves through the pudendal nerves to the dorsal roots of S2, S3 and S4 of the spinal cord. The pudendal nerve has its cell bodies located in Onuf's nucleus, which lies within the spinal cord segments, S2–S4.

It has been customary to differentiate between reflexogenic erections (arising from genital sensation)

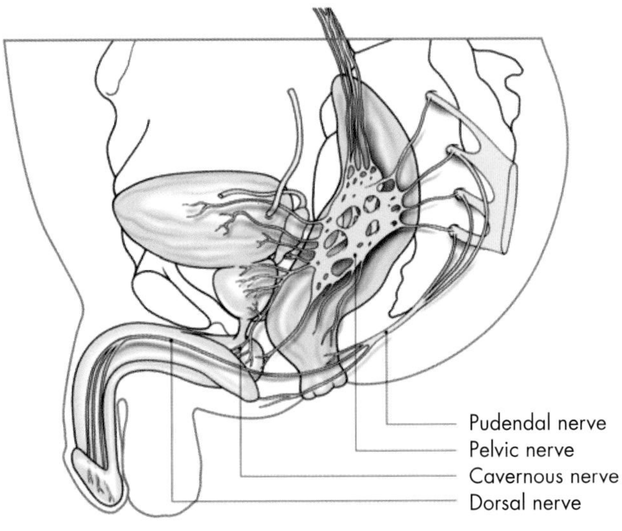

Figure 18.9 *The autonomic and somatic innervation of the penis.*

and psychogenic erections but such a division serves little purpose. It does, however, serve to emphasize that after spinal cord injuries higher than T9, erections are the result of a local reflex arc, and that with lower lesions, erections may occur as a result of efferent impulses through the thoracic sympathetic outflows.

Neurotransmitters involved in penile erection and intracellular pathways (Figure 18.10)

Noradrenaline (norepinephrine)

It is now clear that the main excitatory or antierectile neurotransmitter involved in penile erection is noradrenaline (norepinephrine), while other peptides such as neuropeptide Y may also play a modulatory role. Noradrenaline (norepinephrine) appears to act on both alpha-1 and -2 adrenoreceptors in corporeal tissue, although the alpha-1 subtype appears to be functionally the most important for smooth muscle contraction. The alpha-1 adrenoreceptors have been further typed and it appears that alpha-1A, -1B and -1D are the predominant types present within human corporeal tissue. Beta-adrenoreceptors have also been identified within penile erectile tissue, but they appear to be less abundant than alpha-receptors, and their functional significance is largely unknown, although stimulation of beta-receptors appears to cause relaxation of corporeal smooth muscle.

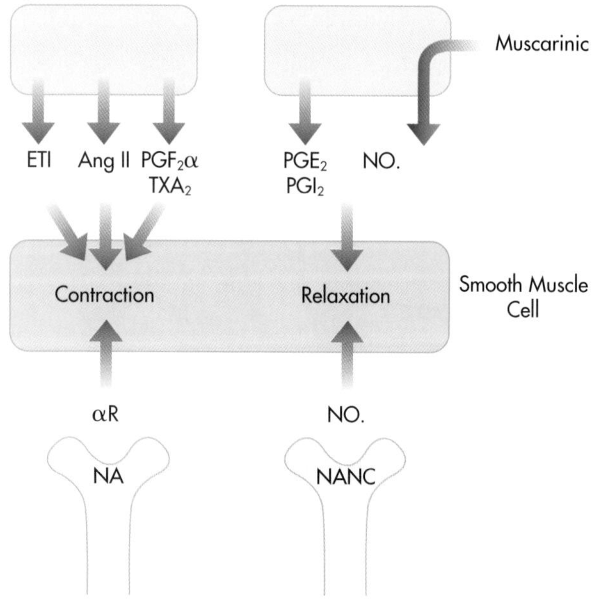

Figure 18.10 *Diagram depicting the functional anatomy of the corpus cavernosum and the main vaso-active factors involved in penile erection.*

Stimulation of alpha-1 receptors by noradrenaline (norepinephrine) leads to activation of phospholipase C. This results in production of the intracellular second messengers inositol triphosphate (IP_3) and diacylglycerol (DAG) from membrane-bound phophatidylinositol 4,5 biphosphate (PIP_2) (see Chapter 1). Both DAG and IP_3 lead to an increase in intracellular calcium levels. IP_3 acts mainly by liberating calcium ions from the endoplasmic reticulum, while DAG activates protein kinase C. Eventually, protein kinase C changes the permeability of membrane-bound calcium channels, resulting in an increase in intracellular calcium. The resultant increase in cytoplasmic calcium levels leads to smooth muscle contraction, through interaction of calcium with the calmodulin and myosin light-chain complex (see Chapter 1). This eventually leads to the actin and myosin cross-bridge formation, leading to corporeal as well as penile arteriolar smooth muscle contraction.

Rho kinase

As discussed above, NA acts on post-junctional alpha-1 adrenoceptors and causes contraction of corporeal smooth muscle. This contraction is dependent on an increase in intracellular calcium. However, activation of receptors coupled to G-proteins may cause contraction of corporeal smooth muscle by increasing Ca^{2+} sensitivity without an increase in intracellular calcium. This pathway is coupled to Rho-A, a small monomeric G protein that activates an enzyme called Rho-kinase. Activated Rho-kinase has the ability to phosphorylate the regulatory subunit of myosin phosphatase, leading to smooth muscle contraction. Rho-kinase inhibitors have been shown to cause corporeal smooth muscle relaxation in vitro and may represent a potential therapeutic target.

Acetylcholine (ACh)

The presence of cholinergic nerve fibres within the penis has been well documented. Muscarinic receptors are localized on corporeal smooth muscle and the endothelium lining the cavernous spaces within the penis. In fact, there are different subtypes of M receptor expressed in human corpus cavernosum (M1–M4), with a predominance of the M3 subtype on the endothelium, while the M2 receptor is mainly found on the corporeal smooth muscle cell. Muscarinic receptor stimulation by acetylcholine (ACh) (termed 'endothelium-dependent relaxation') appears to release nitric oxide (NO) from the endothelium of most vascular tissues, including the corpus cavernosum. However, it is not entirely clear whether NO is released by direct neural stimulation of M receptors or by sheer forces resulting from an increase in blood flow at the start of erection on the endothelium. NO is rapidly diffusible, leading to cGMP formation and eventually corporeal smooth muscle relaxation.

It is important to note that NO is not the only vasoactive factor released by the endothelium in response to ACh, but other factors, including prostaglandins, appear to be produced simultaneously (see below).

Nitric oxide (NO)

NO is the most important non-adrenergic non-cholinergic (NANC) neurotransmitter within the penis. It has been suggested that NO produced from NANC nerves may represent the most important source of NO in the penis. As mentioned, NO is also formed in the endothelial cells surrounding the sinusoidal spaces.

NO is produced from the conversion of the amino acid L-arginine to L-citrulline by the enzyme, nitric oxide synthase (NOS). This chemical reaction also requires NADPH as a co-factor (Figure 18.11). The presence of NOS can be demonstrated on the endothelium and smooth muscle, and within nerve fibres of the cavernosal bodies. Thus, three isoforms of NOS exist, including neuronal (nNOS), endothelial (eNOS) and inducible (iNOS) forms.

NO causes relaxation of corporeal smooth muscle via the production of cyclic GMP, its active intracellular second messenger. NO diffuses across the smooth muscle cell and binds with intracellular, soluble guanylate cyclase. This enzyme converts GTP into cGMP (Figure 18.12). The mechanism by which cGMP results in smooth muscle relaxation is not completely understood (see below). However, a reduction in intracellular calcium levels appears to be paramount to this. A fall in intracellular Ca^{2+} levels suppresses the activity of myosin light-chain (MLC) kinase and increases the intracellular content of dephosphorylated MLC, enabling the corporeal smooth muscle cell to relax.

The activity of cGMP is terminated by its conversion to GMP, which is catalysed by enzymes called phosphodiesterases (PDEs). A number of PDE isoenzymes have now been identified within mammalian tissues, although, functionally the type 5 isoenzyme appears to be the most important in the human penis (Table 18.3). Sildenafil (Viagra) increases the levels of cGMP by selectively inhibiting PDE 5 in the penis.

Other neurotransmitters

NO is by far the most important NANC neurotransmitter involved in the erectile process, although a number of other NANC neurotransmitters may induce corporeal smooth muscle relaxation, including vasoactive intestinal polypeptide (VIP).

Endothelium-derived factors

As with other vascular tissues, the endothelium of the penis has an important functional role in the regulation of corporeal smooth muscle tone. A variety

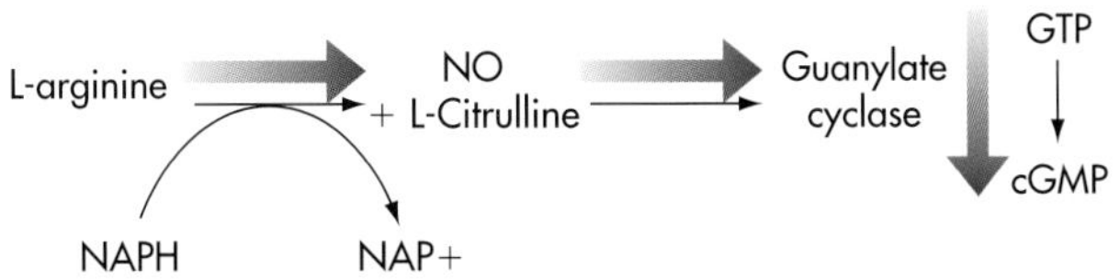

Figure 18.11 *Biosynthesis of prostanoids.*

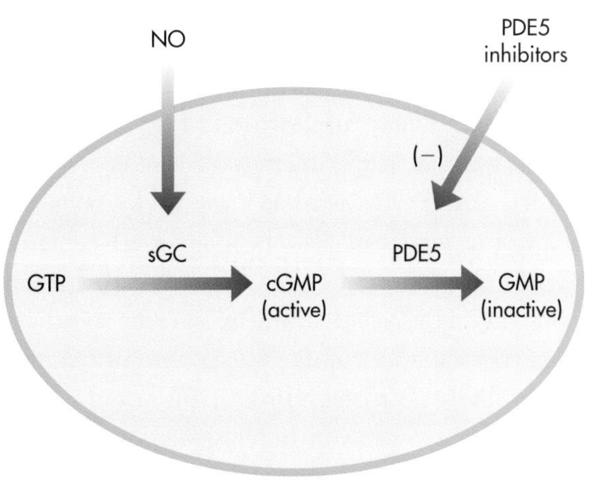

Figure 18.12 *The cellular action of NO incorporal smooth muscle (sGC-soluble guanylate cyclase).*

Table 18.3 Pharmacology and localization of phosphodiesterases. (Reproduced with permission from Brock et al 2002).

Isoenzyme	Substrate	Tissue
PDE 1	cGMP/cAMP	Brain, heart, vascular smooth muscle
PDE 2	cAMP/cGMP	Brain, heart, vascular smooth muscle, skeletal muscle, adrenal cortex
PDE 3	cAMP/cGMP	Smooth muscle, platelets, liver
PDE 4	cAMP	Brain, heart, vascular smooth muscle, skeletal muscle, adrenal cortex, lung, mast cells, thyroid, testis
PDE 5	cGMP	Vascular smooth muscle, platelets
PDE 6	cGMP	Retina
PDE 7	cAMP	Skeletal muscle, heart
PDE 8	cAMP	Testis, ovary, intestinal tract
PDE 9	cGMP	Spleen, intestinal tract
PDE 10	cAMP/cGMP	Brain, testis, thyroid
PDE 11	cAMP/cGMP	Vascular smooth muscle, brain, heart

of endothelium-derived relaxing and contracting factors are produced, including prostaglandins (PGs), endothelins and angiotensins. Both endothelins and angiotensins appear to cause contraction of penile smooth muscle.

Endothelins are produced from vascular endothelium, including the endothelium of the corporeal sinusoids. Endothelin (ET) 1 appears to cause potent corporeal smooth muscle contraction, probably via activation of ETA receptors. This appears to be associated with an increase in intracellular calcium via both IP_3- and DAG-mediated pathways. Endothelins, such as ET2 and ET3 also appear to cause corporeal smooth muscle contraction.

The actions of PGs within the penis are complex and not completely understood. PGs are derived from arachidonic acid. Arachidonic acid is converted to PGH_2 by PGH synthase or cyclo-oxygenase. Arachidonic acid can also be converted to leukotrienes by the action of other enzymes called lipoxygenases. PGH_2 is acted upon by specific synthases, leading to formation of $PGF_{2\text{-alpha}}$, thromboxane A_2 (TXA_2), PGI_2 (prostacyclin), PGE_2 and PGD_2. Prostanoid receptors can be classified according to functional and binding characteristics. For example, PGD_2 acts mainly on the DP receptor, while PGE_2, $PGF_{2\text{-alpha}}$ and TXA_2 act via their respective receptors, namely, EP, FP and TP. These receptors can be further subclassified (Table 18.4). However, the pharmacological effects of PGs appear to be less clear, with some such as PGE_1 causing relaxation, while others, including $PGF_{2\text{-alpha}}$ and TXA_2, mainly producing contraction of corporeal smooth muscle.

PGE_1 stimulates an EP2/EP4 receptor, which is linked to its own G protein. This leads to activation of an enzyme called adenylate cyclase, which con-

Table 18.4 The major prostaglandin receptors and their intra cellular second messengers. Note that the data is derived from a number of animal species and tissues.

Receptor	intracellular second messenger response
DP	↑ cAMP
EP	
EP_1	↑Ca
EP_2	↑ cAMP
EP_3	↑ or ↓cAMP
EP_4	↑ cAMP
FP	PI response
IP	cAMP and PI response
TP	
TP α	PI and ↓cAMP
TP β	PI and ↑cAMP

verts ATP into cAMP. Cyclic AMP is also metabolized to 5-AMP by specific PDEs. The differing effects of PGs on vascular smooth muscle, including the penis appear to depend upon activation of diverse populations of PG receptors. Table 18.4 summarizes the pharmacological effects of PGs on smooth muscles within mammalian tissues.

Human corpus cavernosum has the ability to produce significant amounts of angiotensin. Angiotensin II has been shown to contract corpus cavernosum in vitro and may play a role in detumescence of the penis. This effect may be mediated by the Angiotensin (Ang) II receptor subtype AT1.

Ion channels

Many of the neurotransmitters mentioned so far are able to modulate smooth muscle tone by causing changes in intracellular second messengers. In turn, these intracellular second messengers change the conductivity of membrane-bound ion channels. Ion channels are important for the maintenance of electrical gradients in a variety of smooth muscle cell types. The predominant types of ion channel present within corporeal smooth muscle are the potassium and calcium types. In fact, there are four types of K channels including calcium-sensitive maxi-K channel, the ATP or metabolically regulated K channel, the delayed rectifier K channel and an A type calcium-current channel.

Due to existing transmembrane electrochemical gradients, the opening of K channels leads to efflux of K ions flowing intracellularly to extracellularly. This results in hyperpolarization of the cell membrane and reduces the open probability of the voltage-dependent or L-type calcium channel; thus, the corporeal smooth muscle cell remains in a relaxed state. Conversely, opening of the L-type calcium channel leads to influx of extracellular Ca ions, resulting in depolarization of the cell membrane and corporeal smooth muscle contraction.

Pathophysiology of erectile dysfunction (ED)

ED is defined as the inability to achieve and maintain a penile erection adequate for satisfactory sexual intercourse. Table 18.5 provides a classification of ED, while Tables 18.6–18.9 list the common causes of ED.

Table 18.5 A classification of erectile dysfunction.

Psychogenic	
Endocrine	Diseases of testis, pituitary, hypothalamus, adrenal and thyroid Diabetes mellitus
Vascular	Arteriogenic and venogenic
Neurogenic	Diseases of central and peripheral nervous system
Iatrogenic	Surgical and drug related
Local causes	Peyronie's disease, post-priapism
Miscellaneous	Chronic renal disease, cirrhosis

Table 18.6 Endocrine causes of erectile dysfunction.

Primary hypogonadism	Klinefelter's syndrome Bilateral orchidectomy Testicular maldescent Radiotherapy to testis Mumps orchitis Haemochromatosis
Secondary hypogonadism	Kalmann's syndrome Pituitary tumours Craniopharyngioma Skull fracture Tuberculosis
Hyperprolactinaemia	Prolactinoma Chronic renal impairment Drug-induced
Diabetes mellitus	
Hypothyroidism and thyrotoxicosis	

Table 18.7 Neurogenic causes of erectile dysfunction.

Disease of the central nervous system Spinal cord injury or compression Spina bifida Multiple sclerosis Tabes dorsalis Syringomyelia Transverse myelitis Multiple system atrophy
Disease of the peripheral nervous system Prolapsed lumbar disc Cauda equina lesions Pelvic fracture with damage to sacral nerves Peripheral neuropathy (such as secondary to alcohol or diabetes) Surgical damage to nervi erigentes

Table 18.8 Surgical causes of erectile dysfunction.

Surgery to the central nervous system
Surgery to the spinal cord
Surgery to the cauda equina
Aortofemoral surgery
Radical cystectomy
Radical prostatectomy
Anterior resection of the rectum
Abdominoperineal excision of the rectum
Radical pelvic radiotherapy for carcinoma prostate, bladder or rectum
Surgery for Peyronie's disease
Surgery for priapism
Transurethral prostatectomy

Table 18.9 Drugs which may cause erectile dysfunction.

Psychotropic drugs Benzodiazepines, butyrophenones
Antidepressants Tricyclics, monoamine oxidase inhibitors
Antihypertensives
Endocrine drugs Cyproterone acetate, LHRH analogues, oestrogens
Anticholinergic agents Atropine, propantheline
Others Cimetidine, digoxin, marijuana, alcohol

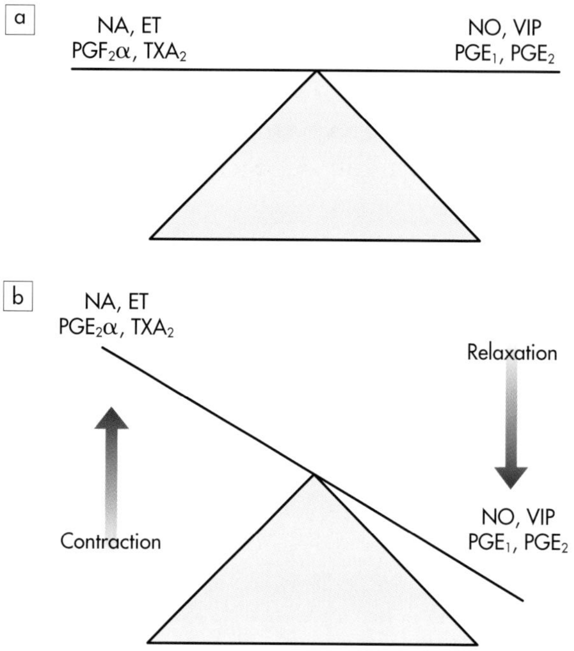

Figure 18.13 *Pathophysiological mechanism of erectile dysfunction. Under physiological conditions, corporeal smooth muscle is maintained by relaxatory factors acting in opposition to contractile factors. In disease states, the balance is tipped to favour contractile factors. This may be secondary to increased formation/uninhibited activity of these factors or secondary to reduced production/activity of relaxatory factors.*

It can be seen that under physiological conditions corporeal smooth muscle tone is maintained by contractile factors acting in opposition to relaxatory factors (Figure 18.13). In the past, there has been a vogue for performing both arterial and venous surgery to treat patients with ED. However, the results of this surgery were shown to be poor in the majority of patients. The reasons for this have become clear, and we now know that the smooth muscle of the corpora is dysfunctional in these patients. Two theories have been proposed to account for the smooth muscle dysfunction seen in patients with ED. The first is that there is heightened corporal smooth muscle tone or impaired smooth muscle relaxation in disease states (Figure 18.13b). The second theory proposes that smooth muscle dysfunction arises from smooth muscle damage secondary to the release of certain growth factors, free radicals species and other cytotoxic agents. It is likely that both theories account for the pathophysiological changes seen in men suffering from ED. We will now examine these factors in greater detail.

Psychogenic ED

In approximately 10–30% of men, there is a major psychogenic component to the aetiology of their ED. Anxiety, marital problems, performance anxiety, depression and a traumatic childhood, as well as previous sexual misadventures, have all been implicated as contributory factors. It has been postulated that overriding psychogenic factors inhibit erection by increasing sympathetic stimulation of the corporeal smooth muscle.

Ageing and ED

The prevalence of ED increases with age from 1.9% at 40 years to 25% at 65 years. After the age of 45 years, there is a gradual decline in the level of plasma-free (bioavailable) testosterone secondary to a rise in sex hormone-binding globulin. In addition to the hormonal factors outlined above, there appear to be age-related pathological changes within penile erectile tissue itself that lead to a reduction in autonomic nerve fibre density. In particular, there is a fall in the amount of NOS in the penises of ageing animals. Furthermore, functional age-dependent changes appear to occur in the human corpus cavernosum that are associated with augmented corporeal smooth muscle contractility in vitro.

It has also been shown in some animal models that androgens directly regulate the expression of NOS, castration resulting in a fall in NOS content within the penile erectile tissues of the rat. Overall, these findings suggest that NO formation may be reduced in the ageing male.

As the prevalence of atherosclerosis increases with age, so the incidence of impaired arterial inflow to the penis rises, and this will inevitably lead to an increased incidence of ED (see later).

Endocrine causes of ED

A number of hormonal disorders have been implicated as causes of ED (Table 18.6). Pituitary dysfunction can result in ED secondary to either hyperprolactinaemia or hypogonadism. While pituitary failure is most commonly due to acquired disease such as tumour, trauma or infection, a number of cases can be congenital in origin. Both hyperthyroidism and hypothyroidism can lead to ED although the mechanism whereby this occurs is unknown.

Diabetes mellitus

Diabetes mellitus requires a special mention as a cause of ED, as the prevalence of ED in diabetic men is high, with up to 35% of diabetics reporting some degree of ED. The pathophysiology of ED in diabetes is multifactorial, with neurological, vascular and endothelial factors all being important. The corporeal tissue of diabetics contains reduced autonomic nerve fibre, including a reduction in acetylcholinesterase and VIP within nerves. Furthermore, and perhaps more importantly, the penile erectile tissues of diabetic animals have reduced NOS expression. This peripheral neuropathy appears to be reflected in vitro, as indicated by the reduced NANC-mediated relaxations of diabetic penile erectile tissues in vitro. Diabetes mellitus also leads to impaired endothelial cell function, which in corporeal tissue is characterized by impaired relaxation to ACh in both human and rabbit diabetic corpus cavernosum in vitro. Thus, it can be seen in diabetes mellitus that there is a reduction in the availability and production of NO within the penis.

Diabetes also increases the production of vasoconstrictor prostanoids and free radicals, which may inactivate or inhibit the activity of NO. Furthermore, diabetes mellitus leads to the deposition of compounds called advanced glycation end products (AGEs). AGEs are formed as a result of a chemical reaction between glucose and tissue proteins and have the ability to inhibit the activity of NO, either directly or by inducing free radical formation. In accordance with these pathophysiological findings, it is interesting to note that antioxidants, high doses of L-arginine (the precursor of NO) and inhibitors of AGE formation can reverse the documented impaired nitrergic responses seen in diabetic penile smooth muscle.

Neurogenic causes of ED

Any disease process or trauma affecting the brain, spinal cord and cavernous nerves can cause ED (Table 18.7) by disruption of the normal neural pathways that control penile erection.

Arteriogenic impotence

Arterial disease can impair arterial inflow into the penis during erection. Thus, hypertension, smoking, hypercholesterolaemia and diabetes mellitus, all of which are implicated in the pathogenesis of atherosclerosis, can result in penile arterial insufficiency.

Atherosclerosis not only affects arteries but can also lead to functional and architectural changes within the corporeal smooth muscle. In a rabbit model of vasculogenic erectile dysfunction, impaired endothelium-dependent relaxation and heightened electrically induced smooth contractions have been documented. In an atherosclerotic rabbit model, NOS immunoreactivity was reduced, and levels of $PGF_{2\text{-alpha}}$ and TXA_2 were increased, suggesting that there is a defect in NO production and increased PG activity in this model of ED.

Hypercholesterolaemia has also been shown to lead to defective endothelium-dependent relaxation in rabbit corpus cavernosum in vitro.

$TGF\beta_1$ has been shown to increase collagen synthesis and thus reduce the quantity of functioning smooth muscle within penile erectile tissues. There appears to be an increase in collagen deposition, with associated fibrosis in the penises of rabbits injected with $TGF\beta_1$, which is similar to that seen in atherosclerotic animals. Therefore, collagen deposition induced by $TGF\beta_1$ may have a primary role in the aetiology of ED, by modulating the structural integrity of the smooth muscle of the penis. Interestingly, PGE_1 can suppress collagen-induced synthesis by $TGF\beta_1$ in human corpus cavernosum.

Iatrogenic causes of ED

Surgical causes of ED

Surgery can cause ED by damaging the nerves or arteries that are essential for normal erection (Table 18.8). The pathophysiology of ED following transurethral resection of the prostate is probably due to diathermy or mechanical injury of the cavernous nerves during surgery. Interestingly, in a rat model, bilateral cavernosal nerve damage induced apoptosis of erectile tissue in the penis of the rat. This may offer some explanation as to why patients develop ED after prostatic surgery.

Drugs and ED

The list of potential drugs that interfere with erectile function is long (Table 18.9). Hypnotics and major tranquillizers may exert their effect by elevating plasma prolactin as well as depressing libido. Drugs which lower or block the action of serum testosterone produce ED, and this group includes oestrogens, spironolactone, digoxin and antiandrogens such as cyproterone acetate. Most antihypertensives produce ED. Centrally acting antihypertensives, such as alpha-methyldopa and clonidine, are thought to exert their effect on erectile function by their central actions on alpha-receptors. Finally, propanolol and other beta-blockers are also associated with ED.

Alcohol has well-known acute effects in ED, but, in addition, chronic alcoholism can cause liver damage and peripheral neuropathy as well as lowering serum testosterone and increasing plasma oestrogen levels.

Other causes of ED

Priapism is often overlooked as a cause of ED. It is defined as a persistent painful erection and may be of a low- or high-flow picture (Table 18.10). There are a number of causes of low-flow priapism, the commonest being intracavernosal injection therapy and sickle-cell disease. A low-flow priapism lasting longer than 4 hours can lead to irreversible necrosis and fibrosis of corpus cavernosal tissue, although the exact time at which this occurs is still debatable. It has also been shown that both hypoxia and acidosis, in vitro, selectively reduce smooth muscle contractility to alpha-agonists, although nitrergic mediated responses appear to be largely unaffected. These findings indicate that there is not only significant ischaemic damage to the smooth muscle under ischaemic conditions, but also underlying smooth muscle dysfunction. The underlying mechanism for this may involve a reduction in transmembrane calcium influx within the corporeal cell during ischaemic conditions.

High-flow priapism is usually the result of trauma to the penis with subsequent development of a fistula, commonly between the cavernosal vessels and corpus cavernosum. However, high-flow priapism may also rarely occur in sickle-cell disease.

Peyronie's disease is another cause of ED, although the exact mechanism for ED in these patients is unclear. Plaque formation may interfere with arterial inflow, resulting in penile flaccidity distal to the plaque, but there may also be abnormalities of

Table 18.10 The biochemical features of low- (ischaemic) and high-flow priapism on blood gas analysis.

	Low flow	High flow (arterial)
Cause	Veno-occlusion	Arterio-lacunar fistula
Aetiology	Drugs, Haematologic (eg sickle cell disease)	Perineal trauma
pH	acidotic	normal
PO_2	low	normal
PCO_2	high	normal

the veno-occlusive mechanism that result in ED secondary to venous leakage. Several theories have been postulated to explain the pathophysiological changes seen in Peyronie's disease. The most widely accepted theory is that the disease process is initiated by tunical mechanical stress and microvascular trauma to the erect penis, which result in aberrant wound healing and fibrosis. Other theories propose that plaque formation is a manifestation of an autoimmune disease initiated by an infectious agent. A genetic predisposition may also occur, as Peyronie's disease is associated with other fibrotic conditions including Dupuytren's contracture and Ledeshore's disease, as well as certain HLA-B7 antigens.

There is increasing evidence for the role of $TGF\beta_1$ in the pathogenesis of Peyronie's disease. Increased expression of $TGF\beta_1$,$TGF\beta_2$ and $TGF\beta_3$ has been found in the plaques and tunica albuginea of patients with Peyronie's disease. It has been suggested that an inflammatory reaction following localized penile trauma may result in excessive generation of reactive oxygen species. Furthermore, $TGF\beta_1$ transcriptionally represses inducible NO synthase (iNOS) production. Both mechanisms would theoretically result in reduced NO production, and this forms the basis for the use of free radical scavengers and antioxidants in the treatment of Peyronie's disease.

Pharmacological treatment of ED

The pharmacological treatment of ED has been revolutionized in recent years, particularly with the introduction of PDE inhibitors. The pharmacotherapy for ED is based on the principles of stimulating central or peripheral proerectile pathways or inhibiting antierectile mechanisms. In particular, drugs enhancing peripheral nitrergic mediated pathways have been developed, and PDE inhibitors, such as Viagra, deserve a special mention (Table 18.11 classifies the drugs currently available for treating ED).

Table 18.11 Currently available pharmacological treatments for male erectile dysfunction.

Oral treatments	Mechanism of action
Sildenafil citrate (Viagra™)	PDE 5 inhibitor
Tadalafil (Cialis™)	PDE 5 inhibitor
Vardenafil hydrochloride	PDE 5 inhibitor
Apomorphine sublingual (Uprima™)	Dopamine agonist
Yohimbine	Alpha-adrenoceptor antagonist
Phentolamine (Vasomax™)	Alpha-adrenoceptor antagonist
Prazosin and Doxazosin	Alpha-adrenoceptor antagonist
L-Arginine	NO precursor
Intra-cavernosal agents	**Mechanism of action**
PGE1 (Alprostadil)	Increase in intracellular cAMP
Papaverine	Non selective PDE inhibitor
Vasoactive intestinal polypeptide	Increase in intracellular cAMP
Linsidomine Chlorhydrate	NO donor
Phentolamine	Alpha adrenoceptor antagonist
Topical agents used for the treatment of MED	**Mechanism of action**
Transdermal nitroglycerin	NO donor
Intra-urethral PGE1 (MUSE)	Increase in intracellular cAMP
Topical PGE1	Increase in intracellular cAMP

PDE-inhibitors

Drugs such as Sildenafil and the novel PDE 5 inhibitors Vardenafil and Tadalafil are referred to as competitive inhibitors of PDE 5, as such, they have a similar chemical structure to cGMP. As mentioned before, PDE inhibitors inhibit the breakdown of cGMP to 5-GMP, leading to an increase in corporeal smooth muscle relaxation.

Pharmacological concepts of potency and selectivity of a drug

An ideal drug for the treatment of a medical condition should be potent and have a high selectivity towards its target tissue. In pharmacological terminology, drug potency is defined as the concentration of a drug required to inhibit an enzyme or receptor in vitro. Potency under these conditions is expressed as the IC_{50} of the drug; that is, the concentration of the drug in vitro required to inhibit 50% of a measured response, such as enzyme activity. Thus, in the case of PDE 5 inhibitors, the lower the IC_{50} value, the more potent the drug is in vitro. This is purely a pharmacological concept meaning that less of the drug is required to produce a desired effect in vitro. In other words, the lower IC_{50} value of a PDE inhibitor, the more potent, theoretically, the drug is. However, a low IC_{50} does not always indicate that a drug is more potent and thus has greater efficacy. The efficacy of a drug is a measure of its clinical or in vivo effects and therefore does depend simply on the potency of the drug in vitro, but also on its pharmacokinetic profile, that is, its absorption, distribution and metabolism within the body (Table 18.12).

The selectivity of a drug is its relative activity between different receptor types or isoenzymes. For competitive antagonists such as the PDE inhibitors, selectivity can be expressed by the ratio of IC_{50} values for each PDE isoenzyme. Selectivity is the main factor determining the side-effect profile of a drug (Table 18.13).

PDE inhibitors used for MED should have a high selectivity for PDE 5, thereby minimizing their side effects on other PDEs present in the body. The side effects of PDE 5 inhibitors are related to their effects on other PDEs around the body. This accounts for the commonly observed adverse events ascribed to these drugs, including headache, facial flushing and dyspepsia.

Table 18.12 Pharmacokinetic profiles of available PDE 5 inhibitors.

	Cmax (ng/ml)	Tmax (h)	t½(h)
Sildenafil	560	0.8	3.7
Vardenafil	209	0.7	3.9
Tadalafil	378	2.0	17.5

FERTILITY

Male fertility depends upon the satisfactory integration of a series of physiological events, starting with sperm production and ending with fertilization of the oocytes (Table 18.14). This process may be interrupted voluntarily by pathological changes or by adverse factors in the female partner. The essence of fertility management is to establish a prognosis, or the chance of the partner's conceiving in a given period of time, and to offer treatment that will increase the chances of conception. To do this, it is necessary to have a sound understanding of the pathophysiology of infertility.

During childhood, the testes are small, and the seminiferous tubules are solid, cord-like structures containing primitive spermatocytes and Sertoli cells. The seminiferous tubules gradually acquire a lumen as

Table 18.13 Properties of the PDE 5 inhibitors. IC_{50} is the concentration of drug required to achieve 50% inhibition of enzyme; the lower the value, theoretically, the more efficacious the drug. The selectivity ratio is represented for PDE 5 over the other PDE isoenzymes; the higher the value, the more specific the drug is for PDE 5 over the other isoenzymes.

	Sildenafil	Tadalafil	Vardenafil
Time to onset	60 min	45 min	25–40 min
Duration of action	4–8 hours	24–36 hours	Not known
IC_{50} PDE 5 (nM)	3.5	0.9	0.7
Selectivity ratio			
PDE 1	80	>10 000	257
PDE 2	1000	>10 000	>10 000
PDE 3	1000	>10 000	>10 000
PDE 4	>10 000	>10 000	>10 000
PDE 5	1	1	1
PDE 6	10	780	16

Table 18.14 Sequence of events leading to fertilisation.

Event	Test (assay)	
Spermatogenesis	Testis biopsy	Semen analysis
Acquisition of mortility	Semen analysis	CASA
Migration through female tract	Penetration tests	
Capacitation Hyperactive motility Membrane integrity	 CASA HSA	 HOPT
Zona pellucida binding	HZA	
Acrosome reaction	HZA	HOPT
Zona pellucida penetration	HZA	HOPT
Sperm head decondensation		HOPT
Fusion with oocyte DNA		

CASA, computer analysis of sperm number and quality test; HOPT, heterologous oocyte penetration test; HSA, hypo-osmotic swelling assay; HZA, hemizoma assay.

the spermatocytes differentiate after the age of 6 years. Testicular and penile sizes increase greatly at puberty, driven by hormonal changes, with an increase in plasma levels of both luteinizing hormone and follicle-stimulating hormone. The hormonal control of the testes has already been mentioned in the control of testosterone secretion. Testosterone is essential for spermatogenesis, but the control of spermatogenesis is by follicle-stimulating hormone, which acts through the Sertoli cells to stimulate the germ cells to manufacture sperm. Inhibin is a glycoprotein produced by the Sertoli cells once spermatogenesis proceeds to the spermatocyte stage and is the feedback mechanism to regulate follicle-stimulating hormone production.

Spermatogenesis is a complex process of cellular changes, which are divided into three groups. The spermatogenic cycle in the testis is about 16 days in duration, but the total time from the commencement of spermatogenesis to the expulsion of spermatozoa in the semen is approximately 72 days. In the first phase of spermatogenesis, the spermatogonia undergo cell division to produce type A spermatogonia, which, in turn, produce intermediate and then type B spermatogonia. Recognition of these spermatogonia is difficult with ordinary light microscopy. In the second phase of spermatogenesis, the spermatogonia divide to produce spermatocytes, which undergo division with halving of the number of chromosomes. The secondary spermatocytes divide in the final stage of spermatogenesis to produce spermatids and then spermatozoa. During spermiogenesis (the third stage), the rounded spermatocytes become elongated and recognizable as sperm, with an acrosomal cap, a midpiece and a tail. The Sertoli, or supporting, cells serve to capture hormones that nourish the germ cells. Sertoli cells rest on the basement membrane of the seminiferous tubules and have multiple cytoplasmic extensions into the lumen of the tubules between the germinal cells. The contents of the seminiferous tubules are outside the body, and special tight cell junctions exist adjacent to the Sertoli cells. These junctions allow passage of fluid into the seminiferous tubules. The Sertoli cell is thought to contribute to the blood–testis barrier.

Spermatogenesis is usually assessed by histological examination of a small portion of the testis with a fixative that does not cause shrinkage of the seminiferous tubules. Bouin's solution is favoured in many centres, and the tissues are sliced and stained according to preference. The histological findings should be described, and there is some merit in using a semiquantitative technique such as the Johnsen score.

Hormonal control of spermatogenesis

The hormonal control of spermatogenesis requires the actions of the pituitary gonadotrophin-luteinizing hormone and the follicle-stimulating hormone (Figure 18.14). There is general agreement that both these hormones are needed for the initiation of spermatogenesis during puberty. However, the specific role and relative contribution of the two gonadotrophins in maintaining spermatogenesis are unclear.

Luteinizing hormone stimulates Leydig cell steroidogenesis, resulting in increased production of testosterone. Normal spermatogenesis is absolutely dependent on testosterone, but its mode of action and the amount required remain uncertain. Specific androgen receptors have not been demonstrated in germs cells, but they are present in Sertoli and peritubular cells. This implies that the actions of androgens on spermatogenesis must be mediated by somatic cells in the seminiferous tubules. The concentration of testosterone in the testis is 50 times higher than that in the peripheral circulation. There is thus a gross excess of testosterone within the normal adult testis, and any T-related abnormalities must be due to defects in steroid utilization rather than supply. Follicle-stimulating hormone initiates function in immature Sertoli cells prior to the onset of spermatogenesis by stimulating the formation of the blood–testis barrier, secretion of tubular fluid and other specific secretory products via follicle-stimulating hormone receptors that activate intracellular cAMP. Once spermatogenesis is established in the adult testis, Sertoli cells become less responsive to follicle-stimulating hormone. It is uncertain whether follicle-stimulating hormone maintains spermatogenesis by increasing spermatogonial mitosis or by decreasing the number of cells that degenerate at each cell division. Testosterone is essential for the subsequent stages from meiosis to spermiogenesis.

Spermatozoa

Spermatozoa have a dense oval head with an acrosomal cap, a midpiece and a tail (Figure 18.15). These highly specialized structural features reflect the unique functional activities of the spermatozoon. The acrosome contains enzymes essential for fertilization and the tail contains the mechanism for motility, and these combine to deliver the paternal contribution of genetic information in the nucleus to the egg to initiate the development of a new

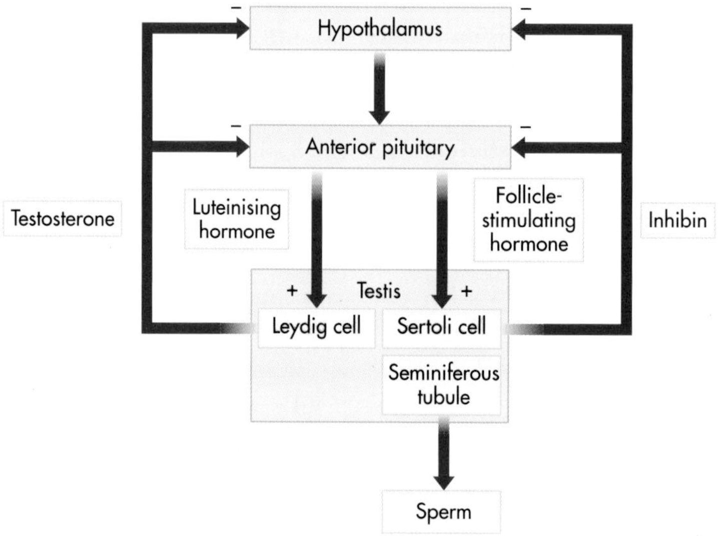

Figure 18.14 *Hormonal regulation of testicular function.*

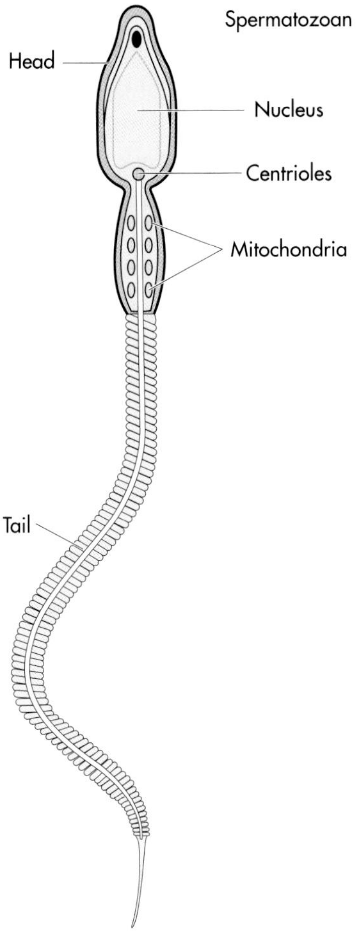

Figure 18.15 *A mature human spermatozoon.*

individual. The head is made up largely of highly condensed nuclear chromatin, constituting the haploid chromosome complement, and it is covered on its anterior half by a membrane-enclosed sac of enzymes, the acrosome. The area of the sperm head immediately behind the acrosome is important, as it is this part that attaches to and fuses with the egg. The motor apparatus of the tail is the axoneme, which consists of a central pair (doublets) of microtubules of non-contractile tubulin protein enclosed in a sheath linked radially to nine outer pairs of microtubules. Each doublet is also joined by nexin bridges to its neighbour via two ATPase-rich dynein protein arms. Lack of these dynein arms is associated with Kartagener's syndrome of bronchiectasis, sinusitis and situs inversus. Energy for sperm motility is provided by the sheath of mitochondria in the midpiece of the tail through a second messenger system involving the calcium-mediated, calmodulin-dependent conversion of ATP to cAMP and interaction with the ATPase of the dynein.

Disorders of spermatogenesis

Patients with testicular failure have impaired or defective spermatogenesis and usually present with azoospermia. Patients with primary testicular failure usually have elevated levels of plasma follicle-stimulating hormone and small testes. Secondary testicular failure is usually characterized by low or sometimes normal levels of follicle-stimulating hormone.

Primary testicular failure (hypergonadotrophic hypogonadism)

This condition is characterized by small testes, impaired spermatogenesis and elevated levels of follicle-stimulating hormone, which may or may not be accompanied by androgen deficiency.

Genetic abnormalities

The overall incidence of chromosome abnormalities is 2.2% in men attending an infertility clinic, but increases to 15.4% of those men with azoospermia. The most common abnormality is Klinefelter's syndrome (XXY), which may account for nearly half of the abnormalities. More recent studies have related defective spermatogenesis to abnormalities of the gene in the Y chromosome, but some spermatogenesis may still occur even in the absence of the AZF gene. The absence of the AZFb gene is thought to be associated with total lack of spermatogenesis.

Testicular maldescent

Argument persists as to whether the failure of testicular descent is due to an intrinsic defect in the testis or to multiple external factors. There is no good evidence that an intra-abdominal testis will make sperm, and the occurrence of spermatogenesis after bilateral orchidopexy for a truly undescended testis is uncertain. Such testes usually have normal numbers of Leydig cells but atrophy and/or fibrosis of the germinal epithelium. The incidence of carcinoma of the testis is increased in adults with undescended testes. Carcinoma is found in 25% of abdominal testes compared to only 0.5–1% of men having a testicular biopsy as part of their evaluation for subfertility/infertility.

Bilateral Sertoli cell-only syndrome

In this condition, seminiferous tubules are lined by Sertoli cells with a complete absence of any spermatogenic epithelium. With the advent of intracytoplasmic sperm injection, it is now realized that even when testicular biopsies show bilateral Sertoli cells only, the patient may have foci of spermatogenesis and may even have sperm in the ejaculate.

Acquired testicular failure

Anoxia, due to testicular torsion or acute epididymo-orchitis, mumps orchitis, radiotherapy or chemotherapy, may damage the testis to a varying extent. The histological appearances vary from focal loss of spermatogenesis, a variable amount of fibrosis or even the appearance of Sertoli cell-only syndrome.

Secondary testicular failure (hypogonadotrophic hypogonadism)

In this condition, the defect is due to a deficiency of hypothalamic-releasing or pituitary hormones. The latter may be part of an overall pituitary deficiency, a loss of both gonadotrophic hormones, a loss of luteinizing hormone (fertile eunuch syndrome) or an isolated deficiency of follicle-stimulating hormone, or may be due to excessive production of prolactin. Recognition of hypogonadotrophic hypogonadism is important, as it is the sole cause of azoospermia that is amenable to hormonal treatment.

Obstructive azoospermia

Men with a FSH level twice normal range are more likely to have smaller testes and lower mean Johnsen scores on subsequent histology at testicular biopsy indicative of primary testicular failure. In contrast, men with azoospermia, normal FSH, LH and testosterone with normal-sized testes are more likely to have obstructive azoospermia. The site of obstruction may be anywhere between the testis and the ejaculatory ducts (Table 18.15).

Congenital bilateral absence of the vas deferens (CBAVD) may be found in men presenting with azooospermia and can be associated with other genitourinary abnormalities. Often, there is hypoplasia or absence of the seminal vesicles or ampullae. Patients may be carriers of the cystic fibrosis gene and should therefore be screened for that gene.

Unilateral vasal aplasia may also occur in men with azoospermia and can be associated with a number of contralateral genitourinary abnormalities.

Congenital obstruction of the ejaculatory ducts can occur as a result of Müllerian duct cysts and Wolffian duct anomalies.

Sperm maturation

Spermatozoa are functionally immature and immotile when they pass from the testis into the caput epididymis, and the maturation process continues as they pass through the epididymis. The epididymis is under adrenergic and androgen control, and the epithelium actively reabsorbs testicular fluid and also secretes a hyperosmolar fluid rich in glycerophosphorylocholine, inositol and carnitine. The specific transport of these compounds across the epithelium creates a favourable fluid environment whereby the progressive motility and fertilizing capacity of the spermatozoa are normally acquired. Thus, the cytoplasmic droplets decrease in size and move distally along the midpiece, the acrosome membrane swells, the epididymal glycoproteins are

Table 18.15 Causes of testicular obstruction (modified from Whitfield).[1]

	% Incidence	Aetiology
Caput epididymis	29	Youngs syndrome
Cauda epididymis	19	Post infective
Empty epididymis	13	Defective Spermatogenesis, Immune Orchitis
Blocked vas	11	Post infective and Post Surgical
Absent vas		
Bilateral	18	Congenital
Unilateral	5	Mixed
Ejaculatory duct obstruction	4	Congenital Traumatic Neoplastic

incorporated into the plasma membrane, S–S bonds are formed in the sperm tail cytoskeleton and cAMP content increases. The normal site of sperm storage is in the cauda epididymis, and spermatozoa are found in the seminal vesicles only in ejaculatory duct obstruction.

Ejaculation

The processes of orgasm and ejaculation are closely associated and usually occur synchronously when sexual activity is associated with a sufficient degree of stimulation. Orgasm is dependent on intact pudendal nerves through which the pelvic floor ischiocavernosus and bulbocavernosus muscles are stimulated to contract rhythmically. This is associated with emotional changes and with the emission of semen into the prostatic urethra, closure of the bladder neck and propulsion of the semen out of the urethra. The bulk of the ejaculate consists of secretions of the seminal vesicles (65%) and prostate (30%). The seminal vesicle secretions are rich in fructose, PGs and coagulates, whereas the prostatic fluid contains protolytic enzymes that liquefy the coagulated proteins of the ejaculated semen and are rich in citric acid, acid phosphatase and zinc. Men with ejaculatory duct obstruction have a characteristically low-volume (0.3–1.0 ml), acid (pH 6.5) semen with an absence of fructose and spermatozoa. Similar semen abnormalities are also found in men with congenital bilateral vasal aplasia.

It is usual to divide ejaculation into three phases. The first phase consists of the emission of seminal fluid into the urethra. This is under sympathetic control, is associated with contraction of the epididymes and vasa, and is followed by contraction of the seminal vesicles and subsequently the prostate. The order of ejaculation may be studied by the split-ejaculate technique, cinephotography, or video. In the second phase of ejaculation, the bladder neck is closed to resist retrograde flow into the bladder, and there is contraction of the posterior urethra. In the third phase, the external sphincter closes, and there is rhythmic contraction of the bulbospongiosus along the urethra. The precise level of the centre controlling ejaculation is uncertain, but it is probably in the hypothalamus. Ejaculation is triggered when the sensory stimuli reach sufficient intensity. The effector mechanism is through the thoracic sympathetic outlets and the sympathetic chains. The preganglionic fibres for the genital system exit via the bifurcation of the aorta to synapses at short adrenergic fibres that terminate in alpha-receptors within the smooth muscle cells of the epididymes, vasa and seminal vesicles.

Seminal analysis

Seminal analysis is an important element of fertility assessment. Routine seminal analysis should be standardized and performed as recommended by the World Health Organization.[2] Unfortunately, there is no agreement as to the criteria for normal fertility, and a man with 5 million sperm of good progression in an ejaculate is probably fertile. It is important to consider all aspects of the semen test while assessing fertility.

Computer analysis of sperm number and quality and other special tests of sperm function (Table 18.16) are valuable research tools but have no place in routine fertility management. The outcome of in vitro fertilization is the best functional assessment of spermatozoa that is currently available.

Table 18.16 Percentage chance of spontaneous conception during the subsequent 12 months of couples attending an infertility clinic.

Motile sperm concentration (million/ml)	Duration of infertility (years)			
	1	2	3	8
0	0	0	0	0
0.5	16	12	9	6
1	25	19	14	9
2	34	26	19	13
5	36	28	21	14
>10	37	28	21	14

[1] See Hargreave and Elton[2].

Fertilization

At the site of fertilization, capacitated sperm with intact acrosomes penetrate the cumulus to reach the outer zona. Mechanical shearing forces generated by the characteristic flagellar movements of the capacitated sperm are probably the main mechanism responsible for cumulus penetration. Surface hyaluronidase (possibly escaping from the acrosomal membrane) may facilitate cumulus penetration but is not essential.

Binding of sperm to zona triggers the acrosome reaction, which is an essential step in the fertilization process because only acrosome-reacted sperm can penetrate the zona pellucida and fuse with the oolemma. During the acrosome reaction, the outer acrosome membrane fuses progressively with the inner plasma membrane at a number of sites and vesiculates, forming exit pores (fenestrations) through which the acrosome enzyme matrix is released.

The proteins contained in semen serve to buffer the acidity of the vaginal secretions. Few, perhaps 200, of the many millions of ejaculated sperm are functionally competent and capable of fertilizing oocytes. Only those sperm with good progressive motility are capable of transversing the cervical canal and entering the uterine cavity to reach the middle third of the fallopian tube, where fertilization usually occurs. In the female genital tract, spermatozoa undergo the process of capacitation whereby the protective coating of proteins on the sperm head, which was acquired during passage through the epididymis, is lost. The plasma membrane of the sperm head is destabilized, and the sperm movement changes, with vigorous beating of the sperm tail, with poor progression and marked undulation of the sperm head. This facilitates the penetration of the cumulus of the egg, which is further aided by surface hyaluronidase of the sperm. Binding of the sperm to the egg triggers the acrosome reaction, which is an essential step in the fertilization process, since only acrosome-reacted sperm can penetrate the zona pellucida and fuse with the oolemma. Defects in the sperm quality and/or fertilizing capacity may be overcome by the direct microinjection of a single sperm into each egg. This technique of intracytoplasmic sperm injection has revolutionized infertility management.

Table 18.17 Aetiologies of male infertility.

Diagnosis	WHO[1] 1979–1982 (%)	Melbourne[2] 1979–1980 (%)
Unrecognized	48.3	47.9
Idiopathic azoo/oligozoospermia	16.1	7.3 (combined)
Idiopathic astheno-teratozoospermia	16.8	
Variococoele	17.2	25
Genital tract infection	4.0	
Sperm autoimmunity	1.6	5
Congenital (crypto-orchidism) chromosomal disorders	2.1	1.9
Genital tract obstruction	1.8	10.8
Systemic/iatrogenic	1.3	1.0
Coital disorders	1.0	0.5
Gonadotrophin deficiency	0.6	0.6

[1] See reference 3.
[2] See reference 4.

Infertility

Infertility occurs when a woman fails to conceive after 12 months of unprotected coitus, and the essence of management is to assess and improve the prognosis (the percentage chance of conception within the next 12 months). The age of the woman and the duration of infertility (Table 18.16) are of as much importance in establishing the prognosis as the diagnosis of specific defects in the female and male partners. Some of the male factors have already been discussed, but others are summarized in Table 18.17.

REFERENCES

1. Whitfield H, Hendry WF, Kirby R, Duchett J, eds. Textbook of Genitourinary Surgery. 2nd edn. Oxford: Blackwell, 1998; 1483 (Table 120.1)
2. Hargreave TB, Elton RA. Is conventional semen analysis of any use? Br J Urol 1983; 55: 780–784
3. Cates W, Farley TMM, Rowe PJ. Worldwide patterns of infertility: is Africa different? Lancet 1985; ii: 596–598
4. Baker HWG. Clinical evaluation and management of testicular disorders in the adult. In: Burger H, de Kretser DM, eds. The Testis. 2nd edn. New York: Raven Press, 1989: 419–440

FURTHER READING

Kalsi JS, Cellek S, Muneer A, Kell PD, Ralph DJ, Minhas S. Current oral treatments for erectile dysfunction. Expert Opin Pharmacother 2002; Nov 3(11): 1613–1629

Andersson KE. Pharmacology of penile erection. Pharmacol Rev 2001; Sept 53(3): 417–450

Serhal P, Overton C. Good clinical practice in assisted reproduction. Cambridge University Press, 2004

19

The prostate and benign prostatic hyperplasia

Mark Emberton and Anthony R Mundy

THE PROSTATE

The average urologist spends about 30% of his or her time dealing with problems related to the prostate. Surprisingly, for a structure that attracts so much of our attention, we know very little about why the prostate is there and what it does. It is one of four accessory sex glands or pairs of glands; the other three are the seminal vesicles, Cowper's glands and the glands of Littre. If we know little about the prostate, we know even less about the others. The seminal vesicles, which are secretory glands, and not storage organs for semen as their name implies, contribute substantially to the volume of seminal fluid and produce one or two substances that we know about, notably fructose and glyceryl phosphocholine. However, the other two structures are something of a mystery.

We do know that the prostate is intimately related anatomically to the bladder neck and plays an integral part in ensuring antegrade ejaculation. We know it contains a substantial amount of smooth muscle as well as glandular tissue and that this smooth muscle is under alpha-adrenergic control and is thought somehow to be involved in the process of seminal emission prior to ejaculation. We know that the prostate contributes various substances to the ejaculate, some of which are present in unusually high concentrations, notably zinc, citrate and polyamines. We know that its development and function are under hormonal control; in other words, it is a secondary sex organ.

We do not know, however, what part if any the prostate plays in continence in normal individuals; the mechanism of emission and ejaculation is uncertain (in humans); and we do not know why the prostatic secretion contains so much zinc, citrate and polyamines, nor what the roles are of these and the various other substances that the prostate secretes.

The structure of the prostate

The prostate has been described as having a lobar structure, firstly, because of the endoscopic appearance of 'lobes' in patients with benign prostatic hyperplasia and in the pathological specimen after retropubic prostatectomy, and secondly, on embryological grounds in which the prostate is seen to develop from five distinct ductal systems.[1] More recently, the morphology of the prostate has been described on the basis of the predisposition of parts of its structure to various pathological processes, and to McNeal we owe our current understanding of the structure of the prostate (Figure 19.1).[2–5]

McNeal noted that the nodules of benign prostatic hyperplasia began in the periurethral glandular area within the collar of the preprostatic sphincter in the supramontanal part of the prostate. Subsequently, he noted that these microscopic nodules were principally concentrated just below the distal margin of the preprostatic sphincter, and he named that area the transitional zone. The transitional zone only accounted for about 2% of the glandular tissue of the normal prostate but accounted for much more as the hyperplastic nodules coalesced, became macroscopic and tended to displace the normal prostate away from the urethra.

McNeal noted that about 25% of prostatic cancer originated within the transitional zone, whereas

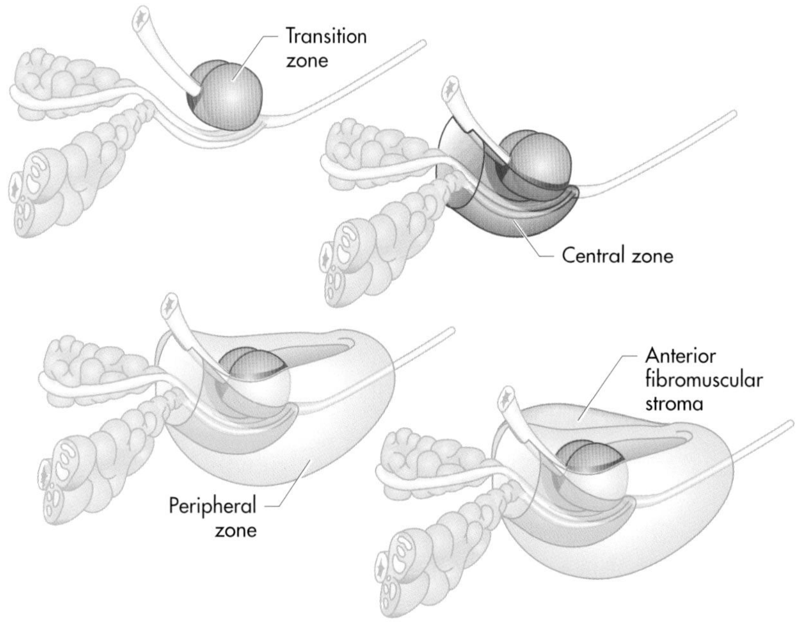

Figure 19.1 *Zones of the prostate.*

75% of cancers and almost all instances of prostatitis arose in the so-called peripheral zone. The peripheral zone forms a posteriorly and inferiorly orientated cup that encloses the central zone, through the centre of which are transmitted the ejaculatory ducts. McNeal noted the comparative absence of disease in the central zone by comparison with the other glandular areas of the prostate and likened it to the seminal vesicles, which are also comparatively free of disease. He speculated further that both these structures might arise embryologically from the Wolffian ducts and he noted some histological similarities between the central zone and the seminal vesicles to support this contention.[5]

Completing the anterior aspect of the substance of the prostate where the peripheral zone peters out on either side is the anterior fibromuscular stroma of the prostate. Most of the glandular tissue of the prostate is in the peripheral zone, which accounts for 65% of the total, the remaining 25% of the glandular tissue of the prostate being in the central zone. It is not known whether the three zones of glandular tissue – transitional, central and peripheral – have different secretory functions.

Embryological development of the prostate

As mentioned above, the seminal vesicles (and possibly the central zone of the prostate) arise from the Wolffian ducts along with the vasa and their ampullae and the epididymes. Their development is under the control of testosterone. However, the prostate develops from urogenital sinus mesenchyme and its development is under the control of dihydrotestosterone. This difference of embryological origin and hormonal control may account for the observation that, whereas the prostate is commonly involved in disease, the structures of Wolffian duct origin rarely are.

Endocrinology of the prostate

The prostate develops and functions in response to dihydrotestosterone, which is produced within the prostate cells themselves from circulating testosterone (Figure 19.2). The circulating testosterone is derived from testicular secretion; the testis produces 6–7 mg a day under the influence of luteinizing hormone, which in turn is produced by the pituitary in response to the pulsatile release of luteinizing hormone-releasing hormone from the hypothalamus. Testosterone is insoluble in water and is carried in the circulation bound principally to sex hormone-binding globulin, with only a tiny free fraction. However tiny it is, the free testosterone is the important component, and because it is a small, lipid-soluble molecule, it transfers across the lipid cell membrane with ease to be converted

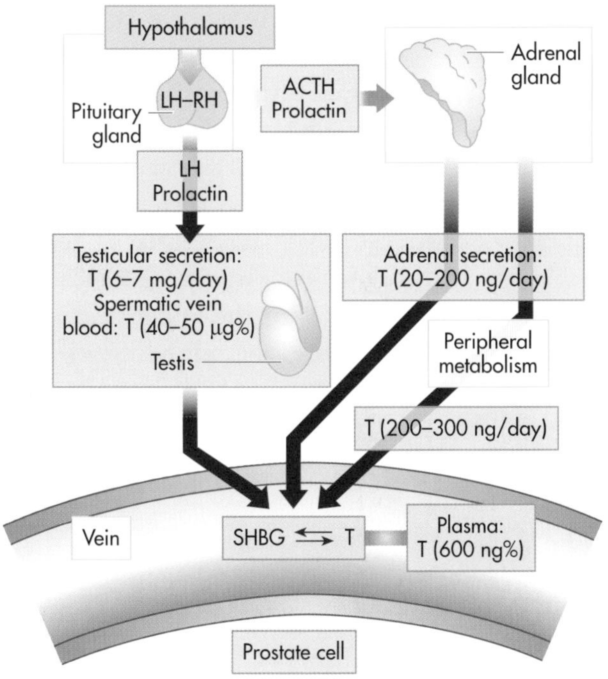

Figure 19.2 *Endocrinological influences on the prostate. Pulsatile release of luteinizing hormone-releasing hormone (LH-RH) from the hypothalamus causes the release of luteinizing hormone (LH) from the anterior pituitary, which circulates to the Leydig cells of the testis, which produce testosterone (T). Testosterone circulates from the testis bound to sex hormone-binding globulin (SHBG) and is available to the prostate. Circulating testosterone has a negative-feedback inhibition of the hypothalamic release of luteinizing hormone-releasing hormone. Adrenal secretion and peripheral aromatization are other sources of circulating androgens.*

by 5-alpha reductase into the active component dihydrotestosterone.

The adrenal produces androgens that can be converted to testosterone, and there is a mechanism for the peripheral conversion of various substrates into testosterone, but the vast majority of testosterone is derived from testicular secretion and without testicular testosterone the prostate undergoes involution.

The enzyme 5-alpha reductase within the prostatic cell is crucial in producing the active androgen, dihydrotestosterone. There are two types of 5-alpha reductase, of which type 2 is the more important, and it is blocked by the 5-alpha reductase inhibitor finasteride, which has recently been introduced therapeutically for the treatment of benign prostatic hyperplasia.[6] It is a deficiency of this enzyme also that is responsible for the intersex state first noted by Imperato-McInley in the Dominican Republic in which apparently normal girls change to boys at puberty.[7]

Dihydrotestosterone exerts its effect by binding to the androgen receptor and then translocating to the nucleus to bind with DNA and initiate transcription. Binding of dihydrotestosterone to the androgen receptor causes a confirmational change of the androgen receptor, thereby exposing its hormone-responsive element, which binds to its target DNA to initiate transcription (Figure 19.3).

Both the epithelial cells and the stromal cells are capable of producing dihydrotestosterone as both contain the 5-alpha reductase enzyme.[8] Similarly, both epithelial and stromal cells contain androgen receptors. However, it appears that dihydrotestosterone is principally formed in epithelial cells and although some of this acts within the epithelial cell nuclei to initiate the transcription of DNA that is responsible for the secretory activity in the prostate, most of the dihydrotestosterone formed in epithelial cells diffuses to the stromal cells where most of the androgen receptors are found. In stromal cells, the binding of dihydrotestosterone to the androgen receptor principally stimulates the stromal nuclei to produce growth factors and these growth factors drive both the epithelial cells and the stromal cells themselves to grow and develop.[9,10]

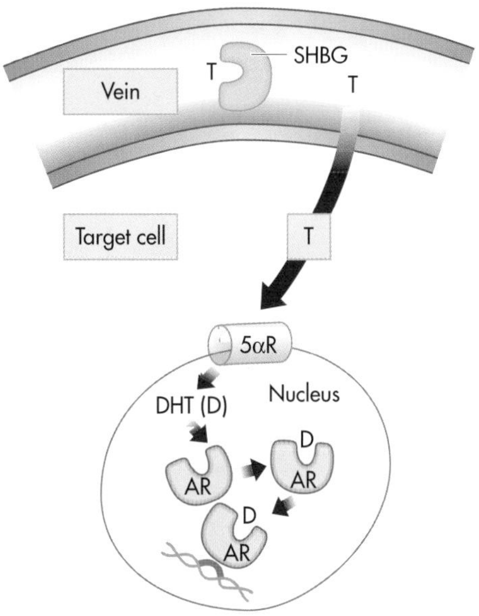

Figure 19.3 *Testosterone (T) dissociates from its protein binding and translocates across the cell membrane. Intracellularly, it is converted to dihydrotestosterone (DHT) and binds to the androgen receptor (AR), from where it translocates to the nucleus.*

It is this interaction between the stroma and the epithelium that is thought to account not only for development and for normal function but also, when the interaction is deranged, for the process leading to benign prostatic hyperplasia.

Thus, several processes are active within the prostate. The endocrine effect of testosterone leads to the intracrine effect of dihydrotestosterone, which generates the autocrine and paracrine effects of growth factors on both the stroma and the epithelium of the prostate (Figure 19.4). These growth factors, responsible for the autocrine and paracrine effects, act principally during the G1 phase of the cell cycle and have various effects, mainly stimulatory but in some instances inhibitory, leading generally to the entry of the cell into the S phase and ultimately then to mitosis.

The normal adult prostate should not be thought of as being an entirely static structure. There is a turnover of cells throughout life and this turnover is heterogeneous.[11] Those glandular cells further out in the periphery of the gland away from the urethra show little in the way of secretion and most in the way of mitotic activity within the prostate, resembling basal or stem cells. At an intermediate level

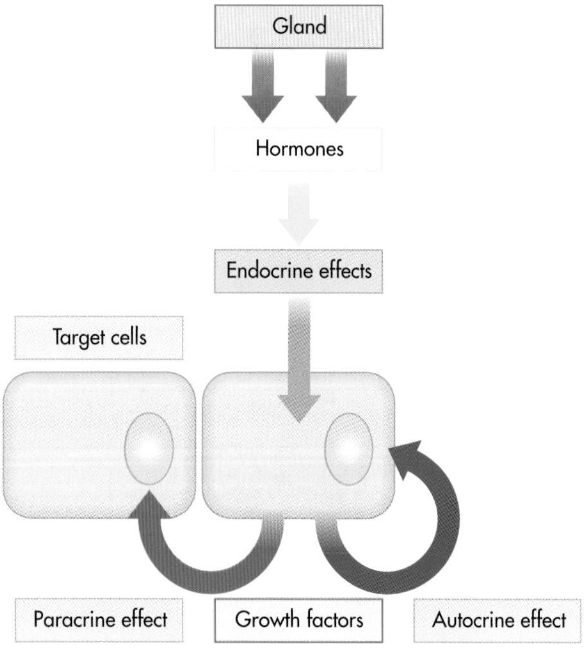

Figure 19.4 *The effect of androgens in the stroma is to cause the release of growth factors that have an autocrine effect on themselves and a paracrine effect on epithelial cells.*

along the prostatic duct, the epithelial cells show less mitosis but almost all of the secretory activity of the prostate. These two types of acinar cells are tall and columnar and show no evidence of cell death. More centrally, close to the urethra, the epithelial cells are lower, flatter and without any secretory activity, and programmed cell death (apoptosis) is readily visible. In relation to these different epithelial cell types there are differences in the underlying extracellular matrix that probably reflect the driving force for epithelial differentiation.[12] In addition, there are the neuroendocrine cells described below.

Growth factors in the prostate

It has been known for many years that prostatic cells could only proliferate in vitro in the presence of serum. The factors that were present in serum were not present in plasma and so it seemed that whatever was necessary to stimulate cell growth in vitro was derived from the process of blood coagulation and most probably liberated from platelets. Thus, one of the first 'growth factors' to be identified was called platelet-derived growth factor. Various other factors were subsequently identified as being 'growth factors' for various different cell types in vitro and have derived their names from the circumstances under which they were isolated. These substances may have effects other than being 'growth factors' and most have many different roles in stimulating cellular growth both in vitro and in vivo (see Chapter 1).

Other factors that are known to be important in the normal growth and development in the prostate have been: (a) derived from the mouse submaxillary gland (epidermal growth factor); (b) shown to have a very characteristic and strong tendency to bind to heparin (fibroblast growth factor, one of the so-called heparin-binding growth factors); or (c) biochemically related to pro-insulin (insulin-like growth factor). Hence the origin of names that are somewhat confusing to the uninitiated.

Typically, growth factors are grouped into families of factors having similar effects and there is an epidermal growth factor family, a fibroblast growth factor family, a transforming growth factor-β family (transforming growth factor-α – somewhat confusingly – is a member of the epidermal growth factor family), and the insulin-like growth factor family. There are other growth factor families as well, but these are the ones that are thought to be important in the normal prostate.

Of these various growth factors, the most important stimulatory ones are epidermal growth factor and transforming growth factor-α, both of which are derived from the epidermal growth factor family, and basic fibroblast growth factor of the fibroblast growth factor family. Of these, basic fibroblast growth factor and epidermal growth factor are thought to account for 80% and transforming growth factor-α for 20% of the stimulatory growth factor effect in health.[13] The other important growth factor is transforming growth factor-β, whose effects are complex but generally inhibitory.[14]

Other growth factors such as insulin-like growth factor are thought to be principally 'permissive' in the same sense that androgens are permissive. Insulin-like growth factor and testosterone have to be present in vivo and in vitro, but adding more and more of either does not produce a corresponding parallel proliferation of the prostate in vitro, whereas adding epidermal growth factor, transforming growth factor or basic fibroblast growth factor does. The effects of some of these factors are only or principally apparent at different stages of development. Epidermal growth factor and basic fibroblast growth factor are predominant in the adult (developed) prostate. On the other hand, transforming growth factor and another member of the fibroblast growth factor family, acidic fibroblast growth factor, are principally evident in fetal life.[15]

The role of the prostate in continence

One could be forgiven for thinking that the prostate has a major role in continence by virtue of its situation around the bladder neck, but of course the female of the species manages perfectly well without it.

In individuals of either sex there is a change in the orientation of the smooth muscle bundles of the detrusor as they approach the region of the bladder neck, with a tendency to become more oblique in disposition, smaller and more finely interspersed in a more dense connective tissue framework (Figure 19.5).[16] In males, but not in females, there is a quite definitely circular/oblique orientation of smooth muscle bundles around the area just below the bladder neck and within the substance of the prostate, with a dense adrenergic innervation that can be demonstrated by immunofluorescence (Figure 19.6).[17] Elsewhere in the bladder in both sexes and in the female urethra, alpha-adrenergic innervation is only seen in relation to blood vessels, although alpha-adrenergic receptors may be more widely distributed. This ring of smooth muscle around the supramontanal prostatic urethra, between the bladder neck and the site of drainage of the prostatic ducts and ejaculatory ducts into the urethra, is called

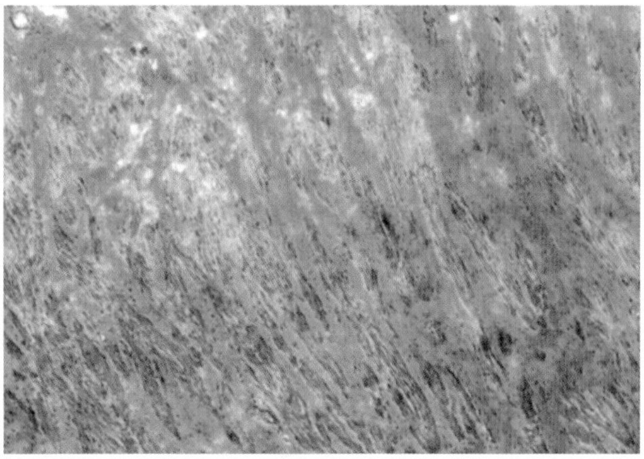

Figure 19.5 *The orientation of smooth muscle bundles at the bladder neck to form the preprostatic sphincter.*

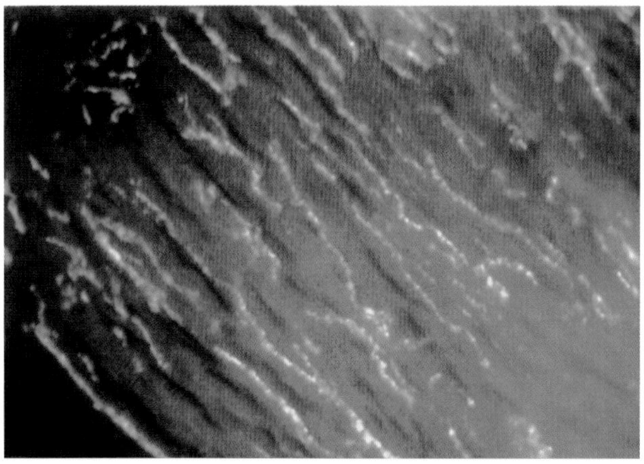

Figure 19.6 *Immunofluorescence photomicrograph to show the presence of noradrenergic nerves interspersed between the smooth muscle bundles at the bladder neck.*

the preprostatic sphincter. It is present to ensure antegrade ejaculation (see below).

Elsewhere within the prostate, particularly within the prostatic capsule but distributed throughout the stroma, there are smooth muscle cells that amount to about 50% of the total mass of the stroma of the prostate.[18] These cells also have (mainly) an alpha-adrenergic innervation.[19]

Classical pharmacological studies were able to distinguish between alpha- and beta-adrenergic activities and, more recently, between alpha-1 receptors (postjunctional alpha adrenoceptors that mediate the effector response) and alpha-2 receptors (prejunctional alpha adrenoceptors that regulate neurotransmitter release). Further, pharmacological alpha-1 subtypes are now distinguished by the selective antagonistic effects of certain blockers. Recently, the International Union of Pharmacology published a new classification of alpha receptors. This was needed to clarify the confusing nomenclature that was being used to describe native as distinct from cloned receptors.[20] Suffice it to say that all three alpha-1 receptor subtypes have been identified in human prostatic stroma but the predominant one is the alpha-1A subtype. Unfortunately, none of the alpha blockers in use today has much selectivity for the alpha-1A subtype. The most selective at present seems to be indoramin,[21] but its other pharmacological effects (antihistaminic, local anaesthetic and cardiodepressant) limit its potential clinical usefulness.

This adrenergic innervation is not the only form of innervation to the prostate, however; it is not even the only innervation of prostatic smooth muscle cells. There is a cholinergic innervation and there are a number of different non-adrenergic non-cholinergic nerve or receptor types as well. The latter include serotonin (5-hydroxytryptamine), dopamine beta hydroxylase, vasoactive intestinal polypeptide, neuropeptide Y, leu-encephalin, met-encephalin, calcitonin gene-related peptide and substance P.[22] What these are all doing is by no means clear.

The majority of the adrenergic receptors are of the alpha adrenergic type, 98% of which are located within the stroma, of which 90% are of the alpha-1 subtype. Only 10% of alpha receptors and neurons are of the alpha-2 subtype. Of the alpha-1, the alpha-1A type accounts for 60%, and it is these that are the cells that have been targeted pharmacologically by drugs such as indoramin, terazosin and doxazosin in an attempt to reverse some of the features of bladder outflow obstruction due to benign prostatic hyperplasia.[21] The cholinergic innervation is thought to control epithelial secretion.[23]

Some of the non-adrenergic non-cholinergic substances listed above are present in so-called 'neuroendocrine cells'.[24] The principal neuroendocrine cell types are cells that secrete serotonin and thyroid-stimulating hormone. Other cells contain calcitonin or the calcitonin gene-related peptide and somatostatin. It is not clear what these do, but they are thought to be involved in the regulation of secretion or cell growth. The function of the other neurons or receptors is completely unknown; they may not actually have any function. As has been pointed out elsewhere in this volume, the presence of neurons does not necessarily imply the presence of receptors for those neurons and vice versa, and even if both are present, that does not necessarily mean that there is a neural pathway, and if there is, it does not necessarily follow that that pathway has a physiological significance even if it has a pathological significance.

Thus, there is no evidence that the prostate plays any active role in continence, although in disease it may interfere with normal continence. There is no evidence that the male bladder neck in the strict sense is any different from the female bladder neck except that it simply has a preprostatic sphincter superimposed on the common bladder neck pattern. All the evidence is that the prostatic smooth muscle and its innervation and the other nerve supply to the prostate are involved in glandular secretion and the process of emission.

EMISSION AND EJACULATION

Ejaculation in human beings remains a mystery, in part as it is so difficult to study because of the problems of sexual sensibilities. In animals this is less of a problem; indeed, because of the financial implications of breeding in animal husbandry, ejaculation in some species has been studied in considerable detail.

We have known for some time from so-called 'split ejaculate' studies in humans that spermatozoa and prostatic fluid are ejaculated first, followed by seminal vesicle fluid later.[25] We also know that ejaculation is antegrade in the presence of a competent bladder neck despite the competence of the urethral sphincter mechanism, which therefore must be overcome actively or reflexly to enable ejaculation to occur. It is also common male experience that voiding is difficult with an erection and for a while after ejaculation.

The latter has been shown to be due to tightening of the 'bladder neck' – more accurately, of the preprostatic sphincter – on erection, which becomes more marked in the period leading up to ejaculation. This has been shown both on urethral pressure profile studies, which show enhancement of the pressure zone produced by the bladder neck (Figure 19.7), and on transrectal ultrasound studies, which demonstrate the preprostatic sphincter quite clearly and which show it to become more marked in the pre-ejaculatory period.[26]

The next step, also shown on transrectal ultrasound[26] (and radiographically in some animal species), is the transportation of spermatozoa from the ampullae of the vasa into the prostatic urethra. This process of filling of the inframontanal prostatic urethra, below the occluding preprostatic sphincter, is known as emission, as distinct from the process by which the seminal fluid is transported to the outside world, which is ejaculation. The mechanism for this is not clear. Once it occurs, ejaculation is imminent. Next is a contraction of the prostatic smooth muscle including the preprostatic sphincter, which is presumably under alpha-1A adrenergic control.

Synchronously but not in any coordinated fashion, there is a sequence of five or six contractions of the bulbo-spongiosus muscle. The first generally occurs before any of the seminal fluid has entered the bulbar urethra, and the last occurs after pulsatile ejaculation ceases. The mechanism for this is not clear either, nor is the means by which the urethral sphincter mechanism is overcome. It used to be thought that it was overcome passively by the sheer pressure that prostatic emission generates. But the

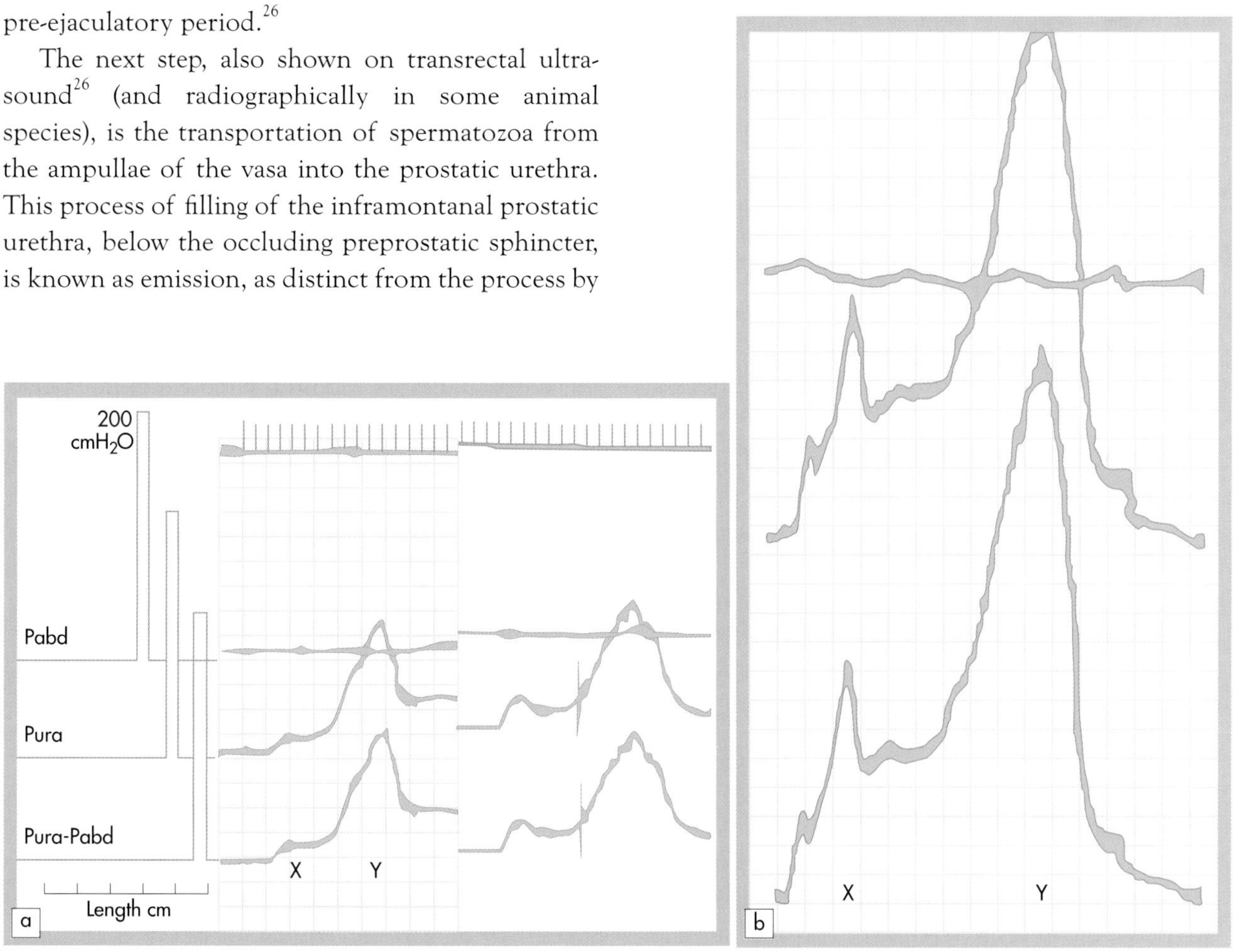

Figure 19.7 *(a) A urethral pressure profile of the bladder neck (where x is the site of the bladder neck and y is the site of the urethral sphincter mechanism). (b) A urethral pressure profile during erection to show the enhanced pressure zone at the bladder neck.*

recent transrectal ultrasound studies referred to above suggest that this is probably not the case. Urethral sphincter studies to look for a relaxation mechanism have not been useful in providing an alternative explanation. In any case, a postulated urethral sphincter relaxation mechanism would tend to flounder on the observation that after transurethral resection, men are not incontinent during sexual activity when the bladder neck mechanism has been ablated.

Once emission and ejaculation have begun, there is further contraction of the prostate and of the seminal vesicles until the process is complete.

There is therefore an important role for the prostate in the process of emission leading to ejaculation, irrespective of the content of prostatic secretion added.

The physiological function of prostatic secretion

In an average ejaculate, 2 ml are contributed by the secretion of the seminal vesicles, 0.5 ml is contributed by the secretion of the prostate, and Cowper's glands and the glands of Littre contribute 0.1 ml.[27] The contribution of the sperm cells themselves is insignificant. Although the function of these various secretions is not clear, epididymal sperm can fertilize an ovum but not as well as ejaculated sperm, so presumably their function is to maximize the potential for fertilization. This may be by having a protective effect during the onward journey of the sperm until its contact with the ovum, or an effect to enhance motility and sperm survival more directly, or a role to increase the fertilizing effect of the sperm when it reaches the ovum. There are various pieces of evidence to support a role in each of these three areas, but details are distinctly lacking.

These various secretions also have a protective role in the lower urinary tract itself. The sheer presence of the fluid provides lubrication both of the urethra itself and, through the pre-ejaculatory fluid, for penetration, although penetration has often occurred long before most human males produce pre-ejaculatory fluid. Nonetheless, this may at least be the role of the glands of Littre. It would be nice to think they were there for some purpose!

A protective effect on the lower urinary tract by the biological effects of some of the components of seminal fluid may be more important, indeed much more important than just the mechanical washing of the urethra. In fact, it has been argued that the principal function of the prostate and the other sexual secondary sex organs is to protect the integrity of the spermatozoa. Zinc has a strong antimicrobial action; spermine less so. Immunoglobulins of various types could have a similar biological role. All this is, however, unproven.

One substance known to enhance the fertilizing capacity of ejaculated sperm cells after ejaculation is fertilization-promoting peptide, which is structurally similar to thyrotrophin-releasing hormone.[28] Its mode of action is unknown, nor is it known whether there are other compounds with a similar action. Epidermal growth factor has a high concentration in seminal fluid, second only to colostrum in fact, and it may be that this reflects a role in fertilization.

Numerous compounds are produced by the prostate, most of which have no obvious function. Acid phosphatase splits glycerylphosphocholine produced by the seminal vesicles to produce glycerylphosphate ultimately and it may be that glycerylphosphate is important in sperm protection. It may be more than just coincidental that in a laboratory setting glycerine is used for this sort of purpose. Polyamines are the strongest known cationic substances in nature and they may have an important role in transcription and translation.[29] Alternatively, these two observations may be no more than just coincidence. Prostate specific antigen is a serine protease that has a role in sperm liquefaction.[30] Sperm coagulation and liquefaction have an important role in small mammals such as rats and mice but their role in humans is unclear.

More interesting perhaps, because of their high concentration within the prostate, are zinc and citrate. Citrate is present in 240–1300 times the concentration found elsewhere,[31] and zinc is present in about 30 times the concentration elsewhere;[32] it seems likely that there is a reason for this and for the uniquely high concentrations of polyamines. There appears to be a close correlation between all three, and it has long been suspected that citrate is there as a ligand for zinc.[33] It is thought that the zinc is there to help maintain the quaternary structure of sperm chromatin[34] in addition to the biological protective effect mentioned above. It now seems likely that the complex of zinc and citrate and polyamines forms a structure that has electrochemical neutrality and therefore buffers the citrate,[35] although this does seem an extremely energy-inefficient way of achieving this effect. An alternative, or additional, explanation is that the complex is there not just to protect the zinc (so to speak) but to hold the citrate there.[36] The optimum pH for the activity of acid phosphatase is much lower than the natural pH of seminal fluid and if acid phosphatase does indeed have an important biological role, this may be facilitated by the availability of large amounts of citrate. This, however, is pure speculation at present.

One of the problems is that most of these substances have only been investigated from the point of view of their concentrations in disease to serve as a marker for a disease state rather than to investigate their physiological role. Until the thrust of research is redirected, the function of these various components of prostatic and seminal vesicular secretion will continue to remain obscure.

BENIGN PROSTATIC HYPERPLASIA

Having discussed some of the aspects of our current understanding of the prostate in health, we now turn to a consideration of the disorders of the prostate seen in benign prostatic hyperplasia.

The general impression generated in many reviews is that benign prostatic hyperplasia is a generalized and diffuse disease of the prostate that occurs as a result of some sort of hormonal derangement that leads to hyperplasia of the prostate producing enlargement of the gland as a whole, which in turn leads to compression of the prostatic urethra and a progressive occlusion of the bladder outflow and the clinical syndrome of 'prostatism'. None of this is true.

Benign prostatic hyperplasia is very unusual in that it only occurs in human beings and dogs. The same is true of carcinoma of the prostate. Despite this and the fact that both diseases are common, most authorities suggest that there is no direct link between the two diseases.[37] Recently, however, there has been a suggestion that the two are related: that a series of genetic 'hits' gives rise to benign prostatic hyperplasia, and further 'hits' to prostate cancer.[38] Benign prostatic hyperplasia is therefore an early stage in the development of prostate cancer in this hypothesis.

Benign prostatic hyperplasia seems to be a disease (also like carcinoma of the prostate) that any human male can expect to get if he lives long enough with functioning testes and if his prostate was normal to start off with. It is clearly important, therefore, to distinguish between the clinical condition associated with the histological disease of benign prostatic hyperplasia and other clinical conditions affecting the lower urinary tract in ageing males.

The recent interest in symptom scores and in the effects of ageing on the bladder in individuals of either sex seems to make it clear that there are symptoms arising from the lower urinary tract, and particularly from the bladder, that are related to ageing that need to be distinguished from those symptoms related to histological benign prostatic hyperplasia in males. Furthermore, many of the features of the benign prostatic hyperplasia clinical symptom complex are difficult to explain in relation to histological benign prostatic hyperplasia alone. Acute retention can be explained when it is secondary to urinary tract infection, severe constipation or sympathetic stimulation in hypothermia and psychological stress, but otherwise its nature is somewhat elusive, although it may be due to prostatic infarction or some other prostatic 'vascular accident'.[39] The 'urge' symptom complex related to secondary detrusor instability is more easy to explain,[40] but bladder decompensation is more difficult given our present knowledge of clinical benign prostatic hyperplasia and the experimental effects of obstruction on bladder function,[41] unless this is related more to the coincidentally ageing bladder than to benign prostatic hyperplasia per se. It is, in fact, difficult to explain how benign prostatic hyperplasia causes obstruction at all. Squeezing on a hosepipe is a very inefficient way of stopping the water emerging from the end, and a very marked restriction of the calibre of the hosepipe has to be produced before there is any overt change in flow. Obstruction by urethral constriction is easily understood in relation to urethral stricture disease but it is much more difficult to argue for a similar effect in the prostatic urethra in benign prostatic hyperplasia when a large resectoscope can be passed through and into the bladder with ease. It may therefore be that it is distortion of the prostatic urethra that is more important in producing outflow obstruction than compression or constriction, as it is distortion of a hosepipe by kinking that is more likely to stop flow.

Aetiology

It has already been mentioned that the only proven risk factors for developing benign prostatic hyperplasia are ageing and the presence of functioning testes,[42] assuming that the prostate was normal to start off with – in other words, if 5-alpha reductase was present to convert testosterone to dihydrotestosterone and there were functioning androgen receptors for the dihydrotestosterone to bind to.

Various factors have been investigated such as dietary factors, alcohol and cirrhosis of the liver,[43] all of which may affect androgen–oestrogen balance, but there is no substantial evidence to support any of these contentions. The only evidence for any other factor is for an inherited predisposition to develop the disease at a younger than usual age, which runs in families.[44]

Pathogenesis

It has also been pointed out that androgens (in other words, functioning testes) were permissive for prostatic growth and development in health, and the same is true for the prostate in vitro. Androgens (and insulin-like growth factor and other 'factors') have to be present for the prostate to grow, but once the critical 'permissive' concentration has been reached, there is no extra growth produced by adding more.

Also discussed above was the concept of a stromal–epithelial interaction in which testosterone production by the epithelial cells leads to the elaboration of growth factors by the stromal cell that act in both an autocrine and paracrine fashion to produce further growth and differentiation in both the stroma and the epithelium. This stromal–epithelial interaction was most clearly demonstrated by Cunha (Figure 19.8), who implanted embryonic urogenital sinus mesenchyme and adult bladder epithelial cells from a normal mouse under the renal capsule of a nude mouse and showed that the urogenital sinus

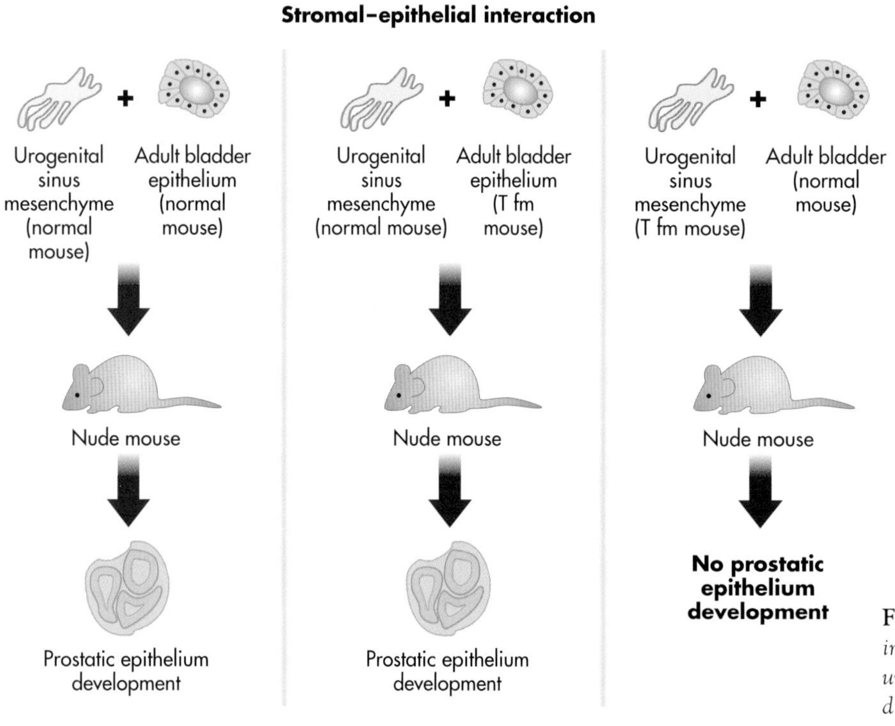

Figure 19.8 *Cunha's experiments showing the importance of stroma (in this case urogenital sinus mesenchyme) in epithelial differentiation.*

mesenchyme induced prostatic epithelial differentiation of the bladder epithelium.[45] Cunha also showed that normal prostatic differentiation could be induced from the bladder epithelium taken from a mouse with androgen receptor deficiency as long as the urogenital sinus mesenchyme was taken from a normal mouse. Prostatic epithelial differentiation did not occur when the urogenital sinus mesenchyme was taken from a mouse with androgen receptor deficiency whatever the androgen receptor status of the bladder epithelium. In this way, Cunha demonstrated the importance of the androgen receptor in the prostatic stroma (derived from urogenital sinus mesenchyme) as well as the importance of the stromal–epithelial interaction in producing epithelial and glandular development.

In benign prostatic hyperplasia, the stromal: epithelial ratio increases.[18] Normally, it is something in the region of 2:1, but in benign prostatic hyperplasia it increases to 3:1 or 4:1. As mentioned above, there is a substantial smooth muscle component to the stroma in health and in benign prostatic hyperplasia, but the majority of the stroma is made up of connective tissue such that about 50% of benign prostatic hyperplasia is connective tissue, 25% is smooth muscle and 25% is epithelium.[19]

The first discernible sign of benign prostatic hyperplasia is the presence of microscopic nodules of fibromuscular hyperplasia with a variable epithelial cell component. These nodules are found initially in the transition zone just below the smooth muscle collar of the preprostatic sphincter (Figure 19.9).[46] The transition zone is found on either side of the urethra, and nodules in this area are a

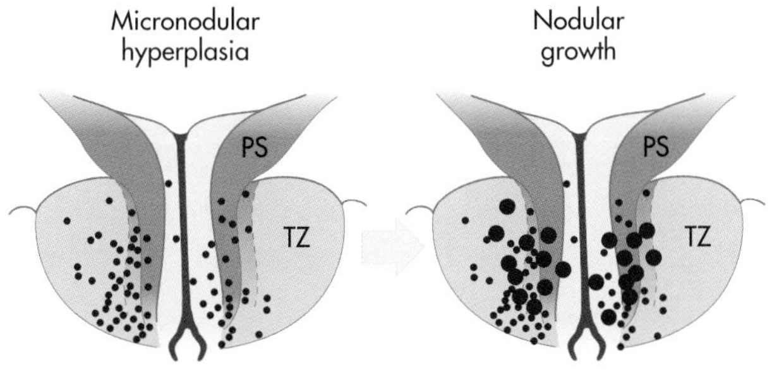

Figure 19.9 *The siting of early nodules in benign prostatic hyperplasia: just below and within the collar of the preprostatic sphincter (PS) in the general area of the transitional zone (TZ).*

mixture of glandular and epithelial hyperplasia. The nodules of benign prostatic hyperplasia also form, with lesser frequency, in the periurethral glandular tissue within the smooth muscle collar of the preprostatic sphincter. Here, they form principally posteriorly and have no epithelial or glandular component;[47,48] they are pure connective tissue nodules. In these nodules, there are changes visible that are most unusual, notably fibroblasts transforming themselves into smooth muscle cells. It was this observation that led McNeal to suggest that the nodules of benign prostatic hyperplasia, wherever they occurred, were the result of an 'embryonic reawakening' as a consequence of localized changes in the normal stromal–epithelial interaction.[46,49]

The so-called lateral lobes of benign prostatic hyperplasia are derived from micronodule formation and coalescence and further growth within the transition zone, whereas the so-called middle lobe is derived from nodule formation and development within the periurethral glandular sleeve posteriorly. The remainder of the prostate – as has been well recognized for many years – is compressed outwards to form a false capsule posteriorly.[50]

In other words, benign prostatic hyperplasia is not a diffuse and generalized disease of the prostate but is a highly localized disease of the smallest area of the prostate (the transition zone and the periurethral gland area). There is no evidence that it is related either directly to a derangement of androgen metabolism or to an androgen–oestrogen imbalance, given that it occurs at a time when serum androgen levels are steadily decreasing and oestrogen levels are steadily increasing, and that only a small proportion of the prostate as a whole is affected.[51]

Whereas the description 'embryonic reawakening' may not be entirely accurate, the disease does seem to be related to an abnormal stromal–epithelial interaction confined to this small area of the prostate, in which both increased cell growth and reduced cell death – that is to say, programmed cell death (apoptosis) – are equally important components.[52] It was mentioned above that along the prostatic duct, from the urethra out to the periphery, the most distal glands were dividing while the most proximal ones (nearest the urethra) were undergoing apoptosis. The epithelial cells of the more distal or peripheral glands, which have been noted to be more mitotically active, seem to be related to underlying smooth muscle cells that are vimentin positive, whereas those that are proximal or central, which tend to show apoptosis, are related to smooth muscles that are actin positive.[12,53] Perhaps vimentin-positive smooth muscle cells tend to be more stimulatory, whereas those that are actin positive produce inhibitory growth factors or growth factors that tend to promote apoptosis. Alterations in growth factor expression have, indeed, been identified in benign prostatic hyperplasia, although it is not yet possible to say with confidence that these growth factors are the cause of this histological condition, that they are confined to the transition zone and are not found elsewhere within the prostate, and that they alone are responsible for the changes seen in benign prostatic hyperplasia.

Most of the work on growth factors in the prostate has been very recent; new work is being published all the time, and the picture is far from clear and is changing. Nonetheless, what follows is a summary of what currently appears to be true at the time of writing.[54]

Most of the growth factors alluded to above act to increase gene expression, although the transforming growth factor beta family is notable for generally producing inhibition. Most growth factors act through single-pass transmembrane receptors with tyrosine kinase activity that, through a transduction pathway, induce mitogen-activated protein kinases, which produce the increase in gene expression.

In the normal prostate, the main stimulatory growth factors are epidermal growth factor and transforming growth factor alpha, the former being principally active in adults and the latter in growth and differentiation of the prostate. Neither of these appears to play any part in benign prostatic hyperplasia, although the epidermal growth factor expression appears to be reduced.[55] Another growth factor family with an important role in the normal prostate is the fibroblast growth factor family. Like transforming growth factor alpha, acidic fibroblast growth factor is predominantly active in growth and differentiation.[15] It is basic fibroblast growth factor that is the main stimulatory growth factor of this group in adults. All members of the fibroblast growth factor family have a variety of actions on a variety of different cell types, including producing angiogenesis and remodelling the extracellular matrix by producing modulating proteases and inducing the synthesis of fibronectin.[14,56] Members of the fibroblast growth factor family are abundant in the extracellular matrix, where they bind heparin avidly. Basic fibroblast growth factor is interesting because it is not secreted; it is only released from cells by injury or cell death, although it may, of course, have intracrine activity.[57] However, there is another member of this family, called keratinocyte growth factor.[58] This is a truly paracrine substance that is secreted only by stromal cells but for which there are only receptors on epithelial cells. It may be that some of the stimulatory activity previously ascribed to basic fibroblast growth factor is, in fact, more related to keratinocyte growth factor. Both basic fibroblast growth factor and keratinocyte growth factor appear to have a role in benign prostatic hyperplasia as both show increased expression.[59]

The transforming growth factor-β family is the family of growth factors that are generally inhibitory for epithelial cells. It is more true to say that they may be inhibitory or stimulatory depending on the cell type, the state of differentiation and the circumstances,[14,60] but in general they are inhibitory for epithelial cells and stimulatory for stromal cells. They also increase angiogenesis and extracellular matrix formation.[61,62] This family is interesting, firstly because these growth factors have receptors that are serine/threonine kinases rather than tyrosine kinases, which are usual with growth factor receptors,[62] and secondly, because they can inhibit the transition from the G1 phase to the S phase of the cell cycle and thereby override the action of mitogens, including the growth factors alluded to above.[14,63]

There are five isoforms of transforming growth factor alpha, but only three have been found in mammals (1–3) and only alpha-1 and alpha-2 have been investigated in benign prostatic hyperplasia. Transforming growth factor alpha-1 is negatively regulated by androgen: a fall in androgen leads to increased expression of the growth factor, and vice versa.[62] It also seems that basic fibroblast growth factor and keratinocyte growth factor expression is regulated by transforming growth factor β.[14] As a result, fibroblast growth factor expression is regulated by androgen indirectly by the androgen effect on transforming growth factor alpha expression.

The fibroblast growth factors – basic fibroblast growth factor and keratinocyte growth factor – are stimulatory growth factors and transforming growth factors alpha-1 and alpha-2 are inhibitory. Stromal cells produce both fibroblast growth factors and transforming growth factor alpha-1.[14,58] Epithelial cells produce transforming growth factor alpha-2.[64] Basic fibroblast growth factor acts on both epithelial cells and stromal cells but principally on stromal cells because that is where it is released. Keratinocyte growth factor, on the other hand, can only act on epithelial cells because only epithelial cells have receptors for it. The transforming growth factors alpha-1 and alpha-2 act on both epithelial and stromal cells (Figure 19.10).

Thus, keratinocyte growth factor stimulates and transforming growth factor beta inhibits epithelial cells, and basic fibroblast growth factor stimulates and transforming growth factor beta inhibits stromal cells, and, in the normal prostate, a steady state exists in which each pair is in balance. It is believed[65] that

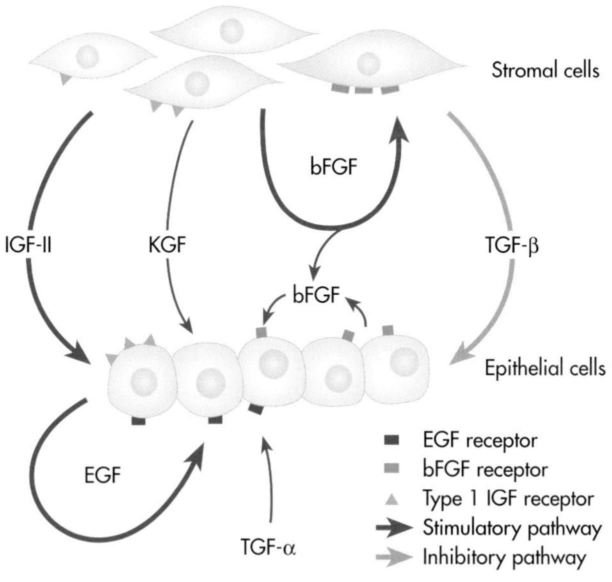

Figure 19.10 *The interaction of growth factors in benign prostatic hyperplasia. bFGF, basic fibroblast growth factor; IGF-II, insulin-like growth factor II; KGF, keratinocyte growth factor; TGF-β, transforming growth factor beta; TGF-α, transforming growth factor alpha; EGF, epidermal growth factor.*

in benign prostatic hyperplasia, the fibroblast growth factors tend to override the transforming growth factor alphas and there is therefore a proliferation of epithelial and stromal cells and, in addition, because of the effect on extracellular matrix components, an increased activity there as well.

If one assumes that this hypothesis is true, there is still a need to identify the cause of the changes outlined above. It has been suggested that declining androgen levels could account for the increasing expression of transforming growth factor alpha,[66] but that would not explain the localized nature of the disease process. An alternative explanation is that repeated microtrauma or inflammation produced by repeated (lifelong) voiding and ejaculation, acting, as they do, on the point of angulation of the prostatic urethra, which is where the transition zone is situated, leads to cell damage at that site, which in turn leads to the release of basic fibroblast growth factor, which starts the whole process off.

Whether or not the details given above and the hypothesis outlined in the last few paragraphs prove ultimately to be true, it is quite clear that benign prostatic hyperplasia is not a diffuse generalized disease of glandular epithelium due to androgen imbalance within the glandular epithelium or due to an altered androgen:oestrogen ratio. It is a focal, stromal-induced disease affecting the transition and periurethral zones, producing micronodule formation by a stromal–epithelial interaction that appears to be mediated by growth factors. Androgen appears to act through transforming growth factor alpha expression to regulate the expression of other growth factors. The micronodules enlarge and coalesce, perhaps with an altered balance between cell growth and programmed cell death, which is also mediated by growth factor activity. This, in turn, produces an effect on the prostatic urethra, possibly by distortion, to produce bladder outflow obstruction. This, however, is only one of the symptom complexes found in ageing patients who have histological benign prostatic hyperplasia, and in some, non-obstructive benign prostatic hyperplasia may well produce symptoms by means that are not entirely clear. Others, possibly as a result of a 'vascular accident' within the prostate, or otherwise due to sympathetic stimulation or superadded obstruction by external compression in constipation, or by epithelial oedema in urinary infection, develop acute retention. Others develop detrusor instability as a consequence of the secondary changes induced by obstruction in the detrusor cells, although many patients with benign prostatic hyperplasia will have detrusor instability coincidentally as a result of this. Still others, possibly as a result of the coincidence of benign prostatic hyperplasia in conjunction with the impaired detrusor contractility that is commonly seen with the ageing bladder, develop detrusor decompensation and the symptom complex that leads ultimately to chronic retention and overflow incontinence. In some of these patients, the obstructive element causes high intravesical pressures, leading to structural and functional abnormalities of the upper urinary tract and thus to renal impairment and renal failure.

It should again be stated that some of the changes outlined in the last paragraph are hypothetical and unproven, but are nonetheless more likely to be accurate than the rather simplistic ideas hitherto promulgated on the basis of 'prostatic enlargement', 'urethral compression' and 'obstruction' leading to 'prostatism'.

Urodynamic aspects

It has already been suggested that benign prostatic hyperplasia may be asymptomatic or symptomatic, and that symptoms may arise purely and simply from the condition itself by virtue of its effects on the prostate alone or from its secondary obstructive effect on the prostatic urethra. Mention has been made of the secondary effects that obstruction can have on the previously normal bladder, leading to detrusor instability, and on the ageing bladder, hastening the process begun by ageing and leading through progressive degrees of detrusor decompensation to chronic retention with overflow; and that in the latter category high intravesical pressures can lead to obstructive changes in the upper tracts leading ultimately to renal failure. Also mentioned have been those factors that can act in benign prostatic hyperplasia to cause acute retention.

Symptom severity, which is increasingly being defined by symptom scores,[67–69] can be used as selection criteria for surgery. When symptom scores are high, 90% of men will experience substantial improvement in symptoms after surgery, even in the absence of proven urodynamic obstruction.[70,71] In addition, the symptoms of benign prostatic hyperplasia in obstructed patients seem to be relieved by thermotherapy and other recent 'alternative treatments' for this condition without any effect on flow.[72]

Urinary symptoms may equally be the result of detrusor instability that has developed as a consequence of obstruction, in which case the patient may have both obstructive and irritative symptoms, and they might equally be relieved by transurethral resection of the prostate if relief of the obstruction causes the detrusor to return to normal function.

Unfortunately, those same urinary symptoms may occur as a result of 'idiopathic' detrusor instability that the patient has developed for some entirely different reason, and the fact that he might coincidentally have histological benign prostatic hyperplasia is irrelevant. Such a patient will not benefit from transurethral resection of the prostate because the instability will persist.

Similarly, a patient with a poorly contractile bladder may have it in association with, or even, perhaps, as a consequence of, outflow obstruction due to benign prostatic hyperplasia and might therefore benefit from transurethral resection of the prostate. But, equally, the poorly contractile bladder may be an age-related phenomenon and coincidental benign prostatic hyperplasia may not be causing any symptoms, in which case transurethral resection of the prostate would not be helpful.[73,74]

Clearly, therefore, benign prostatic hyperplasia is not always obstructive but may nonetheless cause symptoms, generally of an irritative nature, and, equally, those symptoms may occur for other reasons than benign prostatic hyperplasia, generally arising in the bladder smooth muscle as an age-related or other phenomenon causing detrusor instability or impaired detrusor contractility or a combination of the two.

Somehow, these different phenomena have to be dissected out to determine the cause of a patient's symptoms and to decide how best to treat him; and urodynamic studies of various different types are the means by which this is done in clinical practice.

Historically, only bladder outflow obstruction was considered of any significance. Indeed, 50 years ago, treatment was only considered in the presence of urinary retention or when there was evidence of impaired function of the upper urinary tract and kidneys. More recently, detrusor instability has been recognized as an entity, but even so, detrusor instability and bladder decompensation leading to chronic retention and overflow incontinence were both thought of only as consequences of obstruction rather than conditions that might arise per se. Irritative symptoms in the absence of obstructive instability were largely ignored. It is only the recent interest in symptom scores, in alternative treatments for benign prostatic hyperplasia that reduce symptoms without any effect on urodynamic variables, and in the effect of ageing on the bladder that has led to a reconsideration of this historical attitude. Nonetheless, the attitude that only obstruction mattered has established the primacy of the pressure–flow relationship in the objective assessment of benign prostatic hyperplasia in clinical practice.

Urinary obstruction can be regarded as being present when intravesical pressure has to be raised in order to maintain the urinary flow rate. When an elevated intravesical pressure can no longer maintain the urinary flow rate, the flow rate begins to decline. Thus, in the first stage of obstruction, voiding detrusor pressure is raised above the upper limit of normal (which is about 50 cmH_2O), but the peak urinary flow rate is still greater than 15 ml/s, which is the lower limit of normal. In the second stage of obstruction, the peak urinary flow rate drops below 15 ml/s.

This relationship between pressure and flow was likened by Griffiths[75] to the Hill equation, which was a well-established and widely accepted means of describing the relationship between the force of contraction and the speed of shortening of skeletal muscle. Griffiths, by relating detrusor pressure to flow rate in what he called the 'bladder output relation', showed that the two relationships were very similar. He also introduced the concept of the 'urethral resistance relationship' by relating flow rate to detrusor pressure throughout the period of a voiding detrusor contraction.[76] In this way, he was able to distinguish graphically (Figure 19.11) between an obstructed system, in which pressure was high and flow was low, and an unobstructed system, in which pressure was low and flow was high. In practice, rather than plot the continuous relationship graphically, Abrams and Griffiths[77] devised a nomogram on which could be plotted the single point of detrusor pressure at maximum urinary flow rate (Figure 19.12). Several other physicists, notably Schafer, have devised more sophisticated techniques for the analysis of pressure–flow data, but they are all based on the same principles.[78,79]

The two main reasons why physicists are continuing to analyse this pressure–flow relationship are, firstly, to be able to express it in a single term rather

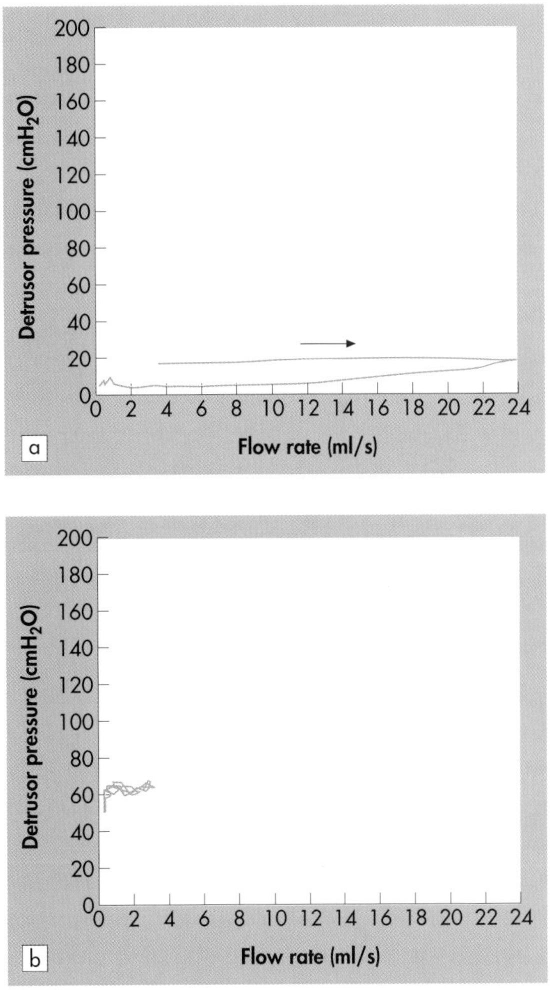

Figure 19.11 *(a) A dynamic pressure–flow plot during voiding to illustrate normal emptying with low pressure and high flow. (b) A dynamic pressure–flow plot of so-called compressive bladder outflow obstruction due to benign prostatic hyperplasia – with high pressure and low flow.*

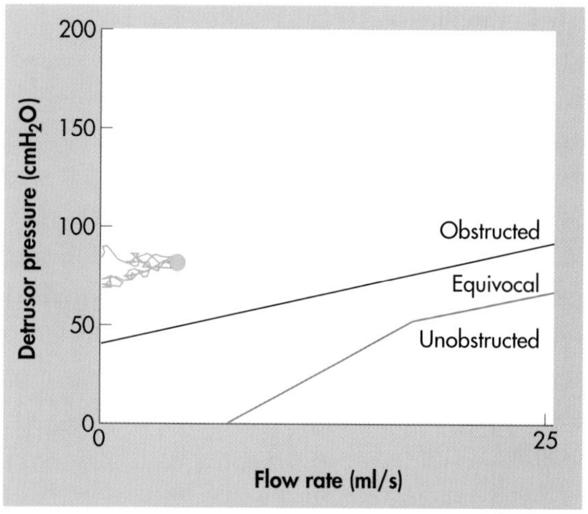

Figure 19.12 *An obstructive pressure–flow plot, similar to Figure 17.11b, superimposed on the Abrams–Griffiths nomogram. Normally, only the detrusor pressure at maximum flow (the dot) would be marked on the plot – this figure illustrates the principle.*

than as a relationship between two variables, particularly if this could be determined non-invasively, and, secondly, to minimize the equivocal zone.

The desire to find a non-invasive way of extrapolating the pressure–flow relationship is obviously commendable but has so far been unsuccessful. Nonetheless, in the interests of patient comfort and as it is a quick, simple, cheap and easy test to use, the problem has been circumvented in routine clinical practice by measuring flow rate alone and by inferring the pressure–flow relationship from this measurement.[77] In this way, most unobstructed patients with normal flow rates can be saved from ineffective and inappropriate obstruction-relieving surgery. Unfortunately, a low flow rate is not exclusively due to high pressure–low flow outflow obstruction; a low flow rate may also be due to a poorly contracting detrusor.

Poor detrusor contractility also accounts for most of the equivocal results on pressure–flow analysis. Poor detrusor contractility characteristically shows normal or low detrusor pressure and low flow, and this is very common, with an incidence that increases with age. Indeed, as a general rule, all men over the age of 80 have a maximum flow rate of less than 10 ml/s.[80]

Thus, we appear to have three independent variables determining the clinical picture – symptoms, benign prostatic hyperplasia and bladder outflow obstruction – each of which, as has been said, may be confounded by two age-related abnormalities of detrusor contractility – impaired detrusor contractility and detrusor instability. Irritative symptoms in men with or without benign prostatic hyperplasia correlate strongly with the presence of detrusor instability on urodynamic evaluation,[81] and this presumably accounts, at least in part, for the observation that symptom scores are the same in an unselected population of elderly women (in whom detrusor instability is equally common) as they are in an unselected population of elderly men.[82] By contrast, objectively demonstrable obstruction correlates poorly with symptoms,[83] presumably because obstructive symptoms are less 'bothersome', although those with bothersome obstructive symptoms who have objectively demonstrable obstruction, rather than low pressure–low flow bladders due to impaired detrusor contractility, do best after transurethral resection of the prostate.[84]

Detrusor instability is clearly an important factor in the patient with benign prostatic hyperplasia, whether it is a secondary consequence of obstruction or coincidental. Nocturia and daytime urgency and frequency are the commonest reasons why elderly men seek medical attention,[85] and although there are other causes of these symptoms, detrusor instability is the commonest reason for all these symptoms being present together.

It is generally thought that most instances of detrusor instability in patients with benign prostatic hyperplasia are secondary to obstruction, and that 70% or so will improve symptomatically after transurethral resection of the prostate because the obstruction has been relieved, allowing the detrusor to recover and the pathophysiological changes to reverse. Various experimental studies support this view,[86] although they have failed to show complete recovery after relief of obstruction, only a tendency to improve. The alternative view is that detrusor instability in these patients is an entirely age-related phenomenon in both sexes that coincidentally develops at the same time as benign prostatic hyperplasia in men, and that the reason why so many men improve after transurethral resection of the prostate is related to denervation (or de-afferentation, to be more accurate) produced by this surgical procedure.[87,88]

Impaired detrusor contractility is more problematic. Like detrusor instability, this is common in the elderly of both sexes and is a regular cause of dissatisfaction in male patients who have undergone transurethral resection of the prostate because they were thought to be obstructed.[89] Unlike detrusor instability, which regularly seems to resolve after this operation, impaired detrusor contractility rarely, if ever, improves. This is the first reason for suggesting that impaired detrusor contractility is an independent age-related condition rather than secondary to obstruction, as has always been assumed. The second reason is that experimental models of obstruction cause a thick-walled, trabeculated, high-pressure, unstable bladder, and not chronic retention.[90] Thus, the view that impaired contractility – causing residual urine initially, progressing eventually to chronic retention with overflow incontinence – arises as a result of decompensation of the detrusor in the face of continuing obstruction after an initial phase of compensation seems flawed. It may be that if obstruction is superimposed on impaired detrusor contractility, the consequences are correspondingly more severe, and it may be that these patients are prone to high-pressure retention and renal impairment as a result. Either way, impaired detrusor contractility is common in elderly men and women, and may be complicated by superadded detrusor instability in some,[91] suggesting that in many, if not all, males with benign prostatic hyperplasia, impaired contractility is an independent variable unrelated to obstruction in its cause.

And so the diagnostic quandary persists. Obstruction is still the only problem that can reliably and predictably be treated, and urodynamic studies that measure both detrusor pressure and urinary flow during voiding are still the only way to diagnose obstruction reliably. With a clinical problem that is so common, this poses logistic problems and, as obstruction is only one part of the picture, the problems are compounded. Nonetheless, a normal flow rate will virtually exclude obstruction, and such patients might be treated by any of the various non-surgical treatments currently available and discussed in detail elsewhere. Otherwise, these patients might benefit from simple reassurance and discussion. Those with a reduced flow rate and a little or no residual urine can confidently be diagnosed as obstructed and treated accordingly. Those with a substantial residual urine volume (250 ml or more on repeated assessment) may have an obstructive component to their symptoms but are more likely to have impaired detrusor contractility, and the likelihood of this increases as the residual urine volume and the patient's age increase, and the likelihood that transurethral resection of the prostate will help these patients symptomatically or objectively decreases accordingly. There are various caveats to these generalizations, but at least they form a basis for considering the problems in clinical practice.

REFERENCES

1. Lowsley O. The development of the human prostate gland with reference to the development of other structures at the neck of the urinary bladder. Am J Anat 1912; 13: 299–346
2. McNeal JE. The zonal anatomy of the prostate. Prostate 1981; 2: 35–49
3. McNeal JE. The prostate gland: morphology and pathology. Monogr Urol 1983; 4: 3–6
4. McNeal JE. The prostate gland: morphology and pathobiology. Monogr Urol 1988; 9: 3–4
5. McNeal JE. Normal histology of the prostate. Am J Surg Pathol 1988; 12: 619–633
6. Gormley G, Stoner E, Bruskewitz R, et al. The effect of finasteride in men with benign prostatic hyperplasia. N Engl J Med 1992; 327: 1185–1191
7. Wilson J, Griffin J, Russell D. Steroid five alpha reductase (II) deficiency. Endocr Rev 1993; 14: 577–593
8. Schweikert H, Totzauer P, Rohr H, Bartschi G. Correlated biochemical and stereological studies on testosterone metabolism in the stromal and epithelial compartment of human benign prostatic hyperplasia. J Urol 1985; 134: 403–407
9. Camps JL, Chang SM, Hsu TC, Freeman MR et al. Fibroblast-mediated acceleration of human epithelial tumour growth in vivo. Proc Natl Acad Sci USA 1990; 87: 75–79
10. Cunha GR, Battle E, Young P, Brody J et al. Role of epithelial–mesenchymal interactions in the differentiation and spacial organisation of visceral smooth muscle. Epithelial Cell Biol 1992; 1: 76–83
11. Bruchovski N, Lesser B, Van Doorn E, Craven S. Hormonal effects of cell proliferation in rat prostate. Vitam Horm 1975; 33: 61–102

12. Lee C, Sensibar JA, Dudek SM, Hiipakka RA, Liao ST. Prostatic ductal system in rats: regional variation in morphological and functional activities. Biol Reprod 1990; 43: 1079–1086
13. Begun FP, Story MT, Hopp KA, Shapiro E, Lawson RK. Regional concentration of basic fibroblast growth factor in normal and benign hyperplastic human prostates. J Urol 1995; 153: 839–843
14. Story MT, Hopp KA, Meier DA, Begun FP, Lawson RK. Influence of transforming growth factor beta 1 and other growth factors on basic fibroblast growth factor level and proliferation of cultured human prostate-derived fibroblasts. Prostate 1993; 22: 183–197
15. Taylor TB, Ramsdell JS. Transforming growth factor alpha and its receptor are expressed on the epithelium of the rat prostate gland. Endocrinology 1993; 113: 1306–1308
16. Gosling JA, Dixon DS. The structure and innervation of smooth muscle in the wall of the bladder neck and proximal urethra. Br J Urol 1975; 47: 549–552
17. Hedlund H, Anderson K, Larsson B. Alpha adrenoceptors and muscarinic receptors in the isolated human prostate. J Urol 1985; 134: 1291–1293
18. Bartsch G, Muller H, Oberholzer M, Rohr H. Light microscopic and stereological analysis of the normal human prostate and of benign prostatic hyperplasia. J Urol 1979; 122: 487–491
19. Shapiro E, Hartanto V, Lepor H. The response to alpha blockade in benign prostatic hyperplasia is related to the percent area density of prostate smooth muscle. Prostate 1992; 21: 297–307
20. Bylund DB, Eikenberg DC, Hieble JP, Langer SZ et al. International Union of Pharmacology nomenclature of adrenoceptors. Pharmacol Rev 1994; 46: 121–136
21. Forray C, Bard JA, Wetzel JM, Chiu G et al. The alpha-1 adrenergic receptor that mediates smooth muscle contraction in the human prostate has the pharmacological properties of the cloned human alpha-1c subtype. Mol Pharmacol 1994; 45: 703–709
22. Gu J, Polak JM, Probert L, Islam KN et al. Peptidergic innervation of the human male genital tract. J Urol 1983; 130: 386–391
23. Lieberman C, Nogimori T, Wu CF, Van Buren T et al. TRH pharmacokinetics and nerve stimulation evoked prostatic fluid secretion during TRH infusion in the dog. Acta Endocrinol (Copenh) 1989; 120: 134–142
24. Crowe R, Chapple C, Burnstock G. The human prostate gland: a histochemical and immunohistochemical study of neuropeptides, serotonin, dopamine beta hydroxylase and acetylcholinesterase in autonomic nerves and ganglia. Br J Urol 1991; 68: 53–61
25. Brindley G. Pathophysiology of erection and ejaculation. In: Hendry W, Whitfield H, eds. A Textbook of Genitourinary Surgery. London: Churchill Livingstone, 1988: 1083–1094
26. Gil-Vernet J, Alvarez-Vijande R, Gil-Vernet J Jr. Ejaculation in men: a dynamic endorectal ultrasonographical study. Br J Urol 1994; 73: 442–448
27. Tauber PF, Zaneveld LJD, Propping D, Schumacher GF. Components of human split ejaculate. J Reprod Fertil 1975; 43: 249–267
28. Kennedy AM, Morrell JM, Siviter RJ, Cockle SM. Fertilisation promoting peptide in reproductive tissues and semen of the male marmoset. Mol Reprod Dev 1997; 47: 113–119
29. Williams-Ashman HG, Cannellakis ZN. Polyamines in mammalian biology and medicine. Perspect Biol Med 1979; 22: 421–453
30. Lilja H. Structure and function of prostatic and seminal vesicle-secreted proteins involved in the gelatin and liquefaction of human semen. Scand J Lab Invest 1988; 48 (Suppl): 13–17
31. Coffey DS. Physiology of male reproduction: the biochemical and physiology of the prostate and seminal vesicles. In: Harrison JH, Gittes RF, Perlmutter AD et al, eds. Campbell's Urology, Vol. 1. 4th edn. Philadelphia: WB Saunders, 1978: 61–94
32. Fair WR, Wehner N. The prostatic antibacterial factor: identity and significance. In: Marberger H, ed. Prostatic Disease, Vol. 6. New York: Alan R Liss, 1976: 383
33. Grayhack JT, Kropp KA. Changes with aging in prostatic fluid: citric acid and phosphatase and lactic dehydrogenase concentration in man. J Urol 1965; 56: 6–11
34. Kvist U. Reversible inhibition of nuclear chromatin decondensation (NCD) ability of human spermatozoa induced by prostatic fluid. Acta Physiol Scand 1980; 109: 73–78
35. Kvist U. Importance of spermatozoal zinc as temporary inhibitor of sperm nuclear chromatin decondensation ability in man. Acta Physiol Scand 1980; 109: 79–84
36. Kvist U, Kjellberg J, Bjorndahl L, Santir JC, Arver S. Seminal fluid from men with agenesis of the Wolffian ducts: zinc binding properties and effects on sperm chromatin stability. Int J Androl 1990; 13: 245–252
37. Greenwald P, Kirmes V, Polan A, Dick V. Cancer of

the prostate among men with BPH. J Natl Cancer Inst 1974; 355: 53–56
38. Carter H, Plantadosi S, Isaacs J. Clinical evidence for and implications of the multistep development of prostate cancer. J Urol 1990; 143: 742–746
39. Spiro L, Labay G, Orkin L. Prostatic infarction: role in acute urinary retention. Urology 1974; 3: 345–347
40. Cuchi A. The development of detrusor instability in prostatic obstruction in relation to sequential changes in voiding dynamics. J Urol 1994; 51: 1342–1344
41. Levin RM, Longhurst PA, Monson FC, Kato K, Wein AJ. Effect of bladder outlet obstruction on the morphology, physiology and pharmacology of the bladder. Prostate 1990; 3 (Suppl): 9–26
42. Glynn R, Campion E, Bouchard G, Silbert J. The development of benign prostatic hyperplasia among volunteers in the normative aging study. Am J Epidemiol 1985; 121: 78–90
43. Adlercreutz H. Western diet and Western diseases: some hormonal and biochemical mechanisms and associations. Scand J Clin Invest 1990; 50 (Suppl): 3–23
44. Sanda M, Beatty T, Stautzman R. Genetic susceptibility of benign prostatic hyperplasia. J Urol 1994; 151: 115–119
45. Cunha GR, Battle E, Young P, Brody J et al. Role of epithelial– mesenchymal interactions in the differentiation and spatial organisation of visceral smooth muscle. Epithelial Cell Biol 1992; 1: 76–83
46. McNeal JE. Origin and evolution of benign prostatic enlargement. Investig Urol 1978; 15: 340–345
47. Eble JN, Tejada E. Prostatic stromal hyperplasia with bizarre nuclei. Arch Pathol Lab Med 1991; 115: 87–89
48. Leong SS, Vogt PF, Yu GM. Atypical stroma with muscle hyperplasia of the prostate. Urology 1988; 31: 163–167
49. McNeal JE. The pathobiology of nodular hyperplasia. In: Bostwick DG, ed. Pathology of the prostate. New York: Churchill Livingstone, 1990: 31–36
50. Franks LM. Benign nodular hyperplasia of the prostate: a review. Ann R Coll Surg Engl 1954; 14: 92–106
51. Partin AW, Oesterling JE, Epstein JI, Horton R, Walsh PC. Influence of age and endocrine factors on the volume of benign prostatic hyperplasia. J Urol 1991; 145: 405–409
52. Isaacs JT. Antagonistic effect of androgen on prostatic cell death. Prostate 1984; 5: 545–547
53. Sensibar JA, Griswold MD, Sylvester SR, Buttyan R et al. Prostatic ductal system in rats: regional variation in localisation of an androgen-repressed gene product, sulphated glycoprotein-2. Endocrinology 1991; 128: 2091–2102
54. Steiner MS. Review of peptide growth factors in benign prostatic hyperplasia and urological malignancy. J Urol 1995; 153: 1085–1096
55. Gregory H, Willshire IR, Kavanagh JP, Blacklock NJ, Chowdury S, Richards RC. Urogastrone-epidermal growth factor concentrations in prostatic fluid of normal individuals and patients with benign prostatic hypertrophy. Clin Sci 1986; 70: 359–363
56. Folkman J, Klagsbrun M, Sasse J, Wadzinski M, Inger D, Vlodavsky I. Heparin-binding angiogenic protein – basic fibroblast growth factor – is stored within the basement membrane. Am J Pathol 1988; 130: 393–400
57. Ku PT, D'amore P. Regulation of fibroblast growth factor (bFGF) gene and protein expression following its release from sublethally injured endothelial cells. J Cell Biochem 1995; 58: 328–343
58. Yan G, Fukaborvi Y, Nikolaropoulos S, Wang F, McKeehan WL. Heparin-binding keratinocyte growth factor is a candidate for stromal to epithelial andromedin. Mol Endocrinol 1992; 6: 2123–2128
59. Yan G, Fukabori Y, McBride G, Nikolaropolous S, McKeehan WL. Exon switching and activation of stromal and embryonic fibroblast growth factor (FGF)–FGF-receptor genes in prostate epithelial cells accompany stromal independence and malignancy. Mol Cell Biol 1993; 13: 4513–4522
60. Sporn MB, Roberts AB. TFT-beta: problems and prospects. Cell Regul 1990; 1: 875–882
61. Brogli E, Wu T, Namiki A, Isner JM. Indirect angiogenic cytokines upregulate VEGF and bFGF gene expression in vascular smooth muscle cells, whereas hypoxia upregulates VEGF expression only. Circulation 1994; 90: 649–652
62. Roberts AB, Sporn MB. Physiological actions and clinical applications of transforming growth factor-beta (TGF-β). Growth Factors 1993; 8: 1–9
63. Timme TL, Truong LD, Merz VW, Krebs T et al. Mesenchymal epithelial interactions and transforming growth factor beta expression during mouse prostate morphogenesis. Endocrinology 1994; 134: 1039–1045
64. Millan FA, Denhez F, Kondaiah P, Akhurst RJ. Embryonic gene expression patterns of TGF beta-1, beta-2 and beta-3 suggest different development functions in vivo. Development 1991; 111: 131–143
65. Sporn MB, Roberts AB. Interactions of retinoids and transforming growth factor beta in regulation of cell

differentiation and proliferation. Mol Endocrinol 1991; 5: 3–7
66. Katz AE, Benson MC, Wise GJ, Olsson CA et al. Gene activity during the early phase of androgen-stimulated rat prostatic regrowth. Cancer Res 1989; 49: 5889–5894
67. Boyarski S, Jones G, Paulson DF, Prout GR. A new look at bladder neck obstruction by the Food and Drug Administration regulators: guidelines for the investigation of benign prostatic hypertrophy. Trans Am Assoc Genitourin Surg 1977; 68: 29–32
68. Madsen PO, Iversen P. A point system for selecting operative candidates. In: Hinman F Jr, ed. Benign prostatic hypertrophy. New York: Springer-Verlag, 1983: 763–765
69. Barry MJ, Fowler FJ, O'Leary MP, Bruskewitz RC et al. The American Urological Association symptom index for benign prostatic hyperplasia. J Urol 1992; 148: 1549–1557
70. McConnell JD, Barry MJ, Bruskewitz RC et al. Benign prostatic hyperplasia: diagnosis and treatment. In: Clinical Practice Guidelines, No. 8. Rockville, MD: US Department of Health and Human Services, 1994: 99–103
71. Emberton M, Neal DE, Black N, Fordham M et al. The effect of prostatectomy on symptom severity and quality of life. Br J Urol 1996; 77: 233–247
72. Tubaro A, Ogden C, de la Rosette J, et al. The prediction of clinical outcome from thermotherapy by pressure flow study. Results of a European multicentre study. World J Urol 1994; 12: 352–356
73. Neal DE, Styles RA, Powell PH, Ramsden PD. Relationships between detrusor function and residual urine in men undergoing prostatectomy. Br J Urol 1987; 60: 560–566
74. George NJR, Feneley RCL, Roberts JBM. Identification of the poor risk patient with prostatism and detrusor failure. Br J Urol 1986; 58: 290–295
75. Griffiths DJ. Urodynamics: the mechanics and hydrodynamics of the lower urinary tract. Medical Physics Handbook 4. Bristol: Adam Hilger, 1980
76. Griffiths DJ. Urethral resistance to flow: the urethral resistance relation. Urol Int 1975; 30: 28
77. Abrams PH, Griffiths DJ. The assessment of prostatic obstruction from urodynamic measurements and from residual urine. Br J Urol 1979; 51: 129–134
78. Van Mastrigt R, Rollema HJ. Urethral resistance and urinary bladder contractility before and after transurethral resection as determined by the computer program CLIM. Neurourol Urodyn 1988; 7: 226–230
79. Schafer W. Principles and clinical application of advanced urodynamic analysis of voiding function. Urol Clin North Am 1990; 17: 553–566
80. Jorgensen JB, Jensen KME, Morgensen P. Age-related variation in urinary flow variables and flow cure patterns in elderly males. Br J Urol 1992; 69: 265–271
81. Olssen CA, Goluboft ET, Chang DT, Kaplan SA. Urodynamics and the etiology of post-prostatectomy incontinence. J Urol 1994; 151: 2063–2065
82. Lepor H, Machi G. Comparison of AUA symptom index in unselected males and females between fifty-five and seventy-nine years of age. Urology 1993; 42: 36–40
83. Barry MJ, Cockett ATK, Holtgrewe HL, McConnell JD et al. Relationship of symptoms of prostatism to commonly used physiological and anatomical measures of the severity of benign prostatic hyperplasia. J Urol 1993; 150: 351–356
84. Abrams P. In support of pressure flow studies for evaluating men with lower urinary tract symptoms. Urology 1994; 44: 153–155
85. Roberts RO, Rhodes T, Panser LA. Natural history of prostatism: worry and embarrassment of firm urinary symptoms and health care-seeking behaviour. Urology 1994; 43: 621–628
86. Malkowiez SB, Wein AJ, Elbadawi A, Van Arsdalen K, Ruggieri MR, Levin RM et al. Acute biochemical and functional alterations in the partially obstructed rabbit urinary bladder. J Urol 1986; 136: 1324–1329
87. Susset JG. The effect of aging and prostatic obstruction on detrusor morphology and function. In: Hinman C, ed. Benign Prostatic Hypertrophy. New York: Springer Verlag, 1985: 653–665
88. Luutzeyer W, Hannapel J, Schafer W. Sequential events in prostatic obstruction. In: Hinman C, ed. Benign Prostatic Hypertrophy. New York: Springer Verlag, 1985: 693–700
89. Schafer W, Rubben H, Noppeney R, Deutz FJ. Obstructed and unobstructed prostatic obstruction. A plea for urodynamic objectivation of bladder outflow obstruction in benign prostatic hyperplasia. World J Urol 1989; 6: 198–203
90. Dixon JS, Gilpin CJ, Gilpin SA, Gosling JA, Brading AF, Speakman MJ. Sequential morphologic changes in the pig detrusor in response to chronic partial urethral obstruction. Br J Urol 1989; 64: 385–390
91. Coolsaet BRLA, Blok C. Detrusor properties related to prostatism. Neurourol Urodyn 1986; 5: 435–441

20

Biology of cancer and metastasis

David E Neal

CANCER

An understanding of cancer is important to the urologist, not only because it is common, but also because its study provides insight into normal and abnormal cellular function. One in five adults die of cancer (Tables 20.1 and 20.2) and about 30–50% of common, solid epithelial tumours are advanced and incurable when first detected clinically. So far as urological tumours are concerned, prostate, bladder and kidney cancers are common, and while testis cancer is rare, it is important because, even when advanced, it is frequently curable and because it occurs in young men with an otherwise full life-expectancy.

It is thought that every individual cancer arises from a single cell following a set of genetically determined events. The evidence for this monoclonal origin lies in findings, firstly, that all cells in a tumour often contain specific point mutations in genes which would be unlikely to arise by chance in several cells, and, secondly, that in women, in whom one X chromosome is inactivated in a mosaic and apparently random fashion throughout the body, one particular X chromosome is inactivated throughout the tumour.

Table 20.1 Common causes of human cancer.

- ionising radiation (haematopoietic cells, bone)
- sunlight (malignant melanoma, squamous cell carcinoma of the skin)
- familial genetic causes (certain types of breast, colon, kidney and prostate cancer)
- familial cancer predispositions due to altered activity in detoxifying or activating enzymes such as *N*-acetyltransferase 2 and glutathione transferase M (bladder, lung and colon cancer)
- chemicals from occupations and smoking (bladder, larynx and lung cancer)
- chronic inflammation (squamous cell carcinoma arising in a chronic ulcer, schistosomal bladder cancer, tumours in ulcerative colitis and adenocarcinoma arising in Barrett oesophagus)
- viral infection: *DNA viruses*: penile and cervical cancer (papovavirus), liver cancer (Hep B and C), Epstein-Barr virus (Burkitt's lymphoma, nasopharyngeal cancer); *RNA viruses*: human T-cell leukaemia (HTLV–1), Kaposi's sarcoma (HIV-1).

CHEMICAL CARCINOGENESIS

Many different chemicals have been shown to be carcinogenic (Table 20.3). The best known historical example is that of scrotal cancer, in which Percival Pott demonstrated through epidemiological observations that boys who had been employed as chimney sweeps were likely to develop this disease as adults. He hypothesized that chemicals in soot caused the problem. Tobacco use (mainly cigarette smoking) was later shown to be clearly associated with cancers of the mouth, larynx, trachea, lung, kidney and bladder.

Further evidence of a chemical cause for bladder cancer was found by Rehn in 1894 when he recorded a series of tumours occurring in workers in aniline dye factories. Huepner was subsequently able to show that 2-naphthylamine was carcinogenic in dogs, and further investigation demonstrated that a variety of chemicals may be carcinogenic.

Common factors in most human cancers include damage to several genes (rather than one) resulting from mutations, insertions or deletions in certain genes known as oncogenes or tumour-suppressor genes.

Table 20.2 Cancer incidence and death in the USA.

Type of cancer	New cases per year	%	Deaths per year	%
Total	1 170 000	100	528 300	100
Mouth and pharynx	29 800	3	7700	1
Colon and rectum	152 000	13	57 000	11
Stomach	24 000	2	13 600	3
Pancreas	27 700	2	25 000	5
Lung	170 000	15	149 000	28
Breast	183 000	16	46 300	9
Malignant melanoma	32 000	3	6800	1
Prostate	185 000	14	35 000	7
Ovary	22 000	2	13 300	3
Cervix	13 500	1	4400	1
Uterus	31 000	3	5700	1
Bladder	52 300	4	9900	2
Kidney	21 200		8300	
Haematopoietic	93 000	8	50 000	9
CNS	18 250	2	12 350	2
Testis	5100		210	
Sarcomas	8000	1	4150	1

Occupations which have been reported to have a significantly excess risk of bladder cancer are shown in Table 20.4.

Historically, chemicals have been classified into those which produced mutations in DNA on first application (initiators), but which of themselves were usually insufficient to cause cancer unless there was further exposure to the initiator or unless initiator application was followed by a promoter. These compounds do not cause cancer, however often they are applied, but they will cause the development of cancer when there has been previous applications of an initiator. Promoters include chemicals such as phorbol esters, which stimulate protein kinase C (PKC). PKC phosphorylates several proteins on serine and threonine residues and activates MAP kinase, which is also activated by the ras pathway (see later under *ras*).

Most carcinogens are genotoxic and cause damage to DNA. It is thought that there is also a class of non-genotoxic carcinogens which, in mice, cause peroxisome proliferation, and which may activate agents which interfere with the cell cycle or apoptosis. It is uncertain whether this mechanism is active in man.

GENETIC POLYMORPHISMS

Many genotoxic carcinogens are inactive and require to be converted into active agents by acetylation or hydroxylation (Figure 20.1). Mammalian cells have developed a complex system for detoxifying external biologically active chemicals known as xenobiotics. These enzymes, which also detoxify drugs and carcinogens, include:

- hydroxylation by means of the cytochrome P450 system (CYP) which are found on the microsomal fraction of cells (mainly in the liver)
- Glutathione transferase, which couples glutathione to water-insoluble chemicals, and which is classified into families (α, β, μ, π)
- *N*-acetyltransferase pathway (NAT-1 and NAT-2).

Table 20.3 Compounds associated with bladder cancer.

2-Naphthylamine	Chlornaphazine	4,4′-Methylene *bis* (2-choloranliline)
4-Aminobiphenyl	4-Chloro-*o*-toluidine	Methylene dianiline
Benzidine	*o*-toluidine	Benzidine-derived azo dyes

Table 20.4 Occupations associated with bladder cancer.

Textile workers	Leather workers	Lorry drivers
Dye workers	Shoe manufacturers and cleaners	Drill press operators
Tyre rubber and cable workers	Painters	Chemical workers
Petrol workers	Hairdressers	Rodent exterminators and sewage workers

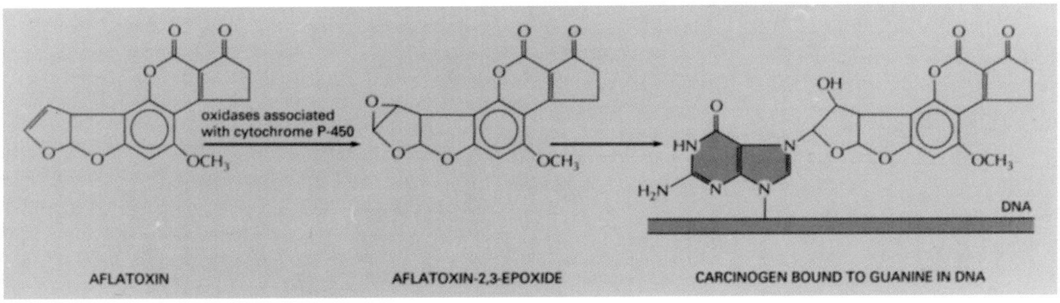

Figure 20.1 *Metabolic activation of a carcinogen. Many chemical carcinogens have to be activated by a metabolic transformation before they will cause mutations by reacting with DNA. The compound illustrated here is aflatoxin B1, a toxin made from a mould (*Aspergillus flavus oryzae*) that grows on grain and peanuts stored under humid tropical conditions. It is thought to be a contributory cause of liver cancer in the tropics and is associated with specific mutations of the* p53 *gene.*

Some individuals are more at risk than others after exposure to a carcinogen because of genetic polymorphisms. This arises because each individual carries two alleles for each gene, but within a population there may be many alleles. Some combinations will lead to an individual's having enzymes which may be more or less active than those found in other individuals. Polymorphic genes of interest in bladder cancer include *N*-acetyltransferase types 1 and 2 (NAT-1, -2), glutathione transferase M1 and π (GSTM1 and GSTπ) and several cytochrome P450s (CYP2D6: debrisoquine hydroxylase; and CYP1A1). Individuals who have high levels of NAT-2 or GSTM1 may be less likely to develop cancer after exposure to smoking because they can detoxify the mutagen, whereas those with high levels of CYP2D6 may be more likely to develop cancer because they convert inactive to active forms of the mutagen. Similarly, some individuals may be generally resistant to carcinoma formation because they have polymorphisms that produce protective compounds. It should be noted that some enzymes will have a dual effect; for instance, NAT-2 in the liver will detoxify some carcinogens, but may activate others. This explains the paradox that fast acetylators are less likely to develop bladder cancer, but may be more likely to develop colon cancer. NAT-1 is found in high levels in the bladder urothelium, and non-toxic metabolites produced by NAT-2 in the liver and excreted in the urine can be taken into the urothelial cells and converted by NAT-1 into active carcinogens that produce genotoxic damage in the bladder cell.

Cancer is a multistep process

Human cancer requires several mutations to occur before a tumour develops clinically. One reason for supporting this view is that cancer incidence increases markedly with age, and this would be unlikely if tumours simply arose from a single gene mutation. Instead, tumourigenesis would be more likely to occur randomly throughout life. Recent molecular biological studies have supported the view that cancer arises only when there has been an accumulation of several genetic events.

Cancer genes

Several tumours have a strong genetic component, including retinoblastoma (Rb gene), Wilms' tumour (WT gene), familial forms of prostate cancer (unknown gene, possibly on chromosome 1), breast cancer (BRCA1 and BRCA2 genes and mutations in p53 in Li-Fraumeni families), familial adenomatosis polyposis (*APC* gene), hereditary non-polyposis colon cancer (HNPCC) (MSH1 gene) and von Hippel-Lindau disease (VHL gene). These tumours have proven to be instructive because in most cases they appeared to be inherited clinically in a dominant fashion. Nevertheless, biochemically, these genes act in a recessive fashion because, although the disease is caused by an inherited mutation in one allele of a tumour-suppressor gene, cancer develops only when the other normal allele becomes deleted

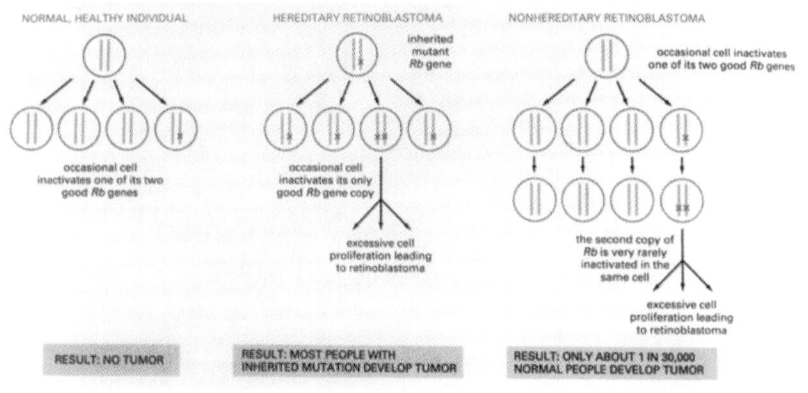

Figure 20.2 *The genetic mechanisms underlying retinoblastoma. In the hereditary form, all cells in the body lack one of the normal two functional copies of a tumour-suppressor gene, and tumours occur where the remaining copy is lost or inactivated by a somatic mutation. In the non-hereditary form, all cells initially contain two functional copies of the gene, and the tumour arises because both copies are lost or inactivated through the coincidence of two somatic mutations in one cell.*

or mutated by chance (Figure 20.2). Why tumours in such patients appear only in certain tissues is uncertain when tumour-suppressor genes are inactivated in most cells.

Other tumours can arise in patients whose DNA-repair machinery is deficient (xeroderma pigmentosa, ataxia telangiectasia and HNPCC).

DNA repair genes

Mismatch repair

Patients with HNPCC have tumours in which there are a large number of microsatellites in the genome of the tumour. Microsatellites are short (2–4 nucleotides: for example, CACA on one strand and GTGT on the other), non-coding, tandem repeats of DNA which are found throughout the genome, and which show pronounced polymorphism. Abnormalities in microsatellites have been found in Huntington's chorea, the fragile X syndrome and spinobulbar atrophy, in which, over several generations, there is a progressive expansion of the nucleotide repeats in the genes of interest. This leads to disease, but it is found that with each succeeding generation there is an increased severity of the disease because the microsatellites become longer. This phenomenon is called genetic anticipation. In HNPCC, microsatellite instability is thought to be the result of failure to correct replication errors that occur during cell division. This failure is caused by hereditary defects in the enzymes responsible for the repair of these replication mismatch errors. These enzymes include MSH2, MLH1, GTBP, PMS1 and PMS1.

Nucleotide excision repair

Abnormal nucleotide insertions can occur during DNA replication and are excised by mechanisms which are deficient in xeroderma pigmentosa.

CELLULAR CHARACTERISTICS OF CANCER

Not all features of cancer cells are caused directly by abnormal genes; some abnormalities are due to failure to regulate genetically normal genes (Table 20.5). These epigenetic events include upregulation of enzymes that can dissolve the basement membrane (such as cathepsins and plasminogen activators) and

Table 20.5 Characteristics of the transformed cell.

Plasma membrane abnormalities
Increased transmembrane transport (as for glucose and calcium)
Excessive endocytosis and blebbing
Increased mobility
Adhesion molecules
Decreased adhesion
Failure of organization of actin into stress fibres
Reduced fibronectin expression
Increased expression of enzymes such as cathepsin and plasminogen activators
Growth
Growth to high density (lack of density-dependent inhibition)
Decreased requirement for added growth factors
Anchorage-independent growth
Immortal
Can cause animal tumours

may predispose the cell to metastasize; changes in expression of cell-surface molecules (such as HLA antigens) that may allow the cancer cell to escape detection by the body's immunosurveillance; loss of molecules responsible for intercellular adherence, leading the cell to be more likely to metastasize (such as E-cadherin); upregulation of growth factors or their receptors, allowing the cell to become self-reliant (such as epidermal growth factor and its receptor, EGFr); and upregulation of molecules that detoxify anticancer drugs (such as the multitumour-suppressor gene – MDR-1).

ANGIOGENESIS

Angiogenesis is the process of new blood-vessel formation, which is found in a number of diseases, including cancer, diabetic retinopathy and the inflammatory arthritides. The initiation of angiogenesis in tumours is dependent on the coordinated expression of several factors (Table 20.6). Angiogenesis requires dilatation of vessels, breakdown of perivascular stroma, migration and proliferation of endothelial cells, and canalization of endothelial buds. Potent inhibitors of angiogenesis include angiostatin (which, paradoxically, is secreted by some primary tumours) and thrombospondin (which is involved in the binding of macrophages to apoptotic cells, and which is also upregulated by normal p53). A potent stimulus of angiogenesis is hypoxia, which upregulates the expression of vascular endothelial growth factor (VEGF). This occurs through the upregulation of the intermediate hypoxia inducible factors (HIF) (Figure 20.3).

Table 20.6 Peptides associated with angiogenesis.

- Vascular endothelial growth factor (VEGF)
- FGFs
- PDGF
- Tumour necrosis factor α
- Angiogenin
- EGF
- TGF α and TGF β
- Platelet-derived endothelial cell growth factor (PDECGF) or thymidine phosphorylase

VEGF is a specific mitogen for endothelial cells. It exists in four forms (121-, 165-, 189- and 206-aa peptides) and is secreted by a number of cell types. VEGFr, which is a tyrosine kinase, is found on endothelial cells in two forms (Flt-1 and Flk-1).

METASTASIS

This is the process by which cells from the primary tumour enter the circulation and seed elsewhere in the body to produce secondary tumours. It is the usual cause of death in cancer. It is a series of linked

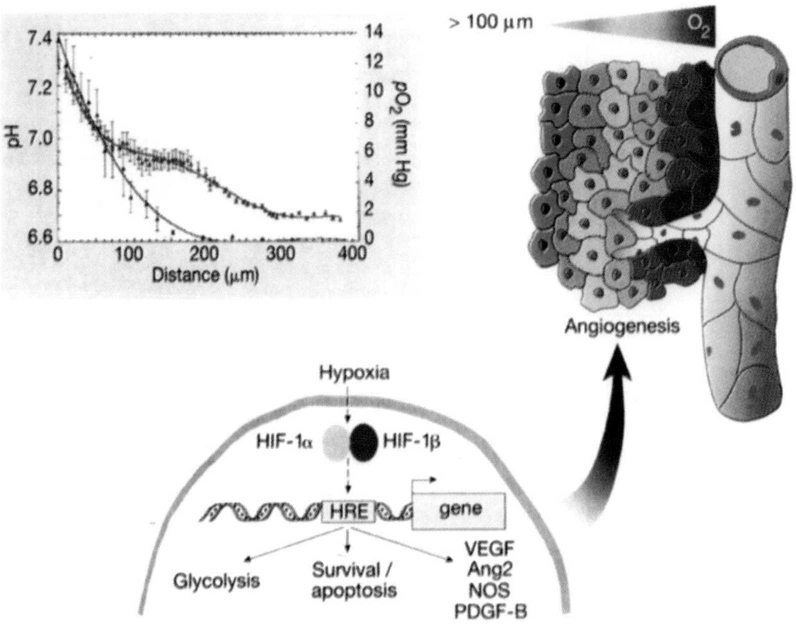

Figure 20.3 *Factors controlling angiogenesis. Hypoxia induces transcription of hypoxia inducible factors (HIF) that act on HIF-responsive elements in the promoter region of genes such as VEGF.*

processes, but it is thought that only some subclones of cells are capable of spreading. Most cells entering the circulation do not survive. There are intriguing features; some tumours have preferential sites for metastasis – the prostate or bone, for example. Experimental data have shown that subclones of cells, produced from the same tumour, may have very different capacities for metastasis (Figure 20.4). The following steps are thought to be important in metastasis:

- angiogenesis
- invasion and degradation
- altered adhesion
- migration and circulation
- tumour cell attachment
- invasion and degradation
- migration
- colonization of the secondary site.

Degradation of extracellular matrix barriers

Metastasis requires cancer cells to penetrate extracellular matrix barriers. This involves the proteolytic degradation of extracellular matrix components. Metalloproteinases (MMPs) are a family of zinc-dependent endopeptidases (gelatinases) known to degrade extracellular matrix components. Their activity is inhibited by tissue inhibitors of metalloproteinases (TIMPs). High levels of TIMP-2 immunoreactivity, detected both in tumour cells and in stroma, have been reported to be associated with cancer-specific death. This is somewhat surprising, given that TIMPs inhibit the degradation of the extracellular matrix. However, recent studies have shown that, under certain circumstances, TIMP-2 can also activate MMP-2. Other enzymes include the plasminogen activators. These enzymes may be expressed by host stromal around a tumour merely as an indicator of tissue remodelling (Figure 20.5). Hence, they have not shown consistent usefulness as prognostic markers.

Altered cell adhesion

Decreased intercellular adhesiveness favours detachment of tumour cells, and this may play a role in regression to metastatic disease. At least four families of cell adhesion molecules are thought to be involved in cell–cell adhesion (cadherins, selectins, immunoglobulins and integrins). The most widely studied have been E-cadherin, a cell-surface glycoprotein restricted to epithelial tissue, which is involved in calcium-dependent homotypic cell–cell adhesion; and the vascular cell adhesion molecules, E-selectin, vascular cell adhesion molecule-1 (VCAM-1) and intercellular adhesion molecule-1 (ICAM-1). The

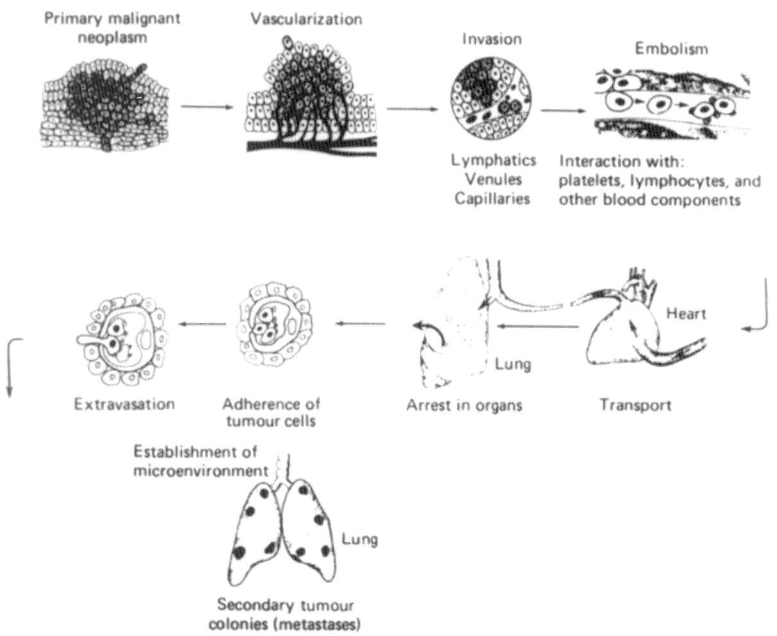

Figure 20.4 *Factors involved in metastasis.*

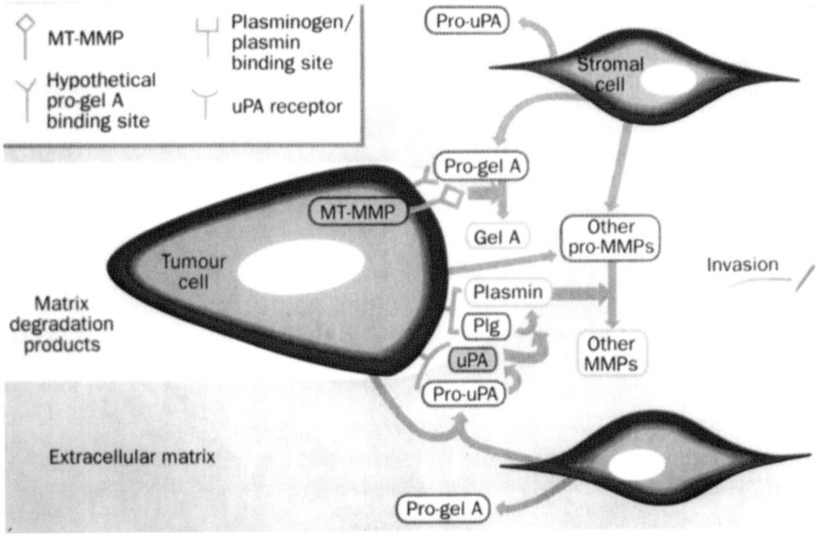

Figure 20.5 *Secretion of proteases (and their inhibitors) by tumour and stroma.*

regulation of the expression of E-cadherin on tumour cells is unclear. Post-translational modification of the protein product may affect function. It is known that three molecules (α, β and γ catenins) form bridges between the cytoplasmic tail of E-cadherin and the cytoskeleton, a bridging which may be necessary for E-cadherin to function normally.

Migration and circulation

Tumour cells have increased motility that allows them to insinuate between the components of the extracellular matrix. They then reach the basement membranes of capillaries or lymph vessels, which they lyse to enter the circulation. This process is likely to be controlled in part by the secretion of cytokines, chemokines and growth factors by tumour or stromal cells.

Attachment and colonization

Most tumour cells do not survive. From experimental studies, we know that less than 1% survive and less than 0.1% will grow and proliferate. We know that growth in animal models is far more complex than that produced by the same cells in tissue culture. Attachment of tumour cells is controlled by various factors. Shear forces at the bifurcation of vessels increase the risk that tumour cells will become attached. Certain tumours may induce the formation of distant fibrin clots that makes it more likely that tumour cells will stick. Tumour cells that possess the capacity to invade and migrate are more likely to spread in secondary sites. Capillaries, lymph vessels and veins are more susceptible than arteries to invasion by tumour cells, as they lack protease inhibitors.

The site of metastasis can be typical. For instance, bone stroma is likely to be the site of secondary spread from prostate cancer. This occurs because of the secretion of particular growth factors that encourage the survival of prostate cells. Other sites, such as the spleen, are very unlikely to be invaded by tumour cells. The immunological factors in tumour control are discussed elsewhere in the book.

ACKNOWLEDGEMENT

Artwork reproduced from Alberts B, Johnson A, Lewis J, Raff M, Roberts K, Walter P (eds), Molecular Biology of the Cell, 4th Edition, New York: Garland Science.

21

Tumour suppressor genes and oncogenes

David E Neal

ONCOGENES

What have sometimes been referred to as 'recessive oncogenes' are now more commonly called tumour suppressor genes. Many DNA viruses produce proteins that directly perturb the function of tumour suppressor genes (for example, large T antigen of SV40 binds p53 and Rb; E6 and E7 of the papilloma virus bind p53 and Rb; the E1A protein of adenovirus binds Rb).

The term 'oncogene' was originally used to describe those genes carried by viruses (most of them being retroviruses) which were found to be the cause of transmissible forms of cancer in animals. These retroviral oncogenes (v-*oncs*) were closely related to normal host cellular genes called proto-oncogenes. Cellular oncogenes found in cancer (c-*oncs*) were shown to be normal proto-oncogenes that had become 'activated' by a variety of mechanisms, including point mutations, deletion, insertional mutagenesis, translocation and overexpression – often associated with gene amplification. The initial techniques involved in identifying these genes (transfection of tumour DNA into NIH 3T3 fibroblasts) tended to select dominantly acting transforming genes, which are now generally known as 'oncogenes'.

As the number of known oncogenes increased and their functions became known, they were classified into families defined by their normal cellular counterparts. The include growth factors and their receptors, nuclear regulators of gene transcription and DNA replication, and signal transduction proteins which couple cell-surface receptors and the nucleus. More than 60 oncogenes have now been identified. The types of oncogenes and some of their functions are shown in Figure 21.1. Their transfection into cells causes transformation (Table 21.1).

A cellular proto-oncogene can be converted to an oncogene in the following ways:

- insertion of a section of DNA into the promoter region of the gene (insertional mutagenesis: for example, Wnt-1)
- deletion (conversion of EGFr to v-erbB-2)

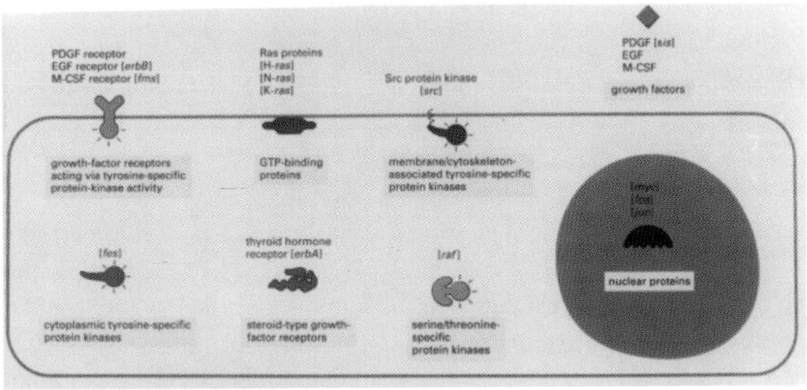

Figure 21.1 *The activities and cellular locations of the products of the main classes of known proto-oncogenes. Some representative proto-oncogenes in each class are indicated in brackets.*

Table 21.1 Some oncogenes.

Oncogene	Proto-oncogene	Source of virus	Virus-induced tumour
abl	Tyrosine kinase	Mouse	Leukaemia
erbB	Tyrosine kinase (EGFr, c-erbB2, etc.)	Chicken	Erythroleukaemia
fes	Tyrosine kinase	Cat	Sarcoma
fms	Tyrosine kinase (M-CSM factor)	Cat	Sarcoma
fos	AP-1 protein	Mouse	Osteosarcoma
jun	AP-1 protein	Chicken	Fibrosarcoma
raf (MAP kinase-kinase-kinase)	Serine kinase activated by ras	Chicken	Sarcoma
myc	Transcription factor	Chicken	Sarcoma
H-ras	GTP (G)-binding protein	Rat	Sarcoma
K-ras	G protein	Rat	Sarcoma
rel	NFκB transcription factor	Turkey	Reticuloendotheliosis
sis	Platelet-derived growth factor (PDGF)	Monkey	Sarcoma
src	Tyrosine kinase	Chicken	Sarcoma

- translocation or chromosomal rearrangement (Philadelphia chromosome) (Figure 21.2)
- point mutation (*H-ras*)
- gene amplification (EGFr in brain tumours).

G proteins and ras

Proteins that bind and hydrolyse guanidine triphosphate (GTP) are found commonly in the cell and play a crucial role in cell signalling. When GTP (which is found in large excess in the cell compared with GDP) is bound to such G proteins, the protein becomes activated and initiates a cascade of events. However, GTP-binding proteins also rapidly hydrolyse GTP to GDP, thereby rendering themselves inactive. Other proteins can control the activity of GTP binding to such proteins, including one called GTPase-activating protein (GAP), which binds to G proteins, inducing them to convert GTP to GDP and become inactive. Another protein called guanine nucleotide-releasing protein (GNRP) binds to G proteins, inducing them to release GDP and bind GTP (which is present in large amounts in the normal cell), converting it into an active form. G proteins are classified into:

- monomeric G proteins (such as ras, rac and rho)
- heterotrimeric G proteins (often directly coupling cell-surface receptors to intracellular receptors, such as adrenoreceptors or muscarinic acetylcholine receptors to adenylcyclase and phospholipase C, respectively).

Ras family

The human *ras* gene family consists of three closely related genes: H-*ras*, K-*ras* and N-*ras*, which encode 21-kDa signal transduction G proteins involved in the transmission of signals from cell-surface receptors. Ras proteins belong to the monomeric family

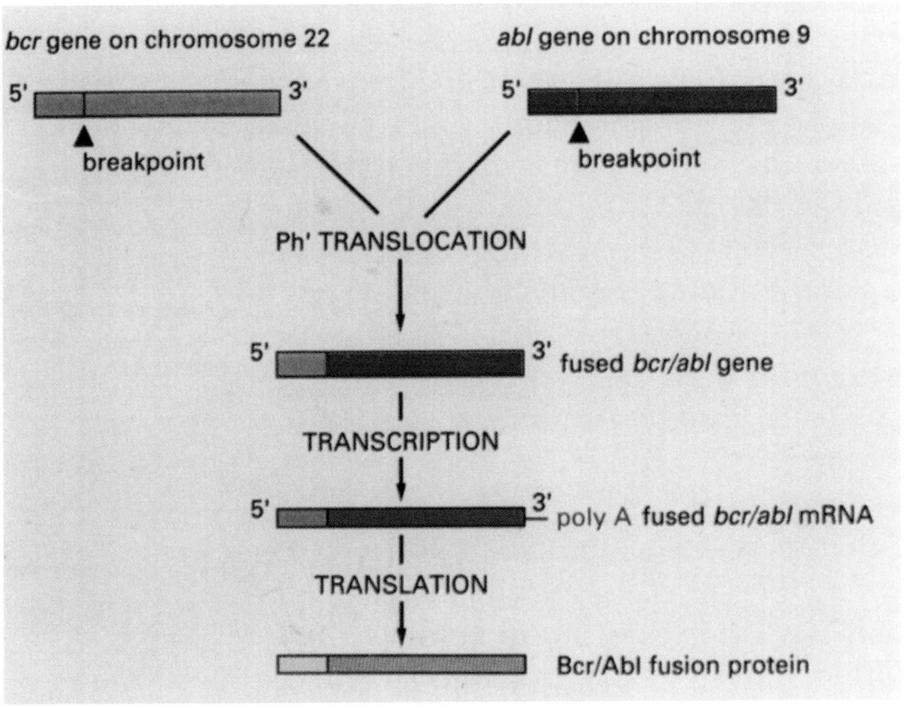

Figure 21.2 *The translocation between chromosomes 9 and 22 responsible for chronic myelogenous leukaemia. The smaller of the two resulting abnormal chromosomes is called the Philadelphia chromosome, after the city where the abnormality was first recorded.*

of G proteins as distinct from the trimeric family that couple cell-surface receptors (such as adrenergic receptors) to intracellular events. Other monomeric G proteins include the rho and rac family which, like ras proteins, are involved in the relay of signals from the cell membrane. Activation of *ras* by mutation occurs as a result of a single amino-acid change as a consequence of single nucleotide mutations. Activated H-*ras* has been found in bladder carcinomas, Ki-*ras* in lung and colon carcinomas, and N-*ras* in haematological malignancies. H-ras is a monomeric G protein. In its mutated (H-*ras*) form, it contains a single-point mutation leading to the conversion of a glycine to a valine residue at codon 12. Mutated H-*ras* is constitutively active whether GTP is bound or not.

Ras helps to link activated tyrosine kinase receptors to downstream events by acting as a molecular switch. It is in the 'off' position when bound to GDP and in the 'on' position when bound to GTP. Some tyrosine kinase receptors phosphorylate themselves on tyrosine residues, which then bind to other proteins that have SH2 domains that dock to phosphorylated tyrosine residues. These proteins with SH2 domains then link to other proteins (such as Sos) that activate ras. Activated ras initiates a serine/threonine phosphorylation cascade, which eventually activates a kinase called mitogen-activated protein kinase (MAP kinase). Eventually, such activation stimulates the action of a number of transcription factors including jun and elk-1 (Figure 21.3). Figure 21.3 shows another important point: namely, that protein kinase C can also activate MAP kinase.

Heterotrimeric G proteins

A large number of membrane-bound receptors function by activating downstream trimeric G proteins, which initiate a phosphorylation cascade stimulating certain enzymes. The trimeric G proteins consist of three parts (α, β and γ) that disassemble when activated. The α-subunit bound to GTP activates nearby enzymes such as adenyl cyclase, which synthesizes cyclic AMP (Figure 21.4), or phospholipase C, which forms inositol triphosphate (IP_3), and diacylglycerol from inositol biphosphate found in the cell membrane (Figure 21.5). IP_3 causes calcium release from various intracellular stores and diacylglycerol activates protein kinase C, which is a serine/threonine kinase (Figure 21.6), that, as pointed out above, can also stimulate MAP kinase.

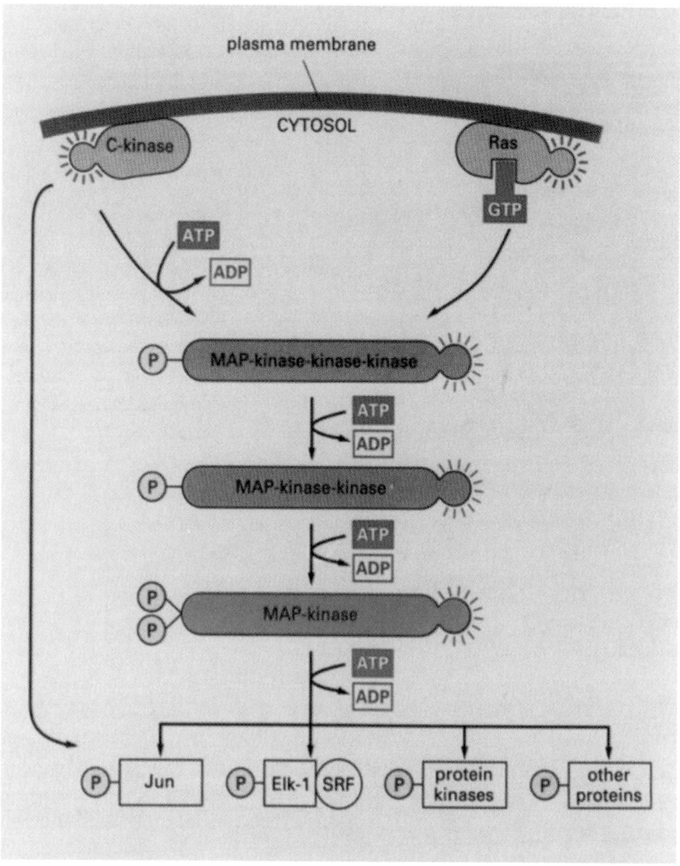

Figure 21.3 *The serine/threonine phosphorylation cascade activated by ras and C-kinase. In the pathway activated by receptor tyrosine kinases via ras, the MAP-kinase-kinase-kinase is often a serine/threonine kinase called Raf, which is thought to be activated by the binding of activated ras. In the pathway activated by G-protein-linked-receptors via C-kinase, the MAP-kinase-kinase-kinase can either be Raf or a different serine/threonine kinase. A similar serine/threonine phosphorylation cascade involving structurally and functionally related proteins operates in yeasts and in all animals that have been studied, where it integrates and amplifies signals from different extracellular stimuli. Receptor tyrosine kinases may also activate a more direct signalling pathway to the nucleus by directly phosphorylating, and thereby activating, gene regulatory proteins that contain SH2 domains.*

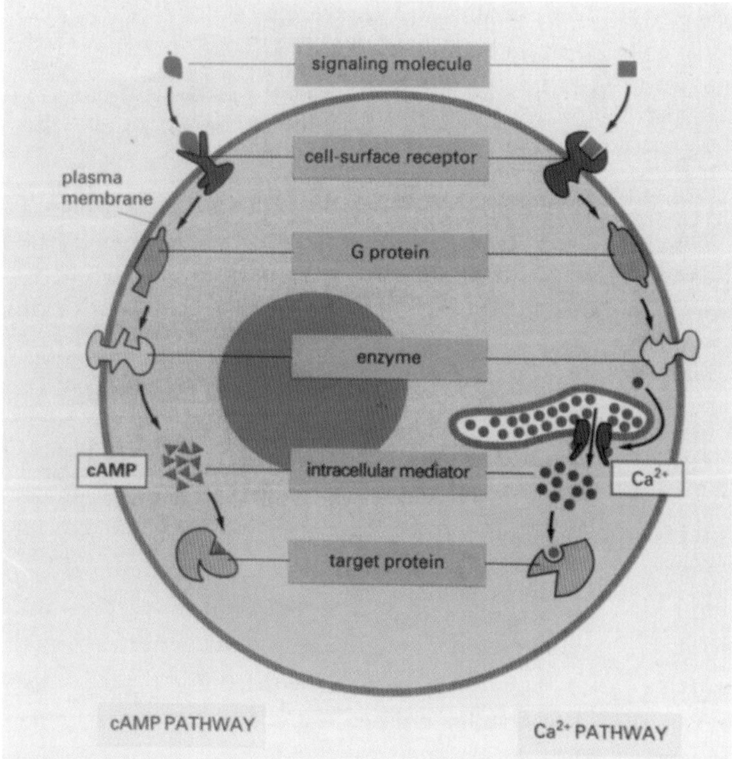

Figure 21.4 *Two major pathways by which G-protein-linked cell-surface receptors generate small intracellular mediators. In both cases, the binding of an extracellular ligand alters the conformation of the cytoplasmic domain of the receptor, causing it to bind to a G protein that activates (or inactivates) a plasma membrane enzyme. In the cyclic AMP (cAMP) pathway, the enzyme directly produces cyclic AMP. In the Ca^{2+} pathway, the enzyme produces a soluble mediator (inositol trisphosphate) that releases Ca^{2+} from the endoplasmic reticulum. Like other small intracellular mediators, both cyclic AMP and Ca^{2+} relay the signal by acting as allosteric effectors: they bind to specific proteins in the cell, altering their conformation and thereby their activity.*

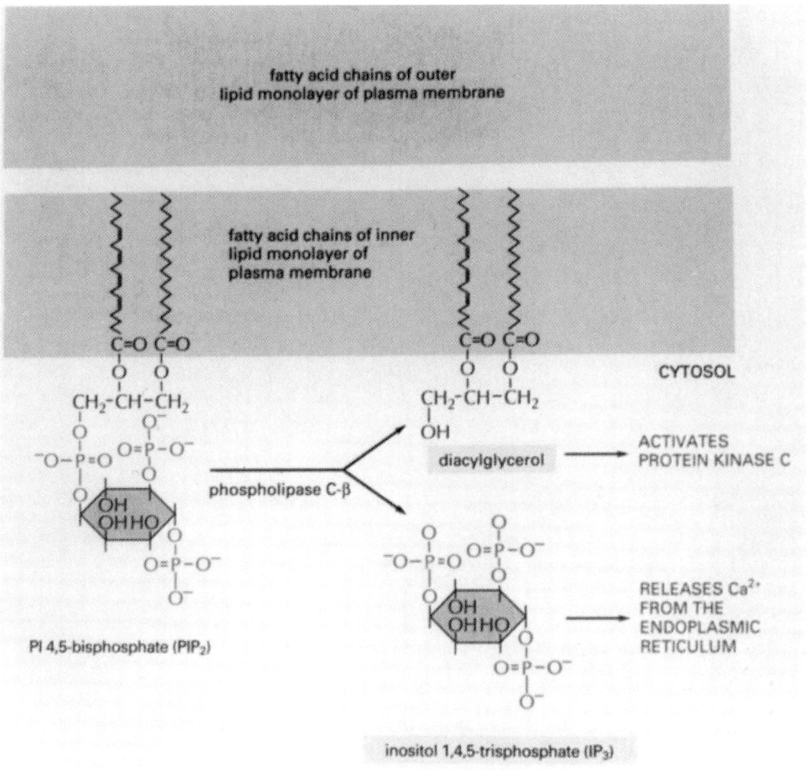

Figure 21.5 *The hydrolysis of PIP_2. Two intracellular mediators are produced when PIP_2 is hydrolysed:* inositol triphosphate *(IP_3), which diffuses through the cytosol and releases Ca^{2+} from the ER, and* diacylglycerol, *which remains in the membrane and helps activate the enzyme protein kinase C. There are at least three classes of phospholipase C-β, γ and δ-, and it is the β class that is activated by G-protein-linked receptors. We shall see later that the γ class is activated by a second class of receptors, called* receptor tyrosine kinases, *that activate the inositol-phospholipid signalling pathway without an intermediary G protein.*

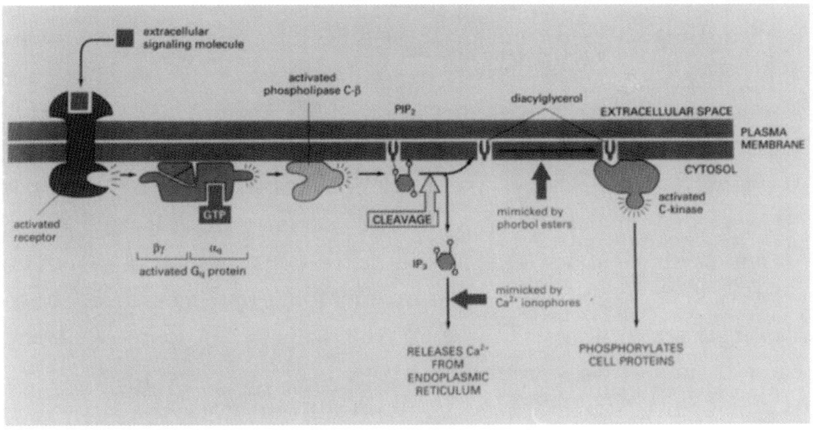

Figure 21.6 *The two branches of the inositol phospholipid pathway. The activated receptor binds to a specific trimeric G protein (G_q), causing the α subunit to dissociate and activate phospholipase C-β, which cleaves PIP_2 to generate IP_3 and diacylglycerol. The diacylglycerol (together with bound Ca^{2+} and phosphatidylserine – not shown) activates C-kinase. Both phospholipase C-β and C-kinase are water-soluble enzymes that translocate from the cytosol to the inner face of the plasma membrane in the process of being activated. The effects of IP_3 can be mimicked experimentally in intact cells by treatment with Ca^{2+} ionophores, while the effects of diacylglycerol can be mimicked by treatment with phorbol esters, which bind to C-kinase and activate it.*

Examples of receptors linked by G proteins to phospholipase C include the muscarinic receptor. Activation of the muscarinic receptor causes an increase in transmembrane calcium flux and also a release of IP_3, which further releases calcium from the endoplasmic reticulum. Receptors linked by G proteins to adenyl cyclase include the β-adrenergic receptor (stimulation of cyclic AMP) and the α_2-receptor (inhibition of cyclic AMP). The α_1-receptor stimulates phospholipase C as well as inhibiting adenylcyclase. Thus, although a wide variety of receptors are coupled to different G proteins, the exact consequences of receptor activation depend on the specific G protein which couples the receptor to downstream intracellular signalling mechanisms.

Tyrosine kinase growth factor receptors

Many cell-surface receptors for growth factors contain a tyrosine kinase domain as part of the protein which is similar to the src family of oncogene tyrosine kinase (including Src, Yes, Fgr, Lck, Lyn, Hck and Blk) and which contain SH2 domains facing the internal portion of the cell. Other growth-factor receptors are closely associated with separate tyrosine kinase proteins that are not an intrinsic part of the receptor protein itself. Most of the transforming growth factor receptors (EGFr, IGF-Ir, NGFr, PDGFr, FGFr and VEGFr [vascular endothelial growth factor]) contain an intrinsic tyrosine kinase domain, with the exception of that for TGFβ, which contains a serine/ threonine kinase. When activated by ligand binding, tyrosine kinase receptors autophosphorylate at several phosphorylation sites and can then act as docking sites for a small set of intracellular proteins that recognize tyrosine-associated phosphate sites *via* their SH2 domains (such as SOS and GrB2). Activation of the EGFr produces dimerization of the receptor, autophosphorylation of tyrosine residues and phosphorylation of target proteins. EGFr activation is linked to the *ras* signal transduction pathway via two proteins (Sos and Grb2), which, when EGFr is activated, link *via* Raf (MAP kinase-kinase-kinase) to the downstream signals of the *ras* pathway such as MAP kinase.

In many growth-factor receptors, ligand binding induces dimerization, a conformational change takes place and the tyrosine kinase domain is activated. Some mutated growth-factor receptors are constitutively active, whereas other receptors can become activated in the absence of ligand if the receptor protein is found at very high levels. Such receptors can also form heterodimers (such as c-erbB-2 with c-erbB-3 or with c-erbB-1 [EGFr]). It should be noted that herceptin has recently been introduced as cancer treatment in advanced breast cancer; it is a 'humanized' antibody against c-erbB2. It is proof of the principle that novel treatments against some of these targets can be clinically useful.

Epidermal growth factor (EGF) and the EGF receptor (EGFR)

EGF is a 53-amino-acid peptide with mitogenic activity whose action is mediated by binding to a membrane-bound receptor. EGF was originally isolated from murine submaxillary gland extracts, and its distribution is widespread, with high levels of milk, prostatic fluid and urine. The detection of high levels of EGF in urine prompted studies of EGFr levels in bladder cancer.

EGFr is a 175-kDa transmembrane protein with an extracellular EGF-binding domain, a small hydrophobic region which spans the plasma membrane, and an intracellular domain which has tyrosine kinase activity as well as target tyrosine residues for autophosphorylation. EGFr (c-*erb*B-1 gene) has considerable sequence homology with the $gp65^{erbB}$ protein from the avian erythroblastosis virus. EGFr is also the target for the peptide growth factor TGF-α, which is synthesized by a wide range of common epithelial tumours, including transitional cell carcinomas (TCC) of the urinary bladder, renal and prostate.

EGFr is distributed throughout the body and is present on normal fibroblasts, corneal cells, kidney cells, basal prostate epithelium and basal urothelium. Increased expression of EGFr protein is transforming in some cell lines, and some human solid tumours, including TCC, have increased levels of EGFr protein. This appears to be achieved by a variety of mechanisms, including gene amplification, upregulation of mRNA, increased translation or post-translational modification of the protein.

C-*erb*B-2

The proto-oncogene c-*erb*B-2 (also known as *neu* or HER-2) encodes a transmembrane glycoprotein which is related to the EGFr. Several groups have reported a candidate ligand for the c-*erb*B-2 receptor, and elucidation of its structure (*neu* differentiation factor [NDF] or heregulin-α [HRG- α]) reveals it to be an additional member of the EGF family. Two further members of the erbB receptor family are HER3/p160^{erbB-3} and HER4/p180^{erb-4}. Recent evidence suggests, however, that heregulin is the physiological ligand for c-erbB-3, and that for c-erbB-2 is as yet unidentified.

Fibroblast growth factors (FGFs)

The FGFs are a family of peptides related by sequence similarity which have been implicated in the regulation of cell proliferation, angiogenesis, embryonal development, differentiation and motility. The family includes fibroblast growth factor (aFGF; FGF1), basic fibroblast growth factor (bFGF; FGF2), *int*2 (FGF3), *hst* (FGF4), FGF5, *hst*2 (FGF6), keratinocyte growth factor (KGF; FGF7), androgen-inducible growth factor (AIGF; FGF8) and FGF9. They bind with varying degrees of specificity to a family of tyrosine kinase receptors (FGFRs). bFGF has been shown to transform mouse fibroblasts in vitro, *int*2 FGF3 is the human homologue of one of the common integration sites of mouse mammary tumour virus (MMTV), and *hst* (FGF4) is the most frequently detected human transforming gene after *ras* in the NIH 3T3 assay. These two genes were reported to be amplified in 3/43 (7%) of bladder tumours and 41/238 (17%) of breast carcinomas.

Basic FGF has been identified in both benign and malignant human prostate. Immunohistochemistry has identified FGF-2 predominantly in prostatic stroma but also epithelial cells. FGF-1 is also present in the prostate but at a lower level than FGF-2. In addition, in a prostate stromal cell culture model, there is evidence for the interaction of FGF-2 and TGF-β_1, resulting in positive and negative proliferative effects, respectively. Besides potential autocrine loop activation, FGFs may also contribute to the pathophysiology of the prostate via paracrine activity. FGF-7, or keratinocyte growth factor (KGF), is synthesized and secreted by stromal cells, being thought to act on FGF-receptor-bearing epithelial cells, resulting in cellular proliferation. It is also interesting to note that, in a transgenic mouse system, overexpression of FGF-3 or *int*-2, alterations to the prostate of the male progeny were dramatic and involved only hyperplasia, without evidence of malignant transformation.

The fibroblast growth factor receptors (FGFRs) share structural similarities in both the extracellular domains that bind FGFs and the intracellular domains that activate the signal transduction pathway. The four FGFRs, FGFR-1 to FGFR-4, display different binding affinities for the different FGFs. FGF-1 binds to all four receptors, while FGF-2 is more restricted and binds only to the first three FGFRs. Receptor–receptor interactions are known to occur and may have a role in the development of both benign hyperplasia and carcinoma of the prostate. To date, the expression of FGFs and their receptors is not fully understood, but there does appear to be a major difference between benign and malignant prostate in the activity of the FGF system. Splice variants occur in the FGFRs. It is likely that subtle changes occur in the FGF system during malignant progression. This has been demonstrated elegantly in a mouse prostate cancer model. During progression from the benign to the malignant phenotype, the prostate epithelial cells display a switch of expression of FGFR splice variants, conferring a switch of high-affinity binding from FGF-7 to FGF-2. FGF-2 was also concomitantly upregulated along with FGF-3 and FGF-5. Further evidence supporting a role for FGFs in the development of malignancy is that transformation of BHK-21 (baby hamster kidney) cells with plasmids carrying the bFGF coding sequence results in cells which exhibit the transformed phenotype. The prostatic cancer cell lines DU145 and PC-3 produce active FGF-2 and express large amounts of FGFR-2. However, only the DU145 cell line, and not the PC-3 cell line, has been shown to respond to exogenous FGF-2.

The interaction between the androgen receptor and growth factor systems is important. It is known that certain growth factors, including FGF-7/KGF, IGFs and EGF, may activate androgen-dependent gene expression in the absence of androgen, and this may represent a mechanism for the development of hormone insensitivity in prostate tumours.

Insulin-like growth factors (IGFs)

Insulin-like growth factor I (IGF-I) is a 70-amino-acid polypeptide with functional homology to insulin. The mitogenic effect of IGF-I is due to its ability to facilitate the transfer of cells from the G1 phase to the S phase in the cell cycle. IGF-I and the closely related IGF-II are present in biological fluids and tissue extracts, and are usually bound to an IGF-binding protein (IGF-BP). There are two types of receptors for the IGFs. The type 1 receptor is a tyrosine kinase and binds both IGF-I and IGF-II. The type 2 receptor is structurally distinct and binds primarily IGF-II. The majority of the mitogenic effects of the IGFs appear to be mediated via the type 1 IGF receptor.

The growth of normal prostatic epithelial cells in culture is dependent on the presence of IGF-I and II. The response is most marked with IGF-I. The type 1 IGF receptor has been identified in normal, benign and malignant prostatic tissues. It is preferentially expressed in the basal cells. Production of IGF-II has been demonstrated by prostatic fibroblasts, but IGF-I has not been identified as being produced by either prostatic fibroblasts or epithelial cells. However, IGF-I mRNA has been identified in stromal cells from benign prostatic hyperplasia (BPH) specimens. The mechanism of IGF-II-mediated stimulation of prostatic epithelial cells in BPH appears to be similar to that in normal prostate, although the expression of IGF-II mRNA is 10-fold higher in fibroblasts from BPH tissues. This led to the hypothesis that such cells may be 'reverting to a fetal-like state', where IGF-II expression is normally high, causing stimulation of proliferation and the development of BPH.

Transforming growth factor-beta (TGF-β)

TGF-β_1 is the predominant species in the TGF-β superfamily, which includes several modulators of growth, differentiation and morphogenesis (including bone morphogenetic proteins). TGF-β_1 is classically regarded as a stimulator for mesenchyme cells and an inhibitor for epithelial cells. Five isoforms of TGF-β have so far been identified, of which only the first three occur in mammals. TGF-β_1 is a homodimer of two 112-amino-acid subunits linked by disulphide bonds. Cellular receptors for TGF-β_1 have been identified in the rat ventral prostate where they are negatively regulated by androgens and involved in the mechanism of castration-induced prostatic cell death. Receptors for TGF-β_1 have been identified in the human prostate cancer cell lines DU145 and PC-3. TGF-β_1 has been shown to have an inhibitory effect on human prostatic fibroblasts and epithelial cells in culture. It has been suggested that TGF-β_1 causes inhibition of proliferation by preventing phosphorylation of the protein product of the retinoblastoma gene (pRB) by upregulation of p15, which is a cyclin-dependent kinase inhibitor, and by stabilization of the p27 protein. The TGFβ receptor is a serine protease and links to downstream signals, including SMAD2.

TUMOUR SUPPRESSOR GENES

Evidence for the existence of tumour suppressor genes has come from several sources, although the significance of the observations was not appreciated at the time. Experiments dating back to the 1960s, involving the fusion of normal and transformed cells, had shown that normal genes can suppress transformation and malignancy in cell lines.

The second line of evidence came from an analysis of the inheritance of rare hereditary childhood cancers. Based on retinoblastoma, Knudson proposed a two-hit inactivation process in which both copies of a critical gene had to be inactivated for the disease to be manifest. That these hereditary cancers are often associated with predisposition to a wide range of sporadic tumours of other tissues led to the further suggestion that somatic mutation or loss of these same genes was probably involved in the genesis of a wide range of cancers, including bladder cancer. This also provided a possible explanation for the observation of the non-random chromosome deletions seen in sporadic tumours. This concept in turn led to the identification of the p53 gene as a tumour suppressor gene.

Cytogenetic studies have shown that frequent non-random chromosome alterations occur in cancer. For instance, in bladder cancer, these involve chromosomes 1p, 3p, 9p, 10q, 11, 13q, 17p and 18q. Loss of one copy of chromosome 9p was found as an early event in low-stage, low-grade tumours, unlike other chromosome losses, which appeared to be more prevalent in advanced tumours. The high frequency of chromosome 9p losses in bladder cancer is not seen in other tumour types, suggesting the possible location of a tumour suppressor gene specific to bladder cancer.

The p53 tumour suppressor gene

The human p53 gene, located on the short arm of chromosome 17, encodes a nuclear phosphoprotein which binds to specific DNA sequences in the human genome and appears to play a key role in the control of DNA replication and hence cellular proliferation. Non-random chromosome 17 losses involving the p53 locus are commonly found in human tumours, including bladder cancer, and the loss of one copy of the p53 gene has been found to be frequently accompanied by mutation of the remaining allele. Transfection studies have shown that the wild-type protein is able to suppress cell proliferation and transformation. It thus acts in such circumstances as a tumour suppressor gene which can contribute to tumour formation by deletions or loss of function mutations. Germ-line mutations of the p53 gene have been found in certain inherited predispositions to cancer (Li-Fraumeni syndrome, in which there is clustering of soft tissue and bone sarcomas at any age; and cancers under the age of 45 in breast, brain, adrenal cortex and lung) and somatic cell mutations have frequently been detected in a wide range of common sporadic tumours, including breast, colon, brain and lung tumours, as well as bladder cancer. These mutations are predominantly of the point mis-sense type and occur at many different locations within four highly conserved regions of the gene (codons 117–142, 171–181, 234–258 and 270–286) located in exons 4 to 9 of the p53 gene.

The p53 protein has three parts: a central DNA-binding domain in which mutations are usually of the mis-sense type, a transcription domain (N terminus) and a regulatory domain (C terminus) in which mutations result in non-sense or stop codons. The protein mdm2 binds near the N terminus of the protein. One of the genes activated by p53 is the p21 protein (WAF1), which inhibits the activity of cyclin-dependent kinases and which also binds to PCNA. Other genes include gadd45 and the protein bax (which promotes apoptosis).

The p53 protein has a short half-life, measured in the order of minutes, and is normally present at low levels not detectable by immunohistochemistry. One of the remarkable features of the p53 gene is that a broad spectrum of mutations can lead to an altered conformation and inactivation of the protein product with an increased cellular half-life, resulting in accumulation in the cell to levels that are readily detectable by immunohistochemical staining. Although this initially led to suggestions that positive detection of p53 by immunohistochemistry was synonymous with the detection of mutations, this is now realized not to be the case. Moreover, some mutations do not result in accumulation of the altered protein product, and these have to be screened for by alternative complementary methods such as single-strand conformation polymorphism (SSCP) assays to obtain a more complete picture. However, even combined, these techniques are, at best, a way of trawling for mutations rather than a way of systematically screening for all possible mutations. The definitive method of establishing the presence of a mutation in a sample is by DNA-sequencing procedures.

Inactivation of normal p53 in tumours

Some proteins have been shown to bind to p53 and inactivate it. For instance, in sarcomas, it has been shown that p53 mutations are rare, but there is increased expression of a protein called mdm-2 which, like the large T antigen of the SV40 virus, binds to p53, inactivates it and stabilizes it. This confirms the frequent involvement of the p53 pathway in many human tumours.

p53 and G1 arrest

Irradiation of cells has been shown to result in marked upregulation of the wild-type p53 protein. It may be that the primary event is DNA repair following radiotherapy, which then activates p53. However, upregulation of p53 switches on downstream genes such as p21, which is a potent inhibitor of cell division, and places them into G1 arrest, allowing completion of DNA repair if this is possible.

p53 and apoptosis

Some authors believe that increased levels of p53 can, if DNA damage is too severe to repair during G1 arrest, force the cell into apoptosis. There is no doubt that with severe DNA damage there is an initial attempt at DNA repair followed by upregulation of p53, stimulation of p21 and cell-cycle arrest. With more severe DNA damage or with less severe damage in certain types of cells (such as thymocytes), this process may be followed by apoptosis, but, currently, it is controversial as to whether p53 is directly responsible for apoptosis in such circumstances. Certainly, p53 can upregulate bax (a promoter of apoptosis), but it is also certain that in some cells apoptosis can occur without recourse to the p53–bax pathway.

mdm-2 oncogene

The *mdm-2* gene (murine double minute-2) is located on chromosome 12q13–14 and encodes a 90-kDa nuclear protein. The *mdm-2* protein may act as an oncoprotein when overexpressed, by binding to the 'guardian of the genome', wild-type p53 protein, and abrogating its functions.

Retinoblastoma gene

The Rb1 gene encodes a 105–115-kDa nuclear phosphoprotein which binds to DNA and appears to be involved in growth regulation in a wide variety of cell types. There are related p107 and p130 proteins, whose function in man has not been elucidated, but which may have overlapping actions. The Rb1 gene product binds to the transforming proteins of several DNA tumour viruses, including adenovirus E1A, SV40 large T antigen and human papilloma virus E7 proteins. Abnormalities in the Rb gene were first reported in patients with inherited retinoblastoma who had one abnormal copy of the gene in all retinal cells; it is thought that subsequent 'spontaneous' alterations in the remaining copy of the Rb gene causes tumour formation.

The Rb protein is central to the function of the cell cycle; it is inactive when phosphorylated or when bound to inactivating proteins. It is the target of cyclin-dependent kinases and cyclin D. When it is activated, it stimulates the E2F family of transcription factors (myc and jun are among them): it is a negative regulator of the cell cycle. Disruption of this pathway is central to many tumours. The cyclin-dependent kinase inhibitor p16 is particularly linked to Rb, so when p16 is upregulated, the activity of cdk2 is inhibited. The Rb protein is not phosphorylated, so it binds to DNA and inhibits transcription, and the E2F family of transcription factors is switched off.

A wider role for the Rb1 gene was suggested by the observation that those who inherit the mutant allele have a higher incidence of a wide range of non-ocular second tumours, particularly osteosarcomas, but also lung melanoma and bladder cancer.

Initial studies with the Rb1 cDNA probe, based mainly on tumour cell lines, reported frequent structural abnormalities of the gene and absence of Rb1 mRNA. Subsequent extensions of these studies with polyclonal antisera indicated that absence or abnormal forms of the Rb protein are almost universal in small cell lung cancer (SCLC) cell lines and present in one-third of bladder carcinoma cell lines, while being infrequent in colonic, breast and melanoma cell lines. Studies on primary bladder tumours have shown that loss of heterozygosity for Rb1-linked markers is associated with the development of invasive lesions. The overall frequency of Rb1 allelic loss in bladder cancer was 3/63 (5%) for superficial (pTa/pT1) and 30/58 (53%) for invasive (T2–T4) tumours. Major rearrangements of the remaining Rb1 gene were detected in only a small proportion of these cases, suggesting that generally more subtle small deletions or point mutations are involved that have yet to be characterized. Altered Rb protein expression is associated with a poor outcome in several tumour types, including bladder.

von Hippel-Lindau (VHL) disease

This is inherited as a dominant abnormality and consists of retinal cysts, cerebellar haemangioblastomas, pancreatic cysts, phaeochromocytomas, renal cysts and renal cancer. The VHL gene is situated on chromosome 3p and also affects many sporadic renal cancers. It encodes a small protein (213 aa) with three exons, and in the human gene there are eight pentapeptide repeats in exon 1. Most mutations in VHL are found at the carboxy-terminus of exon 1 and at the beginning of exon 3. Similar mutations are found in sporadic tumours, but, in addition, mutations are found in exon 2, a rare event in VHL. The VHL protein binds to the elongation factors elongin B and C, which help in the synthesis of mRNA; it is thought that the VHL/elongin B and C complex moves from the nucleus into the cytoplasm as a response to cell/cell contacts. VHL also upregulates the peptide VEGF (see next section): a feature which may be responsible for angiogenesis in renal cancer.

Genes associated with chemoresistance

Chemotherapy with epirubicin or mitomycin C is increasingly used for recurrent superficial papillary tumours. In muscle-invasive disease, adjuvant and neoadjuvant chemotherapy regimens are currently being tested in clinical trials. Molecular mechanisms that mediate cellular drug resistance may play a role in the differential responsiveness of individual bladder tumours to chemotherapy. Transcript levels of the multidrug resistance (*mdr*1) gene have been found to vary 34-fold in high-grade muscle-invasive bladder tumours. In addition, renal cell carcinomas have very high levels of this gene, perhaps explaining why it is chemoresistant.

ACKNOWLEDGEMENT

Artwork reproduced from Alberts B, Johnson A, Lewis J, Raff M, Roberts K, Walter P (eds), Molecular Biology of the Cell, 4th Edition, New York: Garland Science.

22

The molecular genetics and pathology of renal cell carcinoma

Marie O' Donnell, Marie E Mathers, Eamonn R Maher and Steven C Clifford

INTRODUCTION

Renal cell carcinomas (RCC) represent 2–3% of all adult cancers diagnosed. Overall, RCCs account for approximately 24 000 new cases and 10 000 deaths annually in the USA with the highest prevalence observed in the 50–60-year age group, and a male:female ratio of approximately 2:1. Occupational exposure to hydrocarbons (trichloroethylene) has been associated with an increased risk of RCC in large epidemiological studies, whereas cigarette smoking is a positive risk factor for non-occupation-associated RCC development. Additional risk factors include hypertension and obesity, and there is an increased risk in patients with end-stage renal failure.[1,2]

THE PATHOLOGICAL AND GENETIC CLASSIFICATION OF ADULT RENAL EPITHELIAL NEOPLASMS

Recent years have seen considerable reorganization in the histological classification of adult renal epithelial neoplasms, culminating in the publication of generally agreed diagnostic categorizations.[3–5] This classification is based on our increased understanding of the molecular pathology of renal neoplasms, the close correlation between specific genetic abnormalities and identifiable histological subgroups of renal neoplasms, and the prognostic utility of these subgroupings.[6,7]

This new classification has been generally accepted because, in the majority of cases, an accurate pathological diagnosis can be made by routine histopathological techniques, with more specialized molecular genetic studies reserved for a minority of cases. The current classification (summarized in Table 22.1), around which this review is organized, moves away from older classifications of renal epithelial neoplasia, which were essentially a discussion of renal adenocarcinoma and its architectural and cytological subtypes.[8]

Here we review the major clinical and histopathological features of adult renal epithelial neoplasms. We then consider our current understanding of the molecular and genetic basis of renal neoplasm development; the close interplay that exists between genetic, histopathological and clinical features; and how these features underlie the current classification of renal epithelial neoplasia.

Table 22.1 The Heidelberg classification of adult renal epithelial neoplasms.

Benign tumours	Malignant tumours
Papillary renal cell adenoma	Conventional renal cell carcinoma
Metanephric adenoma	Papillary renal cell carcinoma
Oncocytoma	Chromophobe renal cell carcinoma
	Collecting duct carcinoma (including renal medullary carcinoma)
	Renal cell carcinoma, unclassified

THE CLINICAL AND HISTOPATHOLOGICAL FEATURES OF ADULT RENAL EPITHELIAL NEOPLASMS

Benign tumours

Papillary renal adenoma: the macroscopic and microscopic appearances of papillary renal adenoma and its association with papillary adenocarcinoma

Renal adenomas are more common than all other renal neoplasms combined, affecting over 40% of the general population. These are usually seen at autopsy or in nephrectomies removed for papillary RCC. In the latter instance, they are almost always multiple with a mean of 8 lesions seen per kidney.[9,10] They are usually subcapsular in distribution and have a uniform circumscribed, cream-coloured appearance. Adenomas must be less than 5 mm in maximum diameter to fulfil current diagnostic criteria for this entity.[3,4] Lesions greater than this size must be regarded as having definite malignant potential. This reflects a shift away from previous criteria, where neoplasms up to 2–3 cm were regarded as being benign. However, several studies showed that lesions of this diameter are capable of metastasizing.[11] Neoplasms less than 5 mm have not been recorded to behave in a malignant fashion; hence the use of this cutoff point. Histologically, renal adenomas have a tubulopapillary architecture but should not show nuclear pleomorphism, significant mitotic activity or lymphatic/vascular invasion.[12] These tumours exhibit a very similar cytogenetic pattern to papillary renal cell carcinoma, and it is currently felt that these neoplasms exhibit an adenoma–carcinoma sequence with acquisition of additional genetic hits in tumours that acquire the malignant phenotype.[13,14] Currently, it is unclear what percentage of renal adenomata progress to carcinoma in clinical practice.

With increasing use of nephron-sparing surgery for RCC, it is likely that renal adenomas will acquire greater clinical significance in the management of patients with papillary RCC.[15,16] Reduction of diagnostic criteria from 2–3 cm to 5 mm means that these lesions are not identifiable by current radiological methods. They may therefore also prove problematic in the context of renal transplantation, where tumours of just over 5 mm in diameter are discovered at the time of organ retrieval.

Metanephric adenoma: epidemiology, and macroscopic and microscopic appearances

These are rare, recently recognized, neoplasms of the kidney that appear to behave in a benign fashion. They are more common in females, with a 2:1 female to male predominance. They have been described in all age groups but are most often seen in middle-aged adults, with a mean age at presentation of 41 years. In most instances, the tumours are found incidentally during the course of other investigations. However, presentation with pain, haematuria and palpable mass is also described.[12,17] An unusual finding is the association of this entity and polycythaemia which disappears after resection, and which appears to be due to erythropoietin production by the tumour cells.[18,19]

Histologically, these tumours are composed of closely packed tubules, although areas with a tubulopapillary architecture are also recognized. Glomeruloid bodies reminiscent of embryonic metanephric tissue are also seen. These tumours previously were unrecognized by pathologists and were misclassified as Wilms' tumour, nephroblastomatosis or unusual tubular carcinoma of the kidney. Original reports indicated that these tumours had cytogenetic profiles identical to renal adenoma and papillary carcinoma, suggesting a common origin.[20] However, recent evidence suggests that this is erroneous and relates to inclusion of cases of solid variant papillary RCC, with which this tumour can also be confused.[21]

Oncocytoma: epidemiology, macroscopic features and microscopic appearances

Renal oncocytoma is a benign tumour of the renal cortex first reported in 1942 by Zippel[22] and accounting for approximately 2–7% of renal neoplasms in surgical series. This tumour probably arises from the distal convoluted tubule.[23–27] There is a male to female ratio of 2.5:1. Although cases have been described in young adults and adolescents, most cases occur in the elderly, with a mean age of 65 years at presentation. These lesions are usually asymptomatic and are generally found during

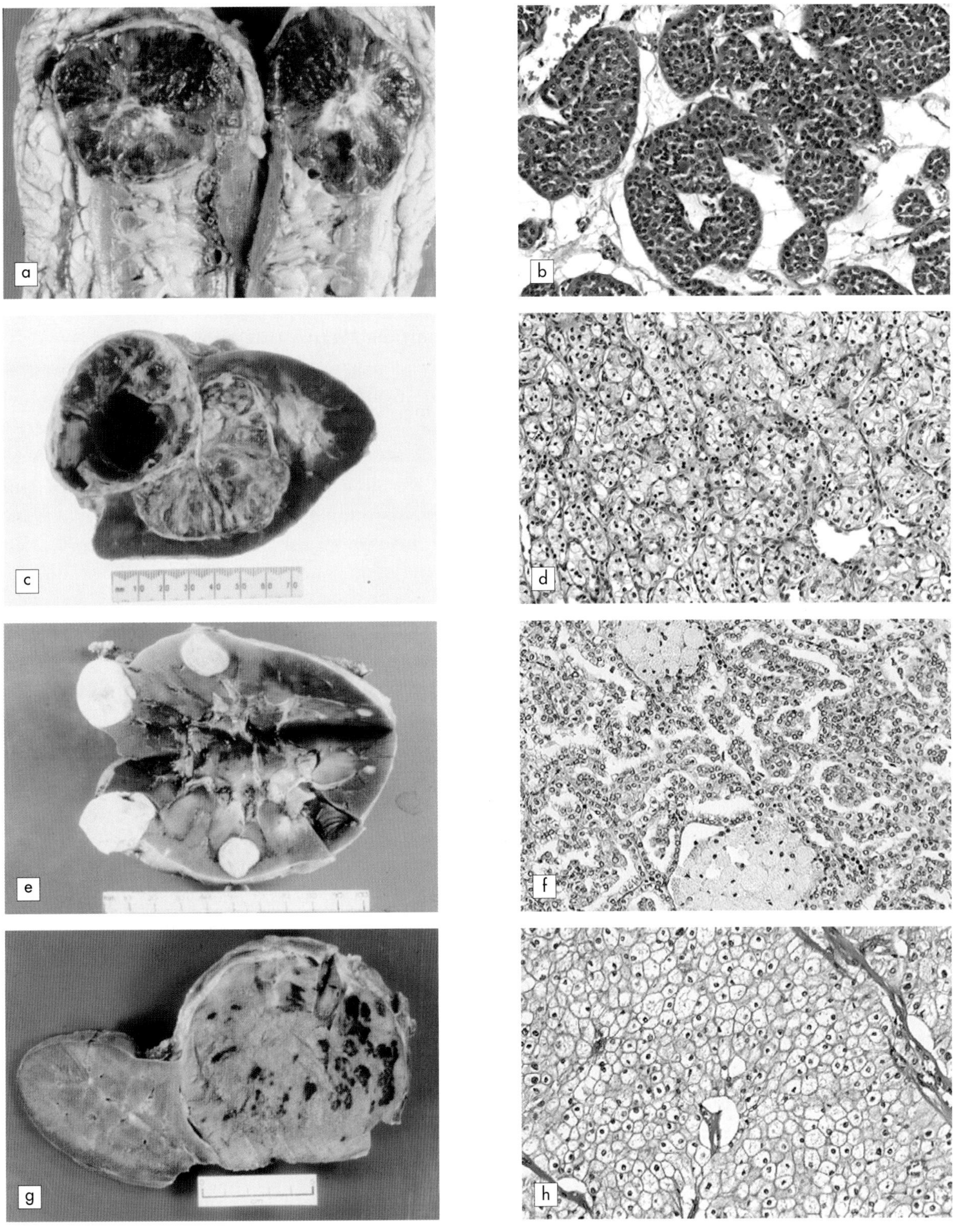

Figure 22.1 *Macroscopic and histological appearances of adult renal epithelial neoplasms. (a) Macroscopic appearance of renal oncocytoma, showing tan-brown cut surface and prominent central fibrous scar. (b) Typical histological appearance of oncocytoma, with nests of eosinophilic cells in hyalinized stroma. (c) Macroscopic appearance of C-RCC with prominent cystic degeneration and haemorrhage. (d) Histology of conventional RCC with clear-cell morphology. (e) Macroscopic image of nephrectomy specimen bearing multiple P-RCCs. (f) Histological appearance of type 1 P-RCC with tubulopapillary architecture. Collections of foamy macrophages were a prominent feature in this case. (g) Macroscopic appearance of chromophobe RCC with a beige cut surface. (h) Chromophobe RCC characterized by large polygonal cells with prominent cell borders.*

investigations for other medical problems.[28,29] These neoplasms are said to have a characteristic radiological appearance and are described as having a cartwheel peripheral vascular arrangement on angiography.[30,31]

Most oncocytomas are discrete unilateral masses but occasional multicentric and bilateral tumours have been described.[29,32,33,33a] Diffuse oncocytosis is also rarely described in the literature.[34] Cases of synchronous or metachronous RCCs in the ipsilateral or contralateral kidney have also rarely been documented.[35,36] Grossly, these tumours are well-circumscribed, unencapsulated, solid, tan-brown, subcapsular masses with a pushing margin that compresses adjacent renal parenchyma, giving the gross impression of encapsulation. They can vary in size, with a range of 0.3–20 cm. The average diameter is approximately 7.5 cm. Larger tumours tend to have a central, stellate, cream-white fibrous scar. Haemorrhage can occasionally be seen, but cystic change and necrosis is most unusual (Figure 22.1a).

Histologically, the tumours are composed of polygonal or round cells with moderate to abundant eosinophilic cytoplasm. The nuclei are round and have evenly dispersed chromatin. The cells are arranged in nests or trabeculae separated by hypocellular, hyalinized stroma (Figure 22.1b). Occasionally, they may adopt a more solid architectural pattern of growth, but definite papillary areas are not allowed. Foci of nuclear pleomorphism are well described and often occur adjacent to the central scarred area. Mitotic activity is minimal. Ultrastructurally, the cytoplasm of the neoplastic cells is packed full of mitochondria, accounting for the eosinophilic appearance of the cells seen on light microscopy.

Some tumours may show atypical features, including extension into perirenal adipose tissue, extension into adjacent renal parenchyma, or lymphatic/vascular invasion. Some authors have termed these lesions 'atypical oncocytoma'.[28,37] Evidence to date suggests that these neoplasms also behave in a benign fashion, although more prolonged follow-up of this subgroup of patients is recommended. Several authors have described malignant variants of oncocytoma over the years.[38] However, most of these case reports predate the recognition of chromophobe carcinoma, and it is likely that the majority of so-called malignant oncocytomas represent eosinophilic variants of chromophobe or conventional RCC (C-RCC).

Malignant tumours (RCC)

Conventional RCC (C-RCC): the macroscopic and microscopic appearances of C-RCC

C-RCC accounts for 70–80% of all surgically excised renal neoplasms.[3] This tumour was previously called 'clear cell carcinoma' or 'hypernephroma', terms that should now be avoided to prevent diagnostic confusion. C-RCC is thought to arise from the proximal renal tubular epithelial cell.[39–42] The male to female ratio is about 2:1. C-RCC most commonly occurs in the sixth decade but has a wide age range. Presentation with abdominal pain, abdominal mass and haematuria is common, but this tumour can also cause a variety of paraneoplastic syndromes, including pyrexia of unknown origin and hypercalcaemia.[43–46]

The macroscopic appearance of C-RCC is well recognized. Smaller tumours may be uniformly yellow/orange, but larger neoplasms have a typical variegated appearance with areas that are yellow, white, red or brown, depending on the percentage of viable tumour, haemorrhage or necrosis present (Figure 22.1c). Most tumours show areas of cystic degeneration, with occasional tumours showing such cystic change that they can mimic benign cysts of the renal cortex macroscopically.[47–49] Tumours tend to infiltrate with a pushing margin and may have a fibrous pseudocapsule. The presence of a less well-defined infiltrative margin is an ominous sign and is suggestive of sarcomatoid transformation.[50]

Most C-RCCs are composed of neoplastic cells that have abundant clear cytoplasm due to the presence of intracytoplasmic lipid and glycogen (Figure 22.1d). Occasional neoplasms are composed predominantly of cells with granular cytoplasm that have less glycogen and lipid than their clear-cell counterparts. Other tumours of this type show a mixed pattern. The cells are usually organized in sheets and trabeculae separated by a rich vascular fibrous stroma, or they are arranged in a pseudoglandular or cystic pattern. As tumour grade increases, the organized tumour pattern may become less obvious. On immunohistochemistry, the neoplastic cells co-express cytokeratin and vimentin in the majority of cases, a finding that can be helpful in the differential diagnosis between different subgroups of RCC.[42,51,52]

Papillary adenocarcinoma: the clinical presentation, macroscopic and microscopic appearances of papillary renal carcinoma

Papillary renal cell carcinoma (P-RCC) is a distinct subgroup of RCC with different cytogenetic abnormalities from C-RCC (see next section).[53–55] Older literature sometimes refers to this variant as 'chromophil carcinoma'.[56] This carcinoma comprises 10–15% of renal tumours in surgical series.[57–59] P-RCC is more common in males, with a male to female ratio of approximately 1.5:1. Most neoplasms of this type occur in the sixth decade, but, as for C-RCC, there is a wide age range. The symptoms are similar to those encountered in C-RCC and include abdominal pain, abdominal mass and haematuria. P-RCCs are often multifocal and bilateral. In most instances, they are accompanied by multiple renal cell adenomata in the ipsilateral or contralateral kidney.[59] This is the type of RCC which most frequently occurs in individuals on haemodialysis with acquired cystic disease of the kidney.[60] P-RCCs tend to be avascular or hypovascular on renal angiography, and hypoechoic on ultrasonography.[61,62] They also show a much higher rate of tumour calcification than other RCCs.

Grossly, P-RCC tumours average 8 cm in diameter and, in general, are circumscribed and more likely to be organ confined at presentation. Smaller tumours tend to have a cream-white appearance with flecks of gold.[59] Larger tumours tend to accumulate serous fluid, necrotic debris and haemorrhage rather than actual tumour mass. In these cases, viable tumour may only be seen in histological sections taken from the periphery of the tumour (Figure 22.1e).[57]

Microscopically, over 70% of the tumour must exhibit papillary or a tubopapillary architecture to sustain the diagnosis of P-RCC (Figure 22.1f).[3,63] Solid variants of this entity have been described, but a compressed papillary architecture is discernible on careful examination.[59] Frequently these tumours show aggregates of foamy macrophages, areas of haemorrhage and necrosis with prominent cholesterol clefts and psammoma bodies. This carcinoma shows strong positive staining of tumour cells with cytokeratin 7, which may be of use diagnostically.[59]

Type 1 versus type 2 P-RCC

Recent studies have identified two distinct histological P-RCC subtypes. Type 1 P-RCC is composed of cuboidal basophilic cells lining the papillary formations, while type 2 shows larger columnar cells with more abundant eosinophilic cytoplasm and larger nuclei.[64] There appears to be correlation between these tumour subtypes and prognosis. Type 1 tumours, which are twice as common, are associated with a better prognosis compared with type 2 neoplasms. Overall, stage for stage and grade for grade, P-RCC appears to have a better 5-year survival than C-RCC.[64a]

Chromophobe RCC: epidemiology, and macroscopic, microscopic and ultrastructural appearances

Thoenes et al first described this variant of RCC in 1985.[65,66] It accounts for 5% of renal neoplasms in surgical series and is thought to arise from the intercalated cells of the nephron.[67] These neoplasms are more likely to be identified incidentally during other medical investigations.[68] Radiologically, they cannot be distinguished from C-RCC; however, they have a better prognosis than C-RCC and are more likely to be organ confined at presentation. There is a very slight male predominance, and there is a mean age at presentation in the sixth decade and an age range of 31–75 years.[68–70]

Grossly, chromophobe RCC resembles C-RCC, averaging 8 cm in size, with a range of 1.3–20 cm. The cut surface is usually more solid and less variegated than C-RCC, and is usually beige or light brown but can be grey (Figure 22.1g). Occasional tumours can mimic oncocytomas, with a central or eccentric, stellate fibrous scar.[50] Ultrastructurally, these tumours have a characteristic appearance. The cytoplasm of the neoplastic cells contain numerous microvesicles 150–300 nm in diameter. These vesicles are round to oval and often have the complex appearance of a vesicle within a vesicle.[71,72]

Classical versus eosinophilic chromophobe RCC variants

Histologically, two variants of chromophobe RCC are recognized: classical and eosinophilic.[69,73] The classical type has a compact solid architecture and is composed of large polygonal cells with abundant finely granular cytoplasm. The cells show condensation of the cytoplasm at the periphery of the cell, resulting in prominent cytoplasmic membranes (Figure 22.1h). The classical form can mimic C-RCC. The eosinophilic variant is composed of cells with abundant eosinophilic granular cytoplasm and can resemble renal oncocytoma. Hales colloidal iron stain is diagnostically useful in this regard, as it stains the cytoplasm of the neoplastic cells blue, a reaction that does not usually occur with other renal neoplasms.[74,75] Cytokeratin 7 immunohistochemistry may also be useful in this context.[76]

Collecting duct carcinoma: epidemiology, and macroscopic and microscopic appearances

Collecting duct carcinoma, as its name implies, is a neoplasm that arises from the collecting duct epithelium.[77,78] It is a rare tumour accounting for approximately 1% of renal neoplasms in surgical series.[3,5] The tumour appears to be more common in males, and while the mean age at presentation is 55 years, several cases have been described in patients in their second and third decades.[77,78] The tumour most commonly presents with haematuria, and urine cytology is more frequently positive for malignant cells than with other renal neoplasms.[79,80]

The tumours are usually smaller than C-RCC with an average diameter of about 5 cm. The mass is usually located within the renal medulla, where it commonly distorts the pelvicalyceal system.[77] Usually, the tumours are uniformly grey-white in colour and generally lack areas of necrosis or haemorrhage. Satellite deposits of tumour may occasionally be seen in a subcapsular position.[77,78]

Histologically, these tumours may have a tubulopapillary architecture. Generally, the bulk of the neoplasm is composed of infiltrating glands lined by pleomorphic cells which lie in a desmoplastic stroma.[5,77] Occasional tumours show dysplastic changes in the cells lining adjacent collecting ducts.[78] These tumours often contain mucicarmine-positive intracytoplasmic mucin and show positive immunoreactivity for both high-molecular-weight cytokeratin and *Ulex europaeus* agglutinin, findings which help distinguish this from other RCC variants.[81]

Collecting-duct RCC are associated with a very poor clinical prognosis, with very few patients alive at 5-year follow-up. At the time of diagnosis, there is often evidence of tumour dissemination and spread to retroperitoneal lymph nodes, an uncommon finding in other forms of RCC.[82,83] Medullary carcinoma, a very poorly differentiated form of collecting-duct carcinoma, has been described in young adults with sickle-cell trait.[83a]

RCC, unclassified

There remains a very rare group of neoplasms that do not neatly fit into the current diagnostic framework, and that are currently included in the unclassified group. In the past few years, this has led to the delineation of new pathological entities reported as single case reports or small case series in pathological journals. Further recognition and characterization of these neoplasms in adjuvant genetic studies should lead to further refinement and modification of RCC classification.

Sarcomatoid change

Older classifications of RCC delineated a separate subgroup of sarcomatoid RCC. The current classification recognizes that sarcomatoid change merely represents dedifferentiation of the carcinoma cells, allowing them to acquire a morphology that is similar to that seen in many soft-tissue sarcomas. This morphology can occur in any form of RCC, and areas of the parent tumour can usually be seen with careful sampling. Although some studies have suggested an increased incidence in chromophobe carcinoma,[4] it is these authors' impression that this morphology occurs more frequently with C-RCC. The importance of sarcomatoid change lies in its association with a poor clinical outcome.[84,85]

THE MOLECULAR GENETICS OF RENAL EPITHELIAL NEOPLASIA DEVELOPMENT

Over the last two decades, significant insights have been gained into the molecular mechanisms underlying the development of renal epithelial neoplasia. Our current understanding is based primarily upon findings gathered from the following three broad but complementary approaches:

1. the study of rare inherited cancer syndromes which predispose to the development of renal neoplasia
2. the identification and further analysis of chromosomal defects in RCC by cytogenetic and molecular cytogenetic methods
3. the analysis in RCC of candidate genes which play defined roles in the development of other malignancies.

In this section, we review the major chromosomal and gene-specific defects detected in adult renal neoplasia, and consider their relevance and contribution to the current histopathological classification.

Inherited cancer predisposition syndromes identify genes involved in RCC development

While the majority of RCCs (~98%) are sporadic in nature, a significant hereditary component of the disease exists (approximately 2% of cases). Genetic investigations of the causes of inherited forms of RCC have provided important insights into the molecular mechanisms of tumourigenesis in both familial and sporadic RCC. In many cases, the underlying genetic defects in these tumour-predisposition syndromes have also been demonstrated to play a significant role in sporadic disease. Notably, the mean age at onset is younger in familial than sporadic RCC cases.[86–88] Familial RCC may be classified by whether (1) RCC is the only feature or (2) whether there are additional features, as in von Hippel-Lindau (VHL) disease. The genetic basis of inherited RCC susceptibility is summarized in Table 22.2.

von Hippel-Lindau (VHL) disease and familial conventional RCC

The most common cause of inherited RCC is von Hippel-Lindau (VHL) disease, a dominantly inherited familial cancer syndrome with a prevalence of approximately 1 in 35 000 live births, which is characterized by a high risk of C-RCC (>70% by age 60 years); retinal and cerebellar haemangioblastomas, phaeochromocytomas and renal, pancreatic and epididymal cysts. Pancreatic islet cell tumours and endolymphatic sac tumours are rare but significant complications. C-RCC is the most common cause of death in VHL disease, and is characterized by a combination of early onset (mean age of onset in VHL patients is in the fifth decade, but C-RCC has been reported in a teenager with VHL disease) and often multiple tumours (>50% of patients have bilateral or multicentric tumours).[89,90]

Identification of the* VHL *tumour-suppressor gene

The gene for VHL disease has been localized to the distal region of the short arm of chromosome 3 (3p25–26), and was isolated in 1993.[91] This has provided opportunities for the management and early diagnosis of VHL patients who do not satisfy the clinical diagnostic criteria. Current *VHL* mutation analysis using a complete range of techniques can provide a detection rate approaching 100% in non-mosaic patients with classical VHL disease.[92] Most families have different mutations in the *VHL* gene, but DNA predictive testing (by direct mutation analysis or linked DNA markers) is possible in the majority of families, so that annual screening can be discontinued in relatives who are shown not to be gene carriers. In addition to identifying gene carriers, the identification of a *VHL* gene mutation may also provide a guide to the likely phenotype. Marked differences in disease phenotype are observed between VHL families such that germline deletions or mutations predicted to cause a truncated protein product are associated with a low risk of phaeochromocytoma, whereas specific amino-acid substitutions can cause a high risk of phaeochromocytoma. Most missense mutations are associated with a high risk of RCC, but some

Table 22.2 The genetic basis of hereditary forms of RCC: genetic defects indentified to date, relationships to histopathological subtypes, and their role in sporadic RCC development.

Inherited RCC predisposition	Syndrome	Genetic defect			Role in sporadic RCC
		Locus	Gene	Function	
Conventional RCC	von Hippel-Lindau disease	3p25	VHL	Tumour suppressor gene	Inactivated in 60–70% of C-RCC cases
Conventional RCC	non-VHL familial C-RCC	? (no linkage to VHL, MET or chromosome 3p loci)	?	?	?
Conventional RCC	Familial C-RCC	Chromosome 3p translocations, e.g. t(3;8), t(3;6) and t(2;3)	?	?	?
Papillary RCC (type 1)	Hereditary papillary RCC type 1 (HPRC1)	7q31.1–34	MET	Oncogene	Activating mutations in 13% of P-RCC cases
Papillary RCC (type 2)	Multiple cutaneous and uterine leiomyomatosis (MCL)	1q42.3–q43	Fumarate hydratase (FH)	? Tumour suppressor gene	?
Papillary RCC	Hyperparathyroidism–jaw tumour syndrome and familial papillary thyroid cancer	1q21–31	?	?	?
Renal oncocytoma/ chromophobe RCC	Birt-Hogg-Dube syndrome	17p11.2	BHD	? Tumour suppressor gene	?
RCC	Tuberose sclerosis	9q34, 16p13	TSC1, TSC2	Tumour suppressor genes	No somatic mutations in RCC cases

missense mutations are associated with a low risk of RCC and a high risk of phaeochromocytoma.[93–97]

The VHL *TSG in sporadic C-RCC tumourigenesis*

The *VHL* gene appears to function as a classic tumour-suppressor gene (TSG) so that inactivation of both alleles is required to initiate tumourigenesis. Thus, in VHL patients, inactivation of one allele by a germline mutation is followed by inactivation (usually loss) of the second allele.[98,99] Importantly, it appears that inactivation of both *VHL* alleles also occurs in the majority of sporadic RCCs, thus establishing that somatic inactivation of the *VHL* gene is a critical event in the pathogenesis of the most common form of non-familial RCC. Somatic *VHL* gene mutations can be identified in approximately 50% of conventional RCCs. A further 15% of tumours display epigenetic *VHL* gene inactivation through promoter hypermethylation and transcriptional silencing. Notably, *VHL* inactivation appears to be specific to the C-RCC subtype. Somatic *VHL* gene mutations have not been identified in sporadic non-C-RCC, supporting the concept that conventional and non-C-RCC have a different genetic basis.[100–104] Chromosome 3p loss also appears to be an early event in tumourigenesis (see next section), an observation compatible with a role for *VHL* inactivation in tumour initiation.[105]

Function of the VHL *TSG product*

The *VHL* TSG encodes two protein products, a full-length 213-amino-acid VHL protein ($pVHL_{29}$) which migrates with an apparent molecular mass of ~29 kDa, and a second product ($pVHL_{19}$) that is generated by internal translation and lacks the first 53 amino acids.[106] Reintroduction of the wild-type

VHL protein into VHL-deficient RCC cells suppresses tumourigenicity both *in vitro* and *in vivo* in nude mice assays, thus confirming its tumour suppressor function.[107,108] No germline or somatic mutations have been reported in the first 53 codons, and $pVHL_{19}$ has been shown to possess tumour suppressor activity.[106] The complex genotype–phenotype associations observed in VHL disease (see above) suggest that the VHL gene product has multiple and tissue-specific functions.[109] pVHL has been reported to bind directly or indirectly a number of proteins, including elongins B and C, Cul2, Rbx1 and fibronectin, and to play roles in the regulation of cell-cycle progression, extracellular matrix assembly and expression of target genes such as vascular endothelial growth factor and carbonic anhydrases.[109]

Critical insights into pVHL function emerged from similarities observed between the VCBC(R) (*V*HL-elongin *C*-elongin*B*-Cul2-*R*bx1) complex and the SCF (*S*kp–1-*C*dc53/Cul1-*F*-box protein) class of E3 ubiquitin ligases,[110] findings further supported by the solving of the three-dimensional structure of the pVHL–elonginB–elonginC complex.[111] Thus, Maxwell et al[112] demonstrated that pVHL is critical for targeting the alpha subunits of the hypoxia-inducible transcription factors HIF-1 and HIF-2 (EPAS) for proteosomal destruction under normoxic conditions. The HIF-1 and HIF-2 transcription factors play a key role in the cellular response to hypoxia (oxygen sensing) and the regulation of genes involved in energy metabolism, angiogenesis and apoptosis, including VEGF. Inactivation of the pVHL TSG (as observed in tumours from VHL patients and most sporadic C-RCC) results in constitutively elevated intracellular levels of HIF-1α and HIF-2α, which correlate with the high levels of VEGF expression and hypervascularity observed in these tumours.[112,113] The VCBCR complex has also been shown to promote HIF-1α ubiquitylation,[114] and pVHL has been demonstrated to act as an adapter protein that recruits specific protein targets for ubiquitylation and proteosomal degradation (reviewed by Kaelin[115]). Disease-causing pVHL mutants are predicted to disrupt the VCBCR complex,[111] and we recently demonstrated that disruption of HIF-1α/2α regulation is characteristic of RCC-associated pVHL mutants.[116] The identification of further protein substrates for pVHL-targeted proteasomal degradation or additional non-SCF-like functions for pVHL may provide further insights into pVHL function, its role in RCC tumourigenesis and genotype–phenotype correlations in VHL disease. The function of the VHL protein is summarized in Figure 22.2.

Chromosome 3 translocations and familial C-RCC

In rare cases, inherited predisposition to C-RCC has been associated with balanced translocations involving the short arm of chromosome 3. Reports of chromosome 3 translocations associated with RCC susceptibility have described a variety of chromosome 3 breakpoints, such as t(3;8)(p14;q24),[117] t(3;6)(p13;q25),[118] t(2;3)(q35;q21)[119] and t(3;12)(q35;q21).[120] Thus, there is no consistent involvement of candidate TSG regions on chromosome 3p, since C-RCC-associated chromosome 3 translocations are contained within the pericentromeric regions of 3p and 3q.[121] Analysis of tumours from patients with the C-RCC-associated translocations t(3;8), t(3;6) and t(2;3) has demonstrated loss of the derivative chromosome. Furthermore, the retained chromosome 3 has been found to harbour a somatic *VHL* gene mutation in tumours from individuals with the t(3;8) and t(2;3) (so the tumours had biallelic *VHL* gene inactivation).[119,122] These findings further implicate *VHL* gene inactivation in the pathogenesis of C-RCC, whereby a model for RCC tumourigenesis in translocation families is (1) inheritance of a pericentromeric chromosome 3 translocation, (2) loss of the derivative chromosome 3 containing a *VHL* gene by random non-disjunction and (3) somatic mutation of the remaining normal *VHL* allele.

Non-VHL familial C-RCC (FCRC)

Familial C-RCC with no additional features of VHL disease occurs, but is uncommon. Prior to 1991, there had been 23 reports of 105 patients with familial C-RCC.[87] Although *VHL* gene mutations have been identified in some cases of familial phaeochromocytoma (without other features),[123,124] to date, germline *VHL* gene mutations have not been reported in familial C-RCC kindreds. The definition of subtypes of familial RCC based on histopathology and the availability of molecular genetic testing

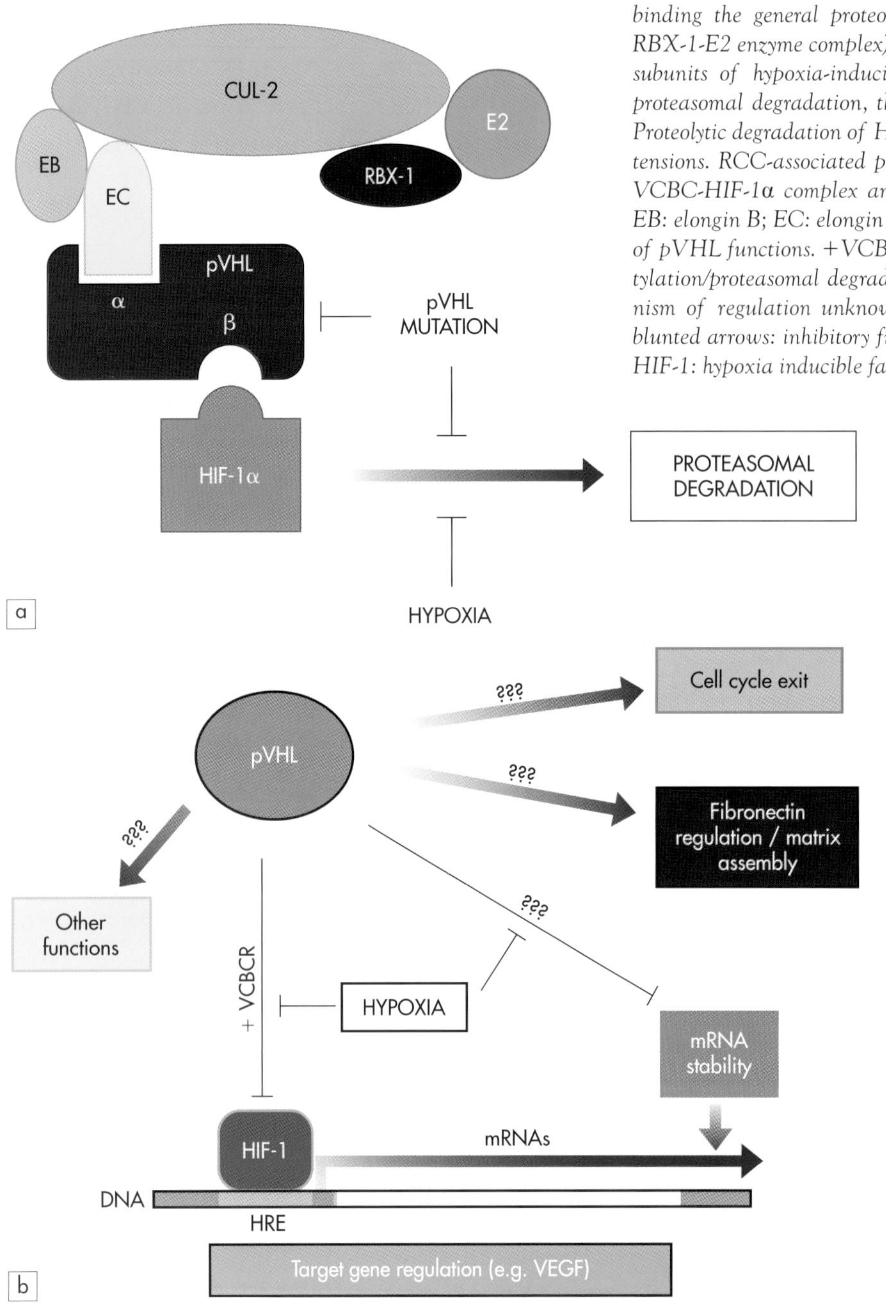

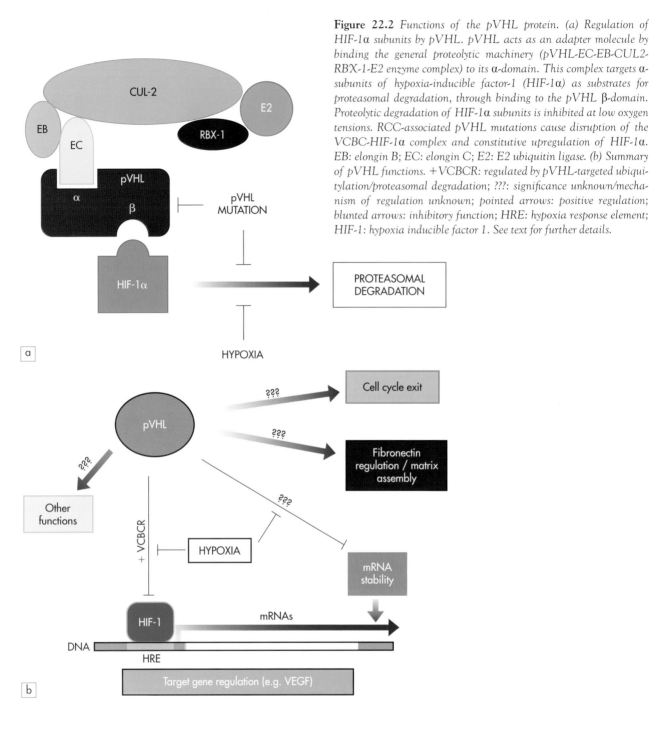

Figure 22.2 *Functions of the pVHL protein. (a) Regulation of HIF-1α subunits by pVHL. pVHL acts as an adapter molecule by binding the general proteolytic machinery (pVHL-EC-EB-CUL2-RBX-1-E2 enzyme complex) to its α-domain. This complex targets α-subunits of hypoxia-inducible factor-1 (HIF-1α) as substrates for proteasomal degradation, through binding to the pVHL β-domain. Proteolytic degradation of HIF-1α subunits is inhibited at low oxygen tensions. RCC-associated pVHL mutations cause disruption of the VCBC-HIF-1α complex and constitutive upregulation of HIF-1α. EB: elongin B; EC: elongin C; E2: E2 ubiquitin ligase. (b) Summary of pVHL functions. +VCBCR: regulated by pVHL-targeted ubiquitylation/proteasomal degradation; ???: significance unknown/mechanism of regulation unknown; pointed arrows: positive regulation; blunted arrows: inhibitory function; HRE: hypoxia response element; HIF-1: hypoxia inducible factor 1. See text for further details.*

for germline *VHL* and *MET* (see next section) gene mutations has led to the recognition of families with dominantly inherited susceptibility to C-RCC who do not have VHL disease or a chromosome 3 translocation.[88,125,126] In the original description of two large kindreds with FCRC, the age at onset was later than in VHL disease (8/9 patients aged >50 years) and usually unilateral. However, a further report identified additional families with FCRC in which there was early onset of RCC (50% diagnosed <50 years of age).[88] To date, there is no evidence of a significantly increased risk of non-renal cancers in FCRC kindreds. The molecular basis of familial non-VHL C-RCC (FCRC) has not been defined, except that it is not linked to *VHL*, *MET* or chromosome 3p.[88,126]

The *MET* proto-oncogene and familial type 1 papillary (P-)RCC (HPRC1)

Zbar et al[125,127] have described kindreds with dominantly inherited P-RCC. Linkage to the *VHL* gene was excluded in families suitable for genetic linkage analysis.[127] Recently, it was suggested that P-RCC can be subdivided into two groups with different histopathologies: type 1 tumours, which are usually multiple and low grade, and type 2, which are single, are of higher grade and have a poorer prognosis.[64]

HPRC1 is caused by mutations in the MET *proto-oncogene*

HPRC1 is a rare dominantly inherited disorder (minimum prevalence 1 per 10 million) characterized by the development of multiple, bilateral type 1 P-RCC. By linkage analysis, the HPRC1 gene was localized to a 27 cM interval contained within chromosome 7q31.1–34 in HPRC1 families. Mutational analysis of candidate genes within this region identified germline mutations in the *MET* proto-oncogene in these families.[128–130] *MET* mutations reported to date in HPRC1 represent missense mutations within its tyrosine kinase domain, and three HPRC1 *MET* gene mutations (H1112R, V1238I, V1110I) have been reported as probable founder mutations. A striking feature of HPRC1 families is non-penetrance, and there is a high frequency of subclinical disease in gene carriers who undergo renal imaging, illustrated by reports that penetrance of the H1112R mutation by abdominal CT scanning is estimated as only 30% at age 50 years.[131] In an effort to understand the relationship between *MET* mutation and the trisomy 7 commonly observed in tumours from HPRC1 patients, Zhuang et al[132] demonstrated that the additional chromosome 7 copy consistently arose from a non-random duplication of the chromosome bearing the mutated *MET*, further implicating this event in tumourigenesis.

MET *mutations in sporadic P-RCC*

Somatic *MET* mutations have been shown to play a role in 13% of sporadic P-RCC cases with no family history of renal tumours. Consistent with the definition of type 1 P-RCC, both familial and sporadic renal tumours with identifiable *MET* mutations show a distinctive P-RCC type 1 phenotype and are thus genetically and histologically different from renal tumours seen in other hereditary renal syndromes and most sporadic renal tumors with papillary architecture. Although all hereditary and sporadic P-RCC with *MET* mutations share P-RCC type 1 histology, not all type 1 sporadic P-RCC carry *MET* mutations, suggesting the involvement of further genetic mechanisms in these tumours.[133]

Function of the MET *proto-oncogene and its role in RCC development*

The *MET* proto-oncogene, primarily expressed in epithelial cells, encodes a cell-surface receptor for hepatocyte growth factor (HGF). Under normal circumstances, signalling through the MET receptor tyrosine kinase requires the presence of its ligand. Normal signalling through the HGF/MET system is involved in cell growth, movement and differentiation and appears to play an important role in the early development of the metanephros and branching tubulogenesis of the developing kidney.[134,135] The impact of the *MET* mutations identified in HPRC1 patients has been studied by introducing these mutations into the mouse *met* gene, and testing their effects on cellular signalling, growth and tumourigenicity. The *MET* mutations identified exhibited increased levels of tyrosine phosphorylation and enhanced kinase activity when compared to wild-type *MET*, and caused the oncogenic transformation of mouse NIH 3T3 cells. Thus, all germline *MET* mutations associated with HPRC1 appear to be activating and tumourigenic;[128,129,136] however, the functional consequences of different *MET* mutations vary, and there is evidence that different *MET* mutations may activate different signalling pathways and display differential effects on tumourigenicity.[137]

The fumarate hydratase (FH) gene and familial type 2 papillary RCC (HPRC2)

Multiple cutaneous and uterine leiomyomatosis (MCL) is an autosomal dominant disease in which affected cases develop benign smooth muscle tumours of the skin (leiomyomata). In a subset of families, predisposition to type 2 P-RCC (HPRC2) is found together with hereditary leiomyomata (HLRCC/MCL). The gene responsible for multiple leiomyomatosis has been mapped to a 14 cM interval on chromosome 1q42.3–q43, and was recently identified as fumarate hydratase (*FH*), a Krebs cycle enzyme.[138] *FH* therefore represents a HPRC2 susceptibility gene. Mutations of *FH* in affected individuals are predicted to be inactivating and include both truncating (deletions, premature termination codons) and non-truncating (missense mutations, in-frame deletions) changes. Moreover, *FH* appears to act as a tumour suppressor gene in HLRCC/MCL, since the majority of tumours from affected individuals also display deletion of the wild-type *FH* allele. These genetic data are further substantiated by the reduced fumarase activity detected in tumours from affected individuals.[138]

The FH gene in sporadic RCC

The role of *FH* mutations in the development of sporadic RCCs remains to be established. Kiuru et al[139] recently reported no evidence of *FH* mutations in a series of 52 RCCs. Although this study ruled out a major role for *FH* mutations in C-RCC development (no mutations were detected in 40 C-RCC tumours), only five type 2 P-RCC cases were investigated. The examination of a more extensive type 2 P-RCC cohort and alternative mechanisms of *FH* inactivation to mutation (such as transcriptional silencing though promoter hypermethylation) will therefore be required to assess comprehensively the role of *FH* in RCC pathogenesis.

Birt-Hogg-Dube syndrome and familial chromophobe RCC/renal oncocytoma

Weirich et al[140] provided evidence that susceptibility to renal oncocytoma/chromophobe RCC may be inherited. Five families were described with multiple members affected with renal oncocytoma. Tumours were often multiple and bilateral in affected family members. Toro et al[141] reported that 3/5 of the kindreds with familial renal oncocytoma contained affected individuals with rare hamartomatous tumours of the hair follicle known as fibrofolliculoma, consistent with a diagnosis of the dominantly inherited skin disorder, Birt-Hogg-Dube (BHD) syndrome.[142] BHD syndrome and renal tumours were observed to segregate together in an autosomal dominant fashion, and patients with BHD and their relatives are thus at risk of development of renal tumours.[141] Renal tumours in BHD may be single or multiple, and the histological appearance of renal tumours in BHD is predominantly that of chromophobe RCC/oncocytoma but variable, although they are histologically distinct from those observed in HPRC1.[143]

BHD (folliculin) mutations in BHD patients

Using a recombination-mapping approach, Nickerson et al[144] narrowed the BHD disease locus to a 4 cM region at chromosome 17p11.2. In BHD families, disease-associated mutations were subsequently identified in a novel gene contained within this region, designated *BHD*, which predisposes to the development of oncocytic and chromophobe renal tumours, BHD skin lesions and collapsed lung/lung cysts. The full-length sequence of the *BHD* gene predicts a novel protein, folliculin, which is highly conserved across species. *BHD* mutations typically result in truncation of the folliculin protein, consistent with its inactivation in RCC pathogenesis and a potential tumour suppressor role.[144] Further studies are required to address the role and relevance of *BHD* mutations in sporadic RCC development, and their functional consequences.

Familial P-RCC and hyperparathyroidism–jaw tumour syndrome/familial papillary thyroid cancer

A familial hyperparathyroidism syndrome associated with jaw cysts (HPT-JT) has been mapped to chromosome 1q21–q31.[145] A further family linked to the HPT-JT region in which renal cysts and a variety of tumours, including renal cortical adenoma and P-RCC, were associated with parathyroid tumours was recently reported.[146] Furthermore, Malchoff et al[147] described a single kindred with familial papillary thyroid cancer susceptibility mapping to chromosome 1q21. Two family members developed P-RCC, suggesting a common link between these tumour types. Taken together, evidence from these two syndromes suggests the presence of a further P-RCC susceptibility locus in the 1q21–31 region, although the gene responsible remains to be identified.

Tuberose sclerosis

This dominantly inherited multiple hamartoma syndrome has been associated with an increased risk of

RCC.[148–150] Tuberose sclerosis is genetically heterogeneous and caused by germline mutations in the *TSC1* and *TSC2* TSGs. In rats, germline mutations in *TSC2* cause the Eker rat model of familial RCC,[151] and heterozygous *Tsc1* and *Tsc2* knockout mice develop a renal cystadenoma/carcinoma phenotype.[151,152] However, in humans, angiomyolipomas are by far the most common renal lesion. Although RCC is infrequent in tuberose sclerosis, several reports have described multifocal and bilateral disease in young patients.[148–150] Although the histological appearances of angiomyolipoma are very variable and some lesions could be mistaken for atypical RCC,[153] the current consensus is that there is a real association between TSC and RCC (of variable histopathology).[154,155] However, it is notable that somatic mutation of either the *TSC1* or *TSC2* genes has not been reported in sporadic human RCC.

Common RCC chromosomal abnormalities are associated with histopathological criteria

The application of cytogenetic and molecular cytogenetic techniques to the analysis of RCC tumours has revealed characteristic patterns of chromosomal aberrations associated with each RCC histopathological subtype (see Table 22.3), suggesting the presence of loci involved in RCC development on these chromosomes. Non-P-RCC (predominantly C-RCC) are characterized by the loss of chromosome 3 sequences, rearrangement of chromosome 5q and loss of chromosome 14q sequences (reviewed by Kovacs[58]). P-RCC are commonly characterized by trisomy of chromosomes 7 and 17, and loss of the Y chromosome (in men), as well as additional trisomies (such as chromosomes 12, 16, 20) (reviewed by Kovacs[58]), but notably, chromosome 3 deletions (which occur in most C-RCC) are uncommon.[125] A specific chromosomal translocation between chromosomes X and 1 (t(X;1)(p11;q21)) has been described for a subgroup of P-RCC,[156] and a fusion gene which is created at the translocation breakpoint has been identified,[157] although its role in P-RCC pathogenesis remains to be elucidated. In a series of chromophobe RCC, Speicher et al[158] reported that losses of entire chromosomes were commonly observed, with underrepresentation of chromosome 1 occurring in most cases and losses of chromosomes 2, 6, 10, 13, 17 and 21 in >65% of cases. Y chromosome loss was also observed in 6 of 13 tumours from male patients. Finally, renal oncocytoma is characterized by both normal and abnormal karyotypes (reviewed by Kovacs[58]). A number of different structural rearrangements/translocations involving the q13 region of chromosome 11 have been reported in these tumours (for example, t(9;11)(p23;q12), t(9;11)(p23;q13) and t(5;11)(q35;q13)) (reviewed by Fuzesi et al[159]).

The mapping and identification of further RCC tumour suppressor genes: correlations with histopathological data

Tumour suppressor genes (TSGs) generally regulate tumour growth and development in a negative fashion, such that both alleles of such genes must be inactivated to promote tumour development. Genetic changes which inactivate TSGs typically involve two types of event; firstly, the loss of large regions of chromosomal DNA encompassing the

Table 22.3 Common chromosomal abnormalities detected in sporadic RCC.

RCC subtype	DNA losses	DNA gains	Chromosomal rearrangements
Conventional	3, 14	–	3p (translocations), 5q (rearrangements)
Papillary	Y	Trisomy 7, 17	t(X;1) translocation
Chromophobe	1, 2, 6, 10, 13, 17, 21, Y	–	–
Oncocytoma	–	–	11q13 region (translocations)

first allele (such as deletion, chromosome loss or elimination through mitotic recombination errors), and, secondly, a smaller mutational event affecting the second allele (such as point mutation, epigenetic modification or smaller deletion). Thus, in tumour samples, chromosomal regions displaying significant DNA losses are suggestive of TSG location and may be detected by cytogenetic/molecular cytogenetic methods or by screening tumours for loss of heterozygosity (LOH) by allelotyping with polymorphic microsatellite markers.

Multiple TSGs on the short arm of chromosome 3 are central to non-P-RCC development

Deletions of the short arm of chromosome 3 are the most common genetic aberration observed in RCC, with 3p LOH reported to occur in 45–90% of sporadic and hereditary RCC, although these changes are specifically associated with non-P-RCC and are not usually observed in papillary tumours.[91,105,160] Furthermore, 3p allele loss is an early event which does not correlate with stage or grade. In addition to the *VHL* TSG locus, several further regions of 3p have been implicated in the development of RCC by LOH studies, suggesting the involvement of multiple tumour suppressor loci on this chromosome arm. The key regions most commonly implicated are 3p21,[161,162] 3p12–14[163,164] and 3p25–26 (*VHL*) (see Figure 22.3). When 3p deletions are detected, the 3p21 region is most consistently included, and LOH at 3p12–21 is observed in both the presence and absence of *VHL* inactivation, suggesting the presence of *VHL*-independent tumour suppressor loci.[104,162,165] These data are supported by functional evidence from gene-transfer experiments, which demonstrate the ability of 3p12–21 elements to suppress tumourigenicity. Firstly, Sanchez et al[166] showed that transfer of the 3p14–q11 region into a highly malignant RCC cell line reduced its tumourigenicity in nude mice. No equivalent suppression was reported upon introduction of a 3p12–q24 fragment, thus functionally defining a tumour suppressor locus between 3p12–14. Secondly, Killary et al[167] introduced a 2 Mb fragment of 3p21 into a mouse fibrosarcoma cell line, which dramatically reduced its tumourigenicity.

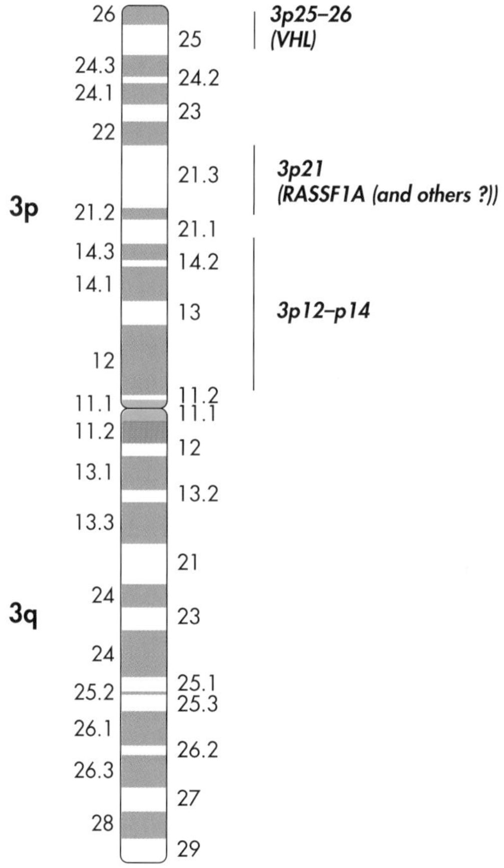

Figure 22.3 *Human chromosome 3 and C-RCC. Idiogram showing the three independent subchromosomal regions harbouring candidate tumour suppressor genes involved in C-RCC development.*

Taken together, these findings indicate that *VHL* inactivation is not sufficient to initiate C-RCC and that loss of gatekeeper 3p12–21 TSG(s) is a crucial event for RCC development in both *VHL*-negative and *VHL*-positive C-RCC. Inactivated genes located within these regions await identification. Recently, the RAS association family 1 gene (isoform *RASSF1A*), located at 3p21.3, was identified as a candidate TSG in lung and breast carcinomas, which display frequent chromosomal losses affecting the 3p21 region.[168,169] Notably, rather than displaying inactivation by genetic mutation, *RASSF1A* is commonly targeted for inactivation by epigenetic mechanisms in conjunction with chromosomal loss. Studies of *RASSF1A* in RCC have demonstrated epigenetic silencing of its expression by promoter hypermethylation in the majority (up to 90%) of C-RCCs, affecting both *VHL*-inactivated and *VHL*-intact (wild-type) C-RCC tumours.[170–172] Interestingly, *RASSF1A* hypermethylation has also been reported in a significant subset of P-RCC (~40%) in the absence of chromosome 3p deletion.[171] Experimental studies have confirmed a tumour suppressor function for the RASSF1A protein in RCC *in vitro*.[170] Together, these data are highly suggestive that *RASSF1A* may represent the candidate renal TSG for the 3p21.3 region, and may play a significant role in the pathogenesis of both C-RCC and P-RCC.

Mapping further RCC TSGs provides insights into RCC pathogenesis

Thrash-Bingham et al[105] surveyed allelic losses across the entire genome in 28 RCC samples (22 non-papillary, 6 papillary). Consistent with previous findings, 3p loss was the most common aberration detected in non-papillary tumours (41%), and was not observed in any P-RCC. Allelic losses on 6q, 8p, 9p, 9q and 14q (18–21%) were also observed in both subtypes. These molecular data show good agreement with previous cytogenetic studies which have shown loss of chromosomes 6p (14%), 8p (22%), 9pq (14%) and 14q (30–50%) in RCC tumours.[58] LOH for chromosomes 11 and 21 was detected in papillary tumours, suggesting the involvement of a TSG on this chromosome in P-RCC. This study also revealed no correlation between disease stage and LOH of any particular chromosome. It is highly significant that 3p loss was never the sole aberration observed in any tumour, and usually occurred in association with losses on 6q, 8p, 9pq and/or 14q. These data further suggest that alterations to genes on 3p are necessary, but not sufficient for the development and/or progression of non-P-RCC and that other TSGs are involved in the tumourigenesis of RCC.

Of the changes described, loss of chromosomes 8p, 9p and 14q may be of particular interest. LOH at these loci has been detected in 18–33% (8p), 21–33% (9p) and 37–45% (14q) of non-P-RCC, and significantly correlate with tumour grade, suggesting that they may be promising markers of adverse prognosis.[58,173,174] These data are consistent with observations by Thrash-Bingham et al[105] that loss of 14q is associated with an elevated level of overall allele loss compared to tumours with 14q retention, suggesting that 14q loss may be associated with aggressive disease, and that a gene on 14q may be involved in the control of genomic stability.

Allelotyping studies have also identified genetic differences between type 1 and type 2 P-RCCs: Significant differences in frequency of allelic loss were noted on 17q (78.6% of type 1 P-RCC versus 12.5% of type 2 tumours, $P = 0.006$) and 9p (0% versus 37.5%).[175] These data reinforce the presence of P-RCC genes at these loci, and support the premise that the two P-RCC subtypes arise from distinct genetic pathways.

Analysis of candidate TSGs in RCC: PTEN, the P53 pathway and RB

The *PTEN (MMAC1)* TSG was recently isolated at chromosome 10q23 and found to be inactivated by point mutation or homozygous deletion in tumour types including glioma, prostatic and breast carcinoma.[176,177] *PTEN* was also identified as the gene predisposing to Cowden's disease, an autosomal dominant cancer predisposition syndrome associated with an increased risk of breast, skin and thyroid tumors and occasional cases of other cancers, including bladder and RCC.[178] Two studies have since reported that *PTEN* mutation is observed in a small subset of sporadic RCCs (~7.5% of cases), with mutations observed in both C-RCC and P-RCC samples.[179,180]

The *P53* TSG at chromosome 17p13.1 encodes a 393-amino-acid protein which plays a specific role in the maintenance of DNA integrity and cell-cycle control. Missense *P53* mutations, the most commonly detected alteration of the *P53* gene, and/or allelic losses occur frequently in diverse human cancers. Indeed, alterations to the *P53* gene have been demonstrated to be one of the most common genetic changes identified in human cancer, detected in most common carcinomas including lung (40–80% of tumours), gastric (30–60%), breast (10–40%), colorectal (40–70%) and bladder (30–60%) (reviewed by Chang et al[181]). LOH studies at the *P53* locus in RCC have demonstrated good concordance (17–21% loss).[182,183] However, in such studies, *P53* mutation rates in RCC are consistently low (in 0–10% of cases),[183–185] with those few mutations detected showing no overall association with any histopathological criteria. Abrogation of P53 function in tumour development may also occur through the genetic disruption of further key proteins in the P53 regulatory pathway including ARF (alternative reading frame; mouse $p19^{ARF}$, human $p14^{ARF}$) and MDM2 (human, HDM2) (reviewed by Sherr[186]). Rare mutations at the *CDKN2A* locus (encoding $p14^{ARF}$) have been reported in a panel of 113 C-RCC (in ~10% of cases), but no homozygous deletions were detected in 54 cases analysed.[187] Similarly, no evidence of *MDM2* amplification was detected in a series of 53 RCC cases.[188] On the basis of this accumulated evidence, genetic disruption of the P53-MDM2-$p14^{ARF}$ axis does not appear to play a major role in RCC pathogenesis.

The retinoblastoma (*RB*) TSG has been localized to chromosome band 13q14, a region frequently deleted in many sporadic cancers. The *RB* gene encodes a nuclear phosphoprotein (pRB) whose normal cellular functions are centred on its ability to regulate the cell cycle through induction of G1 arrest. *RB* loss has been detected in tumour types including small cell lung cancer and osteosarcomas (reviewed by Classon and Harlow[189]). No mutational analyses of the *RB* gene have been reported in RCC; however, studies by Suzuki et al[190] showing no LOH at the *RB* locus in 15 informative RCCs, and by Walther et al[173] demonstrating no loss of RB protein staining by immunohistochemistry in 30 tumours suggest that alterations to the *RB* gene are not central to RCC development.

SUMMARY

Molecular genetic techniques have provided a powerful research tool which has allowed the elucidation of specific genetic alterations involved in the development and progression of RCC. Molecular findings have informed the diagnostic classification for adult renal epithelial neoplasms, which currently groups these tumours into subtypes based on clinical, histopathological and genetic criteria. Recent advances in our understanding of the molecular basis of RCC development have further reinforced the close relationships that exist between specific genetic defects and the different RCC subtypes, and support the concept that each RCC subtype represents a distinct clinical and genetic entity characterized by the dysregulation of specific pathways underlying tumourigenesis. Furthermore, the distinctive pathogenesis of renal cell tumours compared to other major adult tumour types is highlighted and exemplified by the lack of defects affecting the *RB* gene and P53 pathway, and the involvement of multiple TSGs on the short arm of chromosome 3.

Further clarification of the oncogenetic processes involved in RCC development is anticipated over the coming years. For chromosomal defects detected in RCC, the identification of the putative RCC genes harboured within these regions will be of prime importance. Where specific gene defects have been identified, the elucidation of their functional consequences and role in tumourigenesis will be critical. Moreover, the application of new genome-wide technologies (such as gene expression microarrays) is anticipated to affect significantly our understanding of renal neoplasia.

This increased understanding of the molecular basis of RCC development provides the realistic prospect of improved management for RCC patients. Firstly, genetic and molecular markers of RCC development may provide reliable indicators of biological behaviour or therapeutic responsiveness, for use alongside current criteria in the diagnostic and prognostic assessment of RCC patients. Secondly, beyond gene identification, a greater understanding of the molecular pathways in which RCC genes function may highlight specific molecular targets for the development of novel therapeutic strategies in RCC. Meanwhile, the identification of specific genetic defects underlying inherited RCC susceptibility (for example, *VHL*, *MET*, *FH* and *BHD* mutation) has improved the clinical management and support of these families.

REFERENCES

1. Fleischmann J, Huntley NH. Renal tumours. In: Krane RJ, Siroky MB, Fitzpatrick JM, eds. Clinical Urology. Philadelphia: JP Lippincott, 1994; 359–373
2. Chow WH, Gridley G, Fraumeni JF, Jr, Jarvholm B. Obesity, hypertension, and the risk of kidney cancer in men. N Engl J Med 2000; 343: 1305–1311

3. Kovacs G, Akhtar M, Beckwith BJ, Bugert P et al. The Heidelberg classification of renal cell tumours. J Pathol 1997; 183: 131–133
4. Akhtar M, Tulbah A, Kardar AH, Ali MA. Sarcomatoid renal cell carcinoma: the chromophobe connection. Am J Surg Pathol 1997; 21: 1188–1195
5. Storkel S, Eble JN, Adlakha K, Amin M et al. Classification of renal cell carcinoma: Workgroup No. 1. Union Internationale Contre le Cancer (UICC) and the American Joint Committee on Cancer (AJCC). Cancer 1997; 80: 987–989
6. Moch H, Gasser T, Amin MB, Torhorst J et al. Prognostic utility of the recently recommended histologic classification and revised TNM staging system of renal cell carcinoma: a Swiss experience with 588 tumors. Cancer 2000; 89: 604–614
7. Amin MB, Tamboli P, Javidan, J, Stricker H et al. Prognostic impact of histologic subtyping of adult renal epithelial neoplasms: an experience of 405 cases. Am J Surg Pathol 2002; 26: 281–291
8. Thoenes W, Storkel S, Rumpelt HJ, Moll R. Cytomorphological typing of renal cell carcinoma—a new approach. Eur Urol 1990; 18 (Suppl 2): 6–9
9. Xipell JM. The incidence of benign renal nodules (a clinicopathologic study). J Urol 1971; 106: 503–506
10. Ornstein DK, Lubensky IA, Venzon D, Zbar B et al. Prevalence of microscopic tumors in normal appearing renal parenchyma of patients with hereditary papillary renal cancer. J Urol 2000; 163: 431–433
11. Evins SC, Varner W. Renal adenoma—a misnomer. Urology 1979; 13: 85–86
12. Grignon DJ, Eble JN. Papillary and metanephric adenomas of the kidney. Semin Diagn Pathol 1998; 15: 41–53
13. Kovacs G, Tory K, Kovacs A. Development of papillary renal cell tumours is associated with loss of Y-chromosome-specific DNA sequences. J Pathol 1994; 173: 39–44
14. Van Poppel H, Nilsson S, Algaba F, Bergerheim U et al. Precancerous lesions in the kidney. Scand J Urol Nephrol Suppl 2000; 205: 136–165
15. Morgan WR, Zincke H. Progression and survival after renal-conserving surgery for renal cell carcinoma: experience in 104 patients and extended follow-up. J Urol 1990; 144: 852–857; discussion 857–858
16. Fergany AF, Hafez KS, Novick AC. Long-term results of nephron sparing surgery for localized renal cell carcinoma: 10-year follow-up. J Urol 2000; 163: 442–445
17. Davis CJ, Jr, Barton JH, Sesterhenn IA, Mostofi FK. Metanephric adenoma. Clinicopathological study of fifty patients. Am J Surg Pathol 1995; 19: 1101–1114
18. Brisigotti M, Cozzutto C, Fabbretti G, Sergi C et al. Metanephric adenoma. Histol Histopathol 1992; 7: 689–692
19. Jones EC, Pins M, Dickersin GR, Young RH. Metanephric adenoma of the kidney. A clinicopathological, immunohistochemical, flow cytometric, cytogenetic, and electron microscopic study of seven cases. Am J Surg Pathol 1995; 19: 615–626
20. Brown JA, Sebo TJ, Segura JW. Metaphase analysis of metanephric adenoma reveals chromosome Y loss with chromosome 7 and 17 gain. Urology 1996; 48: 473–475
21. Renshaw AA. Basophilic tumours of kidney. J Urol Pathol 1998; 8: 85–101
22. Zippel L. Zur Kenntnis der Onkocyten. Virchows Arch Pathol Anat 1942; 308: 360–382
23. Klein MJ, Valensi QJ. Proximal tubular adenomas of kidney with so-called oncocytic features. A clinicopathologic study of 13 cases of a rarely reported neoplasm. Cancer 1976; 38: 906–914
24. Lieber MM, Tomera KM, Farrow GM. Renal oncocytoma. J Urol 1981; 125: 481–485
25. Merino MJ, Livolsi VA. Oncocytomas of the kidney. Cancer 1982; 50: 1852–1856
26. Choi H, Almagro UA, McManus JT, Norback DH et al. Renal oncocytoma. A clinicopathologic study. Cancer 1983; 51: 1887–1896
27. Alanen KA, Ekfors TO, Lipasti JA, Nurmi MJ. Renal oncocytoma: the incidence of 18 surgical and 12 autopsy cases. Histopathology 1984; 8: 731–737
28. Amin MB, Crotty TB, Tickoo SK, Farrow GM. Renal oncocytoma: a reappraisal of morphologic features with clinicopathologic findings in 80 cases. Am J Surg Pathol 1997; 21: 1–12
29. Perez-Ordonez B, Hamed G, Campbell S, Erlandson RA et al. Renal oncocytoma: a clinicopathologic study of 70 cases. Am J Surg Pathol 1997; 21: 871–883
30. Weiner SN, Bernstein RG. Renal oncocytoma: angiographic features of two cases. Radiology 1977; 125: 633–635
31. Ambos MA, Bosniak MA, Valensi QJ, Madayag MA et al. Angiographic patterns in renal oncocytomas. Radiology 1978; 129: 615–622
32. Hara M, Yoshida K, Tomita M, Akimoto M et al. A case of bilateral renal oncocytoma. J Urol 1982; 128: 576–578

33. Warfel KA, Eble JN. Renal oncocytomatosis. J Urol 1982; 127: 1179–1180
33a. Base J. Bilateral multifocal oncocytoma of the kidney. Rozhl Chir 1996; 75: 573–575
34. Tickoo SK, Reuter VE, Amin MB, Srigley JR et al. Renal oncocytosis: a morphologic study of fourteen cases. Am J Surg Pathol 1999; 23: 1094–1101
35. Amin MB, Tickoo SK, Crotty TB, Farrow GM. Concurrent renal oncocytoma and renal cell carcinoma within the same kidney: diagnostic implications. Am J Surg Pathol 1998; 22: 510
36. Nishikawa K, Fujikawa S, Soga N, Wakita T et al. Renal oncocytoma with synchronous contralateral renal cell carcinoma. Hinyokika Kiyo 2002; 48: 89–91
37. Davis CJ, Mostofi FK et al. Renal oncocytoma. Clinicopathologic study of 166 patients. J Urogen Pathol 1991; 112: 805–808
38. Lewi HJ, Alexander CA, Fleming S. Renal oncocytoma. Br J Urol 1986; 58: 12–15
39. Braunstein H, Adelman JU. Histochemical study of the enzymatic activity of human neoplasms. II. Histogenesis of renal cell carcinoma. Cancer 1966; 19: 935–938
40. Wallace AC, Nairn RC. Renal tubular antigens in kidney tumors. Cancer 1972; 29: 977–981
41. Bennington JL. Proceedings: Cancer of the kidney—etiology, epidemiology, and pathology. Cancer 1973; 32: 1017–1029
42. Fleming S, Lindop GB, Gibson AA. The distribution of epithelial membrane antigen in the kidney and its tumours. Histopathology 1985; 9: 729–739
43. Chisholm GD, Roy RR. The systemic effects of malignant renal tumours. Br J Urol 1971; 43: 687–700
44. Masuda F, Yoshida M, Kondo N, Takahashi T et al. Fever in renal cell carcinoma. Gan No Rinsho 1985; 31: 1293–1296
45. Ueno M, Akita M, Ban SI, Ohigashi T et al. Production of parathyroid hormone-related protein in two new cell lines of renal cell carcinoma. Int J Urol 2001; 8: 549–556
46. Ueno M, Ohigashi T, Nakashima J, Nonaka S et al. Hypercalcemia and acute renal failure caused by production of parathyroid hormone-related protein from renal cell carcinoma. Scand J Urol Nephrol 2002; 36: 149–151
47. Murad T, Komaiko W, Oyasu R, Bauer K. Multilocular cystic renal cell carcinoma. Am J Clin Pathol 1991; 95: 633–637
48. Murphy WM, et al. Tumors of the kidney. In: Murphy WM, ed. Atlas of Tumor Pathology: Tumors of the Kidney, Bladder and Related Urinary Structures. Washington, DC: Armed Forces Institute of Pathology, 1994: 98–100
49. Corica FA, Iczkowski KA, Cheng L, Zincke, H et al. Cystic renal cell carcinoma is cured by resection: a study of 24 cases with long-term follow-up. J Urol 1999; 161: 408–411
50. Fleming S, O'Donnell M. Surgical pathology of renal epithelial neoplasms: recent advances and current status. Histopathology 2000; 36: 195–202
51. Fleming S, Symes CE. The distribution of cytokeratin antigens in the kidney and in renal tumours. Histopathology 1987; 11: 157–170
52. Rahilly MA, Salter DM, Fleming S. Composition and organization of cell-substratum contacts in normal and neoplastic renal epithelium. J Pathol 1991; 165: 163–171
53. Kovacs G. Molecular cytogenetics of renal cell tumors. Adv Cancer Res 1993; 62: 89–124
54. Lager DJ, Huston BJ, Timmerman TG, Bonsib SM. Papillary renal tumors. Morphologic, cytochemical, and genotypic features. Cancer 1995; 76: 669–673
55. Corless CL, Aburatani H, Fletcher JA, Housman DE et al. Papillary renal cell carcinoma: quantitation of chromosomes 7 and 17 by FISH, analysis of chromosome 3p for LOH, and DNA ploidy. Diagn Mol Pathol 1996; 5: 53–64
56. Thoenes W, Storkel S, Rumpelt HJ. Histopathology and classification of renal cell tumors (adenomas, oncocytomas and carcinomas). The basic cytological and histopathological elements and their use for diagnostics. Pathol Res Pract 1986; 181: 125–143
57. Mancilla-Jimenez R, Stanley RJ, Blath RA. Papillary renal cell carcinoma: a clinical, radiologic, and pathologic study of 34 cases. Cancer 1976; 38: 2469–2480
58. Kovacs G. Molecular differential pathology of renal cell tumours. Histopathology 1993; 22: 1–8
59. Renshaw AA, Corless CL. Papillary renal cell carcinoma. Histology and immunohistochemistry. Am J Surg Pathol 1995; 19: 842–849
60. Ishikawa I, Kovacs G. High incidence of papillary renal cell tumours in patients on chronic haemodialysis. Histopathology 1993; 22: 135–139
61. Blei CL, Hartman DS, Friedman AC, Davis CJ, Jr. Papillary renal cell carcinoma: ultrasonic/pathologic correlation. J Clin Ultrasound 1982; 10: 429–434
62. Press GA, McClennan BL, Melson GL, Weyman PJ

et al. Papillary renal cell carcinoma: CT and sonographic evaluation. AJR Am J Roentgenol 1984; 143: 1005–1009

63. Bostwick DG, Murphy GP. Diagnosis and prognosis of renal cell carcinoma: highlights from an international consensus workshop. Semin Urol Oncol 1998; 16: 46–52
64. Delahunt B, Eble JN. Papillary renal cell carcinoma: a clinicopathologic and immunohistochemical study of 105 tumors. Mod Pathol 1997; 10: 537–544

64a. Amin MB, Corless CL, Renshaw AA, Tickoo SK et al. Papillary (chromophil) renal cell carcinoma: histomorphologic characteristics and evaluation of conventional pathologic prognostic parameters in 62 cases. Am J Surg Pathol 1997; 21: 621–635

65. Thoenes W, Storkel S, Rumpelt HJ. Human chromophobe cell renal carcinoma. Virchows Arch B Cell Pathol Incl Mol Pathol 1985; 48: 207–217
66. Bonsib SM, Lager DJ. Chromophobe cell carcinoma: analysis of five cases. Am J Surg Pathol 1990; 14: 260–267
67. Storkel S, Steart PV, Drenckhahn D, Thoenes W. The human chromophobe cell renal carcinoma: its probable relation to intercalated cells of the collecting duct. Virchows Arch B Cell Pathol Incl Mol Pathol 1989; 56: 237–245
68. Akhtar M, Kardar H, Linjawi T, McClintock J et al. Chromophobe cell carcinoma of the kidney. A clinicopathologic study of 21 cases. Am J Surg Pathol 1995; 19: 1245–1256
69. Thoenes W, Storkel S, Rumpelt HJ, Moll R et al. Chromophobe cell renal carcinoma and its variants—a report on 32 cases. J Pathol 1988; 155:277–287
70. Crotty TB, Farrow GM, Lieber MM. Chromophobe cell renal carcinoma: clinicopathological features of 50 cases. J Urol 1995; 154: 964–967
71. Thoenes W, Baum HP, Storkel S, Muller M. Cytoplasmic microvesicles in chromophobe cell renal carcinoma demonstrated by freeze fracture. Virchows Arch B Cell Pathol Incl Mol Pathol 1987; 54: 127–130
72. Tickoo SK, Lee MW, Eble JN, Amin M et al. Ultrastructural observations on mitochondria and microvesicles in renal oncocytoma, chromophobe renal cell carcinoma, and eosinophilic variant of conventional (clear cell) renal cell carcinoma. Am J Surg Pathol 2000; 24: 1247–1256
73. Latham B, Dickersin GR, Oliva E. Subtypes of chromophobe cell renal carcinoma: an ultrastructural and histochemical study of 13 cases. Am J Surg Pathol 1999; 23: 530–535
74. Tickoo SK, Amin MB, Zarbo RJ. Colloidal iron staining in renal epithelial neoplasms, including chromophobe renal cell carcinoma: emphasis on technique and patterns of staining. Am J Surg Pathol 1998; 22: 419–424
75. Skinnider BF, Jones EC. Renal oncocytoma and chromophobe renal cell carcinoma. A comparison of colloidal iron staining and electron microscopy. Am J Clin Pathol 1999; 111: 796–803
76. Mathers ME, Pollock AM, Marsh C, O'Donnell M. Cytokeratin 7: a useful adjunct in the diagnosis of chromophobe renal cell carcinoma. Histopathology 2002; 40: 563–567
77. Fleming S, Lewi HJ. Collecting duct carcinoma of the kidney. Histopathology 1986; 10: 1131–1141
78. Kennedy SM, Merino MJ, Linehan WM, Roberts JR et al. Collecting duct carcinoma of the kidney. Hum Pathol 1990; 21: 449–456
79. Caraway NP, Wojcik EM, Katz RL, Ro JY et al. Cytologic findings of collecting duct carcinoma of the kidney. Diagn Cytopathol 1995; 13: 304–309
80. Nguyen GK, Schumann GB. Cytopathology of renal collecting duct carcinoma in urine sediment. Diagn Cytopathol 1997; 16: 446–449
81. Srigley JR, Eble JN. Collecting duct carcinoma of kidney. Semin Diagn Pathol 1998; 15: 54–67
82. Carter MD, Tha S, McLoughlin MG, Owen DA. Collecting duct carcinoma of the kidney: a case report and review of the literature. J Urol 1992; 147: 1096–1098
83. Dimopoulos MA, Logothetis CJ, Markowitz A, Sella A et al. Collecting duct carcinoma of the kidney. Br J Urol 1993; 71: 388–391

83a. Davis CJ Jr, Mostofi FK, Sesterhenn IA. Renal medullary carcinoma. The seventh sickle cell nephropathy. Am J Surg Pathol 1995; 19: 1–11.

84. Mucci B, Lewi HJ, Fleming S. The radiology of sarcomas and sarcomatoid carcinomas of the kidney. Clin Radiol 1987; 38: 249–254
85. Tomera KM, Farrow GM, Lieber MM. Sarcomatoid renal carcinoma. J Urol 1983; 130: 657–659
86. Maher ER, Yates JR, Ferguson-Smith MA. Statistical analysis of the two stage mutation model in von Hippel-Lindau disease, and in sporadic cerebellar haemangioblastoma and renal cell carcinoma. J Med Genet 1990; 27: 311–314

87. Maher ER, Yates JR. Familial renal cell carcinoma: clinical and molecular genetic aspects. Br J Cancer 1991; 63: 176–179
88. Woodward ER, Clifford SC, Astuti D, Affara NA et al. Familial clear cell renal cell carcinoma (FCRC): clinical features and mutation analysis of the VHL, MET, and CUL2 candidate genes. J Med Genet 2000; 37: 348–353
89. Maher ER, Yates JR, Harries R, Benjamin C et al. Clinical features and natural history of von Hippel-Lindau disease. Q J Med 1990; 77: 1151–1163
90. Choyke PL, Glenn GM, Walther MM, Patronas NJ et al. von Hippel-Lindau disease: genetic, clinical, and imaging features. Radiology 1995; 194: 629–642
91. Latif F, Tory K, Gnarra J, Yao M et al. Identification of the von Hippel-Lindau disease tumor suppressor gene. Science 1993; 260: 1317–1320
92. Stolle C, Glenn G, Zbar B, Humphrey JS et al. Improved detection of germline mutations in the von Hippel-Lindau disease tumor suppressor gene. Hum Mutat 1998; 12: 417–423
93. Crossey PA, Richards FM, Foster K, Green JS et al. Identification of intragenic mutations in the von Hippel-Lindau disease tumour suppressor gene and correlation with disease phenotype. Hum Mol Genet 1994; 3: 1303–1308
94. Chen F, Kishida T, Yao M, Hustad T et al. Germline mutations in the von Hippel-Lindau disease tumor suppressor gene: correlations with phenotype. Hum Mutat 1995; 5: 66–75
95. Brauch H, Kishida T, Glavac D, Chen F et al. Von Hippel-Lindau (VHL) disease with pheochromocytoma in the Black Forest region of Germany: evidence for a founder effect. Hum Genet 1995; 95: 551–556
96. Maher ER, Webster AR, Richards FM, Green JS et al. Phenotypic expression in von Hippel-Lindau disease: correlations with germline VHL gene mutations. J Med Genet 1996; 33: 328–332
97. Zbar B, Kishida T, Chen F, Schmidt L et al. Germline mutations in the Von Hippel-Lindau disease (VHL) gene in families from North America, Europe, and Japan. Hum Mutat 1996; 8: 348–357
98. Tory K, Brauch H, Linehan M, Barba D et al. Specific genetic change in tumors associated with von Hippel-Lindau disease. J Natl Cancer Inst 1989; 81: 1097–1101
99. Crossey PA, Foster K, Richards FM, Phipps ME et al. Molecular genetic investigations of the mechanism of tumourigenesis in von Hippel-Lindau disease: analysis of allele loss in VHL tumours. Hum Genet 1994; 93: 53–58
100. Foster K, Prowse A, van den Berg A, Fleming S et al. Somatic mutations of the von Hippel-Lindau disease tumour suppressor gene in non-familial clear cell renal carcinoma. Hum Mol Genet 1994; 3: 2169–2173
101. Gnarra JR, Tory K, Weng Y, Schmidt L et al. Mutations of the VHL tumour suppressor gene in renal carcinoma. Nat Genet 1994; 7: 85–90
102. Shuin T, Kondo K, Torigoe S, Kishida T et al. Frequent somatic mutations and loss of heterozygosity of the von Hippel-Lindau tumor suppressor gene in primary human renal cell carcinomas. Cancer Res 1994; 54: 2852–2855
103. Herman JG, Latif F, Weng Y, Lerman MI et al. Silencing of the VHL tumor-suppressor gene by DNA methylation in renal carcinoma. Proc Natl Acad Sci USA 1994; 91: 9700–9704
104. Clifford SC, Prowse AH, Affara NA, Buys CH et al. Inactivation of the von Hippel-Lindau (VHL) tumour suppressor gene and allelic losses at chromosome arm 3p in primary renal cell carcinoma: evidence for a VHL-independent pathway in clear cell renal tumourigenesis. Genes Chromosomes Cancer 1998; 22: 200–209
105. Thrash-Bingham CA, Salazar H, Freed JJ, Greenberg RE et al. Genomic alterations and instabilities in renal cell carcinomas and their relationship to tumor pathology. Cancer Res 1995; 55: 6189–6195
106. Schoenfeld A, Davidowitz EJ, Burk RD. A second major native von Hippel-Lindau gene product, initiated from an internal translation start site, functions as a tumor suppressor. Proc Natl Acad Sci USA 1998; 95: 8817–8822
107. Iliopoulos O, Kibel A, Gray S, Kaelin WG, Jr. Tumour suppression by the human von Hippel-Lindau gene product. Nat Med 1995; 1: 822–826
108. Chen F, Kishida T, Duh FM, Renbaum P et al. Suppression of growth of renal carcinoma cells by the von Hippel-Lindau tumor suppressor gene. Cancer Res 1995; 55: 4804–4807
109. Clifford SC, Maher ER. Von Hippel-Lindau disease: clinical and molecular perspectives. Adv Cancer Res 2001; 82: 85–105
110. Lonergan KM, Iliopoulos O, Ohh M, Kamura T et al. Regulation of hypoxia-inducible mRNAs by the von Hippel-Lindau tumor suppressor protein requires binding to complexes containing elongins B/C and Cul2. Mol Cell Biol 1998; 18: 732–741
111. Stebbins CE, Kaelin WG Jr, Pavletich NP. Structure of the VHL-ElonginC-ElonginB complex: implica-

tions for VHL tumor suppressor function. Science 1999; 284: 455–461
112. Maxwell PH, Wiesener MS, Chang GW, Clifford SC et al. The tumour suppressor protein VHL targets hypoxia-inducible factors for oxygen-dependent proteolysis. Nature 1999; 399: 271–275
113. Siemeister G, Weindel K, Mohrs K, Barleon B et al. Reversion of deregulated expression of vascular endothelial growth factor in human renal carcinoma cells by von Hippel-Lindau tumor suppressor protein. Cancer Res 1996; 56: 2299–2301
114. Cockman ME, Masson N, Mole DR, Jaakkola P et al. Hypoxia inducible factor-alpha binding and ubiquitylation by the von Hippel-Lindau tumor suppressor protein. J Biol Chem 2000; 275: 25733–25741
115. Kaelin WG Jr. Molecular basis of the VHL hereditary cancer syndrome. Nat Rev Cancer 2002; 2: 673–682
116. Clifford SC, Cockman ME, Smallwood AC, Mole DR et al. Contrasting effects on HIF-1alpha regulation by disease-causing pVHL mutations correlate with patterns of tumourigenesis in von Hippel-Lindau disease. Hum Mol Genet 2001; 10: 1029–1038
117. Cohen AJ, Li FP, Berg S, Marchetto DJ et al. Hereditary renal-cell carcinoma associated with a chromosomal translocation. N Engl J Med 1979; 301: 592–595
118. Kovacs G, Brusa P, De Riese W. Tissue-specific expression of a constitutional 3;6 translocation: development of multiple bilateral renal-cell carcinomas. Int J Cancer 1989; 43: 422–427
119. Bodmer D, Eleveld MJ, Ligtenberg MJ, Weterman MA et al. An alternative route for multistep tumorigenesis in a novel case of hereditary renal cell cancer and a t(2;3)(q35;q21) chromosome translocation. Am J Hum Genet 1998; 62: 1475–1483
120. Kovacs G, Hoene E. Loss of der(3) in renal carcinoma cells of a patient with constitutional t(3;12). Hum Genet 1988; 78: 148–150
121. van Kessel AG, Wijnhoven H, Bodmer D, Eleveld M et al. Renal cell cancer: chromosome 3 translocations as risk factors. J Natl Cancer Inst 1999; 91: 1159–1160
122. Schmidt L, Li F, Brown RS, Berg S et al. Mechanism of tumorigenesis of renal carcinomas associated with the constitutional chromosome 3;8 translocation. Cancer J Sci Am 1995; 1: 191
123. Crossey PA, Eng C, Ginalska-Malinowska M, Lennard TW et al. Molecular genetic diagnosis of von Hippel-Lindau disease in familial phaeochromocytoma. J Med Genet 1995; 32: 885–886
124. Neumann HP, Eng C, Mulligan LM, Glavac D et al. Consequences of direct genetic testing for germline mutations in the clinical management of families with multiple endocrine neoplasia, type II. JAMA 1995; 274: 1149–1151
125. Zbar B, Glenn G, Lubensky I, Choyke P et al. Hereditary papillary renal cell carcinoma: clinical studies in 10 families. J Urol 1995; 153: 907–912
126. Teh BT, Giraud S, Sari NF, Hii SI et al. Familial non-VHL non-papillary clear-cell renal cancer. Lancet 1997; 349: 848–849
127. Zbar B, Tory K, Merino M, Schmidt L et al. Hereditary papillary renal cell carcinoma. J Urol 1994; 151: 561–566
128. Schmidt L, Duh FM, Chen F, Kishida T et al. Germline and somatic mutations in the tyrosine kinase domain of the MET proto-oncogene in papillary renal carcinomas. Nat Genet 1997; 16: 68–73
129. Schmidt L, Junker K, Weirich G, Glenn G et al. Two North American families with hereditary papillary renal carcinoma and identical novel mutations in the MET proto-oncogene. Cancer Res 1998; 58: 1719–1722
130. Schmidt L, Junker K, Nakaigawa N, Kinjerski T et al. Novel mutations of the MET proto-oncogene in papillary renal carcinomas. Oncogene 1999; 18: 2343–2350
131. Choyke PL, Walther MM, Glenn GM, Wagner JR et al. Imaging features of hereditary papillary renal cancers. J Comput Assist Tomogr 1997; 21: 737–741
132. Zhuang Z, Park WS, Pack S, Schmidt L et al. Trisomy 7-harbouring non-random duplication of the mutant MET allele in hereditary papillary renal carcinomas. Nat Genet 1998; 20: 66–69
133. Lubensky IA, Schmidt L, Zhuang Z, Weirich G et al. Hereditary and sporadic papillary renal carcinomas with *c-met* mutations share a distinct morphological phenotype. Am J Pathol 1999; 155: 517–526
134. Cantley LG, Barros EJ, Gandhi M, Rauchman M et al. Regulation of mitogenesis, motogenesis, and tubulogenesis by hepatocyte growth factor in renal collecting duct cells. Am J Physiol 1994; 267: F271–280
135. Woolf AS, Kolatsi-Joannou M, Hardman P, Andermarcher E et al. Roles of hepatocyte growth factor/scatter factor and the *met* receptor in the early development of the metanephros. J Cell Biol 1995; 128: 171–184

136. Jeffers M, Schmidt L, Nakaigawa N, Webb CP et al. Activating mutations for the met tyrosine kinase receptor in human cancer. Proc Natl Acad Sci USA 1997; 94: 11445–11450
137. Giordano S, Maffe A, Williams TA, Artigiani S et al. Different point mutations in the *met* oncogene elicit distinct biological properties. FASEB J 2000; 14: 399–406
138. Tomlinson IP, Alam NA, Rowan AJ, Barclay E et al. Germline mutations in FH predispose to dominantly inherited uterine fibroids, skin leiomyomata and papillary renal cell cancer. Nat Genet 2002; 30: 406–410
139. Kiuru M, Lehtonen R, Arola J, Salovaara R et al. Few FH mutations in sporadic counterparts of tumor types observed in hereditary leiomyomatosis and renal cell cancer families. Cancer Res 2002; 62: 4554–4557
140. Weirich G, Glenn G, Junker K, Merino M et al. Familial renal oncocytoma: clinicopathological study of 5 families. J Urol 1998; 160: 335–340
141. Toro JR, Glenn G, Duray P, Darling T et al. Birt-Hogg-Dube syndrome: a novel marker of kidney neoplasia. Arch Dermatol 1999; 135: 1195–1202
142. Birt AR, Hogg GR, Dube WJ. Hereditary multiple fibrofolliculomas with trichodiscomas and acrochordons. Arch Dermatol 1977; 113: 1674–1677
143. Pavlovich CP, Walther MM, Eyler RA, Hewitt SM et al. Renal tumors in the Birt-Hogg-Dube syndrome. Am J Surg Pathol 2002; 26: 1542–1552
144. Nickerson ML, Warren MB, Toro JR, Matrosova V et al. Mutations in a novel gene lead to kidney tumors, lung wall defects, and benign tumors of the hair follicle in patients with the Birt-Hogg-Dube syndrome. Cancer Cell 2002; 2: 157–164
145. Szabo J, Heath B, Hill VM, Jackson CE et al. Hereditary hyperparathyroidism-jaw tumor syndrome: the endocrine tumor gene HRPT2 maps to chromosome 1q21-q31. Am J Hum Genet 1995; 56: 944–950
146. Haven CJ, Wong FK, van Dam EW, van der Juijt R et al. A genotypic and histopathological study of a large Dutch kindred with hyperparathyroidism-jaw tumor syndrome. J Clin Endocrinol Metab 2000; 85: 1449–1454
147. Malchoff CD, Sarfarazi M, Tendler B, Forouhar F et al. Papillary thyroid carcinoma associated with papillary renal neoplasia: genetic linkage analysis of a distinct heritable tumor syndrome. J Clin Endocrinol Metab 2000; 85: 1758–1764
148. Bjornsson J, Short MP, Kwiatkowski DJ, Henske EP. Tuberous sclerosis-associated renal cell carcinoma. Clinical, pathological, and genetic features. Am J Pathol 1996; 149: 1201–1208
149. Sampson JR, Patel A, Mee AD. Multifocal renal cell carcinoma in sibs from a chromosome 9 linked (TSC1) tuberous sclerosis family. J Med Genet 1995; 32: 848–850
150. Al-Saleem T, Wessner LL, Scheithauer BW, Patterson K et al. Malignant tumors of the kidney, brain, and soft tissues in children and young adults with the tuberous sclerosis complex. Cancer 1998; 83: 2208–2216
151. Kobayashi T, Hirayama Y, Kobayashi E, Kubo Y et al. A germline insertion in the tuberous sclerosis (Tsc2) gene gives rise to the Eker rat model of dominantly inherited cancer. Nat Genet 1995; 9: 70–74
152. Onda H, Lueck A, Marks PW, Warren HB et al. Tsc2(+/−) mice develop tumors in multiple sites that express gelsolin and are influenced by genetic background. J Clin Invest 1999; 104: 687–695
153. Pea M, Bonetti F, Martignoni G, Henske EP et al. Apparent renal cell carcinomas in tuberous sclerosis are heterogeneous: the identification of malignant epithelioid angiomyolipoma. Am J Surg Pathol 1998; 22: 180–187
154. Robertson FM, Cendron M, Klauber GT, Harris BH. Renal cell carcinoma in association with tuberous sclerosis in children. J Pediatr Surg 1996; 31: 729–730
155. Henske EP, Thorner P, Patterson K, Zhuang Z et al. Renal cell carcinoma in children with diffuse cystic hyperplasia of the kidneys. Pediatr Dev Pathol 1999; 2: 270–274
156. Suijkerbuijk RF, Meloni AM, Sinke RJ, de Leeuw B et al. Identification of a yeast artificial chromosome that spans the human papillary renal cell carcinoma-associated t(X;1) breakpoint in Xp11.2. Cancer Genet Cytogenet 1993; 71: 164–169
157. Sidhar SK, Clark J, Gill S, Hamoudi R et al. The t(X;1)(p11.2;q21.2) translocation in papillary renal cell carcinoma fuses a novel gene PRCC to the TFE3 transcription factor gene. Hum Mol Genet 1996; 5: 1333–1338
158. Speicher MR, Schoell B, du Manoir S, Schrock E et al. Specific loss of chromosomes 1, 2, 6, 10, 13, 17, and 21 in chromophobe renal cell carcinomas revealed by comparative genomic hybridization. Am J Pathol 1994; 145: 356–364

159. Fuzesi L, Gunawan B, Braun S, Bergmann F et al. Cytogenetic analysis of 11 renal oncocytomas: further evidence of structural rearrangements of 11q13 as a characteristic chromosomal anomaly. Cancer Genet Cytogenet 1998; 107: 1–6
160. Presti JC Jr, Rao PH, Chen Q, Reuter VE et al. Histopathological, cytogenetic, and molecular characterization of renal cortical tumors. Cancer Res 1991; 51: 1544–1552
161. van der Hout AH, van der Vlies P, Wijmenga C, Li FP et al. The region of common allelic losses in sporadic renal cell carcinoma is bordered by the loci D3S2 and THRB. Genomics 1991; 11: 537–542
162. van den Berg A, Hulsbeek MF, de Jong D, Kok K et al. Major role for a 3p21 region and lack of involvement of the t(3;8) breakpoint region in the development of renal cell carcinoma suggested by loss of heterozygosity analysis. Genes Chromosomes Cancer 1996; 15: 64–72
163. Yamakawa K, Morita R, Takahashi E, Hori T et al. A detailed deletion mapping of the short arm of chromosome 3 in sporadic renal cell carcinoma. Cancer Res 1991; 51: 4707–4711
164. Lubinski J, Hadaczek P, Podolski J, Toloczko A et al. Common regions of deletion in chromosome regions 3p12 and 3p14.2 in primary clear cell renal carcinomas. Cancer Res 1994; 54: 3710–3713
165. Martinez A, Fullwood P, Kondo K, Kishida T et al. Role of chromosome 3p12-p21 tumour suppressor genes in clear cell renal cell carcinoma: analysis of VHL dependent and VHL independent pathways of tumorigenesis. Mol Pathol 2000; 53: 137–144
166. Sanchez Y, el-Naggar A, Pathak S, Killary AM. A tumor suppressor locus within 3p14-p12 mediates rapid cell death of renal cell carcinoma in vivo. Proc Natl Acad Sci USA 1994; 91: 3383–3387
167. Killary AM, Wolf ME, Giambernardi TA, Naylor SL. Definition of a tumor suppressor locus within human chromosome 3p21-p22. Proc Natl Acad Sci USA 1992; 89: 10877–10881
168. Dammann R, Li C, Yoon JH, Chin PL et al. Epigenetic inactivation of a RAS association domain family protein from the lung tumour suppressor locus 3p21.3. Nat Genet 2000; 25: 315–319
169. Burbee DG, Forgacs E, Zochbauer-Muller S, Shivakumar L et al. Epigenetic inactivation of RASSF1A in lung and breast cancers and malignant phenotype suppression. J Natl Cancer Inst 2001; 93: 691–699
170. Dreijerink K, Braga E, Kuzmin I, Geil L et al. The candidate tumor suppressor gene, RASSF1A, from human chromosome 3p21.3 is involved in kidney tumorigenesis. Proc Natl Acad Sci USA 2001; 98: 7504–7509
171. Morrissey C, Martinez A, Zatyka M, Agathanggelou A et al. Epigenetic inactivation of the RASSF1A 3p21.3 tumor suppressor gene in both clear cell and papillary renal cell carcinoma. Cancer Res 2001; 61: 7277–7281
172. Yoon JH, Dammann R, Pfeifer GP. Hypermethylation of the CpG island of the RASSF1A gene in ovarian and renal cell carcinomas. Int J Cancer 2001; 94: 212–217
173. Walther MM, Gnarra JR, Elwood L, Xu HJ et al. Loss of heterozygosity occurs centromeric to RB without associated abnormalities in the retinoblastoma gene in tumors from patients with metastatic renal cell carcinoma. J Urol 1995; 153: 2050–2054
174. Schullerus D, Herbers J, Chudek J, Kanamaru H et al. Loss of heterozygosity at chromosomes 8p, 9p, and 14q is associated with stage and grade of non-papillary renal cell carcinomas. J Pathol 1997; 183: 151–155
175. Sanders ME, Mick R, Tomaszewski JE, Barr FG. Unique patterns of allelic imbalance distinguish type 1 from type 2 sporadic papillary renal cell carcinoma. Am J Pathol 2002; 161: 997–1005
176. Li J, Yen C, Liaw D, Podsypanina K et al. PTEN, a putative protein tyrosine phosphatase gene mutated in human brain, breast, and prostate cancer. Science 1997; 275: 1943–1947
177. Steck PA, Pershouse MA, Jasser SA, Yung WK et al. Identification of a candidate tumour suppressor gene, MMAC1, at chromosome 10q23.3 that is mutated in multiple advanced cancers. Nat Genet 1997; 15: 356–362
178. Liaw D, Marsh DJ, Li J, Dahia PL et al. Germline mutations of the PTEN gene in Cowden disease, an inherited breast and thyroid cancer syndrome. Nat Genet 1997; 16: 64–67
179. Alimov A, Li C, Gizatullin R, Fredriksson V et al. Somatic mutation and homozygous deletion of PTEN/MMAC1 gene of 10q23 in renal cell carcinoma. Anticancer Res 1999; 19: 3841–3846
180. Kondo K, Yao M, Kobayashi K, Ota S et al. PTEN/MMAC1/TEP1 mutations in human primary renal-cell carcinomas and renal carcinoma cell lines. Int J Cancer 2001; 91: 219–224

181. Chang F, Syrjanen S, Syrjanen K. Implications of the p53 tumor-suppressor gene in clinical oncology. J Clin Oncol 1995; 13: 1009–1022
182. Ogawa O, Habuchi T, Kakehi Y, Koshiba M et al. Allelic losses at chromosome 17p in human renal cell carcinoma are inversely related to allelic losses at chromosome 3p. Cancer Res 1992; 52: 1881–1885
183. Uchida T, Wada C, Shitara T, Egawa S et al. Infrequent involvement of p53 mutations and loss of heterozygosity of 17p in the tumorigenesis of renal cell carcinoma. J Urol 1993; 150: 1298–1301
184. Torigoe S, Shuin T, KubotaY, Horikoshi T et al. p53 gene mutation in primary human renal cell carcinoma. Oncol Res 1992; 4: 467–472
185. Uchida T, Wada C, Wang C, Egawa S et al. Genomic instability of microsatellite repeats and mutations of H-, K-, and N-ras, and p53 genes in renal cell carcinoma. Cancer Res 1994; 54: 3682–3685
186. Sherr CJ. The INK4a/ARF network in tumour suppression. Nat Rev Mol Cell Biol 2001; 2: 731–737
187. Schraml P, Struckmann K, Bednar R, Fu W et al. CDKNA2A mutation analysis, protein expression, and deletion mapping of chromosome 9p in conventional clear-cell renal carcinomas: evidence for a second tumor suppressor gene proximal to CDKN2A. Am J Pathol 2001; 158: 593–601
188. Imai Y, Strohmeyer TG, Fleischhacker M, Slamon DJ, Koeffler HP. p53 mutations and MDM-2 amplification in renal cell cancers. Mod Pathol 1994; 7: 766–770
189. Classon M, Harlow E. The retinoblastoma tumour suppressor in development and cancer. Nat Rev Cancer 2002; 2: 910–917
190. Suzuki Y, Tamura G, Maesawa C, Fujioka T et al. Analysis of genetic alterations in renal cell carcinoma using the polymerase chain reaction. Virchows Arch 1994; 424: 453–457

23

Transitional cell carcinoma of the bladder

T R Leyshon Griffiths and J Kilian Mellon

INTRODUCTION

Each year in England and Wales, approximately 12 000 people are diagnosed with bladder cancer and 4000 people die from the disease; it is three times more common in men than women, and it is the fourth most common cancer after lung, colorectal and prostate/breast cancer.[1]

In the developed world, transitional cell carcinoma (TCC), rather than squamous or adenocarcinoma, is responsible for most bladder carcinoma. About 25% of newly diagnosed cancers are muscle-invasive (T2–T4); the remainder are superficial (70%), classified as limited to the mucosa (pTa) or lamina propria (pT1), or as being in situ changes (Tis – 5%).

AETIOLOGY

The aetiology of bladder cancer is heavily dependent on chemical exposure from smoking and occupation, although genetic polymorphisms for certain enzymes involved in detoxification affect susceptibility. Keratinizing squamous metaplasia induced by stones, strictures and infection by *Schistosoma haematobium* is a risk factor in the development of squamous carcinoma.

Industrial chemicals (Table 23.1)

Occupational exposure to chemicals accounts for up to 20% of bladder cancers. Most carcinogens have a latent period of 15–20 years between exposure and the development of tumours. In 1938, Hueper produced the first experimental evidence showing that the aromatic amine, β-naphthylamine, could induce bladder cancer in dogs.[2] Following this and other reports, a full epidemiological survey conducted by Case showed that exposure to α-naphthylamine, β-naphthylamine or benzidine, rather than to aniline itself, was the main factor associated with the development of bladder cancer.[3] Further evidence suggests that some polycyclic aromatic hydrocarbons can also act as urinary tract carcinogens.[4]

Smoking

Meta-analysis of data from 43 studies reveals that current smokers face a threefold increased risk of developing urinary tract cancer compared with non-smokers.[5] Indeed, approximately two-thirds of all bladder cancers may be related to cigarette smoking. The risk correlates with the number of cigarettes smoked, the duration of smoking, and the degree of inhalation of smoke. Ex-cigarette smokers have a

Table 23.1 Occupations associated with bladder cancer.

Textile workers
Dye workers
Tyre rubber and cable workers
Petroleum workers
Leather workers
Shoe manufacturers and cleaners
Painters/printers
Hairdressers
Lorry drivers
Drill press operators
Rodent exterminators and sewage workers

reduced incidence of bladder cancer compared with active smokers, but the risk does not return to baseline. Within 4 years of quitting, the risk of developing bladder cancer decreases by 30–60%.[6] Nitrosamines, β-naphthylamine and 4-aminobiphenyl are known to be present in smoke.

Drugs

In the 1950s and 1960s, analgesic abuse was rife in Australia and New Zealand. Both upper tract and bladder TCC were linked to the aniline derivative, phenacetin. Cyclophosphamide has also been shown to induce bladder cancer; the increased risk of TCC has been calculated as ninefold.[7] In comparison to other carcinogenic agents, the latency period is relatively short.

Pelvic irradiation

Patients who are treated with pelvic radiotherapy for cervical carcinoma have a two- to fourfold increased risk of developing bladder cancer.[8,9]

Genetic polymorphisms

The predominant role of drug- and carcinogen-metabolizing enzymes is the processing of lipophilic chemicals to products that are more water soluble and can be excreted. These enzyme systems are partly controlled by genetic polymorphism. In the liver, chemicals are oxidized by the cytochrome P450 superfamily and detoxified by *N*-acetylation, predominantly by *N*-acetyltransferases (*NAT*). Aromatic amines are usually detoxified by (*NAT*)2. Certain allelic combinations result in the slow acetylation phenotype. In a meta-analysis of 22 case-control studies conducted in the general population, (*NAT*)2 slow acetylation was associated with a 40% increased risk of bladder cancer.[10] Current results suggest that the risk may be higher in smokers than in non-smokers.[11] Approximately 50% of Caucasians and 25% of Asians are slow acetylators. Among the P450 superfamily, there is a suggestion of increased risk of TCC in subjects with rapid *CYP1A2* activity.[12]

Chemical intermediates generated by the P450 system can also be inactivated by their conjugation with glutathione. This reaction is predominantly catalysed by the glutathione S-transferases (*GST*). The *GSTM1* null genotype in an individual is associated with up to threefold increased risk of TCC.[13]

PATHOLOGY

The calyces, renal pelvis, ureter, bladder and urethra as far as the navicular fossa are lined by transitional cell epithelium. Tumours of the bladder are about 50 times as common as those of the ureter or renal pelvis. Most are TCC (70% pure TCC; 20% TCC with squamous or glandular components). The remainder are rare tumours, including pure squamous cell carcinoma, adenocarcinoma, sarcoma and undifferentiated tumours. Adenocarcinomas of the rectum, uterus, breast, ovary and prosate may metastasize to the bladder, and very rarely, adenocarcinoma may arise in an urachal remnant.

Premalignant conditions

Keratinizing squamous metaplasia, seen in exstrophy, chronic bladder inflammation and schistosomiasis, is premalignant. Urothelial dysplasia is a flat, non-invasive, urothelial lesion recognized at low magnification by the presence of nuclear clustering. Dysplasia has been detected in 20–86% of bladder cancer patients, depending on the extent of the examination. Dysplastic changes are more commonly detected in association with muscle-invasive and high-grade tumours. Investigators supporting dysplasia as a premalignant condition cite the frequent co-existence of dysplastic and neoplastic lesions, the frequency of tumour recurrence and tumour progression among bladder cancer patients with dysplasia,[14] and experimental studies that document a progression of morphological changes from normal through dysplasia to invasive cancer. However, it is not clear whether dysplasia develops before or concomitantly with clinically manifest TCC. Moreover, in clinical studies showing progression, dysplasia is often confused with carcinoma in situ (Tis).

CLINICAL FEATURES

The natural history of bladder cancer can be classified as follows:

- no further recurrence
- local recurrence, which can occur on a single occasion or on multiple occasions; it can involve single or multiple tumour recurrences, but recurrent tumours are usually of the same stage and grade as the primary tumour
- local progression – an increase in local stage with time; the appearance of distant metastases and subsequent death.

Prediction of these events depends strongly on the presenting stage and grade of the primary tumour and whether there is concomitant Tis.

Tumour stage

The TNM staging system provides the basis for assessing the future behaviour of a newly diagnosed tumour (Table 23.2; Figure 23.1).[15] In superficial tumours (pTa and pT1), good data on the pT category should be obtained from histological examination of resection biopsies.

On the basis of resection biopsies, the pathologist can state only that muscle invasion is present or absent. Careful examination under anaesthesia after resection can determine the clinical stage and tumour size. However, of apparently organ-confined (clinical stage T2) tumours, 40–50% are more advanced on histological assessment of the radical cystectomy specimen.

Tumour grade

The favoured grading system in the UK over the last three decades has been the 1973 WHO classification.[16] One concern has been the considerable disagreement in interpretation of histological grade among pathologists using this system.[17] Another has been the heterogeneity in biological activity among, in particular, grade 2 tumours. More recently, several other classifications have been introduced, but, to date, they have not been accepted by most pathologists in the UK. These include a European classification,[18] the 1998 WHO/International Society of Urological Pathology (ISUP) Consensus classification,[19] and the 1999 WHO classification.[20]

In the European classification, grade 2 tumours are subdivided into grade 2a and 2b. Cellular polarity is normal in grade 2a tumours, whereas there is a tendency to loss of cellular polarity in grade 2b tumours. In the 1998 WHO/ISUP consensus, well-differentiated tumours in which nuclei show enlargement but are uniform in size, shape, and chromatin

Table 23.2 TNM classification of bladder cancer (1997).[15]

Ta	Non-invasive papillary carcinoma
Tis	Carcinoma in situ: 'flat tumour'
T1	Tumour invades subepithelial connective tissue
T2a	Tumour invades superficial muscle (inner half)
T2b	Tumour invades deep muscle (outer half)
T3a	Tumour invades perivesical tissue microscopically
T3b	Tumour invades perivesical tissue macroscopically (extravesical mass)
T4a	Tumour invades prostate or uterus or vagina
T4b	Tumour invades pelvic wall or abdominal wall
NX	Regional lymph nodes cannot be assessed
NO	No regional lymph-node metastasis
N1	Metastasis in a single lymph node ≤2 cm in diameter
N2	Metastasis in a single lymph node >2 cm to ≤5 cm in diameter or multiple lymph nodes, none >5 cm in diameter
N3	Metastasis in a lymph node >5 cm in diameter
MX	Distant metastases cannot be assessed
MO	No distant metastases
M1	Distant metastasis

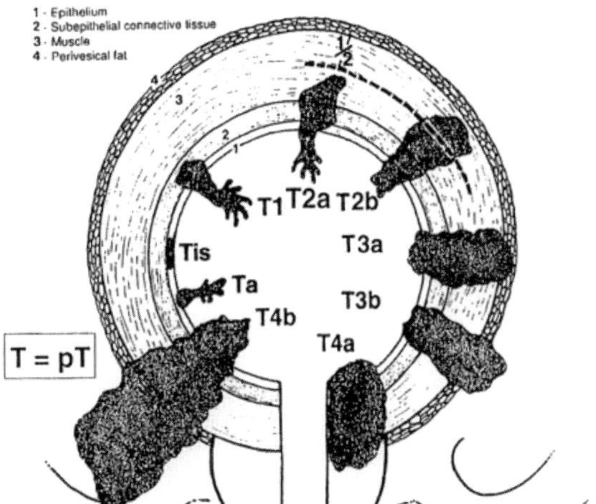

Figure 23.1 *Stage of primary tumour in TNM classification (1997).*[15]

are called 'papillary urothelial neoplasms of low malignant potential'; mitotic figures are not seen. A new 'low-grade' category includes approximately 10% of tumours at the upper end of WHO grade 1 combined with the lower 40% of WHO grade 2 tumours. A 'high-grade' category includes the remaining 50–60% of WHO grade 2 tumours and all grade 3 tumours.

The 1999 WHO classification is similar to the 1998 WHO/ISUP classification except that 'low-grade' tumours are termed grade I, and 'high-grade' tumours are subdivided into grade II and grade III tumours.

Tumour size

Tumours more than 5 cm in diameter have a worse prognosis than smaller tumours. Superficial tumours less than 2 cm in size have a significantly lower risk of recurrence. A simple system has been proposed of stratifying risks of recurrence on the basis of multifocality and recurrence at 3 months (Table 23.3).[21,22]

Abnormalities of urothelium distant from the primary lesion

In the 1998 WHO/ISUP consensus,[19] flat urothelial lesions with atypia include reactive atypia, atypia of unknown significance, dysplasia (low-grade intraurothelial neoplasia) and Tis (high-grade intraurothelial neoplasia). Urine cytology may detect Tis that has not been found by random mucosal biopsies, because surface urothelial cells are not adherent in Tis. The sensitivity and specificity of voided urine cytology in the detection of Tis is >90%. In patients with marked irritative symptoms such as bladder pain, urethral irritation and dysuria, but no abnormal clinical findings, the cytological examination of several specimens of urine is recommended. A biopsy of abnormal mucosa should be performed.

Prognostic factors and natural history (Tables 23.4 and 23.5)

Bladder cancer can be classified into superficial and muscle-invasive tumours, but urologists now prefer to separate pT1 and pTa tumours. Of patients presenting with TCC, 70% have superficial tumours (50% pTa and 20% pT1) not invading detrusor muscle, and 25% have muscle-invasive tumours. The latter account for the majority of deaths from bladder cancer, and such patients have an overall survival of 50% at 5 years. Of newly diagnosed superficial bladder tumours, approximately 30% are multifocal at presentation, 60–70% will recur, and 10–20% will undergo stage progression to muscle-invasive or metastatic disease.[23] Of newly diagnosed muscle-invasive tumours, 50% have occult nodal or systemic metastases that manifest themselves within 12 months.

Table 23.3 Prognostic groups, their relationship to risks of recurrence and recommended management plans for Ta and T1 (G1 and G2) (WHO, 1973) tumours.[21,22]

Prognostic groups	Cystoscopic findings	Management plan
Group 1	Solitary tumour at presentation, no tumour recurrence at 3 months (20% risk of recurrence at 1 year)	Followed up safely by annual flexible cystoscopy
Group 2	Solitary tumour at presentation, tumour recurrence at 3 months; multiple tumours at presentation, no tumour recurrence at 3 months (40% risk of recurrence at 1 year)	Followed up 3-monthly by flexible cystoscopy for the first year; then annually if no recurrence
Group 3	Multiple tumours at presentation, tumour recurrences at 3 months (90% risk of recurrence at 1–2 years)	3-monthly rigid cystoscopic assessment under general anaesthesia for 2 years; then annually if no recurrence

Table 23.4 Risk of recurrence in superficial tumours.[106]

	Number	Recurrence rate (positive cystoscopies per 100 patient months)
Tumour status		
Primary	190	5.2
Recurrent	118	10.4
Number of prior recurrences per year		
None	190	5.2
≤1	38	5.6
1–2	28	12.7
>2	42	12.8
Number of tumours		
1	161	4.8
2–3	71	7.8
>3	68	12.3
Diameter of largest (cm)		
<2	201	6.4
>3	95	7.9
Grade		
1	241	6.4
2–3	60	8.9

Table 23.5 Risk of progression.[23]

	Percentage risk
pTa	10
pT1	24
pT1 (recurrent)	56
Solitary versus multiple	
pTa single	5
pTa multiple	20
pT1 single	33
pT1 multiple	46
Grade	
pTa grade1	None
pTa grade 2	6
pTa grade 3	25
pT1 grade 2	25
pT1 grade 3	50

Superficial tumours

pTa disease

After 5–10 years of follow-up, 50% of patients have no recurrence; 20% have only one recurrence; and 30% have more than one recurrence. Recurrence at 3 months' follow-up is highly predictive of recurrence (90% continue to recur).[24] Small papillary tumours have a significantly lower risk of recurrence (30%) compared with multifocal or large sessile tumours (80%).

Among patients with pTa tumours who develop recurrence, about 15% progress. The survival of patients with pTaG1/G2 disease is similar to that of an age-matched and sex-matched control population.

pT1 disease

About 20% of patients with pT1 disease will die from bladder cancer within 5 years.[25] Moreover, high-grade pT1 tumours managed by immediate radical cystectomy are found to be under-staged in up to one-third of cases.[26] The presence of Tis near the site of the initial tumour is associated with a greater risk of tumour progression.[27]

Grade

Despite inaccuracies in grading, most authors report that tumour grade has a pronounced influence on progression, and the poor prognosis of pT1 grade 3 tumours is well described (50% progression rate if accompanied by Tis).[28,29]

Flow-cytometric DNA analysis correlates in general with grade, recurrence rate, risk of progression and survival. However, it is unclear whether such objective assessments improve prediction over conventional grading.

Carcinoma in situ (Tis)

Carcinoma in situ is classified as primary and secondary. In primary Tis, there is no history of previous or concurrent tumour. 'Concomitant Tis' is a term used when a tumour is present at the same time. In secondary Tis, there is a previous history of bladder tumour.

Primary Tis

Patients presenting with bladder pain, dysuria and positive urine cytology are likely to harbour primary Tis. Around 50% of these patients die of metastatic TCC within a year or two if aggressive treatment with intravesical therapy is not instituted.[30]

Secondary Tis
This can be demonstrated by carrying out random or preselected site biopsies in patients with bladder cancer. However, most authors have found that random biopsies of apparently normal urothelium do not add prognostic information.

Concomitant Tis
Concomitant Tis can be demonstrated in around 40% of patients. It is highly predictive of recurrent disease[31] and also predicts the progression of superficial bladder cancer. Fifty per cent of those with Tis or severe dysplasia progress to muscle invasion. Failure of Tis to respond to intravesical treatment should lead to the consideration of early cystectomy.

Muscle-invasive disease

Tumour stage at presentation is the most useful prognostic indicator associated with outcome. Moreover, a gradually increasing proportion of lymph-node metastases are found with increasing stage. Among patients with muscle-invasive bladder cancer thought to have negative nodes on preoperative computerized tomography, around one-fifth are found to have metastatic nodal disease when managed by means of radical cystectomy and bilateral lymphadenectomy. In these patients, overall 5-year survival rates up to 30% have been reported.[32]

Over 50% of patients with muscle-invasive disease have occult metastatic disease at presentation; its presence is strongly related to initial tumour stage, being most frequent in T4 disease. Other nonspecific features of poor prognosis include signs such as anaemia, renal failure and performance status. The presence of upper tract dilatation in muscle-invasive disease is associated with increased risks of lymph-node metastases, systemic spread and a worse clinical outcome.

MOLECULAR STUDIES AND BLADDER CANCER

For patients with superficial bladder cancer, none of the established prognostic markers are sufficiently sensitive or specific to identify precisely those in whom early radical therapy would be beneficial. For those with muscle-invasive tumours, criteria are needed to distinguish tumours likely to respond to local therapy and those likely to metastasize. It is now clear that the same tumour phenotype can be generated in a variety of ways.

Genetic alterations identified in TCC

The sequence of events leading to cell reproduction is known as the cell cycle. Normal cell proliferation is positively regulated by growth factors, transcription factors, cyclins and cyclin-dependent kinases (cdks). The negative regulatory forces are provided by tumour-suppressor proteins and cdk inhibitors. The major checkpoint is in the G1-to-S phase transition. The culmination of overexpression of positive regulators and inactivation of negative regulators is deregulation of the cell cycle.

In TCC, an extensive repertoire of genes is genetically altered including oncogenes and tumour-suppressor genes.[33] Loss of heterozygosity (LOH) analysis and comparative genomic hybridization have yielded a considerable amount of information.

Oncogenes
Several known oncogenes are altered in TCC. They contribute to the malignant phenotype in a dominant manner. This is achieved either by overexpression of the gene product or, less commonly, by expression of a mutant protein product with altered function. Overexpression may be achieved genetically by gene amplification or chromosome translocation that places the gene downstream of a powerful heterologous promoter.

HRAS
The detection of an activated *Harvey-RAS* (*HRAS*) gene in the bladder tumour cell line EJ/T24 prompted researchers to look for *RAS* mutations in human tumours. The frequency of *HRAS* mutation on chromosome 11 (11p15) in TCC has been controversial. Mutation frequencies of 6–44% have been reported. To date, no clear association of *HRAS* with clinical phenotype has been found.

FGFR3

The fibroblast growth factor receptor 3 (*FGFR3*) gene found on chromosome 4 (4p16) encodes a glycoprotein which belongs to a family of structurally related tyrosine kinase receptors. Mutated *FGFR3* has been detected in more than 30% of TCC,[34] and is associated with pTa TCC[35] and lower bladder cancer recurrence rates.[36]

ERBB2 (HER2)

This gene encodes a 185-kDa cell-surface glycoprotein with extensive homology to the epidermal growth factor receptor (EGFR). The frequency of *ERBB2* gene amplification at 17q21 is 10–14% in high-grade and muscle-invasive TCC.[37] Although *ERBB2* gene amplification is associated with overexpression, alternative mechanisms of overexpression must exist, because overexpression of the protein in the absence of gene amplification has been described.[37] Although associations between gene amplification, protein overexpression and death from bladder cancer have been reported, the prognostic significance of *ERBB2* activation has not been fully explored.

EGFR

The epidermal growth factor receptor (EGFR) is a 175-kDa glycosylated transmembrane protein which is a member of the tyrosine kinase receptor family. The *EGFR* gene is also known as the *ERBB1* or *HER1* proto-oncogene. In epithelial cells, both epidermal growth factor (EGF) and its structural homologue, transforming growth factor-α (TGF-α), can bind to and stimulate the activity of the EGFR. With the R1 monoclonal antibody, approximately 50% of bladder tumours demonstrate strong staining for EGFR, and this is associated with high stage and grade.[38] A prospective study found that tumour stage and histological grade did not overshadow the importance of EGFR positivity in predicting stage progression to muscle-invasive TCC and survival.[39] Mechanisms underlying EGFR overexpression in bladder cancer are not clear, although gene amplification is not the principal mechanism. Furthermore, despite the absence of altered gene copy numbers or chromosomal translocations, elevated levels of EGFR messenger RNA have been detected in tumours compared with normal urothelium.[40]

CCND1

The *CCND1* gene located on chromosome 11 (11q13) encodes cyclin D1, a pivotal cyclin in the early G1 phase, which, through interaction with its corresponding cyclin-dependent kinase (cdk), is essential for G1/S phase progression. Gene amplification of *CCND1* has been detected in up to 20% of TCC.[41] Overexpression of cyclin D1 is significantly higher in low-stage, well-differentiated TCC.[42] The independent prognostic significance of cyclin D1 in bladder cancer is currently unclear.

MDM2

The *MDM2* gene is a proto-oncogene located on chromosome 12 (12q13–14) that encodes a 90-kDa nuclear protein. Gene amplification has been detected in up to 5% of bladder tumours.[43] The MDM2 protein binds to p53, inhibiting its transcriptional activity and targeting it for degradation through the proteosome. MDM2 overexpression does not appear to have independent prognostic value in bladder cancer. Patients with bladder tumours exhibiting an altered p53 pathway, including MDM2 overexpression, TP53 gene mutation, p53 protein accumulation and loss of p21 (WAF1) nuclear expression, have significantly reduced survival.[44]

Tumour-suppressor genes

In the mammalian cell cycle, functional inactivation of these genes either by mutation, deletion or DNA hypermethylation contributes to the development of cancer. Several known tumour-suppressor genes are altered in TCC.

RB1

The *RB1* gene located at chromosome 13q14 was the first tumour-suppressor gene isolated. Structural alterations to the *RB1* gene by mutation or deletion are associated with muscle-invasive TCC and have been reported in up to half of these tumours.[45] Three patterns of retinoblastoma protein (pRb) nuclear immunostaining are seen in bladder cancer: absent, heterogeneous and homogeneous. Studies differ, however, in their definition of normal pRb staining patterns. In some, this is defined as homogeneous expression; in others, it is the heterogeneous expression pattern. The cooperative effects of altered pRb and p53 expression on progression and early death are discussed later.

TP53

The *TP53* gene has been mapped to chromosome 17q13. *TP53* gene mutations are associated with high-grade and high-stage TCC. Around 50% of muscle-invasive TCCs harbour *TP53* gene mutations.[46] Overall, p53 protein accumulation is associated with *TP53* gene mutation. Mutant p53 has an increased half-life and can be detected with ease, whereas normal physiological concentrations of the wild-type protein are undetectable. Most studies have therefore used immunohistochemical detection of p53 protein as a surrogate for gene activation by mutation. However, microdissection studies of p53-immunopositive and -immunonegative regions have demonstrated that p53 accumulation is not a reliable method of screening for *TP53* gene mutations in TCC.[47] Clearly, p53 accumulation can arise by alternate methods of p53 inactivation or by upregulation of functional wild-type p53. Studies are consistent with the MDM2 protein as a mediator of p53 inactivation in TCC. Nevertheless, more than 20% staining of tumour cell nuclei for p53 with the antibody 1801 is an independent predictor of progression in patients with pT1 TCC.[48,49] Although there is a clear association with outcome, use of p53 as a single marker lacks predictive power on which to base decisions for individual patients.

INK4A-ARF and INK4B

This complex genomic region at chromosome 9p21 encodes three distinct proteins (p16, p14ARF and p15, respectively). p16 and p15, together with p18 and p19, are members of the INK4 family of cyclin-dependent kinase (cdk) inhibitors. Loss of heterozygosity of INK4A-ARF has been demonstrated in 60% of bladder tumours in all grades and stages.[50] It is now clear that homozygous deletion is the common mechanism of inactivation at this locus.[51] Loss of expression of p16 is associated with immortalization in TCC cell cultures.[52] The potential prognostic implications of gene inactivation at this locus have not yet been studied in detail.

PTEN

The gene *PTEN* has recently been located at chromosome 10q23. *PTEN* encodes a protein which acts as a phosphatidylinositol phosphatase; this implies a role in cell signalling. One-third of muscle-invasive TCCs demonstrate LOH in the region of this gene compared with only 6% of superficial TCCs.[53] However, very few tumours have been identified with mutation of the retained allele or homozygous deletion of the gene.[54]

PTCH

Loss of heterozygosity encompassing the Gorlin syndrome gene locus (*PTCH*) at 9q22.3 has been detected in 60% of bladder tumours and is found in all grades and stages.[55] The mutation frequency in the retained allele is very low. Functional analyses to assess the effect of introduction of wild-type *PTCH* into bladder tumour cell lines which show no gene expression are awaited.

TSC1

The *TSC1* gene is one of the genes for the familial hamartoma syndrome, tuberous sclerosis. The *TSC1* gene locus was mapped in 1997 to 9q34. In 60% of bladder tumours, LOH encompassing this locus has been demonstrated; it is found in all grades and stages.[56] The mutation frequency in the retained allele is very low. Functional analyses are awaited.

DBCCR1

Loss of heterozygosity encompassing 9q32–33 has been detected in 60% of bladder tumours and is found in all grades and stages.[57] A single candidate gene has been identified in this relatively gene-poor region and has been designated *DBCCR1* (*deleted in bladder cancer candidate region gene* 1).[58] However, no tumour-specific mutations have been detected to date. In bladder tumour cell lines with no expression of DBCCR1, the likely mechanism of gene inactivation appears to be gene methylation in the promoter of the gene.

DCC/SMAD

Loss of heterozygosity of 18q has been shown in 30% of muscle-invasive TCCs.[59] This encompasses the candidate gene, *DCC/SMAD*. Mutational analyses have not been published to date.

TP53-related proteins

Recently, two members of the p53 family, termed p73 and p63, have been identified at 1p36.3 and 3q27–29, respectively. p73 and p63 share remarkable sequence identity to the DNA-binding, transactivation and oligomerization domains of p53. Unlike p53, however, p73[60] and p63[61] are not targets of genetic alteration in TCC. Despite this, elevated expression of p73[60] and p63[61] is demonstrated in approximately 40% and 60%, respectively, of TCCs. Taken together, these data suggest that p73 and p63 are unlikely to act as tumour-suppressors.

Kip/cip family of cyclin-dependent kinase inhibitors

The Cip/Kip family of cdk inhibitors includes p27, p57 and p21 (WAF1). The p27 protein appears to be the major regulator of cyclin E, a late G1 cyclin. The activation of the cyclin E/cdk2 complex is the rate-limiting step for transition into the S phase. Regulation of p27 and p21 occurs at the post-translational level in human primary tumours, because alterations to these genes are rare. Low protein levels of p27 and cyclin E correlate with high-grade TCC and reduced survival.[62,63] More than one-third of primary muscle-invasive bladder tumours demonstrate reduced expression of p57 mRNA compared with that expressed in morphologically normal urothelium.[64] The frequency of LOH in the chromosome 11p15.5 region was similar, consistent with p57 acting as a tumour-suppressor protein.

The p21 protein appears to be the main regulator of cyclin D1, an early G1 cyclin which complexes with cdk4 and cdk6. The action of p53 on the cell cycle is mediated in part through expression of p21. Controversy exists regarding the prognostic significance of p21 in bladder cancer. In patients with TCC undergoing cystectomy, loss of p21 expression (≤10% p21 immunopositivity) is an independent predictor of reduced survival.[65] In contrast, a Finnish study utilizing the same cutoff failed to demonstrate an association between p21 expression and survival.[66] With muscle-invasive bladder tumours treated by radical radiotherapy, p21+p53+ tumours are associated with the best survival and p21–p53+ the worst.[67]

Genetic model of tumour progression

Current evidence suggests that LOH of chromosome 9 is an early event in bladder tumour formation. It is the only event found at high frequency (60%) in superficial, low-grade papillary tumours. Of interest, it has also been identified in hyperplastic urothelium[68] and in morphologically normal urothelium taken from tumour-bearing bladders.[69] Genetic events identified at lower frequency in both superficial and invasive tumours include *CCND1* amplification, 11p LOH and 4p LOH.

In contrast, most genetic events detected to date have been identified in high-grade and muscle-invasive tumours. These include mutations of *TP53*, *RB*, *CDKN2/ARF*, *HRAS*, amplification and over-expression of *ERBB2* and LOH of 3p, 8p, 10q and 18q. Many of these events are also found in Tis, confirming the likely progression to muscle-invasive TCC via Tis.

pRb and p53 pathways (Figure 23.2)

Two interrelated pathways, commonly referred to as the pRb and p53 pathways, maintain G1 checkpoint control.[70] Cyclin-dependent kinase (cdk)/cyclin complexes act to phosphorylate the Rb protein. Phosphorylated pRb can no longer bind the transcription factor E2F1, and the released E2F1 initiates the transcription of genes required for progression into the S phase.

In one pathway, the p16 protein encoded by the *INK4A* gene acts as a CDK inhibitor and therefore induces G1 arrest. In the second pathway, the p14 protein encoded by the *ARF* gene upregulates p53, which in turn upregulates p21 (WAF1), an inhibitor of the CDK4/cyclinD1 complex. In this pathway, the mechanism of p53 stabilization via p14 appears to be through binding to and promoting degradation of MDM2. Moreover, the two pathways are interlinked; expression of p14 is regulated by E2F1.

The first prediction of this model is that complete dysregulation of these pathways requires

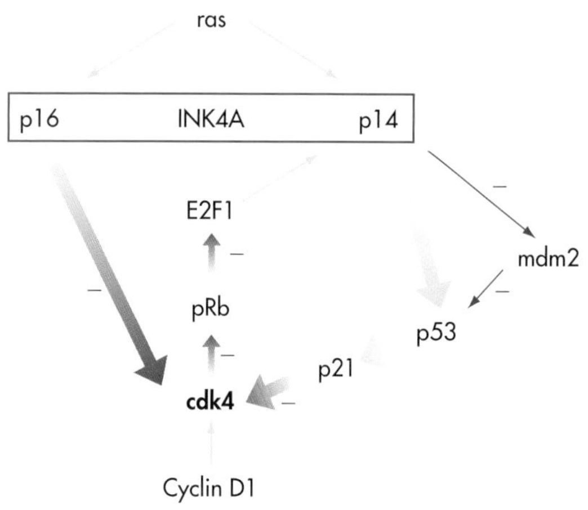

Figure 23.2 *p53 and pRb pathways*

inactivation of *RB* or *INK4A* and *p14/ARF* or *TP53*. The second prediction is that alterations in either pathway alone will generate a phenotype which is less aggressive than if both pathways were altered. Three retrospective studies of TCC have confirmed these predictions.[71–73]

Genetic model of tumour recurrence

This is less well studied than the model for progression. Genetic alterations associated with tumour recurrence include monosomy 9 and polysomy 7 and 17.

Adhesion molecules

As an initial step, cancer cells must detach from their original site before they can invade the surrounding tissue and metastasize to distant organs. The main families of adhesion molecules are the cadherins, integrins, members of the immunoglobulin superfamily, and selectins. This diverse system of transmembrane glycoproteins mediates cell–extracellular matrix adhesion and intercellular matrix adhesion.

The cadherins are the most studied adhesion molecules in TCC. They are the prime mediators of cell–cell adhesion involved in calcium-dependent, homotypic interactions: a cadherin molecule on one cell binds to a cadherin molecule of the same type on another cell to form a homodimer. E-cadherin is expressed on all epithelial tissue. E-cadherin interacts with cytoskeletal proteins through the catenin complex. The catenin complex consists of α-catenin, β-catenin, γ-catenin and p120. In cases where E-cadherin is downregulated at the protein level, expression of α-catenin and, to a lesser extent, of β- or γ-catenin is also reduced.[74]

The adhesive counterreceptor for the α(E)β(7)-integrin of intraepithelial T lymphocytes is E-cadherin. However, the degree of infiltration of tissue by these lymphocytes does not appear to be related to the intensity of E-cadherin expression.[75] In patients treated with cystectomy, aberrant E-cadherin expression is associated with advanced tumour stage, lymph-node metastasis, dedifferentiation and increased risk of death from bladder cancer, and is an independent predictor of disease progression.[76] In this study, metastatic lesions exhibited a higher frequency of E-cadherin-positive cells than primary tumours. It may be that after losing E-cadherin expression temporarily in the primary tumour mass, the tumour cells may metastasize and then once in the new organ environment, may express E-cadherin, which may aid in establishing a viable metastatic deposit.

An 80-kDa, soluble form of E-cadherin (sE-cadherin) has been detected in the urine[77] and sera[78] of healthy individuals and patients with bladder cancer. In superficial TCC, elevated levels of sE-cadherin in sera correlate with high-grade, multifocal tumours at presentation and tumour recurrence at 3 months.

Angiogenesis

Angiogenesis, the growth of new blood vessels from existing vessels, is essential to meet the metabolic requirements for tumour growth. The microvessel density of advanced TCC, a histological surrogate for angiogenesis correlates with reduced survival.[79] A number of angiogenic factors are expressed in TCC, including vascular endothelial growth factor (VEGF), thymidine phosphorylase (TP), acidic and basic fibroblast growth factor (bFGF), hepatocyte growth factor, interleukin-8 (IL-8) and transforming growth factor-alpha (TGF-α).

A key angiogenic stimulator in TCC is VEGF. High VEGF mRNA levels in pT1 TCC predict earlier tumour recurrence and stage progression.[80] Elevated urinary VEGF protein levels provide similar prognostic information.[81] Transcription factors such as hypoxia-inducible factor-1α (HIF-1α) and HIF-2α are key components in the hypoxic upregulation of VEGF.[82]

Another major angiogenic stimulatory factor is the intracellular enzyme, thymidine phosphorylase (TP), also called platelet-derived endothelial cell growth factor. Messenger RNA levels of TP are 33-fold higher in invasive TCC than in superficial TCC and 260-fold higher than in normal bladder.[83] Protein levels of TP are also highest in invasive tumours.[84] The functional role of TP has been demonstrated in an *in vitro* study in which the wild-type RT112 cell line did not invade stroma, whereas transfection of RT112 with a TP clone enabled stromal invasion.[85] Preliminary results in superficial (Ta/T1) TCC suggest that time to first tumour recurrence is significantly earlier in patients with high tumour TP levels than in those in whom TP levels are lower.[86]

Cyclo-oxygenase (COX) is a key enzyme in the synthesis of prostaglandins from arachidonic acid. The inducible form of COX, COX-2, produces prostaglandins E_1 and E_2, which are considered to be angiogenic stimulators. COX-2 is rarely detected in normal urothelium. Elevated expression of COX-2 correlates with high-grade TCC,[87] but in a recent study was not an independent predictor of survival.[88]

Thrombospondin-1 is an important component of the extracellular matrix and is known to be a potent inhibitor of angiogenesis both *in vitro* and *in vivo*. In patients with bladder cancer treated by radical cystectomy, low thrombospondin-1 expression is an independent predictor of early disease recurrence and reduced survival.[89]

Invasion of normal tissues

The ability of tumour cells to degrade tissue extracellular matrix and basement membrane components is a prerequisite for invasion and metastasis. Such functions can be performed by a family of zinc-dependent proteolytic enzymes called matrix metalloproteinases (MMPs). Of this family, MMP-2 and MMP-9 (type-4 collagenases) are particularly important in superficial TCC. Recent studies have revealed that membrane-type matrix metalloproteinase-1 (MT1-MMP) induces specific activation of the MMP-2 precursor.[90] Protein expression of MMP-2 and MMP-9 correlates with higher stage and grade of TCC,[91] and high tumour mRNA levels of MMP-2 and MMP-9 levels are associated with early tumour recurrence in superficial TCC.[92] Elevated MMP-2 and MT1-MMP mRNA levels are independent prognostic predictors of survival in patients with TCC.[93] Metalloproteinases are inhibited by a family known as tissue inhibitors of metalloproteinases (TIMPs). TIMP-1 inactivates MMP-2 and MMP-9, whereas TIMP-2 specifically inhibits MMP-2 activity. Higher expression of TIMP-1 mRNA correlates with higher grade and stage of TCC and is associated with early death.[94] High urinary levels of TIMP-1 protein are associated with early progression.[95] Although this positive relationship of TIMP-1 expression with cancer seems paradoxical, this may be only in response to higher MMP activity.

Defects in mismatch repair mechanisms

The activity of DNA repair genes such as the mismatch repair genes have been assessed in bladder cancer. Early results suggest changes in the ratio of expression of the Mut S and Mut L homologues in muscle-invasive TCC compared with superficial TCC and normal urothelium.[96] Loss of hMSH2 (human mut S homolog-2) protein expression may be a useful predictor of tumour recurrence in bladder cancer.[97]

Immortalization

The genetically determined lifespan of somatic cells is controlled not only by regulators of the cell cycle but also by the progressive erosion of chromosomal ends during each cell division. These ends, called telomeres, are formed by an array of tandem repeats of the sequence TTAGGG. Their main function is to protect chromosomes from the activity of DNA-degrading enzymes such as exonucleases and ligases. All chromosomes lose a small amount of telomeric DNA (50–100 bp) during each cell division as a consequence of the inability of DNA polymerase to replicate the 3′ end of the lagging strand in the replicative fork.

Cell senescence is triggered when telomeres lose a critical number of repeats.

Telomerase is a ribonucleoprotein that compensates for the progressive erosion of telomeres. It is usually suppressed in normal somatic cells, but, in cancers, telomerase represents an important step in immortalization. Telomerase is expressed in 90% of bladder cancers but does not appear to be associated with tumour stage or grade.[98] The prognostic value of telomerase in bladder cancer has not been fully explored. In patients with upper tract TCC, expression of the telomerase RNA subunit hTR was associated with significant decreases in disease-free and overall survival rates.[99]

Apoptosis

Apoptosis is a unique form of cell death in which the cell activates a self-destruct mechanism, causing its death. Suppression of apoptosis can facilitate accumulation of gene mutations. Genes responsible for the regulation of apoptosis interact in a cascade which can be divided into initiation, regulation and degradation phases. Initiators include p53 and cytokines such as tumour necrosis factor-α and fas ligand (FasL). The key regulators are the bcl-2 family of proteins, which are located on intracellular membranes and the endoplasmic reticulum. They can dimerize with one another, with one monomer antagonizing or enhancing the function of the other. Bcl-2, bcl-x_L, bcl-w and mcl-1 inhibit apoptosis. Conversely, bax, bik, bak, bad and bcl-x_S activate apoptosis. There is now a body of data showing that bcl-2 promotes chemoresistance and radioresistance in TCC. In one study, bcl-2 positivity was an independent indicator of reduced survival in patients with muscle-invasive TCC treated by combined transurethral resection, chemotherapy and radiotherapy.[100]

The degradation stage of apoptosis is primarily mediated by a family of 10 or more proteolytic enzymes termed 'caspases'. They are expressed as precursors which are activated when cleaved. Caspases target proteins which are integral to the cell structure and repair processes. Activated caspase 3 can inhibit the cyclin-dependent kinase activity of p27 by cleaving it into two fragments. In patients with Tis of the bladder, loss of p27 nuclear immunostaining accompanied by elevated expression of activated caspase 3 is associated with the development of muscle-invasive TCC.[101]

MOLECULAR BASIS OF SYNCHRONOUS AND METACHRONOUS TCC

Patients with bladder cancer often present with metachronous tumours, presenting at different times and different sites in the bladder. Some investigators attribute this observation to a 'field defect' such as dysplasia or Tis in the bladder that allows the individual transformation of epithelial cells at a number of sites. In contrast, recent reports based on molecular biological studies have added a new dimension, suggesting a common clonal origin for concomitant urothelial tumours, at least in some cases. Cells of adult tissues in females have either one of the two X chromosomes randomly inactivated by methylation. Therefore, if cells are individually transformed, multiple tumours would be heterogeneous with respect to which chromosomes remained active. For each of four female patients with multiple tumours, it was found that all the tumours from a given individual had inactivation of the same X chromosome.[102] Lunec reported identical TP53 mutations and ERBB2 gene amplification in a case of concomitant TCC of the renal pelvis and urinary bladder.[103] Lateral intraepithelial spread of transformed cells from the origin of a bladder carcinoma and dispersal of tumour cells are possible mechanisms underlying multifocal disease. In support of these theories, a single instillation of intravesical epirubicin[104] or mitomycin C[105] immediately following transurethral resection increases recurrence-free intervals.

NEW THERAPIES UTILIZING MOLECULAR TARGETS

Novel therapeutic options are currently undergoing clinical assessment in patients with bladder cancer. Examples include an EGFR-selective tyrosine kinase inhibitor (Iressa), an antagonist (monoclonal antibody) to HER2 (Herceptin), non-steroidal anti-inflammatory agents (Piroxicam) and a potent inhibitor of MMP-2 (Halofuginone).

REFERENCES

1. OPCS (2001). Cancer statistics registration: OPCS – A Publication of the Government Statistical Service
2. Hueper WC, Wiley FH, Wolfe HD. Experimental production of bladder tumours in dogs by administration of beta-naphthylamine. J Indust Hyg Toxicol 1938; 20: 46–84
3. Case RAM, Hosker ME. Tumour of the urinary tract as an occupational disease in the rubber industry in England and Wales. Br J Prev Soc Med 1954; 8: 39–50
4. BAUS Subcommittee on Industrial Bladder Cancer. Occupational bladder cancer: a guide for physicians. Br J Urol 1988; 61: 183–191
5. Zeegers MP, Tan FE, Dorant E, van Den Brandt PA. The impact of characteristics of cigarette smoking on urinary tract cancer risk: a meta-analysis of epidemiologic studies. Cancer 2000; 89: 630–639
6. Hartge P, Silverman D, Hoover R, Schairer C et al. Changing cigarette habits and bladder cancer risk: a case-control study. J Natl Cancer Inst 1987; 78: 1119–1125
7. Fairchild WV, Spence CR, Solomon HD, Granger MP. The incidence of bladder cancer after cyclophosphamide therapy. J Urol 1979; 122: 163–164
8. Duncan RE, Bennett DW, Evans AT, Aron BS et al. Radiation-induced bladder tumours. J Urol 1977; 118: 43–45
9. Sella A, Dexeus FH, Chong C, Ro JY et al. Radiation therapy-associated invasive bladder tumours. Urology 1989; 33: 185–188
10. Marcus PM, Vineis P, Rothman N. NAT2 slow acetylation and bladder cancer risk: a meta-analysis of 22 case-control studies conducted in the general population. Pharmacogenetics 2000; 10: 115–122
11. Green J, Banks E, Berrington A, Darby S et al. *N*-acetyltransferase 2 and bladder cancer: an overview and consideration of the evidence for gene–environment interaction. Br J Cancer 2000; 83: 412–417
12. Lee SW, Jang IJ, Shin SG *et al*. CYP1A2 activity as a risk factor for bladder cancer. J Korean Med Sci 1994; 9: 482–489
13. Filiadis IF, Geogiou I, Alamanos Y, Kranas V et al. Genotypes of *N*-acetyltransferase-2 and risk of bladder cancer: a case-control study. J Urol 1999; 161: 1672–1675
14. Cheng L, Cheville JC, Neumann RM, Bostwick DG. Natural history of urothelial dysplasia of the bladder. Am J Surg Pathol 1999; 23: 443–447
15. Hermanek P, Hutter RVP, Sobin LH, Wagner G et al. TNM Atlas. 4th edn. UICC: Springer, 1997
16. Mostofi F. International histologic classification of tumours. A report by the Executive Committee of the International Council of Societies of Pathology. Cancer 1973; 33: 1480–1484
17. Ooms EC, Anderson WA, Alons CL, Boon ME et al. Analysis of the performance of pathologists in the grading of bladder tumours. Hum Pathol 1983; 14: 140–143
18. Pauwels RP, Smeetes AW, Schapers RF, Geraedts JP et al. Grading in superficial bladder cancer. (I). Morphological criteria. Br J Urol 1988; 61: 135–139
19. Epstein JI, Amin MB, Reuter VR, Mostofi FK and the Bladder Consensus Conference Committee. World Health Organization/International Society of Urological Pathology Consensus Classification of Urothelial (Transitional Cell) Neoplasms of the Urinary Bladder. Am J Surg Pathol 1998; 22: 1435–1448
20. Mostofi FK, Davis CJ, Sesterhenn IA in collaboration with Sobin LH and pathologists in 10 countries. World Health Organization International Histological Classification of Tumours. 2nd edn. Histological typing of urinary bladder tumours. Springer, 1999
21. Parmar MK, Freedman LS, Hargreave TB, Tolley DA. Prognostic factors for recurrence and follow-up policies in the treatment of superficial bladder cancer: report from the British Medical Research Council Subgroup on Superficial Bladder Cancer (Urological Cancer Working Party). J Urol 1989; 142: 284–288
22. Hall RR, Parmar MK, Richards AB, Smith PH. Proposal for changes in cystoscopic follow-up of patients with bladder cancer and adjuvant intravesical chemotherapy. BMJ 1994; 308: 257–260
23. Lutzeyer W, Rubben H, Dahm H. Prognostic parameters in superficial bladder cancer: an analysis of 315 cases. J Urol 1982; 127: 250–252
24. Fitzpatrick JM, West AB, Butler MR, Lane V, O'Flynn JD. Superficial bladder tumours (stage pTa, grades 1 and 2): the importance of recurrence pattern following initial resection. J Urol 1986; 135: 920–922
25. Anderstrøm C, Johansson S, Nilsson S. The significance of lamina propria invasion on the prognosis of patients with bladder cancer. J Urol 1980; 124: 23–26
26. Freeman JA, Esrig D, Stein JP, Simoneau AR et al. Radical cystectomy for high risk patients with superficial bladder cancer in the era of orthotopic urinary reconstruction. Cancer 1995; 76: 833–839

27. Flamm J, Havelec L. Factors affecting survival in primary superficial bladder cancer. Eur Urol 1990; 17: 113–118
28. Heney NM, Ahmed S, Flanagan MJ, Frable W et al. Superficial bladder cancer: progression and recurrence. J Urol 1983; 130: 1083–1086
29. Jakse G, Loidl W, Seeber G, Hofstadter F. Stage T1 grade G3 transitional cell carcinoma of the bladder: an unfavourable tumour? J Urol 1987; 137: 39–43
30. Utz DC, Farrow GM. The management of carcinoma in situ of the urinary bladder: the case for surgical management. Urol Clin North Am 1980; 7: 533–541
31. Wolf H, Olsen PR, Fischer A, Højgaard K. Urothelial atypia concomitant with primary bladder tumour. Incidence in a consecutive series of 500 unselected patients. Scand J Urol Nephrol 1987; 21: 33–38
32. Mills RD, Turner WH, Fleischmann A, Markwalder R et al. Pelvic lymph node metastases from bladder cancer: outcome in 83 patients after radical prostatectomy and pelvic lymphadenectomy. J Urol 2001; 166: 19–23
33. Knowles M. The genetics of transitional cell carcinoma: progress and potential clinical application. BJU Int 1999; 84: 412–427
34. Cappellen D, De Oliveira C, Ricol D et al. Frequent activating mutations of FGFR3 in human bladder and cervix carcinomas. Nat Genet 1999; 23: 18–20
35. Sibley K, Cuthbert-Heavens D, Knowles MA. Loss of heterozygosity at 4p16.3 and mutation of FGFR3 in transitional cell carcinoma. Oncogene 2001; 20: 686–691
36. van Rhijn BW, Lurkin I, Radvanyi F, Kirkels WJ, van der Kwast TH, Zwarthoff EC et al. The fibroblast growth factor receptor 3 (FGFR3) mutation is a strong indicator of superficial bladder cancer with low recurrence rate. Cancer Res 2001; 61: 1265–1268
37. Sauter G, Moch D, Moore P et al. Heterogeneity of erbB-2 gene amplification in bladder cancer. Cancer Res 1993; 53: 2199–2203
38. Neal DE, Sharples L, Smith K, Fennelly J, Hall RR, Harris AL. The epidermal growth factor receptor and the prognosis of bladder cancer. Cancer 1990; 65: 1619–1625
39. Mellon K, Wright C, Kelly P et al. Long-term outcome related to epidermal growth factor receptor status in bladder cancer. J Urol 1995; 153: 919–925
40. Wood DP Jr, Fair WR, Chaganti RS. Evaluation of epidermal growth factor receptor, DNA replication and mRNA expression in bladder cancer. J Urol 1992; 147: 274–277
41. Proctor AJ, Coombs LM, Cairns JP, Knowles MA. Amplification at chromosome 11q13 in transitional cell tumours of the bladder. Oncogene 1991; 6: 789–795
42. Tut VM, Braithwaite KL, Angus B, Neal DE et al. Cyclin D1 expression in transitional cell carcinoma of the bladder: correlation with p53, waf1, pRb and Ki67. Br J Cancer 2001; 84: 270–275
43. Simon R, Struckmann K, Schraml P, Wagner U et al. Amplification pattern of 12q13-q15 genes (MDM2, CDK4, GLI) in urinary bladder cancer. Oncogene 2002; 21: 2476–2483
44. Lu ML, Wikman F, Orntoft TF, Charytonowicz E et al. Impact of alterations affecting the p53 pathway in bladder cancer on clinical outcome, assessed by conventional and array-based methods. Clin Cancer Res 2002; 8: 171–179
45. Cairns P, Proctor AJ, Knowles MA. Loss of heterozygosity at the RB locus is frequent and correlates with muscle-invasion in bladder carcinoma. Oncogene 1991; 6: 2305–2309
46. Spruck CHR, Ohneseit PF, Gonzalez-Zulueta M, Esrig D et al. Two molecular pathways to transitional cell carcinoma of the bladder. Cancer Res 1994; 54: 784–788
47. Abdel-Fattah R, Challen C, Griffiths TRL, Robinson MC et al. Alterations of TP53 in microdissected transitional cell carcinoma of the human bladder: high frequency of TP53 accumulation in the absence of detected mutations is associated with poor prognosis. Br J Cancer 1998; 77: 2230–2238
48. Sarkis AS, Dalbagni G, Cordon-Cardo C, Zhang ZF et al. Nuclear overexpression of p53 protein in transitional cell carcinoma: a marker for disease progression. J Natl Cancer Inst 1993; 85: 53–59
49. Serth J, Kuczyk MA, Bokemeyer C, Hervatin C et al. p53 immunohistochemistry as an independent prognostic factor for superficial transitional cell carcinoma of the bladder. Br J Cancer 1995; 71: 201–205
50. Williamsom MP, Elder PA, Shaw ME, Devlin J et al. p16 (CDKN2) is a major deletion target at 9p21 in bladder cancer. Hum Mol Genet 1995; 4: 1569–1577
51. Orlow I, Lacombe L, Hannon GJ, Serrano M et al. Deletion of the p16 and p15 genes in human bladder tumours. J Natl Cancer Inst 1995; 87: 1524–1529
52. Yeager TR, De Vries S, Jarrard DF, et al. Overcoming cellular senescence in human cancer pathogenesis. Genes Dev 1998; 12: 163–174
53. Aveyard JS, Skilleter A, Habuchi T, Knowles MA. Somatic mutation of PTEN in bladder carcinoma. Br J Cancer 1999; 80: 904–908

54. Cairns P, Evron E, Okami K, Halachmi N et al. Point mutation and homozygous deletion of PTEN/ MMAC1 in primary bladder tumours. Oncogene 1998; 16: 3215–3218
55. McGarvey TW, Maruta Y, Tomaszewski JE, Linnenbach AJ, Malkowicz SB. PTCH gene mutations in invasive transitional cell carcinoma of the bladder. Oncogene 1998; 17: 1167–1172
56. Hornigold N, Devlin J, Davies AM, Aveyard JS, Habuchi T, Knowles MA. Mutation of the 9q34 gene TSC1 in bladder cancer. Oncogene 1999; 18: 2657–2661
57. Habuchi T, Yoshida O, Knowles MA. A novel candidate tumour suppressor locus at 9q32–33 in bladder cancer: localization of the candidate region within a single 840 kb YAC. Hum Mol Genet 1997; 6: 913–919
58. Habuchi T, Luscombe M, Elder PA, Knowles MA. Structure and methylation-based silencing of a gene (DBCCR1) within a candidate bladder cancer tumour suppressor region at 9q32-q33. Genomics 1998; 48: 277–288
59. Brewster SF, Gingell JC, Browne S, Brown KW. Loss of heterozygosity on chromosome 18q is associated with muscle-invasive transitional cell carcinoma of the bladder. Br J Cancer 1994; 70: 697–700
60. Chi S-G, Chang S-G, Lee S-J et al. Elevated and biallelic expression of p73 is associated with progression of human cancer. Cancer Res 1999; 59: 2791–2793
61. Park B-J, Lee S-J, Kim JI, et al. Frequent alteration of p63 expression in human primary bladder carcinomas. Cancer Res 2000; 60: 3370–3374
62. Del Pizzo JJ, Borkowski A, Jacobs SC, Kyprianou N. Loss of cell cycle regulators p27 and cyclin E in transitional cell carcinoma of the bladder correlates with tumour grade and patient survival. Am J Pathol 1999; 155: 1129–1136
63. Kamai T, Takagi K, Asami H, Ito Y et al. Decreasing of p27 and cyclin E protein levels is associated with progression from superficial into invasive bladder cancer. Br J Cancer 2001; 84: 1242–1251
64. Oya M, Schulz WA. Decreased expression of p57 mRNA in human bladder cancer. Br J Cancer 2000; 83: 626–631
65. Stein JP, Ginsberg DA, Grossfeld GD, Chatterjee SJ et al. Effect of p21 WAF1/CIP1 expression on tumour progression in bladder cancer. J Natl Cancer Inst 1998; 90: 1072–1079
66. Lipponen P, Aaltomaa S, Eskelinen M, Ala-Opas M et al. Expression of p21 (waf1/cip1) protein in transitional cell bladder tumours and its prognostic value. Eur Urol 1998; 34: 237–243
67. Qureshi KN, Griffiths TR, Robinson MC, Marsh C et al. Combined p21WAF1/CIP1 and p53 overexpression predict improved survival in muscle-invasive bladder cancer treated by radical radiotherapy. Int J Radiat Oncol Biol Phys 2001; 51: 1234–1240
68. Hartmann A, Moser K, Kriegmair M, Hofstetter A, Hofstaedter F, Knuechel R. Frequent genetic alterations in simple urothelial hyperplasias of the bladder in patients with papillary urothelial carcinoma. Am J Pathol 1999; 154: 721–727
69. Pycha A, Mian C, Hofbauer J, et al. Multifocality of transitional cell carcinoma results from genetic instability of entire transitional epithelium. Urology 1999; 53: 92–97
70. Scherr CJ. Cancer cell cycles. Science 1996; 274: 1672–1677
71. Grossman HB, Liebert M, Antelo M, et al. p53 and RB expression predict progression in T1 bladder cancer. Clin Cancer Res 1998; 4: 829–834
72. Cote RJ, Dunn MD, Chatterjee SJ, Stein JP et al. Elevated and absent pRb expression is associated with bladder cancer progression and has co-operative effects with p53. Cancer Res 1998; 58: 1090–1094
73. Cordon-Cardo C, Zhang ZF, Dalbagni G, Drolonjak M et al. Cooperative effects of p53 and pRB alterations in primary superficial bladder tumours. Cancer Res 1997; 57: 1217–1221
74. Bringuier PP, Giroldi LA, Umbas R, Shimazui T et al. Mechanisms associated with abnormal E-cadherin immunoreactivity in human bladder tumours. Int J Cancer 1999; 83: 591–595
75. Cresswell J, Robertson H, Neal DE, Griffiths TR, Kirby JA. Distribution of lymphocytes of the alpha (E) beta (7) phenotype and E-cadherin in normal human urothelium and bladder carcinomas. Clin Exp Immunol 2001; 126: 397–402
76. Byrne RR, Shariat SF, Brown R, Kattan MW et al. E-cadherin immunostaining of bladder transitional cell carcinoma, carcinoma in situ and lymph node metastases with long-term follow-up. J Urol 2001; 165: 1473–1479
77. Banks RE, Porter WH, Whelan P, Smith PH, Selby PJ. Soluble forms of adhesion molecule E-cadherin in urine. J Clin Pathol 1995; 48: 179–180
78. Griffiths TR, Brotherick I, Bishop RI, White MD et al. Cell adhesion molecules in bladder cancer: soluble serum E-cadherin correlates with predictors of recurrence. Br J Cancer 1996; 74: 579–584

79. Bochner BH, Cote RJ, Weidner N, Groshen S et al. Angiogenesis in bladder cancer: relationship between microvessel density and tumour prognosis. J Natl Cancer Inst 1995; 87: 1603–1612
80. Crew JP, O'Brien T, Bradburn M, Fuggle S et al. Vascular endothelial growth factor is a predictor of relapse and stage progression in superficial bladder cancer. Cancer Res 1997; 57: 5281–5285
81. Crew JP, O'Brien T, Bicknell R, Fuggle S et al. Urinary vascular endothelial growth factor and its correlation with bladder cancer recurrence rates. J Urol 1999; 161: 799–804
82. Jones A, Fujiyama C, Blanche C, Moore JW et al. Relation of vascular endothelial growth factor production to expression and regulation of hypoxia-inducible factor-1α and hypoxia-inducible factor-2α in human bladder tumours and cell lines. Clin Cancer Res 2001; 7: 1263–1272
83. O'Brien T, Cranston D, Fuggle S, Bicknell R, Harris AL. Different angiogenic pathways characterise superficial and invasive bladder cancer. Cancer Res 1995; 55: 510–513
84. O'Brien TS, Fox SB, Dickinson AJ, Turley H et al. Expression of the angiogenic factor thymidine phosphorylase/platelet derived endothelial cell growth factor in primary bladder cancers. Cancer Res 1996; 56: 4799–4804
85. Jones A, Fujiyama C, Turner K, Cranston D et al. Role of thymidine phosphorylase in an in vitro model of human bladder cancer invasion. J Urol 2002; 167: 1482–1486
86. Mizutani Y, Wada H, Ogawa O, Yoshida O et al. Prognostic significance of thymidylate synthase activity in bladder carcinoma. Cancer 2001; 92: 510–518
87. Yoshimura R, Sano H, Mitsuhashi M, Kohno M et al. Expression of cyclooxygenase-2 in patients with bladder carcinoma. J Urol 2001; 165: 1468–1472
88. Shirahama T, Arima J-I, Akiba S, Sakakura C. Relation between cyclooxygenase-2 expression and tumour invasiveness and patient survival in transitional cell carcinoma of the urinary bladder. Cancer 2001; 92: 188–193
89. Glossfeld GD, Ginsberg DA, Stein JP, Bochner BH et al. Thrombospondin-1 expression in bladder cancer: association with p53 alterations, tumour angiogenesis, and tumour progression. J Natl Cancer Inst 1997; 89: 219–227
90. Stanton H, Gavrilovic J, Atkinson SJ, d'Ortho MP et al. The activation of ProMMP-2 (gelatinase A) by HT1080 fibrosarcoma cells is promoted by culture on a fibronectin substrate and is concomitant with an increase in processing of MT1-MMP (MMP-14) to a 45 kDa form. J Cell Sci 1998; 111: 2789–2798
91. Papathoma AS, Petraki C, Grigorakis A, Papakonstantinou H et al. Prognostic significance of matrix metalloproteinases 2 and 9 in bladder cancer. Anticancer Res 2000; 20: 2009–2013
92. Hara I, Miyake H, Hara S, Arakawa S et al. Significance of matrix metalloproteinases and tissue inhibitors of metalloproteinase expression in the recurrence of superficial transitional cell carcinoma of the bladder. J Urol 2001; 165: 1769–1772
93. Kanayama H, Yokota K, Kurokawa Y, Murakami Y et al. Prognostic values of matrix metalloproteinase-2 and tissue inhibitor of metalloproteinase-2 expression in bladder cancer. Cancer 1998; 82: 1359–1366
94. Yano A, Nakamoto T, Hashimoto K, Usui T. Localization and expression of tissue inhibitor of metalloproteinase-1 in human urothelial cancer. J Urol 2002; 167: 729–734
95. Durkan GC, Nutt JE, Rajjayabun PH, Neal DE et al. Prognostic significance of matrix metalloproteinase-1 and tissue inhibitor of metalloproteinase-1 in voided urine samples from patients with transitional cell carcinoma of the bladder. Clin Cancer Res 2001; 7: 3450–3456
96. Thykjaer T, Christensen M, Clark AB, Hansen LR et al. Functional analysis of the mismatch repair system in bladder cancer. Br J Cancer 2001; 85: 568–575
97. Leach FS, Hsieh JT, Molberg K, Saboorian MH et al. Expression of the human mismatch repair gene hMSH2: a potential marker for urothelial malignancy. Cancer 2000; 88: 2333–2341
98. Orlando C, Gelmini S, Selli C, Pazzagli M. Telomerase in urological malignancy. J Urol 2001; 166: 666–673
99. Nakanishi K, Kawai T, Hiroe S, Kumaki F et al. Expression of telomerase mRNA component (hTR) in transitional cell carcinoma of the upper urinary tract. Cancer 1999; 86: 2109–2116
100. Kaufman DS, Shipley WU, Griffin PP, Heney NM et al. Selective bladder preservation by combination treatment of invasive bladder cancer. N Engl J Med 1993; 329: 1377–1382
101. Burton PB, Anderson CJ. Caspase 3 and p27 as predictors of invasive bladder cancer. N Engl J Med 2000; 343: 1418–1419
102. Sidransky D, Von Eschenbach A, Oyasu R, Preisinger AC et al. Clonal origin bladder cancer. N Engl J Med 1992; 326: 737–740
103. Lunec J, Challen C, Wright C, Mellon K et al. C-erb-

B2 amplification and identical p53 mutations in concomitant transitional carcinomas of renal pelvis and urinary bladder. Lancet 1992; 339: 439–440

104. Oosterlinck W, Kurth KH, Schroder F, Bultinck J et al. A prospective European Organization for Research and Treatment of Cancer Genitourinary Group randomised trial comparing transurethral resection followed by a single intravesical instillation of epirubicin or water in single stage Ta, T1 papillary carcinoma of the bladder. J Urol 1993; 149: 749–752

105. Tolley DA, Parmar MKB, Grigor KM, Lallemand G and the Medical Research Council Superficial Bladder Cancer Working Party. The effect of intravesical mitomycin C on recurrence of newly diagnosed superficial bladder cancer: a further report with 7 years follow-up. J Urol 1996; 155: 1233–1238

106. Dalesio O, Schulman CC, Sylvester R, De Pauw M et al. Prognostic factors in superficial bladder tumours. A study of the European Organization for Research on Treatment of Cancer: Genitourinary Tract Cancer Cooperative Group. J Urol 1983; 129: 730–733

24

Prostate cancer

Freddie C Hamdy, Mark I Johnson and Craig N Robson

As the eyes grow dim, the trunk bends, the cartilages ossify, and the arteries change in their coats, so the prostate is supposed to grow large and hard.

James Miller, 1864

INTRODUCTION

Prostate cancer is the second leading cause of cancer-specific death in the USA and the UK.[1] The increased awareness of this disease, in combination with serum testing for prostate-specific antigen (PSA), has led to an increase in the use of radical prostatectomy as a treatment for clinically organ-confined prostate cancer in the USA and elsewhere in the Western world.[2] In England and Wales, the age-specific incidence peaked in 1994, with the subsequent rate decreasing towards the underlying trend in most age groups.[3] Public awareness of the disease is clearly on the increase, partly because of media interest and growing general interest in men's health issues.

Evidence of carcinoma has been found in post-mortem studies in approximately 30% of men aged 50 years, and 70% of men over the age of 80 years,[4,5] but only a small proportion of these tumours progress to become clinically significant. With well-conducted screening programmes, it is now possible to detect small-volume tumours amenable to cure. However, clinicians are still unable to predict which tumour is likely to progress and which will remain quiescent.

AETIOLOGY

Prostate cancer results from a complex and yet unclear interaction between ageing, genetic factors, hormones, growth factors and the environment, including an increasing body of evidence incriminating dietary fat.[4–7]

Prostate cancer can be sporadic; it may be familial, with clustering of disease within families and exposure to common risk factors, or hereditary, with typical characteristics of early age onset and an autosomal-dominant inheritance pattern. The latter is likely to be triggered by a single gene passed along families, yet to be discovered and possibly located in chromosome 1.[8] It has been estimated that men who have three first-degree relatives affected have a 10.9-fold increase in risk of developing the disease.[9] An increased risk of prostate cancer has also been associated with familial breast cancer.[7] It is generally accepted that prostate cancer is not divided into latent and clinically significant tumour, but that its very long natural history, coupled with cumulative genetic and biological changes eventually leads to progressive disease. It is the length of this natural history which allows more men to die *with* the disease than *from* it.

PATHOLOGY

Adenocarcinoma arising from the prostatic epithelium accounts for about 95% of prostatic malignancies and is usually composed of small glandular acini which infiltrate in an irregular, haphazard manner.[10] The critical feature in prostatic adenocarcinoma is absence of the basal cell layer (Figure 24.1), which may be detected immunohistochemically by using monoclonal antibodies against high-molecular-weight cytokeratin. Perineural and microvascular invasion may be seen, the latter correlating with histological grade.

Prostatic adenocarcinoma originates in the peripheral zone in approximately 75% of cases, with the rest originating in the transition zone.[11] The

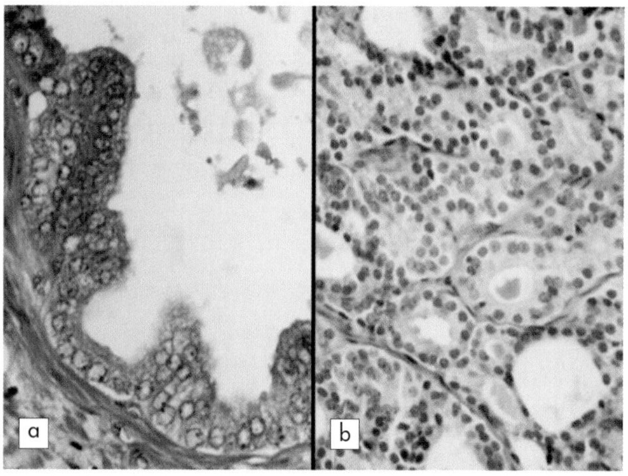

Figure 24.1 *(a) A photomicrograph of the prostate demonstrating high-grade prostatic intraepithelial neoplasia with dysplastic changes, nuclear enlargement, hyper chromatism, prominent nuclei, cellular crowding, overlapping nuclei and epithelial hyperplasia. *H & E staining; magnification approximately ×400.) (b) A photomicrograph of the prostate demonstrating adenocarcinoma with small glandular acini infiltrating in an irregular haphazard manner. The acini are composed of a single layer of cells showing nuclear enlargement with prominent nucleoli. the critical diagnostic feature in prostatic adenocarcinoma is absence of the basal layer. (H & E staining; magnification approximately ×400.)*

tumours arising from these separate zones have different pathological features and clinical behaviour. Transition zone tumours arise in or near foci of benign prostatic hyperplasia (BPH) and are usually smaller and better differentiated (Gleason patterns 1 and 2). Peripheral zone cancers are often less well differentiated (Gleason patterns 2, 3 or 4) and larger in volume than transition zone tumours, and are frequently associated with greater stromal fibrosis, extracapsular extension, seminal vesicle invasion and lymph-node metastases.[12]

Histological grading

There are numerous grading systems, but the accepted standard is that developed by Gleason.[13] The system is based on the degree of architectural differentiation, and individual cell cytology does not play a role. The system identifies five patterns which are often seen in prostatic adenocarcinoma, and to accommodate this, a primary and secondary pattern are assigned, and the Gleason score is given as their sum, ranging from 2 to 10, with the dominant pattern recorded first; for example, 3 + 4 = 7 (Figure 24.2). The Gleason score correlates strongly with crude survival, tumour-free survival and cause-specific survival, and is a significant predictor of time to recurrence after radical prostatectomy.[14]

Grading errors are common in needle-biopsy specimens of the prostate, with underestimation of the grade in 40% of cases, and overestimation in 25% when compared with the whole specimen following prostatectomy. This occurs more readily in

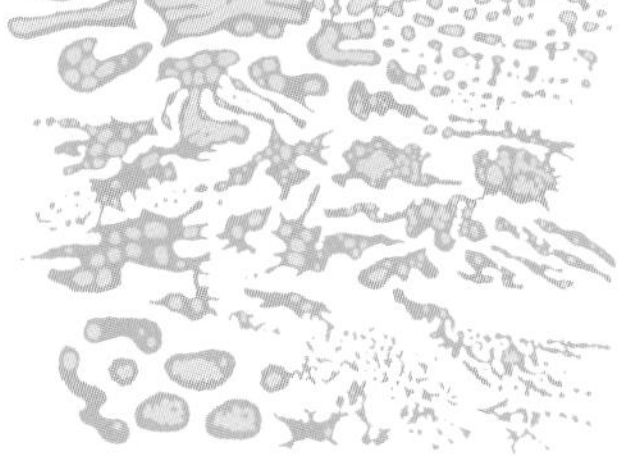

Grade	Margins	Gland pattern	Gland size	Gland distribution
1	Well defined	Single, separate, round	Medium	Closely packed
2	Less defined	Same as one but more variable	Medium	Spaced up to one gland apart
3	Poorly defined	Single, separate, irregular rounded masses of cribriform epithelium	Small, medium or large	Spaced more than one gland apart, rarely packed
4	Ragged infiltrating	Fused glandular masses	Small	Fused ragged masses
5	Ragged infiltrating. Poorly defined	Almost absent, few tiny glands or signet ring cells	Small	Ragged anaplastic masses of epithelium

Figure 24.2 *The Gleason system of grading adenocarcinoma of the prostate.*

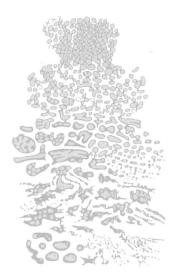

biopsies containing small foci and low-grade cancers, reflecting sampling error and tumour heterogeneity. Nevertheless, useful predictive information can be provided by Gleason grading of needle biopsies.[15]

Tumour staging

The TNM system, recently modified,[16] is the most common classification used worldwide (Table 24.1). Clinical staging is limited by a number of factors, including clinical under-staging with digital rectal examination (DRE) and transurethral resection of the prostate (TURP) specimens, limited accuracy of imaging, and the wide pathological variation of tumours identified on needle biopsy (stage T1c). The inaccuracy of clinical staging is especially important when comparing non-surgical treatment methods (observation or radiotherapy) with pathologically staged disease following radical prostatectomy.

Prostate cancer commonly spreads to the pelvic lymph nodes; bones, especially the axial skeleton; and lung. Unlike most other malignancies, skeletal metastases from prostate cancer are osteoblastic in over 80% of cases, and despite the increase in bone formation, they lead to disturbance in the normal skeletal architecture and subsequent pathological fractures if left untreated.

Putative premalignant lesions of the prostate

Prostatic intraepithelial neoplasia

Prostatic intraepithelial neoplasia (PIN) is believed to be the preinvasive end of a morphological continuum of cellular proliferation affecting prostatic ducts, ductules and acini. It tends to be multifocal and occurs in the peripheral zone, as does prostate cancer. PIN is divided into two groups: low-grade and high-grade. The continuum from normal prostatic epithelium through low-grade and high-grade PIN to invasive cancer is characterized by increased epithelial dysplasia within the luminal secretory cell layer. The dysplastic changes with increasing grade

Table 24.1 TNM classification of prostate cancer.

Tumour	Tx		Primary tumour cannot be assessed
	T0		No evidence of primary tumour
	T1		Tumour clinically inapparent, not palpable nor visible by imaging
		T1a	Incidental finding following TURP in up to 5% of tissue
		T1b	Incidental finding following TURP in more than 5% of tissue
		T1c	Tumour identified by needle biopsy (e.g. because of elevated PSA)
	T2		Tumour confined to the prostate, palpable or visible by imaging
		T2a	Tumour involves one lobe
		T2b	Tumour involves both lobes
	T3		Locally advanced tumour
		T3a	Extracapsular extension
		T3b	Invasion of the seminal vesicle
			Invasion into the prostatic apex or into (but not beyond) the prostatic capsule is not classified as T3, but as T2
	T4		Tumour is fixed or invades adjacent structures other than seminal vesicles; i.e. bladder neck, external sphincter, rectum, levator muscles, and/or pelvic wall
Nodes	Nx		Regional lymph nodes cannot be assessed
	N0		No regional lymph node metastases
	N1		Regional lymph node metastases
Metastasis	Mx		Presence of distant metastases cannot be assessed
	M0		No distant metastases
	M1		Distant metastases present
		M1a	Non-regional lymph nodes
		M1b	Skeletal metastases
		M1c	Other sites

of PIN include nuclear enlargement, hyperchromatism, prominent nucleoli, cellular crowding with overlapping nuclei and epithelial hyperplasia (Figure 24.1). The basal cell layer remains intact though there may be some disruption in high-grade PIN. There is strong clinical, histological and molecular evidence linking high-grade PIN with prostate cancer.[17] High-grade PIN is seen in up to 16% of needle biopsies in men over 50 years of age. In malignant prostates, PIN is more frequent and of higher grade than in glands without cancer. The incidence of PIN increases with age, with low-grade PIN occurring in men in their third and fourth decade, and high-grade PIN occurring in their fifth decade.[18–20]

Atypical adenomatous hyperplasia

Atypical adenomatous hyperplasia (AAH) is a small acinar proliferation which may be confused histologically with low-grade prostatic adenocarcinoma. AAH consists of crowded small glands with a predominantly lobular growth pattern. Basal cells are never seen in carcinoma, but are distributed in a patchy discontinuous manner in AAH. AAH is characteristically found near the apex, in the transition zone and periurethral region, and therefore is most commonly seen in TURP specimens. It has been suggested that AAH may be a precursor of low-grade transition zone cancer, though the data linking them together are inconclusive.[21]

Prostate-specific antigen (PSA)

PSA is a serine protease and organ-specific glycoprotein (molecular weight 34 000) which originates in the cytoplasm of ductal cells of the prostate. It is responsible for liquefaction of seminal coagulation. The measurement of serum PSA concentrations is now well established as a useful investigation in the diagnosis and follow-up of patients with prostate cancer.[22] The greatest limitation of PSA is that it is *tissue*, and not *tumour*, specific in the prostate. However, PSA concentrations are the best overall predictor of bone-scan findings and can be used as a screening test for prostate cancer.[23,24] PSA circulates in blood mainly bound to protease inhibitors, including alpha-1-antichymotrypsin (ACT) and alpha-2-macroglobulin (AMG); only a small fraction of the total PSA exists in a free state. While AMG encapsulates all epitopes of the PSA protein, ACT leaves some exposed; therefore, immunoassay techniques have been developed to assess free PSA and PSA bound to ACT, but not to AMG.[25] Reports suggest that the f/tPSA ratio in patients with BPH is significantly higher than in prostate cancer, but its role is not yet fully established in diagnosing the disease. Several studies report various optimal cutoff levels, largely due to the different nature of assays used.[26] A large study using the Hybritech assay (Hybritech Inc, USA), demonstrated a sensitivity of 90% in diagnosing prostate cancer in the total PSA range of 2.6–4.0 ng/ml, while sparing approximately 18% of patients from having prostatic biopsies.[27] The use of free/total PSA ratios in routine clinical practice remains to be determined.[28]

Circulating PSA-positive cells in prostate cancer

Clinically localized prostate cancers are frequently under-staged in over 50% of cases, with resulting positive surgical margins, extracapsular extension and potential treatment failure. This has stimulated researchers to detect circulating micrometastases prior to the establishment of overt secondaries, to avoid unnecessary radical treatment. Metastasis does not rely on the random survival of cells released from the primary tumour, but on the selective growth of specialized subpopulations of highly metastatic cells endowed with properties which will allow them to complete successfully each step of the metastatic cascade.[29,30] In recent years, new technology, including flow cytometry and the reverse transcription polymerase chain reaction (RT-PCR), has given researchers the opportunity of detecting circulating tumour cells with high levels of sensitivity. In that sense, prostate cancer has a significant advantage over other malignancies, due to the specificity of PSA as a reliable marker. However, it has to be emphasized again that PSA is not tumour specific, a major drawback of all techniques attempting to detect circulating tumour cells. Therefore, a PSA-positive cell in the peripheral blood, does not necessarily mean a prostate tumour cell, but a cell expressing PSA, which is likely to be of prostatic origin, particularly if the cell is found to express the gene constitutively; that is, with mRNA for PSA. Based on these principles, analytical flow cytometry and RT-PCR have been used in an attempt to detect and isolate circulating tumour cells from patients with prostate cancer. Studies have shown that although quantification of circulating PSA-positive cells by FC was a better predictor of skeletal metastases than isotope bone scanning, the majority of these cells were not of prostatic origin, raising important questions regarding the role of non-prostatic circulating PSA-positive cells in patients with prostate cancer.[31,32] RT-PCR methods, on the other hand are considerably more sensitive in detecting circulating PSA-positive cells, relying on the identification of mRNA for PSA, an unequivocal proof that the cells are of prostatic origin. A number of studies demonstrated the ability of RT-PCR to detect circulating prostate cells in patients with apparently localized disease who were undergoing radical prostatectomy, and some found a strong correlation between a positive PCR reaction, capsular tumour penetration and positive surgical margins, suggesting the potential of this technique to be used for 'molecular staging' of prostate cancer.[33] Other workers used nested RT-PCR to compare the sensitivity of PSA with a more recently identified marker, prostate-specific membrane antigen (PSMA) in the detection of circulating prostatic cells.[34] The authors of all these studies assume that circulating PSA-positive cells are endowed with metastatic propensity despite the fact that the results demonstrate only the presence of cells of prostatic origin. Furthermore, the specificity of PSA mRNA in identifying cells of prostatic origin has been questioned in a recent study.[35] The role of detecting circulating PSA-positive cells in the circulation of patients with prostate cancer remains unclear.[36]

SCREENING FOR EARLY PROSTATE CANCER

Primum non nocere.

Hippocrates

There is an apparent consensus, based on the evidence, that there is no justification to introduce population screening for prostate cancer. The classic triad of screening tests consists of serum PSA measurement, digital rectal examination (DRE) and transrectal ultrasound (TRUS) of the prostate, and biopsy, which detect up to 6% of a screened population as having prostate cancer. A number of groups are addressing this issue, particularly in Europe. These studies will utilize mortality from prostate cancer as their end point in the screened compared with the unscreened population, indirectly revealing whether treating the disease early may improve survival.[37] However, methods of screening are changing rapidly, and when the results of these studies are available, it may well be that urologists will be detecting a different category of disease altogether compared with current screening modalities.[38]

CLINICAL PRESENTATION

We found the patient complaining of excruciating pains in various parts of the body, which could be compared to nothing except the pains under which persons afflicted with carcinoma occasionally labour. He could void no urine without the assistance of a catheter. The prostate gland, examined by the rectum, was found to be much enlarged and of a stony hardness. I continued to visit him in consultation for nearly a year, at the end of which time he suddenly lost the use of the muscles of his lower limbs and died a fortnight afterwards.

Sir Benjamin Brodie, 1842

Early prostate cancer is asymptomatic. The above description by Benjamin Brodie, over 160 years ago, illustrates all the relevant symptoms of advanced prostate cancer. Patients with symptomatic disease can present in a variety of ways, including bladder outflow obstruction, irritative bladder symptoms secondary to trigonal involvement and haematuria. Metastatic disease may present with skeletal pain, spinal cord compression secondary to collapsed vertebrae and pathological fractures; or with general systemic manifestations, including weight loss, weakness and anorexia. With locally advanced disease, prostate cancer may manifest itself as renal failure secondary to involvement of bilateral ureteric orifices.

TREATMENT

The more resources we have, and the more complex they are, the greater are the demands on our clinical skill. These resources are calls upon our judgement, and not substitutes for it.

Sir Francis Walsh

For the sake of simplicity, prostate cancer can be classified into early organ-confined, and advanced disease when treatment is dicussed.

Organ-confined prostate cancer

Conventional 'curative' treatments of localized disease include surgery in the form of radical prostatectomy through the retropubic or perineal routes, or radiotherapy with its variations, including conformal approaches and radioactive seed implantation, otherwise known as brachytherapy. These treatments carry relatively low morbidity in experienced hands, and a high cure rate. Watchful waiting, on the other hand, remains a reasonable option in men with low-grade, small-volume tumours and a life expectancy of less than 10 years. Evidence concerning the effectiveness of treatments is limited to observational studies with the full range of well-described limitations of such material, including differences in patient selection criteria, operative techniques, post-operative assessments, variable definitions and lengths of follow-up, and methods of data analysis. Survival following treatment for localized prostate cancer is good for all modes of treatment: 85–90% for radical prostatectomy, 65–90% for radiotherapy, and 70–90% for conservative management. A randomized trial comparing radical prostatectomy with watchful waiting, in Scandinavian patients recruited prior to the widespread use of PSA testing, demonstrated a reduction in disease-specific mortality, but no improvement in overall survival at a median follow-up of 6.2 years.[39] Radical interventions are not recommended for men who are likely to have a life expectancy of less than 10 years. Studies indicate that selected groups of men may benefit from radical intervention, particularly those who are youngest and fittest, and have high-grade tumours. However, problems with the accuracy of clinical staging by the classical triad of serum PSA levels, DRE and TRUS of the prostate mean that up to 50% of men with apparently localized tumours are found to have extracapsular disease and positive margins following radical prostatectomy. This major issue of treatment efficacy in early prostate cancer can be resolved only by well-conducted, randomized, controlled trials, some of which are underway in the USA and the UK, but will take a number of years to yield any significant results.

Advanced prostate cancer

Locally advanced disease

External beam irradiation is widely accepted in treating locally advanced prostate cancer. There is evidence, however, that a large number of clinicians adopted the policy of no treatment in the absence of symptoms. This problem was addressed recently by the Medical Research Council trial of immediate versus deferred treatment, and the results suggest that there is a small but significant advantage in treating these patients early, albeit to delay or prevent the advent of serious morbidity and complications from progressive disease.[40] Downstaging of extracapsular disease has also been attempted in a number of studies, whereby androgen ablation is performed for 3–6 months prior to radical prostatectomy. Although the incidence of positive margins decreases in clinically T2 tumours, there is no apparent change in T3 disease, and disease-free survival is not affected.[41,42]

Metastatic disease

In 1940, Charles Huggins discovered the beneficial effects of androgen deprivation in patients with metastatic prostate cancer.[43] Since then, hormonal manipulation has remained the mainstay of treatment in advanced stages of the disease. It is still expected that about 80% of all patients with advanced prostate cancer will respond to androgen blockade. Patients will show both subjective and objective responses, manifested by considerable and rapid symptomatic improvement, particularly in metastatic skeletal pain, together with local and distant regression of the disease. This is complemented by normalization of serum tumour markers. Relapse, however, is common at a mean interval of 2 years following initiation of treatment. The disease is then hormone resistant and the prognosis becomes extremely poor. Methods of hormonal manipulation include bilateral orchidectomy, and oestrogen preparations, which are rarely prescribed nowadays, in view of the serious cardiovascular side effects encountered with the recognized 3-mg daily dose, in order to achieve castrate levels. The use of the smaller dose of 1 mg daily remains controversial, as castrate levels are not reached in 30% of patients. Alternative therapy includes the use of analogues of the hypothalamic luteinizing hormone-releasing hormone (LHRH). These occupy the receptors of LHRH in the pituitary, initially stimulating the release of luteinizing hormone and then blocking the subsequent stimulation of the receptors by the endogenous pulsatile secretion of luteinizing hormone. Finally, synthetic antiandrogens are also being used. They all act by competing with androgen receptors in hormone-sensitive prostatic cells, benign or malignant. In the late 1980s, total androgen blockade was advocated to prevent the effect of the non-testicular circulating testosterone formation by the adrenals. After initial enthusiasm, recent studies have failed to show any survival advantage in patients treated with maximum androgen blockade.[44,45]

Novel therapies in prostate cancer

The development of new therapeutic approaches in prostate cancer will rely on continuing progress made in three specific areas: (1) imaging of the prostate and identification of cancerous lesions; (2) the delivery of different forms of energy to achieve safe and targeted tissue ablation; and (3) understanding the biology of prostate cancer from its early genetic alterations to the molecular changes responsible for tumour progression. Based on modern TRUS technology, two distinct modes of energy delivery systems for tissue ablation have been revived in recent years: cryotherapy and high-intensity, focused ultrasound (HIFU).

Cryotherapy

The in situ destruction of tumours by the application of low temperatures was first developed in the 1970s to treat localized prostate cancer, and it had reasonable success. Cryoablation had a number of advantages over other forms of treatment, but suffered from many limitations. Equipment was cumbersome, probes were placed mostly transurethrally under digital rectal guidance, temperature control was poor, and damage to adjacent tissue was common. The ability of real-time TRUS to guide cryoprobe placement and accurately monitor the freezing process, in addition to the development of urethral warming devices encouraged clinicians to attempt again the destruction of prostate cancer by freezing. A number of studies on humans followed the animal work, and results are slowly emerging.[46,47]

High-intensity focused ultrasound (HIFU)

HIFU consists of delivering ultrasonic energy with resultant heat and tissue destruction to a discrete point without damaging intervening tissue. Much higher temperatures are generated at the focal point by HIFU (approximately 98°C) than by diffuse ultrasound hyperthermia (approximately 42°C), leading to complete tumour necrosis. After evaluation of the technique, initially in animal models and in vitro in cell lines, its use was reported in the treatment of benign prostatic hyperplasia without significant side effects as a minimally invasive therapeutic option in symptomatic patients. The relative safety of HIFU coupled with its documented ability to cause targeted tissue necrosis prompted researchers to extrapolate its application to the treatment of prostate cancer, as an alternative to surgery and radiotherapy.[48,49]

Gene therapy

Since the discovery of DNA and its structure by James Watson and Francis Crick in 1953, our knowledge of the molecular basis of human genetics in health and disease has made giant steps forward, bringing closer the 'double helix' to the bedside of patients where every other conventional treatment may be failing. Advances in molecular biology, particularly in recombinant DNA technology, have paved the way to unlimited possibilities in predicting, controlling and preventing disease at its molecular origin.

The prostate is a prime target in the development of successful gene therapy for the following reasons:

1. Prostate cancer is slow growing.
2. Tumour burden can be significantly reduced by surgery.
3. The prostate expresses unique antigens, including PSA and PSMA.

The most significant limitation of gene therapy is the difficulty in gene delivery to the relevant cells. Gene transfer can be achieved in vitro or in vivo. In vitro methods can be chemical, through calcium-phosphate transfection; physical, through electroporation or microinjection, by fusion with liposomes, through receptor-mediated endocytosis, or using recombinant viruses. In vivo methods include direct injection of DNA either naked, contained in liposomes, conjugated to a carrier (such as antibodies to a specific cell-surface protein, or by particle bombardment.[50]

Gene-directed enzyme prodrug therapy (GDEPT) is based on the potential use of prodrugs which are essentially inert, but can be converted in vivo to highly toxic active species with the aim of specifically destroying tumour cells. Activation can be the result of metabolism by an enzyme which is either unique to the target organ, or present at much higher concentrations compared with other tissues. Tumour destruction involves two essential steps: (1) specific targeting of malignant cells with the gene-encoding enzyme, which can also be under the control of a specific promoter (such as PSA or PSMA in the prostate); (2) administration of the prodrug, which will be activated into its toxic derivative by the appropriate enzyme *within* the target tissue concerned, with little or no systemic consequences.[51]

Tumour vaccines represent a potentially new and different treatment modality. There are three basic approaches to construct cancer vaccines:

1. whole tumour cells or non-purified cellular extract preparations, in an attempt to include relevant tumour antigens which can stimulate protective immune responses
2. partially purified preparations, enriched in the cellular fraction most likely to contain relevant tumour antigens
3. preparations from highly purified tumour antigens.

The development of these 'vaccines' depends on expression of a family of genes reported to encode antigens recognized by autologous cytotoxic T lymphocytes (CTLs). Such genes have now been identified in melanoma cells *(MAGE-1, MAGE-3, BAGE* and *GAGE)* as well as in head and neck tumours, non-small-cell lung cancers and bladder carcinomas. Recent work from Chen et al[52] demonstrated the presence of two new genes *(PAGE* and *GAGE-7)*, expressed in the LNCaP cell line, which may be specific to prostate cancer and serve as a potential target for tumour immunization.

Every technique mentioned above has specific advantages and disadvantages, the details of which are beyond the scope of this chapter. Experimental studies of gene therapy in prostate cancer are emerging in the literature at an increasing frequency.

APOPTOSIS-REGULATING GENES IN PROSTATE CANCER

Apoptosis

Hormone ablation in prostate cancer achieves its effect by activation of apoptosis (programmed cell death),[53,54] which is a distinct mode of cell death occurring in both normal physiological conditions and disease such as cancer.[55] Apoptosis is an active process characterized by distinct morphological changes in single cells, with compaction and margination of nuclear chromatin, cytoplasmic condensation and convolution of nuclear and cell outlines. Later changes involve nuclear fragmentation and budding of the cell with the development of membrane-bound apoptotic bodies, which are removed by phagocytosis.[55] In contrast to necrosis, which is a passive process, there is no associated inflammation.

It is now apparent that there is a common final pathway, which ultimately leads to DNA fragmentation and apoptotic cell death. This process is mediated by a family of cysteine proteases named caspases, which have the ability to cleave aspartic acid.[56] Caspase activation by an apoptotic signal initiates a cascade, with proteolytic activation of further caspases. The end point of this cascade is the activation of the endonuclease CAD (caspase-activated DNase) by activated caspase-3 within cytoplasm. CAD then enters the nucleus, leading to degradation of chromosomal DNA.[57] There are several ways in which the caspase cascade can be activated. Firstly, there is an inductive mechanism in which cytokines mediate caspase activation. Tumour necrosis factor (TNF-) α acts through its receptor (TNFR) and Fas ligand through the Fas receptor. Both these receptors have a cytoplasmic 'death domain' that, on the binding of the appropriate ligand, leads to activation of caspase 8, which then activates other caspases.[58]

An alternative mechanism appears to centre on the normal function of mitochondria. Apoptosis appears to be initiated when cytochrome *c* relocalizes from the mitochondria to the cytosol. In the cytosol, cytochrome *c* binds to the protein Apaf-1 (apoptotic protease-activating factor-1). This complex then binds to caspase-9, leading to its activation.[59] This results in the activation of caspase-3 with subsequent CAD activation.[60,61]

Numerous genes are involved in the control of apoptosis, including the proto-oncogene bcl-2 on chromosome 18, region 18q21,[62,63] and the tumour suppressor gene p53 on chromosome 17, region 17p13.[64]

bcl-2

The bcl-2 gene was initially identified in B-cell lymphomas,[65] and the gene product acts by inhibiting apoptosis, but has no direct effect on cell proliferation.[62] A rapidly expanding group of genes showing homology to bcl-2 have been described and named the bcl-2 gene family, forming two functionally antagonistic groups controlling the balance between cell death and survival. Bax accelerates apoptotic cell death by forming heterodimers, with bcl-2 leading to suppression of apoptosis.[63–65] The molecular mechanisms by which the bcl-2 protein suppresses apoptosis remain unresolved. High levels of bcl-2 may act by preventing the release of cytochrome *c* from mitochondria.[59] In the prostate, bcl-2 is normally expressed in basal epithelial cells, seminal vesicles and ejaculatory ducts.[63]

In primary prostate cancer, bcl-2 is expressed in around 25% of cases. Bcl-2 overexpression is associated with increasing tumour stage and the development of hormone refractory disease.[66,69]

In high-grade prostatic intraepithelial neoplasia (HGPIN), the reported expression of bcl-2 has shown a wide variation from 0 to 100%.[70,71] The largest study reported bcl-2 expression in 17% of cases of HGPIN.

p53

Inactivation of the tumour suppressor gene p53 is presently the most common mutation identified in human cancers.[72] Functional (wild-type) p53 protein has DNA-binding properties and forms a key part of the mechanism by which mammalian cells undergo growth arrest or apoptosis in response to DNA damage. Mutation of p53 may result in loss of its normal function.[73] Mutations in the p53 gene commonly occur in the highly conserved exons 5, 6, 7 and 8. In most cases, one allele is completely deleted with a missense mutation in the remaining allele. Mutant p53 protein has a prolonged half-life compared to the wild-type p53 protein, and its nuclear accumulation is detectable by immunohistochemistry.

In benign prostatic epithelium, p53 positivity is absent. In primary prostate cancer, p53 nuclear positivity is present in around 20% of cases.[74,75] p53 protein accumulation appears to be a late event, being associated with advanced stage, high Gleason tumour grade, hormonal resistance, poor survival, DNA aneuploidy and high cell-proliferation rate.[76–79] A good correlation is seen between p53 immunoreactivity in prostate cancer and direct evidence of gene mutation using the polymerase chain reaction, single-strand conformational polymorphism and direct sequencing.[80] p53 positivity is infrequent in high-grade, prostatic-intraepithelial neoplasia, the largest study showing strong nuclear staining in 22%.[81]

Wild-type p53 may participate with bcl-2 and bax in a common pathway regulating cell death by decreasing the expression of bcl-2 while simultaneously increasing the expression of bax, resulting in apoptosis.[82]

The combination of bcl-2 overexpression and p53 nuclear protein accumulation in human prostate cancer has been shown to correlate with the development of hormone refractory disease,[68] and these two factors are independent prognostic markers for post-radical prostatectomy recurrence.[83]

ANGIOGENESIS

Microvessel density (MVD)

The ability of a tumour to grow and metastasize depends on tumour angiogenesis. The quantification of new microvessels within a tumour is commonly performed using antibodies against factor VIII to identify endothelial cells. Increasing MVD correlates with increasing Gleason score and presence of metastases, and it is an independent predictor of progression after radical prostatectomy for Gleason scores 5–7 tumour.[84,85]

Vascular endothelial growth factor

Angiogenesis is controlled by a group of substances known as angiogenic factors. Vascular endothelial growth factor (VEGF) is a potent inducer of endothelial cell growth and is expressed in a variety of tumours. In prostate cancer, VEGF expression is increased in prostate cancer compared to benign prostatic epithelium.[86]

GROWTH FACTORS

Growth factors may act as positive or negative effectors of various cellular processes, including proliferation, differentiation and cell death. Interaction occurs with specific membrane receptors, resulting in the transmission of signals through an intracellular protein cascade and the activation or repression of a number of target genes. Several growth factors have been associated with prostatic growth, including transforming growth factors α and β, fibroblast growth factors, insulin-like growth factors, epidermal growth factor, nerve growth factor and various cytokines.

Growth factors act primarily over short distances in either an autocrine or paracrine manner. In addition, growth factors may act through an endocrine pathway affecting target cells at distant sites. Many growth factors possess a mitogenic activity which is mediated through a membrane-bound receptor. Interaction occurs with an extracellular ligand-binding domain, leading to a change in receptor conformation and resulting in the activation of an intracellular tyrosine kinase domain. Tyrosine phosphorylation of specific intracellular proteins is responsible for the mitogenic signal. In many cases, the protein components of the intracellular cascade remain to be elucidated. Aberrant signalling may result from mutation in growth factors or their downstream effector proteins, leading to either loss of growth factor function, that is, switching off the signalling pathway, or to uncontrolled expression or activation, that is, a permanently switched-on signalling pathway. Such changes are commonly associated with the malignant state and the aggressive phenotypes of cancer cells.

Transforming growth factor-beta 1 (TGF-β1)

TGF-β1 belongs to a superfamily of structurally related regulatory polypeptides that includes activins/inhibins and bone morphogenetic proteins (BMPs). TGF-β1 is a multifunctional cytokine that acts through type I and II receptor kinases to regulate positively or negatively the proliferation of various cell types. Generally, TGF-β1 functions as a mitogen for various mesenchymal cells and a potent growth inhibitor of lymphoid, endothelial and epithelial cells. TGF-β1 and -2 have been implicated in the development of prostatic disease. TGF-β1 has been detected immunohistochemically in both human prostatic stromal and epithelial cells, and TGF-β2 mRNA has been identified in normal and malignant human prostate. Addition of TGF-β1 to cultured prostatic epithelial and stromal cells inhibits proliferation.[87]

Bone morphogenetic proteins (BMPs)

The term 'bone morphogenetic protein' (BMP) refers to an activity derived from bone that induces ectopic bone formation in vivo.[88] The proteins belong to the TGF-β superfamily and, to date, 13 BMPs have been identified. Since their discovery in 1965, researchers have focused on identification of these proteins and, more recently, on understanding the role of BMPs in normal human embryonic development. To date, very few efforts have been made to link BMP activity with the development and progression of cancer. This is not surprising because the majority of bony secondaries result in osteolytic lesions, with increased bone resorption and osteoclastic activity, unlike prostatic secondaries, which are mostly osteoblastic. A number of studies have shown an association between BMP expression and skeletal metastases in prostate cancer. BMP-6, in particular, is expressed in the majority of primary prostate cancers with established skeletal secondaries, and rarely in localized disease. Primary and secondary prostate cancer expresses BMP-6, which is found infrequently in skeletal metastases from other human malignancies. BMP-6 may have a role in the initiation of skeletal secondaries, and the osteoblastic reaction commonly seen in these deposits.[89]

Fibroblast growth factors (FGFs)

The FGF family of polypeptide growth factors has diverse physiological and pathological functions, including development, wound healing, angiogenesis and tumourigenesis.[90] In man, the FGFs comprise at least 10 genes, and the receptor family comprises four members. Multiple ligands and receptors allow interaction between a single receptor and several ligands, and between different receptor monomers through heterodimerization after activation by FGF.[91]

Basic FGF (FGF-2) is secreted by prostatic fibroblasts in response to androgen and acts in an autocrine fashion to stimulate fibroblast cell growth.[92] Stromal-derived keratinocyte growth factor (KGF/FGF-7) is upregulated in hormone-resistant prostate cancer and has a role as a potential paracrine growth factor on epithelial cells.[93] KGF has a potent mitogenic action on epithelial cells and has been proposed to act as an androgen-regulated mediator of epithelial cell growth. A similar paracrine action applies to FGF-8 (androgen-induced growth factor), which is secreted in response to androgens and can stimulate growth of epithelial and fibroblast cells.[94]

Insulin-like growth factors (IGFs)

IGF-1 and -2 are important mitogens that mediate normal and neoplastic cell growth. The IGFs bind to specific receptors, designated types I and II IGF receptors (IGFR). Type I IGFR is a transmembrane heterotetramer tyrosine kinase, which primarily mediates the mitogenic actions of IGFs. IGFs are two of the most abundant growth factors in bone,[95] the preferential site for metastatic prostate cancer. Type I IGFR is expressed by prostate cancer cells, and this could facilitate the development of bone metastases.

IGFs also have high affinity for a family of at least 6 IGF-binding proteins (IGFBPs), which act to regulate their bioavailability.[96] The level of circulating IGFBPs is regulated by endocrine factors and by specific proteases that cleave IGFBPs to small inactive peptides. IGFBPs are believed to modulate the proliferative and mitogenic effects of IGFs, as well as modulating cell growth independently of IGF. Although all IGFBPs have a high affinity for IGFs, IGFBP-3 is the major transporter of IGFs in serum. A number of studies have suggested that IGFBPs may be involved in the growth modulation of prostate malignancy. One study showed elevated IGFBP-2 and decreased IGFBP-3 in patients with prostate cancer.[97]

Epidermal growth factor (EGF)

Binding of EGF to the extracellular domain of its receptor, EGFR, results in activation of the receptor's cytoplasmic tyrosine kinase, phosphorylation of substrate proteins and stimulation of cell proliferation. Members of the EGF family play a role in modulation of prostatic growth. Withdrawal of androgen from the rodent prostate leads to reduced expression of EGF, which is a potent mitogen for epithelial cells.[98]

Thus, the continued presence of androgens within the prostate helps maintain epithelial cell proliferation mediated through the expression of EGF.

CELL ADHESION

Cell adhesion is of fundamental importance in establishing and maintaining tissue form and function. Several molecules, including cadherins, integrins, selectins and members of the immunoglobulin superfamily, are involved in the mechanisms by which a cell maintains contact with other cells and interacts with the extracellular matrix. Fibronectin, collagen, laminin and vitronectin, major components of this complex extracellular matrix, interact with their cognate receptors, most of which are integrins. Integrins function as heterodimeric membrane glycoproteins, the combination of α and β subunits determining the ligand specificity. Differential expression of members of the large integrin family allows the cell to modulate its interaction with other cells and the extracellular matrix. Integrins are important components of cellular signal transduction, mediating cell–matrix interactions, while cadherins principally mediate intercellular interactions.

Cadherins are a large family of calcium-dependent morphoregulatory proteins. The best-studied proteins in this family are E- and N-cadherin. Membrane-associated cadherins require members of the catenin family of proteins to mediate their interaction with the cytoskeleton. Catenins probably act by oligomerizing proteins to which they bind or attach them to the actin cytoskeleton.

E-cadherin

The E-cadherin gene plays a critical role in embryogenesis and organogenesis through mediating epithelial cell–cell recognition and adhesion processes.[99] E-cadherin protein is frequently found reduced or absent in cancer cell lines. Experiments performed with the Dunning rat model for prostate cancer showed a correlation between a lack of E-cadherin and tumour invasion, demonstrated by the progession of a non-invasive, E-cadherin-positive tumour to an invasive, E-cadherin-negative tumour. Immunocytochemistry performed on human prostate cancer samples showed a general reduction of E-cadherin expression in high-grade tumours associated with aberrant staining. This aberrant E-cadherin staining is proving to be a powerful predictor of poor outcome, in terms of both disease progression and patient survival.[100]

CD44

The CD44 gene is an integral transmembrane glycoprotein involved in specific cell–cell and cell–extracellular matrix interactions.[101] The gene is encoded by 20 exons, at least 10 of which are differentially expressed due to alternative splicing of mRNA. CD44 is expressed on the plasma membrane of prostatic glandular cells. It is involved in cell adhesion since it acts as a receptor for the extracellular matrix components hyaluronic acid and osteopontin. CD44 is believed to play a major role in tumour metastases, and alternative splice variants of the receptor differ in their capacity to enhance or decrease metastatic potential. In human prostate cancer, CD44 down-regulation is correlated with high tumour grade, aneuploidy and distant metastases.[102]

PROLIFERATION

The hallmark of malignancy is uncontrolled growth. It is therefore logical to assume that measuring proliferative activity within a tumour may indicate its invasive potential, and capacity to progress. Several methods are available to assess proliferation, including determination of S-phase fraction by flow cytometry, labelling of replicating DNA with bromodeoxyuridine (BrdU), and immunohistochemistry with antibodies against proliferation-related antigens (Ki67 and MIB-1).[103,104] Their use in clinical practice, however, remains to be determined.

TUMOUR PLOIDY AND NUCLEAR MORPHOMETRY

Nuclear DNA content, otherwise known as ploidy, can be studied by flow cytometry and image or static cytometry. Tumours can be broadly classified as diploid, tetraploid or aneuploid, with accompanying variations in view of the well-documented heterogeneity of prostatic adenocarcinoma. Several reports emerged in the last three decades, correlating DNA ploidy with prognosis in prostate cancer. The results are conflicting, and only half the studies published confirm ploidy to be an independent prognostic marker.[105] A more modern and sensitive method of assessing ploidy has been developed recently, using fluorescent (FISH) and non-fluorescent DNA in situ hybridization of interphase cells. These techniques visualize individual chromosomes by specific binding of a labelled probe to a particular DNA sequence, mostly localized at the centromere region. There is good correlation with flow cytometry, but FISH appears to be more sensitive.[106] If these methods are to have an impact on clinical practice, large studies analysing ploidy determination in biopsy specimens must be conducted.

ANDROGEN REGULATION

Androgens are important male sex hormones which, in addition to being essential for the growth and differentiation of all male sex accessory organs, are strongly associated with the development and progression of prostate cancer. Androgen action in prostate cancer is mediated throught the androgen receptor (AR), a ligand-dependent transcription factor which is a member of the steroid/thyroid hormone receptor gene superfamily. The mitogenic effects of androgens on prostatic growth appear to be mediated through the action of soluble peptide growth factors, acting in either an autocrine or paracrine manner. Various model systems for prostate cancer have shown FGF-7 and TGF-β1 to be paracrine mediators of androgen action and FGF-2 to be an androgen-mediated autocrine growth factor.

Androgen depletion prolongs the disease-free interval for prostate cancer patients, indicating that the cancer cells are androgen sensitive. However, this treatment is only palliative since androgen-independent clones of cancer cells expand and progress. This observation has been made in almost every case of prostate cancer. These androgen-independent cells acquire the ability to proliferate in the absence of androgen through genetic mutations. Mutations may result in changes in the function or expression of AR protein or growth factors and their receptors.

Androgen receptor (AR)

The AR can be structurally divided into three domains, a transcriptional activation domain, a DNA-binding domain and a ligand-binding domain (Figure 24.3).[107] Cellular signalling occurs following androgen binding to the AR and translocation to the nucleus. This activated complex associates with androgen-responsive elements contained in the DNA sequence of a number of target genes to affect their transcriptional activity. The possible presence in vivo of alternate AR isoforms, the extent of AR phosphorylation, the association with other proteins and the presence of polymorphic glutamine and glycine regions may provide additional levels of control for AR action.

Radioligand binding studies and immunohistochemistry have been used to detect AR protein expression. Both primary and metastatic prostate cancer have shown elevated AR by ligand-binding assays when compared to non-malignant prostate tissue.[108] Immunohistochemistry supports elevated AR in prostate cancer with strong nuclear staining, mostly of a heterogeneous nature, in hormone-relapsed and

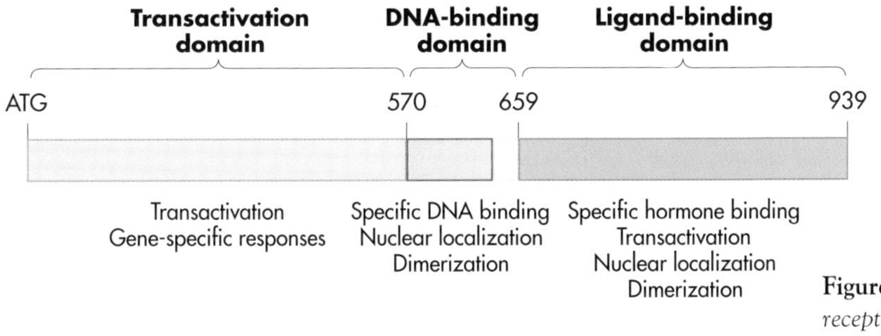

Figure 24.3 *Functional organisation of the androgen receptor.*

in primary and metastatic hormone-refractory prostate cancer.[109]

A number of recent studies have suggested that a high frequency of amino-acid substitutions occur in the AR protein (25–50%) in untreated advanced prostate cancer and in hormone-relapsed tumours from primary and metastatic sites. Functional analysis of these mutations has revealed alterations in ligand binding and transcriptional activation. Additionally, AR gene amplification has been identified in 30% of recurrent prostate tumours.[110] Examination of the corresponding primary tumour prior to initiation of hormone therapy showed no evidence of amplification, suggesting that amplification occurred during androgen deprivation and conferred a growth advantage on the prostate cancer cells. Variation in the length of a polyglutamine stretch in the N-terminal domain of the AR protein, causing an alteration in AR function, has been suggested as a contributory factor to an increased lifetime risk of the development of prostate cancer.

GENETIC FACTORS

Genetic alterations are important contributory events in neoplasia. A variety of genes have been identified that are associated with predisposition or progression for most of the common epithelial neoplasms, with the exception of prostate cancer. Most known oncogenes and suppressor genes have been screened for their importance in primary prostate cancer, but no common mutations have been identified. p53 mutations are rare in early prostate cancer but have been observed in almost 50% of advanced, metastatic disease.[82] Mutations in the retinoblastoma (Rb) gene and deletion or methylation of $p16^{INK4a}$ (CDKN2), two genes intimately linked to cell-cycle progression, have been described in a few prostate tumours and cell lines.

Allelic loss, defined by the absence of one of the two copies of an autosomal locus present in somatic cells, commonly occurs in prostate cancer. Loss of heterozygosity (LOH) and comparative genomic hybridization analyses have revealed frequent loss of genetic material from chromosome regions 7q, 8p, 10pq, 13q, 16q, 17p and 18q in primary and metastatic prostate cancer. More recently, specific gene loci have been identified as metastatic suppressors in prostate cancer. Introduction of the genes for KAI1 (chromosome 11p11.2), E-cadherin (chromosome 16q22) or CD44 (chromosome 11p13) into prostate cancer cells have been shown to suppress metastatic ability.

A number of studies revealed a familial clustering for prostate cancer. A risk factor of between 2 and 3 has been indicated for a relative of a prostate cancer patient acquiring the disease. This risk factor depends on the relationship within the family; a first-degree relative (such as brother or father) presents the highest risk. Moreover, the risk factor increases if two or more family members have the disease.

Hereditary prostate cancer, which can be separated from familial prostate cancer, has been reported to account for some 9% of all prostate cancer and more than 40% of early-onset disease.[111] Further work provides strong evidence for a major susceptibility locus for prostate cancer on chromosome 1 (1q24–25).[112,113,114]

MATRIX METALLOPROTEINASES (MMPS) AND THEIR INHIBITORS

Tumour invasion and metastasis represent key events in the natural history of cancer. To complete the different steps involved in the metastatic cascade of events, a malignant cell has to overcome a number of natural barriers, including extracellular matrix and basement membranes. This can be partly achieved through excess production of proteolytic enzymes either by the tumour cells themselves, or through stimulation of surrounding stromal cells to secrete such enzymes.[115] The matrix metalloproteinases (MMPs) are extracellular zinc enzymes that mediate a number of tissue-remodelling processes, and have been heavily incriminated in cancer progression. A number of malignancies, including prostate cancer, have been shown to express differentially MMPs that correlated strongly with aggressive disease.[116–118] More recently, a new membrane-type MMP (MT-MMP) has been found to be specifically expressed in fibroblastic cells of human carcinomas and in prostate cancer.[119] MMPs are tightly regulated by their inhibitors called TIMPs (tissue inhibitors of metalloproteinases). Synthetic TIMPs have been developed recently, and may represent a novel therapeutic approach in prostate cancer.

IN VITRO AND IN VIVO MODELS OF PROSTATE CANCER

In order to investigate the biology of prostate cancer, a number of models have been developed over the years. The three most widely used cell lines are LNCaP, an AR-positive epithelial prostate cancer cell line originating from a metastatic lymph node; DU-145, an AR-negative epithelial prostate cancer line originating from metastatic bone secondaries; and PC-3, an AR-negative epithelial prostate cancer line originating from metastatic brain secondaries.[120–122] Animals used for in vivo experiments include spontaneous models (canine and Lobund-Wistar rat); inducible cancer models (Noble and Lobund-Wistar rat); transplantable cancer models (Dunning R-3327 rat, Pollard rat, Shain rat and Noble rat); and xenograft nude and transgenic mice models.[123–127] These models are extremely useful in studying a variety of factors thought to affect the development and progression of prostate cancer, but suffer from limitations in terms of reproducibility in humans.

REFERENCES

1. Shibita A, Whittemore AS. Prostate cancer incidence and mortality in the United States and the United Kingdom. J Natl Cancer Inst 2001; 93: 1109–1110
2. Lu-Yao GL, Greenberg ER. Changes in prostate cancer incidence and treatment in USA. Lancet 1994; 343: 251–254
3. Quinn M, Babb P. Patterns and trends in prostate cancer incidence, survival, and mortality. Part II: individual countries. BJU Int European Urology Update Series 2002; 90: 174–184
4. Pienta KJ. The epidemiology of prostate cancer: clues for chemoprevention. In Vivo 1994; 8: 419–422
5. Muir CS, Nectoux J, Statzsewski J. The epidemiology of prostatic cancer. Acta Oncol 1991; 30: 133–140
6. Whitmore WF. Localised prostate cancer: management and detection issues. Lancet 1994; 343: 1263–1267
7. Pienta KJ, Esper PS. Risk factors for prostate cancer. Ann Intern Med 1993; 118: 793–803
8. Smith JR, Freije D, Carpten JD, Gronberg H et al. Major susceptibility locus for prostate cancer on chromosome 1 suggested by a genome-wide search. Science 1996; 274: 1371–1374
9. Bova GS, Beaty TH, Steinberg GD, Childs B et al. Hereditary prostate cancer: epidemiologic and clinical features. J Urol 1993; 150: 797–802
10. Bostwick DG. Neoplasms of the prostate. In: Bostwick DG, Eble JN, eds. Urologic Surgical Pathology. St Louis, MO: Mosby, 1997: 343–421
11. McNeal JE, Redwine EA, Frieha FS, Stamey TA. Zonal distribution of prostatic adenocarcinoma: correlation with histologic pattern and direction of spread. Am J Surg Pathol 1988; 12: 897–906
12. Bostwick DG, Cooner WH, Denis L, Jones GW et al. The association of benign prostatic hyperplasia and cancer of the prostate. Cancer 1992; 70: 291–301
13. Gleason DF. Histologic grading of prostate cancer: a perspective. Hum Pathol 1992; 23: 273–279
14. Humphrey PA, Frazier HA, Vollmer RT, Paulson DF. Stratification of pathologic features in radical prostatectomy specimens that are predictive of elevated initial postoperative serum prostate-specific antigen levels. Cancer 1993; 71: 1821–1827
15. Bostwick DG. Gleason grading of prostatic needle biopsies; correlation with grade in 316 matched prostatectomies. Am J Surg Pathol 1994; 18: 796–803
16. Schröder FH, Hermanek P, Denis L, Fair MK et al. The TNM classification of prostate cancer. Prostate 1992; 4 (Suppl): 129–138
17. Bostwick DG. Prospective origins of prostate carcinoma. Prostatic intraepithelial neoplasia and atypical adenomatous hyperplasia. Cancer 1996; 78: 330–336
18. Helpap B, Bonkhoff H, Cockett A, Montironi R et al. Relationship between atypical adenomatous hyperplasia (AAH), prostatic intraepithelial neoplasia (PIN) and prostatic adenocarcinoma. Pathologica 1997; 89: 288–300
19. Sakr WA. Haas GP, Cassin BF, Pontes JE et al. The frequency of carcinoma and intraepithelial neoplasia of the prostate in young male patients. J Urol 1993; 150: 379–385
20. Häggman MJ, Macoska JA, Wojna KJ, Oesterling JE. The relationship between prostatic intraepithelial neoplasia and prostate cancer: critical issues. J Urol 1997; 158: 12–22
21. Epstein JI, Armas OA. Atypical basal cell hyperplasia of the prostate. Am J Surg Pathol 1992; 16: 1205–1214
22. Oesterling JE. Prostate specific antigen: a critical assessment of the most useful tumour marker for adenocarcinoma of the prostate. J Urol 1991; 145: 907–923
23. Chybowski FM, Larson Keller JJ, Beerstralh EH, Oesterling JE. Predicting radionuclide bone scan findings in patients with newly diagnosed, untreated prostate cancer: prostate specific antigen is superior to all other clinical parameters. J Urol 1991; 145: 313–318

24. Catalona WJ, Ritchie JP, Ahmann FB, Hudson MA et al. Comparison of digital rectal examination and serum prostate specific antigen in the early detection of prostate cancer: results of a multicentre clinical trial of 6,630 men. J Urol 1994; 151: 1283–1290
25. Christensson A, Bjork T, Nilsson O, Dahlen U et al. Serum prostate specific antigen complexed to alpha-1-antichymotrypsin as an indicator of prostate cancer. J Urol 1993; 150: 100–105
26. Leung H, Lai L, Day J, Thomson J et al. Serum free PSA in the diagnosis of prostate cancer. Br J Urol 1997; 80: 256–259
27. Catalona WJ, Smith DS, Ornstein DK. Prostate cancer detection in men with serum PSA concentrations of 2.6 to 4.0 ng/ml and benign prostate examination: enhancement of specificity with free PSA measurements. JAMA 1997; 227: 1452–1455
28. Woodrum DL, Brawer MK, Partin AW, Catalona WJ et al. Interpretation of free prostate specific antigen clinical research studies for the detection of prostate cancer. J Urol 1998; 159: 5–12
29. Fidler IJ. Metastasis: quantitative analysis of distribution and fate of tumour emboli labelled with ^{125}I-5-iodo-2′-deoxyuridine. J Natl Cancer Inst 1970; 45: 773–782
30. Fidler IJ, Hart IR. Biological diversity in metastatic neoplasms: origins and implications. Science 1982; 217: 998–1003
31. Hamdy FC, Lawry J, Anderson JB, Parsons MA et al. Circulating prostate-specific antigen-positive cells correlate with metastatic prostate cancer. Br J Urol 1992; 69: 392–396
32. Fadlon EJ, Rees RC, Lawry J, McIntyre C et al. Detection of circulating PSA-positive cells in patients with prostate cancer by flow cytometry and reverse transcription polymerase chain reaction. Br J Cancer 1996; 74: 400–405
33. Katz AE, Olsson CA, Raffo AJ, Cama C et al. Molecular staging of prostate cancer with the use of an enhanced reverse transcriptase-PCR assay. Urology 1994; 43: 765–774
34. Israeli RS, Miller WH, Su SL, Powell T et al. Sensitive nested reverse transcription polymerase chain reaction detection of circulating prostatic tumor cells: comparison of prostate-specific membrane antigen and prostate-specific antigen-based assays. Cancer Res 1994; 54: 6306–6310
35. Smith MR, Biggar S, Hussain M. Prostate specific antigen messenger RNA is expressed in non-prostate cells: implications for the detection of micrometastases. Cancer Res 1995; 55: 2640–2644
36. Gomella LG, Ganesh VR, Moreno JG. Reverse transcriptase polymerase chain reaction for prostate specific antigen in the management of prostate cancer. J Urol 1997; 158: 326–337
37. Schröder FH. Detection of prostate cancer. BMJ 1995; 310: 140–141
38. Hamdy FC, Neal DE. Screening for prostate cancer: methods are changing rapidly. BMJ 1995; 310: 1139–1140
39. Holmberg L, Bill-Axelson A, Helgesen F, Salo JO et al. A randomized trial comparing radical prostatectomy with watchful waiting in early prostate cancer. New Engl J Med 2002; 347: 781–789
40. Adib RS, Anderson JB, Ashken MH, Baumber CD et al. Immediate versus deferred treatment for advanced prostatic cancer: initial results of the Medical Research Council trial. Br J Urol 1997; 79: 235–246
41. Abbas F, Scardino PT. Why neoadjuvant androgen deprivation prior to radical prostatectomy is unnecessary. Urol Clin North Am 1996; 23: 587–604
42. Witjes WP, Schulman CC, Debruyne FM. Preliminary results of a prospective randomized study comparing radical prostatectomy versus radical prostatectomy associated with neoadjuvant hormonal combination therapy in T2-T3 N0 M0 prostatic carcinoma. European Study Group on Neoadjuvant Treatment of Prostate Cancer. Urology 1997; 49 (Suppl. 3A): 65–69
43. Huggins C, Hodges CV. Studies on prostate cancer. The effect of castration, of oestrogen and of androgen injection on serum phosphatase in metastatic carcinoma of the prostate. Cancer Res 1941; 1: 293–297
44. Maximum androgen blockade in advanced prostate cancer: an overview of 22 randomised trials with 3283 deaths in 5710 patients. Prostate Cancer Trialists' Collaborative Group. Lancet 1995; 346: 265–269
45. Caubet JF, Tosteson TD, Dong EW, Naylon EM et al. Maximum androgen blockade in advanced prostate cancer: a meta-analysis of published randomized controlled trials using nonsteroidal antiandrogens. Urology 1997; 49: 71–78
46. Onik GM, Cohen JK, Reyes GD, Rubinsky B et al. Transrectal ultrasound-guided percutaneous radical cryosurgical ablation of the prostate. Cancer 1993; 72: 1291–1299
47. Wieder J, Schmidt JD, Casola E, van Sonnenberg E et al. Transrectal ultrasound-guided transperineal cryoablation in the treatment of prostatic carcinoma: preliminary results. J Urol 1995; 154: 435–441

48. Gelet A, Chapelon JY, Bouvier R, Souchon R et al. Treatment of prostate cancer with transrectal focused ultrasound: early clinical experience. Eur Urol 1996; 29: 174–183
49. Madersbacher S, Pedevilla M, Vingers L, Susani M et al. Effect of high-intensity focused ultrasound on human prostate cancer in vivo. Cancer Res 1995; 55: 3346–3351
50. Culver KW. Gene Therapy. A Handbook for Physicians. New York: Liebert, MA, 1994
51. Connors TA. The choice of prodrugs for gene directed enzyme prodrug therapy of cancer. Gene Ther 1995; 2: 702–709
52. Chen ME, Sikes RA, Troncoso P, Lin S-H et al. PAGE and GAGE-7 are novel genes expressed in the LNCaP prostatic carcinogenesis model that share homology with melanoma associated antigens. J Urol 1996; 155: 642A
53. Kyprianou N, English HF, Isaacs JT. Programmed cell death during regression of PC-82 human prostate cancer following androgen ablation. Cancer Res 1990; 50: 3748–3753
54. Colombel M, Symmans F, Gil S, O'Toole KM et al. Detection of the apoptosis-suppressing oncoprotein bcl-2 in hormone-refractory human prostate cancers. Am J Pathol 1993; 143: 390–400
55. Kerr JFR, Winterford CM, Harmon BV. Apoptosis. Its significance in cancer and cancer therapy. Cancer 1994; 27: 2013–2026
56. Alnemri ES, Livingston DJ, Nicholson DW, Salvesen G et al. Human ICE/CED-3 protease nomenclature. Cell 1996; 87: 171
57. Enari M, Sakahira H, Yokoyama H, Okawa K et al. A caspase-activated DNase that degrades DNA during apoptosis, and its inhibitor ICAD. Nature 1998; 391: 43–50
58. Boldin MP, Goncharov TM, Goltsev YV, Wallach D. Involvement of MACH, a novel MORT1/FADD-interacting protease, in Fas/APO-1- and TNF receptor-induced cell death. Cell 1996; 85: 803–815
59. Reed JC. Cytochrome c: can't live with it—can't live without it. Cell 1997; 91: 559–562
60. Wyllie A. An endonuclease at last. Nature 1998; 391: 20–21
61. Li P, Nijhawan D, Budihardjo I, Srinivasulasm et al. Cytochrome c and dATP-dependent formation of Apaf-1/caspase-9 complex initiates an apoptotic protease cascade. Cell 1997; 91: 479–489
62. Hockenbery D, Nunez G, Milliman C, Schreiber RD et al. Bcl-2 is an inner mitochondrial membrane protein that blocks programmed cell death. Nature 1990; 348: 334–336
63. Lu QL, Abel P, Foster CS, Lalani EN. Bcl-2: role in epithelial differentiation and oncogenesis. Hum Pathol 1996; 27: 102–110
64. Lane DP. p53, guardian of the genome. Nature 1992; 358: 15–16
65. Kroemer G. The proto-oncogene Bcl-2 and its role in regulating apoptosis. Nat Med 1997; 3: 614–620
66. Bauer JJ, Sesterhenn IA, Mostofi FK, Mcleod DG et al. Elevated levels of apoptosis regulator proteins p53 and bcl-2 are independent prognostic biomarkers in surgically treated clinically localised prostate cancer. J Urol 1996; 156: 1511–1516
67. McDonnell TJ, Troncoso P, Brisbay SM, Logothetis C et al. Expression of the proto-oncogene bcl-2 in the prostate and its association with emergence of androgen-independent prostate cancer. Cancer Res 1992; 52: 6940–6944
68. Apakama I, Robinson MC, Walter NM, Charlton RG et al. bcl-2 overexpression combined with p53 protein accumulation correlates with hormone-refractory prostate cancer. Br J Cancer 1996; 74: 1258–1262
69. Krajewski M, Krajewski S, Epstein JI, Shabaik A et al. Immunohistochemical analysis of bcl-2, bax, bcl-X and mcl-1 expression in prostate cancers. Am J Pathol 1996; 148: 1567–1576
70. Stattin P, Damber J-E, Karlberg L, Nordgren H et al. Bcl-2 immunoreactivity in prostate tumourigenesis in relation to prostatic intraepithelial neoplasia, grade, hormonal status, metastatic growth and survival. Urol Res 1996; 24: 257–264
71. Johnson MI, Robinson MC, Marsh C, Robson CN et al. Expression of Bcl-2, Bax and p53 in high-grade prostatic intraepithelial neoplasia and localized prostate cancer: relationship with apoptosis and proliferation. Prostate 1998; 37: 223–229
72. Vogelstein B, Kinzler KW. p53 function and dysfunction. Cell 1992; 70: 523–526
73. Levine AJ, Momand J, Finlay CA. The p53 tumour suppressor gene. Nature 1991; 351: 453–456
74. Mellon K, Thompson S, Charlton RG, Marsh C et al. p53, c-erbB-2 and the epidermal growth factor receptor in the benign and malignant prostate. J Urol 1992; 147: 496–499
75. Thomas DJ, Robinson M, King P, Hasan T et al. p53 expression and clinical outcome in prostate cancer. Br J Urol 1993; 72: 778–781
76. Visakorpi T, Kallioniemi OP, Heikkinen A, Koivula T et al. Small subgroup of aggressive, highly

proliferative prostatic carcinomas defined by p53 accumulation. J Natl Cancer Inst 1992; 84: 883–887
77. Myers RB, Oelschlager D, Srivastava S, Grizzle WE. Accumulation of the p53 protein occurs more frequently in metastatic than in localized prostatic adenocarcinomas. Prostate 1994; 25: 243–248
78. Kallakury BV, Figge J, Ross JS, Fisher HA et al. Association of p53 immunoreactivity with high Gleason tumor grade in prostatic adenocarcinoma. Hum Pathol 1994; 25: 92–97
79. Heidenberg HB, Sesterhenn JP, Gaddipati JP, Weghorst CM et al. Alteration of the tumour suppressor gene p53 in a high fraction of hormone refractory prostate cancer. J Urol 1995; 154: 414–421
80. Navone NM, Troncoso P, Pisters LL, Goodrow TL et al. p53 protein accumulation and gene mutation in the progression of human prostate carcinoma. J Natl Cancer Inst 1993; 85: 1657–1669
81. Humphrey PA, Swanson PE. Immunoreactive p53 protein in high-grade prostatic intraepithelial neoplasia. Pathol Res Pract 1995; 191: 881–887
82. Miyashita T, Reed JC. Tumor suppressor p53 is a direct transcriptional activator of the human bax gene. Cell 1995; 80: 293–299
83. Moul JW, Bettencourt M-C, Sesterhenn IA, Mostofi FK et al. Protein expression of p53, bcl-2 and KI-67 (MIB-1) as prognostic biomarkers in patients with surgically treated, clinically localized prostate cancer. Surgery 1996; 120: 159–166
84. Weidner N, Carroll PR, Flax J, Blumenfield W et al. Tumour angiogenesis correlates with metastasis in invasive prostate carcinoma. Am J Pathol 1993; 143: 401–409
85. Silberman MA, Partin AW, Veltri RW, Epstein JI. Tumour angiogenesis correlates with progression after radical prostatectomy but not with pathologic stage in Gleason sum 5 to 7 adenocarcinoma of the prostate. Cancer 1997; 79: 772–779
86. Ferrer FA, Miller LJ, Andrawis RI, Kurtzman SH et al. Vascular endothelial growth factor (VEGF) expression in human prostate cancer: in situ and in vitro expression of VEGF by human prostate cancer cells. J Urol 1997; 157: 2329–2333
87. Byrne RL, Leung H, Neal DE. Peptide growth factors in the prostate as mediators of stromal epithelial interaction. Br J Urol 1996; 77: 627–633
88. Urist MR. Bone formation by autoinduction. Science 1965; 150: 893–899
89. Hamdy FC, Autzen P, Wilson Horne CH, Robinson MC et al. Immunolocalization and mRNA expression of bone morphogenetic protein-6 in human benign and malignant prostate tissue. Cancer Res 1997; 57: 4427–4431
90. Basilico C, Moscatelli D. The FGF family of growth factors and oncogenes. Adv Cancer Res 1992; 59: 115–165
91. Leung HY, Hughes CM, Kloppel G, Williamson RCN et al. Expression and functional activity of fibroblast growth factors and their receptors in human pancreatic cancer. Int J Oncol 1994; 4: 1219–1223
92. Story MT. Regulation of prostate growth by fibroblast growth factors. World J Urol 1995; 13: 297–305
93. Leung HY, Mehta P, Gray LB, Collins AT et al. Keratinocyte growth factor expression in hormone insensitive prostate cancer. Oncogene 1997; 15: 1115–1120
94. Tanaka A, Miyamoto K, Matsuo H, Matsumoto K et al. Human androgen-induced growth factor in prostate and breast cancer cells: its molecular cloning and growth properties. FEBS Lett 1995; 363: 226–230
95. Yoneda T, Sasaki A, Mundy GR. Osteolytic bone metastasis in breast cancer. Breast Cancer Res Treat 1994; 32: 73–84
96. Jones JI, Clemmons DR. Insulin-like growth factors and their binding proteins: biological actions. Endocr Rev 1995; 16: 3–34
97. Kanety H, Madjar Y, Dagan Y, Levi J et al. Serum insulin-like growth factor-binding protein-2 (IGFBP-2) is increased and IGFBP-3 is decreased in patients with prostate cancer: correlation with serum prostate-specific antigen. J Clin Endocr Metab 1993; 77: 229–233
98. Denmeade SR, Lin XS, Isaacs JT. Role of programmed (apoptotic) cell death during the progression and therapy for prostate cancer. Prostate 1996; 28: 251–265
99. Takeichi M. Cadherin cell adhesion receptors as a morphogenetic regulator. Science 1991; 251: 1451–1455
100. Umbas R, Isaacs WB, Bringuier PB, Schaafsma HE et al. Decreased E-cadherin expression is associated with poor prognosis in patients with prostate cancer. Cancer Res 1994; 54: 3929–3933
101. Gunthert U, Stauder R, Mayer B, Terpe H et al. Are CD44 variant isoforms involved in human tumour progression? Cancer Surv 1995; 24: 19–42

102. Kallakury BVS, Yang F, Figge J, Smith K et al. Decreased levels of CD44 protein and mRNA in prostate carcinoma. Correlation with tumor grade and ploidy. Cancer 1996; 78: 1461–1469
103. Cattoretti G, Becker MHG, Key G, Duchrow M et al. Monoclonal antibodies against recombinant parts of Ki-67 antigen detect proliferating cells in microwave-processed formalin-fixed paraffin sections. J Pathol 1992; 168: 357–363
104. Noordzij MA, van der Kwast TH, van Steenbrugge GJ, van Weerden WM et al. Determination of Li-67 in formalin-fixed, paraffin-embedded prostatic cancer tissues. Prostate 1995; 27: 154–159
105. Adolfsson J. Prognostic value of deoxyribonucleic acid content in prostate cancer: a review of current results. Int J Cancer 1994; 58: 211–216
106. Persons DL, Takai K, Gibney DJ, Katzmann JA et al. Comparison of fluorescence in situ hybridisation with flow cytometry and static image analysis in ploidy analysis of paraffin-embedded prostate adenocarcinoma. Hum Pathol 1994; 25: 678–683
107. O'Malley B. The steroid receptor superfamily: more excitement predicted for the future. Mol Endocr 1990; 4: 363–369
108. Brolin J, Skoog L, Elman P. Immunohistochemistry and biochemistry in detection of androgen, progesterone, and estrogen receptors in benign and malignant human prostatic tissue. Prostate 1992; 20: 281–295
109. Masai M, Sumiya H, Akimoto S, Yatani R et al. Immunohistochemical study of androgen receptor in benign hyperplastic and cancerous human prostates. Prostate 1990; 17: 293–300
110. Visakorpi T, Hyytinen E, Koivisto P, Tanner M et al. In vivo amplification of the androgen receptor gene and progression of human prostate cancer. Nat Genet 1995; 9: 401–406
111. Carter BS, Beaty TH, Steinberg GD, Childs B et al. Mendelian inheritance of familial prostate cancer. Proc Natl Acad Sci USA 1992; 89: 3367–3371
112. Smith JR, Freije D, Carpten JD, Gronberg H et al. Major susceptibility locus for prostate cancer on chromosome 1 suggested by a genome-wide search. Science 1996; 274(5291): 1371–1374
113. Gronberg H, Isaacs SD, Smith JR, Carpten JD et al. Characteristics of prostate cancer in families potentially linked to the hereditary prostate cancer 1 (HPC1) locus. JAMA 1997; 278(15): 1251–1255
114. Berry R, Schaid DJ, Smith JR, French AJ et al. Linkage analyses at the chromosome 1 loci 1q24-25 (HPC1), 1q42,2-43 (PCAP), and 1p36 (CAPB) in families with hereditary prostate cancer. Am J Hum Genet 2000; 66(2): 539–546
115. Liotta LA. (1986) Tumor invasion and metastases. Role of the extracellular matrix: Rhoads Memorial Award Lecture. Cancer Res 1986; 46: 1–7
116. Hamdy FC, Fadlon EJ, Cottam DW, Lawry J et al. Matrix metalloproteinase-9 expression in human prostatic adenocarcinoma and benign prostatic hyperplasia. Br J Cancer 1994; 69: 177–182
117. Wood M, Fudge K, Mohler JL, Frost AR et al. In situ hybridization studies of metalloproteinases 2 and 9, and TIMP-1 and TIMP-2 expression in human prostate cancer. Clin Exp Metastasis 1997; 15: 246–258
118. Still K, Robson C, Neal DE, Hamdy FC. The ratio of tissue matrix metalloproteinase-2 (MMP-2) to tissue inhibitor of matrix metalloproteinase (TIMP-2) is increased in high grade prostate cancer. J Urol 1997; 157: 25A
119. Bates TS, Armstrong J, Perry A, Gingell C. Increased expression of membrane-type matrix metalloproteinase in malignant prostate compared with paired benign tissue and specimens of benign prostatic hyperplasia. J Urol 1996; 155: 515A
120. Kaighn ME. Establishment and characterization of a human prostatic carcinoma cell line (PC-3). Investig Urol 1979; 17: 16–23
121. Stone KR, Mickey DD, Wunderli H, Mickey GH, Paulson DF. Isolation of a human prostate carcinoma cell line (DU–145). Int J Cancer 1978; 21: 274–281
122. Horoszewicz JS, Leong SS, Kawinski E, Karr JP et al. LNCaP model of tumor prostatic carcinoma. Cancer Res 1983; 43: 1809–1818
123. Buttyan R, Slawin K. Rodent models for targeted oncogenesis of the prostate gland. Cancer Metastasis Rev 1993; 12: 11–19
124. Pugh TD, Chang C, Uemura H, Weindruch R. Prostatic localization of spontaneous early invasive carcinoma in Lobund-Wistar rats. Cancer Res 1994; 54: 5766–5770
125. Royai R, Lange PH, Vessella R. Preclinical models of prostate cancer. Semin Oncol 1996; 23: 35–40
126. Klein KA, Reiter RE, Redula J, Moradi H et al. Progression of metastatic human prostate cancer to androgen independence in immunodeficient SCID mice. Nat Med 1997; 3: 402–408
127. Gingrich JR, Barrios RJ, Morton RA, Boyce BF et al. Metastatic prostate cancer in a transgenic mouse. Cancer Res 1996; 56(18) 4096–4102

25

Testis cancer

Alex Freeman and Stephen J Harland

During the twentieth century, the incidence of testis cancer rose at a dramatic rate in most Western countries. The reason for this is unknown. Denmark, which saw the highest national prevalence, has seen a steady increase from 3 to 9/100 000 person years between 1945 and 1990.[1] In six countries around the Baltic Sea, the annual increase between the early post-war period and 1990 varied from 2.3% in Sweden to 5.2% in the former East Germany.[2] Notable, then, are populations where the incidence of testis cancer has not increased. These include North American Blacks where the incidence is low (1 per 100 000) and Switzerland where it is high (6 per 100 000).[3]

These rapid changes in the incidence of testis cancer are a persuasive argument for environmental factors being a major cause in its development. In fact, analysis of the data from the Baltic countries shows that birth cohort is a stronger determinant of testis cancer prevalence than time period.[3] It was of particular interest when it was shown that the upward trend in incidence by year of birth was interrupted in the years before and during the war years in Denmark (1935–45),[1] a finding that was subsequently found to be true of Norway (1935–45) and Sweden (1930–40),[3] but not of the former East Germany, Finland or Poland[3] (Figure 25.1). The implication was that if it was the wartime conditions which affected the testis cancer incidence in the early 1940s cohorts, these conditions must have been operating in the early years of life, if not in utero.

The age distribution for testis cancer is unique (Figure 25.2). The sharp rise in incidence after the onset of puberty indicates the importance of factors which become operative in tumour development at this time. For the steep fall in the incidence curve after the mid-thirties, two explanations are offered. The first is that all those pre-cancers that have been initiated prior to adolescence progress during adolescent and adult life until there are none left (Figure 25.3a). Alternatively, testicular tumours may be initiated by an adolescence-specific factor (such as rapid testicular growth) and present after a limited interval afterwards (Figure 25.3b). Both epidemiological and histopathological studies might shed light on this issue (see below).

EPIDEMIOLOGY

Testicular maldescent

The association of testicular maldescent with testis cancer is well established. Although only 1–2% of cryptorchid boys develop testis cancer, the relative risk for the condition is increased, a figure of 4.7 being typical.[4] The question of whether early correction of maldescent can prevent tumour development is one which may have a bearing on the age of tumour initiation. Comparison of the age of correction for a population of cryptorchid subjects who had developed testis cancer with a population who had not, led to the conclusion that early correction was ineffective in this regard.[5] Two large recent case-control studies – one in Denmark,[6] the other in the UK[7] – have provided persuasive evidence that the reverse is the case (Table 25.1). The data shown suggest that there

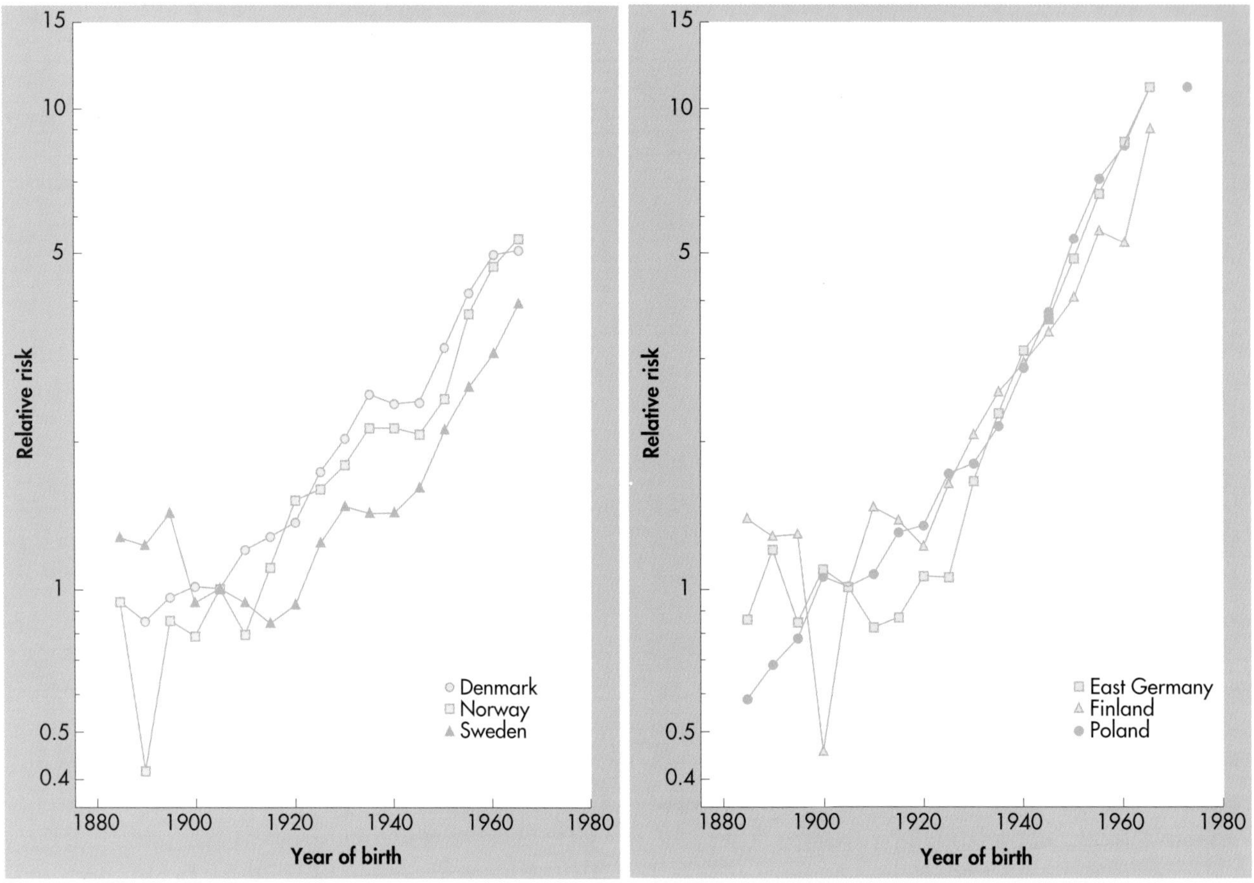

Figure 25.1 *Relative risk of developing testicular cancer by country and birth cohort using men from between 1900 and 1909 as the reference. (Reproduced from* Journal of the National Cancer Institute *with permission.*[2]*)*

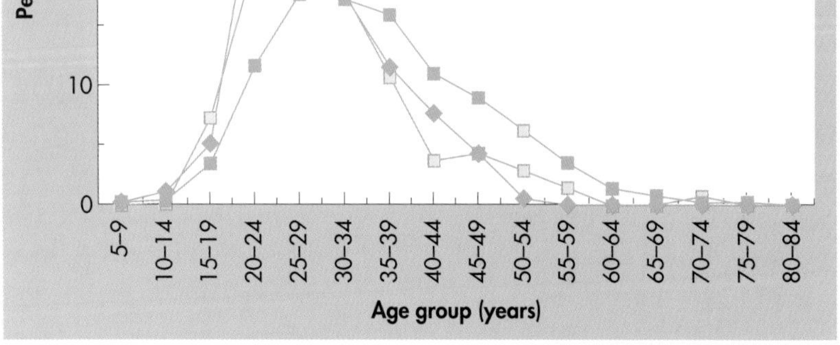

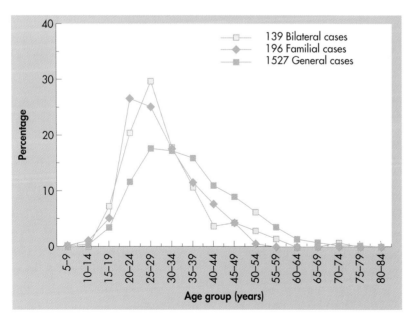

Figure 25.2 *Distribution of age of presentation of 1527 general cases of testicular germ cell cancer (Pugh),*[110] *together with 139 bilateral cases (first tumour) and 196 familial cases. (Reproduced from* British Journal of Cancer *with permission.*[33]*)*

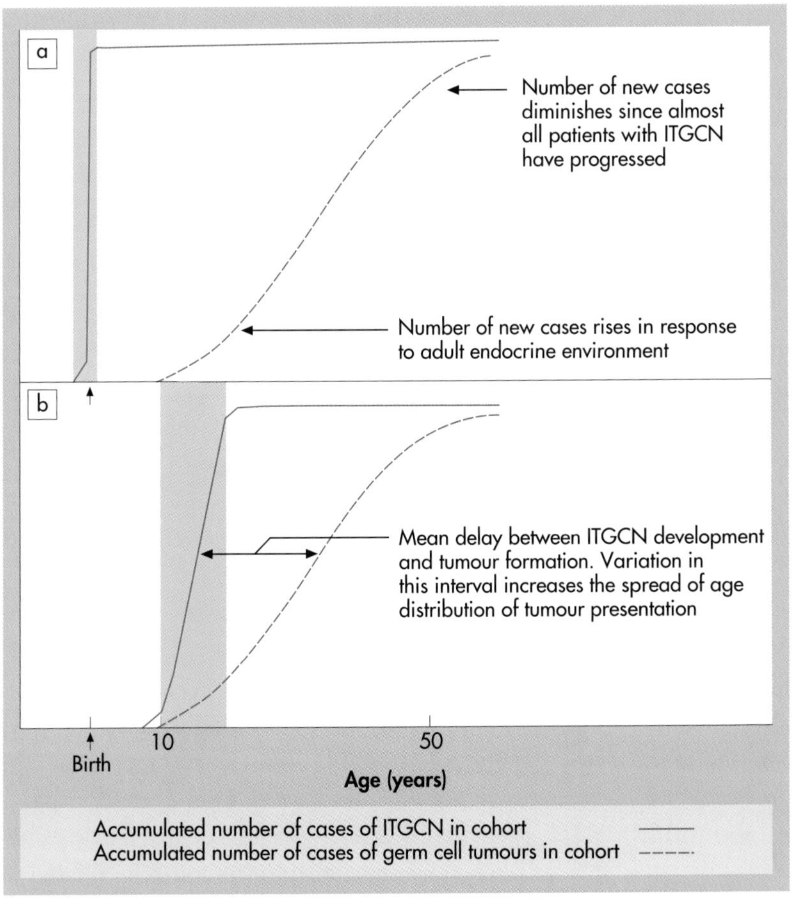

Figure 25.3 *Two hypotheses to account for the age distribution of testis cancer. (a) ITGCN develops in utero (shaded); (b) ITGCN develops in adolescence.*

Table 25.1 Two large case-control studies comparing the age of correction of cryptorchidism with testis cancer incidence.

	Denmark[6]			UK[7]		
	Cases	Controls	OR[a]	Cases	Controls	OR[a]
n	514	720		794	794	
Treated or persisting cryptorchidism	6.6%	1.8%	3.6 (1.8–6.9)	8.2%	2.1%	3.8 (2.2–6.5)
Bilateral	2.1%	0.4%	4.9 (1.3–18.1)			
Unilateral	4.1%	1.4%	2.9 (1.3–6.3)			
Age at treatment (years)						
0–9	0.4%	0.3%	1.1 (0.2–8.2)	0.8%	1.3%	0.6 (0.2–1.7)
10–14	3.1%	1.0%	2.9 (1.2–7.1)	2.9%	0.4%	7.7 (2.3–26)
15+	1.4%	1.4%	3.5 (0.9–14)	0.6%	0%	inf[b] (1.2–inf[b])
Persisting	1.8%	0.1%	14.4 (1.8–115)	1.5%	0.5%	3 (0.97–9.3)

[a] Odds ratio (95% confidence interval).
[b] Infinity.

are biological events which occur in an undescended testis between the ages of 10 and 14 years which can cause subsequent tumour development.

Social class

The association of testis cancer with high social class is well established.[8] In more recent times, the relationship has diminished in the West, an effect which has been well studied in Finland. Whereas in the early 1970s there was a fivefold risk for social class 1 over social classes 4 and 5, this ratio has now dropped to 2.[9] An association between cryptorchidism and social class has been found in Denmark, but it is in the other direction: there is a threefold risk in the lower social classes.[6] The risk of testis cancer is only moderately associated with higher social class in Denmark and only with that of the mother. A dietary basis for the secular trend in the social-class relationship is possible. In Finland, studies on food consumption have shown that the dietary pattern of lower social classes follows that of upper social classes with a lag time of about 10 years.[10]

Social class effects are of interest in the developing world where dietary variation may be very great. In Bombay, testis cancer incidence, which has been rising for the last 30 years, was associated with higher educational level.[11] In Japan, where the highest increase in testis cancer incidence has been found, there is a correlation with intake of cheese (r = 0.8), followed by animal fats and milk.[12] Diet, however, may only be acting as a marker of Westernized lifestyle.

Other factors

Factors favouring the importance of environmental factors during adolescence

The recent British and Danish studies both found significant associations between young age of onset of puberty and testis cancer. The difference in testis cancer incidence between the oldest and youngest age group for onset of puberty was 1.5–2.0-fold depending on the pubertal indicator used. Other studies[6,13] have also suggested a protective effect of late puberty. The onset of puberty in men is gradual and memory of the age at which it occurs is often poor. Furthermore, early onset of puberty brings forward the years at risk of testicular cancer, so confounding results can be obtained if a disproportionate number of younger age tumours are collected. Nevertheless, the fall in age of onset of puberty that has been seen over the last century has been dramatic. Accurate figures for boys are not available, but the fall in girls has been from a mean age of 16.5 in 1885 to 13.4 years in 1965.[14] The time frame seems to correspond to the observed increase in testicular cancer incidence and makes age of onset of puberty a good candidate for further study.

Intensive physical exercise (over 15 hours per week at the age of 20) has been shown to be associated with protection from testicular cancer (35% less compared with a no-exercise group). Similarly, the number of hours seated during the day was strongly associated with increased risk of testis cancer.[7] This effect was seen even after correction for social class. It is therefore possible that a reduction in the amount of activity associated with certain occupations over the course of the last century (for example, as a result of mechanization) could be related to the change in testis cancer incidence that has been seen during this time.

The same study also found that increased sexual activity, using 20 years as the reference age, was slightly but significantly associated with an increased risk of testis cancer.

Testis biopsy carried out during orchidopexy in boys with undescended testis at Great Ormond Street was associated with an increased risk of testis cancer. Compared with a man in the general population, the relative risk was 67 when a biopsy was performed and 6.7 when it was not.[15] However, a Danish study where all boys underwent a simultaneous biopsy at the time of surgery for cryptorchidism found relative risk to be only in the range 2–4.[16] It seems likely therefore that biopsy does not cause neoplasia, but that surgeons can identify those testes at high risk, and these they choose to biopsy.

Factors favouring the importance of the intrauterine environment

Being a later sibling – that is, being the fourth or fifth child in a family – is associated with a lower risk of testis cancer.[7] It has been suggested that this reflects differences in maternal physiology between early and late pregnancies.

The use of exogenous oestrogens during early pregnancy was fairly common in the USA in the 1940s and 1950s. Three studies have related its usage to testis cancer incidence (Table 25.2). All three studies show a trend in favour of oestrogen exposure in the cases, though only one shows a significant difference. In some cases, the exposure amounted to a single injection given as a pregnancy test. The history of exposure depended on the mother's memory of it. The possibility has been raised that this may have been subject to recall bias, given the publicity associated with the link between oestrogens and cancer.[17]

It has been noted that gonatrophin and oestrogen levels are higher in women who have had a dizygotic (DZ) twin pregnancy than in controls,[18] so if maternal oestrogen levels are an important determinant of testicular cancer, a difference in incidence should be detected. In fact, two studies on the Swedish Twin Registry have found a rate of 1.4 × that of the general population for all twins[19] and 2.3 × for DZ twins.[20] In the UK, DZ twins were found to have 1.5 × the incidence of monozygotic (MZ).[21]

Oestrogen exposure in pregnancy has been thought to be the link between testicular maldescent, testis cancer, low birth weight and an absence of acne in later years.[22] The recent European case-control studies have made no contribution to this question since so few mothers were exposed. However, no relationship between acne and testis cancer was found.[23]

The discovery that certain water pollutants can act as weak oestrogens has led to the hypothesis that these may be the cause both of the increase in testis cancer incidence and the apparent decline in sperm density in semen in male populations.[24] The relationship between intrauterine exposure to exogenous oestrogens is unproven however and exposure to environmental oestrogens has yet to be related to either low sperm density in man or testicular cancer.

HEREDITARY FACTORS

Studies on migrating populations have suggested the importance of genetic factors in determining susceptibility to testis cancer. Thus, both in Africa and the USA, black populations have a low prevalence. Again in the USA, those of northern European descent ("Protestants") have a higher prevalence than those of southern European descent ("Catholics"), reflecting the situation on the eastern side of the Atlantic. It is of interest that the UK Testicular Cancer Study Group found that the two strongest associations with testis cancer were having a brother (relative risk 8) and having a father (relative risk 4) with the condition. Similar levels of risk have been found by other groups (Table 25.3). A positive family history is not common in testis cancer, however, first-degree relatives being affected in only 1.0–2.8% of cases.[25] Furthermore, it is rare, unlike other types of familial cancer, for there to be more than two cases in a family.[26,27]

The paradox of a strong genetic influence on the development of testicular cancer, but infrequent positive family histories, may have been explained by studies on bilateral testicular cancer. Prolonged follow-up of testis cancer patients[28–30] has found that 5% of patients develop a tumour of the contralateral testis – a figure identical to the prevalence of contralateral intratubular germ-cell neoplasia (ITGCN) at the time of first presentation with testicular cancer.[31,32] This is a much higher incidence

Table 25.2 Exposure of mothers of testis cancer patients and of controls to oestrogens during pregnancy.

Author	Cases	Controls	Relative risk
Henderson et al, 1979[165]	6/78	1/78	5 (*P* 0.11)
Shottenfeld et al, 1980[166]	11/190	3/141[a]	2.6 (*P* > 0.10)
Depue et al, 1983[11]	9/97	2/105	8 (*P* 0.02)

[a]Only 48% of cases had neighbourhood controls.

Table 25.3 Relative risk to first-degree relatives of testis cancer patients.

Country	All 1st degree	Brothers	Fathers	Sons	Reference
USA	6				168
W. Germany	3.1 (.77–18)				169
UK		8	4		26
Norway, S. Sweden		10.2 (6.2–16)	4.3 (1.6–9.3)	5.7 (0.7–23)	27
Denmark		12.3 (3.3–32)	2.0 (1.0–3.4)		170
Netherlands		9–13	2		171
Sweden		8.3	3.8		172

than would be expected from chance alone. Analogy with bilateral tumours of other paired organs, such as retinoblastoma and Wilms' tumour, suggests that they are all of hereditary origin – that is, that a susceptibility is carried in the germ line of these patients, as is the case in patients with familial disease. Familial retinoblastoma is carried as a dominant gene with high penetrance: 50% of the offspring of an affected parent would carry the predisposition, which would give rise to tumour development in nearly all and bilateral disease in the majority. Familial testis cancer stands in marked contrast to this. Not only is it rare for the offspring of familial cases to be affected, but also bilateral disease in familial cases is uncommon, probably in the region of 14%.[27,33]

If one makes the assumption that all bilateral cases (5% of all cases) are of hereditary origin and that these represent only 14% of the hereditary cases, the conclusion is reached that 33% of all cases are of hereditary origin.[33] The similarity in age distribution between hereditary cases and bilateral cases (Figure 25.1) is evidence that the underlying assumption is correct. From the prevalence of testis cancer and the known risk to fathers and brothers of patients, the best fit genetic model is one in which the inherited susceptibility is carried as a recessive gene, and an individual who is homozygous for this susceptibility has a 45% chance of developing a tumour.[33] This model is conjectural but a subsequent segregation analysis on a large population of Norwegian and Swedish patients arrived at one very similar (Table 25.4).[34]

The classical way of determining the importance of hereditary factors is with twin studies where one would expect the risk to the co-twin of a proband should be higher in MZ than in DZ twins. The relative risks (95% confidence interval) to the co-twin of a testis cancer patient has been found to be 77 (11–518) for MZ twins and 36 (5–245) for same-sex DZ twins.[21] As can be seen by the overlap in confidence intervals, insufficient cases were found to give the required answer. It was estimated, however, that the risk to an identical twin of a testis cancer patient is 14% by the age of 40.[21]

The contribution heredity to the increase in testis cancer incidence is almost nil – there is no suggestion that the genetic make-up of the populations in question has altered appreciably over the last 100 years. It would seem likely, however, that the penetrance of the genotype has increased during this time.

IDENTIFYING A TESTIS CANCER GENE

The search for a predisposing gene in a heritable condition has used two methods. The first depends on the identification of a chromosomal abnormality present in one or more individuals who develop the condition. This abnormality – for example, a break point or a site of chromosomal translocation – may point to the site of DNA mutations in the germ line of predisposed individuals. This approach led to the discovery of the Rb gene in familial retinoblastoma. No suitable chromosomal abnormality has been associated with individuals with testis cancer.

Table 25.4 Hereditary testicular cancer – two analyses compared.

Authors	Nicholson and Harland, 1995[33]	Heimdal et al, 1997[34]
Source of information	British Testicular Tumour Panel Danish and German testis biopsy series[31,32] Published case reports	978 testis cancer patients treated in Oslo and Lund
Major gene effect	Assumed	Favoured by analysis
Proportion of general cases attributable to genotype	33%	19% (proband generation); higher in parental generation
Type of inheritance	Recessive	Recessive
Risk to homozygotes	45%	43%
Gene frequency	5%	3.8%

The second method, linkage analysis, depends on the overrepresentation within families of chromosomal regions in those who have developed the heritable condition. In the case of affected siblings, there is a 50% chance that a chromosome region will be shared whether it is responsible for the condition or not. Only when there is a significant excess of affected relatives sharing a chromosomal region can one say that there is a probability that a particular region is likely to bear the offending gene. This probability is measured by a 'LOD score' (*l*ogarithm of the *od*ds ratio). LOD scores above 1.0 are regarded as interesting. Scores above 2.0 are considered suggestive; scores above 3.0, conclusive. The statistical calculations are sophisticated and take into account the large number of chromosomal regions examined and the possibility that some of the affected relatives will be chance associations – not dependent on a shared gene. Moreover, when more than one family is considered, there may be more than one gene involved.

The above method was used successfully in the identification of the familial breast cancer genes BRCA1 and BRCA2. Familial breast cancer is particularly amenable to linkage analysis because large pedigrees are found containing many affected individuals. The process was made more difficult, however, by the fact that breast cancer is a common disease, so relatives may not have had the heritable form, and to a lesser extent by the appearance of disease in the later decades of the current generation. These two last problems do not apply to the search for testis cancer genes, but a much greater problem is the small size of affected kindreds. The International Testis Cancer Linkage Consortium, having collected 193 kindreds, found only 17 which contained more than two cases (Table 25.5).[35] With this number of pedigrees, however, there would be sufficient power (over 90% chance) to identify a locus with a LOD score of over 3.0 if there was a single dominant gene accounting for all familial testis cancer. If two dominant genes were contributing equally, the power to identify these genes would fall to 45%.[35]

In fact, when all families are analysed together, there is no site on the genome which gives a LOD score of >1.94 if dominant inheritance is assumed, or 2.29 if recessive inheritance is assumed. This is

Table 25.5 International Testis Cancer Linkage Consortium.[35]

	Affected kindreds
Sib pairs	105
Sib trios	5
Father–son	26
Cousins	
– maternal	4
– paternal	7
– other	10
Uncle–nephew	
– maternal	7
– paternal	9
Other pairs	3
Large pedigrees	17
Total	193

good evidence against a single gene's accounting for the great majority of pedigrees.[35]

When linkage on the X chromosome was considered, families where the inheritance was obligatorily through the father (such as paternal uncle–nephew pairs) were excluded. A LOD score of 2.01 was then obtained for the region Xq27 with an estimate (alpha) that 32% of affected kindreds could be linked by a gene at this site. When the families were subdivided into those where one individual had bilateral testis cancer or where there was a history of undescended testis, LOD scores of 4.76 and 2.5, respectively, were obtained (Table 25.6).[35] This is very good evidence for a familial testis cancer gene at Xq27, although limited by the small number of patients in the subgroups. There is another reason for questioning this result. Xq27 is a gene-poor area. The two genes known to be present at that site have been examined for mutations, but none has been found.

It has to be stressed that if a cancer-predisposing gene, TGCT1, is found at Xq27, it could account only for the minority of testis cancer families. While an X-linked gene may account for the paucity of father–son pairs in the consortium kindreds, there is no excess of maternal over paternal cousins or uncle–nephew pairs.

Cytogenetic analysis has not been helpful in testicular cancer as a result of the high frequency of chromosomal abnormalities. The commonest finding is the presence of the isochromosome i(12p), present in 80% of cases. In fact, fluorescent labelling of the short arm of chromosome 12 shows that, even in those tumours which do not have the isochromosome, material from 12p is overrepresented.[36] Despite the universal abnormalities in the short arm of chromosome 12 in testicular cancer, no consistent break point has been identified which might lead to the discovery of a cancer-inducing or -suppressing gene. Among the genes mapped to 12p is that which encodes cyclin D2, a positive regulator of cell-cycle progression. This gene was found to be deregulated in a panel of germ-cell tumour (GCT) cell lines.[37]

INTRATUBULAR GERM-CELL NEOPLASIA (ITGCN)

ITGCN – also known as carcinoma in situ – is very commonly found in testes containing a GCT. Cytological abnormalities involving spermatogonia in tubules adjacent to such tumours were recognized by Wilms in 1896.[38] But the suggestion that these atypical cells were a form of preinvasive malignancy was made by Skakkebaek in 1972[39] when he noted that two infertile men who developed GCT had had atypical germ cells in their preceding biopsies. This relationship was supported by extensive retrospective reviews of archival testicular biopsies from the infertile population associated with patient follow-up.[40–42] Subsequently, the prevalence of ITGCN in normal men and various abnormal conditions was established (Table 25.7) and has remained similar in a recent review.[43]

Morphology and distribution

The diagnosis of ITGCN is best made on biopsies fixed in Stieve's, Cleland's or Bouin's fluid and stained with haematoxyin and eosin. Interpretation of biopsies fixed in formal saline is hampered by diminution of nuclear detail.

Microscopically, ITGCN is composed of atypical germ cells situated at the periphery of seminiferous

Table 25.6 Evidence for a testis cancer gene on the X chromosome:[35] maximum HLOD* Scores at Xq27.

Family characteristics	*n*	Max HLOD	Proportion of families linked (alpha)
All families	99	2.01	0.32
Bilateral testis cancer	15	4.76	1.00
Undescended testis	19	2.50	0.74

* HLOD – LOD score under heterogeneity

Table 25.7 The prevalence of ITGCN in various groups.

General Danish population	< 0.8%
Cryptorchidism	2.3%
Infertility	0.4–1.1%
Contralateral testis in men with unilateral germ cell tumours (GCT)	5.6%
Androgen insensitivity	33% (4/12)
Gonadal dysgenesis	high (4/4)
Extragonadal GCT	
Retroperitoneal	42%
Mediastinal	low (0/8)
Central nervous system	? low (0/2)

Taken from Giwercman et al, 1993[73] and Daugaard et al, 1992[167].

tubules. It is rarely demonstrated immunocytochemically in tubules showing spermatogenesis, presumably reflecting 'pagetoid spread' – that is, along the basement membrane (also seen in the rete). The abnormal germ cells comprising ITGCN have ballooned clear cytoplasm (containing fat and glycogen) and a large hyperchromatic nucleus which may show mitotic figures (infrequently seen in benign tubules). These morphological appearances are identical in ITGCN adjacent to seminomas and non-seminomatous GCT.

ITGCN is closely associated with atrophy (narrow tubules lacking spermatogenesis). Thus, in the context of biopsies during investigation of infertility, ITGCN is associated with a Johnsen score of <4.[41] In orchidectomy performed for palpable tumour, ITGCN is also seen within atrophic tubules, but it may be focal, and in adjacent lobules, tubules of normal diameter showing spermatogenesis may be seen.[44,45] This contrasts with the long-standing assumption that ITGCN is diffuse, based on the pick-up rate achieved in simulated biopsies on four orchidectomies following a biopsy diagnosis of ITGCN.[46] However, it must be noted that even in these four cases, the distribution of ITGCN in the testis whole mounts varied widely.

Biomarkers of ITGCN

Biomarkers are relevant in a variety of contexts:

- diagnostic
- pathogenetic – emphasizing the similarity to fetal germ cells
- biological
- heterogeneity related to different categories of GCT
- changes associated with invasion.

Placental alkaline phosphatase (PLAP) and CD 117 (c-kit) are used in diagnostic histopathology.[42,47] Positive staining is seen in a paranuclear and cytoplasmic membrane distribution, providing useful confirmation in most circumstances.

TRA-1-60 and M2A are two markers of pathogenetic interest, as they may also be found in normal fetal germ cells.[48] This may imply that ITGCN arises from fetal germ cells or that such fetal antigens are re-expressed in ITGCN arising post-natally. Ultrastructural studies also support similarity between ITGCN and germ cells in the early stage of differentiation. A major difference between these two cell types is the limited development of ultrastructural cell contacts in ITGCN.[49]

ITGCN is aneuploid,[50] with an average nuclear DNA content of about 4C.[51] The DNA content of ITGCN is similar to that of classical seminoma, which is significantly higher than that seen in non-seminomatous GCT.[52] The high proliferative activity of ITGCN is reflected in AgNOR counts per nucleus[53] and MIB-1 positivity.[54] In the majority of cases, p53 glycoprotein has been identified immunocytochemically,[55–57] but its significance is uncertain. The data on p53 gene mutations are conflicting. Mutations were found in ITGCN adjacent to 12 of 18 GCT; in one instance, an identical p53 mutation was identified in both ITGCN and the neighbouring tumour.[58] However, mutations were not found in 22 invasive GCTs.[59]

Evidence for the heterogeneity of ITGCN is suggested by immunocytochemical studies demonstrating differences in the extent of PLAP and TRA-1-60 expression adjacent to seminoma and non-seminomatous GCT.[60] Furthermore, a higher copy number of chromosome 15 is found adjacent to seminoma than non-seminomatous GCT.[61]

Progression from ITGCN to invasive GCT is associated with loss of p21 (a cell-cycle-dependent kinase inhibitor) and gain of mdm-2 (ubiquitin ligase mouse double-minute-2). These results are evidence for disruption of the p53 regulatory pathway in the progression to invasive tumour.[57] Isochromosome 12p, formerly thought to be present in ITGCN, has more recently been shown to be a late event and present only in invasive GCT.[37,62] Similarly, progression of ITGCN to invasive seminoma is also marked by the loss of $\alpha3$ integrin subunit expression.[63]

Association with microlithiasis (microcalcification)

The term 'microlithiasis' is used in both the histopathological and imaging literature. Microscopically, microliths are seen within seminiferous tubules, some of which are the site of ITGCN. In a study of 36 specimens showing ITGCN, microlithiasis was identified in 39% compared to an incidence of 2% in 429 non-malignant testicular disorders.[64] Two further series describe the presence of a GCT in association with micolithiasis in 17 out of 42 and 6 out of 16 cases.[65,66]

A recent sonographic series of 528 symptomatic patients found that 48 (9%) had microlithiasis; of these, 13 (27%) had testicular cancer. Of the remaining 480 patients without microlithiasis, 38 (8%) had cancer.[67] Thus, of those with cancer, about 25% have microlithiasis, and of those with microlithiasis, a similar proportion (about 25%) will have cancer.

However, the situation in healthy men is different. A prospective study of testicular sonography on 1504 healthy men aged 18–35 years revealed microlithiasis in 84 (5.6%). For black Americans, this prevalence was 14%, and this higher proportion in a low-risk population would seem to deny a close association between microlithiasis and cancer.[68]

The value of ultrasonography in a screening context is unproven, although a case may be considered for its value in the investigation of the atrophic testis.[69] The question of whether the incidental finding of testicular microlithiasis on ultrasound justifies a biopsy is still unanswered. This issue is further confused by the fact that histopathological and sonographic microliths are not identical, and there is a 10-fold difference in size between these two lesions.[70]

Type of biopsy

The biopsy used in most studies has been the 'open biopsy', where a 3-mm stab incision is made through the tunica. Needle biopsy of the testis with a biopty-gun has been used in Norway.[71] The pick-up rates of ITGCN in a series of 92 open and 93 needle biopsies were 12% and 15%, respectively.[72] This seems surprising, as needle biopsies are sometimes distorted and contain fewer tubules. Follow-up of this series will give useful data on the false-negative rates of the two biopsy techniques. A needle biopsy has the advantage that it can be performed under local anaesthetic and would be expected to cause less trauma to the gonad. Efforts to diagnose ITGCN on cytological features of seminal fluid have had some success in a research setting but are not used routinely.[73]

Significance of the presence of ITGCN

Two series of infertile men with ITGCN have both demonstrated that 50% of these patients developed an invasive GCT within 5 years of the biopsy. Patients followed beyond 5 years continued to develop invasive tumours.[73,74] There are no data as yet to suggest that ITGCN may lie 'dormant' for decades, nor that it is a condition which only sometimes progresses to invasive tumour.

When patients with ITGCN of a testis contralateral to an established GCT have been managed by surveillance alone, the rate of tumour development has been identical to that seen in the infertile patients with ITGCN.[31]

Significance of the absence of ITGCN on biopsy

The interpretation[75] and observation[44] that ITGCN may be diffuse or focal relates to the findings in infertile men and those with an established GCT, respectively. The validity of applying either of these observations to the biopsy of the atrophic contralateral gonad in men with GCT could be questioned.

Of greater value, perhaps, in providing information on the sensitivity of testis biopsy in detecting ITGCN are the several series of patients with biopsies negative for this condition who have been followed up from 3 to 35 years. The number of cases of GCT developing were 2 out of 718,[51] 1 out of 1500,[73] 3 out of 863[74] and 5 out of 1859.[32,43]

A high-risk group for ITGCN of contralateral testis in testicular cancer

The overall prevalence of ITGCN of the contralateral testis in testicular cancer is 5%,[31,32] but within this population is a group of patients at particularly high risk. Two studies have now confirmed contralateral testicular atrophy and age at orchidectomy as independent risk factors for contralateral ITGCN.[32,41] Thus, of 53 testis cancer patients who had a small (less than 12 ml) contralateral testis and who were aged 30 or less, 18 (34%) had a contralateral testis biopsy positive for ITGCN. The combination of small contralateral testis and age over 30 was associated with a corresponding figure of only 4 out of 59 (7%). It is estimated that a policy of confining contralateral testicular biopsy to this very high-risk group, which comprises 6% of all testis cancer patients, would detect approximately 40% of all patients with contralateral ITGCN.[41]

Sensitivity of ITGCN to radiotherapy and chemotherapy

There is good evidence that radiotherapy can destroy ITGCN. Most telling is the experience of the Christie Hospital, Manchester, where the practice was to include the contralateral testis in the radiation field given as adjuvant therapy to stage 1 seminoma of testis. Of over 1000 patients treated, none developed a second tumour where 30–50 would have been expected.[76] Repeat testicular biopsies carried out 24 months after administering 20 Gy in 10 fractions for ITGCN showed only Sertoli cells present within tubules.[77] Testicular irradiation usually allows at least some preservation of Leydig cell function, and doses as low as 16–20 Gy have been shown to achieve histological remission from ITGCN over a 5-year follow-up period.[78] Loss of libido is uncommon and may be dose related. Basal testosterone levels usually remain within normal limits, though LH levels may be raised.[77,79] The testosterone response to human chorionic gonadotrophin (HCG) is usually impaired.[77]

A small fraction of ITGCN may be radioresistant, however, as exemplified by the occasional case of invasive GCT reported after treatment of ITGCN by radiotherapy.[80]

The efficacy of chemotherapy is much less certain. Both biopsies positive for ITGCN and tumours have been reported to follow platinum-based chemotherapy.[81–83] In one series of orchidectomies performed a median of 22 weeks after such chemotherapy for metastatic testicular cancer, 8 out of 23 (35%) were positive for CIS.[84] Furthermore, in a large population of testis cancer patients, the proportion developing second tumours did not appear to be diminished in those who had received chemotherapy.[30]

Age of onset of ITGCN

The age at which the morphological features constituting ITGCN can be commonly recognized is controversial. The question is of interest because of its pathogenetic significance. Furthermore, the value of performing a testicular biopsy to exclude ITGCN in younger age groups needs to be clarified.

In adults, clear information on the precursor relationship of ITGCN to invasive GCTs and the range of time intervals between these two lesions is available from testicular biopsies in the infertile population[38,74,85] and patients with a contralateral GCT.[31] The fact that ITGCN in adults displays markers and some ultrastructural features seen in fetal germ cells has been interpreted as evidence that ITGCN originates in the fetus. However, markers seen in the fetus may be displayed in adult tumours in the absence of intervening lesions (for example, carcinoembryonic antigen in colon cancer). Furthermore, in contrast to the high incidence of ITGCN adjacent to adult GCTs, it is the subject of only occasional case reports in childhood[86,87] and was not identified morphologically or immunocytochemically in the orchidectomy specimens from pubertal GCT patients.[88,89] Similarly, in a series of children and adolescents with intersex syndrome (known to be at high risk of developing invasive GCT), ITGCN was found in only 2 of 87 in the prepubertal age group but 4 of 23 pubertal patients.[90]

The sequential information available in adults relating ITGCN on biopsy to subsequent invasive GCT is rarely available in childhood.[91] In a review of biopsies from maldescent testes, ITGCN was identified only in the testis of a 16-year-old and not from biopsies taken from children aged 9, 10 and 14 years in whom GCT subsequently developed.[92]

DIAGNOSIS OF GCT

Role of intraoperative cryostat section diagnosis

Unilateral testicular mass

Intraoperative frozen section diagnosis has a limited contribution to make to the management of a testicular mass, as clinical diagnosis is usually sufficiently accurate to support orchidectomy. Testicular tumours frequently have a mixed morphology; therefore, restricted sampling reduces the certainty with which the tumour type can be stated, and opportunities for misinterpretation abound. For example, especially when normal anatomy is distorted, hyperkeratotic squamous epithelium may have originated from metaplasia in the epididymis or an encysted hydrocele, in addition to an area of differentiated teratoma. A chronic granulomatous inflammatory response may later prove to be within a seminoma. However, intraoperative confirmation of the neoplastic nature of a mass in a solitary testis may be valuable if the clinical findings are equivocal.

Bilateral testicular masses

There are rare instances of bilateral testicular swelling in which the diagnosis may be strongly suspected and intraoperative confirmation preclude bilateral orchidectomy. Lymphoma, bilateral in 13–50% of cases, may be suspected clinically because it usually occurs in men over 60 years of age, in contrast to the younger age group, in whom germ-cell tumours present.[93–95] Hamartomas are seen in up to 25% of post-pubertal juveniles and adults with androgen insensitivity. These may present a management problem in those patients raised as males, but, in phenotypic females, bilateral orchidectomy will be the treatment of choice after puberty.[96] The tumours associated with undiagnosed or inadequately treated adrenogenital syndrome may arise from Leydig cells, adrenal rests or pluripotential stromal cells stimulated by ACTH and suppressed by adequate steroid replacement.[97–99] Papillary cystadenomas occur within the epididymis and efferent ducts associated with von Hippel-Lindau syndrome. These tumours are benign, but their clear-celled nature may raise the possibility of metastatic renal parenchymal carcinoma, which also occurs in von Hippel-Lindau syndrome. Orchitis as a localized event or part of a systemic disorder occasionally causes diagnostic difficulty, as for example, in lepromatous leprosy.[100]

Immunocytochemistry as an adjunct to morphology in clinically relevant differential diagnosis

Immunocytochemistry is rarely necessary in the diagnosis of testicular GCT but is helpful in certain differential contexts. As a result of their rarity, Leydig and Sertoli cell tumours are occasionally misdiagnosed as seminoma[101] – the former when the cytoplasm is so vacuolated that it appears clear, and the latter when tubules resemble the tubular variant of seminoma.[102–104] Placental alkaline phosphatase and CD 117 (c-kit) in a diffuse membranous distribution with a paranuclear dot are components of the seminoma immunotype;[105,106] whereas inhibin and calretinin are demonstrated in both Leydig and Sertoli cell tumours. Tumour metastatic to the testis may resemble undifferentiated teratoma. With the exception of melanoma and sarcoma, metastases usually occur in older patients, and show an interstitial, infiltrative (in contrast to an ablative) growth pattern, frequently involving paratesticular structures and lacking ITGCN. In addition, undifferentiated teratomas are commonly CD 30 and PLAP positive.[105] In contrast EMA and CEA are commonly seen in metastatic carcinoma, and more specific markers, such as HMB 45 and PSA, are available for certain primary sites.

Lymphoma may occasionally be confused with classical seminoma with a marked lymphocytic infiltrate. Both of these neoplasms may occur in older men. Lymphoma leaves the tubular testicular architecture intact, whereas this is destroyed by seminoma. Tubular invasion by lymphoma may mimic ITGCN. Seminoma cells and ITGCN are easily identified by PLAP and CD 117 positivity. Lymphomas of the testis are most commonly of B-cell origin, although examples of T-cell lymphomas and plasmacytomas have also been reported in rare cases. As such, they are commonly positive for lymphoid markers such as CD 20, CD 79a (B cell), CD 3, CD 5 (T cell) or CD 138 (plasma cell).

Undifferentiated teratoma may resemble the so-called atypical or anaplastic seminoma enhanced by the lymphocytic and granulomatous infiltrate rarely seen in the former. CD 30, pancytokeratin and CK 19 are seen more frequently and with a diffuse distribution in undifferentiated teratoma compared with seminoma. Conversely, CD 117 and PLAP are more commonly seen with a diffuse distribution in seminoma. The phenotypes CD 117 positive/CD 30 negative and CD 117 negative/CD 30 positive are very suggestive of seminoma and undifferentiated teratoma, respectively.[106] Of recent interest are a small group of morphologically atypical seminomas which are CD 117 negative but CD 30 and CAM 5.2 positive.[107] A uniform approach to diagnosis and treatment of such cases has not been established.

Classical seminoma occurs over a wide age range and therefore may present in the older age group in whom spermatocytic seminoma is typically diagnosed. The latter are distinguished from classical seminomas by their lack of a fibrous stroma and associated lymphocytic and granulomatous infiltrate. The nuclei of spermatocytic seminoma vary in size and texture, whereas those in classical seminoma are uniform to the point of monotony. In classical seminoma, CD 117 and PLAP show a diffuse membranous reaction,[107,108] in which membrane and dot positivity for cytokeratins are seen far less frequently and in a focal distribution.[105,107] Recently, CD 143 (angiotension 1-converting enzyme) has been identified in classical seminoma,[109] but it is not yet in widespread diagnostic use. In spermatocytic seminoma, PLAP, CD 117, CD 143 and cytokeratins are reported as either negative or focally positive in a minority of cases.[108,109]

Classification of testicular tumours and histological predictors of metastatic spread

After orchidectomy for testicular tumour, the histopathological features of direct relevance to clinical management include the tumour cell type and its extent (stage), including vascular invasion. Up to the age of 60, GCT is the most frequent diagnosis, neoplasms arising from Sertoli or Leydig cells accounting for less than 5% of cases, and mesothelioma, rete carcinoma, metastases and intratesticular neoplasms of mesenchymal origin (such as leiomyoma) are rarities.

Nomenclature relating to GCT is governed by the two classifications.[110,111] These systems have far more similarities than differences. Equivalence in nomenclature is easily demonstrated (Table 25.8), and synonyms are given in the most recent WHO publication on histological typing of testis tumours.[112,113] Disagreements on the minutiae of histopathological detail have ceased to be clinically relevant. However, when interpreting publications, the most important difference to note is that the term 'teratoma' in the British classification is applied to all non-seminomatous tumours, but it is restricted in the WHO system to neoplasms composed entirely of differentiated somatic elements that may be mature or immature. Both classifications have persisted predominantly as a means of communication. In therapeutic trials, their use enables the tumour populations in different studies to be compared.

The management and prognosis for patients with GCT has been completely changed by improvements in clinical staging and cisplatin-based chemotherapy. Following the operation of a high-surveillance regimen for patients with stage I teratoma treated by orchidectomy, the subgroups of the British classification were associated with significantly different relapse-free rates on univariate analysis.[114] However, on multivariate analysis, the features predicting relapse which have stood the test of prospective studies with a reproducibility analysis are undifferentiated teratoma (embryonal carcinoma), vascular

Table 25.8 Classification of testicular germ cell tumours (GCT).

British Testicular Tumour Panel and Registry; Pugh et al, 1976[110]	World Health Organization (WHO) Mostofi and Sobin, 1977[111]
Seminoma Classical Spermatocytic	Seminoma Classical Anaplastic Spermatocytic
Teratoma differentiated (TD) Mature Immature	Teratoma Mature Immature With malignant transformation
Malignant teratoma intermediate (MTI)	Embryonal carcinoma and teratoma
Malignant teratoma undifferentiated (MTU)	Embryonal carcinoma
Malignant teratoma trophoblastic (MTT) Teratoma trophoblastic (pure form)	Choriocarcinoma ± teratoma, embryonical carcinoma Choriocarcinoma
Yolk-sac tumour/orchioblastoma (predominantly a tumour of childhood)	Yolk-sac tumour/embryonal carcinoma, infantile type

invasion by tumour and the absence of yolk-sac tumour.[115–117] These features have been further refined by quantification of the undifferentiated teratoma (embryonal carcinoma), but this is not standardized or universally applied.

In studies of prognostic factors in metastatic GCT, trophoblastic teratoma was a significant prognostic factor on multivariate analysis,[118] and the presence of undifferentiated and trophoblastic teratoma was associated with a significantly worse 3-year survival rate on univariate analysis.[119] However, the prognostic features seen consistently and incorporated into an international consensus classification reflect the volume and site of metastases. Thus, a large mediastinal mass; degree of elevation of alpha fetoprotein (AFP), HCG and lactate dehydrogenase (LDH); and the presence of non-pulmonary visceral metastases are all poor prognostic factors.[120]

Morphological prognostic features in seminoma are not uniformly accepted and their incorporation into clinical management varies. Some studies indicate the importance of vascular invasion as a predictor of relapse in stage I disease,[121,122] but this has not been a consistent finding.[123,124] The indication that primary tumour size might be of prognostic value[121] has been confirmed in patients with stage I disease treated by orchidectomy and high surveillance.[124,125]

ASSESSMENT OF EXCISED TUMOUR MASSES AFTER CHEMOTHERAPY

After chemotherapy for metastatic non-seminomatous GCT, if markers are within normal limits but residual masses remain, resection is performed as a diagnostic and therapeutic procedure. The following features are related to the post-operative disease course: number and site of metastases, the mediastinum being an adverse location;[126,127] completeness of resection as assessed intraoperatively;[128–130] the content of the mass; and the presence of viable malignant GCT (undifferentiated teratoma/embryonal carcinoma, yolk-sac tumour and trophoblastic tumour) predicting progressive disease.[129–131]

In nine series each reporting residual masses from over 50 patients, malignant GCT components were found in 6–28% (mean 17%), fibrosis and necrosis only in 22–65% (mean 45%) and differentiated teratoma (plus or minus necrosis/fibrosis) in 22–57% (mean 36%).[130] The 2-year progression-free survival rate for patients whose masses included malignant GCT elements was 12.5% compared with 88% in patients where these components were absent.[130] As decisions on further chemotherapy are based on the contents of the mass, non-operative predictors of morphology have been sought with a view to leaving necrotic masses in situ. It has been shown that shrinkage of the mass during chemotherapy to a size of ≤1.5 cm, high serum LDH and normal serum AFP and HCG levels before chemotherapy, and absence of differentiated teratoma from the primary are indicative of necrotic tissue only in the residual mass.[132,133]

Whether the morphological features of one resected mass can safely be assumed to reflect the findings at other sites remains controversial.[130,134–136]

Case reports draw attention to the development of non-GCT malignancies (such as sarcoma, adenocarcinoma and squamous carcinoma) in residual masses associated with a poor prognosis. Although these tumours were found in up to 6.6% of post-chemotherapy retroperitoneal lymph-node dissections in 557 patients with testicular teratomas at the Indiana University Medical Center,[137] they were not identified in sections from a series of 163 residual masses reviewed recently in the UK.[130] These differences may have occurred by chance or may reflect referral of malignancies to highly specialized centres.

TUMOUR MARKERS

Testicular tumours have been strongly associated with the release of proteins into the plasma. Some of these, notably alpha fetoprotein (AFP) and human chorionic gonadotrophin (HCG), are found in only very low concentrations in the plasma of healthy adult males, and their presence in the context of a testicular tumour is strong evidence of the persistence or recurrence of viable tumour; hence, they are considered to be tumour markers. Furthermore, although the capacity for a mass of given size to produce marker substances is very variable, fluctuations within an individual in marker levels usually reflect changes in the total body tumour mass. Marker substances can therefore be a sensitive measure of response to treatments.

The secretion of marker substances, particularly hormones, by tumours is often described as ectopic – that is, involving the expression of genes normally suppressed by the cell of origin. In the case of testicular tumours, the secretion of substances is frequently appropriate to the tissue present within the tumours. Thus, the presence of AFP in the plasma usually implies the presence of yolk-sac elements within the tumour. The secretion of HCG by a testicular tumour indicates the presence of syncytiotrophoblasts, most frequently as single cells, and is rarely associated with cytotrophoblast in trophoblastic teratoma (choriocarcinoma).

The sensitivity of tumour markers is proportional to the magnitude of the fluctuations that are seen. For a tumour composed of pure choriocarcinoma, it would not be unknown for a patient to present with an HCG level in excess of 10^6 iu/l. At this stage, the patient may have 10^{12} cells of tumour, implying that the HCG level will not return to normal until there are only 10^6 cells present. This would correspond to a viable tumour volume of 10 mm^3.[138]

Human chorionic gonadotrophin (HCG)

Intact HCG comprises an alpha (larger) and a beta subunit. The alpha subunit is identical to that of luteinizing hormone, follicular-stimulating hormone and thyroid-stimulating hormone. Though it has 80% homology with the alpha subunit, the beta subunit is specific to HCG, and it is this which provides the epitope for modern radioimmunoassays for HCG in serum. Free beta HCG is also secreted, but, as its clearance rate is high – 33 ml/min compared to 3.3 ml/min for intact HCG – it usually contributes little to the measured level.[139]

Elevations of serum HCG are seen in 55% of non-seminomatous germ-cell tumours (NSGCTs), depending on the stage[140] and in 19% of seminomas.[141] Trophoblastic tumour is likely to be present in the neoplasm only when higher serum levels are found. The secretion of HCG by a tumour of uncertain type is often considered to be evidence of a germ-cell origin. It must be realized, however, that this hormone is secreted by other tumour types, notably colon, bladder and pancreatic cancers. Occasionally, HCG is secreted in inflammatory bowel disease.

In patients with localized seminoma of testis, production of HCG is of no prognostic significance.[141] In patients with metastatic NSGCT, prognosis worsens with increasing levels of HCG. The prognostic significance of serum levels is shown in Table 25.9.

Table 25.9 Prechemotherapy serum levels of tumour markers in metastatic non-seminomatous germ cell tumour (NSGCT): frequency and relation to prognosis.

	% of patients with metastatic NSGCT	Progression-free at 5 years	Survival at 5 years
AFP: (mg/ml)			
<1000	84%	79%	83%
1000–10 000	12%	59%	68%
>10 000	4%	51%	57%
HCG (iu/l)			
<5000	86%	79%	84%
5000–50 000	7%	59%	66%
>50 000	7%	43%	51%
LDH (xULNR)[a]			
<1.5	67%	84%	88%
1.5–10	32%	63%	69%
>10	1%	37%	47%

Taken from International Germ Cell Cancer Collaborative Group (1997).[120]
[a]Upper limit of normal range.

As the trophoblastic elements of testis tumours have a tendency to metastasize to brain, measurement of HCG levels in cerebrospinal fluid (CSF) can be of value in the detection of this complication. The CSF level of HCG is normally less than 1/60 of that of the plasma, except when the plasma level is falling rapidly.[142]

Alpha fetoprotein (AFP)

Within a GCT of testis, it is the yolk-sac elements which are associated with AFP production.[143] Raised serum levels of AFP are found in 60% of NSGCT patients.[140] Under physiological conditions, large amounts of AFP are produced by the yolk sac and the liver during gestation. It is the major plasma protein in the fetus. After birth, very little is produced so that low 'adult' levels are reached within a few months. Liver disease can produce a modest elevation of plasma AFP levels. Hepatocellular carcinoma and occasional gastrointestinal tumours can be associated with high levels. Few other tumours which occur commonly in young men produce AFP, so a raised level can be of diagnostic value in a patient with metastatic disease of unknown type. Although raised AFP levels have on rare occasions been associated with pure seminoma,[144] the treatment of metastatic seminoma with radiotherapy in the presence of a raised AFP has been disastrous,[145] suggesting that in the majority of these cases, covert NSGCT is also present. In metastatic NSGCT, very high levels of AFP may be found. Prognosis relates to serum AFP level (Table 25.9).

Lactate dehydrogenase (LDH)

A raised level of LDH is frequently found in advanced cancer. It is specific neither for testis cancer nor for neoplastic disease in general. Furthermore, unlike HCG and AFP, elevations over 10-fold above normal are uncommon, so its sensitivity is low. Its interest in testis cancer is its very strong association with prognosis (Table 25.9).

Placental alkaline phosphatase (PLAP)

Malignant teratoma undifferentiated (MTU) (embryonal carcinoma), seminoma and ITGCN both give a positive stain in histological sections for PLAP. Modestly elevated levels of serum PLAP are seen in over 50% of patients with metastatic seminoma.[146] It is neither sensitive nor specific – elevations are seen in smokers – and PLAP levels are little used clinically.

BASIS OF THE SENSITIVITY OF TESTICULAR TUMOUR TO DNA-DAMAGING AGENTS

The efficacy of both radiotherapy and cytotoxic chemotherapy in metastatic testicular neoplasia is well known. Seminoma metastatic to para-aortic nodes is usually cured with radiotherapy. Disease beyond this site is usually treated, as with NSGCTs, with chemotherapy, and this again usually produces long-term cure. Radiotherapy is seldom used in metastatic NSGCT, as much because of the likelihood of latent disease outside the irradiated areas as its lack of efficacy against bulky tumour. However, the ability of moderate doses of radiotherapy to prevent the development of metastatic disease within an irradiated area is established.[147]

New light has been shed on the reason for the exquisite sensitivity of GCT to genotoxic agents by studies on human testis cancer cell lines. Compared to bladder cell lines, a given concentration of etoposide produced a 16-fold loss of clonogenicity. The DNA damage produced showed a difference of only twofold, but testis cancer cell lines showed five times as much apoptosis as those from bladder tumours. When an equivalent frequency of strand breaks was produced, the testicular cell lines died more readily.[148]

Normal tissues react to DNA damage by increasing the amount of p53 glycoprotein in cells. This induces the transcription of other proteins, notably Waf-1 and Mdm-2. Waf-1 is a potent inhibitor of cyclin-dependent kinases[149,150] and can cause cell-cycle arrest in G1 – that is, before the phase of DNA synthesis. G1-arrested cells have the opportunity to recover from genotoxic damage. Alternatively, particularly when myc, myb or E2F are overexpressed, an elevated p53 expression may lead to apoptosis (Figure 25.4).[151–153]

Normal germ cells contain high levels of wild-type p53. GCT are similar[154] and do not have mutations in the *p53* gene.[155–157] When GCT lines are exposed to etoposide, p53 protein is increased, but Waf-1 only modestly so, and apoptosis ensues.[148] Bladder carcinoma cell lines show two patterns of response. Either the p53 protein remains at low level, possibly because of the presence of a *p53* mutation, or p53 induction takes place and the associated Waf-1 induction causes G1 arrest. The sensitivity of GCT to genotoxic agents is therefore associated with the apoptotic response to genotoxic damage. This, in turn, is in part attributed to the high levels of wild-type p53, the absence of *p53* mutations and only a modest level of Waf-1 induction.

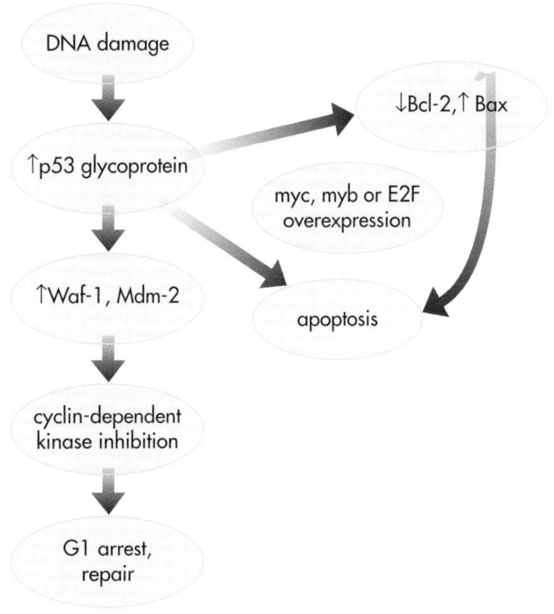

Figure 25.4 *Pathways for repair or apoptosis following DNA damage.*

GCT cell lines have higher levels of the apoptosis-promoting proteins Bax than bladder-cancer cell lines and lower levels of the suppressor of apoptosis, Bcl-2.[148] The Bax:Bcl-2 ratio may be of importance in determining whether the response to cell damage is apoptosis or repair. The role of p53 in affecting this ratio in GCTs is uncertain. Whereas p53 in certain cells has been shown to upregulate Bax and to downregulate Bcl-2[158–160] and that Bax upregulation has been observed to follow genotoxic damage,[161] perturbations of the Bax:Bcl-2 ratio were not seen in the GCT lines after etoposide exposure.[148]

Since cisplatin has such a dominant role in the successful management of metastatic GCT, there has been much interest in the reason for sensitivity to this agent. Work has not so far been supportive of the p53 hypothesis. Sensitive testis cancer cells do not have higher levels of p53 than resistant ones,[162] though, since it is likely that the resistant cell lines had been derived from tumours heavily exposed to chemotherapeutic agents in vivo, other – acquired –

resistance mechanisms may be operative. More difficult to explain away is the observation that partial inactivation of p53 in sensitive cells did not make them resistant.[162]

Exposure of cells to cisplatin causes crucial intrastrand cross-links, and this is followed by nuclear excision repair (NER). Testis cancer cells have been shown to be deficient in this process. NER is complex and includes the recognition of DNA damage by high-mobility group (HMG) proteins. There is a testis-specific HMG protein. When this has been transfected into HeLa (cervical cancer) cells, the amount of apoptosis following cisplatin exposure was increased in some cases.[163] Of the other proteins involved in NER, the xeroderma pigmentosum group A (XPA) protein and the ERCC1-XPF endonuclease complex are present in low levels in testis cancer cells. When these proteins were added to testis tumour cell extracts, full NER capacity was restored,[164] suggesting a pivotal role for these proteins.

REFERENCES

1. Moller H. Clues to the aetiology of testicular germ cell tumours from descriptive epidemiology. Eur Urol 1993; 23: 8–15
2. Bergstrom R, Adami HO, Mohner M, Zatonski W et al. Increase in testicular cancer incidence in 9 European countries: a birth cohort phenomenon. J Natl Cancer Inst 1996; 88: 727–733
3. Ekbom A, Akre O. Increasing incidence of testis cancer: a birth cohort effect. In: Rajpert-De Meyts E, Grigor KM, Skakkebaek NE, eds. Neoplastic Transformation of Testicular Germ Cells. APMIS 1998; 106: 225–229
4. Giwercman A, Grindsted J, Hansen B, Jensen OM, Skakkebaek NE. Testicular cancer risk in boys with maldescended testis: a cohort study. J Urol 1987; 138: 1214–1216
5. Pike MC, Chilvers C, Peckham MJ. Effect of age at orchiopexy on risk of testicular cancer. Lancet 1986; 1(8492): 1246–1248
6. Moller H, Skakkebaek NE. Risks of testicular cancer and cryptorchidism in relation to socio-economic status and related factors: case control studies in Denmark. Int J Cancer 1996; 7: 264–274
7. Forman D, Pike MC, Davey G et al. Aetiology of testicular cancer – association with congenital abnormalities, age of puberty, infertility and exercise. BMJ 1994; 306: 1393–1399
8. Ross RK, McCurtis JW, Henderson BE, Merick HR, Mack TM, Martin SP. Descriptive epidemiology of testicular and prostatic cancer in Los Angeles. Br J Cancer 1979; 39: 284–292
9. Pukkala E, Wiederpass E. Socio-economic differences in incidence rates of cancers of the male genital organs in Finland, 1971–95. Int J Cancer 2002; 102: 643–648
10. Prattala R, Berg MA, Puska P. Diminishing or increasing contrasts? Social class variation in Finnish food consumption patterns, 1979–1990. Eur J Clin Nutr 1992; 46: 279–287
11. Yeole BB, Jussawalla DJ. Descriptive epidemiology of the cancers of male genital organs in greater Bombay. Indian J Cancer 1997; 34: 30–39
12. Ganmaa D, Li XM, Wang J, Qin LQ, Wang PY, Sato A. Incidence and mortality of testicular and prostatic cancers in relation to world dietary practices. Int J Cancer 2002; 98: 262–267
13. Swerdlow AJ, Huttly SR, Smith PG. Testis cancer: postnatal hormone factors, sexual behaviour and fertility. Int J Cancer 1989; 43: 549–553
14. Tanner JM. Trend towards earlier menarche in London, Oslo, Copenhagen, The Netherlands and Hungary. Nature 1973; 243: 96–97
15. Swerdlow AJ, Higgins CD, Pike MC. Risk of cancer in cohort of boys with cryptorchidism. BMJ 1997; 314: 1507–1511
16. Moller H, Cortes D, Engholm G, Thorup J. Risk of testicular cancer with cryptorchidism and with testicular biopsy: cohort study. BMJ 1998; 317: 729–730
17. Senturia Y. The epidemiology of testicular cancer. Br J Urol 1987; 60: 285–291
18. Martin NG, Olsen ME, Theile H, El Beaini JL, Handelsman D, Bhatnagar AS. Pituitary-ovarian function in mothers who have had 2 sets of dizygotic twins. Fertil Steril 1984; 41: 878–880
19. Hemminki K, Li X. Cancer risks in twins: results from Swedish family-cancer database. Int J Cancer 2002; 99: 873–878
20. Braun MM, Ahlbom A, Floders B, Brinton LA et al. Effect of twinship on incidence of cancer of the testis, breast and other sites (Sweden). Cancer Causes Control 1995; 6: 519–552
21. Swerdlow AJ, De Stavola BL, Swanwick MA, Maconochie NE. Risks of breast and testicular cancers in young adult twins in England and Wales: evidence on prenatal and genetic aetiology. Lancet 1997; 350: 1723–1728
22. Depue RH, Pike MC, Henderson BE. Estrogen expo-

sure during gestation and the risk of cancer of the testis. J Natl Cancer Inst 1983; 71: 1151–1155
23. Chilvers CED, Forman D, Oliver RTD et al. Social behavioural and medical factors in the aetiology of testicular cancer – results from the UK study. Br J Cancer 1994, 70: 513–520
24. Carlsen E, Giwercman A, Keiding N, Skakkebaek NE. Evidence for decreasing quality of semen during past 50 years. BMJ 1992; 305: 609–613
25. Dieckmann K-P, Pichlmeier U. The prevalence of familial testicular cancer. Cancer 1997; 80: 1954–1960
26. Forman D, Oliver RTD, Brett AR, Marsh SG et al. Familial testicular cancer: a report of the UK family register, estimation of risk and an HLA class 1 sib-pair analysis. Br J Cancer 1992; 65: 255–262
27. Heimdal K, Olsson H, Tretli S, Flodgren P, Borresen AL, Fossa SD. Familial testicular cancer in Norway and southern Sweden. Br J Cancer 1996; 73: 964–969
28. Osterlind A, Berthelsen JG, Abildgaard N, Hansen SO et al. Risk of bilateral testicular germ cell cancer in Denmark: 1960–1984. J Natl Cancer Inst 1991; 83: 1391–1395
29. Colls BM, Harvey VJ, Skelton L, Thompson PI, Frampton CM. Bilateral germ cell testicular tumours in New Zealand: experience in Auckland and Christchurch 1978–1994. J Clin Oncol 1996; 14: 2061–2065
30. Wanderas EH, Fossa SD, Tretlis S. Risk of a second germ cell cancer in 2201 Norwegian male patients. Br J Cancer 1997; 33: 244–252
31. von der Maase H, Rorth M, Walbom-Jorgensen S, Sorensen BL et al. Carcinoma in situ of contralateral testis in patients with testicular germ cell cancer: study of 27 cases in 500 patients. BMJ 1986; 293: 1398–1401
32. Dieckmann K-P, Loy V. Prevalence of contralateral testicular intraepithelial neoplasia in patients with testicular germ cell neoplasms. J Clin Oncol 1996; 14: 3126–3132
33. Nicholson PW, Harland SJ. Inheritance and testicular cancer. Br J Cancer 1995; 71: 421–426
34. Heimdal K, Olsson H, Tretli S, Fossa SD, Borrensen AL, Bishop DT. A segregation analysis of testicular cancer based on Norwegian and Swedish families. Br J Cancer 1997; 75: 1084–1087
35. Rapley EA, Crockford GP, Easton DF, Stratton MR et al. The genetics of testicular germ cell tumours. In: Harnden P, Joffe JK, eds. Germ Cell Tumours V. London: Springer-Verlag, 2002
36. Geurts van Kessel A, Suijkerbuijk RF, Sinke RJ, Looijenga L et al. Molecular cytogenetics of human germ cell tumours: i(12p) and related chromosomal abnormalities. Eur Urol 1993; 23: 23–29
37. Chaganti RS, Houldsworth J. The cytogenetic theory of the pathogenesis of human adult male germ cell tumours. Review article. APMIS 1998; 106: 80–83
38. Sigg C, Hedinger C. Atypical germ cells in testicular biopsy in male sterility. Int J Androl 1981; Suppl. 4: 163–171
39. Skakkebaek NE. Possible carcinoma in situ of the testis. Lancet 1972; 2: 516
40. Pryor JP, Cameron KM, Chilton CP, Ford TF et al. Carcinoma in situ in testicular biopsies from men presenting with infertility. Br J Urol 1983; 55; 780–784
41. Harland SJ, Cook PA, Fossa SD, Horwich A et al. Intratubular germ cell neoplasia of the contralateral testis in testicular cancer: defining a high risk group. J Urol 1998; 160: 1353–1357
42. Jacobsen GK, Norgaard-Pedersen B. Placental alkaline phosphatase in testicular germ cell tumours and in carcinoma in situ of the testis. Acta Pathol Microbiol Scand Sect A 1984; 92: 323–329
43. Dieckmann KP, Skakkebaek NE. Carcinoma in situ of the testis: a review of biological and clinical features. Int J Cancer 1999; 83: 815–822
44. Loy V, Wigand I, Dieckmann KP. Incidence and distribution of carcinoma in situ in testes removed for germ cell tumour: possible inadequacy of random testicular biopsy in detecting the condition. Histopathology 1990; 16: 198–200
45. Cappelen D, Fossa ST, Stenwig AE, Aass N. False-negative biopsy for testicular intraepithelial neoplasia and high risk features for testicular cancer. Acta Oncol 2000; 39: 105–109
46. Berthelsen JG, Skakkebaek NE. Value of testicular biopsy in diagnosing carcinoma in situ testis. Scand J Urol Nephrol 1981; 15: 165–168
47. Rajpert-De Meyts E, Skakkebaek NE. Expression of the c-*kit* protein product in carcinoma in situ and invasive testicular germ cell tumours. Int J Androl 1994; 17: 85–92
48. Jorgensen N, Rajpert-De Meyts E, Graem N, Muller J, Giwercman A, Stakkebaek NE. Expression of immunohistochemical markers for testicular carcinoma in situ by normal human foetal germ cells. Lab Invest 1995; 72: 223–231
49. Gondos B. Ultrastructure of developing and malignant germ cells. Eur Urol 1993; 23: 68–75
50. Moller J, Skakkebaek NE. Microspectrophotometric DNA measurements of carcinoma in situ germ cells in the testis. Int J Androl 1981; Suppl. 4: 211–221

51. Nistal M, Codesal J, Paniagua R. Carcinoma in situ of the testis in infertile men. A histological, immunocytochemical and cytophotometric study of DNA content. J Pathol 1989; 159: 205–210
52. el-Naggar AK, Ro JY, McLemore D, Ayala AG, Batsakis JG. DNA ploidy in testicular germ cell neoplasms. Histogenetic and clinical implications Am J Surg Pathol 1992; 16: 611–618
53. Moller J, Lauke H, Hartmann M. The value of the AgNOR staining method in identifying carcinoma in situ testis. Pathol Res Pract 1994; 120: 429–435
54. Ball RY, Sandison A, Areas AM et al. DNA ploidy and proliferation fraction in classical seminoma and intratubular germ cell neoplasia. J Urol Pathol 1998; 78: 141–155
55. Bartkova J, Bartek J, Lukas J, Vojtesek B et al. p53 protein alterations in human testicular cancer including pre-invasive intratubular germ cell neoplasia. Int J Cancer 1991; 49: 196–202
56. Moore BE, Banner BF, Gokden M, Woda B et al. p53: a good diagnostic marker for intratubular germ cell neoplasia, unclassified. Appl Immunohistochem Mol Morphol 2001; 9: 203–206
57. Datta MW, Macri E, Signoretti S, Renshaw AA, Loda M. Transition from in situ to invasive testicular germ cell neoplasia is associated with the loss of p21 and gain of mdm-2 expression. Mod Pathol 2001; 14: 437–442
58. Kuczyk MA, Serth J, Bokemeyer C, Jonassen J et al. Alterations of the p53 tumour suppressor gene in carcinoma in situ of the testis. Cancer 1996; 78: 1958–1966
59. Peng HQ, Hogg D, Malkin D, Bailey D et al. Mutations of the p53 gene do not occur in testicular cancer. Cancer Res 1993; 53: 3574–3578
60. Rajpert-De Meyts E, Kvist M, Skakkebaek NE. Heterogeneity of expression of immunohistochemical tumour markers in testicular carcinoma in situ: pathogenetic relevance. Virchows Arch 1996; 428: 133–139
61. Oosterhuis JW, Gillis AJ, van Putten WJ, de Jong B, Looijenga LH. Interphase cytogenetics of carcinoma in situ of the testis. Numerical analysis of the chromosomes 1, 12 and 15. Eur Urol 1993; 23: 16–21
62. Rosenberg C, Van Gurp RJ, Geelen E, Oosterhuis JW, Looijenga LH. Overrepresentation of the short arm of chromosome 12 is related to invasive growth of human testicular seminomas and nonseminomas. Oncogene 2000; 19: 5858–5862
63. Timmer A, Oosterhuis JW, Koops HS, Sleijfer DT et al. The tumour micro-environment: possible role of integrins and the extracellular matrix in tumour biological behaviour of intratubular germ cell neoplasia and testicular seminomas. Am J Pathol 1994; 144: 1035–1044
64. Kang J-L, Rajpert-De Meyts W, Giwercmann A, Skakkebaek NE. The association of testicular carcinoma in situ with intratubular microcalcifications. J Urol Pathol 1994; 2: 235–242
65. Backus ML, Mack LA, Middleton WD, King BF et al. Testicular microlithiasis: imaging appearances and pathological correlation. Radiology 1994; 192: 781–785
66. Hobarth K, Szabo N, Klingher HC, Kratzik C. Sonographic appearance of testicular microlithiasis. Eur Urol 1993; 24: 251–255
67. Bach AM, Hann LE, Hadar O, Shui W et al. Testicular microlithiasis: what is its association with testicular cancer? Radiology 2001; 220: 70–75
68. Peterson AC, Bauman JM, Light DE, McMann LP, Costabile RA. The prevalence of testicular microlithiasis in an asymptomatic population of men 18 to 35 years old. J Urol 2001; 166: 2061–2064
69. von Eckardstein S, Tsakmakidis G, Kamischke A, Rolf C, Nieschlag E. Sonographic testicular microlithiasis as an indicator of premalignant conditions in normal and infertile men. J Androl 2001; 22: 818–824
70. Freeman A, Rowbotham C, Parkinson MC. Re: The prevalence of testicular microlithiasis in an asymptomatic population of men 18 to 35 years old. J Urol 2003; 169: 1474
71. Heikkila R, Heilo A, Stenning AE, Fossa SD. Testicular ultrasonography and 18G Biopty biopsy for clinically undetected cancer or carcinoma in situ in patients with germ cell tumours. Br J Urol 1993; 71: 214–216
72. Harland SJ, Nicholson PW. Implications of a hereditary model for testis cancer. In: Appleyard I, Harnden P, Joffe JK, eds. Germ Cell Tumours IV. John Libbey, 1998: 19–27
73. Giwercman A, von der Maase H, Skakkebaek NE. Epidemiological and clinical aspects of carcinoma in situ of the testis. Eur Urol 1993; 23: 104–114
74. Bettocchi C, Coker CB, Deacon J, Parkinson C, Pryor JP. A review of testicular intratubular germ cell neoplasia in infertile men. J Androl 1994; 15: 14S–16S
75. Berthelsen JG, Skakkebaek NE. Distribution of carcinoma in situ in testes from infertile men. Int J Androl 1981; Suppl. 4: 172–184
76. Read G. Carcinoma in situ of the contralateral testis. BMJ 1987; 294: 121

77. Giwercman A, von der Maase H, Berthelsen JG, Rorth M et al. Localised irradiation of testes with carcinoma in situ: effects on Leydig cell function and eradication of malignant germ cells in 3 patients. J Clin Endocr Metab 1991; 73: 596–603
78. Petersen PM, Giwercman A, Daugaard G, Rorth M et al. Effect of graded testicular doses of radiotherapy in patients treated for carcinoma in situ in the testis. J Clin Oncol 2002; 20: 1537–1543
79. Shalet SM. Effect of irradiation treatment on gonadal function in men treated for germ cell cancer. Eur Urol 1993; 23: 148–152
80. Dieckmann KP, Lauke H, Michl U, Winter E, Loy V. Testicular germ cell cancer despite previous local radiotherapy to the testis. Eur Urol 2002; 41: 643–650
81. Fossa SD, Aass N. Cisplatin-based chemotherapy does not eliminate the risk of secondary testicular cancer. Br J Urol 1989; 63: 531–534
82. Von der Maase H, Meinecke B, Skakkebaek NE. Residual carcinoma in situ of contralateral testis after chemotherapy. Lancet 1988; 1(8583): 477–478
83. Von Ostau C, Krege S, Hartmann M, Rubben H. Metachronous contralateral germ cell tumour 7 years after management of testicular intraepithelial neoplasia by chemotherapy and multiple control biopsies. Scand J Urol Nephrol 2001; 35: 430–431
84. Bottomley D, Fisher C, Hendry WF, Horwich A. Persistent carcinoma in situ of the testis after chemotherapy for advanced testicular germ cell tumours. Br J Urol 1990; 66: 420–424
85. Skakkebaek NE, Berthelsen JG, Lisfeidt J. Clinical aspects of testicular carcinoma in situ. Int J Androl 1981; Suppl 4: 153–162
86. Hu LM, Phillipson SH. Intratubular germ cell neoplasia in infantile yolk sac tumour: verification by tandem repeat sequence in-situ hybridization. Diagn Mol Pathol 1992; 1: 118–128
87. Stamp IM, Barlebo H, Rix M, Jacobsen GK. Intratubular germ cell neoplasia in an infantile testis with immature teratoma. Histopathology 1993; 22: 69–72
88. Manivel JC, Simonton S, Wold LE, Dehner LP. Absence of intratubular germ cell neoplasia in testicular yolk sac tumours in children. Arch Pathol Lab Med 1988; 112: 641–645
89. Soosay GN, Bobrow L, Happerfield L, Parkinson MC. Morphology and immunohistochemistry of carcinoma in situ adjacent to testicular germ cell tumours in adults and children: implications for histogenesis. Histopathology 1991; 19: 537–544
90. Ramani P, Yeung CK, Habeebu SSM. Testicular intratubular germ cell neoplasia in children and adolescents with intersex. Am J Surg Pathol 1993; 17: 1124–1133
91. Moller J, Skakkebaek NE, Nielsen OH, Graem N. Cryptorchidism and testis cancer. Atypical infantile germ cells followed by carcinoma in situ and invasive carcinoma in adulthood. Cancer 1984; 54: 629–634
92. Parkinson MC, Swerdlow AJ, Pike MC. Carcinoma in situ in boys with cryptorchidism: when can it be detected? Br J Urol 1994; 73: 431–435
93. Duncan PR, Checa F, Gowing NFC, McElwain TJ et al. Extranodal non-Hodgkin's lymphoma presenting in the testicle. Cancer 1980; 45: 1578–1584
94. Turner RR, Colby TV, MacKintosh FR. Testicular lymphomas: a clinicopathologic study of 35 cases. Cancer 1981; 48: 2095–2102
95. Lagrange JL, Ramaioli A, Theodore CH, Terrier-Lacombe MJ et al. Non-Hodgkin's lymphoma of the testis: a retrospective study of 84 patients treated in the French anticancer centres. Ann Oncol 2001; 12: 1313–1319
96. Rutgers JL, Scully RE. Pathology of the testis in intersex syndromes. Semin Diag Pathol 1987; 4: 275–291
97. Witten FR, O'Brien BP, Sewell CW, Wheatley JK. Bilateral clear cell papillary cystadenoma of the epididymes presenting as infertility: an early manifestation of von Hippel-Landau's syndrome. J Urol 1985; 133: 1062–1064
98. Rutgers JL, Young RH, Scully RE. The testicular 'tumour' of the adrenogenital syndrome. Am J Surg Pathol 1988; 12: 503–513
99. Knudsen JL, Savage A, Mobb GE. The testicular 'tumour' of adreno-genital syndrome – a persistent diagnostic pitfall. Histopathology 1991; 19: 468–470
100. Akhtar M, Ali MA, Mackey DM. Lepromatous leprosy presenting as orchitis. Am J Clin Pathol 1980; 73: 712–715
101. Lee AH, Mead GM, Theaker JM. The value of central histopathological review of testicular tumours before treatment. Br J Urol Int 1999; 84: 75–78
102. Zavala-Pompa A, Ro JY, El-Naggar AK. Tubular seminoma. An immunohistochemical and DNA flow-cytometric study of four cases. Am J Clin Pathol 1994; 102: 397–401
103. Ulbright TM. Morphologic variation in seminoma. Am J Clin Pathol 1994; 102: 395–396
104. Henley JD, Young RH, Ulbright TM. Malignant Sertoli cell tumour of the testis: a study of 13 examples of a neoplasm frequently misinterpreted as seminoma. Am J Surg Pathol 2002; 26: 541–550

105. Cheville JC, Rao S, Iczkowski KA, Lohse CM, Pankratz VS. Cytokeratin expression in seminoma of the human testis. Am J Clin Pathol 2000; 113: 583–588
106. Leroy X, Augusto D, Leteurtre E, Gosselin B. CD30 and CD117 (c-*kit*) used in combination are useful for distinguishing embryonal carcinoma from seminoma. J Histochem Cytochem 2002; 50: 283–285
107. Tickoo SK, Hutchinson B, Bacik J, Mazumdar M et al. Testicular seminoma: a clinicopathologic and immunohistochemical study of 105 cases with special reference to seminomas with atypical features. Int J Surg Pathol 2002; 10: 23–32
108. Kraggerud SM, Berner A, Bryne M, Petterson EO, Fossa SD. Spermatocytic seminoma as compared to classical seminoma: an immunohistochemical and DNA flow cytometric study. APMIS 1999; 107: 297–302
109. Franke FE, Pauls K, Kerkman L, Sterger K et al. Somatic isoform of angiotensin I-converting enzyme in the pathology of testicular germ cell tumours. Hum Pathol 2000; 31: 1466–1476
110. Pugh RCB. Testicular tumours – introduction. In: Pugh RCB, ed. Pathology of the Testis. Blackwell Scientific, Oxford: 139–159
111. Mostofi FK, Sobin LH. Histological typing of testis tumours. International Histological Classification of Tumours, No. 16. Geneva: World Health Organization, 1977
112. Mostofi FK, Sesterhenn IA in collaboration with Sobin AH and pathologists in 9 countries. World Health Organization International Histological Classification of Tumours. Histological Typing of Testis Tumours. 2nd edn. Berlin: Springer-Verlag, 1998
113. IARC classification, 2003, in press
114. Freedman LS, Parkinson MC, Jones WG, Oliver RT et al. Histopathology in the prediction of relapse of patients with stage I testicular teratoma treated by orchidectomy alone. Lancet 1987; 2(8554): 294–298
115. Read G, Stenning SP, Cullen MH, Parkinson MC et al. Medical Research Council prospective study of surveillance for stage I testicular teratoma. J Clin Oncol 1992; 10: 1762–1768
116. Cullen MH, Stenning SP, Parkinson MC, Fossa SD et al. Short course adjuvant chemotherapy in high risk stage I non-seminomatous germ cell tumours of the testis: a Medical Research Council report. J Clin Oncol 1996; 14: 1106–1113
117. Parkinson MC, Harland SJ, Harnden P, Sandison A. The role of the histopathologist in the management of testicular germ cell tumours in adults. Histopathology 2001; 38: 183–194
118. Stoter G, Sylvester R, Sleijfer DT, ten Bokkel Huinink WW et al. Multivariate analysis of prognostic factors in patients with disseminated non-seminomatous testicular cancer: results from a European Organization for Research on Treatment of Cancer Multiinstitutional Phase III Study. Cancer Res 1987; 47: 2714–2718
119. Mead GM, Stenning SP, Parkinson MC, Horwich A et al. The second Medical Research Council study of prognostic factors in non-seminomatous germ cell tumours. J Clin Oncol 1992; 10: 85–94
120. International Germ Cell Cancer Collaborative Group. International germ cell consensus classification: a prognostic factor-based staging system for metastatic germ cell cancers. J Clin Oncol 1997; 15: 594–603
121. Marks LB, Rutgers JL, Shipley WU, Walker TG et al. Testicular seminoma: clinical and pathological features that may predict para-aortic lymph node metastases. J Urol 1990; 143: 524–527
122. Horwich A, Alsanjari N, A'Hern R, Nicolls J, Dearnaley DP, Fisher C. Surveillance following orchidectomy for stage I testicular seminoma. Br J Cancer 1992; 65: 775–778
123. Hoeltl W, Kosak D, Pont J, Hawel R et al. Testicular cancer: prognostic implications of vascular invasion. J Urol 1987; 137: 683–685
124. Jacobsen GK, von der Maase H, Specht L et al. Histopathological features of stage I seminoma treated with orchidectomy only. J Urol Pathol 1995; 3: 85–94
125. Warde P, Specht L, Horwich A, Oliver T et al. Prognostic factors for relapse in stage I seminoma managed by surveillance: a pooled analysis. J Clin Oncol 2002; 20: 4448–4452
126. Loehrer PJ, Hui S, Clark S, Seal M et al. Teratoma following cisplatin-based combination chemotherapy for non-seminomatous germ cell tumours: a clinicopathological correlation. J Urol 1986; 135: 1183–1189
127. Steyerberg EW, Keizer HJ, Zwartendijk J, Van Rijk GL et al. Prognosis after resection of residual masses following chemotherapy for metastatic non-seminomatous testicular cancer: a multivariate analysis. Br J Cancer 1993; 68: 195–200
128. Hendry WF, A'Hern RP, Hetherington JW, Peckham MJ, Dearnaley DP, Horwich A. Para-aortic lym-

phadenectomy after chemotherapy for metastatic non-seminomatous germ cell tumours: prognostic value and therapeutic benefit. Br J Urol 1993; 71: 208–213
129. Gerl A, Clemm C, Schmeller N, Djenemann H et al. Outcome analysis after post-chemotherapy surgery in patients with non-seminomatous germ cell tumours. Ann Oncol 1995; 6: 483–488
130. Stenning SP, Parkinson MC, Fisher C, Mead GM et al. Postchemotherapy residual masses in germ cell tumour patients: content, clinical features, and prognosis. Medical Research Council Testicular Tumour Working Party. Cancer 1998; 83: 1409–1419
131. Hendry WF. Decision-making in abdominal surgery following chemotherapy for testicular cancer. Eur J Cancer 1995; 31A: 649–650
132. Toner GC, Panicek DM, Heelan RJ, Geller NL et al. Adjunctive surgery after chemotherapy for non-seminomatous germ cell tumours: recommendations for patient selection. J Clin Oncol 1990; 8: 1683–1694
133. Steyerberg EW, Keizer HJ, Stoter G, Habbena JDF. Predictors of residual mass histology following chemotherapy for metastatic non-seminomatous testicular cancer: a quantitative overview of 996 resections. Eur J Cancer 1994; 30A: 1231–1239
134. Gerl A, Clemm C, Schmeller N, Dienemann H et al. Sequential resection of residual abdominal and thoracic masses after chemotherapy for metastatic non-seminomatous germ cell tumour. Br J Cancer 1994; 70: 960–965
135. Brenner PC, Herr HW, Morse MJ, Sheinfeld J et al. Simultaneous retroperitoneal, thoracic and cervical resection of post-chemotherapy residual masses in patients with metastatic non-seminomatous germ cell tumours of the testis. J Clin Oncol 1996; 14: 1765–1769
136. Steyerberg EW, Keizer HJ, Messemer JE. Residual pulmonary masses after chemotherapy for metastatic non-seminomatous germ cell tumour prediction of histology. Cancer 1997; 79: 345–355
137. Little JS, Foster RS, Ulbright TM, Donohue JP. Unusual neoplasms detected in testis cancer patients undergoing post-chemotherapy retroperitoneal lymphadenectomy. J Urol 1994; 152: 1144–1149
138. Bagshawe KD, Rustin GDS. Circulating tumour markers. In: Peckham M, Pinedo HM, Veronesi U, eds. Oxford Textbook of Oncology, vol. 1. Oxford: Oxford Medical Publications, 1995: 412–420
139. Wehmann RE, Nisula BC. Metabolic and renal clearance rates of purified human chorionic gonadotrophin. J Clin Invest 1981; 68: 184–193
140. Rustin GJS, Vogelzang NJ, Sleijfer DT, Nisselbaum SN. Consensus statement as circulating tumour markers and staging of patient with germ cell tumours. In: Prostate Cancer and Testicular Cancer, EORTC Genitourinary Group Monograph 7. New York: AR Liss, 1990
141. Schwartz BF, Auman R, Peretsman SJ, Moul JW et al. Prognostic value of BHCG and local tumour invasion in stage I seminoma of the testis. J Surg Oncol 1996; 61: 131–133
142. Bagshawe KD, Harland S. Immunodiagnosis and monitoring of gonadotrophin producing metastases in the central nervous system. Cancer 1976; 38: 112–118
143. Teilum G, Albrechtsen R, Norgaard-Pedersen B. Immunofluorescent localization of alpha-fetoprotein synthesis in endodermal sinus tumor (yolk sac tumor). Acta Pathol Microbiol Scand 1974; 82A: 586–588
144. Oliver RTD. A comparison of the biology and prognosis of seminoma and non-seminoma. In: Horwich A, ed. Testicular Cancer, Investigation and Management. Chapman and Hall Medical, 1991
145. Lange PH, Nochomovitz LE, Rosai J, Fraley EE et al. Serum alpha-fetoprotein and human chorionic gonadotrophin in patients with seminoma. J Urol 1980; 124: 472–478
146. Lange PH, Millan JL, Stigbrand T, Vessella RL, Ruoslahti E, Fishman WH. Placental alkaline phosphatase as a tumor marker for seminoma. Cancer Res 1982; 42: 3244–3247
147. Rorth M, Jacobsen GJ, von der Maase H, Madsen EL et al. Surveillance alone versus radiotherapy after orchiectomy for clinical stage I non-seminomatous testicular cancer. J Clin Oncol 1991; 12: 1543–1547
148. Chresta CM, Masters JR, Hickman JA. Hypersensitivity of human testicular tumours to etoposide-induced apoptosis is associated with functional p53 and a high Bax: Bcl-2 ratio. Cancer Res 1996; 56: 1834–1841
149. el-Deiry WS, Harper JW, O'Connor PM, Velculescu VE et al. WAFI/CIPI is induced in p53-mediated G_1 arrest and apoptosis. Cancer Res 1994; 54: 1169–1174
150. Canman CE, Gilmer TM, Coutts SB, Kastan MB. Growth factor modulation of p53-mediated growth arrest versus apoptosis. Genes Dev 1995; 9: 600–611

151. Wagner AJ, Kokontis JM, Hay N. *myc*-mediated apoptosis requires wild-type p53 in a manner independent of cell cycle arrest and the ability of p53 to induce p21wafl/cipl. Genes Dev 1994; 8: 2817–2830
152. Lin D, Fiscella M, O'Connor PM, Jackman J et al. Constitutive expression of B-myb can bypass p53-induced Wafl/Cip1-mediated G_1 arrest. Proc Natl Acad Sci USA 1994; 91: 10079–10083
153. Wu X, Levine AJ. p53 and E2F-1 cooperate to mediate apoptosis. Proc Natl Acad Sci USA 1994; 91: 3602–3606
154. Bartek J, Bartkova J, Vojtesek B, Staskova Z et al. Aberrant expression of the p53 oncoprotein is a common feature of a wide spectrum of human malignancies. Oncogene 1991; 6: 1699–1703
155. Peng HQ, Hogg D, Malkin D, Bailey M et al. Mutations of the p53 gene do not occur in testis cancer. Cancer Res 1993; 53: 3574–3578
156. Heimdal K, Lothe RA, Lystad S, Holm R, Fossa SD, Borresen AL. No germline TP53 mutations detected in familial and bilateral testicular cancer. Genes Chromosomes Cancer 1993; 6: 92–97
157. Fleischhacker M, Strohmeyer T, Imai Y, Slamon DJ et al. Mutations of the p53 gene are not detectable in human testicular tumours. Mod Pathol 1994; 7: 435–439
158. Miyashita T, Harigai M, Hanada M, Reed JC. Identification of a p53-dependent negative response element in the Bcl-2 gene. Cancer Res 1994; 54: 3131–3135
159. Miyashita T, Krajewski S, Krajewska M, Wang HG et al. Tumour suppressor p53 is a regulator of Bcl-2 and bax gene expression in vitro and in vivo. Oncogene 1994; 9: 1799–1805
160. Selvakumaran M, Lin HK, Miyashita T, Wang HG et al. Immediate early up-regulation of bax expression by p53 but not TGF B1: a paradigm for distinct apoptotic pathways. Oncogene 1994; 9: 1791–1798
161. Zhan Q, Fan S, Bae I, Guillouf C et al. Induction of bax by genotoxic stress in human cells correlates with normal p53 status and apoptosis. Oncogene 1994; 9: 3743–3751
162. Kersemaekers AMF, Mayer F, Molier M, van Weeren PC et al. Role of P53 and MDM2 in treatment response of human germ cell tumours. J Clin Oncol 2002; 20: 1551–1561
163. Zamble DB, Mikata Y, Eng CH, Sandeman KE et al. Testis-specific HMG-domain protein alters the responses of cells to cisplatin. J Inorg Biochem 2002; 91: 451–462
164. Köberle B, Masters JRW, Hartley JA, Wood RD. Reduced repair of cisplatin-induced DNA damage in testicular germ cell tumours due to a specific protein defect. Curr Biol 1999; 9: 273–276
165. Henderson BE, Benton B, Jing J, Yu MC, Pike MC. Risk factors for cancer of the testis in young men. Int J Cancer 1979; 23: 598–602
166. Shottenfeld D, Warshauer ME, Sherlock S. The epidemiology of testicular cancer in young adults. Am J Epidemiol 1980; 112: 232–246
167. Dugaard G, Rorth M, von der Maase H, Skakkebaek NE. Management of extragonadal germ cell tumours and the significance of bilateral testicular biopsies. Ann Oncol 1992; 3: 283–289

26

Radiotherapy: scientific principles and practical application in urological malignancies

Mary McCormack, Richard S D Brown and Heather A Payne

INTRODUCTION

Radiotherapy is the therapeutic use of ionizing radiation. X-rays were first used in the treatment of cancer over 100 years ago by Freund, a German surgeon. Since that time, our understanding of the effects of ionizing radiation on malignant and normal tissues has progressed through the field of radiobiology. In parallel with this, our knowledge of radiation physics has advanced together with significant technological developments in treatment planning and delivery.

This chapter outlines the underlying physical and radiobiological principles of radiotherapy and discusses the scientific practice of radiotherapy as applied to urological tumours.

RADIATION PHYSICS

Radiation used therapeutically is called ionizing radiation, as it causes its effects through the ionization of intracellular molecules. Ionizing radiation can be classified as electromagnetic or particulate.

Electromagnetic radiation

The two types of electromagnetic radiation used in radiotherapy are X-rays and gamma rays. They are physically identical, but known by different names to distinguish their means of production. Gamma rays are produced from the nuclear decay of radioactive isotopes. X-rays are produced by interactions that occur outside the nucleus. Both types of radiation have short wavelengths, high frequencies and carry high energies that enable them to break chemical bonds and produce biological effects. The term 'photon' is another name that can be used to describe both X-rays and gamma rays.

X-rays are usually produced artificially by electrical means, accelerating electrons to a high energy and then abruptly stopping them in a heavy metal target. Part or all of the kinetic energy of the electrons is converted into X-rays. The energies necessary to generate therapeutic X-ray beams capable of penetrating human tissues are in the megavoltage (MV) range and usually produced by a machine called a linear accelerator. This type of treatment is an example of teletherapy, where the source of radiation is distant from the body, and is often referred to as 'external beam radiotherapy'.

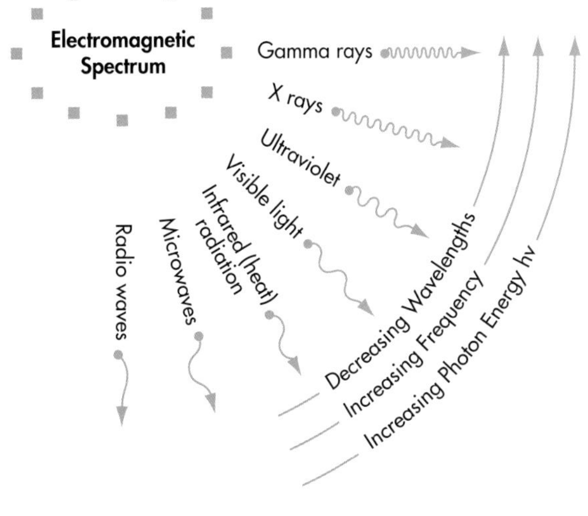

Figure 26.1 *Illustration of the electromagnetic spectrum*

As the energy of the treatment beam increases, so does the penetration depth, as the X-rays are less able to interact with superficial tissues. Modern radiotherapy techniques use megavoltage photons with beam energies typically greater than 8 MV to treat urological tumours such as carcinoma of the prostate or bladder. Prior to the introduction of megavoltage treatment (cobalt machines and linear accelerators), the only available treatment energies were up to 300 kV, which gave inadequate penetration for the treatment of deep target tissues. The term 'deep X-ray therapy' (DXT) is often mistakenly applied to all radiotherapy but historically refers specifically to energies in the 250–300-kV range. These beams deposit their maximum dose in the skin and have a therapeutic penetration of only 3–4 cm. Lower energy beams (90–300 kV) are now used mainly to treat lesions in the skin and superficial tissues.

The other common type of therapeutic radiation, gamma rays, are produced by the nuclear decay of radioactive elements and represent the excess energy that is emitted as an unstable nucleus decays into a more stable form. The higher energy gamma rays emitted from isotopes such as cobalt (^{60}Co) or caesium (^{137}Cs) can be used therapeutically if harnessed into beams for external radiotherapy treatment. Cobalt machines are still used in some centres, but since they produce a relatively low-energy beam, their uses are limited for urological treatments.

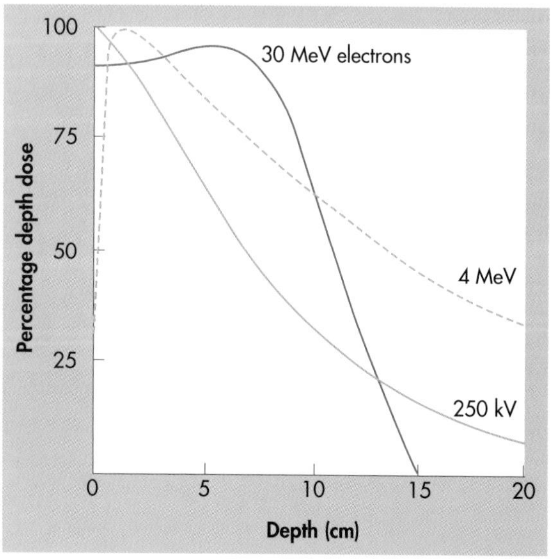

Figure 26.2 *Depth-dose curves for SXR and photons and electrons.*

Other isotopes such as radium (^{226}Ra), iridium (^{192}Ir) and iodine (^{125}I) can be used as temporary or permanent implants, a process known as brachytherapy. Sealed isotope sources may be placed into body cavities (intracavity brachytherapy) or directly into tissues (interstitial brachytherapy).

The main physical advantage of brachytherapy is that it allows a high tumour dose and considerable sparing of surrounding normal tissues. This occurs because of the inverse square law that governs the intensity of all electromagnetic radiation. As the distance from a radiation source doubles, the intensity falls to one-quarter, producing a rapid decline in effect that can be exploited therapeutically in brachytherapy.

The isotopes used in brachytherapy are known as sealed sources because they are contained within protective coverings to stop physical contact between the body and the radioactive material while still allowing the radiation to escape. Radium is now no longer used due to the difficulty of ensuring adequate radiation protection. It decays into radon gas, which is difficult to contain and emits alpha particles, a highly damaging form of particulate radiation (see below).

A third therapeutic use for gamma rays is as 'unsealed sources' in which an isotope is exploited because of its metabolic effect on biological tissues. The isotope is usually incorporated into tissues because of its physical properties, radioactivity being released as the isotope decays. An example of this is administration of radioactive strontium for the palliation of painful bone metastases in metastatic prostate cancer. Strontium is taken up into bone, and the radioactive decay produces local tumour cell kill, resulting in pain relief.

Particulate radiation

Particulate radiation consists of subatomic particles, including electrons, neutrons, protons and alpha particles. In current radiotherapy, electrons are the only commonly used type of particulate radiation. Electrons are also generated by a linear accelerator, but instead of the beam hitting a target to generate X-rays, the electrons are allowed to penetrate directly into the tissues to produce the therapeutic effect.

Electron beams differ from those of photons in that there is a much sharper decline in radiation dose (see Figure 26.2), sparing any underlying tissues. These properties make electron beams ideal for treating superficial tumours where a high dose is needed at or just below the skin surface, but it is necessary to spare the underlying tissues.

Linear accelerators are usually able to produce a range of electron beam energies of 4–20 MeV. The effective treatment depth in centimetres is about one-third of the beam energy in MeV (for example, 4 cm for a 12-MeV electron beam). The electron energy used for treatment is chosen so that the tumour will typically receive 90% of the maximum dose (known as the 90% isodose). This allows for the best homogeneity of treatment dose across the tumour.

Interactions of X-rays with matter

The process by which photons are absorbed depends principally on their energy and the chemical composition of the absorbing material. Three distinct absorption mechanisms are recognized: the photoelectric effect, the Compton effect and pair production. As energy is being absorbed in these interactions, the SI unit of dose in radiotherapy measures amount of energy in joules absorbed per unit mass in kilograms. This unit is the gray, and 1 Gy is equal to 1 J of energy absorbed per kilogram of mass. To illustrate the amount of radiation energy absorbed in biological tissues, Hall has calculated that the same amount of energy is transferred in drinking one sip of hot coffee as is absorbed in a lethal 4-Gy dose of whole-body radiation![1]

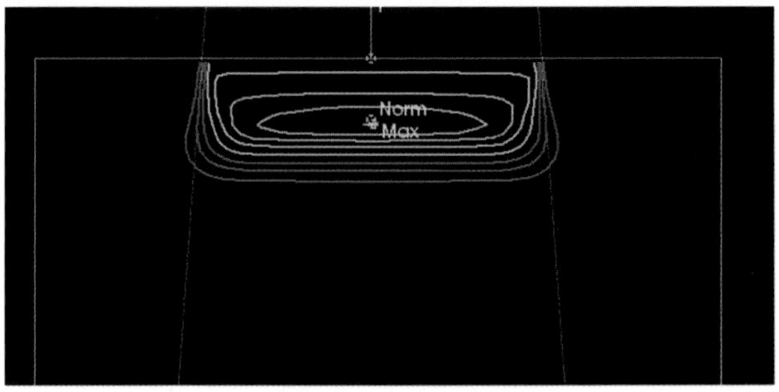

Figure 26.3 *Electron isodose chart.*

The absorption process for low-energy X-rays is called the photoelectric effect. The incident X-ray interacts with an inner orbital electron shell of an atom within the absorbing material. The energy of the X-ray is transferred to the electron as kinetic energy that causes the electron to be ejected from its orbit shell, and the X-ray to be dissipated. The ejected electron is now known as a 'fast electron'. These fast electrons can ionize other atoms in the absorbing material, breaking chemical bonds and initiating a sequence of changes that is ultimately expressed as biological damage. Mathematically, in this interaction, the energy absorbed is proportional to the cube of the atomic number (Z) of the material through which the beam passes.

The photoelectric effect is the major X-ray absorption process for diagnostic radiology. Absorption is preferential in bone because of its relatively high atomic number (Z), and this gives the characteristic white X-ray appearance of bone on standard diagnostic films (as X-rays fail to reach and blacken the photoemulsion). This characteristic of the photoelectric effect is a disadvantage when used for radiotherapy, as bone and cartilage have a relatively high Z, and preferential absorption in these structures can cause radionecrosis. Due to the combination of poor penetration in tissue, the maximum deposition of energy in the skin and the preferential absorption in bone and cartilage, these lower energy X-rays are no longer routinely used except for the treatment of some skin and superficial cancers.

The absorption interaction for photons in the commonest therapy range of 1–10 MV is the Compton effect. In this interaction, the incident photon interacts with a more loosely bound outer electron in the atoms of the absorbing material. The photon gives up part of its energy to the electron as kinetic energy as before, and, deflected from its original path, proceeds through the material with corresponding decreased energy. The result of this interaction is also an ejected fast electron, which can ionize other atoms in the absorber. The deflected photon continues on its new path, interacting with further outer orbital electrons until all its energy is dissipated. Unlike the photoelectric effect, the Compton process is independent of the atomic number of the absorbing material, and photons are not preferentially absorbed in bone and cartilage.

At treatment energies in excess of 10 MV, pair production predominates. The incident photon interacts with the nucleus of an atom, giving up all its energy in the process. This results in the production of a positron and a fast electron. The fast electron can go on to produce tissue ionizations, and the positron is quickly annihilated. Positron annihilation occurs as a further interaction with an adjacent electron of the absorbing material. This creates two new photons of 0.51 MeV energy each, both capable of producing additional tissue ionizations. Pair production, like the photoelectric effect, is also dependent on atomic number.

The resultant biological damage from fast electrons produced by all three different processes occurs in two ways. Direct ionization of atoms within target molecules may be produced, leading to chemical bond breakage and initiating the chain of events which leads to biological change. This is the dominant process when neutrons or alpha particles are used to irradiate tissues. X-rays and gamma rays interact mainly with target biological molecules in an indirect way. The interaction is initially with other atoms and molecules within the cells to produce free radicals. These are highly reactive molecules with an unpaired electron in the outer orbital shell and are

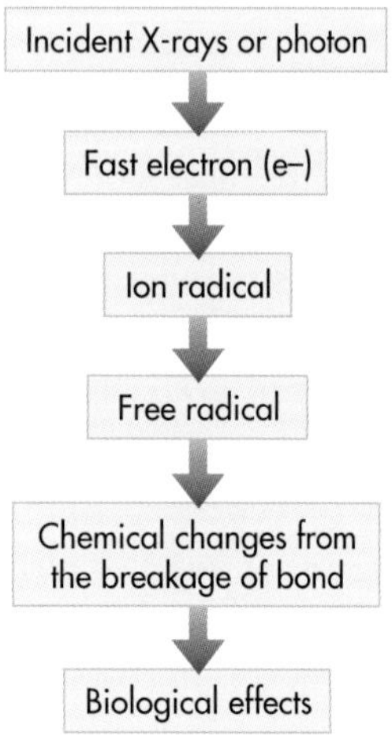

Figure 26.4 *Adapted from Hall*[1].

able to diffuse far enough to reach and damage the critical targets.

Since approximately 80% of a cell is composed of water, it is necessary to consider what happens when radiation interacts with a water molecule. As a result of the interaction with a photon, the water molecule may become ionized:

$$H_2O \rightarrow H_2O^+ + e^-$$

H_2O^+ is an ion radical – it is an ion because it is charged, and a free radical because it has an unpaired electron in its outer shell. It is a highly reactive species with a very short lifespan in the order of nanoseconds. The ion radical can then interact with another water molecule to form the highly reactive hydroxyl radical (OH):

$$H_2O^+ + H_2O \rightarrow H_3O^+ + OH^\bullet$$

It is estimated that about two-thirds of the damage to biological targets from X-rays is produced by hydroxyl radicals. Free radicals can be inactivated by combining with sulphydryl molecules, or they may interact with oxygen and form a highly reactive product, and by so doing, the damage may be fixed (that is, made permanent). The interaction process is summarized in Figure 26.4.

Regardless of whether radiation effects occur due to the direct or indirect interaction, the main biological target in tissues is believed to be DNA. Such interactions result in changes in DNA chemistry, leading to breaks within one or both helical strands. A single-strand break within DNA may be recognized and repaired, as the complementary DNA strand is still present to act as a template. When several ionizations occur in close proximity, a double-strand DNA break may occur. It is thought that double-strand breaks are the lethal lesions that result in cell kill due to the inability of the cell to repair both damaged strands of DNA simultaneously.

Apart from the physical characteristics of radiation beams, there are a number of other important features relating to cells and tissues themselves that influence their response to radiotherapy. These features are discussed below.

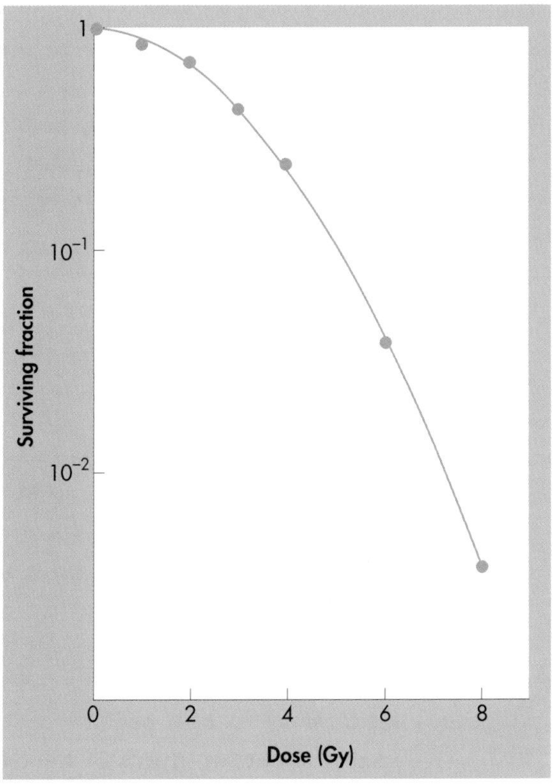

Figure 26.5 *Clonogenic cell survival curve following radiation. A typical surviving fraction at 2 Gy is 0.6 with higher doses producing a lower surviving fraction (courtesy of Dr Gillian Duchesne).*

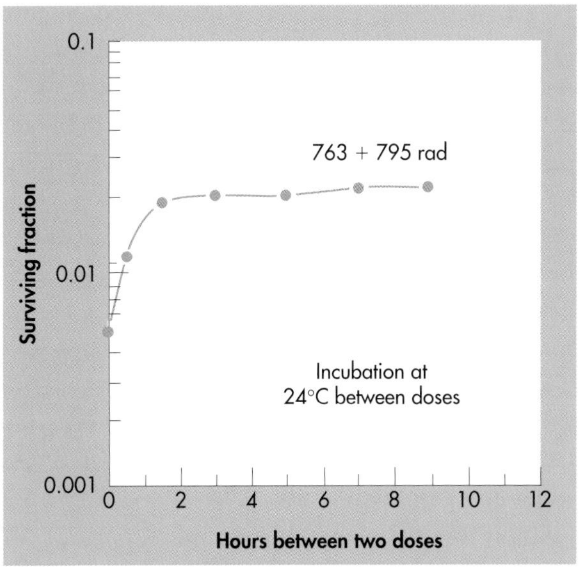

Figure 26.6 *Survival of Chinese hamster cells exposed to two fractions of X-rays with various time intervals between the two and incubated at room temperature. As the time interval is increased, the surviving fraction increases until at about 2 hours, a plateau is reached corresponding to a surviving fraction of 0.02 * (from Elkind et al[3]).*

RADIOBIOLOGY

Radiobiology is the study of the actions of ionizing radiation on living things. The effects of radiation on both normal and malignant tissues evolve through a series of steps. This begins with the physical absorption of energy and ends with the biological effect, which results principally from damage to DNA. Classical radiobiology promotes the 'four Rs' of the radiation response: *r*epair, *r*eoxygenation, *r*eassortment and *r*epopulation.[2]

The development of tissue culture techniques has contributed enormously to our understanding of radiobiology in ways that are not possible to achieve in patients. With such techniques, it is possible to observe the effects of radiation on cells in vitro. The cell survival curve is a cornerstone of in vitro radiobiology and describes the relationship between radiation dose and the proportion of cells surviving. Survival refers to the ability of a single cell to proliferate indefinitely to produce a large clone or colony. Such a cell is said to be clonogenic. Tumour cells are clonogenic, and if one cell survives after a course of radiotherapy, this may be sufficient for the tumour to regrow.

Repair

Radiation damage to mammalian cells can be divided into the following three categories:

1. Lethal damage – this is irreversible and irreparable, leading irrevocably to cell death.
2. Sublethal damage (SLD) – this is damage that under normal circumstances can be repaired over a number of hours. SLD repair is inferred by the increase in survival observed when a dose of radiation is split into two fractions separated by a time interval.
3. Potentially lethal damage (PLD) – this refers to the component of radiation damage that can be modified by post-irradiation environmental conditions.

The ability of cells to repair SLD was recognized by Elkind and colleagues, who demonstrated that the survival of Chinese hamster cells treated with a single dose of radiation was lower than that of cells given the same total dose of radiation, but split into two fractions separated by 30 minutes.[3]

The radiosensitivity of cells also varies with the phases of the cell cycle (as illustrated in Figure 26.7). Cells located in the S phase of the cell cycle are said to be relatively radioresistant, while those in the G2 or M phase are said to be radiosensitive. In the experiments by Elkind et al[3] described above, most of the surviving cells from the first dose of radiation were located in the S phase. When a second dose of radiation was given after an interval of 6 hours, this cohort of cells had progressed around the cell cycle and was now in the G2 or M phase (more sensitive) at the time of the second dose (reassortment). If the increase in radiosensitivity in moving from late S to the G2-M period exceeds the effect of SLD repair, the surviving fraction will fall. In human tissues, the time intervals for cell cycles and SLD repair are generally less well defined, but maximal recovery appears to be complete after 4–6 hours.

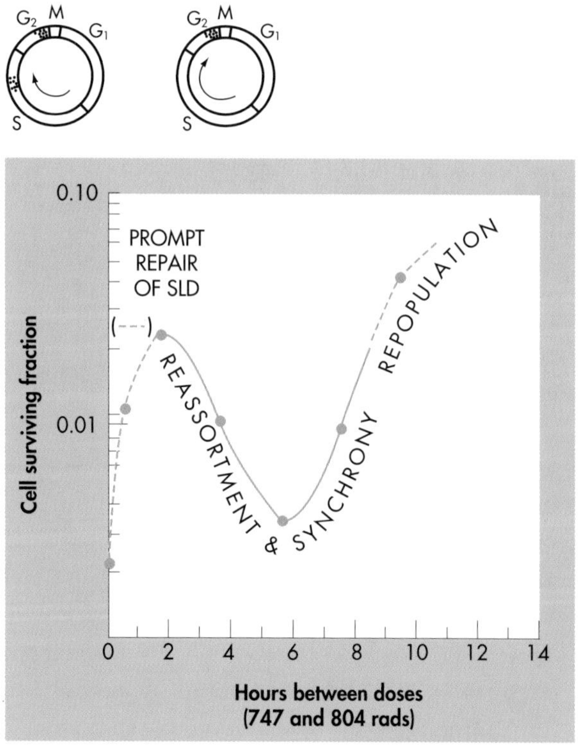

Figure 26.7 *Survival of Chinese hamster cells exposed to two fractions of X-rays with various time intervals between the two doses. This also illustrates three of the four Rs of radiobiology (courtesy of Hall[1] and redrawn from Elkind et al[3]).*

When the interval between the split doses is 10–12 hours, there is an increase in the surviving fraction due to cell division (repopulation) because this time interval exceeds the length of the cell cycle of these rapidly growing cells. This simple in vitro experiment illustrates three of the four 'Rs of radiobiology': *r*epair, *r*eassortment and *r*epopulation.

The duration of the cell cycle and the ability of cells to repair SLD varies not only between different normal tissues but also between normal tissues and tumours. Normal tissues may be divided into those that are considered 'early responding', such as skin, mucosal epithelium and bone marrow and those that are 'late responding', such as the spinal cord and central nervous system tissue. Most tumours behave as early-responding tissues. Early-responding tissues are triggered to proliferate within a few weeks of starting a fractionated course of radiotherapy and the tissue damage, such as skin desquamation or tumour shrinkage, will become apparent during the course of treatment. However, a conventional course of radiotherapy of 6–7 weeks is never long enough to trigger proliferation in late-responding tissues; consequently, radiation effects on these tissues may not become apparent for months to years after the treatment.

Various mathematical models have been used to describe the shape of the cell-survival curve and are useful for the theoretical interpretation of observed experimental changes. The linear-quadratic (α/β) model is one model where alpha (α) measures the probability of causing lethal damage by a single event (such as a double-stranded DNA break), and β estimates the probability of cell death from the interaction between two separate sublethal events. (α is a measure of the width of the shoulder of the curve while β (beta) indicates the curviness of the curve). It is the ratio of α/β (that is, the dose at which cell killing by linear [α] and quadratic [β] components is equal), rather than the individual values of each, which determines how tissues behave to changes in fractionation. Early-responding tissues and most tumours have a high α/β ratio (10–30 Gy), indicating that they are relatively insensitive to changes in radio-

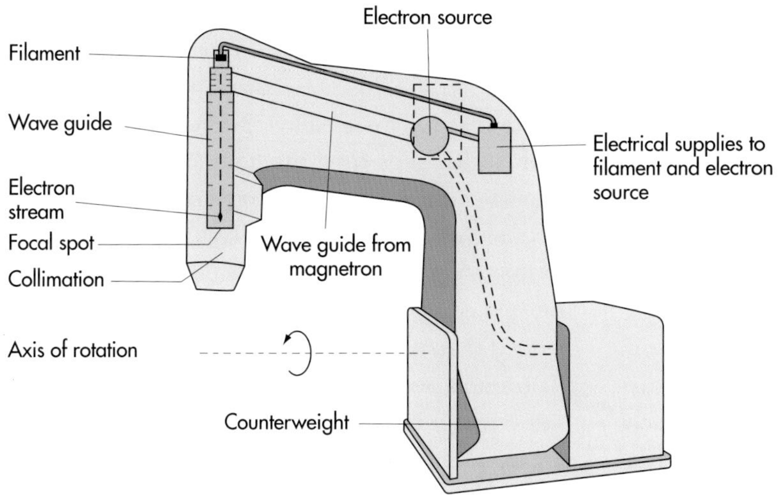

Figure 26.8 *A simulator. This is a diagnostic X-ray unit which has an image intensifier linked to a closed-circuit television for the purpose of screening. It can reproduce treatment conditions.*

therapy fractionation. Late-responding tissues have a low α/β ratio (1–4 Gy), indicating a higher degree of sensitivity to fractionation changes. By altering fractionation, it is possible to produce a differential in cell kill between tumours and late-responding normal tissues, modifying the therapeutic index (that is, the tumour response for a fixed level of normal-tissue damage).

Most tumours arise from epithelial cells and have a fairly high α/β ratio (10–25 Gy). Tissues which give rise to late reactions (months or years) in radiotherapy have relatively low α/β ratios, and changes in fractionation can be made that improve the therapeutic ratio.

Reoxygenation

The importance of a good blood supply for radiosensitivity was first recognized by Mottram in 1924.[4] Further work by Thoday and Reed[5] demonstrated that the proportion of chromosome aberrations resulting from irradiation of root tips in oxygen was three times greater than those seen when irradiation was carried out in nitrogen. They concluded that the availability of oxygen is a very important factor in the production of radiation-induced chromosome aberrations. Experiments by Thomlinson and Gray[6] and Tannock[7] led to the conclusion that cells were present in only two states which have radiobiological significance – oxygenated and hypoxic. Tumour cells closest to blood vessels are generally well oxygenated, and those at a distance greater than the oxygen-diffusion capacity are hypoxic.

Acute as well as chronic hypoxia occurs within tumours; intermittent blood flow within abnormal tumour vasculature was shown to be a cause of acute hypoxia and variability in radiation response by Chaplin et al in 1986.[8] The proportion of hypoxic cells within solid tumours may vary considerably, depending on the tumour type. Although a dynamic process, the hypoxic fraction is thought to remain relatively constant within a given tumour. Immediately after a radiation exposure, remaining viable cells are more likely to be hypoxic, as the well-oxygenated cells die. Over the following hours, oxygen diffuses into these previously hypoxic areas and reoxygenation occurs. The cells are now more sensitive to the next radiation exposure, and the whole process is repeated again. Over a fractionated radiotherapy schedule of several weeks, it is likely that most cells will receive some radiation exposure while in the oxygenated state. Efforts to overcome tumour hypoxia have dominated radiobiological research for the past 40 years. The approaches investigated have included hyperbaric oxygen and hypoxic-cell radiosensitizing drugs, such as misonidazole, but they have met with only limited success.

Reassortment

Cellular radiosensitivity varies with the phase of the cell cycle, as discussed earlier. Radiation damage to DNA is frequently not expressed until cell division. Cells which are in the G0 (resting) phase or only in a very slow cell cycle will not express damage immediately. The length of the cell cycle for most rapidly dividing tumours is approximately 24 hours. In such tumours, the interval between fractions of radiation may be critical to the cell kill achieved, as radiation sensitivity varies by at least twofold through the cycle. A single radiation exposure will eliminate the sensitive cells (G2 and M phase) while the survivors are predominantly in a resistant phase of the cycle (late S).

During the interval between fractions, this surviving cohort will move into G2 and M (that is, more sensitive), a process termed 'reassortment'. While this is relatively easy to demonstrate and manipulate in vitro, it has been difficult to exploit in routine clinical practice.

Repopulation

During a course of fractionated radiotherapy, viable tumour cells continue to divide and repopulate the tumour. Repopulation is an important process for early-responding normal tissues, such as the gut and bone marrow. A protracted, fractionated regimen helps to spare these normal tissues but may compromise tumour cure. Treatment with radiation or cytotoxic drugs can trigger surviving clonagens in a tumour to divide faster than tumour cells in an unperturbed state. This is known as accelerated repopulation. There is evidence that this phenomenon may occur in human tumours. Withers et al[9] used the published literature on radiotherapy for head and neck cancer to estimate the dose of radiation required to achieve local control in 50% of cases (tumour control dose$_{50}$ [TCD$_{50}$]). The analysis suggests that clonogen repopulation in this type of cancer accelerates at about day 28 after treatment begins. A dose increment of about 0.6 Gy per day is thought to be required to compensate for this repopulation. In clinical practice, the dose of radiation per fraction is not usually increased after day 28, provided there are no unscheduled gaps over the course of the treatment. Cancers of the bladder, head and neck, and cervix are tumours where gaps or delays in treatment are thought to have considerable significance for overall tumour control probability. It has been recommended that, if gaps in treatment occur in these types of tumours, some form of compensation is required to ensure tumour control is not compromised.[10] This may involve increasing the dose per fraction for part or all of the remaining treatment or hyperfractionation, where two fractions are given on the same day with an interfraction interval of at least 6 hours.

PRINCIPLES OF RADIOTHERAPY TREATMENT

Radiation is an important modality for the treatment of cancer and can be used with radical, adjuvant or palliative intent. The principles of radiotherapy treatment planning and delivery are discussed below, with examples relevant to urology.

Radical radiotherapy aims to deliver a tumouricidal treatment dose to a well-defined target volume with curative intent, sparing the surrounding normal tissues as much as possible. A fractionated course of radical radiotherapy is usually given over 6–7 weeks for early tumours of the bladder or prostate.

Adjuvant radiotherapy is used to reduce the risk of tumour recurrence after primary surgery. The aim of treatment is to eradicate occult micrometastatic disease that cannot be demonstrated on imaging, as occurs in a significant percentage of patients. An example of this is prophylactic para-aortic radiotherapy after orchidectomy for stage I seminoma. Adjuvant treatment in this setting reduces relapse rates from approximately 20% to 3–4%.[11]

Palliative radiotherapy can be used to alleviate symptoms of local disease (such as haematuria) or distant metastases (such as bone pain). Treatment is usually given with a small number of fractions, and effective results can also be achieved with a single fraction of radiotherapy.

RADIOTHERAPY PLANNING

The initial phase of any radiotherapy is treatment planning, during which the following parameters are defined:

- patient position and immobilization
- definition of treatment volumes
- choice of technique
- calculation of dose distribution.

Patient position and immobilization

The treatment position of the patient must be accurately reproducible throughout radiotherapy. Variation in daily positioning can alter external and internal anatomy of the patient, leading to underdosage of the tumour or overdosage of the surrounding normal tissues.

Accurate patient set-up on the planning machine is achieved by aligning fixed, wall-mounted lasers to certain anatomical reference points such as bony landmarks or permanent skin tattoos applied during planning. An identical alignment system is then used on the treatment machine, ensuring that patient set-up is fully reproducible. Treatment position varies with different tumour sites, but, for urological tumours, the patient is usually supine. Tumours of the prostate are usually treated with a full bladder to keep the small intestine out of the field. Bladder tumours are treated with the bladder empty to keep the treatment volume as small as possible.

A range of immobilization devices are available to prevent patient movement during treatment. These include perspex masks for tumours of the head or neck and vacuum-moulded bags of polystyrene beads for trunk immobilization.

Definition of treatment volumes

In delivery of radiotherapy treatment, parameters such as volume and dose have to be specified for the purposes of prescription, recording and reporting. This has been standardized by the International Committee of Radiation Units and Measurements (ICRU), allowing national and international comparison of treatments between different centres.[12] This report defines the concepts of GTV (gross tumour volume), CTV (clinical target volume) and PTV (planning target volume).

The GTV is the demonstrable macroscopic extent of the tumour. To encompass subclinical or microscopic disease, one adds a margin to the GTV, and this volume is defined as the CTV. During a course of radiotherapy, there may be technical and physiological variations which can cause movement of the CTV. In order to ensure that the prescribed dose is delivered to the CTV for every fraction of treatment, a further margin is added to form the PTV. This is a combination of a set-up margin (SM) to allow for variation in patient positioning and an internal margin (IM) to account for normal organ movement.

Localization of the target volume

The target volume for internal tumours is usually localized by plain X-rays on a machine called a simulator (conventional planning) or a computerized tomography (CT) scanner with an integrated computerized planning system (CT planning). A simulator is a diagnostic X-ray machine used to reproduce the exact treatment arrangement for any megavoltage therapy machine. It has the facility for screening by an image intensifier linked to a closed-circuit television. In the simulator, the target volume is localized by using both clinical information (staging results, surface anatomy and palpable masses) and radiological information (image intensifier views and staging diagnostic X-rays). The conventional method of planning a bladder cancer, for example, involves the introduction of contrast into the bladder through a

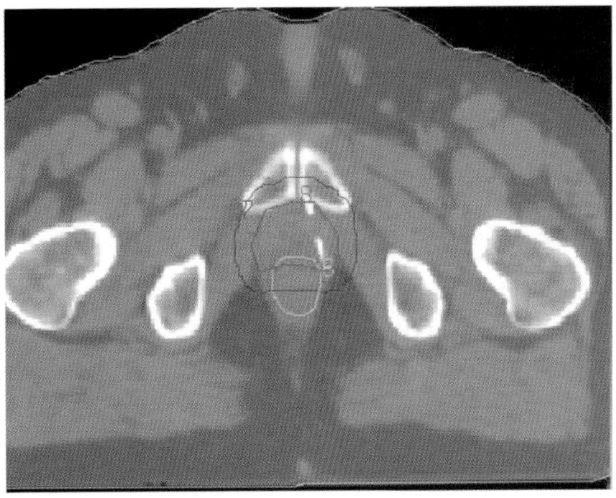

Figure 26.9 *A CT slice through the centre of the target volume of a prostate, showing the GTV, PTV and rectum.*

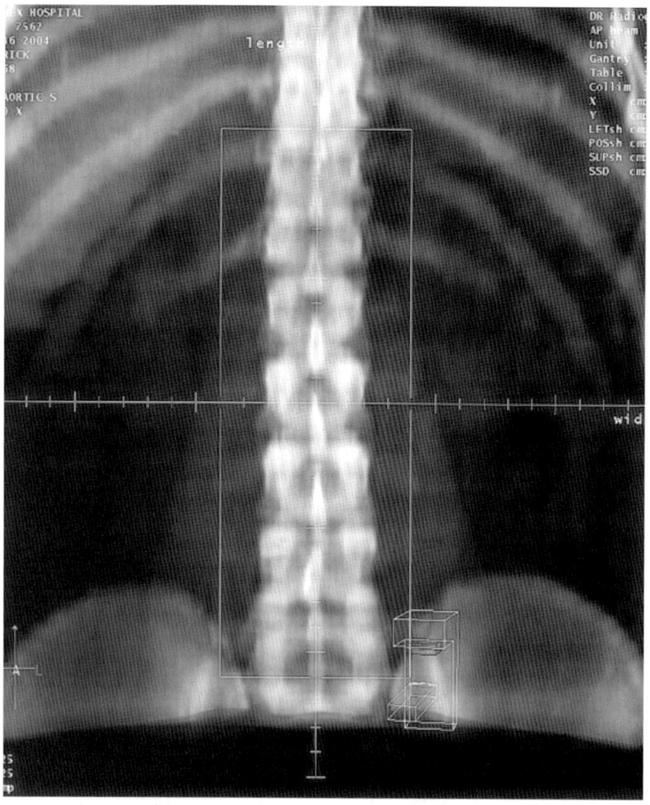

Figure 26.10 *An AP film from the planning CT scanner, showing field margins for para-aortic lymph-node irradiation.*

urinary catheter. Anteroposterior and lateral X-ray films are then taken on the simulator, and these are then used to outline the target volume.

The principles of CT planning are the same as conventional planning, but there is the added advantage of providing more anatomical detail about the tumour and surrounding normal tissues. This can increase the accuracy of the target volume definition, and up to 80% of patients may benefit from this approach. CT localization is now widely used for planning of prostate and bladder tumours.

Choice of technique

In addition to the target volumes defined above, the other important considerations in the choice of technique are the types of normal tissues within the proposed treatment volume. During a course of radiotherapy, it is inevitable that both the tumour and normal tissues will be irradiated. There is considerable variation in the tolerance of different normal tissues to radiotherapy, and this is a major determinant of both the total dose that can be delivered and the treatment technique. It is also usual to outline and identify the important normal tissues within the target volume as well as the tumour.

The simplest technique for treatment is a single radiation field (see isodose chart, Figure 26.3). This is often used for palliative therapy, such as treatment of bone metastases. Another simple arrangement is the use of two opposing parallel fields (anterior and posterior or two lateral fields). This produces a more even dose distribution throughout the irradiated area than a single field, and the combination of fields allows greater penetration at depth. This technique is used for the prophylactic treatment of the para-aortic lymph nodes in stage 1 seminoma (Figure 26.11).

For radical treatment of the prostate or bladder, it is necessary to use higher treatment doses than for seminoma, which is a very radiosensitive disease. More complex beam arrangements are required (often three or four fields) to allow the greatest sparing of normal tissues while maximizing the tumour dose.

Recent technological developments have led to the introduction of conformal radiotherapy, which allow closer, more accurate irradiation of irregularly shaped tumour volumes. Treatment beams are produced within the machine that conform much more closely to the shape of the target volume. This produces greater sparing of normal tissues, and higher doses of radiation can be delivered to the tumour without increasing side effects.[13]

Another recent development is intensity-modulated radiotherapy (IMRT), which allows closer matching of treatment doses to tumour volumes. Rather than having a single or a few radiation beams, the radiation with IMRT is effectively broken into thousands of tiny, pencil-thin beams. These enter the body from many different angles and all converge on the tumour. This produces a high tumour dose and a lower dose to surrounding normal tissues.

Calculation of the dose distribution

Once the PTV and important normal organs are localized, a dose distribution across the target volume is calculated. This is usually now done with computer software that manipulates dose data measured directly from treatment machines. ICRU 50 specifies a maximum variation of dose distribution of from –5% to 7% in dose across the PTV. The dose to the normal tissues is also checked to ensure their tolerance is not exceeded.

Treatment delivery

Once an acceptable treatment plan has been agreed upon, planning information is transferred to the treatment machine, and therapy is started. An essential part of all treatment is verification of the planning set-up, which is achieved by comparison of X-rays taken during simulation and treatment. Therapy doses may also be checked directly during treatment by measurements from the patient. The entire process from planning to verification of treatment delivery is governed by the principles of quality assurance. These define procedures that test all the technical aspects of radiotherapy systems in order to eliminate any inaccuracy or deficiency leading to suboptimal treatments, and must be a routine part of treatment.

Side effects of treatment

The side effects of radiotherapy may be divided into those that occur during or within a few weeks of treatment (acute reactions) and those that occur months to years later (late reactions). The severity of side effects depends principally upon the normal tissues present in the treatment field, total dose and dose per fraction of treatment given. It is important to realize that the radiobiological principles defined in the previous section of the chapter are the basis for both the desirable therapeutic effects and the undesirable side effects that occur during a course of treatment.

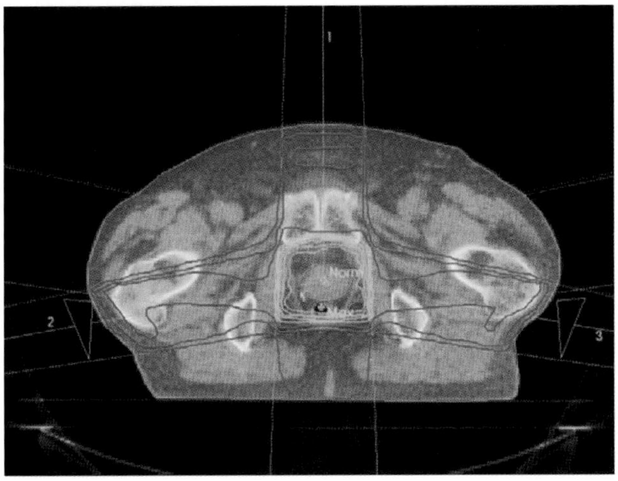

Figure 26.11 *A three-field plan of the prostate showing an anterior and two posterior oblique wedged fields.*

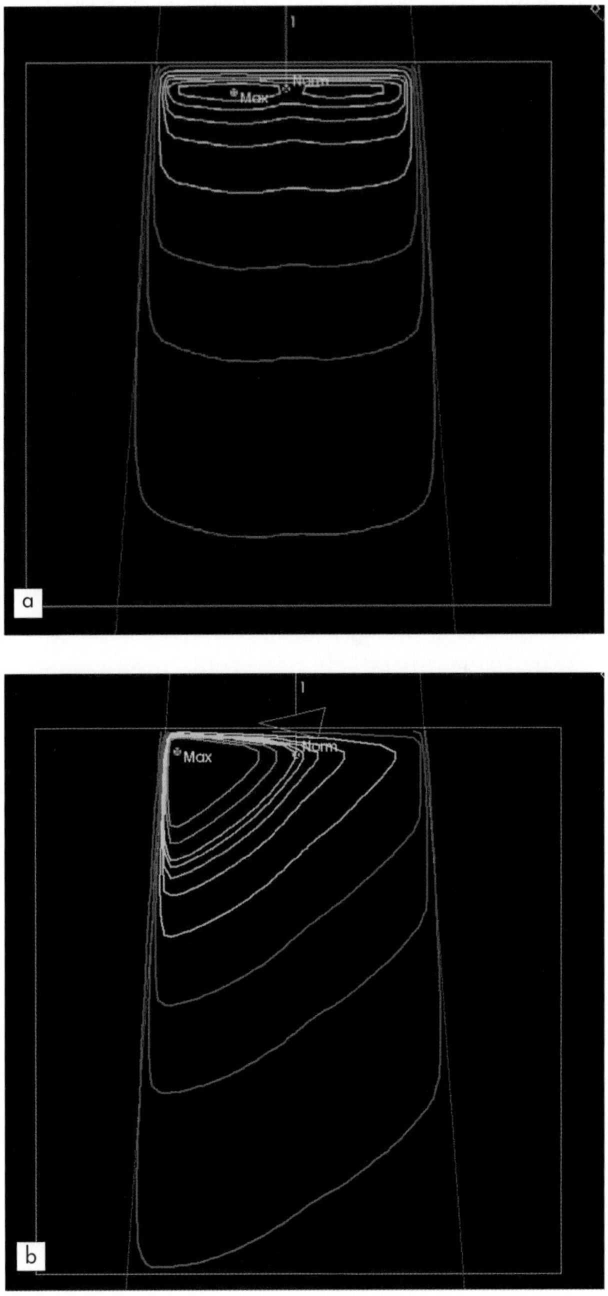

Figure 26.12 *Isodose curves for a 6 MV linear accelerator: (a) open field; (b) wedged field.*

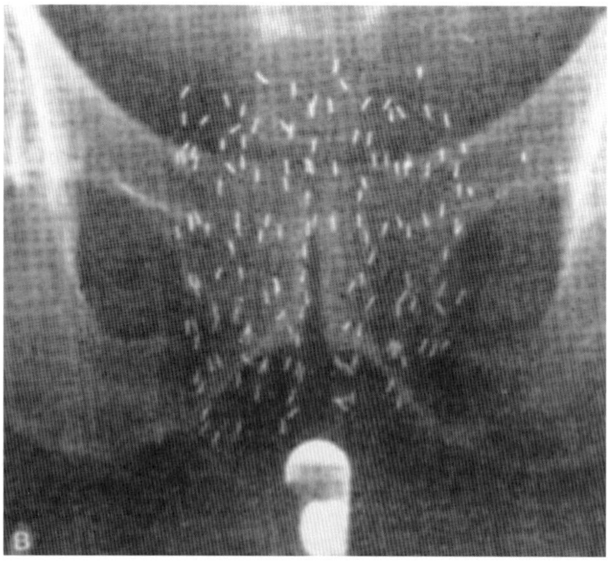

Figure 26.13 *AP simulator film showing the distribution of iodine 125 seeds within the prostate.*

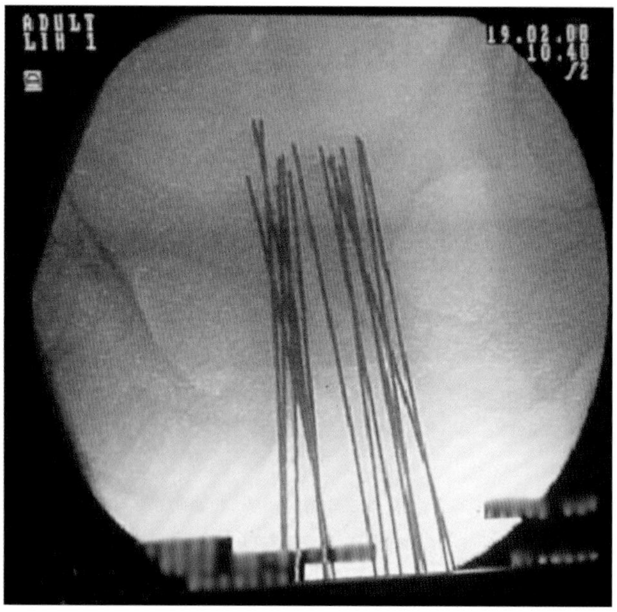

Figure 26.14 *AP film of needles implanted in the prostate for irridium 192 high-dose rate after loading brachytherapy.*

During radical radiotherapy for prostate or bladder cancer, patients principally experience a range of side effects from the normal bladder and bowel within the treatment volume. These may include deterioration of urinary outflow symptoms, haematuria, proctitis and diarrhoea. They are generally the effects of radiation on the normal acute-reacting tissues in the treatment volume. Acute side effects such as these are usually self-limiting, and generally resolve within 6–8 weeks after completing treatment. They can usually be successfully managed with supportive care during radiotherapy.

The late effects of radiotherapy are usually more serious and may be irreversible. For pelvic radiotherapy, these local late effects include bladder fibrosis, chronic proctitis and impotence. Radiation carcinogenesis is another late effect that occurs within the site of the treatment volume and is believed to be due to radiation-induced genetic damage to normal tissues. It tends to occur after other late effects and often carries a poor prognosis. In all radiotherapy treatments, the balance to be achieved lies between the desired beneficial effects (cure or palliation) and the level of acute and late effects that can be tolerated by the treated individual.

Brachytherapy

Brachytherapy has been used in the treatment of urological cancer for over 90 years, but it experienced a renaissance for the treatment of prostate cancer in the 1980s.[14] This was due to improved prostatic imaging with transrectal ultrasound and technological advances in computerized planning systems, allowing better dosimetry and more accurate treatment.

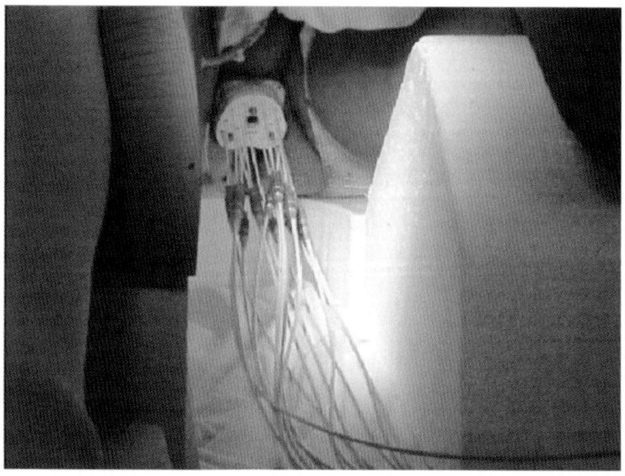

Figure 26.15 *A patient in the lithotomy position attached to the microselectron unit while undergoing irridium 192 high-dose rate after loading brachytherapy.*

The planning principles for brachytherapy are the same as for external beam treatments (that is, patient immobilization, definition of treatment volumes, choice of technique and calculation of the dose distribution).

Brachytherapy can be used as a single modality to deliver a radical treatment alone (such as low-dose-rate ^{125}I seed brachytherapy) or in combination with external beam radiotherapy to deliver a boost treatment (such as high-dose-rate ^{192}Ir brachytherapy).

Permanent iodine seed brachytherapy

Treatment with ^{125}I seeds is indicated for patients with low-grade, organ-confined tumours with a small volume (less than 50 cm^3) and no previous transurethral surgery. Treatment has two stages, planning and therapy, both carried out with the patient in the lithotomy position under anaesthetic. Planning involves a transrectal, ultrasound-guided, prostatic volume study that is done with reference to a fixable perineal positioning template. The relationship of the prostate to the surface template allows the exact number and position of each iodine seed to be planned and calculated with precision. In the second stage of the treatment, applicator needles are inserted transperineally through the template into the corresponding planned position within the prostate. The iodine seeds are then inserted and the applicator needles withdrawn. A typical implant involves 60–120 seeds, depending on prostatic volume and individual seed activity. The aim of treatment is to deliver a dose of 160 Gy to the volume before the radioactivity of the seeds falls to very low levels.

High-dose-rate ^{192}Ir brachytherapy

Temporary ^{192}Ir implants can be used in combination with external beam radiotherapy to escalate the dose to the prostate without significantly increasing normal tissue morbidity.[15] The aim is improved local tumour control, and this treatment is mainly used for higher-grade or locally advanced tumours. The implant procedure is similar to iodine seed therapy with a perineal template and applicator needles. In this case, instead of iodine seeds which deliver the dose of radiation over many days, a very high-activity (high-dose-rate) radioactive iridium source is used to deliver treatment over a period of minutes. Flexible tubes link the template and applicator needles to a remote after-loading machine containing the iridium source.

The iridium is driven under computer control into each successive applicator needle and moved within the needle in small steps for predetermined time periods. This allows the total dose of treatment to the prostate to be built up over three to four fractionated treatments, usually given over 2 days. There is also an advantage in allowing the dose to be optimized for the final resting position of each applicator needle in relation to all the others. At completion of treatment, the needles and template are removed, and the patient proceeds to external beam radiotherapy after a 2-week break.

REFERENCES

1. Hall EJ. The physics and chemistry of radiation absorption. In: Hall EJ. Radiobiology for the Radiologist. Philadelphia: Lippincott, Williams and Wilkins, 1994: 1–14
2. Withers HR. The four R's of radiotherapy. Adv Radiat Biol 1975; 5: 241–247
3. Elkind MM, Sutton-Gilbert H, Moses WB, Alescio T et al. Radiation response of mammalian cells in culture. V. Temperature dependence of the repair of X-ray damage in surviving cells (aerobic and hypoxic). Radiat Res 1965; 25: 359–376
4. Mottram JC. On the skin reactions to radium exposure and their avoidance in radiotherapy: an experimental investigation. Br J Radiol 1924; May: 1–8
5. Thoday JM, Reed J. Effect of oxygen on the frequency of chromosome aberrations produced by X-rays. Nature 1947; 160: 119
6. Tomlinson RH, Gray LH. The histological structure of some human lung cancers and the possible implications for radiotherapy. Br J Cancer 1955; 9: 539–549
7. Tannock IF. The relation between cell proliferation and the vascular system in a transplanted mouse mammary tumour. Br J Cancer 1968; 22: 258–273
8. Chaplin DJ, Durand RE, Olive PL. Acute hypoxia in tumours: implications for modifiers of radiation effects. Int J Radiat Oncol Biol Phys 1986; 12: 1279–1282
9. Withers HR, Taylor JMG, Maciejewski B. Treatment volume and tissue tolerance. Int J Radiat Oncol Biol Phys 1988; 14: 751–759

10. Royal College of Radiologists. Guidelines for the Management of the Unscheduled Interruption or Prolongation of a Radical Course of Radiotherapy. London: 1996
11. Fossa SD, Horwich A, Russell JM, et al. Medical Research Council Testicular Tumour Working Party. Optimal planning target volume for stage I testicular seminoma; an MRC randomised trial. J Clin Oncol 1999; 17: 1146–1154
12. International Commission on Radiation Units and Measurements. Prescribing, recording and reporting photon beam therapy. ICRU 50. Washington, DC: International Commission on Radiation Units and Measurements, 1993
13. Dearnaley DP, Khoo VS, Norman AR, Mayer L et al. Comparison of radiation side-effects of conformal and conventional radiotherapy in prostate cancer: a randomised trial. Lancet 1999; 353: 267–272
14. Holm HH, Juul N, Pedersen JF. Transperineal 125-iodine seed implantation in prostatic cancer guided by transrectal ultrasonography. J Urol 1983; 130: 283–286
15. Mate TP, Gottesman JE, Hatton J, Gribble M et al. High dose-rate after loading irridium 192 prostate brachytherapy: feasibility report. Int J Radiat Oncol Biol Phys 1998; 41: 525–533

FURTHER READING

Radiation physics

Williams JR, Thwaite DI, eds. Radiotherapy Physics in Practice. Oxford: Oxford University Press, 2000

Radiobiology

Steel GG. Basic Clinical Radiobiology. London: Arnold, 1997

Radiotherapy planning

Dobbs J, Barrett A, Ash D. Practical Radiotherapy Planning. London: Arnold, 1999

27

Principles of chemotherapy

Judith Gaffan and John Bridgewater

INTRODUCTION

Two-thirds of patients with cancer will develop metastatic or advanced disease during their illness. The most appropriate management for metastatic disease is systemic treatment, and this is most commonly chemotherapy. The possibility of a systemic therapy for cancer has been observed anecdotally for some time – in 1875, Cutler and Bradford induced remission in a patient with chronic myeloid leukaemia by treatment with arsenic.[1] During World War I, soldiers who died of mustard gas poisoning (Figure 27.1) were noted to have aplastic bone marrow, suggesting a cytotoxic effect of mustard,[2] and, in 1946, Goodman and colleagues[3] successfully demonstrated that the cytotoxic effects of the nitrogen mustard could be put to therapeutic use, in the treatment of a mouse transplanted with lymphosarcoma. The first cancer to be cured by chemotherapy was choriocarcinoma, which has been cured with single-agent methotrexate since the 1950s.

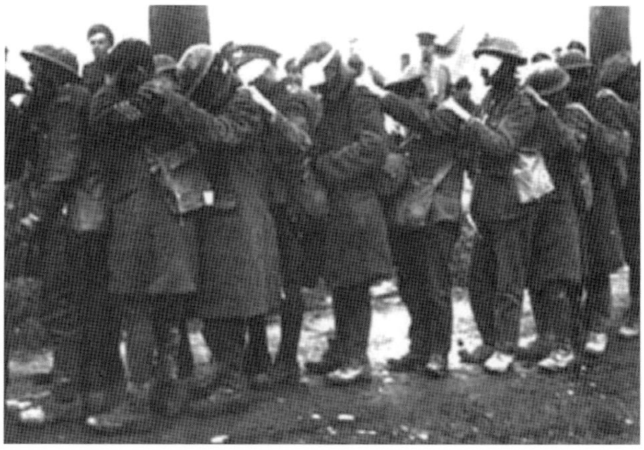

Figure 27.1 *Soldiers suffering from mustard gas poisoning in World War I. Photograph courtesy of the Imperial War Museum, London (IWM Q 11586).*

In this chapter, the pharmacological, molecular, and biological basis of systemic anticancer treatment will be discussed, as well as some of the practical issues surrounding the administration of chemotherapy. Recent research has concentrated on improving response rates by the development of new drugs and better supportive care.

CYTOKINETICS

The study of cytokinetics is central to oncological practice, because attempts to control or eradicate malignant cells are based on the central dogma that cells which are dividing more rapidly are usually more sensitive to chemotherapy.[4] Choriocarcinomas and teratomas double in cell number in under 1 month and are cured in more than 80% of cases, but colonic carcinomas double in over 3 months and are often resistant to chemotherapy.[5–7] The relationship between cell-doubling time and prognosis is not simple. For many types of tumour, markers of high cell proliferation correlate with poor prognosis, possibly because faster-growing cells repopulate rapidly between treatments.

Tumour growth

The relationship between cell-cycle time and tumour-doubling time is complex (see Figure 27.2). A proportion of cells will be in the G0 or resting phase, because they have differentiated into non-dividing cells, because they are necrotic or apoptotic,

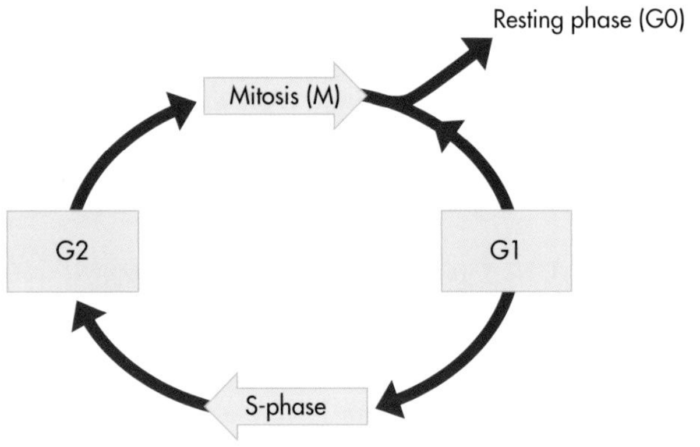

Figure 27.2 *The cell cycle. Cells cycle between synthesis of DNA (S phase) and mitosis or M phase with variable gaps between protein synthesis and cell division (Gap 1 or G1 and Gap 2 or G2). Withdrawal into resting phase (G0) can be reversible or permanent. Progression around the cell cycle is dependent on cyclins and cyclin-dependent kinases.*

or because they are resting. Doubling time is therefore influenced by the growth fraction, the cells lost, and the cell-cycle time.

Tumour growth has been modelled in tissue cultures and animals. The simplest model of tumour growth is exponential cell growth, which assumes that tumour-doubling time is constant, and that, therefore, tumour size will increase exponentially with time (Figure 27.3). An alternative model is gompertzian growth. In this the growth fraction decreases as the tumour size increases, taking into account the effect of increased tumour size on blood supply, nutrients, physical constraints, etc. A gompertzian growth curve is sigmoid in shape[8] and more often accurately reflects the clinical scenario.

Cell killing

There are numerous models of cell killing by treatment, and these are relevant to therapeutics. The first model is fractional cell kill, also known as the Skipper–Schabel–Wilcox model.[9] Assuming that all cells in a tumour are equally sensitive to chemotherapy, and that the tumour is growing exponentially, a given dose of a given drug will kill a constant fraction of the cells. If the treatment is repeated, or if another drug is given alongside the first drug, the two fractional cell kills will be additive (see Figure 27.4). Adjuvant treatment (see later) of micrometastases after surgical removal of primary tumours is based on this hypothesis – the less the tumour load at the start of chemotherapy, the higher is the possibility of eradicating all the tumour and therefore curing patients.

Unfortunately, apparently adequate doses of chemotherapy do not eradicate all tumour cells. The failure to sterilize even small tumours with chemotherapy is largely due to drug resistance. If

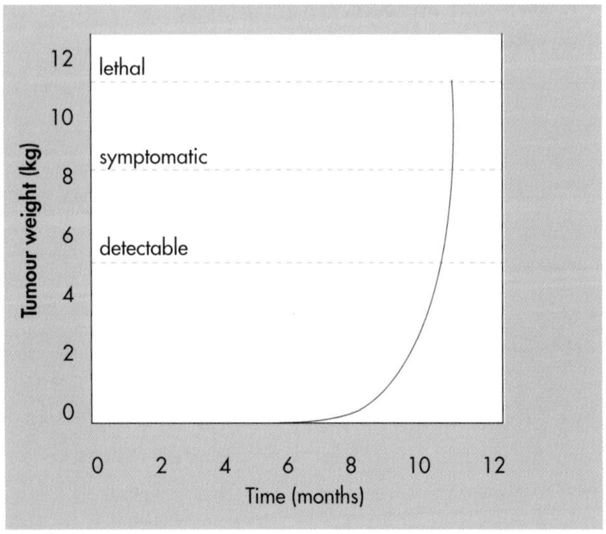

Figure 27.3 *Exponential tumour growth.*

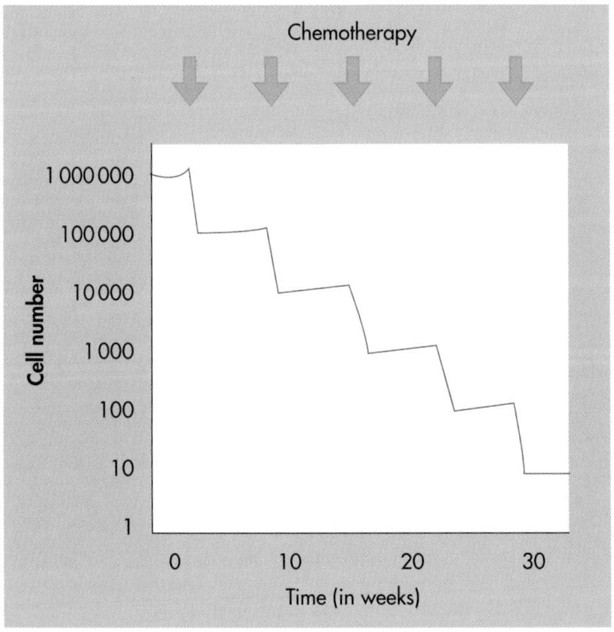

Figure 27.4 *Cell kill.*

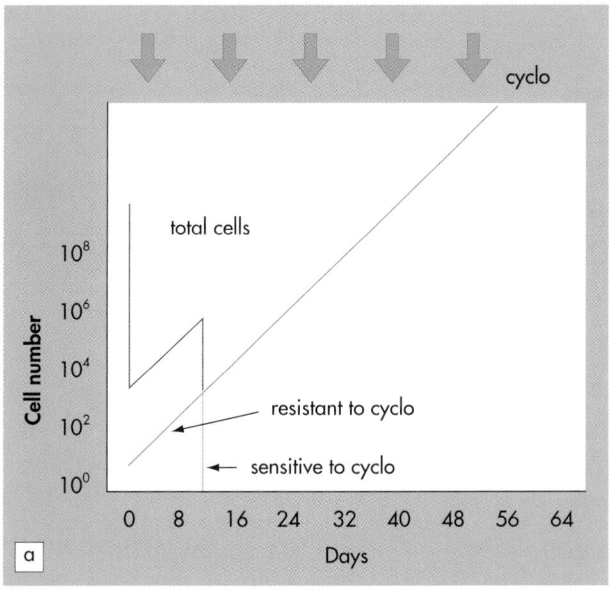

Figure 27.5a *Selection of a resistant clone by single-agent cyclophosphamide chemotherapy (from Goldie and Coldman 1984).*

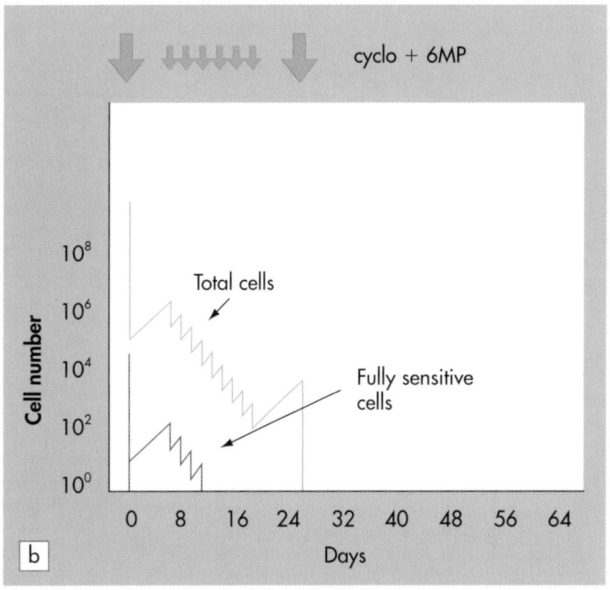

Figure 27.5b *Use of combination chemotherapy to overcome drug resistance.*

all cancers are clonal in origin,[10] one would expect uniform sensitivity to drugs. However, as a tumour grows, spontaneous mutations occur, and some of the cells develop drug resistance. Since this theory was suggested by Goldie and Coldman,[11,12] most chemotherapy regimens include combinations of drugs in an attempt to avoid selecting out resistant cells from a heterogeneous tumour (Figure 27.5).

PHARMACOLOGY

Scheduling and combining drugs correctly is crucial to the success of chemotherapy regimens. For example, some drugs work better when intermittently dosed than when given as continuous infusions.[13–16] Intermittent dosing also allows time for normal tissue recovery between doses, and is therefore both effective and practical. Other drugs, such as 5-fluorouracil (FU), appear to be more effective when given as a long infusion. Toxicity also changes with scheduling. When 5-FU is given as a bolus, is toxicity is predominantly mucositis and neutropenia, whereas as an infusion, it is primarily hand-and-foot syndrome. When combination regimens are being designed, drugs with different mechanisms of action/resistance and dose-limiting toxicities should be combined. All drugs in a regimen should be active as single agents, and interactions should be considered.

Cytotoxic drugs have various mechanisms of action, and some of these are listed in Table 27.1. Some drugs act only on cells which are cycling, and may even be specific to cells in a particular phase of the cell cycle. For example, microtubule poisons such as taxanes act during mitosis and cause metaphase arrest, but alkylating agents are cell-cycle independent. Drug action is not always confined to one class; for example, mitomycin C is primarily an antitumour antibiotic, but it can also alkylate DNA.

DRUG RESISTANCE

Tumour cells may be resistant to drugs for reasons relating to the tumour, the drug, or the host. Some parts of a tumour may have such a poor blood supply that adequate doses of drug cannot reach the cells, and non-cycling cells may escape the cytotoxic effects of some drugs. There are 'sanctuary sites' in the body where cytotoxic drugs cannot penetrate; classically, the central nervous system and the testes. Host characteristics can also cause tumour resistance;[17] for example, if drugs are metabolized very efficiently or not absorbed adequately, the dose

Table 27.1 Mechanisms of action of chemotherapy.

Class of drug	Examples	Target	Mechanism of action
Alkylating agents	Cyclophosphamide, thiotepa, carmustine, cisplatin	DNA	Donate alkyl groups and create DNA cross-links which prevent separation, replication and RNA transcription
Antimetabolites	Methotrexate, cytarabine, fluorouracil, fludarabine	Antifolates; purine and pyrimidine analogues	Resemble normal metabolites for RNA and DNA synthesis; cell cannot differentiate between drug and metabolite, and incorrect formation of RNA/DNA and proteins leads to cell death
Mitotic inhibitors	Vinca alkaloids Taxanes	Microtubules	Disrupt/stabilize microtubules, leading to metaphase arrest
Topoisomerase drugs	Irinotecan/topotecan	Topoisomerase I	Binds to topoisomerase I-DNA cleaveable complex and prevents re-ligation after cleavage
	Etoposide	Topoisomerase II	Produces single-strand breaks in DNA and prevents entry of cells into mitosis
L-asparaginase	L-asparaginase	Protein synthesis	Some tumour cells require l-asparagine, and this enzyme deaminates asparagine
Antibiotics	Doxorubicin (and other anthracyclins)	DNA	Intercalation of drugs into DNA causes untwisting of DNA helix and strand breaks
	Bleomycin	DNA	Single- and double-strand DNA breaks
	Mitomycin	DNA	Cross-links DNA preventing function

reaching the tumour will not be effective. Inability of the patients to tolerate sufficient doses of drugs due to co-morbidity may also lead to ineffective dosage and lack of efficacy.

True resistance to adequate concentrations of drug can be either germline or acquired, and resistance is thought to arise from spontaneous mutations. If drug therapies are being given at the time resistance develops, resistant clones will be selected out. This is often clinically relevant, and the patient will develop progressive disease while undergoing treatment.

Multidrug resistance

Once a tumour is resistant to one drug, it is often also resistant to many other drugs. This discovery has led to the concept of 'multidrug resistance', the best studied mechanism of which is P-glycoprotein overexpression. P-glycoprotein is a cell-membrane glycoprotein pump coded for by the mdr-1 gene, which removes drugs from the cell.[18] It is a naturally occurring glycoprotein which forms part of secretory epithelial structures – for example, the biliary canaliculi. Increased expression of mdr1[19] occurs when cells are cultured in the presence of cytotoxic drugs. Mdr1a knockout mice, who cannot produce P-glycoprotein, have tumours that do not readily develop drug resistance. P-glycoprotein overexpression in vivo correlates with reduced responsiveness to drugs and reduced survival in some series.[20]

It is possible to block P-glycoprotein and prevent the transmembrane protein from pumping drugs out of cells. Drugs available for this purpose include verapamil, quinidine, and ciclosporin A. Clinical trials using these drugs have demonstrated some success in altering the clinical course of drug resistance,[21] but, not improving survival. It is likely that overexpression of P-glycoprotein is only one of many mechanisms involved in multidrug resistance.[22–24]

There are other mechanisms of multidrug resistance, including multidrug resistance protein 1 (MRP1) and lung resistance protein (LRP). MRP1 is also an ATP-dependent transmembrane protein, which results in resistance to a slightly different array of drugs to P-glycoprotein. LRP is a vault protein which is present in many normal cells as well as malignant cells, and it is associated with multidrug resistance.[25]

Reduced apoptosis of DNA-damaged cells may be an important mechanism of drug resistance. Apoptosis in tumour cells is under the control of a complex pathway, which includes p53 and the Bcl-2 family of proteins.[26] Cells with mutant p53 are more likely to be drug resistant than those with wild-type p53,[27–29] and there is interest in restoring wild-type p53 to cells in order to try to stimulate apoptosis after chemotherapy. Overexpression of the antiapoptotic protein Bcl-2 also contributes to chemoresistance, and modulation of Bcl-2 function may increase chemosensitivity.[30] Bcl-2 antisense oligonucleotide therapy has also been tested in patients with non-Hodgkin's lymphoma.[31]

Resistance to specific drugs

Resistance mechanisms can be specific to a particular drug, and a selection of these are outlined in Table 27.2. For example, anthracyclines, epidophyllotoxins, and some other drugs act in various ways to stabilize the cleavable complex formed by topoisomerase II and DNA. Topoisomerase II expression can be upregulated or topoisomerase II can mutate and change its intracellular location to avoid this effect.[32,33] These mechanisms collectively are known as Topo II-related drug resistance.

TOXICITY

Toxicities are generally divided into early and late, and while the majority of early toxicities, such as hair loss, are entirely reversible, some late toxicities are not. The toxicity of a treatment often defines the doses at which a drug can be given, and therefore can be a key factor in limiting efficacy. Management of toxicity is clearly vital to the optimal delivery of chemotherapy.

Early toxicity

Since stem cells in the bone marrow are dividing rapidly, chemotherapy drugs have the potential to cause bone-marrow suppression. Marrow toxicity is very often the dose-limiting factor for chemotherapeutic agents, and or high-dose prolonged chemotherapy can cause anaplastic marrow.

Most chemotherapy regimens are given once every 3 weeks, and, in general, bone-marrow stem cells will recover within 10 days to 3 weeks of the dose being given. Because the lifespan of a circulating white blood cell is 4–5 days, the effects of bone-marrow suppression on the peripheral blood

Table 27.2 Mechanisms of resistance to chemotherapy.

Drug class	Examples	Method of resistance
Topoisomerase I inhibitors	Irinotecan	Decreased expression of topoisomerase I (sometimes compensated for by increased topoisomerase II); mutated topoisomerase I
Spindle poisons	Vinca alkaloids Taxanes	Reduced binding to microtubules
Platinum	Cisplatin	Conjugation with glutathione Increased expression of multidrug resistance protein 2 Increased DNA repair/increased tolerance to DNA damage
Alkylating agents	Cyclophosphamide	Drug inactivation by aldehyde dehydrogenase Increased DNA repair
Antimetabolites	Methotrexate 5-Fluorouracil	Decreased reduced folate carrier expression, and decreased uptake Altered dihydrofolate reductase with reduced affinity for methotrexate Increased production of dihydrofolate reductase Increased thymidylate synthase levels

are seen 4–12 days after the dose is given (the 'nadir' or low point). Platelet nadirs are drug specific, but since the lifespan of platelets is longer (9–10 days), they tend to occur later in the chemotherapy cycle. Red blood cells survive in the peripheral circulation for about 3 months, and so anaemia is usually seen only with prolonged courses of chemotherapy, primarily with platinum-based compounds.

During periods of neutropenia patients are prone to bacterial infections.[34] Many studies have shown that broad-spectrum antibiotics covering aerobic Gram-negative bacilli, especially *Pseudomonas aeruginosa*, should be introduced at the first sign of fever. Treatment should not be delayed until physical signs of infection are present or an organism is identified.[35] The use of prophylactic oral quinolones has been shown to reduce the incidence of infections.[36] Injection of recombinant granulocyte colony-stimulating factors (G-CSF) will reduce the duration and level of the neutropenia and the risk of developing a fever while neutropenic. To date, studies have failed to prove a survival advantage or reduction in significant infection rates for the use of G-CSF.[37] Other early side effects of chemotherapy are shown in Table 27.3.

Cytotoxic drugs are all potentially teratogenic, especially if given in the first trimester. Folate antagonists such as methotrexate have the most consistently poor record.[38] Observational studies of patients given chemotherapy during pregnancy reveal that chemotherapy can be administered relatively safely in the second and third trimester, but it is possible that miscarriage, intrauterine growth retardation, and premature labour may be increased.[39] The incidence of long-term side effects such as carcinogenesis, cardiotoxicity, and neuropsychiatric effects among adults who have received chemotherapy while in utero are not known.

Late toxicity

Male and female fertility is commonly reduced after chemotherapy,[40] and there is a substantial literature on the effects of individual drugs.[41] In the male, sperm production takes place constantly, and chemotherapy reduces or stops production by damaging the germinal epithelium. Azoospermia is therefore not always associated with diminished or absent hormone production. During intensive treatment, 96% of men will become azoospermic.[42] Depending on the regimen, a proportion of them will regain testicular function after chemotherapy. In women, since ovarian germ cells are present at birth, the mechanism of infertility is different. Oestrogen levels are depleted by treatment, and an early menopause can be induced. The extent of the toxicity is related to the underlying diagnosis, dose and type of drugs used, and age of patient at time of treatment.[41]

Because chemotherapeutic drugs work by damaging DNA, they carry a risk of latent carcinogenesis. Alkylating agents are associated with a high risk of

Table 27.3 Early toxicities of chemotherapy.

Toxicity	Drugs	Comments
Alopecia	Especially anthracyclines and taxanes	Starts 2–3 weeks after chemotherapy initiated; reversible, usually starts growing back within 1–2 months of end of treatment
Mouth ulcers	Especially bolus 5-fluorouracil	Can be exacerbated by fungal or viral infections
Diarrhoea	Capecitabine	Often associated with ulceration anywhere in the GI tract
Constipation	Vinca alkaloids	Antiemetics can cause constipation, or vinca alkaloids can cause gut neuropathy
Nausea	Most	Chemotherapy drugs can be directly emetogenic, but constipation and GI ulceration can exacerbate this; usually well controlled with serotonin subtype 3 receptor blockers

myelodysplasia and acute myeloid leukaemia,[43] and after combination chemotherapy, the risk of many solid malignancies is increased: After treatment for Hodgkin's disease, the relative risk of any cancer is 6.4, and the relative risk of acute myeloid leukaemia (AML) is 144.[44,45] The risk of second malignancy is highest when chemotherapy and radiotherapy are used in combination.

Drug-specific toxicities

All chemotherapy drugs have specific side effects in addition to the generic effects described (see Table 27.4). Specific side effects can either be related to cumulative dose (for example, anthracyclines and cardiac toxicity) or be idiosyncratic. The mechanisms vary widely, but are not necessarily directly related to the cytotoxic action of the drugs. As management of toxicity improves, for example, with the use of peripheral blood stem-cell rescue, bone-marrow suppression is less likely to be the dose-limiting toxicity, and some of the toxicities mentioned in Table 27.4 may become dose limiting.

Table 27.4 Drug-specific toxicities.

Drug	Examples of toxicities
Anthracyclines	Cardiotoxicity
Cytosine arabinoside	Cerebral/cerebellar dysfunction
Methotrexate	Hepatitis Nephrotoxicity
Vinca alkaloids	Neurotoxicity Constipation
5-Fluorouracil	Palmar–plantar erythrodysaesthesia
Taxanes	Neurotoxicity Hypersensitivity or anaphylaxis
Bleomycin	Pulmonary fibrosis Skin pigmentation
Cyclophosphamide	Haemorrhagic cystitis due to excretion of metabolites Bladder tumours
Cisplatin	Nephrotoxicity Deafness

This list is not intended to be comprehensive, but to indicate the wide range of possible side effects of chemotherapy.

The toxicity of certain drugs can be reduced by techniques to protect normal tissue. For example, cyclophosphamide and ifosfamide produce acrolein, which is an irritant metabolite excreted through the bladder. Mesna is a thiol compound that acts as a reducing agent, and, when given with cyclophosphamide, reacts with acrolein in the urinary tract and helps prevent chemical cystitis.[46] It has also been found that by altering a regimen to limit the peak concentration of an anthracycline, toxicity will be reduced.[47,48] Dezrazoxone has been shown to reduce the cardiotoxicity of anthracylines,[49] and can be given to patients with pre-existing cardiac impairment. The concern about the strategy of protecting normal tissue is that the tumour will also be protected.

MEASURING EFFICACY

Before prescription of a course of chemotherapy, a method of assessing the success or failure of the treatment should be identified. The method will obviously depend upon the tumour type and site. For tumours which produce markers (for example, prostate-specific antigen for prostate cancer and alpha fetoprotein for germ-cell tumours), serum levels can be readily measured. Symptomatic improvement can also often indicate response, as for example, by a reduction of analgesic requirement by the patient. However, even in the palliative setting, symptomatic improvement alone is rarely considered adequate to prove response, and for solid tumours demonstration of radiological response is the 'gold standard'.

The common practice in assessing radiological response is to obtain an image of a measurable tumour site before and after treatment. The World Health Organization, the National Cancer Institute, and the European Organization for Research and Treatment of Cancer have issued guidelines for tumour response criteria.[50]

Although reduction in tumour mass is the gold standard for measuring treatment efficacy in an individual, survival is the ultimate measure of efficacy. For palliative treatments, quality of life is also an important end point to measure.

Minimal residual disease (MRD)

At a complete radiological response (or after radical surgery), there will be no evidence of disease as measured by any standard marker. Unfortunately, there will often be residual viable tumour cells present in these patients (see Figure 27.6). Currently, imaging does not allow us to detect microscopic disease, but with real-time quantitative polymerase chain reactions (PCR), residual disease at the molecular level can be detected. The absence of minimal residual disease (MRD) could theoretically be used as an end point for radical therapy. In acute promyelocytic leukaemia (APML), evidence of MRD in the bone marrow correlates well with outcome.[51] It is likely that the absence of evidence of t15:17 (the chromosomal abnormality associated with APML) in the bone marrow, as measured by real-time PCR, also correlates with long-term survival after chemotherapy.

INTENSIFYING TREATMENT

In vitro evidence suggests that for some drugs, such as cisplatin, there is a clear relationship between dose of chemotherapy and proportion of cells killed.[17,52] In potentially curable tumours, there has been a great deal of interest in escalating treatment doses in order to improve survival, but as mentioned above, dose is commonly limited by bone-marrow suppression. Supportive care has improved significantly in recent years, and since the 1970s, it has been possible to perform peripheral blood stem-cell rescue.[53,54] This is a procedure whereby the patient's stem cells are collected from the peripheral blood and stored so that they can be returned after a high dose of chemotherapy, thus shortening the duration of neutropenia. The introduction of 5-HT3 antagonists has enabled nausea to be controlled more effectively. For some drugs, the use of colony-stimulating factors alone is enough to increase significantly the tolerated dose.[55]

An absolute survival advantage to dose intensification without stem-cell rescue has yet to be formally demonstrated. There is some evidence that, at standard doses, dose intensity affects the outcome of patients with solid tumours,[56] but not all trials have had the same findings. Modest escalation of dose in testicular cancer, transitional cell carcinoma and ovarian carcinoma has not been shown to be beneficial.[57–59]

There is clear evidence of a benefit from high-dose regimens with stem-cell rescue when treating haematological malignancies, but, for solid tumours, there is still no conclusive evidence that high-dose regimens are beneficial. For example, in germ-cell tumours, preliminary results comparing high-dose

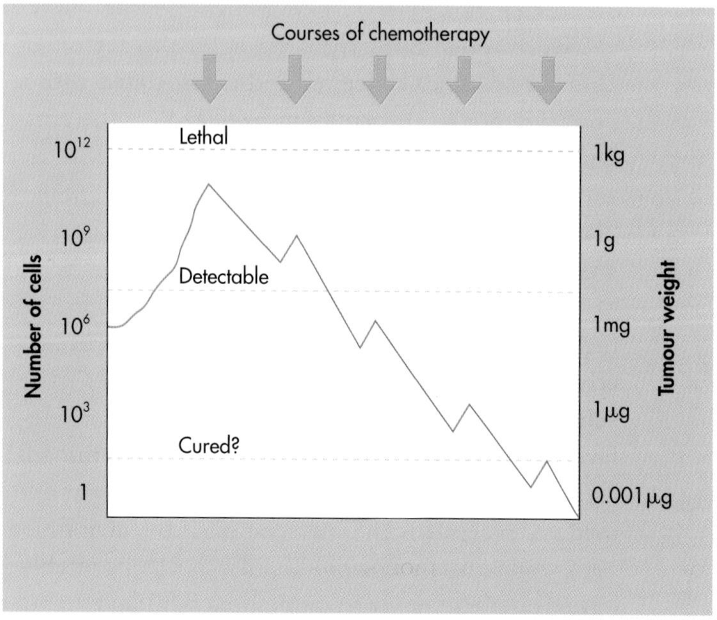

Figure 27.6 *Minimal residual disease (modified from Skipper[9]).*

patients with historical controls were promising,[60,61] but, more recently, a prospective, randomized, controlled trial of high-dose chemotherapy in salvage of patients with advanced germ-cell tumours failed to show an improvement in event-free survival.[62]

There are many potential reasons why these trials have failed to show benefit from dose escalation. In vitro, large dose escalations are required (of the order of a log) to change cell kill. It may be that the doses it is possible to give in vivo are just not high enough to result in a clinical benefit. It may also be that the optimal nature and timing of the dose escalation have not yet been determined.

NEW ANTICANCER DRUGS

Understanding of the molecular biology of malignant cells has increased dramatically in recent years. Therefore, there is scope for developing drugs which are targeted at malignant cells.[63,64] The principle is that drugs are developed that target abnormal biology specific to tumours, thus increasing efficacy and reducing normal tissue damage. This section aims to mention some of the new drugs which are either in use in the clinic or are undergoing trials, in order to illustrate the range of possible new therapeutic strategies becoming available.

Immune modulators

Immune modulation is an attractive anticancer therapeutic option. It has been noted that prolonged periods of immunosuppression predispose to malignancies,[65] and also that spontaneous regression of metastatic tumours (classically renal cell cancers) can occur.[66] What is more, regression of tumours has occasionally been induced by deliberate inoculation with pus or bacterial toxins.[67] The immune system can be stimulated non-specifically or by generation of specific antitumour immunity.

Cytokines

The immune system can be non-specifically stimulated with supraphysiological doses of naturally occurring cytokines. Examples include tumour necrosis factor (TNF), interferons, and interleukins. This method has been shown to have some efficacy in the treatment of renal cell carcinoma, melanoma, and chronic leukaemia.[68–70] Bone-marrow transplants lead to graft-versus-tumour effect, after which the transplanted immune system recognizes the tumour cells as foreign and destroys them. Unfortunately, the graft-versus-tumour effect cannot be achieved without simultaneous graft-versus-host disease. The strategy of allogeneic bone-marrow transplant is commonly used in the treatment of haematological malignancies, but a pilot study in patients with renal cell carcinoma showed some promising results,[71] and this may be an area for future developments in solid tumour oncology.

Antibody therapy

In the nineteenth century, investigators attempted to treat patients with the sera of animals which had been inoculated with human cancers,[72] and since the discovery of the monoclonal antibody in 1975[73] it has been possible to produce antibodies to specific tumour antigens. Monoclonal antibodies can be used to target radiation or prodrugs.[74]

The exact means by which monoclonal antibodies mediate cell killing is complex and not completely understood. Nevertheless, significant advances have been made with the recent introduction of anti-c-erbB2 (Herceptin/Trastuzumab) for breast cancer and anti-CD20 (Rituximab) for B-cell lymphoma.[75] The human epidermal growth factor receptor 2 (or c-erbB2) antigen is overexpressed on the cell surface of 25–30% of breast cancers,[76] and is associated with a poor prognosis.[77] Patients can be tested for the presence of c-erbB2 on the tumour cell surface. If the antigen is found, anti-c-erbB2 antibodies induce responses in some patients who have failed treatment with conventional chemotherapy, or in whom conventional chemotherapy is contraindicated.[78,79] There is a higher response rate to chemotherapy plus anti-c-erbB2 antibodies than to chemotherapy alone.[80] The side-effect profile of monoclonal antibodies is very favourable when compared with conventional chemotherapy, and antibodies to other cell-surface markers are under investigation. Unfortunately, resistance to monoclonal antibodies invariably develops, and discovering the mechanism of this resistance is going to be vital in terms of improving immune-based therapies.

Targeting mediators of malignancy

Receptors on the cell surface require intracellular signalling pathways to translate receptor ligand binding into cell proliferation or other end points. These intracellular signalling pathways are potential targets for anticancer drugs. For example, the epidermal growth factor receptor (EGFR) (also known as HER-1) is overexpressed in many cancers, and seems to be responsible for the malignant behaviour of tumour cells.[81–83] The EGFR has an intracellular tyrosine kinase domain which is activated by phosphorylation. Tyrosine kinase activation can be blocked by specially designed small molecules, one example of which is ZD1839, or Iressa. This has been found to have activity in a number of EGFR-positive tumours and is currently under investigation.[84]

A potential problem with blocking intracellular signalling pathways is that the effect may be short-lived if the cell can bypass the point in the intracellular pathway cascade at which the drug is acting. This can occur either by upregulation of alternative pathways or by mutation of target proteins. The target for the small molecules will also be present in normal tissue. In the case of Iressa, this is manifest by an acneiform skin rash, thought to be due to the fact that epidermal keratinocytes express EGFR and are targeted by the small molecules. This effect is also seen with monoclonal antibodies.

Antiangiogenesis agents

The ability to metastasize is a defining feature of malignant tissue, and metastasis cannot occur without angiogenesis. Angiogenesis is under the control of multiple cytokines, enzymes and proteins.[85] The concept of angiogenesis as a therapeutic target was suggested by Folkman in 1972.[86] Thalidomide is one antiangiogenesis drug currently in use. Thalidomide was first marketed as a sedative but was withdrawn due to teratogenic effects, primarily amelia and phocomelia. It was proposed that these effects were due to degeneration of major limb arteries,[87] and it was subsequently found that thalidomide inhibits the angiogenic cytokines, basic fibroblast growth factor (bFGF) and vascular endothelial growth factor (VEGF).[88,89] Clinical efficacy has been variable.[90,91]

VEGF has been identified as a particularly important angiogenic cytokine.[92] Attempts to block production of VEGF in renal cell carcinoma cell lines have been successful: administration of antisense phosphorothioate oligodeoxynucleotides targeted at VEGF mRNA reduced the growth of renal cell carcinoma cell lines injected into nude mice.[93] Clinical trials of antisense oligonucleotides are not yet available.

CONCLUSION

Conventional chemotherapy along with radiotherapy has formed the mainstay of curative and palliative treatment of solid malignancies in the past 40 years. All conventional cytotoxic drugs damage normal tissue as well as having a therapeutic effect by killing tumour cells. Combining different types and doses of cytotoxic drugs has led to significant improvements in survival from some important cancers in the last 50 years. Recently, novel agents have emerged consequent on improved techniques in molecular medicine. These novel agents are in the early stages of development, and few of them are currently in routine use. It is hoped that in the future, systemic treatment of cancer will be more targeted and therefore not only more successful but less toxic.

REFERENCES

1. Burchenal JH. The historical development of cancer chemotherapy. Semin Oncol 1977; 4: 135–146
2. Krumbhaar EB, Krumbhaar HD. The blood and bone marrow in yellow gas (mustard gas) poisoning: changes produced in the bone marrow of fatal cases. J Med Res 1919; 40: 497
3. Goodman LS, Wintrobe MM, Dameshek W, Goodman MJ et al. Nitrogen mustard therapy: use of methyl-bis(beta-chloroethyl)amine hydrochloride and tris(beta-chloroethyl)amine hydrochloride for Hodgkin's disease, lymphosarcoma, leukemia and certain allied and miscellaneous disorders. JAMA 1946; 132: 126–132

4. Twentyman PR, Bleehen NM. Changes in sensitivity to cytotoxic agents occurring during the life history of monolayer cultures of a mouse tumour cell line. Br J Cancer 1975; 31: 417–423
5. Steel GG. Growth Kinetics of Tumours. Oxford: Oxford University Press, 1977
6. Shackney SE, McCormack GW, Cuchural GJ Jr. Growth rate patterns of solid tumours and their relation to responsiveness to therapy: an analytical review. Ann Intern Med 1978; 89: 107–121
7. The Advanced Colorectal Cancer Meta-Analysis Project. Modulation of fluorouracil by leucovorin in patients with advanced colorectal cancer: evidence in terms of response rate. J Clin Oncol 1992; 10: 896–903
8. Schabel FM Jr. The use of tumour growth kinetics in planning curative chemotherapy of advanced solid tumours. Cancer Res 1969; 29: 2384–2389
9. Skipper HE. Biochemical, biological, pharmacologic, toxicologic, kinetic and clinical relationships. Cancer 1968; 21: 600–610
10. Friedman JM, Fialkow PJ. Cell marker studies of human tumorigenesis. Transplant Rev 1976; 28: 17–33
11. Goldie JH, Coldman AJ. A mathematic model for relating the drug sensitivity of tumours to their spontaneous mutation rate. Cancer Treat Rep 1979; 63 (11–12): 1727–1733
12. Goldie JH, Coldman AJ. Application of theoretical models to chemotherapy protocol design. Cancer Treat Rep 1986; 70: 127–131
13. Selawry OS, Hananian J, Wolman IJ, et al. New treatment schedule with improved survival in childhood leukemia. Intermittent parenteral vs daily oral administration of methotrexate for maintenance of induced remission. Acute leukaemia group B. JAMA 1965; 194: 75–81
14. Reiter A, Schrappe M, Ludwig WD, Hiddemann W et al. Chemotherapy in 998 unselected childhood acute lymphoblastic leukemia patients. Results and conclusions of the multicentre trial ALL-BFM 86. Blood 1994; 84: 3122–3133
15. Devita VT Jr, Serpick AA, Carbone PP. Combination chemotherapy in the treatment of advanced Hodgkin's disease. Ann Intern Med 1970; 73: 881–895
16. Wolfrom C, Hartmann R, Fengler R, Bruhmuller S et al. Randomised comparison of 36-hour intermediate-dose versus 4-hour high-dose methotrexate infusions for remission induction in relapsed childhood acute lymphoblastic leukaemia. J Clin Oncol 1993; 11: 827–833
17. Teicher BA, Herman TS, Holden SA, Wang YY et al. Tumour resistance to alkylating agents conferred by mechanisms operative only in vivo. Science 1990; 247(4949 Pt1): 1457–1461
18. Riordan JR, Deuchars K, Kartner N, Alon N et al. Amplification of P-glycoprotein genes in multidrug-resistant mammalian cell lines. Nature 1985; 316(6031): 817–819
19. Gottesman MM, Hrycyna CA, Schoenlein PV, Germann UA et al. Genetic analysis of the multidrug transporter. Annu Rev Genet 1995; 29: 607–649
20. Pogliani EM, Belotti D, Rivolta GF, Maffe PF et al. Anthracycline drugs and MDR expression in human leukaemia. Cytotechnology 1996; 19: 229–235
21. Belpomme D, Gauthier S, Pujade-Lauraine E, Facchini T et al. Verapamil increases the survival of patients with anthracycline-resistant metastatic breast carcinoma. Ann Oncol 2000; 11: 1471–1476
22. Solary E, Witz B, Caillot D, Moreau P et al. Combination of quinine as a potential reversing agent with mitoxantrone and cytarabine for the treatment of acute leukemias: a randomised multicenter study. Blood 1996; 88: 1198–1205
23. Wilson WH, Bates SE, Fojo A, Bryant G et al. Controlled trial of dexverapamil, a modulator of multidrug resistance, in lymphomas refractory to EPOCH chemotherapy. J Clin Oncol 1995; 13: 1995–2004
24. Wishart GC, Bissett D, Paul J, Jodrell D et al. Quinidine as a resistance modulator of epirubicin in advanced breast cancer: mature results of a placebo-controlled randomised trial. J Clin Oncol 1994; 12: 1171–1177
25. Scheffer GL, Wijngaard PL, Flens MJ, Izquierdo MA et al. The drug resistance-related protein LRP is the human major vault protein. Nat Med 1995; 1: 578–582
26. Reed JC. Bcl-2 family proteins. Oncogene 1998; 17: 3225–3236
27. Cho Y, Gorina S, Jeffrey PD, Pavletich NP. Crystal structure of a p53 tumor suppressor-DNA complex: understanding tumorigenic mutations. Science 1994; 265(5170): 346–355
28. Chin KV, Ueda K, Pastan I, Gottesman MM. Modulation of activity of the promoter of the human MDR1 gene by Ras and p53. Science 1992; 255(5043): 459–462
29. Lowe SW, Ruley HE, Jacks T, Housman DE. P53 dependent apoptosis modulates the cytotoxicity of anticancer agents. Cell 1993; 74: 957–967

30. Konopleva M, Zhao S, Hu W, Jiang S et al. The anti-apoptotic genes Bxl-X_L and Bcl-2 are over-expressed and contribute to chemoresistance of non-proliferating leukaemic $CD34^+$ cell. Br J Haematol 2002; 118: 521–534
31. Waters JS, Webb A, Cunningham D, Clarke PA et al. Phase I clinical and pharmacokinetic study of bcl-2-antisense oligonucleotide therapy in patients with non-Hodgkin's lymphoma. J Clin Oncol 2000; 18: 1812–1823
32. Pommier Y, Leteurtre F, Fesen MR, Fujimori A et al. Cellular determinants of sensitivity and resistance to DNA topoisomerase inhibitors. Cancer Invest 1994; 12: 530–542
33. Beck WT, Danks MK, Wolverton JS, Chen M et al. Resistance of mammalian tumour cells to inhibitors of DNA topoisomerase II. Adv Pharmacol 1994; 29B: 145–169
34. Bodey GP, Buckley MB, Sathe YS, Freireich EJ. Quantitative relationships between circulating leukocytes and infection in patients with acute leukaemia. Ann Int Med 1966; 64: 328–340
35. Schimpff S, Satterlee W, Young VM, Serpick A. Empiric therapy with carbenicillin and gentamicin for febrile patients with cancer and granulocytopenia. N Engl J Med 1971; 284: 1061–1065
36. Engels EA, Lau J, Barza M. Efficacy of quinolone prophylaxis in neutropenic cancer patients: a meta-analysis. J Clin Oncol 1998; 16: 1179–1187
37. Messori A, Trippoli S, Tendi E. G-CSF for the prophylaxis of neutropenic fever in patients with small cell lung cancer receiving myelosuppressive antineoplastic chemotherapy: meta-analysis and pharmacoeconomic evaluation. J Clin Pharm Ther 1996; 21: 57–63
38. Doll DC, Ringenberg QS, Yarbro JW. Antineoplastic agents and pregnancy. Semin Oncol 1989; 16: 337–346
39. Berry DL, Theriault RL, Holmes FA, Parisi VM et al. Management of breast cancer during pregnancy using a standardized protocol. J Clin Oncol 1999; 17: 855–861
40. Chapman RM, Sutcliffe S. The effects of chemotherapy and radiotherapy on fertility and their prevention. In: Williams CJW, Whitehouse JMA, eds. Recent Advances in Clinical Oncology. Edinburgh: Churchill Livingstone, 1986: 239–251
41. Sieber SM, Adamson RH. Toxicity of antineoplastic agents in man, chromosomal aberrations anti-fertility effects, congenital malformations and carcinogenic potential. Adv Cancer Res 1975; 22: 57–155
42. Dragsa RE, Einhorn LH, Williams SD, Patel DN et al. Fertility after chemotherapy for testicular cancer. J Clin Oncol 1983; 1: 179–183
43. Reimer RR, Hoover R, Fraumeni JF Jr, Young RC. Acute leukemia after alkylating-agent therapy of ovarian cancer. N Engl J Med 1977; 297: 177–181
44. Tucker MA. Solid second cancer following Hodgkin's disease. Haematol Oncol Clin North Am 1993; 7: 389–400
45. Henry-Amar M, Dietrich PY. Acute leukaemia after the treatment of Hodgkin's disease. Haematol Oncol Clin North Am 1993; 7: 369–387
46. Brock N, Pohl J, Stekar J. Detoxification of urotoxic oxazaphosphorines by sulfhydryl compounds. J Cancer Res Clin Oncol 1981; 100: 311–320
47. Shapira J, Gotfried M, Lishner M, Ravid M. Reduced cardiotoxicity of doxorubicin by a 6-hour infusion regime. Cancer 1990; 65: 870–873
48. Torti FM, Bristow MR, Howes AE, Aston D et al. Reduced cardiotoxicity of doxorubicin delivered on a weekly schedule. Assessment by endomyocardial biopsy. Ann Intern Med 1983; 99: 745–749
49. Speyer JL, Green MD, Kramer E, Rey M et al. Protective effects of the bispiperazinedione ICRF-187 against doxorubicin-induced cardiac toxicity in women with advanced breast cancer. N Engl J Med 1988; 319: 745–752
50. Therasse P, Arbuck SG, Eisenhauer EA, Wanders J et al. New guidelines to evaluate the response to treatment in solid tumours. J Natl Cancer Inst 2000; 92: 205–216
51. Venditti A, Buccisano F, Del Poeta G, Maurillo L et al. Level of minimal residual disease after consolidation therapy predicts outcome in acute myeloid leukemia. Blood 2000; 96: 3948–3952
52. Skipper HE, Schabel FM. Quantitative and cytokinetic studies in experimental tumour systems. In: Holland J, Frei FE, eds. Cancer Medicine. Philadelphia: Lea and Febiger, 1988: 663–684
53. Gorin NC, Najman A, Salmon C, Muller JY et al. High dose combination chemotherapy (TACC) with and without autologous bone marrow transplantation for the treatment of acute leukaemia and other malignant diseases: kinetics of recovery of haemopoiesis. A preliminary study of 12 cases. Eur J Cancer 1979; 15: 1113–1119
54. Appelbaum FR, Deisseroth AB, Graw RG Jr, Herzig GP et al. Prolonged remission following high dose chemotherapy of Burkitt's lymphoma in relapse. Cancer 1978; 41: 1059–1063

55. Gianni AM, Bregni M, Siena S, Magni M et al. Granulocyte-macrophage colony-stimulating factor or granulocyte colony-stimulating factor infusion makes high-dose etoposide a safe outpatient regimen that is effective in lymphoma and myeloma patients. J Clin Oncol 1992; 10: 1955–1962
56. Tannock IF, Boyd NF, DeBoer G, Erlichman C et al. A randomised trial of two dose levels of CMF chemotherapy for patients with metastatic breast cancer. J Clin Oncol 1988; 6: 1377–1387
57. Ozols RF, Ihde DC, Linehan WM, Jacob J et al. A randomised trial of standard chemotherapy versus a high-dose chemotherapy regime in the treatment of poor prognosis nonseminomatous germ-cell tumours. J Clin Oncol 1988; 6: 1031–1040
58. Seidman AD, Scher HI, Gabrilove JL, Bajorin DF et al. Dose-intensification of MVAC with recombinant granulocyte colony-stimulating factor as initial therapy in advanced urothelial cancer. J Clin Oncol 1993; 11: 408–414
59. Gore M, Mainwaring P, A'Hern R, MacFarlane V et al. Randomized trial of dose-intensity with single-agent carboplatin in patients with epithelial ovarian cancer. London Gynaecological Oncology Group. J Clin Oncol 1998; 16: 2426–2434
60. Motzer RJ, Mazumdar M, Gulati SC, Bajorin DF et al. Phase II trial of high-dose carboplatin and etoposide with autologous bone marrow transplantation in first-line therapy for patients with poor-risk germ cell tumours. J Natl Cancer Inst 1993; 85: 1828–1835
61. Motzer RJ, Mazumdar M, Bosl GJ, Bajorin DF et al. High-dose carboplatin, etoposide, and cyclophosphamide for patients with refractory germ cell tumours: treatment results and prognostic factors for survival and toxicity. J Clin Oncol 1996; 14: 1098–1105
62. Rosti G, Pico JL, Wandt H, Koza V et al. High-dose chemotherapy (HDC) in the salvage treatment of patients failing first-line platinum chemotherapy for advanced germ cell tumours (GCT); first results of a prospective randomised trial of the European Group for Blood and Marrow Transplantation (EBMT): IT-94 study. American Society of Clinical Oncology Abstracts 2002
63. Garrett MD, Workman P. Discovering novel chemotherapeutic drugs for the third millennium. Eur J Cancer 1999; 35: 2010–2030
64. Gibbs JB. Anticancer drug targets: growth factors and growth factor signalling. J Clin Invest 2000; 105: 9–13
65. Penn I. Cancers complicating organ transplantation. N Engl J Med 1990; 323: 1767–1769
66. Oliver RT, Nethersell AB, Bottomley JM. Unexplained spontaneous regression and alpha-interferon as treatment for metastatic renal carcinoma. Br J Urol 1989; 63: 128–131
67. Coley-Nauts HC, Fowler GA, Bogatko RN. A review of the influence of bacterial infection and of bacterial products (Coley's toxins) on malignant tumours in man. Acta Med Scand Suppl 1953; 274–277: 29–97
68. Rosenberg SA, Yang JC, Topalian SL, Schwartzentruber DJ et al. Treatment of 283 consecutive patients with metastatic melanoma or renal cell cancer using high-dose bolus interleukin 2. JAMA 1994; 271: 907–913
69. Bukowski RM, Goodman P, Crawford ED, Sergi JS et al. Phase II trial of high-dose intermittent interleukin-2 in metastastic renal cell carcinoma: a Southwest Oncology Group study. J Natl Cancer Inst 1990; 82: 143–146
70. Quesada JR, Reuben J, Manning JT, Hersh E et al. Alpha interferon for induction of remission in hairy cell leukaemia. N Engl J Med 1984; 310: 15–18
71. Childs R, Chernoff A, Contentin N, Bahceci E et al. Regression of metastatic renal-cell carcinoma after nonmyeloablative allogeneic peripheral-blood stem-cell transplantation. N Engl J Med 2000; 343: 750–758
72. Hericourt J, Richet C. De la sérothérapie dans le traitement du cancer. C R Acad Sci (Paris) 1895; 121: 567–569
73. Kohler G, Milstein C. Continuous cultures of fused cells secreting antibody of predefined specificity. Nature 1975; 256(5517): 495–497
74. Napier MP, Sharma SK, Springer CJ, Bagshawe KD et al. Antibody-directed enzyme prodrug therapy: efficacy and mechanism of action in colorectal carcinoma. Clin Cancer Res 2000; 6: 765–772
75. Coiffier B, Lepage E, Briere J, Herbrecht R et al. CHOP chemotherapy plus rituximab compared with CHOP alone in elderly patients with diffuse large-B-cell lymphoma. N Engl J Med 2002; 346: 235–242
76. Hynes NE, Stern DF. The biology of erbB-2/neu/HER-2 and its role in cancer. Biochim Biophys Acta 1994; 1198(2–3): 165–184
77. Slamon DJ, Godolphin W, Jones LA, Holt JA et al. Studies of the HER-2/neu proto-oncogene in human breast and ovarian cancer. Science 1989; 244(4905): 707–712

78. Cobleigh MA, Vogel CL, Tripathy D, Robert NJ et al. Multinational study of the efficacy and safety of humanized anti-HER2 monoclonal antibody in women who have HER2-overexpressing metastatic breast cancer that has progressed after chemotherapy for metastatic disease. J Clin Oncol 1999; 17: 2639–2648
79. Vogel CL, Cobleigh MA, Tripathy D, Gutheil JC et al. Efficacy and safety of trastuzumab as a single agent in first-line treatment of HER2-overexpressing metastatic breast cancer. J Clin Oncol 2002; 20: 719–726
80. Slamon DJ, Leyland-Jones B, Shak S, Fuchs H et al. Use of chemotherapy plus a monoclonal antibody against HER2 for metastatic breast cancer that overexpresses HER2. N Engl J Med 2001; 344: 783–792
81. Aaronson SA. Growth factors and cancer. Science 1991; 254(5035): 1146–1153
82. Salomon DS, Brandt R, Ciardiello F, Normanno N. Epidermal growth factor-related peptides and their receptors in human malignancies. Crit Rev Oncol Hematol 1995; 19: 183–232
83. Tysnes BB, Haugland HK, Bjerkvig R. Epidermal growth factor and laminin receptors contribute to migratory and invasive properties of gliomas. Invasion Metastasis 1997; 17: 270–280
84. Herbst RS, Maddox A-M, Rothenberg ML, Small EJ et al. Selective oral epidermal growth factor receptor tyrosine kinase inhibitor ZD1839 is generally well-tolerated and has activity in non-small-cell lung cancer and other solid tumours: results of a phase I trial. J Clin Oncol 2002; 20: 3815–3825
85. Risau W. Mechanisms of angiogenesis. Nature 1997; 386(6626): 671–674
86. Folkman J. Anti-angiogenesis: new concept for therapy of solid tumours. Ann Surg 1972; 175: 409–416
87. Parman T, Wiley MJ, Wells PG. Free radical-mediated oxidative DNA damage in the mechanism of thalidomide teratogenicity. Nat Med 1999; 5: 582–585
88. D'Amato RJ, Loughnan MS, Flynn E, Folkman J. Thalidomide is an inhibitor of angiogenesis. Proc Natl Acad Sci USA 1994; 91: 4082–4085
89. Kruse FE, Joussen AM, Rohrschneider K, Becker MD et al. Thalidomide inhibits corneal angiogenesis induced by vascular endothelial growth factor. Graefes Arch Clin Exp Ophthalmol 1998; 236: 461–466
90. Baidas SM, Winer EP, Fleming GF, Harris L et al. Phase II evaluation of thalidomide in patients with metastatic breast cancer. J Clin Oncol 2000; 18: 2710–2717
91. Figg WD, Dahut W, Duray P, Hamilton M et al. A randomised phase II trial of thalidomide, an angiogenesis inhibitor, in patients with androgen-independent prostate cancer. Clin Can Res 2001; 7: 1888–1893
92. Ferrara N. Vascular endothelial growth factor: molecular and biological aspects. Curr Top Microbiol Immunol 1999; 237: 1–30
93. Shi W, Siemann DW. Inhibition of renal cell carcinoma angiogenesis and growth by antisense oligonucleotides targeting vascular endothelial growth factor. Br J Cancer 2002; 87: 119–126

28

Embryology

David F M Thomas

INTRODUCTION

Embryology provides an essential key to understanding the structure and function of the normal urinary tract and the origins of the congenital anomalies encountered in urological practice. The conventional study of embryology, supplemented by additional information from scanning electron microscopy and immunocytochemistry, has provided us with a detailed picture of the developmental anatomy of the embryo and fetus. Now, equipped with the powerful new research methods of molecular biology, notably polymerase chain reaction and fluorescent in situ hybridization, researchers can study the genetic mechanisms regulating this complex and tightly ordered anatomical sequence. As well as mapping and sequencing genes, research is under way to isolate the many gene products responsible for implementing the genetic 'programme' encoded on DNA at a cellular and molecular level. Moreover, the function of specific genes is being extensively documented by studying the consequences of experimentally induced null or 'knockout' gene deletions in experimental rodents. The successful culture of pluripotent embryonic stem cells,[1] coupled with changes in the law permitting research into therapeutic cloning of early embryonic tissue, may ultimately pave the way to the use of a wide range of human cells for tissue reconstruction or regenerative repair. Advances in the new science of developmental biology will create new opportunities for the diagnosis, prevention and possible treatment of inherited disorders and genetically determined anomalies of the genitourinary system. However, these opportunities will also bring new responsibilities and ethical dilemmas. Much of this chapter is devoted to a practical, clinically orientated account of developmental anatomy, but it would be incomplete without some consideration of genetics and the rapidly advancing field of developmental biology.

FERTILIZATION AND EARLY DEVELOPMENT OF THE HUMAN EMBRYO

Human gestation spans the period from fertilization to birth, which averages 38 weeks. Obstetricians conventionally subdivide pregnancy into three, 3-month trimesters. Embryogenesis, the formation of organs and systems, occurs principally between the third and tenth weeks. Subsequent development throughout the rest of fetal life is characterized by the processes of differentiation, branching, maturation and growth.

Fertilization is defined by fusion of the nuclear material of the fertilizing spermatozoon and the oocyte. The process of gametogenesis, whereby spermatozoa and oocytes develop from their germ-cell precursors, is considered below. In males, spermatogenesis is a continuing process initiated at puberty. In contrast, the initial phase of female gametogenesis occurs in fetal life, and primary oocytes remain dormant in the prophase of the first meiotic division until the onset of puberty. During each ovulatory cycle, under the influence of follicle-stimulating hormone, a small number of primary oocytes resume meitoic activity, but, of these, only one usually progresses to maturity as a graafian follicle. At the mid-point of the menstrual cycle, the primary oocyte destined for ovulation transforms into a secondary oocyte by proceeding into the remaining phases of the long-arrested first meiotic division. Protected by the zona pellucida, the secondary oocyte is extruded from the surface of the ovary, from where it is drawn into the reproductive tract by the fimbriae of the fallopian tube. Of an ejaculate totalling perhaps 40–100 million spermatozoa, only a few hundred are destined to complete the journey up the female reproductive canal to come into potential contact with the ovulated oocyte.

Penetration by the fertilizing spermatozoon of the zona pellucida surrounding the secondary oocyte triggers the second meiotic division, which results in the formation of the definitive oocyte and an aggregate of non-functional DNA known as a polar body.

The normal human karyotype comprises a total of 23 pairs of chromosomes, that is, 22 pairs of autosomes and one pair of sex chromosomes, either XX (female) or XY (male). As a result of the two meiotic divisions, each gamete (the spermatozoon or definitive oocyte) carries only half the normal complement of chromosomes, that is, 22 unpaired autosomes and either an X or Y sex chromosome. Fusion of the haploid nuclei of the two gametes at the time of fertilization imparts diploid status (that is, 22 pairs of autosomes plus two sex chromosomes) to the nucleus of the fertilized zygote. From the time of fertilization, the journey down the fallopian tube to the site of implantation in the primed uterine endometrium takes 5–6 days (Figure 28.1). During this journey, the fertilized zygote undergoes a series of cell divisions termed cleavage. By the fourth day, sequential cleavage has created a 32-cell embryo, classically likened to a mulberry (hence the Latin-derived term 'morula'). Further cell division is accompanied by structural differentiation and the formation of a sphere-like blastocyst. It is at this stage in development that the embryo is implanted into the uterine endometrium, 6 days after fertilization.

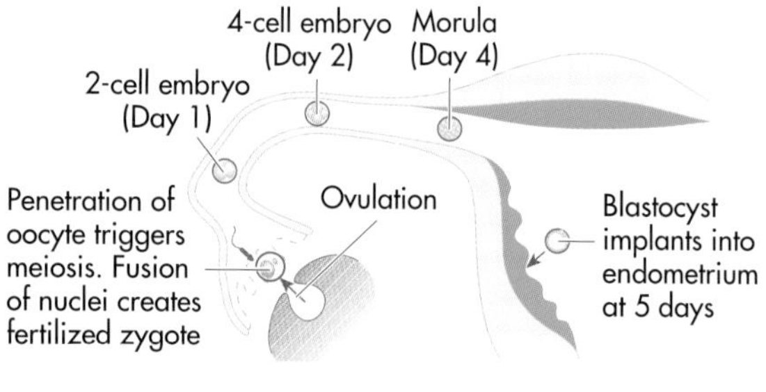

Figure 28.1 *Key stages in the five to six days from fertilization to implantation.*

CHROMOSOMAL ABNORMALITIES: CLINICAL CONSIDERATIONS

A detailed account of the pathogenesis and clinical manifestations of chromosomal abnormalities arising during gametogenesis and cleavage is beyond the scope of this chapter. Major chromosomal abnormalities are common, but most result in the death of the embryo and spontaneous abortion at an early stage in pregnancy. The most serious chromosomal abnormalities consistent with survival to term are the trisomies, notably trisomy 21 – Down's syndrome. The trisomy state occurs when an additional chromosome or portion of a chromosome becomes incorporated into the nucleus of a gamete by non-disjunction or translocation. Non-disjunction refers to the faulty separation of a pair of chromosomes during meiotic or mitotic cell division. In translocation, paired chromosomes separate completely, but one of the pair, or a fragment thereof, becomes inadvertently attached to another unrelated chromosome and is thus retained within the haploid nucleus. Non-disjunction of the X and Y sex chromosomes during gametogenesis accounts for a number of genetically determined syndromes, notably Turner's syndrome (45 X0 karyotype) and Klinefelter's syndrome (47 XXY). Not surprisingly, the gross genetic imbalance created by the presence of so much additional replicated DNA within the zygote nucleus is reflected in profound disturbances of embryogenesis across a number of systems, including the genitourinary tract. The incidence of coexistent renal anomalies ranges from approximately 5% in Down's syndrome (trisomy 21) to 75% in Turner's syndrome (45 X0) (Table 28.1).

Non-disjunction and translocation anomalies are not confined to gametogenesis, but can also arise during the early mitotic cell divisions in the process of cleavage. In the resulting state, termed

Table 28.1 Chromosome defects associated with urinary tract anomalies.

Chromosome defect or syndrome	Frequency (%)	Genitourinary anomalies
Turner's syndrome 45X	60–80	Horseshoe kidney Duplication
Trisomy 18 (Edwards' syndrome)	70	Horseshoe kidney Renal ectopia Duplication Hydronephrosis
Trisomy 13 (Patu syndrome)	60–80	Cystic kidney Hydronephrosis Horseshoe kidney Ureteric duplication
4p (Wolf–Hirschorn syndrome)	33	Hypospadias Cystic kidney Hydronephrosis
Trisomy 21 (Down's syndrome)	3–7	Renal agenesis Horseshoe kidney

'mosaicism', the embryonic tissues contain a varying ratio of cell lines with differing karyotypes depending on the phase of cleavage at which non-disjunction occurred, such as two-cell, four-cell, eight-cell embryo, etc. Abnormalities of the sex chromosomes are often found in mosaic form. True hermaphroditism can be explained on this basis. Affected individuals possess both ovarian (XX) and testicular (XY) tissue, co-existing in streak-like ovotestes. Gonadal mesenchyme carrying a Y chromosome differentiates as testicular tissue, whereas tissue derived from the original population of non-Y embryonic cells differentiates passively down the female (ovarian) pathway. Karyotypes show a varied pattern, including 45 X/46 XY, 46 XX/47 XXY, etc. Turner's syndrome and Klinefelter's syndrome are often associated with mosaic karyotypes.

IMPLANTATION AND EARLY EMBRYONIC DEVELOPMENT

On the fifth or sixth day after fertilization, having travelled down the fallopian tube, the blastocyst implants itself into the endometrium of the uterine cavity, which has been primed by progesterone. Over the ensuing 10 days, two cavities are formed within the spherical mass of rapidly proliferating embryonic cells. The embryonic disc, from which the embryo itself originates, develops in the three-layered interface between the amniotic cavity and definitive yolk sac. The amniotic surface of the trilaminar embryonic disc gives rise to the ectodermal tissues of the embryo, whereas the endodermal derivatives originate from the yolk sac-derived surface. The intraembryonic mesoderm is formed by the inpouring of cells on the amniotic surface of the disc via the primitive streak (Figure 28.2). The layer of intraembryonic mesoderm created by the inpouring process soon subdivides into three components, that is, paraxial mesoderm, intermediate mesoderm and lateral plate mesoderm. It is from this intermediate mesoderm that much of the genitourinary tract is ultimately derived. The third and fourth weeks of gestation are dominated by the processes of segmentation and somite formation that characterize all vertebrate embryogenesis. At this stage, folding of the expanding embryonic disc imparts recognizable shape to the growing embryo.

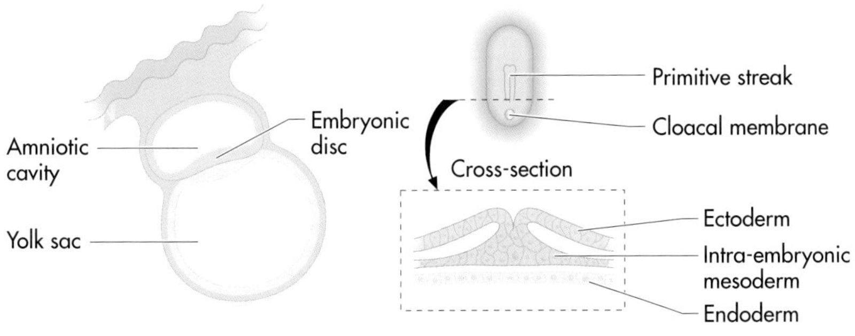

Figure 28.2 *The embryonic disc at 16 days. Inpouring of cells at the primitive streak creates the intra-embryonic mesoderm from which the genitourinary tract is formed.*

EMBRYOLOGY OF THE UPPER URINARY TRACT

The kidneys are derived from the caudal zones of the paired columns of intermediate mesoderm flanking the midline. The emergence of the metanephros, the precursor of the definitive kidney, is preceded by the formation of the pronephros and mesonephros – primitive kidney-like structures. During the fourth week of gestation, the primitive pronephros appears in the cervical portion of the intermediate mesoderm but rapidly undergoes regression. Later in the fourth week, nephron-like tubular structures appear in the mid-section of intermediate mesoderm – the mesonephros (Figure 28.3a).

Concurrently, condensations of mesenchyme lying lateral to the developing mesonephros become the mesonephric ducts. These advance caudally to fuse with the cloaca (the terminal portion of hindgut destined to give rise to the bladder by the process of subdivision). Canalization of the mesonephric duct creates a patent excretory unit, which is believed to function briefly by producing very small quantities of urine. The beginning of the fifth week sees the appearance of the ureteric buds (Figure 28.3b), arising from the most distal portion of the paired mesonephric ducts. Recent research has identified an important and hitherto unrecognized role of the renin angiotensin system in regulating early differentiation and development of the urinary tract.[2] Two types of receptor are responsible for mediating the actions of angiotensin II in target tissues. Stimulation of the angiotensin 1 (AGTR 1) receptor in the embryo promotes cellullar proliferation, matrix deposition and the release of growth factors in the mesenchymal precursors of the kidney and ureter. In contrast, the angiotensin 2 (AGTR2) receptor, which is expressed principally in the embryo and fetus, is responsible for inducing apoptosis and decreased cell growth. 'Knockout' deletions of the AGTR1 and AGTR2 genes in mice result in different patterns of urinaty tract malformations. While deletion of the AGTR1 gene is characterized by progressive dilatation of the collecting system in postnatal life, deletion of AGTR2 gene gives rise to varying degrees of congenital renal hypoplasia, dysplasia and ureteric dilatation.

At around 32 days, the advancing ureteric bud makes contact with the metanephros, and the interactive process of nephrogenesis commences (Figure 28.4). During the sixth to ninth weeks, the lobulated embryonic kidneys ascend up the posterior abdominal wall from their caudal sites of origin to their definitive lumbar position.

The process whereby nephron units are created within the embryonic and fetal kidney spans a period of approximately 30 weeks, from weeks 6 to 36 of gestation. The ureteric bud and the metanephric mesenchyme each make specific contributions to the definitive structure of the kidney. Sequential branching of the ureteric bud gives rise to the renal pelvis, the major calices, the minor calices and the collecting ducts. Within the metanephric mesenchyme, differentiating cells aggregate to form the glomeruli, convoluted tubules and loop of

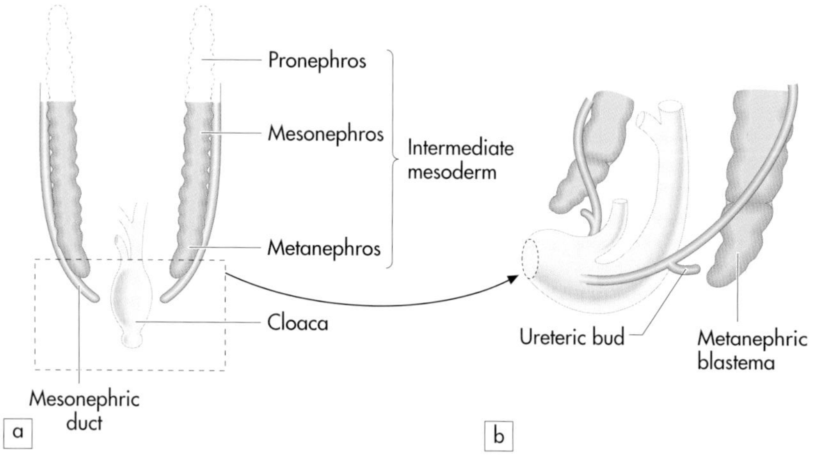

Figure 28.3 *(a) Following the regression of the pronephros, the mesonephros assumes prominence before the emergence of the metanephros as the definitive embryonic kidney. (b) At around 28 days, the ureteric buds appear and advance towards the metanephric mesenchyme.*

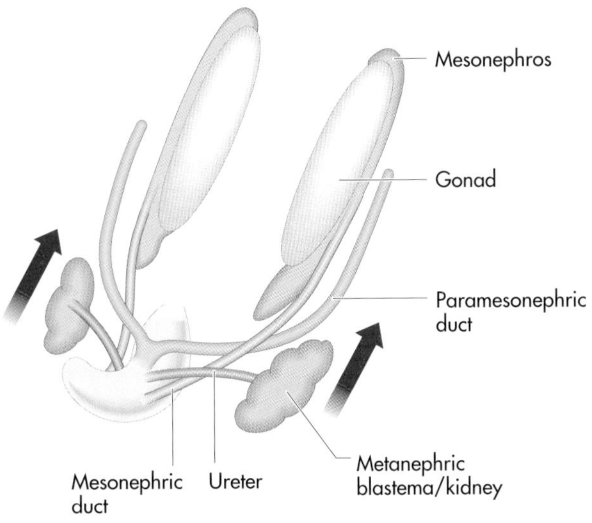

Figure 28.4 *Five to seven weeks: penetration of the metanephric mesenchyme promotes nephrogenesis by a process of mutual induction. Mesonephric tissues support the development of the embryonic gonads in the genital ridges. The paramesonephric ducts develop in the mesenchyme adjacent to the mesonephric ducts.*

Henle. At around the 10th week, the distal convoluted tubules (derived from metanephric mesenchyme) establish continuity with the collecting ducts (of ureteric bud origin) to form functional excretory units. Branching and budding of the ureteric bud derivatives cease at around 15 weeks, but, within the fetal renal cortex, new generations of nephrons continue to appear until the cessation of nephrogenesis at 36 weeks. The process of tubular differentiation within the metanephric mesenchyme is initiated by contact with the ureteric bud. Similarly, proliferative budding and branching of the ureteric bud tissues are dependent upon induction by the metanephric mesenchyme. When grown in tissue culture in isolation, neither of these embryonic tissues has the capacity to differentiate into nephron-like structures. However, when cultured together, nephrogenesis is observed.

The identity of the gene products responsible for mediating the cell-to-cell signalling at a molecular level is being extensively studied in tissue culture, organ culture and genetically engineered transgenic mice. A large number of signalling molecules have already been demonstrated to play a role in regulating the different phases of nephrogenesis.[3,4] The actions of positive growth factors, such as fibroblast growth factor 2 and glial cell line-derived neurotrophic factor (GDNF), are balanced by other substances, such as tumour necrosis factor, which act as negative growth factors by promoting apoptosis (programmed cell death).

Transcription factors constitute another important group of signalling molecules. These DNA-binding proteins are involved in regulating gene expression. Examples of transcription factors closely involved in nephrogenesis include the gene products of the Pax2 gene and Wilms' tumour suppressor gene (WT1 gene), both of which play a central role in branching of the ureteric bud and induction of metanephric mesenchyme. Other signalling molecules include those responsible for cell-to-cell adhesion and cell-to-cell matrix adhesion, such as laminins and integrins.

CONGENITAL RENAL MALFORMATIONS: CLINICAL CONSIDERATIONS

The following four broad morphological categories can be defined:

1. renal agenesis – total absence of the kidney
2. renal dysplasia – a kidney is present, although it is often abnormal in size. The internal architecture is disordered and the histological appearances typically include areas of immature, primitive, 'undifferentiated' tubules, and the inappropriate presence of tissues such as cartilage and fibromuscular tissue within the renal parenchyma
3. cyst formation
4. gross developmental anomalies, such as duplication, horseshoe kidney and pelvic kidney.

Ureteric duplication is readily explained on the basis of bifurcation of the ureteric bud.[5] Depending on the level of the original bifurcation, the duplication may be complete or incomplete. In cases of complete ureteric duplication, the upper pole ureter paradoxically joins the urinary tract more distally than the lower pole ureter. This anatomical pattern (described by the Meyer Weigert law) occurs when the mesonephric duct separates from the embryonic ureter and its terminal portion descends towards the primitive posterior urethra (with a tendency to take the upper pole ureter with it). Gross renal anomalies, such as horseshoe kidney, pelvic kidney and crossed ectopia, date from the period of ascent, during which embryonic kidneys may fuse (horseshoe kidney), cross the midline (crossed fused ectopia) or fail to ascend (pelvic kidney).

PATHOGENESIS OF RENAL MALFORMATIONS

Various mechanisms or aetiological insults have been invoked to explain the patterns of renal malformations described above. The adult and infant forms of polycystic renal disease provide the most convincing examples of genetically determined structural renal disease. Genetic factors have also been implicated in the aetiology of renal agenesis, vesicoureteric reflux and upper tract duplication. In the majority of instances, however, renal malformations are believed to occur on a sporadic basis. Malformations of the upper tract may be the result of an intrinsic abnormality of the metanephros, defects of the ureteric bud, or exposure of the embryonic or fetal kidney to the mechanical effects of obstruction or reflux.

EMBRYOLOGY OF THE LOWER URINARY TRACT (BLADDER AND URETHRA)

The bladder and urethra originate from the anterior portion of the cloaca, the common terminal section of hindgut into which the mesonephric ducts and embryonic ureters drain. The cloaca also contributes the urogenital sinus – which in turn contributes to the vagina. Between the fourth and sixth weeks of gestation, the urorectal septum descends in a shutter-like fashion to subdivide the cloaca into the urogenital canal anteriorly and the anorectal canal posteriorly (Figure 28.5). The process of compartmentalization initiated by the urorectal septum is aided by the lateral in-growth of the folds of Rathke. When the bladder is taking shape in the upper portion of the urogenital canal, the points of entry of the ureter and mesonephric ducts begin to separate (Figure 28.6). As the distance between them increases, the

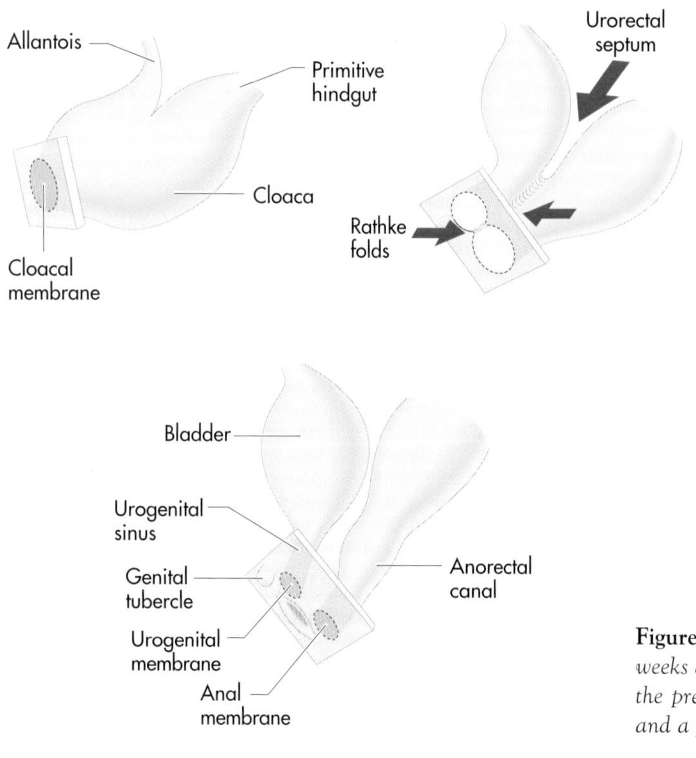

Figure 28.5 *Descent of the urorectal septum between four and six weeks divides the cloaca into an anterior urogenital compartment, the precursor of the bladder, urethra, prostate and distal vagina, and a posterior anorectal canal.*

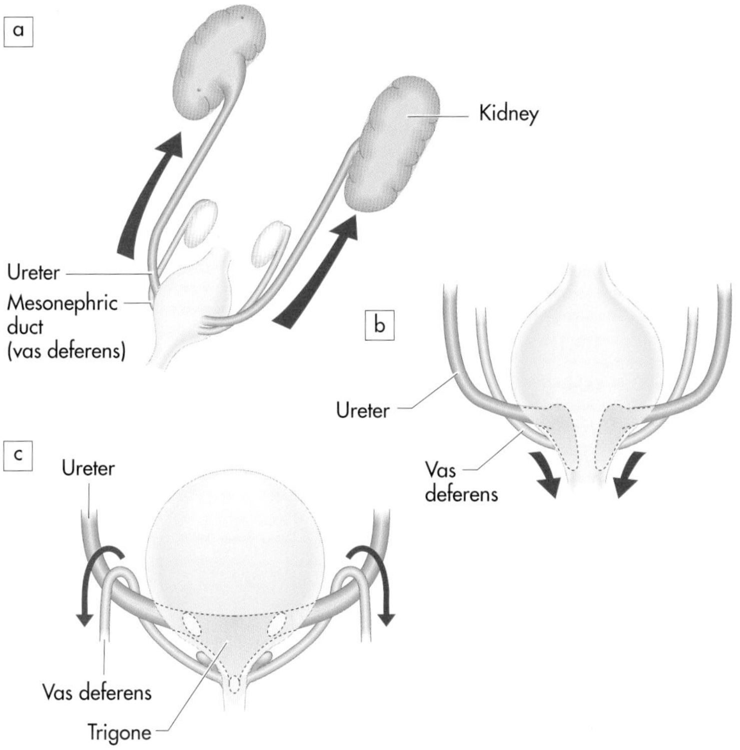

Figure 28.6 *(a) and (b) Although the ureters maintain their position in relation to the developing bladder, the mesonephric ducts are drawn distally to enter the proximal urethra. (c) Tesicular descent causes the mesonephric ducts (vasa deferentia) to loop over the ureters.*

mesonephric ducts descend caudally to open into the developing posterior urethra. In contrast, the ureters retain their original position with respect to the developing bladder. Although the triangular plate of mesoderm enclosing the ureteric orifices and openings of the mesonephric ducts is covered by the endodermal lining of the urogenital canal, its outline is retained as the trigone. The most distal (perineal) portion of the urogenital canal gives rise to the entire length of the female urethra and to the posterior urethra in the male. The anterior portion of the male urethra is created by closure of the urogenital groove, described below. The allantois, an elongated diverticulum, protruding from the dome of the fetal bladder into the umbilicus, is gradually obliterated but persists as the median umbilical ligament.

CLINICAL CONSIDERATIONS

Failed or incomplete descent of the urorectal septum results in a spectrum of anomalies ranging from urogenital sinus to a complete, persistent cloaca.[6] The aetiology of bladder exstrophy and epispadias is incompletely understood, but these anomalies are believed to reflect underlying defects of the cloacal membrane. Persistence of all or part of the allantois gives rise to the various urachal abnormalities.

FUNCTIONAL DEVELOPMENT OF THE FETAL URINARY TRACT

From the ninth or 10th week of gestation, fetal urine is excreted into the amniotic cavity. Initially, the composition of fetal urine closely resembles that of plasma filtrate. In intrauterine life, the excretory and homeostatic functions of the kidney are fulfilled by the placenta, and the principal role of the fetal kidneys is to contribute urine to amniotic fluid. The volume of amniotic fluid reaches its maximum of around 1000 ml at 38 weeks' gestation – at which point, fetal urine comprises 90% of the amniotic fluid. As well as providing a protective fluid environment for the fetus, amniotic fluid plays a vital role in fetal lung development. When fetal urine output is reduced, as a result of either renal agenesis or infravesical obstruction, the resulting oligohydramnios is associated with pulmonary hypoplasia. Moulding or compression deformities can be produced by the compressive effect of the surrounding uterus.

GENITAL TRACTS

The internal and external genitalia of both sexes are formed from identical embryonic precursors, and it is only from the sixth week onwards that differences begin to appear. In both sexes, the formation of the gonads and genital tracts is initiated by the migration of primordial germ cells from the base of the yolk sac, across the coelomic cavity to condensations of mesenchyme flanking the midline of the lumbar region of the embryo (Figure 28.7). The arrival of the primordial germ cells in these zones of mesenchyme stimulates the formation of the paired genital ridges. By a process of mutual induction (analogous to nephrogenesis), the interaction of the germ cells and surrounding mesenchyme results in the formation of the primitive sex cords within the embryonic gonad. It is around this time that a second pair of potential genital ducts (the paramesonephric ducts) makes its appearance. Derived from condensations of coelomic epithelium and lying lateral to the mesonephric ducts, these ducts fuse distally at their point of attachment to the urogenital canal. From the sixth week onwards, the paths of male and female differentiation diverge.

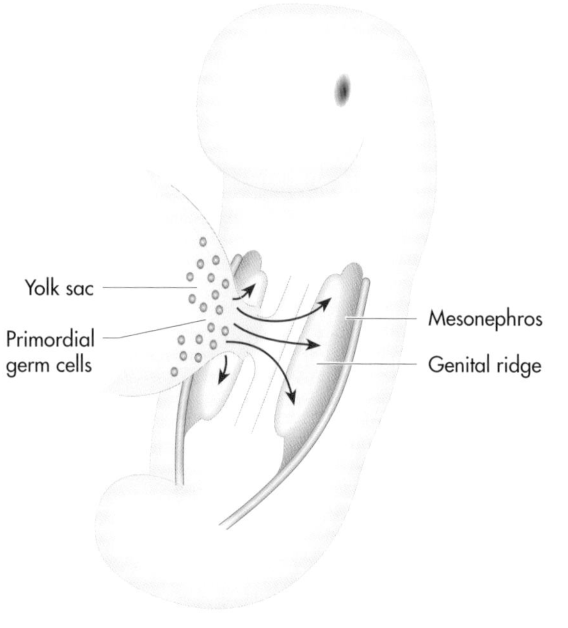

Figure 28.7 *Migration of the primordial germ cells from the yolk sac across the coelomic cavity to colonize the mesoderm of the genital ridges during the fifth week.*

Female

It is widely accepted that unless the genetic information carried by the testis-determining gene (SRY) is present, the gonads and genital tract of the embryo are programmed to differentiate down a female pathway. The primitive sex cords degenerate, but secondary sex cords derived from genital ridge mesoderm enclose the primordial germ cells to form the primitive follicles. However, it may be oversimplistic to view female gonadal differentiation as an entirely passive or 'default' process. For example, the occurrence of dysplastic or streak gonads in females with an XO karyotype (Turner's syndrome) suggests that normal ovarian development is not simply dependent on the absence of the genetic material carried on the Y chromosome but requires the presence of two X chromosomes to permit normal ovarian development. In the female, gametogenesis commences in intrauterine life with the transition from primordial germ cell to primary oocyte being completed in the fetal ovary. The primary oocytes then proceed to the first phase of meiosis before entering a long phase of arrested division, which only resumes again after puberty (Figure 28.8). Without the influence of testosterone, the mesonephric ducts regress (with the exception of vestigial remnants of the epoöphoron and paroöphoron and Gartner's cysts). The paramesonephric ducts persist and develop to become the fallopian tubes. Their merged distal portions give rise to the uterus and upper two-thirds of the vagina (Figure 28.9). At their point of attachment to the urogenital sinus, the fused tips of the paramesonephric ducts induce a condensation of tissue – the sinuvaginal bulb. Downward growth of the sinuvaginal bulb in the direction of the fetal perineum between weeks 10 and 20 has the effect of separating the vagina from the urethra. The vagina is initially represented by a solid plate of paramesonephric tissue, but a lumen develops before week 20. The distal third of the vagina is derived from the urogenital sinus (endoderm), whereas the introitus and external genitalia are ectodermal in origin (Figure 28.10).

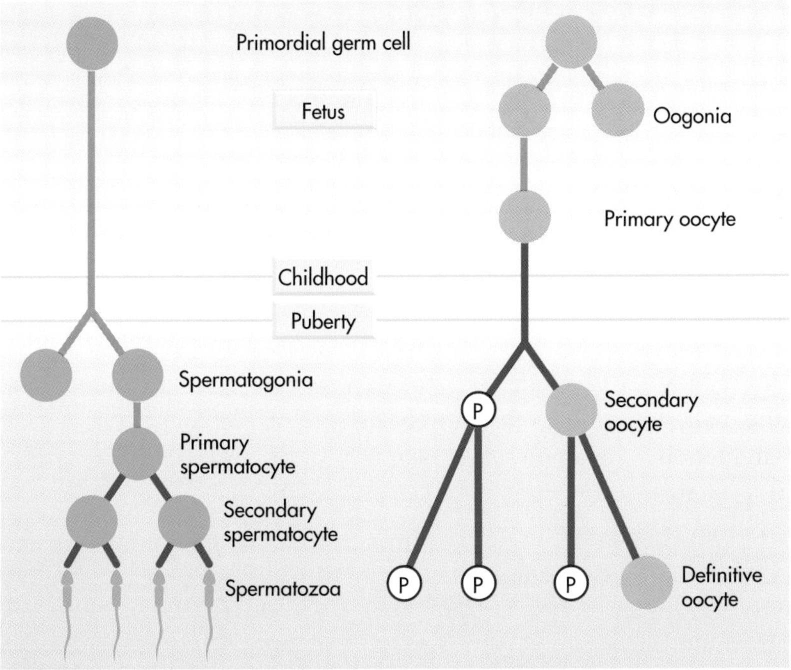

Figure 28.8 *Gametogenesis. Mitotic division of the primordial germ cells in the male embryo is suppressed by the Sertoli cells of the embryonic germinal epithelium. Gametogenesis recommences at puberty. The gametes (spermatoza) are the product of two meiotic divisions, i.e. primary spermatocyte to secondary spermatocyte to spermatoza. Immediately after the second meiotic division, the immature haploid gametes are termed spermatids. The morphological maturation to spermatoza occurs during passage through the seminiferous tubule. In the female, the initial phases of gametogenesis occur in the first five months of fetal life. Primary oocytes remain in arrested meiotic division until meiosis recommences in the maturing Graafian follicle. The two meiotic divisions culminate in the production of a single definitive oocyte and three polar bodies (P).*

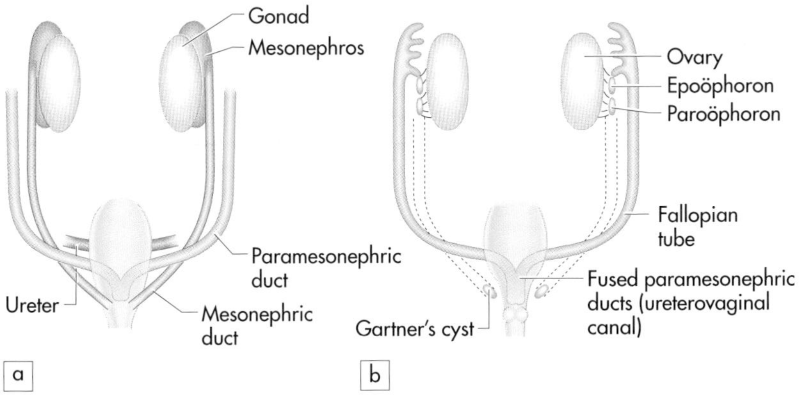

Figure 28.9 *(a) The genital tract of both male and female embryos remains in the same undifferentiated state until the sixth week of gestation. (b) Paramesonephric duct derivatives in the female embryo.*

External genitalia

The external genitalia of the embryo and fetus are 'programmed' to differentiate down a female pathway unless exposed to androgenic stimulation. Thus, the genital tubercle forms the clitoris, the urogenital sinus contributes the vestibule of the vagina, the urogenital folds evolve into the labia minora, and the labioscrotal folds persist as the labia majora.

Male

Many aspects of the male differentiation pathway are mediated by 'downstream' genes located on the Y chromosome and on autosomes, but the process is initiated by the testis-determining gene (SRY) located on the Y chromosome.[7] It is believed that the testis-determining factor encoded on this gene stimulates the medullary sex cords of the embryonic gonad to differentiate into secretory Sertoli cells. From the seventh week onwards, the Sertoli cells secrete a glycoprotein – antiMüllerian hormone or Müllerian-inhibiting substance – which switches differentiation down the male pathway. At least three key functions have been ascribed to Müllerian-inhibiting substance:[8]

1. It causes regression of the paramesonephric ducts: with the exception of vestigial remnants (the appendix, testis and the utriculus), the paramesonephric ducts disappear completely in the male.

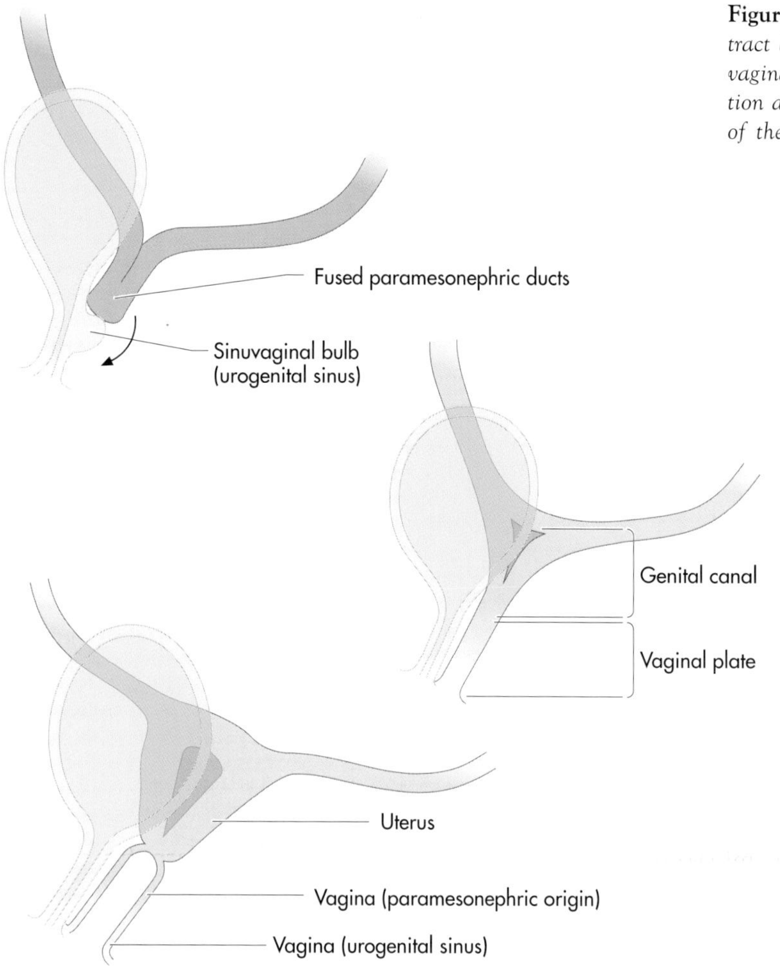

Figure 28.10 *Development of the lower female genital tract between 10 and 20 weeks. Migration of the sinuvaginal bulb towards the fetal perineum results in formation and elongation of the vaginal plate and separation of the vagina from the urethra.*

2. It stimulates the production of testosterone by the Leydig cells of the embryonic testis from the ninth week of gestation.
3. It induces the first stage of testicular descent by its action on the gubernaculum, which anchors the testis in the vicinity of the developing inguinal canal.

Further division of the primordial germ cells is inhibited in the male embryonic gonad. Until recently, it was believed that the testis is quiescent throughout childhood and that the subsequent sequence of gametogenesis is resumed again only at puberty. This concept is now being challenged by evidence pointing to the occurrence of two maturational steps in the prepubertal testis. The first, at around 2–3 months of age, consists of the switch from gonocytes (fetal stem cells), to adult type spermatogonia (the adult stem cell pool). The second step, at approximately 5 years of age, is marked by a transient phase of meiosis, which can be detected histologically by the appearance of primary spermatocytes. The data derived from these biopsy studies of undescended testes have revealed that cryptorchidism has a major impact on the prepubertal maturational process. Although much work has yet to be done, it is already apparent that these new findings have important implications for the management of undescended testes.

Regression of the paramesonephric ducts in response to Müllerian-inhibiting substance is accompanied by the development of mesonephric duct derivatives under the influence of testosterone secreted by the fetal testis (Figure 28.11a). In a process spanning weeks 8–12 of gestation, the mesonephric ducts give rise to the epididymis and rete testis, vas deferens, ejaculatory ducts and seminal vesicles (Figure 28.11b). Within the testis, the

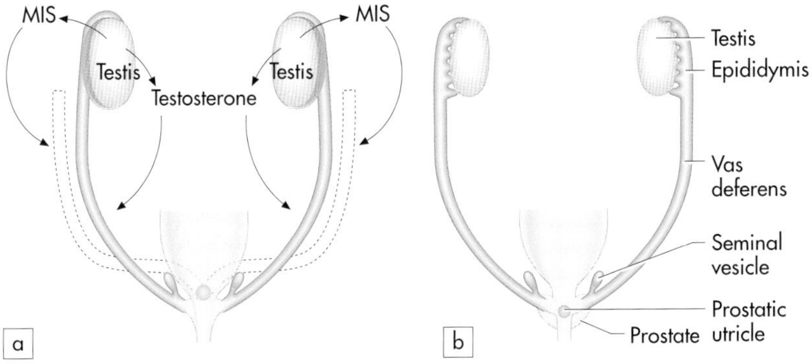

Figure 28.11 *(a) Differentiation of male internal genitalia. Secretion of Müllerian-inhibiting substance (MIS) by pre-Sertoli cells induces regression of the paramesonephric ducts between eight and ten weeks. (b) MIS also stimulates the embryonic Leydig cells to secrete testosterone, which in turn stimulates the mesonephric ducts to differentiate into the definitive male internal genitalia.*

seminiferous tubules take their origin from the primitive sex cords of the genital ridge mesoderm.

The development of the prostate gland[9] provides another example of reciprocal induction. At around week 12, in response to androgenic stimulation, a condensation of mesenchyme in the fetal pelvis induces the outgrowth of endodermal buds on the adjacent region of the developing urethra. Interestingly, in the experimental setting, transitional epithelium from the adult rat can be induced to differentiate into prostatic glandular epithelium when cultured, in contact with the appropriate embryonic mesenchyme. In normal fetal development, however, the endodermal proliferation and branching that give rise to the ducts and glandular acini of the prostate gland are switched off after week 15 of gestation. The glandular tissue of the prostate is derived from urethral (urogenital sinus) endoderm, and the capsule and smooth muscle are mesenchymal in origin, whereas the mesonephric ducts form the intraprostatic vas deferens and ejaculatory ducts.

External genitalia (Figure 28.12)

Prior to the compartmentalization of the cloaca into the urogenital and anorectal canals between the sixth and seventh weeks, the primitive perineum consists of little more than the cloacal membrane and genital tubercle. Separation of the cloaca into the urogenital canal and anorectal canal is accompanied by subdivision of the cloacal membrane into the urogenital membrane anteriorly and the anal membrane posteriorly. Urogenital folds surround the urogenital membrane, flanked by the labioscrotal folds. From the seventh week onwards, the urogenital sinus advances onto the perineum anteriorly and onto the penis as the urethral groove. In-growth of the urethral groove creates a solid urethral plate, which subsequently canalizes to form the definitive urethra. The differentiation of the male external genitalia is dependent, firstly, on the enzymatic conversion of testosterone to dihydrotestosterone and, secondly, on the presence of the appropriate receptors in the target tissues. During weeks 12–14, exposed to increasing androgenic stimulation, the external genitalia begin to adopt a distinctively male configuration. Closure of the urethra is complete by around 15 weeks, the terminal portion being formed by in-growth of ectoderm from the tip of the glans.

The testis

As described above, the fetal testis originates from the interaction of primordial germ cells, the mesenchyme of the genital ridge and mesonephric duct derivatives. Testicular descent occurs in two phases, the first prompted by Müllerian-inhibiting substance, the second under the stimulus of testosterone. In both phases, the endocrine influences are mediated via the gubernaculum. Between weeks 8 and 15, the cord-like gubernaculum extending down from the testis enlarges at its distal end in the region of the labioscrotal swellings (Figure 28.13a). Because the length of the gubernaculum remains relatively fixed during a period of active fetal growth, the effect is to anchor the testis in the region of the future inguinal canal (Figure 28.13b). The second, more active, phase of testicular descent is delayed until weeks 25–30 of gestation when testosterone causes the gubernaculum to shrink and contract, thus guiding the testis down the inguinal canal into its final scrotal position (Figure 28.13c). On its route of descent, the testis is preceded

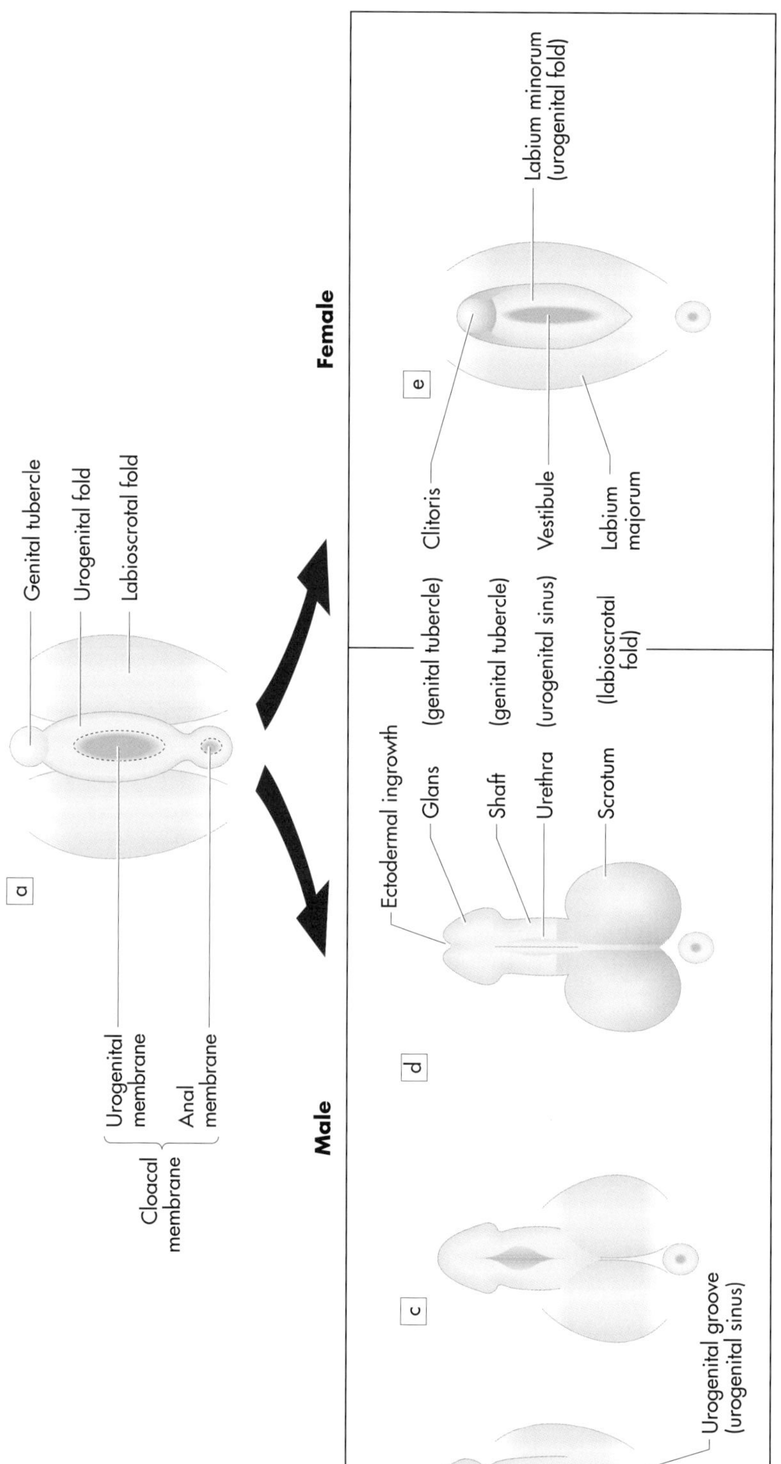

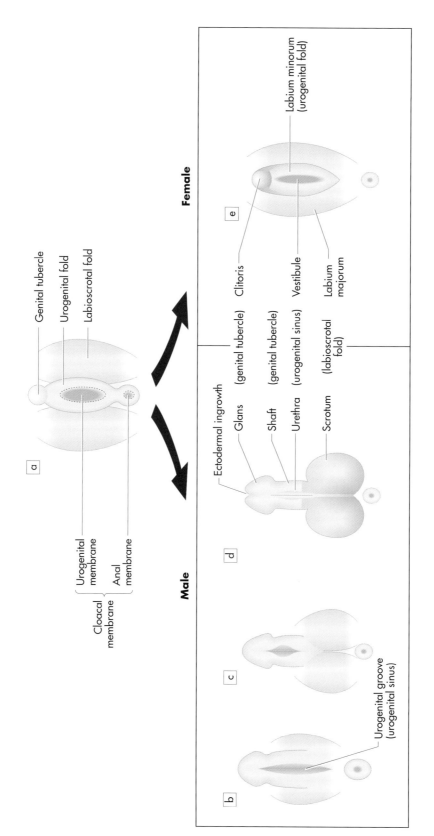

Figure 28.12 *(a) Undifferentiated precursors of male and female external genitalia. (b), (c) and (d) Androgen (testosterone-derived dihydrotestosterone) induced differentiation of the male external genitalia between 12 and 16 weeks. (e) In the absence of androgenic stimulation, the external genitalia are programmed to differentiate along a female pathway.*

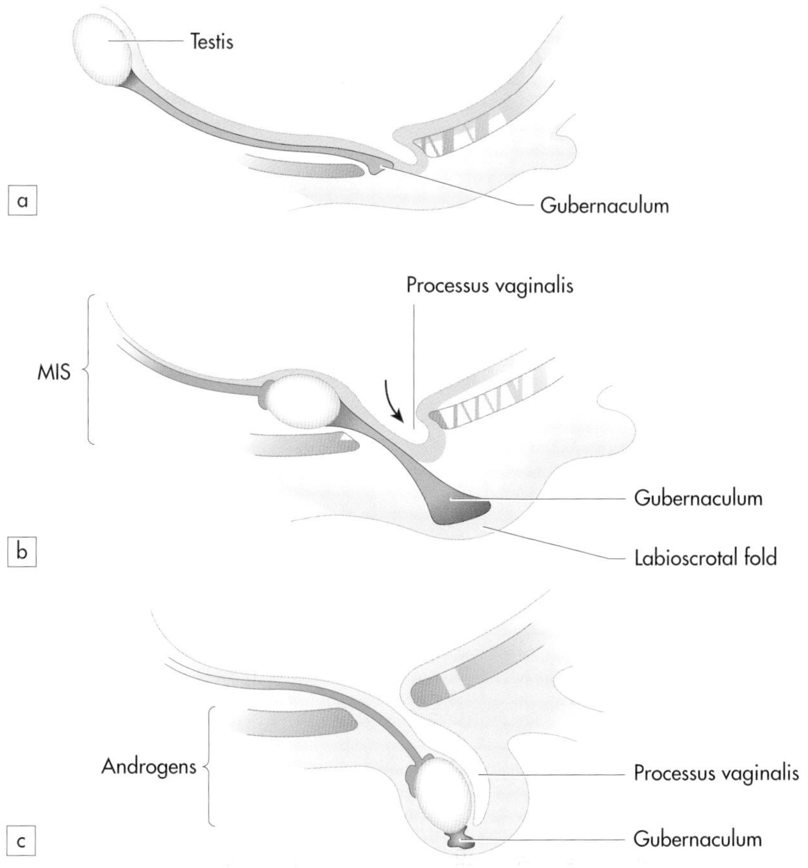

Figure 28.13 *(a) Formation of the gubernaculum. (b) 10–15 weeks: enlargement of the caudal end of the gubernaculum (in response to Müllerian-inhibiting substance) anchors the fetal testis at the developing inguinal canal. (c) 25–30 weeks: testosterone-induced second stage of testicular descent.*

by a sac-like protrusion of peritoneum, the processus vaginalis, which normally closes spontaneously prior to delivery or in the early months of life.

GENITAL ANOMALIES: CLINICAL CONSIDERATIONS

Defects occurring in the development of the paramesonephric duct system result in a variety of clinical manifestations. The occurrence of unilateral renal agenesis in conjunction with complete absence of the ipsilateral paramesonephric duct derivatives points to a fundamental defect at the level of the original intermediate mesoderm.

Congenital absence or atresia of the vagina is a rare anomaly. Total agenesis (Rokitansky syndrome) is thought to result from failure of the paramesonephric ducts to make contact with the urogenital sinus.

Virilization of the external genitalia in the 46 XX female with congenital adrenal hyperplasia accounts for 80% of infants with ambiguous genitalia.[10] In these patients, the internal reproductive tract develops normally along female lines, but the external genitalia differentiate down a male pathway under the influence of high levels of circulating androgens of adrenal origin. In androgen-insensitivity syndrome (testicular feminization syndrome), the external genitalia of 46 XY males fail to virilize despite the production of Müllerian-inhibiting substance and testosterone by the fetal testes. The explanation lies in a genetically determined peripheral receptor insensitivity to dihydrotestosterone.

Incomplete closure of the urethral groove accounts for moderate and severe forms of hypospadias, while distal (glanular) hypospadias probably represents failure of ectodermal in-growth from the glanular tip. Although severe hypospadias, particularly when associated with cryptorchidism and an enlarged utriculus (Müllerian remnant), is probably the manifestation of a more generalized virilization defect, attempts to identify a specific endocrinopathy in such cases have generally proved unrewarding.

The incidence of hypospadias and cryptorchidism appears to be increasing, and exposure of male fetuses to oestrogenic or antiandrogenic environmental pollutants has been implicated as one of the possible causes. Although other explanations have also been postulated, the possibility that environmental factors may be having an impact on genital differentiation is sufficiently alarming to merit serious consideration and further research.

Congenital disorders of the testis and its descent are common. Cryptorchidism affects 1–2% of the male infant population.[11] In the rare, genetically determined syndrome of Müllerian-inhibiting substance deficiency, intra-abdominal testes are found in association with persistent paramesonephric duct structures, including fallopian tubes and uterus. Virilization defects (such as androgen-insensitivity syndrome and 5-alpha ·-reductase deficiency) account for some cases, and cryptorchidism also forms a well-recognized component of many syndromes. Simple mechanical factors provide the most obvious explanation for unilateral cryptorchidism, but the reported finding of histological abnormalities in the contralateral descended testis suggests that endocrinopathy may also play a role in unilateral cryptorchidism. The presence of a blind-ending vas and spermatic vessels in most cases of testicular 'agenesis' is widely interpreted as evidence of intrauterine testicular torsion rather than a defect of embryogenesis.

THE GENETIC BASIS OF GENITOURINARY MALFORMATIONS

Malformations of the urinary and genital tracts are estimated to account for one-third of all congenital anomalies. Although most are believed to represent sporadic, that is, 'one-off', anomalies resulting from defective embryogenesis or faulty development in fetal life, the importance of genetic factors is being increasingly recognized (Table 28.2). Moreover, in conditions with a well-established inherited aetiology, molecular biology is beginning to identify the faulty chromosome(s) and pinpoint the site(s) of mutation. Those genitourinary malformations which have a genetic basis are most commonly inherited as autosomal traits of variable penetrance and expression.

Although some conditions may have their origins in a single gene mutation, our current state of knowledge suggests that the aetiology of most renal anomalies will prove to be more complex. This fact is illustrated by the observation that upper tract anomalies are often expressed unilaterally or asymmetrically even when genetic factors are clearly

Table 28.2 The genetic basis of common urinary tract abnormalities.

Adult polycystic kidney disease	Autosomal dominant	Chromosome 16p Chromosome 4
'Infantile' polycystic kidney disease	Autosomal recessive	
Vesico-ureteric reflux	Autosomal dominant, variable penetrance and expression	(*Pax-2* gene in renal–coloboma syndrome)
Renal agenesis	Various, i.e. autosomal dominant, recessive and X-linked patterns identified	
Ureteric duplication	Autosomal dominant – variable penetrance and expression	
Pelvi-ureteric junction obstruction	When familial behaves as autosomal dominant	Documented familial evidence as isolated anomaly or pelvi-ureteric junction obstruction in association with specific syndromes (e.g. Schinzel Gideon and Johanson Blizzard syndromes)

implicated. In general, the complex process of embryogenesis reflects the regulated, sequential expression of a number of genes. Where genitourinary anomalies constitute one part of a recognized syndrome, it is likely that the affected gene (or genes) encodes for gene products that play a fundamental molecular role in the regulation and development of a number of systems. For example, the KAL gene implicated in X-linked Kallmann's syndrome (microphallus, renal agenesis and anosmia) is known to code for an adhesion molecule implicated in the migration of olfactory neurons in the brain and also in the process of nephrogenesis. Other examples include renal–coloboma syndrome (vesicoureteric reflux and the ophthalmic anomaly, coloboma),[12] which has been attributed to a mutation of the PAX-2 gene encoding for a transcription factor. A detailed account of this exciting and rapidly expanding field is beyond the scope of this chapter. It is already apparent, however, that research in genetics and molecular biology is destined to make a major contribution to our understanding of the normal and abnormal development of the urinary and genital tracts.

FUTURE APPLICATIONS OF DEVELOPMENTAL BIOLOGY

Successful reproductive cloning by using the nucleus of an adult mammalian somatic cell was first achieved by the Roslin Institute in Scotland with the birth of the celebrated sheep 'Dolly'. The feasibility of reproductive cloning has subsequently been confirmed by reports from other centres, raising the highly controversial prospect that human reproductive cloning might be attempted in the future. Initially, the heated ethical debate surrounding reproductive cloning largely overshadowed the excitement generated within the scientific community by the potential applications of therapeutic cloning and 'stem-cell technology'. Clinical indications envisaged for such forms of treatment include tissue reconstruction and the treatment of degenerative disease – particularly neurodegenerative disorders such as Parkinson's disease. For the purposes of therapeutic cloning, it is envisaged that pluripotent embryonic stem cells would be extracted from the cloned blastocyst at around 6 days. While it seems certain that human reproductive cloning will be legally proscribed for the foreseeable future, legislation has been passed in the UK to permit research into the cloning of early human embryonic tissue for certain therapeutic applications (subject to the existing 14-day limit).

Both reproductive and therapeutic cloning share the same initial laboratory methodology termed 'nuclear transfer', which has the following stages:

1. The nucleus of a harvested or donated oocyte is removed by micropuncture. A diploid nucleus extracted from a somatic cell is then injected into the enucleated oocyte. For the purposes of therapeutic cloning, it is envisaged that the somatic cell would be derived from the patient.
2. The cell thus created is induced to divide, as for example, by an electrical charge.
3. A sequence of doubling divisions then ensues which mirrors that of the fertilized zygote. Proteins within the cytoplasm of maternal oocyte are thought to be responsible for inducing the cloned cell to behave as a fertilized zygote rather than the mature somatic cell from which its nucleus was derived (Figure 28.14).

In reproductive cloning, the early embryo is then implanted by standard techniques of in vitro fertilization.

The concept of therapeutic cloning centres principally on the potential use of pluripotent embryonic stem cells derived from cloned embryonic tissue. Tissue derived by therapeutic cloning of a patient's cell would share the same genetic identity and would therefore not provoke rejection by the immune system when reintroduced into the patient for the purposes of treatment. Embryonic stem cells are the precursors of many different definitive cell types. If they could be 'programmed' to differentiate into cells such as neurons, muscle cells and haematopoietic tissue, their use could open up a wide range of therapeutic opportunities. Human embryonic stem cells have already been successfully isolated and grown in tissue culture. Moreover, the methodology needed to induce embryonic stem cells to differentiate down 'programmed' pathways to generate specific cell types is already under

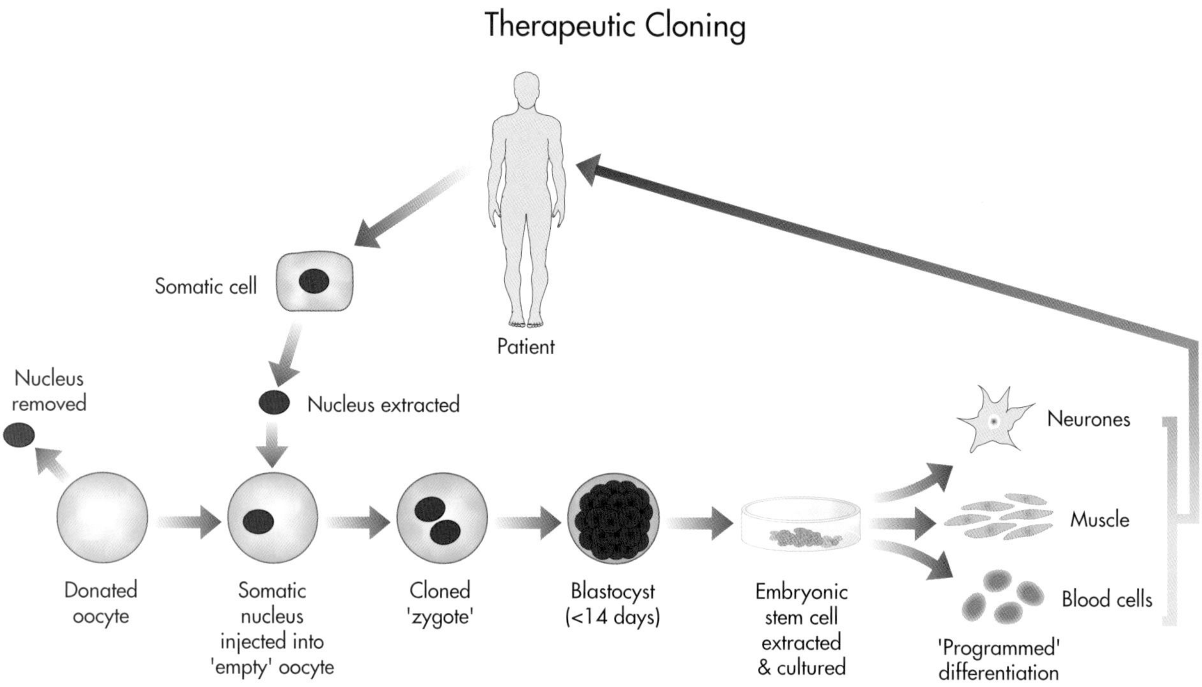

Figure 28.14 *Concept of Therapeutic Cloning. The diploid nucleus of a somatic cell derived from the patient is injected into an 'enucleated' donated oocyte from which the maternal nuclear DNA has been extracted. ('Nuclear transfer') This 'zygote' is then induced to undergo mitotic cell division to form a 'blastocyst' with an identical genetic make up to the patient. Embryonic stem cells are extracted and induced to differentiate down the appropriate pathway to produce the required cell line. Cloned cells or tissue which have been produced in vitro are then reintroduced into the patient for indications such as the treatment of neurodegenerative disorders or a variety of types of tissue repair.*

development. Understanding and regulating differentiation has been described as 'the last great challenge of developmental biology'.

Yet, even when the hurdle of controlling differentiation has been overcome, the scope of therapeutic cloning within clinical practice would be severely limited by practical considerations such as the scarcity of donated oocytes and the invasive nature of oocyte donation. Moreover, cloning of embryonic tissue remains a highly inefficient process. Despite extensive experience with mouse embryonic stem cells, researchers are still required to create scores of embryos in order to establish a single line of cultured pluripotent stem cells. Hopes that reliance on embryonic stem cells could be circumvented by developing strategies based on the plasticity of adult stem cells have unfortunately been undermined by recent work indicating that adult stem cells fuse with other cell types to create hybrid cells with abnormal karyotypes rather than creating new lineages by transdifferentiation.

Thus, in the light of current knowledge, the development and application of therapeutic cloning in urology (as for the treatment of congenital or degenerative renal diseases by inducing new nephron formation in postnatal life, innovative treatments for male infertility and, ultimately, tissue-engineered kidneys for transplantation) must still be viewed as a highly futuristic prospect.

REFERENCES

1. Thomson JA, Itskovitz-Eldor J, Shapiro SS, Waknitz MA et al. Embryonic stem cell lines derived from human blastocysts. Science 1998; 282: 1145–1147
2. Yerke EB. The new renal angiotensin system and its impact on upper urinary tract development. Dialogues Pediatr Urol 2000; 23: 4–5
3. Abidari JM, Baker LA. Overview of the molecular basis of ureteral budding and metanephros differentiation. Dialogues Pediatr Urol 2000; 23: 5–7
4. Wolfe AS. Molecular control of nephrogenesis. Br J Urol 1998; 81(Suppl. 2): 1–7

3. Stephens FD, Smith DE, Hutson J. Congenital Anomalies of the Urinary and Genital Tracts. Oxford: Isis Medical Media, 1996: 222–234
4. Thomas DFM. Cloacal malformations: embryology, anatomy and principles of management. In: Spitz et al. eds. Progress in Paediatric Surgery. Vol. 23. Berlin: Springer-Verlag, 1989: 135–143
5. Larsen WJ. The search for the testis-determining factor. In: Larsen WJ, ed. Human Embryology. Edinburgh: Churchill Livingstone, 1993: 276–279
6. Hutson JM, Terada M, Baiyun Z, Williams MPL. Normal Testicular Descent and the Aetiology of Cryptorchidism. Advances in Anatomy, Embryology and Cell Biology. Vol. 132. Berlin: Springer, 1996: 8–6
7. McNeal JE. Anatomy and embryology. In: Fitzpatrick JM, Kane RJ, eds. The Prostate. Edinburgh: Churchill Livingstone, 1989: 3–9
8. Whitaker RH, Williams DM. Post-natal investigation and management of genital intersex anomalies. In: Thomas DFM, ed. Urological Disease in the Fetus and Infant. Oxford: Butterworth Heinemann, 1997: 279–292
9. John Radcliffe Cryptorchidism Study Group. Cryptorchidism: a prospective study of 7,500 consecutive male births, 1984–8. Arch Dis Child 1992; 67: 892–899
10. Feather S, Woolf AS, Gordon, Risdon RA et al. Vesicoureteric reflux – is it all in the genes? Lancet 1996; 348: 725–728R

29

Urological and biochemical aspects of transplantation biology

David Talbot and Naeem Soomro

INTRODUCTION

The first successful human renal allograft was performed in Boston by Merrill and Murray on 23 December 1954. Preceding this had been many unsuccessful animal and even human transplants. Only two things had been learned from this early work; firstly, how vessels could be successfully anastomosed, and, secondly, that transplantation between non-related individuals was impossible. The Boston transplant was successful because it was between identical twin brothers, and it was not until immunosuppressive drugs became available that transplantation could really develop.

ORGAN DONATION

The early transplants were all performed from live donors; then, with the advent of immunosuppression, non-related cadaver donors could be used. These initially were simply cadavers and therefore were 'non-heart-beating' donors, but later, with legislation and acceptance of brain death, heart-beating but brain-dead donors were used. More recently, with the limited supply of brain-dead donors, there has been significant expansion of both live donation and non-heart-beating donation.

BRAINSTEM DEATH

Though death is an unavoidable aspect of life, all countries have their own procedures and legislation connected with it. With the advent of transplantation and possible use of organs, most countries were forced to consider and thereby distinguish between cardiac and brain death. In some countries, such as Austria, donation was extremely easy because, since the days of the bubonic plague, legislation had made post-mortems compulsory; therefore, donation was the next step. In many countries, criteria were established for the diagnosis of brain death. In the UK, the tests had to be performed on two occasions by two experienced medical practitioners. Certain prerequisite conditions had to be fulfilled; namely, normothermia and absence of sedative drugs. Furthermore, the subject had to be shown to be ventilator dependent and have absent cranial nerve reflexes, notably the gag, corneal and vestibulocochlear reflexes, by two experienced medical practitioners on two occasions.[1] When the patient was diagnosed as being brain dead, the issues of donation and transplant could be discussed with the relatives. The posts of transplant coordinators evolved in the mid-1980s, in part to act as bereavement counsellors and to coordinate the multiple teams involved in a multiorgan donor. Their role has been essential in maintaining donor numbers in the face of reduced death rates from road traffic accidents and improved outcome of neurosurgery.

NON-HEART-BEATING DONATION

Due to the increasing shortage of kidneys for donation, there is a need to increase the pool of organs. Therefore, the option of non-heart-beating donors, which had been utilized before brain-death legislation, was explored again. These donors have been subjected to a varying amount of primary warm ischaemia, during the time between cardiac arrest and perfusion with cold preservation solution. Different categories can be defined which have implications for the degree of warm ischaemia, simply these cover controlled (awaiting cardiac arrest) and those uncontrolled (failed resuscitation in the emergency setting).[2] Because there is damage to the organs after cardiac arrest, care must be taken to establish which kidneys are safe to transplant.[3] If such steps are taken and the kidneys are used, delayed graft function is common.[4] However, after a time, the function recovers, and the long-term outlook is the same as for kidneys transplanted from brain-dead donors.[4,5] Livers and pancreata have all been transplanted from such donors, but greater care must be taken, as delayed graft function, if it occurs, in a liver transplant is usually fatal.[6]

LIVE RELATED AND UNRELATED DONATION

As cold ischaemia is considerably reduced in live donation, the long-term graft survival is better than with cadaveric donor kidney grafts. Formerly, centres with large cadaver-kidney programmes have generally had small live-donor programmes, presumably indicating that supply is sufficient for demand. However, with the generally declining cadaver programmes, live-donor numbers have increased. Commercialization of transplantation has created a huge ethical issue, and many countries have 'solved' this by banning the practice. This means that transplantation from first-degree relatives that can be confirmed by DNA typing is easily regulated. Second- degree relatives and non-related live donors can be controlled by third-party review and committee approval. Though this appears to work in the UK with regulation by ULTRA (Unrelated Live Transplant Regulatory Authority), similar mechanisms are difficult to maintain in developing countries. In these countries, renal failure has a very high mortality rate without a transplant, and a desperate person with wealth can be quite resourceful.

Kidney donation from live donors carries a low mortality rate and formerly was conducted in parallel with the recipient by open surgery. This approach minimizes cold and warm ischaemia, but the donor has the complications of an open wound. An increasingly popular approach is to use laparoscopic donation, which, though it entails some increased primary warm ischaemia, is considerably better for the donor of the left kidney. However, laparoscopic right-kidney donation carries some risk of caval or duodenal injury and should be done routinely only after considerable experience has been obtained from left-kidney donation.

ORGAN PRESERVATION

In the early days of renal transplantation, there was considerable uncertainty as to how to store the organ. The two methods were simple static cold storage and dynamic machine perfusion, which was also performed at cold temperature. Most groups stopped machine preservation when it was discovered that, generally, the longer the kidney remained in storage, the worse was the outcome.[7] Certain groups, principally Belzer et al from the USA, persisted with machine perfusion, and when the solutions were improved, it was found that the kidney preservation was better with this method than with static storage.[8] This was principally the case with marginal donor kidneys, and this method had the added benefit of allowing the surgeons to improve their viability assessment by assessing the resistance and flow through the kidney.[3,9]

The 'holy grail' of preservation, however, is being able to do it at normal temperature, as this allows more accurate viability assessment and recovery of the organ. However, it is extremely difficult due to the metabolic demands of the organ, and only limited success has been possible so far.[10]

PRESERVATION SOLUTIONS

The first aim of preservation fluid is to replace blood, which, if allowed to stand within the organ, will clot and thereby render it useless. The second aim is to reduce the temperature of the organ to near freezing point to minimize the metabolic demands of the organ (hence, the solutions are kept cold). At cold temperatures, the normal cell-membrane electrolyte pumps fail, and cellular swelling occurs. The early solutions were essentially hyperosmolal mannitol, and though they prevented swelling, the intracellular electrolyte concentrations changed; therefore, acute tubular necrosis was common, particularly when cold storage was prolonged. The solutions were therefore modified to preserve the intracellular milieu; hence, Marshalls, Collins and Euro-Collins were developed. Though acute tubular necrosis still occurred with these solutions, it was not as common. However, other organs, notably the liver, that had to work immediately on transplantation had to have a very restricted cold ischaemic time with these solutions. This improved with the development of University of Wisconsin, or Belzer I, solution, which contained the inert sugar lactobionate and starch that are very effective in preventing cell swelling.[11] Both kidneys and livers preserved with this solution could be cold stored for longer with an increased chance of primary function on reperfusion.[12] After cold storage, reperfusion with blood generates oxygen free radicals, and these further damage the graft. Though the University of Wisconsin solution contains glutathione, which is a free radical scavenger, its slightly acid pH means that the glutathione is not stable, and so damage on reperfusion is a problem. Other solutions have been developed, notably histidine, tryptophane-ketoglutarate and Celsior, all of which contain inert buffers and free radical scavengers that could confer some advantages on reperfusion.[13]

ASSESSMENT OF LIVE DONOR

Live donation in the UK is governed by the 1989 Human Organ Transplant (HOT) Act and associated regulations which provide for the establishment of ULTRA. In the UK, it is illegal to undertake a living donor transplantation unless (1) the claimed genetic relationship between the donor and the recipient falls within that specified in the HOT Act and has been established by an approved tester, or (2) ULTRA has approved the transplant combination.

The perioperative mortality rate for living donor nephrectomy is reported as between 1 in 1600 and 1 in 3300. The major perioperative complication rate for donor nephrectomy is 2%.

Informed consent is undertaken with discussion about the potential risks of donor nephrectomy, including death and the general complications of surgery with specific mention of venous thromboembolism, intra-abdominal bleeding and infection, chest complications, urinary tract infections and the possible need for blood transfusion.

The primary aim of the donor evaluation process is to ensure the suitability, safety and well-being of the patient. All potential donors have their ABO and HLA compatibility with the donor checked. In addition, the recipient's serum is tested against the donor cells by cross-match.

In the past, renal anatomy was defined in the donor by abdominal ultrasound, intravenous urography and renal angiography. This meant several hospital visits with potential morbidity from anaphylaxis and vascular damage from angiography. Now, in most centres, either spiral computerized tomography (CT) or magnetic resonance (MR) angiography with 3-D reconstruction has replaced the need for all these tests. The procedure requires one visit to the hospital, and the visualization of the renal venous anatomy is excellent (Figure 29.1).

Assessment of glomerular function rate (GFR) is done in all the potential donors. Serum creatinine is often used as a surrogate marker and the Cockcroft–Gault equation is widely used:

$$\text{Male GFR (ml/min)} = (140 - \text{age}) \times \text{ideal body weight (kg)}/0.8 \times \text{serum creatinine } (\mu\text{mol/l})$$
$$(\text{Female GFR} \times 0.85)$$

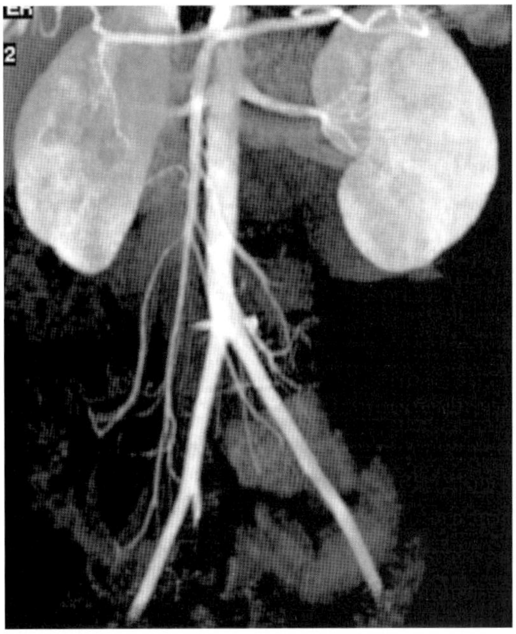

Figure 29.1 *Magnetic resonance angiography for donor vessel assessment.*

A creatinine clearance of 80 ml/min per 73 m^2 is a reasonable lower limit for kidney donation. The radioisotope glomerular filtration rate obtained with ^{51}Cr EDTA is a more reliable measure, and this test can also provide information about split renal function. A minimum level of acceptable GFR is stipulated to prevent the donor from being put at risk. This level depends on the age, and it has to be above two standard deviations below the mean for the age (BTS guidelines).

The absolute and relative contraindications for live donations are tabulated in Table 29.1.[14–16]

ASSESSMENT OF CADAVERIC DONOR

In the UK, cadaveric donor rates are 24 per million population. This is the largest source of kidneys for transplantation. The number of potential donors is much higher, but lack of awareness among the staff and donors' relatives about donation means that these numbers have not increased.

The two main goals of donor evaluation are to exclude donors with severe disease which can be transmitted to the recipient and to exclude kidneys with severe anatomical or functional changes which could compromise allograft function.

Table 29.1 Contraindications to renal transplantation.[15]

Absolute contraindications
Evidence of coercion
Inability to give informed consent
Most malignancies
HIV
Major respiratory or cardiovascular disease
Hypertensive end-organ damage
Body-mass index > 35 kg/m^2
Pregnancy
Intravenous drug use
Thrombophilia
Renal disease
Relative contraindications
Age below 18 years
Age over 70 years
Body-mass index of 30–35 kg/m^2
Cigarette smoking
Psychiatric disorder
Risk factors for type 2 diabetes
Hepatitis B infection
Hypertension

All donors with malignancy are excluded except those who have cutaneous basal-cell carcinoma or primary brain tumours with no metastases. Because of the risk of transmitting choriocarcinoma, chorionic gonadotrophin is estimated in all females of childbearing age who have died from cerebral haemorrhage.

The presence of HIV should preclude the use of organs. Donors with active hepatitis B and C infection are generally excluded, although organs can be transplanted safely into recipients who have already been exposed to these viruses. Measuring viral gene loads can be useful to assess the donor's infectivity. Any possibility of new variant Creutzfeldt–Jacob disease always precludes donation. Donors who have had adequate treatment of bacterial or fungal infection can be used, but a cautious approach is mandatory.

Kidneys from old (>70 years) or young (<2 years) donors or those with a body weight of less than 15 kg perform poorly. Prolonged hypotension, profound use of inotropic drugs, disseminated intravascular coagulation and diabetes mellitus in donors are relative contraindications. Those with high serum creatinine levels can be used safely as kidney donors provided they have a reversible cause of their kidney failure, such as hepatorenal failure.

ASSESSMENT OF THE RECIPIENTS

Ideally, patients with chronic renal failure should receive a transplant at precisely the time that they require a transplant. Unfortunately, this is rarely possible. The timing of the transplant work-up is based on the assumption that most patients would wait for cadaveric transplant for up to 2 years, and it takes approximately 3 months to prepare for a living donor transplant.

The assessment aims to look at recipient suitability to undergo a surgical procedure, and to identify any underlying disease or condition that may delay or would need to be rectified prior to transplantation. It is also an opportunity for the recipient to know what transplantation involves and the pitfalls and possible side effects of immunosuppression.

Cancer is generally a contraindication to immunosuppression, and patients who have active or recent evidence of malignancy, except for some skin cancers, may need to postpone or cancel transplant evaluation. It would be prudent to wait for some time to exclude patients who would develop a recurrence. Delay of longer than 5 years would exclude 87% of patients who would develop a recurrence, whereas a 2-year wait would eliminate about 53% of recurrences. Generally, in most malignancies, patients should be free from recurrence for 2 years before transplantation, but a longer waiting time is required for malignant melanomas, breast cancer and colorectal cancer. No waiting time may be necessary in most skin cancers.

Cardiovascular disease is one of the leading causes of death after renal transplantation. Specific indicators of underlying cardiac disease are a definite history of acute myocardial infarction within the past 6 months, angina, ventricular arrhythmia, or left bundle branch block. Unfortunately, the ability of these indicators to predict a post-surgical cardiac event is not reliable.

The accepted risk factors for cardiovascular disease are as follows:

1. family history of premature coronary artery disease
2. hypertension
3. diabetes
4. men over the age of 45
5. women over the age of 55
6. decreased high-density lipoprotein
7. increased low-density lipoprotein.

For asymptomatic patients who are at high risk or have a history of IHD, a non-invasive test is quite useful to screen patients who might require coronary artery angiography. Thallium scintigraphy and dobutamine echocardiography have been used to screen such patients. All patients who have critical lesions on coronary angiography should undergo revascularization before transplantation.

Patients with a history of transient ischaemic attacks or other evidence of cerebral vascular disease within the previous 6 months should have further evaluation. Patients with autosomal dominant polycystic kidney disease (ADPKD) have an increased risk of ruptured intracranial aneurysms. They should have MR angiography, and patients who have an aneurysm larger than 7 mm would probably benefit from prophylactic surgery.

Hepatitis A and E are not known to cause chronic liver disease in renal transplant recipients. However, recipients who are hepatitis B surface antigen positive, or are e antigen positive (HbeAG), or who have serological evidence of active viral replication are at a higher risk of disease progression in the post-transplant period. Patients who are hepatitis C positive have an increased incidence of chronic active hepatitis.

Extensive work-up is recommended for children and also adults who have a history of urological abnormalities or urinary tract infections. Renal ultrasonography and video-urodynamic studies may be indicated to look into the possibility of reflux and bladder physiology.

The risk of recurrent disease to the transplant kidney is real, but only around 5% graft loss is attributed to recurrent disease. There is a 10–25% risk of recurrence of haemolytic uraemic syndrome and 10–30% risk of recurrence of focal segmental glomerulosclerosis; 40–50% of patients with recurrence will experience graft loss, and there is a 10–25% risk of recurrence in recipients whose original disease was membranous glomerulonephritis. In some cases, the type of immunosuppression used can affect the probability of disease recurrence; for example, calcineurin antagonists (ciclosporin and tacrolimus) promote recurrence of haemolytic uraemic syndrome.

When recipients have met the criteria, they are put on the waiting list to receive a cadaveric organ through the national sharing scheme. At the time of the availability of a suitably matched kidney, a final cross-match is done before transplantation.

MATCHING DONOR AND RECIPIENTS

From the first successful renal transplant, it has been known that for the best results the recipient should have tissue similarities with the donor. Though this was not precisely understood at the time, this tissue similarity is controlled by the ABO blood group and the major histocompatibility complex carried by chromosome 6. For matching by the major blood group, the same rules apply as to blood transfusion, as the endothelium is thrombogenic in an ABO mismatched combination. The major histocompatibility complex is subdivided into classes I and II, which, in man, comprise the human leucocyte antigens (HLA) A, B, C (I) and D (II), respectively. Though class I is expressed by all cells, the role of the professional antigen-presenting cells is more important, and these express class II. Therefore, matching for class II between donor and recipient is more important. Matching has a significant impact on long-term graft survival; therefore, most organ-sharing schemes have this as the principal philosophy. However, paradoxically, in live unrelated donation, usually spouse to spouse, where cold ischaemic time is minimized, the normal milieu of the kidney has minimal disruption, and therefore the recipient's immune system does not become aware that any change has occurred. As a consequence, maximal mismatched kidney transplants can be tolerated without inevitable rejection.

Prior to transplantation, the recipients are tested for their immune sensitivity to the donor. This is done by incubating the donor lymphocytes with the recipients' sera to determine whether or not antibodies are present. This is usually detected by the addition of complement and viability stains for cell death. Flow cytometry can also be used to detect lower concentrations of antibody and to determine the type of antibody. When present, IgG is suggestive of memory and therefore has alloreactive potential, whereas IgM is more non-specific. To transplant in the face of a positive cytotoxic cross-match carries the risk of hyperacute rejection when intravascular thrombosis can occur within minutes of reperfusion.

RENAL TRANSPLANTATION

The surgical technique of transplantation is quite standard and uses the extraperitoneal iliac fossa approach. The vessels are accessible at this point, and the ureter can be kept short, thereby minimizing the risk of ischaemia. With careful surgical technique, no ureteric stent is required, but in large transplant units with many surgeons of different grades, most units utilize a ureteric stent, as it guarantees at least a minimal level of anastomotic technique. It also means the incidence of leak is extremely low. The external iliac artery is the commonest artery used, but the internal and common iliac arteries are also used (see Figures 29.2 and 29.3). In children with small vessels, it is important to utilize the common iliac artery or aorta to ensure a good pressure inflow, as arterial thrombosis is a common reason for graft failure. In those recipients of numerous previous renal allografts, an intraperitoneal approach and even an orthotopic approach with native nephrectomy at the time of transplant have been used successfully.

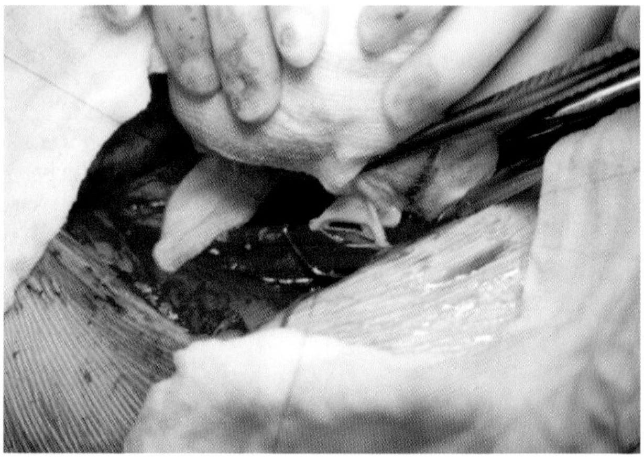

Figure 29.2 *Anastomosing the transplant renal vein to the recipient external iliac vein.*

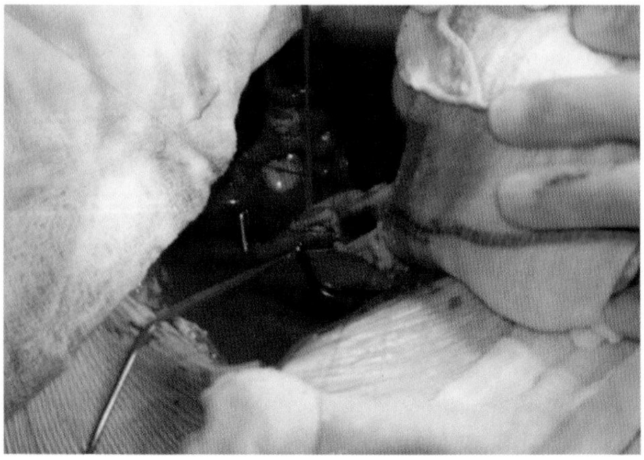

Figure 29.3 *Anastomosing the transplant renal artery to the recipient external iliac artery.*

IMMUNOSUPPRESSION

Transplantation could not develop until the immune system was tamed by drugs. These initially were very unspecific – radiotherapy, steroids and 6-mercaptopurine – but when used in conjunction with good donor–recipient matching, they produced 10-year graft survival not dissimilar to those achieved today. Azathioprine, derived from 6-mercaptopurine, was developed in the 1960s. It is an antimetabolite and therefore produces marrow suppression. Antithymocyte globulin is a polyclonal antibody initially derived from the horse and later from the rabbit. This antibody was introduced in 1968; it lyses human leucocytes and thereby produces a cytokine 'storm', giving the recipient a self-limiting temperature and rigors. This was found to be of particular benefit in steroid-resistant rejection. OKT3, which is a monoclonal antibody directed against T lymphocytes, was developed to supersede ATG. Lymphoma, recognized as a particular problem of strong immunosuppression, was slightly more common with OKT3. The calcineurin antagonists ciclosporin and later tacrolimus were derived from soil organisms and were found to be very effective in minimizing the immunological response; that is, IL2 production was inhibited. These drugs produced a spectacular improvement in graft survival up to 5 years. Beyond this, chronic graft dysfunction produced steady graft attrition, so that at 10 years, graft survival was similar to that seen with the more primitive agents. Mycophenolate mofetil and mycophenolic acid inhibit the purine pathway most cells except lymphocytes have an escape pathway, so lymphocyte proliferation is inhibited. Animal work has suggested that these agents have benefit in chronic graft dysfunction, though human data have not yet confirmed this. Rapamycin, which is also derived from soil organisms, downregulates IL2 production, but in a slightly different way from ciclosporin and tacrolimus, and it therefore is not complicated by the calcineurin nephropathy that may in part contribute to chronic graft dysfunction. Rapamycin could possibly also have benefits for long-term graft function.

In most transplant units combination therapies of the above agents are used; increasingly popular is antibody induction using IL2 receptor blockers, which allows the oral medication to be used more sparingly.

Serious bacterial infection is not a common problem now as it was in early transplant experience, where excessive immunosuppression was common. Viraemia is now more of an issue as a consequence of immunosuppression, particularly with Epstein–Barr virus or herpes 6, the former giving rise to neoplasia and the latter to Karposi's sarcoma. BKV and JCV, which are related to SV40, and belong to the polyoma virus group, can be troublesome after transplant. BKV causes interstitial nephritis and ureteric strictures, while JCV can cause leucoencephalopathy in the immunosuppressed patient.

POST-TRANSPLANT MANAGEMENT

In the early postoperative period, fluid management and blood pressure are the most important aspects, as vascular thrombosis and pulmonary oedema are serious consequences of both extremes of fluid state. Immunosuppression should be modified to obtain suitable levels of calcineurin antagonists. The patients have generally been on antihypertensive agents, and these may not be suitable after a transplant. ACE inhibitors can often be used safely later, but renal impairment at this time complicates the recipients' management. Antiviral prophylaxis is common for cytomegalovirus (CMV), especially if the donor has been exposed to this infection before and the recipient has not. Gangciclovir, valacyclovir or valganciclovir can be used in this situation, though many units choose to monitor for CMV by PCR and treat only when viraemia develops.

The recipients are supported until such time as the kidney starts to work, and graft dysfunction is monitored by graft biopsy in order to identify acute rejection early. Acute rejection is usually treated by augmented steroids, with or without altering the baseline regimen. Steroid-resistant rejection is still often managed by poly- or monoclonal antibody therapy. Urinary tract infections are managed with appropriate antibiotics, and the ureteric stent is often removed early in this situation.

LONG-TERM MANAGEMENT

This is essentially a balancing act, retaining renal function while trying to minimize potentially harmful medication and avoiding rejection. Early after transplantation, immunosuppression is maximal. The primary aim at this time is to reduce steroid augmentation without incurring rejection to baseline levels. Fluid management is usually only relevant in the first few weeks before it stabilizes, unless other problems arise. Blood pressure needs to be optimized initially by non-ACE inhibitor drugs, though they can be used later, especially if proteinuria is detected.

Hypercholesterolaemia can be a problem, particularly in recipients receiving ciclosporin or rapamycin, and they may require treatment with statins. Diabetes mellitus, if present, usually worsens with steroids. In addition, diabetes can develop where it was not present before; this is especially the case with tacrolimus, and it can be reversed by switching immunosuppression to rapamycin. There is a great propensity in the early phase for recipients to put on weight by excessive eating. This occurs because they are suddenly recovering from renal failure and feel fitter, and the dietary restrictions of fluid and potassium are lifted. In addition, steroids increase their appetites. Good dietary care is needed in this early phase because reversing excessive weight gain later is difficult.

The renal function must be monitored together with immunosuppressive drug levels. Graft dysfunction must be investigated after elimination of obvious courses by ultrasound scans and biopsy. Ureteric stenosis should be managed appropriately, usually by, initially, ureteric stent and later ureterotomy or reimplantation, though there is a role for revolving ureteric stents.

Acute rejection should be managed by steroid augmentation and drug manipulation if necessary. Consideration should always be given to patient compliance with immunosuppression, as this is a significant cause of graft failure, particularly in child recipients that are graduating to adult clinics. Osteoporosis and atherosclerosis from protracted steroid use give rise to significant morbidity later; therefore, steroids should be limited as much as is safe to do.

Vigilance for skin tumours, cervical cancer, Karposi's sarcoma, and hypernephroma, particularly in polycystic kidneys and post-transplant lymphoproliferative disease, should always be practised.

RESULTS

In the early days of renal transplantation in the 1950s, the only successful transplants were those between identical twins, obviously a very select group. With the advent of azathioprine and steroid, 1-year outcome was of the order of 35–40%. This figure improved dramatically with the advent of ciclosporin. Since that time, a 1-year recipient death rate of 5% and graft survival of greater than 80% have become usual. These improved figures extend to 10 years after the transplant, but due to a steady attrition rate from chronic rejection, the outcome after 10 years is similar with modern immunosuppressive agents to that seen in the pre-ciclosporin era[17] at 40%. The best results are generally seen in the recipients of live-donor kidneys with minimal cold ischaemia, among whom there is a graft half-life of 15 years. Those grafts which experience initial delayed function have a significantly worse long-term outcome. In addition, donor morbidity, such as hypertension, and death from cerebrovascular disease have a negative impact on graft survival. Poor tissue match between donor and recipient, and recipient hypertension and smoking habits all have a negative impact on outcome. The hidden issues of non-compliance with immunosuppressive medication could potentially have an enormous impact on outcome,[18] though one can take the contrary view that certain drugs promote the cytokine TGFβ, which promotes fibrosis and therefore chronic rejection.[19]

REFERENCES

1. Security DoHaS. Cadaveric organs for transplantation. A code of practice including the diagnosis of brain death. London: Health Departments of Great Britain and Northern Ireland, 1983
2. Transplantation. EBPGfR. Nephrol Dial Transplant 2000; 15(Suppl. 7): 46–47

3. Balupuri S, Buckley P, Snowden C, Sen B et al. The trouble with kidneys derived from the non heart beating donor: a single centre 10 year experience. Transplantation 2000; 69: 842–846
4. Gok M, Buckley P, Shenton B, Balupuri S et al. Long-term renal function in kidneys from non-heart-beating donors: a single-center experience. Transplantation 2002; 74: 664–669
5. Nicholson M, Metcalfe MS, White SA, Waller JR et al. A comparison of the results of renal transplantation from non-heart-beating, conventional cadaveric and living donors. Kidney Int 2000; 58: 2585–2591
6. D'Alessandro A, Hoffmann R, Knechtle S, Eckhoff D et al. Successful extrarenal transplantation from non-heart-beating donors. Transplantation 1995; 59: 977–982
7. Newman C, Baxby K, Hall R, Taylor R. Machine-perfused cadaver kidneys. Lancet 1975; 2: 614
8. Burdick J, Rossendale J, McBride M, Kauffman M et al. National impact of pulsatile perfusion on cadaveric kidney transplantation. Transplantation 1997; 64: 1730
9. Light J. Viability testing in the non-heart-beating donor. Transplant Proc 2000; 32: 179–181
10. Brasile L, Stubenitsky B, Booster M, Lindell S et al. Overcoming severe renal ischemia: the role of ex vivo warm perfusion. Transplantation 2002; 73: 897–901
11. Hoffman R, Stratta R, D'Alessandro A, Sollinger H et al. Combined cold storage-perfusion preservation with a new synthetic perfusate. Transplantation 1989; 47: 32–37
12. Groenewoud A, Thorogood J. Current status of the Eurotransplant randomized multicenter study comparing kidney graft preservation with histidine-tryptophane-ketoglutarate, University of Wisconsin and EuroCollins. Transplant Proc 1993; 25: 1582–1585
13. Muhlbacher F, Langer F, Mittermayer C. Preservation solutions for transplantation. Transplant Proc 1999; 31: 2069–2070
14. Association BTSaR. United Kingdom Guidelines for Living Donor Kidney Transplantation, 2000
15. Kasiske B, Ravenscraft M, Ramos E, Gaston R et al. The evaluation of living renal transplant donors: clinical practice guidelines. J Am Soc Nephrol 1996; 7: 2288–2313
16. Kasiske B, Ramos E, Gaston R, Bia M et al. The evaluation of renal transplant candidates. Clinical practice guidelines. Patient Care and Education Committee of the American Society of Transplant Physicians. J Am Assoc Nephrol 1995; 6: 1–34
17. Beveridge T, Calne R. Cyclosporin (Sandimmun) in cadaveric renal transplantation. Ten-year follow up of a European multicenter trial group. Transplantation 1995; 59: 1568–1570
18. de Geest S, Borgermans L, Gemoets H, Abraham I et al. Incidence, determinants, and consequences of subclinical noncompliance with immunosuppressive therapy in renal transplant recipients. Transplantation 1995; 59: 340–347
19. Mohamed M, Robertson H, Booth T, Balupuri S et al. TGF-b expression in renal transplant biopsies. A comparative study between cyclosporin-A and tacrolimus. Transplantation 2000; 69(5): 1002–1005

30

Tissue transfer in urology

S N Venn and Anthony R Mundy

Two types of tissue transfer are common in urology, firstly, the use of skin and buccal mucosa for urethral reconstruction and, secondly, the use of bowel for bladder reconstruction. The three factors that require some consideration in relation to the subject of tissue transfer in these contexts are the general subject of wound healing, the use of grafts and flaps, and the consequences of incorporating bowel into the urinary tract.

WOUND HEALING

This is the replacement of destroyed tissue by living tissue. In certain reptiles, it includes the ability to replace a tail or limb. This occurs due to the ability of cells to dedifferentiate and then redifferentiate, which does not occur in human adults. Healing in adults is limited to the fibrous obliteration of dead space and limited regeneration. In the embryo, scarless healing has been noted and this is currently the focus of intense research.[1]

The phases of wound healing

Wound healing is traditionally divided into three phases – an inflammatory phase, a proliferative phase and a maturation phase. These phases overlap to some degree, but as a general rule the inflammatory phase lasts for about the first 5 days, the proliferative phase lasts from about day 3 to about day 14, and the maturation phase starts on about day 8 and lasts about 3 months. Each of these phases is controlled and regulated by growth factors.

The first phase of wound healing is the haemostatic response to the injury itself and the inflammation that follow immediately afterwards. At the site where blood vessles and the surrounding tissues are injured, circulating blood comes into contact with extracellular collagen, and platelets aggregate and are activated and the intrinsic component of the coagulation cascade is activated as well. The platelets release the contents of their granules, including cytokines, growth factors, fibronectin, thromboxane and serotonin. The thromboxane and serotonin promote vasoconstriction at the site of the injury, whereas vasodilatation occurs around that site to allow other important healing factors to get to the wound. The vasodilatation is mediated by histamine, which is also released from platelets but other cells as well such as mast cells and basophils.

At the same time, both the intrinsic and the extrinsic coagulation systems are activated, leading to the formation of a fibrin clot. This serves as a scaffolding to allow inflammatory cells such as neutrophils, macrophages and lymphocytes to move into the injured area. The neutrophils arrive first. Selectin receptors on the endothelial cell surface cause neutrophil adhesion to the endothelium, and integrin receptors on the neutrophil cell surface bind to the extracellular matrix, thus bringing the neutrophils into the damaged area. Neutrophils, however, are not essential to wound healing except to deal with bacterial contamination when that exists. The next cells to arrive, the macrophages, are essential. They arrive on about the third day after injury and act as the principal cell controlling the wound-healing process. The main functions are as follows:

1. an antimicrobial effect caused by the release of oxygen radicals and nitric oxide, and by phagocytosis
2. wound debridement by phagocytosis and by the release of varous enzymes
3. matrix synthesis regulation by the release of growth factors, cytokines, enzymes and prostaglandins
4. cell recruitment and activation by the release of growth factors, cytokines and fibronectin
5. angiogenesis by the release of growth factors and cytokines.

The principal cells recruited and activated are fibroblasts and lymphocytes, which migrate in towards the end of the inflammatory phase. The principal enzyme released is collagenase. The principal growth factors released are TGF-β, EGF, PDGF and the angiogenesis growth factors bFGF and VEGF. The principal cytokines are TNF-α, IL-1, IFN-γ and ILC.

Lymphocytes are attracted by the cytokines released by activated macrophages, and these in turn release interferons and interleukins. They also produce nitric oxide. The arrival of the fibroblasts heralds the second, or 'proliferative', phase. Their number increases, so the number of neturophils decreases. Fibroblasts, together with macrophages, then start the process of matrix formation and collagen synthesis. At the same time, endothelial cells proliferate from the margin of the wound to form new capillaries by the process of angiogenesis. At this stage, the inflammatory phase is over, and any remaining inflammatory mediators are inactivated and removed from the wound by diffusion or by the macrophages. The fibroblasts are activated by PDGF and FGF, and also by complement and fibronectin, which binds fibroblasts and helps them to move into the wound in the same way that integrins in the extracellular maxtrix bound neutrophils in the early inflammatory phase.

As activated fibroblasts begin the process of matrix deposition, largely by replacing the fibrin and fibronectin originating from haemostasis and macrophages with collagen, epithelial cells start to proliferate from the wound edges. Again, macrophages are important, producing appropriate cytogrines and growth factors. As the proliferative phase comes to an end and the maturation phase becomes established, macrophages (and neurophils) start to leave the area.

The cardinal feature of the maturation phase is the deposition of collagen. It is the rate, quality and total amount of collagen deposition that determine the strength of the scar, and most of the problems of healing that arise are secondary to poor collagen deposition.

Initially, in the inflammatory phase, the matrix deposited in the wound was composed principally of fibrin and fibronectin that originated from haemostasis and from macrophages, respectively. Other extracellular micoproteins, such as glycosaminoglycans and proteoglycans, come next. Collagen follows after this.

In the intact dermis, collagen I predominates, forming 80–90% of the total collagen. The remaining 10–20% is collagen III. In the granulation tissue of the maturation phase, there is rather more type III collagen – as much as 30% – although this reduces in time to about 10%. Collagen III production actually peaks during the inflammatory phase, while collagen I production, which starts about the first day after injury, continues for about 4–5 weeks. Initially, the collagen is laid down in thin collagen fibres, parallel to the skin and organized along the stress line of the wound. In time, the collagen fibres become thicker, but they never develop the basket-weave-like pattern characteristic of normal dermis. It is perhaps for this reason that the breaking strength of a scar never quite equals the breaking strength of normal skin. At 1 week, the breaking strength of a wound is about 3–5% of its final strength; by 3 weeks, it has reached 20% of its final strength; by 3 months, it reaches 80% of the strength of unwounded skin, and this is about as strong as it ever gets.

Wound contraction is the name given to the final approximation of the wound edges and the shortening of the scar that is typically seen. In the process of healing by first intention – which is what we have been describing so far – contraction is less marked than in healing by second intention. In both circumstances, the process is the same and poorly understood. One theory proposes that the myofibroblast – a special type of fibroblast – is responsible for this. The other main theory is that the movement of cells with reorganization of the cellular cytoskeleton is responsible for contraction. In summary, the exact mechanism is not clear.

Healing by secondary intention (where the wound edges are widely separated) differs in two respects.

1. Epithelialization occurs from the basal cells of the epidermis at the margins of the wound. These cells lose their attachment to the basement membrane and send out cytoplasmic projections, becoming flatter as they do so. As they change, they become more like phagocytes in appearance. Within a day or two of injury, the basal cells show mitosis at an increasing rate and continue to replicate until the defect is covered. When coverage is complete and the epidermis (or other epithelium) has reconstituted itself, the basal cells regain their normal appearace and synthesize their own basement membrane constitutents.
2. Contraction plays a far more important role in healing by secondary intention. Animal models have demonstrated contraction of up to 80%.[6] However, the pathological process involved in contraction is the same.

Complications of wound healing

Complications include infection, wound dehiscence, excessive granulation, keloid, pigmentation, pain, weak scars, circatrization, implantation cyst and neoplasia. Factors influencing healing are listed in Table 30.1.

Table 30.1 Factors influencing wound healing.

Local factors	Poor blood supply Adhesion to underlying structures Direction of wound Infection/foreign body Movement Drying Neoplasia
General	Age Nutrition (protein, vitamin C, zinc) Hormones Temperature

GRAFTS AND FLAPS

Most surgical trainees gain their first experience of grafting in the use of thin split skin grafts to cover a granulating open wound. The open wound, which is secreting collagen and actively generating small new vessels, is covered by a nutrient-rich layer of serum, from which the thin split skin graft gains its nutrition by a process known as 'imbibition'. This is sufficient to nourish a split skin graft for a day or two, but to nourish it beyond that time, as well as to fix it and incorporate it into the healing wound, there must be a link-up between the capillary bed on the undersurface of the graft and the developing capillaries in the open wound, together with interlinking of collagen, and this process is known as 'inosculation'. During the 48 hours of imbibition and the 48 hours of inosculation, the graft must be immobilized and, if it is immobilized and the host bed is well vascularized, then the graft will 'take'. At the end of 96 hours, blood flow into the graft should be established. Eventually, lymphatics will grow in as well.

Immobilization in this context should not be taken to mean simply pressure, although the 'tie-over' dressing commonly used for immobilizing a small skin graft clearly produces some pressure. The intention, though, is to immobilize the graft. Pressure sufficient to inhibit the formation of small haematomas and seromas would probably be sufficient to impair blood flow in the host bed.[7,8]

Thus far, we have been considering the simple split skin graft, and at this stage we should draw attention to the difference between grafts and flaps. A graft is tissue transferred from a donor site to a recipient site without a blood supply, whereas a flap is tissue that is transferred from a donor site with its own blood supply intact, although one type of flap is the free flap, in which tissue is transferred with its blood supply disconnected and then reconnected by means of microvascular surgery at the recipient site. In urology we are principally concerned with split-thickness skin grafts, full-thickness skin grafts, buccal mucosal grafts, bladder epithelial grafts and flaps of local genital skin for urethral reconstruction. In addition, the urologist may wish to use a dermal graft for the correction of Peyronie's disease, and some have used a graft of tunica vaginalis for this purpose.[9,10]

Other than the use of genital skin flaps for urethral reconstruction, simpler advancement, rotation and transposition flaps are commonly used for wound closure, although we do not often think of them as such, except in the specific case of the Z-plasty. Less commonly, flaps may be used for perineal and genital reconstruction, and in this way a simple scrotal flap may be used to cover a perineal defect, or the infinitely more complex radial or ulnar forearm flap may be transferred by microvascular techniques for phalloplasty.[11]

Grafts

Skin has an epidermal layer and a dermal layer, under which lies a subcutaneous, fatty layer. At the interface between the dermis and the subcutaneous layer is the subdermal plexus, which is fed from deeper segmental vessels and which in turn feeds the dermal and epidermal layers above through a second, more superficial, plexus within the dermis itself, called the intradermal plexus (Figure 30.1). The outermost layer of the epidermis is the cornified layer, and the inner layer – the epidermis proper – contains the skin appendages, some of which extend into the dermal layer. The principal skin appendages are the sweat glands, sebaceous glands and hair follicles, and in urological practice it is worth noting that the glans and prepuce in the male and the skin of the labia minora and introitus in the female are free of skin appendages. The same areas also have skin in which the dermis is thin. The dermis consists of the more superficial 'papillary' or 'adventitial' dermis and the deeper 'reticular' dermis. The papillary dermis has a fairly constant thickness, and fibroblasts and capillaries predominate. The deeper reticular dermis is thicker but more variable and here collagen and elastin predominate. The subdermal plexus lies on the deep aspect of the reticular dermis, and the intradermal plexus lies between the reticular and the papillary dermis.

A full-thickness skin graft includes both the epidermis and the dermis with the vessels of the subdermal plexus exposed on its undersurface, and it is to these vessels that the new vessels developing within the host bed must connect by inosculation.

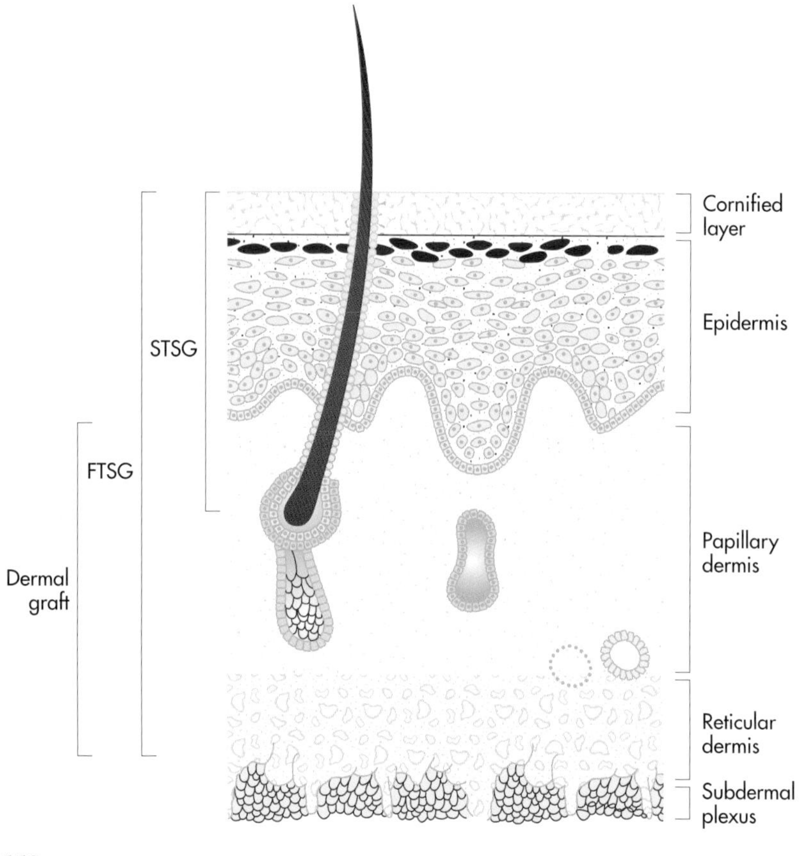

Figure 30.1 *Cross-sectional diagram of the skin. STSG, split-thickness skin graft; FTSG, full-thickness skin graft.*

Full-thickness skin grafts, because of their high content of dermal collagen, contract very little during healing and tend to give the most satisfactory long-term results as a consequence, but there are two problems associated with their use. Firstly, the amount of suitable skin is restricted and, secondly, the subdermal plexus is less extensive than the intradermal plexus and, because of this and also because the graft is relatively thick, it is only slowly revascularized and takes only under the most favourable conditions.

The split-thickness skin graft contains the epidermis and a portion of the adventitial dermis with the vessels of the intradermal plexus exposed on its undersurface. The graft is thinner and the vessels of the intradermal plexus are more plentiful, and so a split-thickness graft is more likely to take, and will do so under less favourable circumstances than a full-thickness skin graft. On the other hand, because there is less dermal collagen, a split-thickness graft tends to contract and, lacking the collagen and elastin of the reticular dermis, the graft tends to be more brittle and fragile than a full-thickness graft.

Bladder epithelial grafts and buccal mucosal grafts are harvested and behave as full-thickness grafts. Bladder epithelium has the disadvantage that it is very prone to desiccation, which leads to hypertrophic changes when, for example, it is used at the urethral meatus.[12] Buccal mucosa is far more resistant to desiccation, and there is the additional advantage that it is easier to open the mouth than the bladder, although this advantage is offset by the greater amount of bladder mucosa available than buccal mucosa. The particular advantages of buccal mucosa are its thickness and toughness (which contrast markedly with the thinness and fragility of bladder epithelium), and the density of the intradermal and subdermal plexuses.[13]

Grafts were the first sort of tissue to be used for urethral reconstruction but fell into disfavour because of their unpredictability until just recently, with the advent of buccal mucosal grafting for 'patch' urethroplasty of strictures that are too long for excision and end-to-end anastomosis.[14] Until then, grafts had become virtually restricted to the use of meshed split-skin grafts for the salvage repair of extensive urethral strictures.[15] This is a technique that is only rarely indicated nowadays. A free preputial skin graft might be used by specialist reconstructive surgeons for anterior urethroplasty, particularly for hypospadias repair, but grafting had become almost entirely superseded by the use of flaps for hypospadias repair and for urethroplasty in the penile urethra, largely under the influence of Duckett.[16] Preputial and postauricular full-thickness skin grafts are now being used more frequently again, particularly for the two-stage reconstruction of the penile urethra.[17] Postauricular full-thickness skin grafts have a particularly rich subdermal plexus and, although the amount of tissue is relatively restricted, the take is far more predictable than with other extragenital skin. Thus, preputial or postauricular full-thickness skin grafts may be used to reconstruct the anterior urethra, usually in two stages, and buccal mucosal grafts, which behave as full-thickness grafts, may be used for the repair of more proximal urethral strictures. Buccal mucosal grafts and bladder epithelial grafts have also been used as tube grafts in the anterior urethra.[18] Only in extreme cases, for extensive urethral salvage procedures, is split-thickness skin used, and then only after it has been meshed, as described by Schreiter.[19]

Flaps

Flaps consist of skin, muscle, bone, fascia, omentum, intestine or combinations of these, but in urology we are principally concerned with skin flaps for urethral and genital reconstruction, omental flaps to help support vesico-vaginal fistula closure, and intestinal flaps for bladder reconstruction.

Flaps may be classified in two ways.[7,8] Firstly, according to their method of elevation, into peninsular flaps, in which the base of the flap remains in continuity; island flaps, in which the flap is only in continuity through the arteriovenous pedicle; and free flaps, in which all continuity of the flap is interrupted but the vascularity is re-established at the recipient site. The second way of classifying flaps is by vascular classification (Figure 30.2), which distinguishes between random flaps, in which there is no identifiable arteriovenous pedicle and survival is dependent entirely on the dermal and intradermal plexuses; axial flaps, which have an identifiable artery and vein entering through the base; and two special

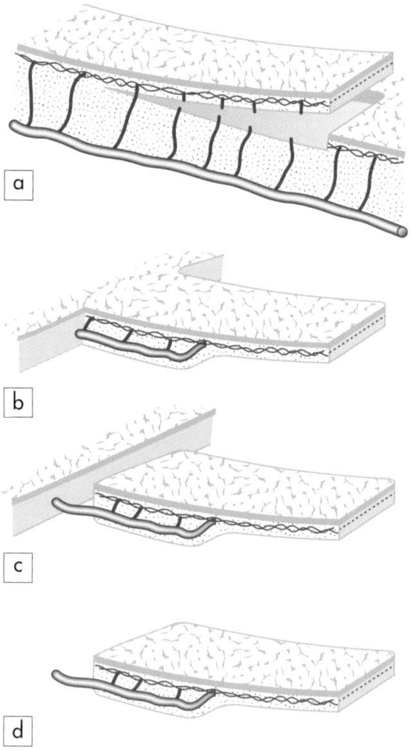

Figure 30.2 *Diagrammatic representation of: (a) a random peninsular flap; (b) an axial peninsular flap; (c) an axial island flap; and (d) a free microvascular flap.*

forms of axial flap known as myocutaneous and fasciocutaneous flaps. Random flaps are restricted in use by a length to width ratio whereas axial flaps are not, being restricted in length only by the nature of the feeder vessels. A peninsular flap may be either a random or an axial flap, but island flaps are all axial flaps. Peninsular flaps are used for advancement, rotation and transposition but are relatively restricted in scope. Axial island flaps have a much greater range of application. Island flaps are somewhat fragile and have to be handled with care, as the vascular pedicle provides both structural and vascular continuity – with such a fragile structure that vascular continuity is threatened unless great care is taken. Sometimes, however, the continuity of an island flap is maintained through a muscle or fascial flap, giving rise to the two particular forms of axial flap referred to above. In the myocutaneous flap, the arteriovenous pedicle is within the muscle itself and the skin island (or 'paddle') retains its attachment to the muscle. Examples include gracilis and rectus abdominis muscle flaps, both of which have applications in urology.[20,21] Similarly, the fasciocutaneous flap transmits the arteriovenous pedicle in close relation to a defined layer of fascia to which the skin paddle is attached. In both the myocutaneous and the fasciocutaneous flaps, the muscle and fascia, respectively, support and protect the arteriovenous pedicle, making the flap more robust.

Free flaps, to be transferred by microvascular anastomoses to the recipient site, can be elevated as axial cutaneous, axial myocutaneous, or axial fasciocutaneous flaps and are the most versatile flaps of all because they can be transferred anywhere. The limitations in their use are firstly technical – they are difficult to learn how to perform – and they tend to leave large donor sites that may leave ugly scars,[22] although this is usually more than offset by a satisfactory end result from the flap itself. Most flaps are mobilized with a defined sensory nerve to provide sensibility to the flap. The best example of the use of a free flap in urology is the radial or ulnar forearm flap used for phalloplasty.[11] The radial artery flap is easier to raise but has considerable donor-site morbidity because the many tendons in the forearm are exposed and, even if these can be covered, the donor site leaves an unsightly scar. The ulnar forearm flap exposes fewer, if any, tendons and the donor site is more easily concealed and has the additional advantage that the skin on the ulnar side of the forearm is much less hirsute, but the flap is more difficult to raise. Both flaps are innervated by the lateral and medial antibrachial cutaneous nerves, which are easily identified and mobilized with the flap to provide sensibility.

Gracilis and rectus myocutaneous flaps have also been used for phallic reconstruction, but are more commonly used for covering large skin defects in and around the groins and perineum. The gracilis muscle can also be used purely as a muscle flap for filling dead space and holding suture lines apart, in the same way that the labial fat pad and omentum are used.

Intestinal flaps in bladder reconstruction

There are more urologists using bowel for bladder reconstruction or replacement by continent or conduit urinary diversion than there are urologists using skin for urethral reconstruction. Bowel is always carried on its blood supply and, as long as there is no undue tension on the vascular pedicle, the bowel heals well in its new circumstances and ischaemia is rare, except when the bowel and its blood supply are compromised by previous radiotherapy. The purpose of this section is not to discuss the more technical aspects related to mobilizing gut segments for use in the urinary tract, but to discuss the metabolic, infective, histological and other consequences of incorporating the gut into the urinary tract. Such matters have been extensively studied by certain groups in experimental models[23] and the clinical consequences have been extensively scrutinized by other groups in humans, but it is still not yet clear how we should apply the theoretical knowledge gleaned from such studies in clinical practice, as that knowledge is currently very incomplete.

Bowel has been used in urology for many years and this has engendered an attitude that it can be freely deployed within the urinary tract without significant consequence. On the other hand, intestine was never meant to serve either as a conduit for urine or as a storage vessel for it, and a more likely explanation for the fact that it appears to be capable of being used freely without complication is that in most circumstances only a small section of bowel is incorporated and, in most patients in whom such procedures are performed, there are compensatory mechanisms to deal with any adverse consequences that might otherwise result. Furthermore, many of these patients have only a short life expectancy, as when an ileal conduit or substitution cystoplasty is used after cystectomy for bladder cancer, and the short duration of use in a patient who is expected to die before long in any case might lead one to overlook consequences that might be apparent in younger patients with longer to live.

Even with this proviso, it was recognized many years ago that patients with uretero-sigmoidostomy were prone to the specific metabolic problem of hyperchloraemic acidosis from the absorption of urinary constituents by the colon,[24] and prone also to the development of tumours at the site of implantation of the ureters into the colon.[25] For these reasons, uretero-sigmoidostomy fell into relative disuse some years ago, although it is undergoing something of a resurrection at present .[26]

Other than the consequences of incorporating a segment of gut into the urinary tract, there may be consequences from removing it from its natural situation. In practice, the only problem that commonly arises is a degree of bowel dysfunction,[27] although it is not clear whether this arises because the bowel has been removed or because the functional status quo has been disturbed by the process of bowel preparation and the starvation associated with the perioperative period and the time that it takes thereafter for normal function to be restored. There is, in any case, a strong association between detrusor instability and the irritable bowel syndrome[28] and neuropathic bowel and neuropathic bladder dysfunction,[29] and it is these two groups that are most prone to notice disturbance of bowel function after augmentation cystoplasty. Bowel dysfunction is far less commonly noted after substitution cystoplasty for conditions such as bladder cancer.

Removal of the terminal ileum or of the ileocaecal valve can interfere with the absorption of bile salts[30] and lead to bacterial colonization of the terminal ileum, both of which may give rise to diarrhoea. For this reason, the terminal ileum is avoided whenever possible during such surgery. There has been concern that the removal of the terminal ileum can give rise to vitamin B_{12} deficiency and other forms of anaemia, but these rarely seem to occur in practice. It is not clear how much ileum has to be removed from the intestinal tract before bile acid malabsorption is sufficiently severe to cause malabsorption of fat and fat-soluble vitamins, but malnutrition and steatorrhoea are rarely, if ever, seen in clinical practice. Such problems might occur, and diarrhoea undoubtedly does occur in people who have had enterocystoplasty, ileal conduit diversion or continent diversion after previous bowel excision or when the bowel is diseased or deficient in any other way.

Removing the right side of the colon may cause diarrhoea, although this does not seem to be a long-term problem. Removal of the sigmoid colon may be a problem in neuropathic patients in whom the sigmoid colon is an important storage organ, but it does not usually cause bowel problems otherwise.

In short, other than in those with previously abnormal bowel, problems rarely arise from taking the bowel out of continuity, and all we need really consider are the problems that arise from incorporating it into the urinary tract.

THE CONSEQUENCES OF INCORPORATING THE BOWEL INTO THE URINARY TRACT

The first point to make is that bowel continues to behave like bowel even when it is in the urinary tract and has been there for many years. It continues to produce mucus – the only overt abnormality that most patients are aware of – and it continues to secrete and absorb just as it does in its natural situation. There is a tendency for both the ileal and colonic epithelium to atrophy with time,[31] and it is not clear whether this represents the consequence of loss of the normal stimulation that it receives during faecal transport in its normal situation or whether, alternatively, it represents some toxic effect of urine. However, the atrophy is less when the intestine is in contact with urine than when it is not in contact with anything at all, so it appears that urine tends to maintain ileal integrity, if anything, albeit less so than does the faecal stream. The atrophic appearance is therefore likely to represent a true, albeit partial, atrophy rather than a toxic effect.

Metabolic changes

The principal metabolic abnormality is a tendency to a respiratory-compensated metabolic acidosis, usually of mild degree.[32] This may influence bone metabolism to a sufficient degree to cause demineralization of the skeleton in growing children.[33] Changes otherwise tend to be subtle, particularly, it is thought, if renal function is normal. Thus, only young patients are prone to any sort of problems in most circumstances.

Why people seem to suffer less from metabolic acidosis these days with a substituted intestinal bladder than they used to suffer with a uretero-sigmoidostomy is almost certainly related, at least in part, to the recurrent sepsis that they also suffered with refluxing uretero-sigmoidostomies.[34]

The nature and severity of the electrolyte anomalies that patients can suffer from depend on the segment of bowel used in the urinary tract. If stomach is used, hypochloraemic metabolic alkalosis can occur. This is rarely significant in the presence of normal renal function, but may be when renal function is severely limited.

When jejunum is used, hyponatraemic, hyperchloraemic, hyperkalaemic metabolic acidosis occurs, and this is both common and potentially serious, resulting in lethargy, nausea, vomiting, dehydration, muscular weakness and an elevated body temperature and, if uncorrected, death. This is the 'jejunal conduit syndrome'.[35]

If ileum or colon is used, hyperchloraemic acidosis may occur. The reported incidence varies and to a certain extent depends on how it is looked for. If the plasma chloride level is the parameter used to make the diagnosis, then about 15% of patients suffer; if arterial blood gas analysis is performed, then a respiratory-compensated metabolic acidosis is found far more commonly – indeed, in the majority.[32] The mechanism of the metabolic acidosis when ileum or colon is interposed in the urinary tract is not entirely clear. What is known is largely derived from the work of McDougall and co-workers.[36]

Water transport across the intestinal epithelium normally follows its osmotic gradient and is dependent upon the permeability of the intercellular junctions of the luminal cells. If these junctions are tight, there is very little leakage; when they are not so tight, water follows its osmotic gradients. Generally, the tightness of the intercellular junctions increases the further down the intestinal tract the segment is taken from. Stomach is very leaky, but there are bidirectional fluxes that cancel each other out. Jejunum is leaky and jejunal conduits lose large amounts of water. Ileum is better but is still somewhat leaky. Colon is the most efficient segment of gut because its intercellular junctions are tighter, and colon segments therefore have a much lower tendency to lose water.

Most electrolyte shifts in the gut are transcellular, although paracellular movement of ions does occur. Furthermore, most electrolyte movements in one direction are coupled with movement of other electrolytes in the opposite direction. Thus, when sodium is absorbed, hydrogen is excreted and when chloride is absorbed, bicarbonate is excreted. Under certain circumstances, these transport processes can be reversed.

Sodium absorption is much the same in the ileum and in the colon and, in general, ileum absorbs less chloride but more potassium than colon. In neither ileal nor colonic segments is either sodium or potassium loss a problem, although in extreme metabolic acidosis, hypokalaemia can occur, as can hypocalcaemia and hypomagnesaemia.

The mechanism for the development of hyperchloraemic acidosis appears to be primarily because of ammonia absorption. Ammonium ions may dissociate into ammonia and hydrogen, in which case the ammonia diffuses into the cell and the hydrogen ion is actively absorbed in exchange for sodium. Alternatively, ammonium may be absorbed as a substitute for potassium through potassium channels. Either way, ammonium enters the ileal or colonic luminal cell and this is balanced by chloride absorption in exchange for bicarbonate secretion. Thus, ammonium and chloride are absorbed, causing hyperchloraemic acidosis, and bicarbonate is lost.

When hypokalaemia does occur it is usually in uretero-sigmoidostomy[37] or as a result of osmotic diuresis. Hypocalcaemia is usually due to bone demineralization. Hypomagnesaemia may be associated with hypocalcaemia but is more commonly due to nutritional depletion or renal wasting.

In most patients, this metabolic acidosis is of little consequence, but in growing children it may be a particular problem as it appears to cause a reduction in growth potential.[38] Children with intestine incorporated into the urinary tract are more prone to orthopaedic problems and pathological fractures, and there is a tendency for them to drop off the growth curve that they were previously following. Exactly why acidosis should lead to skeletal demineralization in growing children and not in anybody else is not clear, but post-menopausal women who might also be prone to skeletal demineralization do not show this abnormality after enterocystoplasty or urinary intestinal diversion.

Again, the mechanism by which acidosis causes demineralization of the skeleton is not clear, but chronic acidosis is buffered predominantly by muscle protein and by bone. In bone, in chronic metabolic acidosis, hydrogen ions are buffered in exchange for calcium. The main buffer is thought to be bicarbonate or carbonate derived from skeletal carbon dioxide stores, and the utilization of this buffer system is accompanied by an efflux not only of calcium but of divalent phosphate as well, due to dissolution of the mineral phase. Calcium efflux is dependent on the bicarbonate concentration as well as on the pH, and compensated chronic metabolic acidosis, in which there is a systemically reduced bicarbonate concentration, will have an adverse effect on skeletal mineralization even though the pH is within the normal range because of the compensation mechanism.

It should again be emphasized that it is growing children who are vulnerable to skeletal demineralization in this way. Once the skeleton has reached maturity, it appears to be resistant to this mechanism. In practice, it means that growing children should have any identifiable metabolic acidosis corrected, but in adults it need not be corrected if it is asymptomatic.[33]

It is frequently reported that patients with renal function below a certain level should not undergo any form of enterocystoplasty or urinary intestinal diversion because metabolic problems are far more likely. Although frequently reported, there is little evidence to support this except in uretero-sigmoidostomy patients who have continuing faecal reflux to contend with as well as hyperchloraemic acidosis. In practice, most patients with impaired renal function undergoing enterocystoplasty or urinary diversion have an obstructive nephropathy, either due to frank outflow obstruction at sphincter level or to high intravesical pressure. If these two problems are eliminated by enterocystoplasty, whatever the level of renal function, there will be at least a temporary stabilization, if not an overt improvement in renal function, and this usually amounts to a window of 18 months to 2 years before intrinsic renal disease causes further deterioration in renal function on the downward slope to renal replacement therapy.

Urinary infection and malignant transformation

Bacterial colonization of the urinary tract is very common after bowel interposition. Although one or two authors report sterile urine in their patients, the majority of surgeons find that the urine is usually, if not always, colonized.

Very often this is with a mixed growth of bacteria and less than the usual 100 000 organisms per ml associated with a 'classic' urinary infection. Not only is this bacteriuria common, there is also an increased incidence of both local and systemic infection in such patients. Average reported figures are that 80% of patients suffer bacteriuria[39] with a diverse bacterial flora and that 15% of patients will suffer acute pyelonephritis at some stage.[40] The highest incidence appears to be during the first year. This incidence is higher than in those who are on clean, intermittent self-catheterization with a normal bladder.[38]

Unlike urothelium, bowel does not attempt to sterilize its luminal content. When bowel is distended, it becomes relatively ischaemic and the mucosal barrier preventing bacterial translocation from mucosa to blood is disrupted. Urine from a substitute bladder is less bacteriostatic because the concentration of urea is lower and the pH higher than in normal urine. These three points probably account for the increased incidence of infection in such patients.

This infection is difficult, if not impossible, to eliminate and most patients suffer asymptomatic bacteriuria even if they are completely unaware of it. Although asymptomatic, it may be nonetheless important in the long run as there is a theoretical link between infection and cancer.

Patients with uretero-sigmoidostomy were noted to have an incidence of cancer at the uretero-intestinal anastomosis of between 6% and 29%, with a mean of 11%.[25] Generally speaking, there is a lag time of 10 to 20 years between the surgery and the development of the tumour. These tumours are extremely aggressive and one-third of patients die from them. They appear to be adenocarcinomas in the main, although other histological types have been reported. Overall, this represents a 500-fold increase in the incidence of tumours in the sigmoid colon in this patient group, and it has been reported that, in patients diverted by this means before the age of 25, the increased risk is 7000-fold.[41]

The aetiology of these tumours is not clear. Presumably, as most are adenocarcinomas, they arise in intestinal epithelium adjacent to the anastomosis, although adenocarcinoma has been shown to arise from transitional epithelium exposed to faeces in experimental animals.[42] Furthermore, histological assessment of the ureters in patients with uretero-sigmoidostomies shows a high incidence of dysplasia as judged by biopsies or surgical specimens from close to the anastomosis.[43] Stewart suggested that these tumours arose as a result of the conversion of nitrates and secondary amines in the urine into nitrosamines due to the action of faecal bacteria.[44] Nitrosamines are known carcinogens and certainly patients with uretero-sigmoidostomies show high concentrations of nitrosamines in the faecal/urinary slurry that they pass.

Patients with enterocystoplasties or urinary diversions show dysplastic changes, and malignant change has been reported, albeit infrequently.[45] Most patients show chronic inflammatory changes in their bladder on biopsy, and nitrosamines are present in the urine, in this case produced by the bacteriuria that they have rather than by exposure to faeces. The greater the degree of the bacteriuria, the greater the degree of the pyuria associated with it, the higher the nitrosamine levels in the urine and the higher the incidence of histological changes, which in some instances would be classified as premalignant if they were found in the bowel in its natural situation. Such changes include keratinizing squamous metaplasia and transitional epithelial mucin distribution – changes similar to the alterations in colonic mucin secretion demonstrated in patients with uretero-sigmoidostomy.

Other factors have been suggested for the development of these tumours, including superoxide radicals and epidermal growth factor receptor proliferation, induced by the urothelial–colonic juxtaposition. Whatever the cause, there seems to be little doubt that some patients, at least, will develop tumours in the long run. Patients should therefore not be lost to follow-up so that such tumours can be detected at the earliest possible moment.

Stones

Patients with ileal conduits were found to have a 20% incidence of renal calculus formation if followed for more than 20 years.[38] Up to one-third of patients with Kock pouches were found to have stones in their pouch, in this instance related to non-resorbable staples. More recently, stones have been noted in the absence of foreign material in patients with diversions and orthotopic substitutions and these have been attributed to acid renal tubule fluid, an increased excretion of calcium, and a high incidence of infection with urease-producing bacteria, as well as to the presence of mucus and almost universal bacteriuria.

However, it should be noted that patients with ileal conduits and with orthotopic substitution cystoplasties that empty spontaneously have a low incidence of stone formation. An orthotopic substitution that has to be emptied by clean, intermittent self-catheterization has a higher incidence. But the highest incidence of all occurs in patients with continent diversions being emptied by clean, intermittent self-catheterization – generally from the top of the bladder, rather than from the bottom – suggesting that stagnation is the most important factor, with mucus presumably acting as a nidus and bacterial colonization as the catalyst.

Other problems

It has already been noted, when discussing metabolic abnormalities, that the primary abnormality leading to acidosis is the increased absorption of ammonia. This ammonia is normally converted into urea by the liver. If the liver is in any way abnormal, then hyperammonaemic encephalopathy may result,[46] and is particularly common in patients with chronic liver disease such as cirrhosis. The hepatic reserve to clear ammonia in this way is great, so this is not a common problem unless liver disease is fairly advanced.

Certain drugs may be absorbed from the urine when bowel is interposed, and phenytoin[47] and certain antimetabolites such as methotrexate[48] have been reported to reach toxic levels in such patients.

Perhaps more importantly, glucose can be reabsorbed from the urine in diabetic patients and control of their diabetes may be made more difficult as a result.[49]

REFERENCES

1. Adzick NS, Harrison MR. The fetal surgery experience. In: Adzick NS, Longaker MT, eds. Fetal Wound Healing. New York: Elsevier, 1992: 1–23
2. Skalli O, Gabbiani G. The biology of the myofibroblast relationship to wound contraction and fibrocontractive disease. In: Clark RAF, Henson PM, eds. The Molecular and Cellular Biology of Wound Healing. New York: Plenum Press, 1988: 373
3. Stewart RJ, Duley JA, Dewdney J, Allardyce RA, Beard ME, Fitzgerald PH. Wound fibroblast and macrophage II. Their origin studied in the human after bone marrow transplantation. Br J Surg 1981; 68: 129–131
4. Kingsnorth AN, Slavin J. Peptide growth factors and wound healing. Br J Surg 1991; 78: 1286–1290
5. Furcht LT. Critical factors controlling angiogenesis: cell products, cell matrix and growth factors. Lab Invest 1986; 55: 505–509
6. Blair GH, Slome D, Walter JB. Review of experimental investigations on wound healing. In: Ross JP, ed. British Surgical Practice: Surgical Progress. London: Butterworth, 1961
7. Converse JM, McCarthy JG, Brauer RO, Ballentyne DL. Transplantation of skin. Grafts and flaps. In: Reconstructive Plastic Surgery, Vol. 1, 2nd edn. Philadelphia: WB Saunders, 1977: 152–182
8. Grabb WC, Smith JW. Plastic Surgery. 2nd edn. Boston: Little Brown, 1973: 1–122
9. Devine CJ Jr, Horton CE. Surgical treatment of Peyronie's disease with dermal graft. J Urol 1989; 142: 1223–1226
10. Perlmutter AD, Montgomery BT, Steinhardt G. Tunica vaginalis free graft for the correction of chordee. J Urol 1985; 134: 311–313
11. Gilbert DA, Horton CE, Terzis J, Devine CJ Jr, Winslow BH, Devine P. New concepts in phallic reconstruction. Ann Plast Surg 1987; 18: 128–136
12. Ehrlich RM, Reda EF, Koyle MA, Kogan SJ, Levitt SB. Complications of bladder mucosal graft. J Urol 1989; 142: 626–627
13. Baskin LS, Duckett JW. Mucosal grafts in hypospadias and stricture management. AUA Update Series 1994; XIII, 34: 270–275
14. Burger RA, Muller SC, El-Damanhoury H, Tschakaloff A, Riedmiller H, Hohenfellner R. The buccal mucosal graft for urethral reconstruction: a preliminary report. J Urol 1992; 147: 662–664
15. Horton CE, Devine CJ Jr. A one stage repair of hypospadias cripples. Plast Reconstr Surg 1970; 45: 425–430

16. Duckett JW. The island flap technique for hypospadias repair. Urol Clin North Am 1981; 8: 503–511
17. Morehouse DD. Current indications and technique of two stage repair for membraneous urethral strictures. Urol Clin North Am 1989; 16: 325–328
18. Mundy AR. Results and complications of urethroplasty and its future. Br J Urol 1993; 71: 322–325
19. Schreiter F, Noll F. Meshgraft urethroplasty using split thickness skin graft of foreskin. J Urol 1989; 142: 1223–1226
20. McCraw J, Massey F, Shaiklin K, Horton C. Vaginal reconstruction with gracilis myocutaneous flaps. Plast Reconstr Surg 1976; 58: 176–183
21. Horton CE, Sadore RC, Jordan GH, Sagher U, et al. Use of the rectus abdominis muscle and fascia flap in reconstruction of epispadias/exstrophy Clin Plast Surg 1988; 15: 393–397
22. Taylor GI, Daniel RK. The anatomy of several free flap donor sites. Plast Reconstr Surg 1975; 56: 243–253
23. Koch MO, McDougal WS, Thompson CO. Mechanisms of solute transport following urinary diversion through intestinal segments: an experimental study with rats. J Urol 1991; 146: 1390
24. Fern DO, Odel HM. Electrolyte pattern of the blood after bilateral ureterosigmoidostomy. JAMA 1949; 142: 634–641
25. Zabbo A, Kay R. Ureterosigmoidostomy and bladder extrophy: a long-term follow-up. J Urol 1986; 136: 396
26. Fisch M, Wammack R, Muller SC, Hohenfellner R. The Mainz 11 (sigma rectum pouch). J Urol 1993; 149: 258–263
27. Singh G, Thomas DG. Bowel problems after enterocystoplasty. Br J Urol 1997; 79: 328–332
28. Whorwell PJ, Lupton EW, Erdiran D, Wilson K. Bladder smooth muscle dysfunction in patients with irritable bowel syndrome. Gut 1986; 27: 1014–1017
29. Spirnak SP, Caldamone AA. Ureterosigmoidostomy. Urol Clin North Am 1986; 13: 285
30. Durrans D, Wujanto R, Carrol RN, Torrance HD. Bile acid malabsorption: a complication of conduit surgery. Br J Urol 1989; 64: 485–488
31. Dean AM, Woodhouse CRJ, Parkinson MC. Histological changes in ileal conduits. J Urol 1984; 132: 1108
32. Nurse DE, Mundy AR. Metabolic complications of cystoplasty. Br J Urol 1989; 63: 165–170
33. Mundy AR, Nurse DE. Calcium balance, growth and skeletal mineralisation in patients with cystoplasties. Br J Urol 1992; 69: 257–259
34. Wear JB Jr, Barquin OP. Ureterosigmoidostomy. Urology 1973; 1: 192
35. Klein EA, Montie JE, Montague DK, Kay R et al. Jejunal conduit urinary diversion. J Urol 1989; 64: 412
36. Koch MO, McDougall WS, Thompson CO. Mechanisms of solute transport following urinary diversion through intestinal segments: an experimental study with rats. J Urol 1991; 146: 1390–1394
37. Geist RW, Ansell JS. Total body potassium after ureteroileostomy. Surg Gynaec Obstet 1961; 113: 585–589
38. McDougall WS, Koch MO. Impaired growth and development and urinary intestinal interposition. Trans Am Assoc Genitourin Surg 1991; 105: 3
39. Guinan PD, Moore RH, Neter E, Murphy GP. The bacteriology of ileal conduit urine in man. Surg Gynaec Obstet 1972; 134: 78–82
40. Schwarz GR, Jeffs RD. Ileal conduit urinary diversion in children: computer analysis of follow-up from 2 to 16 years. J Urol 1975; 114: 285
41. Husmann DA, Spence HM. Current status of tumour of the bowel following ureterosigmoidostomy: a review. J Urol 1990; 144: 607–610
42. Aaronson IA, Constantinides CG, Sallie LP, Sinclair-Smith CC. Pathogenesis of adenocarcinoma complicating ureterosigmoidostomy. Experimental observations. Urology 1987; 29: 538
43. Aaronson IA, Sinclair-Smith CC. Dysplasia of ureteric epithelium: a source of adenocarcinoma in ureterosigmoidostomy? Z Kinderchir Grenzgeb 1984; 39: 364–367
44. Stewart M, Hill MJ, Pugh RC, Williams JP. The role of N-nitrosamine in carcinogenesis at the uretero-colic anastomosis. Br J Urol 1981; 53: 115–118
45. Filmer RB, Spencer JR. Malignancies in bladder, augmentations and intestinal conduits. J Urol 1990; 143: 671–678
46. McDermott WV Jr. Diversion of urine to the intestines as a factor in ammoniagenic coma. N Engl J Med 1957; 256: 460
47. Savarirayan F, Dixey GM. Synope following ureterosigmoidostomy. J Urol 1969; 101: 844–845
48. Bowyer GW, Davies TW. Methotrexate toxicity associated with an ileal conduit. Br J Urol 1987; 60: 592
49. Sridhar KN, Samuell CT, Woodhouse CRJ. Absorption of glucose from urinary conduits in diabetics and nondiabetics. BMJ 1983; 287: 1327–1329

31

Energy sources in urology

Jeremy Elkabir and Ken M Anson

INTRODUCTION

In every operating theatre around the world, an energy source of some description will be available to help the surgeon perform procedures with as limited morbidity as possible. The move toward less invasive therapeutic interventions has also resulted in energy sources moving out of the operating theatre into the outpatient department. Advances in energy delivery have arisen alongside and often in tandem with advances in surgery. The introduction of extracorporeal lithotripsy remains the most potent example of the impact of technology upon surgical practice. The liaison between industry and health-care professionals remains critically important both to the understanding of present-day devices, and for the development of the surgical tools of the future.

Many medical devices have been introduced in recent years throughout the whole field of urology. Some have become accepted treatments while others have fallen by the wayside. Their rapid introduction into everyday urological practice underlines the importance of understanding the basic principles behind their use. It is our aim in this chapter to present the physical principles that underpin the various energy sources that are currently commercially available to urologists. It is hoped that this will provide a 'working knowledge' that will help the clinician not only to choose the tool best suited to the job at hand, but also to be able to use it appropriately and safely. We have divided the energy sources into three broad families: electromagnetic, acoustic and mechanical (Table 31.1). We shall examine the physical characteristics of each, explain their tissue interactions, outline the delivery systems available and provide a brief description of their clinical applications. Electrosurgical energy (such as diathermy) and ionizing radiation will not be considered here, as they appear in detail elsewhere in this book.

Table 31.1 Energy sources in urology.

Electromagnetic energy (non-ionizing)
Radio waves
Microwaves
Lasers
Acoustic energy
Extracorporeal shock-wave lithotripsy
Ultrasound
Mechanical energy
Ballistic energy
Water jet

ELECTROMAGNETIC ENERGY

Many urological instruments use sources that provide energy in the form of electromagnetic radiation (EMR). At first sight, they appear to be very disparate devices with varied delivery systems, but, on closer inspection, they share many common principles that arise from the use of the electromagnetic wave source. Their tissue effects may also seem unrelated but in fact are similar (namely, the deposition of heat within tissues), and often they can be separated only by the speed and depth of energy absorption. However, some of these sources (particularly lasers) have very specific tissue effects which are wavelength dependent and vary greatly from one wavelength to another.

General principles

Visible light, X-rays, microwaves, radio waves and invisible laser wavelengths are all part of the electromagnetic spectrum and are members of the same family. All travel through space at the same enormous velocity (v) of 3×10^8 m/s, the speed of light (c): about 186 000 miles per second. When they travel through a material medium, their speed is reduced but with no evidence of movement of the medium to indicate their passage. There is a constant relationship between velocity (v = c, the speed of light through an empty space), wavelength (λ) and frequency (f), such that $v = f\lambda$. It follows that the relationship between wavelength and frequency is inversely proportional. The electromagnetic spectrum is divided into bands for convenience, as outlined in Figure 31.1.

Quantum physics

Up until the twentieth century, an argument raged as to whether light was a wave form or particulate matter. In the early 1900s, it began to emerge that light exhibited particulate properties. Experimental evidence led to three main observations (the photoelectric effect, Figure 31.2): firstly, when light was directed at a metal surface, electrons were instantaneously ejected; secondly, when light intensity was increased, more electrons were ejected, but their velocity remained the same; and, finally, changing the colour of the light towards the blue end of the visible spectrum (increasing the frequency) increased the maximum velocity of the ejected electrons. The wave theory of light could not explain these phenomena, as metals would have to reach high temperatures before electrons were ejected, and some time delay would be required to allow sufficient energy transfer. Similarly, increasing the intensity would increase the speed of the ejected electrons, and the frequency of light would not be expected to change the findings, since intensity, and not colour, determines the energy of waves.

These findings led to the quantum theory of light, which states that light (or any other EMR) exists in the form of quanta known as photons, which are tiny 'packets' of energy with no mass travelling through space at a velocity of 3×10^8 m/s. The energy of each photon is given as $E = hf$, where E is the energy in joules, f is the frequency and h is a universal constant (Planck's constant = 6.63×10^{-34} J/s). The fundamental concept that energy is dependent upon the frequency of the radiation applies to all parts of the electromagnetic spectrum. Therefore, it can be seen that as the frequency increases, so does the energy of the EMR. Thus, microwaves and radio waves are of low energy while X-ray photons have a high energy enabling them to ionize matter that they come into contact with.

The effect of EMR upon living tissue

Although electromagnetic waves share many physical characteristics, varying only in frequency and wavelength, their effect upon living tissue is very different. For example, the human body is transparent to radio waves, opaque to visible light, and mostly transparent to X-rays. The quantum theory states that to raise an atom from ground to excited state, a photon of a given frequency and hence given energy

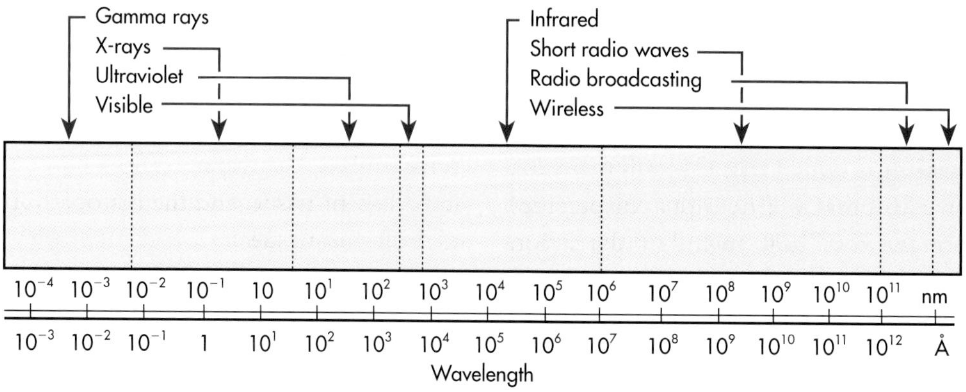

Figure 31.1 *The electromagnetic spectrum.*

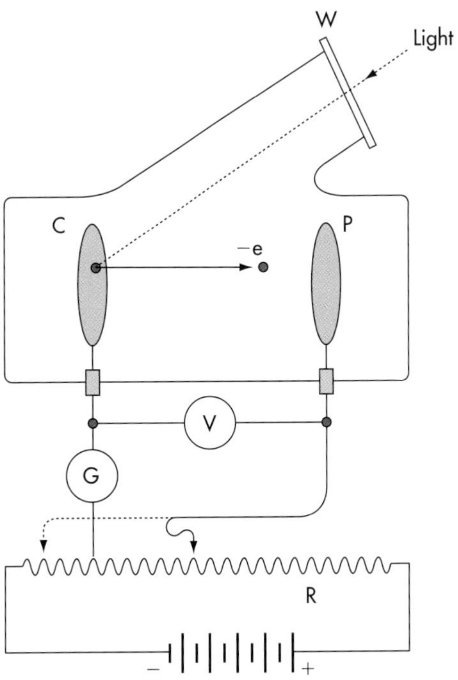

Figure 31.2 *Experimental set-up for observing the photoelectric effect. G - galvanometer, V - voltage, C - cathode, P - plate, W - quartz window*

($\Delta E = hf$, where ΔE is the energy difference) is required. Thus, for a photon to be absorbed (to transfer its energy), it must interact with an atom that will be excited only by that corresponding packet of energy. Radio waves can pass through the body with little effect, while microwaves cause molecular rotation and torsion, and induce tissue heating. The infrared band causes molecular vibration, and X-rays cause tissue ionization.

At the microscopic level, the electrical response of soft tissues to EMR is dependent on the frequency of the energy. This phenomenon is known as the dielectric property of tissues. At low frequencies (that is, below several hundred kilohertz [kHz]), conductivity is determined by electrolytes in the extracellular space, and tissues have a high permeability to EMR at these frequencies. In the low kilohertz range, tissues exhibit a dispersion (the alpha dispersion) due to several processes. These include polarization of counterions near charged surfaces and membrane-bound structures within tissues. In the radio frequency (RF) band, the tissues exhibit a dispersion (the beta dispersion) centred on the 0.1–10-MHz range, due to charging of cell membranes through the intracellular and extracellular media. At microwave frequencies (above 1 GHz and centred around 20 GHz), gamma dispersion occurs due to rotational relaxation of tissue water.

Thermal tissue interactions

In urological practice, non-laser EMR is commonly used to induce thermal damage in tissues. Radiowave and microwave generators have been designed to 'heat the prostate' to different temperatures in order to achieve varying degrees of tissue damage. Some laser techniques have also been developed to obtain similar thermal effects. In each case, the energy inherent within the EMR is converted to heat within tissues. Each different energy source will vary between the amount of energy that can be delivered and the depth to which that energy can reach, but the basic tissue effect desired is the same. The response of tissues to heating varies with the temperature achieved at the target area. At temperatures around 45°C, tissue retracts due to macromolecular conformational changes, bond destruction and membrane alterations. Beyond 60°C, protein denaturation occurs, and this is commonly called 'coagulation' and results in coagulative necrosis. Carbonization of tissues occurs at approximately 80°C along with membrane permeabilization and collagen denaturation. Finally, at temperatures in excess of 100°C, vaporization of water occurs, and in combination with carbonization, yields decomposition of tissue constituents. Below temperatures of 45°C, there is virtually no histological change in tissue following heating. The World Health Organization (WHO) has defined heat treatments as hyperthermia for temperatures of 37–45°C, and as thermotherapy when temperatures exceed 45°C.

It should be noted at this point that many other factors influence the degree of heat deposition at a particular area, and these include the locoregional blood supply, the thermal conductivity of the target and adjacent tissue, and the histopathological nature of the target tissue.

Radio frequency (RF)

Radio-frequency radiation (RFR) is defined by the Institute of Electrical and Electronics Engineers

(IEEE) as extending from 3 kHz to 300 GHz, but this band is commonly divided into a lower-frequency RF band of 3 kHz–300 MHz and a higher-frequency microwave band of 300 MHz–300 GHz. As a result of its low energy, RF, unlike other forms of non-ionizing EMR, requires direct contact with tissues to exert an effect. As the RF energy attempts to pass into tissue, transference of energy occurs in a concentrated area. Typical devices use RF in the range 465–490 kHz delivered transurethrally into the prostate. RF energy is efficient with minimal wastage; consequently, low-wattage energy (up to 15 W) can achieve temperatures approaching 100°C within a short time (typically <5 min) without the need for interruption and cooling. RF devices are therefore often small and compact. Due to the low energy of RF, the prostatic capsule, urethra, external sphincter, neurovascular bundles and rectum are said to be spared from heat dissipation.

Transurethral needle ablation (TUNA) of the prostate

The TUNA device consist of an RF generator and monitor where energy, ablation time, lesion temperature, urethral temperature and tissue impedance are displayed. In this device, the 465–490 kHz RF signal is transmitted directly into the prostate via two needles delivered via the TUNA catheter (Figure 31.3). The generator has a cut-out mechanism to prevent excessive tissue temperatures by monitoring tissue impedance (typically, cut-out of >450 Ω) and urethral temperature (typically, cut-out of >46°C). The delivery system has a disposable cartridge, a resterilizable hand-piece and a zero-degree fibre-optic lens. The TUNA cartridge contains two retractable needles, each surrounded by a protective retractable Teflon shield, except at the needle tips. When extended, the needles leave the body of the catheter and diverge at an angle of 40° between each other and perpendicular to the catheter. Thermocouples are located at the tips of the protective shields and near the tip of the catheter for temperature monitoring of the lesion and prostatic urethra, respectively. The catheter tip is clear in order to allow visualization of the needles during penetration into the prostate.

The procedure can be performed under local anaesthesia and sedation.[1] Lesions produced by the TUNA device are well-defined, ellipsoid necrotic lesions as a result of coagulative necrosis. The exact mechanism whereby relief of symptoms occurs is debated. The concept of anatomical debulking is flawed, as prostate volume changes following TUNA treatment are minimal. Physiological alteration of the dynamic component of voiding is more likely[2,3] or as a result of neural ablation.[4] Long-term data are still awaited, but there has been concern about the durability of this procedure, with up to 20% of patients requiring a TURP within 2 years.[5]

Microwaves

Microwaves occupy the electromagnetic band at frequencies of 300 MHz–300 GHz. These higher frequencies result in higher energy, and therefore greater tissue penetration than RF. The effect of microwave energy on tissue is predominantly due to

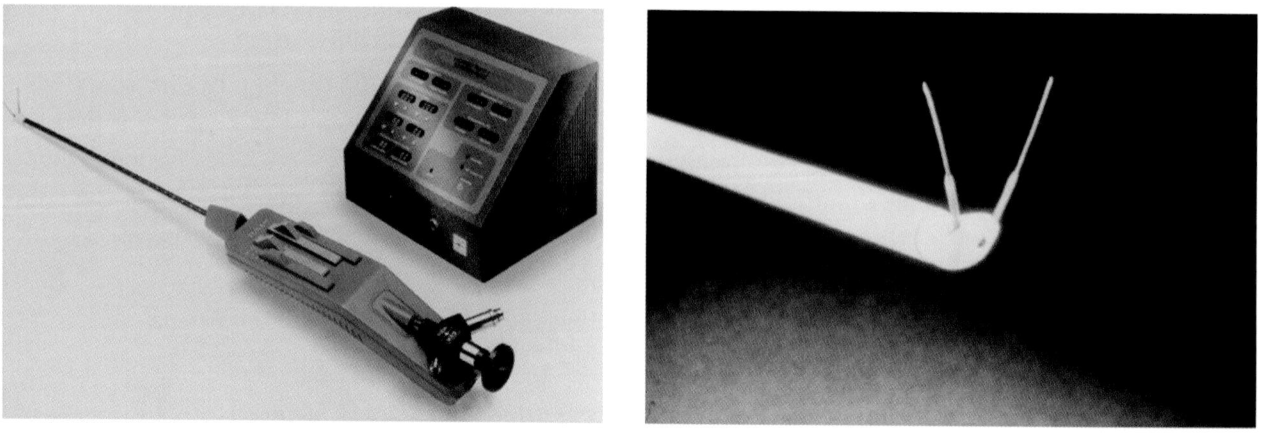

Figure 31.3 *TUNA catheter with retractable sheaths and needles.*

molecular torsion and rotation (oscillation) and polarization of small molecules, especially water, resulting in tissue heating. In clinical practice, frequencies of 915 MHz or 1296 MHz are used, and microwaves are used predominantly in urology for prostatic therapies.

Microwave prostatic therapies

Microwave energy may be applied transrectally and transurethrally, and may induce hyperthermia or thermotherapy, depending on the target tissue temperature. Transrectal hyperthermia was originally described in the treatment of prostate cancer[6] and, with the introduction of rectal cooling, for BPH.[7] Objectively, prostate volume and serum PSA remain unchanged, indicating limited cellular disruption, and placebo-controlled (sham) studies have failed to show relief of the obstructive component of BPH.[8] Its use therefore has largely been abandoned.

Microwave thermotherapy, which is usually achieved by treating the prostate transurethrally, aims to achieve higher temperatures (45–80°C). Objectively, no significant reduction in prostatic volume is reported, although serum PSA rises following this treatment, indicating release from damaged tissue. Return of PSA to its pretreatment value suggests no significant reduction in prostatic volume.[8] Modest reductions in peak flow rate (PFR) following treatment are also observed. Increasing the intraprostatic temperature by changing machine software improves efficacy,[9,10] although the incidence of adverse events, including acute urinary retention and patient discomfort, is also increased. However, other authors have failed to demonstrate objective improvement with high-energy software.[11]

The microwave devices currently in clinical and investigational use are listed in Table 31.2. Most microwave devices apply energy transurethrally, generating high intraprostatic temperatures. The Prostatron™ device will be described here. Water-conductive cooling allows preservation of the urethral mucosa and allows decreased anaesthetic requirement. The microwave antenna produces the microwave field, with a maximum penetration of <2 cm. Superior results are said to occur in larger prostates due to reduced vascular density that reduces heat conduction away from the target lesion. A microwave radiometer measures 'thermal noise', which is directly related to temperature. The prostatic urethra must be at least 35 mm in length for the lower-energy software, that is, Prostatron v.2.0, and 25 mm for the high energy Prostatron v.2.5. The therapy is contraindicated in patients with claudication, prostate or bladder cancer, urethral stricture, or in patients with a pacemaker, defibrillator or other metallic implants. Rectal temperature is monitored, and an alarm system is set which causes a cut-out if excessive rectal temperatures occur. Treatment is commenced at 20 W and increased by 5 W every 2 minutes until the maximum level is reached (60 W for v.2.0 and 70 W for v.2.5), and treatment sessions are usually of 1 hr duration. There have been

Table 31.2 Microwave devices in clinical and investigational use.

Device	Microwave frequency	Software	Comment
Prostatron (EDAP-Technomed)	1296 MHz	v2.0 (standard) v2.5 (high energy)	Original machine Largest evidence base
Maxis (EDAP-Technomed)	1296 MHz	v2.0 (standard) v2.5 (high energy)	More compact
Praktis (EDAP-Technomed)	1296 MHz	v2.0 (standard) v2.5 (high energy)	Second-generation compact device
T3 (Urologix)	915 MHz	Standard	FDA approved
Urowave (Donier)	915 MHz	Standard	Recent FDA approval
ProstaLund (Dantec), ProstCare (Bruker Spectospin) LEO Microtherm (Laser ElectroOptics)			Investigational

concerns regarding clinical durability. Data are available for the v.2.0 software, and in one study with 4 years post-treatment follow-up, two-thirds of TUMT-treated patients required additional treatment, with only 23% patients satisfied with the result,[12] while another showed a clinical efficacy rate of 39% at 50 months.[13] In addition, a randomized trial compared to sham treatment demonstrated no clinically significant difference between the two treatment arms.[14]

Lasers

The term *laser* is an acronym for '*l*ight *a*mplification by the *s*timulated *e*mission of *r*adiation'. Prior to Einstein's pioneering work in 1913, it was thought that a photon could interact with an atom in only one of two ways; it was either absorbed, thus leading to the elevation of an electron to a higher energy orbit, or emitted as the atom dropped to a lower energy level (spontaneous emission). Einstein, however, suggested that a third possibility existed, which he described as 'stimulated emission'. His theoretical model postulated that when a photon (with an energy level corresponding to that of an energy-level transition) interacted with an excited atom, another photon would be released with identical wavelength. It was 50 years later that the first laser was developed by Theodore Maiman in California. He used a ruby rod excited by a helical flash-lamp, to produce a beam of red laser light.[15] A number of lasers were subsequently produced in the 1960s with a variety of different laser mediums. The first gas laser was the helium neon laser manufactured at the Bell Laboratories in New Jersey.[16] The first neodymium:YAG laser was demonstrated in 1964,[17] while the first semiconductor lasers appeared in 1962. In 1964, Patel described the first carbon dioxide laser,[18] and it and the neodymium:YAG laser remain the most popular lasers used in medicine today.

The properties of laser light

The three unique properties of laser light (beam coherence, collimation and monochromaticity), (Table 31.3) separate it from the widely divergent, confused and multiple wavelength light emitted from conventional light sources. Due to the high spatial coherence of laser light, the beam is remarkably collimated and therefore of low divergence. This property allows the full power of the generated light energy to be coupled into, and transmitted down, fine fibre-optic cables to the operative site. As a result, very high power densities (power per unit cross-sectional area) can be achieved at the tissue surface. Furthermore, the beam can be focused to produce even greater power densities with more pronounced tissue effects.

Table 31.3 Properties of laser light.

Coherent (in phase)
Collimated (non-divergent)
Monochromatic (of a single wavelength)

The monochromaticity of laser light means that it consists of a single wavelength. However, some lasers may produce light of one or more wavelengths (the argon laser may produce up to 10 wavelengths of 437–529 nm). The interaction of the light with tissue is dependent both on the laser wavelength and the colour of the tissue irradiated; thus, the single wavelength nature of the beam confers a high selectivity of action. One single laser will not be suitable for all clinical applications. Prior to any treatment, the clinician should ensure that the laser provided is of a suitable wavelength to produce the tissue interaction desired. A number of different laser wavelengths are available for clinical use. They are named after the medium used to generate the laser energy (Table 31.4).

The active medium, composed of the lasing material, is subjected to some form of energy (light, heat or electrical energy). This results in a large number of atoms absorbing enough energy to enter an excited state in which electrons change their orbit. This situation is unstable, and atoms quickly revert to their original energy state, releasing energy in the form of photons of light. The released photons may be reflected by the mirrors, escape as laser light, excite other ground-state atoms to the excited state, or displace higher-energy-state atoms to their ground state with the release of similar photons. The wavelength of each individual laser is identical, but varies from laser to laser and is dependent on the active medium deployed. Amplification is achieved by bouncing the photons back and forth between two mirrors (Figure 31.4).

Table 31.4 Characteristics of medical lasers.

Laser type	Mode	Wavelength (nm)	Visibility*	Tissue penetration (mm)	Tissue absorption	Effects	Clinical uses
Carbon dioxide	CW	10 600	Invisible*	0.1	Water, proteins, nucleic acids and fat	Intense carbonization and vapourization Minimal penetration	Superficial skin lesions, such as penile warts, Bowen's disease Laser scalpel'
Argon	CW	488 + 514 (dual wavelength)	Blue	1	Haemoglobin, melanin	Tissue coagulation and vapourization	Nephron-sparing surgery; laparoscopy; pigmented lesions and lesions with high blood flow
Neodymium: yttrium aluminium garnet (Nd:YAG)	CW/P	1064	Invisible*	3–8	Protein	Protein denaturation Minimal carbonization and vapourization Coagulative necrosis	Treatment of BPH and TCC Interstitial laser therapy of solid tumours
KTP-532	CW/P	532	Green	0.3–1	Haemoglobin	Tissue coagulation and vapourization	Uses similar to argon Posterior urethral valves
Holmium:YAG	P	2100	Invisible*	0.5	Water	Mechanical pressure-wave fragmentation ?Thermal effect	Urinary tract calculi Enucleation of prostate
Pulsed dye laser (coumarin green)	P	504	Green	Minimal	Haemoglobin, but pulses (5–10 Hz) too short (1 ms) for Hb to absorb	Stone fragmentation Pressure effects and plasma formation Minimal damage to urothelium; little thermal effect	Urinary tract calculi
Semiconductor diode lasers	CW	800–890	Invisible*	3–7	Protein	Protein denaturation with coagulative necrosis Some vapourization	Treatment of BPH Interstitial laser therapy of solid tumours

CW: continuous wave; P; pulsed.
*Invisible beams are 'marked' with a low-power helium neon aiming beam.

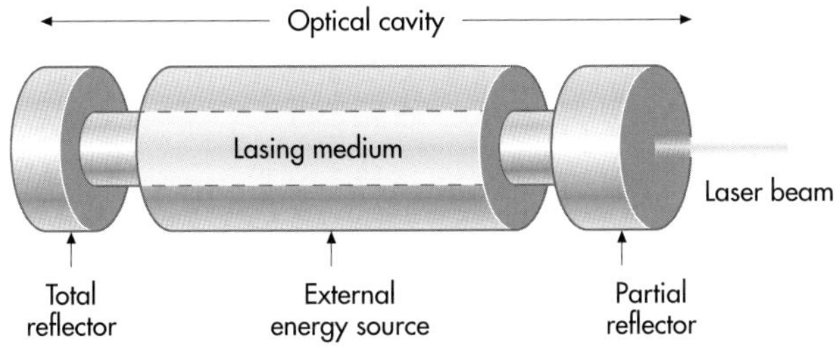

Figure 31.4 *Basic laser design.*

Laser energy can be continuous or pulsed. Pulsing of lasers delivers a higher peak power, the maximum rate of energy delivery during the time of the pulse, and is commonly used to fragment calculi (that is, pulsed dye, holmium:YAG and frequency-doubled KTP/Nd:YAG). Pulsing is achieved either by applying intermittent energy to the active medium or by a process known as Q-switching, in which a fast shutter is placed between the active/using medium and the exit mirror (partial reflector). When the shutter is closed, the photons are trapped within the active medium, resulting in a rapid build-up of energy. When the shutter opens, there is an instantaneous release of energy with a very large peak power.

Originally, lasers were housed in large machines that were noisy, required three phased electrical supplies and were notoriously unreliable and fragile. As technology has developed, few lasers now require water-cooling, and many run on normal electrical supplies. The semiconductor lasers are certainly the smallest and tidiest machines of all. They are robust, lightweight and very portable. They are generally smaller than an average diathermy unit and are likely to be integral parts of most operating theatres in the future.

Laser–tissue interactions

Boulnois has proposed a classification for the possible types of 'photomedical processes' that can occur when laser light interacts with biological tissue.[19] The four photobiological laser processes are thermal, photochemical, electromechanical and photoablative. As with the use of microwaves and RF, the predominant tissue effect with lasers in urology is thermal. The photochemical process is used in photodynamic therapy and involves the interaction of light with a photosensitizing substrate, and the short-pulse regimens of electromechanical and photoablative protocols are concerned with high-power densities delivered in short pulses to produce either stone fragmentation or fine photoablative incisions.

Thermal interactions

When laser light interacts with tissue, it is reflected, transmitted, scattered or absorbed. Transmission results in light passage through the tissue with little or no interaction with the molecules. In contrast, reflection results in deflection of the light away from the surface of the tissue. When absorbed, the electromechanical energy of the incident beam is converted into thermal energy within the tissues. Scattering of the beam results in widespread distribution of the energy at all angles to the incident beam; the energy is subsequently absorbed and converted into thermal energy.

Both the wavelength of the interacting light and the colour of the tissue irradiated determine the relative amount of absorption and scattering within tissue components (Figure 31.5). For example, the blue-green light of the argon laser is readily absorbed by haemoglobin but is transmitted through the dermis and epidermis. These properties allow the successful coagulation of port-wine stains, as the abnormal capillaries absorb most of the energy with little effect on the surrounding skin.[20]

The CO_2 laser has a wavelength of 10 600 nm and is therefore highly absorbed by water, proteins, nucleic acids and fat; thus, its depth of penetration is very small at 0.1 mm. The high absorption by water makes this laser light unsuitable for endoscopic procedures,[21] and it is used for the treatment of superficial lesions (as on skin or external genitalia). There is intense and instantaneous tissue vaporization and carbonization with a very shallow thermal damage front, and healing is therefore achieved with minimal scarring. CO_2 lasers have also been described in vasovasostomy.[22] The stated advantages include complete sealing of the anastomosis with no sperm leakage and therefore granuloma. Albumin may be used as a tissue solder.

In contrast, the neodymium:YAG wavelength (1064 nm) has little effect on water, but proteins

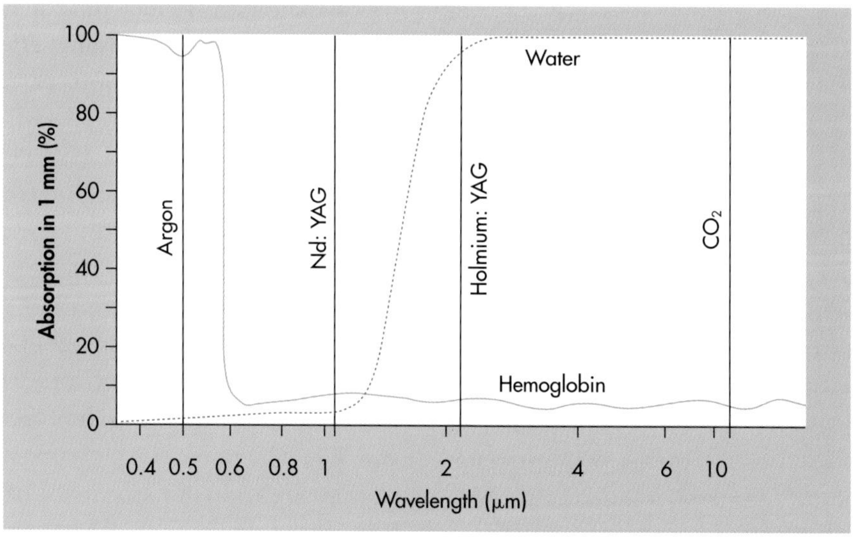

Figure 31.5 *Laser wavelength absorption by haemoglobin and water.*

absorb it. It is therefore widely scattered to a depth of up to 0.8 cm, as the predominantly water-containing tissue is transparent. The scattering results in a wider distribution of the energy at all angles away from the incident beam. The energy is therefore absorbed within a larger volume of tissue. This laser has therefore been used to cause widespread coagulative necrosis within the benign prostate (*e*ndoscopic *l*aser *a*blation of the *p*rostate [ELAP]),[23] and it can also be used to coagulate superficial bladder tumours. The 805-nm semiconductor diode laser has similar properties to Nd:YAG when used for side-fire laser ablation of the prostate.[24,25] Q-switching of Nd:YAG lasers may be used to fragment calculi. Addition of a KTP-532 crystal doubles the frequency (therefore halving the wavelength). This results in more energy delivered at shallower penetrations. It also causes the beam to become visible in the green band of visible light. Its uses are similar to the argon laser and include posterior urethral valve ablation in children.[26]

The power of a laser is related to the power density, that is, the power per surface area, and is given as $PD = W/\pi r^2$ (W [watts] is the power emitted from the laser). The total energy delivered multiplies the power density by duration of exposure; thus, total energy $= Ws/\pi r^2$, and this is measured in joules. It can be seen that doubling of the spot size reduces the power fourfold. The rate of ablation varies with the total energy delivered; the higher the total energy, the faster is the ablation. At low powers, there is time for heat conduction into deeper tissues; therefore, the higher the power density, the less is the thermal damage to underlying tissues. A highly focused beam results in a shallow zone of thermal damage, that is, beneath the lesion's surface, known as the thermal damage front, and results in minimal scarring. A defocused beam results in a reduction of power density at the lesion, but a thick zone of thermal damage front beneath the lesion's surface.

Photoablative and electromechanical interactions

Pulsing of lasers (such as holmium:YAG and pulsed dye lasers) has the additional benefit of a very high peak pressure, causing fragmentation by erosion, shattering and plasma bubble formation with cavitation. This effect is electromechanical or photoablative. When the pulse is very short (that is, 1 ms in the pulsed dye laser), there is insufficient time for haemoglobin to absorb the energy; thus, adjacent tissue such as the ureter will remain undamaged.[21] Unfortunately, the pulsed dye lasers are very expensive and have high running costs. In contrast, the holmium:YAG laser will damage ureteric tissue if in contact, as its effect is thought to be mainly thermal.[27] However, this property endows the laser with a dual purpose, as it can be used to incise tissue such as the prostate and bladder neck (HoLEP).[28]

Photochemical effects – photodynamic therapy

Low-power laser light can photochemically activate a photosensitizing dye such as a haematoporphyrin derivative. This dye is chemically inert until exposed to specific laser wavelengths; this exposure results in energy release in the form of free radicals that are cytotoxic. Tissues that take up these dyes can be destroyed when laser energy is directed at them. Endothelial cells are most sensitive to the effects of free radicals and have increased density within tumours. The injured endothelium also releases interleukin and tumour necrosis factor, causing additional damage to malignant epithelium. This technique is being used in the treatment of carcinoma in situ of the bladder and is being investigated in the treatment of both benign and malignant prostatic disease.

Tissue-welding effects

Laser energy can induce interdigitation of collagen, resulting in a tissue-welding effect. Albumin has been used as a tissue solder, particularly in vasovasostomy.

Laser delivery systems

Laser light can be focused to diameters near 50% of its wavelength. This allows laser light to be transmitted along single quartz fibre-optic fibres. Laser energy is conducted along the fibre by a process known as internal reflection where the light is reflected from one side to the other, as the beam travels along the fibre. The beam must be reflected at a specific angle, known as the critical angle of reflection. If the fibre is displaced, or bent too far, the beam will no longer strike the side wall at the critical angle and will escape from the fibre, causing injury to the user, the endoscope or both. Once the beam exits the fibre tip, it is no longer coherent, as it is driven out of phase during internal reflection, and divergence occurs (about 17%, assuming a flat fibre tip). Therefore, the highest power density is at the tip of the fibre. At present, the CO_2 laser cannot be transmitted by fibres due to the absorption of the energy by the fibre itself. However, CO_2-'friendly' fibres will soon be available.

Laser safety

Strict protocols regarding the use of lasers in the theatre are mandatory. All personnel in the theatre must wear protective goggles. Different goggles are required for different wavelengths, and the wearer should check that the goggles protect against the wavelength in use. The area where the laser is being used must be clearly marked with warning notices and the theatre doors locked when the laser is in use. An illuminated light must be on during laser firing. Black curtains should be applied above eye level to all windows. The retina is susceptible to laser light in the range 400–1400 nm. Accidental exposure can lead to injury, ranging from small scotomata to optic nerve burns. Wavelengths beyond 1400 nms may cause corneal injuries. There is a greater chance of an accidental burn to the skin than the eye. Laser safety rules should be available in all areas where lasers are in use, and the local laser safety officer will be able to advise on these.

ACOUSTIC ENERGY

General principles

Unlike electromagnetic waves, acoustic or sound waves require a medium through which to travel. They are best described as a travelling pressure wave and cannot travel through a vacuum. The audible range is normally 20–20 000 Hz. Waves below this range are termed 'infrasonic'; those above it, 'ultrasonic'. Sound waves are generated by a displacement of an object. A single displacement, such as the energy source of a lithotriptor, will generate a single pressure wave, whereas vibration, such as pulses of electric current applied to piezoceramic crystals, generates a continuous wave form; in this case, ultrasound. Following the initial displacement, the wave is propagated through gas or fluid by successive molecular collisions in the medium through which the sound wave travels. Sound waves are longitudinal, and their speed is dependent on the medium through which they travel and its temperature. Acoustic velocity is independent of pressure, frequency and amplitude of the sound wave.

Acoustic shock waves are complex and have non-linear pressure characteristics. There is an immediate rise in pressure followed by a sudden fall, resulting in a period of negative pressure (Figure 31.6). The focused shock wave generates positive and negative pressures up to 114 and 10 Mpa, respectively.[29] When applied to a stone, the positive pressure phase part of the shock wave is reflected at the stone surface, causing erosion at the entry and exit points due to a high-pressure gradient. A compressive wave continues through the stone causing shattering (Figure 31.7a). During the negative-pressure phase cavitation occurs,[29] causing rapid expansion of gas bubbles in the liquid medium at the stone surface (Figure 31.7b). This phenomenon occurs when a negative pressure greater than the ambient pressure exists in a liquid which then fails under stress.[30] These unstable bubbles collapse, forming microjets that strike the stone surface[31] (Figure 31.7b). Microjet velocities range from 130 to 170 m/s.

There are two mechanisms for the generation of these acoustic shock waves. Supersonic sources release energy in a finite space, producing an explosive plasma and acoustic shock wave (as in spark-gap,

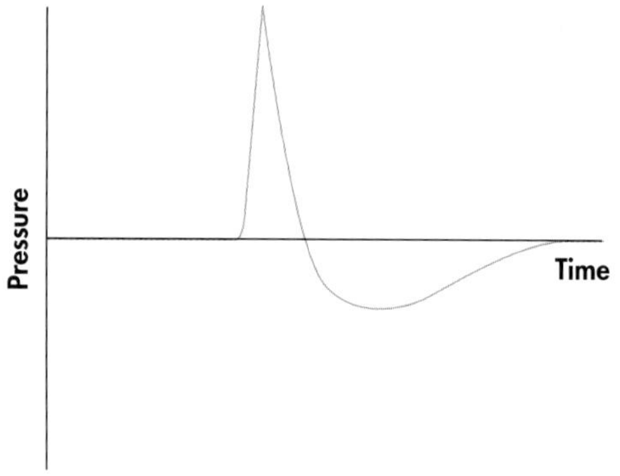

Figure 31.6 *Acoustic shock wave.*

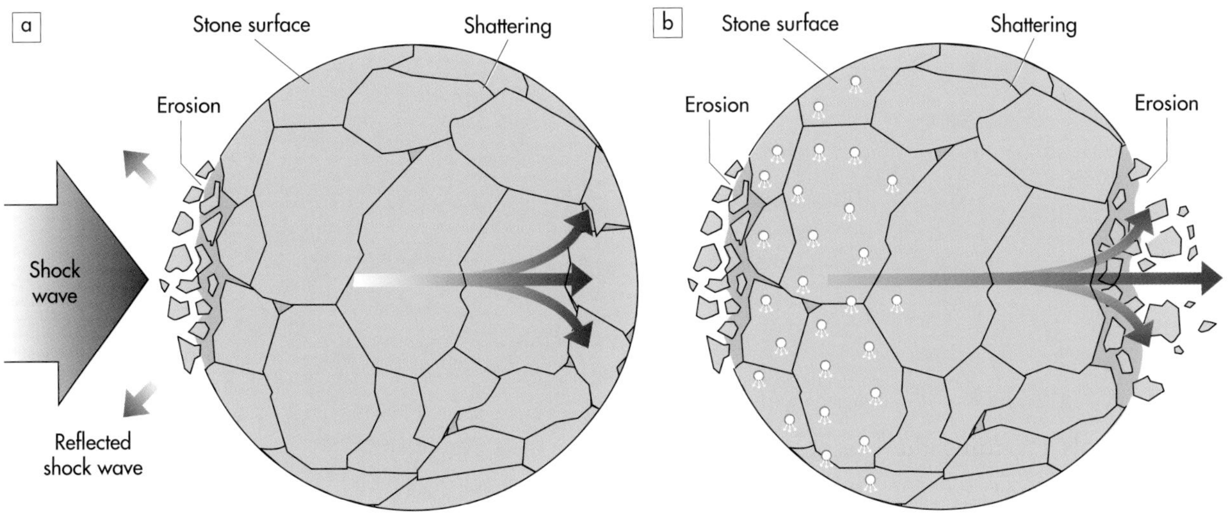

Figure 31.7a *Positive pressure phase effect of a shock wave upon a calculus. (1) The high-pressure gradient generated between the ongoing and reflected shock wave causes surface erosion at the entry and exit points. (2) The forward compression wave traverses the stone causing shattering.*

Figure 31.7b *Negative pressure phase effect of a shock wave upon a calculus. Cavitation occurs with formation of microbubbles, which subsequently collapse, generating microjets which strike the stone surface.*

microexplosive and locally delivered electrohydraulic lithotriptors [EHL]). Fixed-amplitude sources create acoustic shock waves by the sudden displacement of a surface (as in electromagnetic and piezoceramic lithotriptors). The power of a lithotriptor is related to the volume and peak pressure at the focal point. The energy delivered is measured in joules and is greatest for spark-gap lithotriptors due to their large focal points and high peak pressures.[32] Surrounding tissues are spared, as they are not brittle and lie outside the target area.

Extracorporeal shockwave lithotripsy (ESWL)

The first observations of the effect of acoustic energy were made in the USSR in the 1950s, but it was Dornier, an aircraft manufacturer in Germany, who pioneered this medical therapy following observations of damage to metallic components of aircraft resulting from shock waves. The first clinical experience in the human kidney was published in 1980.[33] Modifications were made to the original machine, the HM-1 (Human Model-1), and, in 1983, the HM-3 was widely introduced and still remains in use today in many units. Many ESWL machines have since been developed (Table 31.5) using a variety of energy sources, and these will be discussed later in the text.

Lithotriptor design

All lithotriptors require an energy source, a focusing mechanism for the shock wave, a coupling medium and a stone localization system. Spark-gap lithotriptors (such as Dornier HM-3) utilize an underwater spark that results in instantaneous water vaporization, generating a hydrodynamic pressure wave. The point of spark generation, known as F1, is placed in front of an ellipsoid reflector where pressure waves are focused at a set distance to the target area, known as F2 (Figure 31.8). This type of shock wave is the least consistent energy source from shock to shock.[34] Following repeated spark discharge, the distance between the positive and negative electrodes increases, significantly affecting the geometry of the ellipsoidal reflector. A 1-mm increase in the spark gap at F1 can result in a 1-cm increase in the size of F2. This problem is overcome by frequent changing of the electrodes or by adjusting the electrode tips.

Table 31.5 Classification and properties of ESWL machines.

Lithotriptor class	Focusing mechanism	Peak pressure (bar)	F2 distance (cm)	Focal zone (mm)	Localization
Spark gap lithotriptors					
HM-3 (Dornier)	Ellipsoid reflector	1300	13	15 × 90	F
STS (Medstone)	Ellipsoid reflector	900–1200	15	13 × 50	F, U/S
Tripter X1 (Direx)	Ellipsoid reflector	700–900	13.5	10 × 34	F
MPL-9000 (Dornier)	Ellipsoid reflector	1300	14	3 × 20	U/S
Multimed 2001 (ELMED)	Ellipsoid reflector	1200	13.5	7.5 × 22	F, U/S
Sonolith Praktis (EDAP Technomed)	Ellipsoid reflector	1300	14	12 × 23	F, U/S
LithoTron (Healthtronics)	Ellipsoid reflector	530	15	8 × 38	F
Lithocut C3000S (Comair)	Ellipsoid reflector	1200	13	3.5 × 12	F
Econolith (Medispec)	Ellipsoid reflector	726	13.5	13 × 60	F
MPL 5000 (Dornier)	Ellipsoid reflector	1000	13	10 × 40	F
Electromagnetic lithotriptors					
Lithostar (Siemens)	Acoustic lens	380	11.3	11 × 90	F
Lithostar Modularis (Siemens)	Acoustic lens	500	12	8 × 100	F
Modulith (Storz)	Parabolic reflector	1056	16.5	3 × 37	F, U/S
Piezoelectric lithotriptors					
Piezolith 2300 (Wolf)	Concave dish	1200	12	3 × 11	U/S
Piezolith 2500 (Wolf)	Concave dish	1500	15	3 × 11	F, U/S
LT.01 (EDAP Technomed)	Spherical dish	1144	14	5 × 23	U/S
LT.02 (EDAP Technomed)	Spherical dish	1400	15.5	1.8 × 29	F, U/S

F: fluoroscopy; U/S: ultrasound.

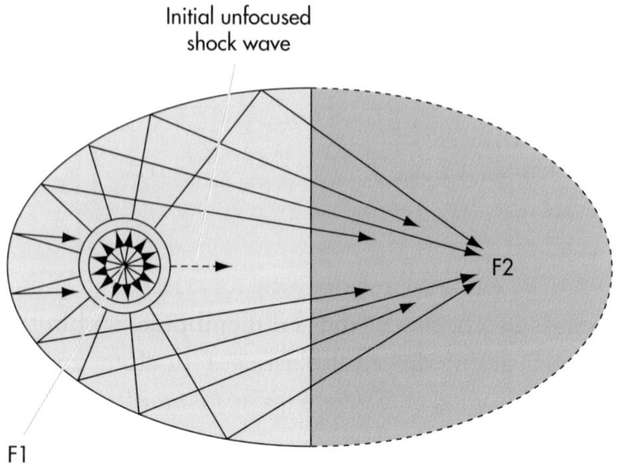

Figure 31.8 *Spark-gap lithotriptor. A spark, generated at F1, causes a hydrodynamic pressure wave that is focused at a set distance to the target area (F2) by an ellipsoid reflector.*

Electromagnetic lithotriptors require the application of an electric current to a coil. This generates a strong magnetic field that repels and thrusts a metallic disc upwards to strike a fixed metallic plate, thus generating an acoustic shock wave (Figure 31.9). The shock waves are focused either by an acoustic lens

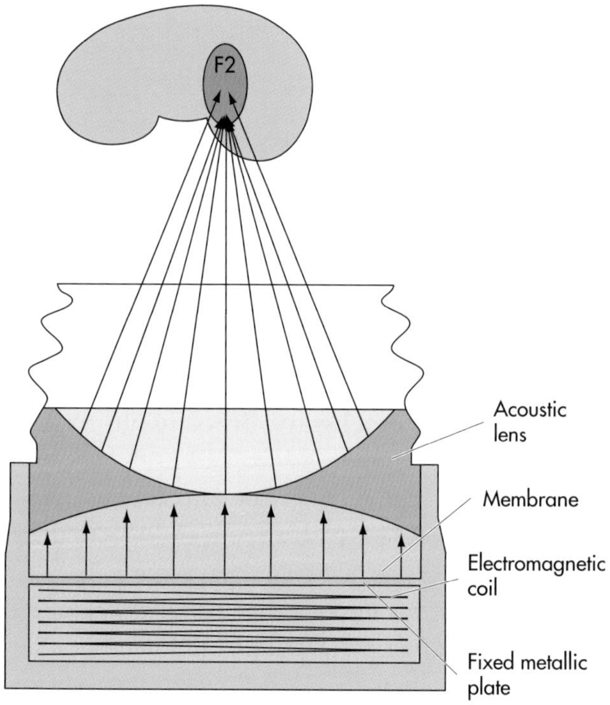

Figure 31.9 *Electromagnetic coil and metallic disc. Application of an electric current to the coil results in a strong magnetic field that repels a metallic disc upwards to strike a fixed metallic plate. Shock waves are focused by an acoustic lens or parabolic reflector.*

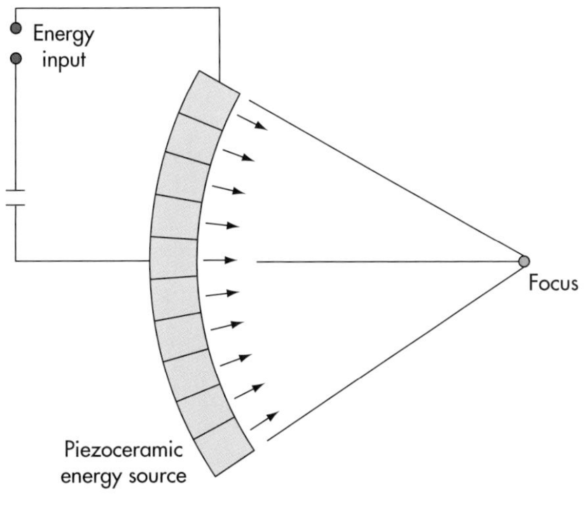

Figure 31.10 *Piezoceramic lithotriptor. Application of an electric current to piezoceramic crystals causes a sudden conformational change, resulting in the generation of an acoustic shock wave.*

(such as the Siemens Lithostar) or by a parabolic reflector (such as the Storz Modulith). Electromagnetic shock wave sources can deliver several hundred thousand shock waves before servicing, in contrast to spark-gap machines. Piezoceramic lithotriptors have a number of piezoceramic crystals aligned on a fixed metallic concave surface (Figure 31.10). The application of simultaneous high-voltage electrical current to the piezoceramic crystals causes a sudden conformational change that generates an acoustic shock wave. As a result of the focusing mechanism, piezoceramic lithotriptors produce shock waves with a very high peak pressure at F2 but also with small focal points. This type of lithotriptor is said to be safe for use in patients with pacemakers.

Imaging is an essential component of lithotriptor machines, and all use ultrasound, fluoroscopy or both. Advantages of ultrasound include the imaging of radiolucent stones (including biliary calculi), real-time imaging and minimization of radiation exposure. Piezoceramic lithotriptors require ultrasound, as continuous monitoring is required for accuracy, given the small focal point of this type of machine. Two types of ultrasound imaging exist: the coaxial unit is aligned with the shock-wave generator and the articulating arm or lateral unit, with a mobile transducer. However, ultrasound imaging in obese patients is suboptimal, and visualization of ureteric stones is more difficult than with fluoroscopy.

Application of ESWL

As is the case with other forms of acoustic energy, coupling is required from the point of shock-wave generation (F1) to the target area (F2). This is achieved by using degassed water within the apparatus (or by submerging the patient in a water bath, as with the Dornier HM-3) and the application of a coupling gel between the patient and the machine. Body tissue, which is 75% water, has acoustical impedance similar to that of water. The focal length of the acoustic shock wave is known as the F2 distance and varies between machines (Table 31.5). This is important, as an exponential decline in energy is observed such that if the F2 point is 2 cm away from the stone, only 20% of power is delivered. Calculi composed of cysteine, calcium oxalate monohydrate and calcium phosphate are very hard and are known to be resistant to fragmentation. In order to prevent cardiac arrhythmia, shock waves are discharged in the refractory period of the cardiac cycle, usually 20 ms after the QRS complex.

ESWL is well described in the fragmentation of urinary calculi, but its effect on both benign and malignant tissue has also been studied. The effects of ESWL on in vitro and in vivo tumour cell lines,[35–37] and, in particular, whether enhancement of chemotherapeutic effect occurs on ESWL-treated tissue, have been the subject of much study.[38,39] ESWL has been shown to cause cellular damage regardless of the cell's doubling time. The mitochondria are most sensitive to its effect,[39] although damage also occurs at the cell membrane, within the nucleus, along the endoplasmic reticulum and in other cell organelles (such as lysosomes). Cellular damage may be mechanical or due to the generation of free radicals[40,41] caused by homolytic cleavage of the molecule within the collapsing bubble.[42] Extracorporeal shock-wave techniques have recently been described in the treatment of Peyronie's plaques[43] and are being investigated in the treatment of malunion of bone fractures. There is evidence that patients with impaired renal function treated with ESWL may experience late-onset hypertension and worsening of renal function,[44] and this is the subject of an ongoing Food and Drug Administration (FDA)-sponsored multicentre study.

High intensity focused ultrasound (HIFU)

HIFU was first developed in the 1940s[45] and is a potential energy modality for non-invasive thermotherapy of lesions located within the body. An ultrasound source is focused at a selected depth within the body to deliver an area of high energy density in which predictable and sharply demarcated areas of tissue can be destroyed while preserving the overlying and surrounding tissue. Initial clinical studies were performed within the cranium.[46] This energy source is derived from a piezoceramic transducer, which rapidly changes its physical configuration in response to an applied electrical potential. This sudden change results in the generation of an acoustic ultrasonic wave where the frequency is directly proportional to the voltage applied. The frequencies used in HIFU therapy are in the range 0.5–10 MHz,[47,48] and the power density at the target area ranges from 750 to 4500 W/cm^2. Temperatures of 80–100°C are generated in the focal zone in a short exposure of 1–10 s. The size and shape of the lesions are dependent on the power density and the area and duration of exposure. In addition to the thermal effect, there is an additional pressure-related effect where a cavitation phenomenon occurs (see section above on ESWL). Intracellular water is forced into gas, creating bubbles within the tissue, and these bubbles collapse, causing coagulative necrosis and cavitation. The acoustic wave is focused either with a concave transducer or by placing a lens in front of the transducer. As with other forms of acoustic energy, the energy pathway must exclude air to avoid dispersion of energy and damage to normal tissues, a process known as coupling.

Although HIFU has not yet been widely accepted in clinical practice, there remain two types of HIFU devices – transrectal and extracorporeal. Extracorporeal HIFU has been extensively used in the treatment of glaucoma,[49] but its use in urology has so far been limited. Several different ultrasonic sources have been described in different animal models. With a 1.69-MHz transducer, the target areas at a depth of 40 mm of 13/18 porcine kidneys were successfully ablated.[50] Other authors have reported success with other frequencies, resulting in different target power densities. A 1.65-MHz transducer delivered a target power density of 4200 W/cm^2 in a canine model,[51] and 1-MHz and 2.25-MHz transducers delivered target power densities of 2750 and 3200 W/cm^2 respectively.[52]

Transrectal HIFU has been used in a clinical setting in the treatment of benign prostatic enlargement and localized prostate cancer. Transrectal probes may incorporate two transducers, for example, Ablatherm™, Technomed, France, uses a 7.5-MHz transducer for imaging and a 2.25-MHz transducer for energy delivery. This system has a focal length of 3.5 cm with target power densities ranging from 700 to 2200 W/cm^2. Alternatively, the same transducer may be used for imaging and therapy; for example, Sonablate™, Focal Surgery Inc., USA, uses the same 4-MHz transducer. Air-free coupling is achieved by covering the probe with a degassed, water-filled condom after insertion into the rectum. The focal length is dependent on the crystal used and the concavity of the transducer or power of the lens, whichever is deployed. Prostate ablation is performed by sequentially moving the target area, thus creating multiple lesions. Histological analysis in a canine model consistently showed intraprostatic coagulative necrosis.[53] However, long-term data in the treatment of BPH suggest that this therapy is not durable, with up to 43% of patients requiring a TURP within 4 years.[54] Its use in the treatment of localized prostate cancer is too unreliable at present, with several studies showing residual disease following HIFU therapy.[55,56] However, there may be additional benefits, as HIFU primarily induces an influx of CD4$^+$ peripheral cells, and tumour growth after a second tumour challenge in previously HIFU-cured animals was significantly reduced.[57]

Ultrasound probes

The ultrasound probe used to fragment calculi consists of an ultrasound energy source coupled to a long metal probe (Figure 31.11). The application of about 100 W to the piezoceramic elements results in oscillation at a frequency of 23–27 MHz.[58] The probe oscillates in both a transverse and longitudinal direction with a displacement of 20 μm. At displacements of >50 μm, soft-tissue disintegration occurs, and such machines may be useful in renal sparing

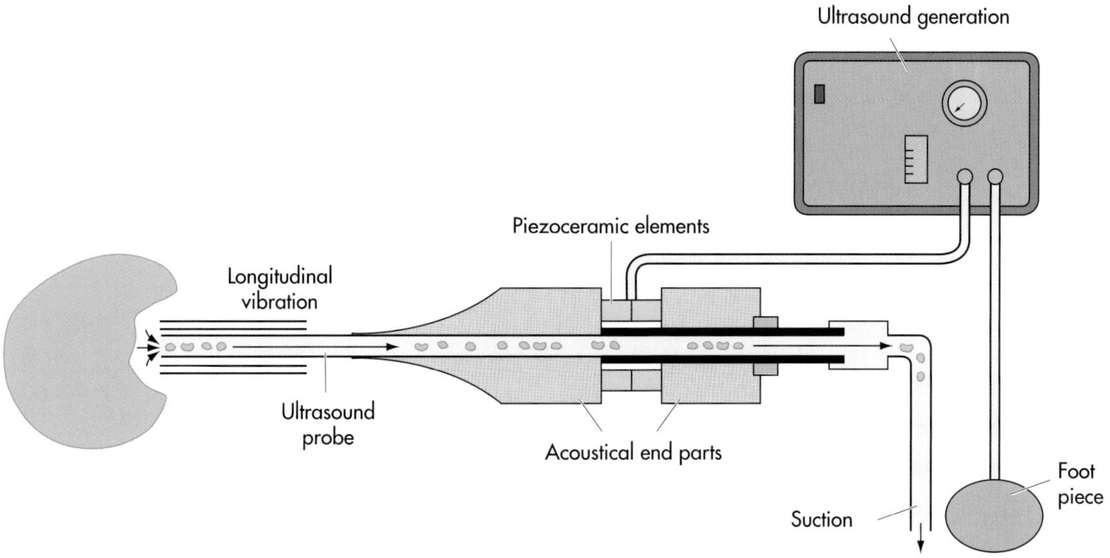

Figure 31.11 *Ultrasound probe. Piezoceramic elements oscillate, causing longitudinal and transverse vibration of the probe.*

surgery. Heat is generated at the point of stone disintegration, and therefore irrigation is required for cooling. This heat can reach temperatures of >50°C; therefore, ultrasound contact lithotripsy is unsuitable for use in the ureter, although its direct effects on tissue are minimal. The metal probe is usually hollow to allow suction of irrigant and small stone fragments. Some hard stones are resistant to ultrasound lithotripsy, but it appears particularly useful for soft stones that are difficult to treat with mechanical intracorporeal lithotripters. The Harmonic Scalpel™ is a device consisting of an ultrasonic source that causes vibration of forceps or a blade. Typically, the displacement is 50–80 μm, and the vibrational frequency approaches 55 500 Hz.[59] This results in predominantly thermal energy generation, with tissue temperatures of about 60°C and a depth of penetration of 1–2 mm. Originally, vessels of >500 μm were skeletonized, but newer machines cause coagulation of vessels up to 3 mm, resulting in relatively bloodless cutting of tissue.

MECHANICAL ENERGY

The number of medical devices that utilize this type of energy source is limited. However, one of the most widely available is the user-friendly Swiss Lithoclast™.

Mechanical lithotripsy

The Swiss Lithoclast™ was developed by the departments of medical electronics and urology at the University Teaching Hospital in Lausanne, Switzerland.[60] The device utilizes compressed air, derived from the operating theatre supply.[61,62] This pressure, in the range 3–5 bar, is delivered in a pneumatic blast of short duration to the inside of a hollow metal cylinder. This causes a metal projectile to be rapidly fired to the opposite end of the cylinder, where it collides and transfers kinetic energy to a metal probe (Figure 31.12).[63] The distal end of the probe is in direct contact with the stone. Transference of kinetic energy from probe to stone causes highly effective fragmentation. Analogy has been made with the jackhammer used to fragment parts of the pavement during road construction. The device is simple, cheap and very effective. One major problem is the propulsion effect upon stones, which is much more marked with this form of energy than with laser lithotripsy. Most stones are amenable to fragmentation, and recently a semiflexible probe has

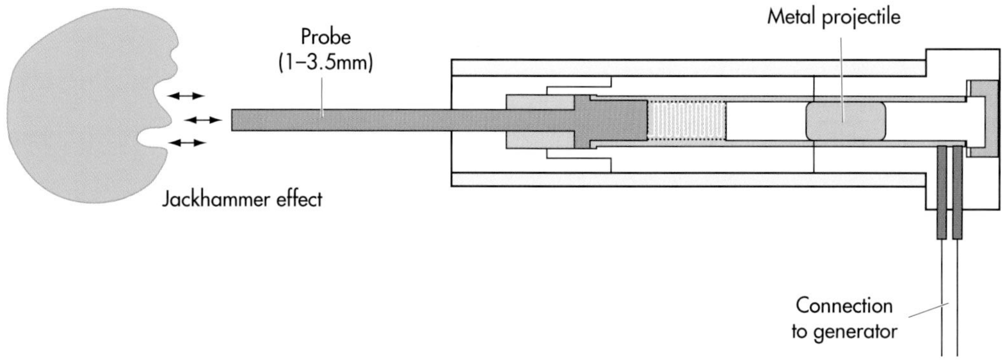

Figure 31.12 *Mechanical lithotripsy. A compressed-air jet propels the metal projectile to strike the base of the probe (pneumatic lithotripsy). An electromagnetic field may be substituted for compressed air (electrokinetic lithotripsy).*

been introduced which may allow limited use via a flexible ureterorenoscope. Similar devices are being developed that use electromagnetic propulsion systems instead of compressed air.[63]

Water-jet scalpel

In this form of mechanical energy, tissue may be separated or cut by the application of a fine water-based jet under high pressure. The apparatus consists of a pump, generating pressures of 10–50 kg/cm^2, connected to a flexible hose with an adjustable pinhole aperture of 0.3 mm.[64] The jet velocity is in the range 0–43 ml/min. Tissue effects are dependent on the pressure and nozzle size selected. A jet of low intensity separates structures, but at higher pressures, parenchymal tissue is selectively cut without damage to vascular or nervous structures. When directed at blood vessels of >200 μm within tissue, the jet temporarily compresses the vessel and flows around and eliminates tissue behind it.[65] This results in skeletonization of vascular structures and therefore allows improved haemostasis with diathermy or suturing. In clinical practice, normal saline is usually substituted for water and, like the Harmonic Scalpel™, this device is an attractive tool for use in nephron-sparing surgery.[66,67]

REFERENCES

1. Issa MM. Transurethral needle ablation of the prostate: report of initial United States clinical trial. J Urol 1996; 157: 413–419
2. Perachina M, Bozzo W, Puppo P, Vitali A et al. Does transurethral thermotherapy induce a long-term alpha blockade? An immunohistochemical study. Eur Urol 1993; 23: 299–301
3. Issa MM, Wojno KJ, Oesterling JE, Pilat MJ et al. Histopathologic and biochemical study of the prostate following transurethral needle ablation (TUNA): insights to the mechanism of improvement in BPH symptoms. J Endourol 1996; 10: 109
4. Schulman CC, Zlotta AR. Possible mechanism of action of transurethral needle ablation of the prostate on benign prostatic hyperplasia: a neurohistochemical study. J Urol 1997; 157: 894–899
5. Schatzl G, Madersbacher S, Djavan B, Lang T et al. Two-year results of transurethral resection of the prostate versus four 'less invasive' treatment options. Eur Urol 2000; 37: 695–701
6. Mendecki J, Friedenthal E, Bostein C et al. Microwave applicators for localized hyperthermia treatment of cancer of the prostate. Int J Radiat Oncol Biol Phys 1980; 6: 1583–1589
7. Yerushalmi A, Fishelovitz Y, Singer D et al. Localized deep microwave hyperthermia in the treatment of poor operative risk patients with benign prostatic hyperplasia. J Urol 1985; 133: 873–876
8. Le Duc A. Microwave and RF wave heat therapy. In: Marberger M ed. Application of Newer Forms of Therapeutic Energy in Urology. Oxford: Isis Medical Media, 1995: 87–97

9. Carter S, Ogden C. Intraprostatic temperature v. clinical outcome in TUMT: is the response heat-dose dependent? J Urol 1994; 151: 756A
10. De la Rosette JJ, De Wildt MJ, Alvizatos G et al. Transurethral microwave thermotherapy in benign prostatic hyperplasia: placebo versus TUMT. Urology 1994; 44: 58–63
11. Ahmed M, Bell T, Lawrence WT, Ward JP et al. Transurethral microwave thermotherapy (Prostatron version 2.5) compared with transurethral resection of the prostate for the treatment of benign prostatic hyperplasia: a randomized, controlled, parallel study. Br J Urol 1997; 79: 181–185
12. Hallin A, Berlin T. Transurethral microwave thermotherapy for benign prostatic hyperplasia: clinical outcome after 4 years. J Urol 1998; 159: 459–464
13. Lau KO, Li MK, Foo KT. Long-term follow-up of transurethral microwave thermotherapy. Urology 1998; 52: 829–833
14. Nawrocki JD, Bell TJ, Lawrence WT, Ward JP. A randomized controlled trial of transurethral microwave thermotherapy. Br J Urol 1997; 79: 389–393
15. Maiman T. Stimulated optical radiation in ruby. Nature 1960; 187: 493–494
16. Javan A, Bennet Jr W, Herriott D. Population inversion and continuous optical laser oscillation in a gas discharge containing a He-Ne mixture. Phys Rev Letters 1961; 6: 106–110
17. Geusic J, Marcos H, Van Uitert L. Laser oscillation in Nd-doped yttrium aluminium, yttrium gallium and gadolinium garnets. Appl Phys Lett 1964; 4: 182–184
18. Patel C. Continuous-wave laser action on vibrational-rotational transmissions of CO_2. Phys Rev 1964; 136A: 1187
19. Boulnois JL. Photophysical processes in recent medical laser developments: a review. Lasers Med Sci 1985; 1: 47–66
20. Anderson R, Levins C, Grevelink J. Lasers in dermatology. In: Fitzpatrick T, Eisen A, Wolff K, Freedberg I et al, eds, Dermatology in General Medicine. McGraw-Hill, 1993: 1755–1766
21. Dretler SP. Laser lithotripsy: a review of 20 years of research and clinical applications. Lasers Surg Med 1998; 8: 341–356
22. Shanberg A, Tansey L, Baghdassarian R, Sawyer D et al. Laser-assisted vasectomy reversal: experience in 32 patients. J Urol 1990; 143: 528–529
23. Anson KM, Nawrocki JD, Buckley J et al. A multicentre, randomised, prospective study of endoscopic laser ablation versus transurethral resection of the prostate. Urology 1995; 46: 305–310
24. Pow-Sang M, Cowan D, Orihuela E et al. Thermocoagulation effect of diode laser radiation in the human prostate: acute and chronic study. Urology 1995; 45: 790–794
25. Judy M, Matthews J, Aronoff B, Hults D. Soft tissue studies with 805 nm diode laser radiation: thermal effects with contact tips and comparison with effects of 1064 nm Nd:YAG laser radiation. Lasers Surg Med 1993; 13: 528–536
26. Gholdoian CG, Thayer K, Hald D, Rajpoot D, Shanberg AM. Applications of the KTP laser in the treatment of posterior urethral valves, ureteroceles and urethral strictures in the pediatric patient. J Clin Laser Med Surg 1998; 16: 39–43
27. Zorcher T, Hochberger J, Schrott KM, Kuhn R et al. In vitro study concerning the efficiency of the frequency-doubled double-pulse neodymium:YAG laser (FREDDY) for lithotripsy of calculi in the urinary tract. Laser Surg Med 1999; 25: 38–42
28. Dushinski JW, Lingeman JE. Urologic applications of the holmium laser. Tech Urol 1997; 3: 60–64
29. Coleman AJ, Saunders JE. A survey of the acoustic output of commercial extracorporeal shock wave lithotriptors. Ultrasound Med Biol 1989; 15: 213–227
30. Crum LA. The tensile strength of water. Nature 1979; 278: 148
31. Crum LA. Cavitation microjets as a contributory mechanism for renal calculi disintegration in shock wave. J Urol 1988; 140: 1587–1590
32. Coleman AJ, Saunders JE. Comparison of extracorporeal shock wave lithotriptors. In: Copcoat MJ, Miller RA, Wickham JE, eds. Lithotripsy II. London: BDI Publishing, 1987
33. Chaussy C, Brendel W, Schmiedt E. Extracorporeally induced destruction of kidney stones by shock waves. Lancet 1980; 2: 1265–1268
34. Cathignol D, Mestas JL, Gomez F et al. Influence of water conductivity on the efficiency and the reproducability of electrohydraulic shock wave generation. Ultrasound Med Biol 1991; 17: 819
35. Russo P, Stephenson RA, Mies C et al. High energy shock waves suppress tumor growth in vitro and in vivo. J Urol 1986; 135: 626–628
36. Randazzo RF, Chaussy CG, Fuchs GJ et al. The in vitro and in vivo effects of extracorporeal shock waves on malignant cells. Urol Res 1988; 16: 419–426
37. Kohri K, Uemura T, Iguchi M et al. Effect of high energy shock waves on tumor cells. Urol Res 1990; 18: 101–105

38. Berens ME, Welander CE, Griffen AS et al. Effect of acoustic shock waves on clonogenic growth and drug sensitivity of human tumour cells in vitro. J Urol 1989; 142: 1090–1094
39. Clayman RV, Long S, Marcus M. High-energy shock waves: in vitro effects. Am J Kidney Dis 1991; 17: 436–444
40. Morgan TR, Laudone VP, Heston WD. Free radical production by high energy shock waves – compaction with ionising radiation. J Urol 1988; 139: 186–189
41. Suhr D, Bruemmer F, Huelser DF. Cavitation-generated free radicals during shock wave exposure: investigations with cell-free solutions and suspended cells. Ultrasound Med Biol 1991; 17: 761–768
42. Kuwahara M. Tissue injuries during extracorporeal shock wave lithotripsy from the standpoint of physics and experimental pathophysiology. Jpn J Endourol ESWL 1993; 6: 5–21
43. Abdel-Salam Y, Budair Z, Renner C et al. Treatment of Peyronie's disease by extracorporeal shockwave therapy: evaluation of our preliminary results. J Endourol 1999; 13: 549–552
44. Bataille P, Cardon G, Bouzernidj M et al. Renal and hypertensive complications of extracorporeal shock wave lithotripsy: who is at risk? Urol Int 1999; 62: 195–200
45. Lynn GR, Zwemer RL, Chick AJ, Miller AF. A new method for the generation and use of focused ultrasound in experimental biology. J Gen Physiol 1942; 26: 115–136
46. Fry WJ, Barnard JW, Fry FJ et al. Ultrasonic lesions in the mammalian central nervous system. Science 1955; 122: 517–518
47. Fry FJ. Intense focused ultrasound in medicine. Eur Urol 1993; 23: 2–7
48. ter Haar GR. Focused ultrasound therapy. Curr Opin Urol 1994; 4: 89–92
49. Silvermann RH, Vogelsang B, Rondeau MJ, Coleman DJ. Therapeutic ultrasound for the treatment of glaucoma. Am J Ophthalmol 1991; 111: 327–337
50. Watkin NA, Morris SB, Rivens IH, ter Haar GR. High-intensity focused ultrasound ablation of the kidney in a large animal model. J Endourol 1997; 11: 191–196
51. Ioritani N, Sirai S, Taguchi et al. Effects of high intensity ultrasound heating on the normal and cancer tissue. Jap J Endourol ESWL 1994; 7: 299
52. Chapelon JY, Margonari J, Theillere Y et al. Effects of high-energy focussed ultrasound on kidney tissue in the rat and the dog. Eur Urol 1992; 22: 147–152
53. Foster RS, Bihrle R, Sanghvi NT et al. Production of prostatic lesions in canines using transrectally administered high intensity focused ultrasound. Eur Urol 1993; 23: 330–336
54. Madersbacher S, Schatzl G, Djavan B, Stulnig T et al. Long-term outcome of transrectal high-intensity focused ultrasound therapy for benign prostatic hyperplasia. Eur Urol 2000; 37: 687–694
55. Beerlage HP, van Leenders GJ, Oosterhof GO et al. High-intensity focused ultrasound (HIFU) followed after one to two weeks by radical retropubic prostatectomy: results of a prospective study. Prostate 1999; 39: 41–46
56. Chaussy CG, Thuroff S. High-intensive focused ultrasound in localized prostate cancer. J Endourol 2000; 14: 293–299
57. Yang R, Reilly CR, Rescorla FJ et al. Effects of high-intensity focused ultrasound in the treatment of experimental neuroblastoma. J Pediatr Surg 1992; 27: 246–251
58. Marberger M. Disintegration of renal and ureteral calculi with ultrasound. Urol Clin North Am 1983; 10: 729–742
59. Lee SJ, Park KH. Ultrasonic energy in endoscopic surgery. Yonsei Med J 1999; 40: 545–549
60. Lanquetin JM, Jichlinski P, Favre R, von Niederhausern W. The Swiss Lithoclast. J Urol 1990; 143: 179A
61. Denstedt JD, Eberwein PM, Singh RR. The Swiss Lithoclast: a new device for intracorporeal lithotripsy. J Urol 1992; 148: 1088–1090
62. Schulze H, Haupt G, Piergiovanni M et al. The Swiss Lithoclast: a new device for endoscopic stone disintegration. J Urol 1993; 149:15–18
63. Vorreuther R, Klotz T, Heidenreich A, Nayal W et al. Pneumatic v electrokinetic lithotripsy in the treatment of ureteral stones. J Endourol 1998; 12: 233–236
64. Penchev RD, Losanoff JE, Kjossev KT. Reconstructive renal surgery using a water jet. J Urol 1999; 162: 772–774
65. Higashihara E. Mechanical energy in urology for non-lithiasis treatment. In Marberger M, ed. Application of Newer Forms of Therapeutic Energy in Urology. Oxford: Isis Medical Media, 1995: 1–13
66. Tomita Y, Koike H, Takahashi K, Tamaki M et al. Use of the harmonic scalpel for nephron sparing surgery in renal cell carcinoma. J Urol 1998; 159: 2063–2064
67. Shekarriz H, Shekarriz B, Upadhyay J et al. Hydro-jet assisted laparoscopic partial nephrectomy: initial experience in a porcine model. J Urol 2000; 163: 1005–1008

32

Urological instrumentation

Hugh N Whitfield and Suresh K Gupta

Although open surgery still plays a significant and important role in urological practice, there is an ever-increasing emphasis on endoscopic techniques in both diagnosis and therapy. Urologists need to understand the workings of the instruments that they use in order to realize fully the potential and the limitations of the sophisticated technology that is available. An historical perspective is invaluable in the appreciation of what exists today.

HISTORY OF UROLOGICAL ENDOSCOPES

Those with innovative and inquisitive minds have, for centuries, searched for ways of exploring the workings of the human body. Hippocrates (460–377 BC) has been credited with designing a speculum that could be used to examine the rectum. A three-bladed vaginal speculum was found in the ruins of Pompeii.[1] After such early attempts, there was an interval of many centuries until significant advances were made. Gynaecologists have played a prominent role in the development of endoscopy to the benefit of many other medical and industrial fields. At the beginning of the nineteenth century, Philip Bozzini (1773–1809) designed an elongated funnel in different sizes with which to inspect various orifices. The problem that faced all endoscope designers was how to provide illumination at the site being inspected. Bozzini used a candle. A Viennese instrument maker, Nitze (1848–1906), used a heated platinum wire with a water-cooling system. A much improved light source became available, thanks to the invention of the incandescent light bulb by Thomas Edison (1847–1931). Small, battery-driven light bulbs, mounted at the end of the endoscope, were used for many years. These were unreliable and provided only a low level of light intensity. The range of procedures that could be performed safely and effectively was correspondingly limited.

There are many who deserve to be given some credit for the evolution of endoscopy (Table 32.1), and more details can be read in a recent comprehensive review by Shah.[2] The one name that stands out above all others, the man who was responsible for the revolution that occurred in endoscopy, is that of Harold Hopkins (1918–1994). He was an optical physicist in Reading, England. Apart from designing the zoom lens for cameras, he set about reconfiguring

Table 32.1 The names of some of those who had a significant role in the development of urological endoscopy.

Date	Name	Country
1806	Philip Bozzini	Italy
1826	Pierre Segalas	France
1827	John Fisher	USA
1853	Antonin Desormeaux	France
1865	Francis Cruise	Britain
1866	Maximillian Nitze	Germany
1880	Thomas Edison	Britain
1883	David Newman	Britain
1889	Boisseau du Rocher	France
1960	Harold Hopkins	Britain

Table 32.2 The names of some of those who worked with Harold Hopkins in the development of endoscopic imaging.

Name	Speciality	Country
Hugh Gainsborough	Gastroenterologist	Britain
H.S. Kapani	Physicist	Britain
Basil Hirschowitz	Gastroenterologist	South Africa
William Peters	Physicist	USA
Jim Gow	Urologist	Britain
Karl Storz	Instrument manufacturer	Germany

the basic telescope that was in use. He also pioneered the use of fibre-optic technology. He was working with others (Table 32.2), but it would be disingenuous to suggest that he was anything other than the prime mover. Hopkins was an amusing and a modest man, who made relatively little personal gain from his inventions. He teamed up with Karl Storz, an instrument maker from Tuttlingen in southern Germany, and, in 1967, the first Storz–Hopkins instrument was introduced.

Telescope design

The original telescopes that were used from the end of the nineteenth century until the 1970s consisted of long, thin tubes in which lenses were fixed at intervals. The lenses were separated by spacers, and there were air gaps between the lenses (Figure 32.1).

The quality of the image depended on the accurate grinding of the lenses, not a simple task, but without which the image quality easily became degraded. To overcome these problems, Hopkins used a solid rod within the telescope which could be ground much more accurately and reliably and fixed within the telescope more easily. The interspersing air gaps were, in effect, the lenses (Figure 32.2). Definition was improved still further by a double layer of antireflective coating at each end of the rod. The result was that the amount of light at the eyepiece was increased by a factor of 80. This was more than adequate not only for endoscopy but also for endoscopic photography.

Contemporary telescope design

The optical performance of a lens or optical system is affected both by its design and by the quality of its manufacture. The measurement of optical performance is necessary to permit the relative assessment of different designs, and to measure how well a manufactured lens or system meets the theoretical design performance.

The overall optical performance of an optical instrument has been traditionally assessed subjectively by measuring the resolving power or resolution of the instrument. The fine detail normally takes the form of a pattern of closely spaced, uniform, black-and-white bars, called a resolution test pattern. The observer determines the spacing of the finest black-and-white bars when the individual bars

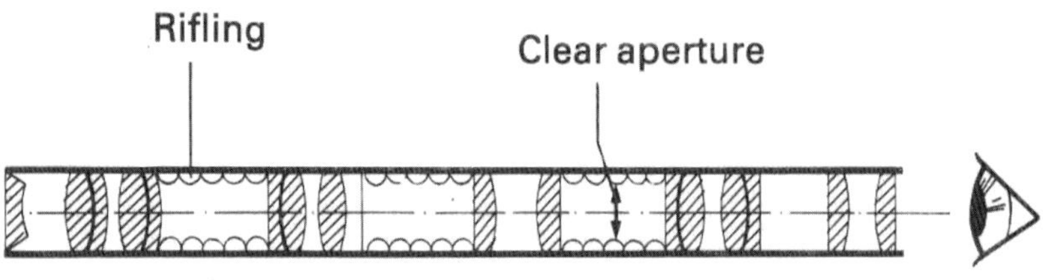

Figure 32.1 *The original design of the telescope used for cystoscopy, with a series of lenses mounted within the telescope with long interspersing air gaps. (Reproduced with permission from Vale J. In: Fundamentals of endoscopic design. Whitfield HN, ed. Genitourinary Surgery. 4th edn. Vol. 3. Rob and Smith Operative Surgery Series. London: Butterworth-Heinemann, 1994).*

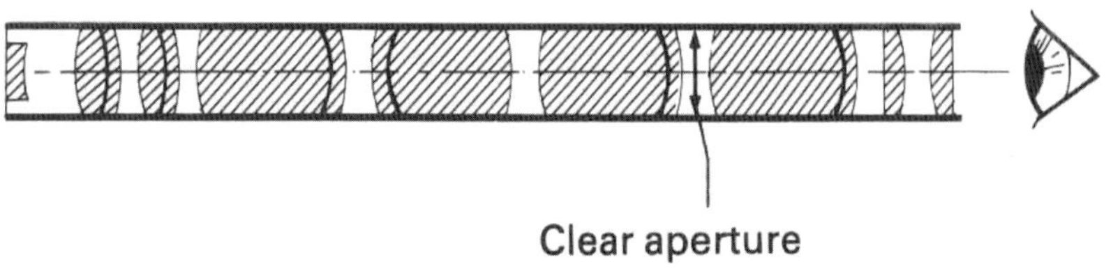

Figure 32.2 *The Hopkins rod lens system. (Reproduced with permission from Vale J, Fundamentals of endoscope design. In: HN Whitfield ed. Genitourinary Surgery, 4th edn., Vol. 3. Rob and Smith Operative Surgery Series. London: Butterworth-Heinemann, 1994).*

can still be seen clearly. Such a measurement depends on the acuity and judgement of the observer. However, experience has shown that results are seldom reproducible, either between different observers, or indeed when made by one observer at different times. After several hours of testing optical instruments, observers tire, and visual abilities may deteriorate.

In recent years, there has been a move away from this subjective method of assessing optical performance to objective methods in which electro-optic techniques are used. The techniques commonly in use include measurement of line-spread function and point-spread function and also optical transfer function.

The basic principle of optical transfer function (OTF) testing is to set up a sinusoidal test pattern (that is, a bar pattern having a sinusoidal variation between the light and dark bars) and to use the lens or optical system under test to form an image of the test pattern. The pitch or spatial frequency of the test pattern is then varied, and a measure is made of the change of contrast in the image, and also of any phase shift in the image, as a result of the change of spatial frequency of the object. The spatial frequency is the reciprocal of the wavelength of the test pattern, and is normally expressed in terms of cycles/mm.

The OTF consists of two components, the modulation transfer function (MTF), and the phase transfer function (PTF). The former is a measure of the reduction in contrast from an object to its image; the latter is the corresponding lateral shift of the image.

Starting off with a test pattern consisting of bars varying sinusoidally between perfect black and full white (that is, with 100% contrast), the image of that pattern formed by an optical system will also have a sinusoidal intensity variation, but will be affected by diffraction and aberration effects inherent in the design of the optical system, and by imperfections caused by manufacturing tolerances. Some of the light will be scattered and deflected to that part of the image which ought, in a diffraction-free system, to be perfectly black. In the image, the white is very slightly dimmed, and the black is very slightly illuminated. The contrast of the image will be less than 100%. The ratio of these two contrasts, that of the image and that of the object, is the MTF of the optical system at one particular spatial frequency. This loss of image contrast generally becomes greater at higher spatial frequencies.

Consider an optical system forming an image of a sinusoidal pattern of a particular spatial frequency. The modulation transfer factor of the optical system at that spatial frequency is defined as the ratio of the image to object contrast (or modulation). The contrast (or modulation) is given by:

$$\text{contrast} = \frac{I_p - I_t}{I_p + I_t}$$

where I_p is the intensity of the peak of the sinusoid and I_t is the intensity of the trough of the sinusoid.

The MTF curve is a plot of the modulation transfer factor against spatial frequency, and gives the relationship between MTF and spatial frequency. MTF is normalized to unity at zero spatial frequency, and the curve tends to drop at higher spatial frequencies.

The PTF is the measure of positional variation between object and image, as this varies with spatial frequency. The units used are units of phase shift, usually degrees, and 360° corresponds to a shift of one complete cycle of the sinusoid. PTF is normalised to zero at zero spatial frequency. PTF is a little-used component of the OTF. It is rarely, if ever, quoted in performance specifications for lenses or optical systems.

Fibre-optic technology

While redeveloping the optical system for cystoscopes, Hopkins was also investigating how to provide reliable, high-intensity illumination. Some years earlier, he had been working with fibre-optic technology, stimulated by a gastroenterologist called Hugh Gainsborough from London to improve the gastroscope that was in use at that time. In 1954 two groups, led respectively by van Heal from the Netherlands and Hopkins and Kapani from the UK, described how images could be transmitted down a bundle of transparent fibres.[3]

The transmission of images and light through a fibre-optic cable depends on the propagation of light

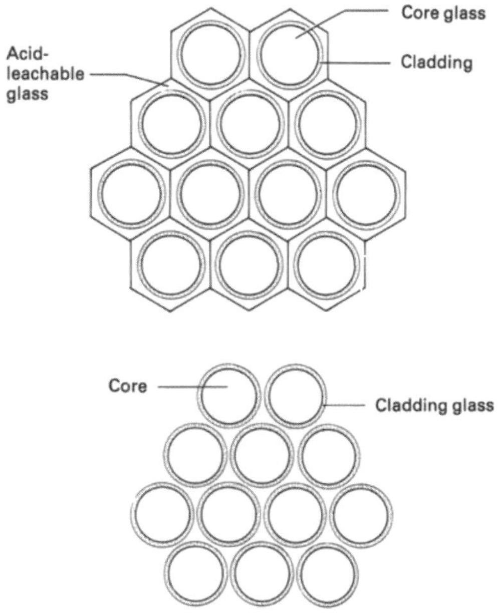

Figure 32.3 *A diagrammatic representation of the acid-leachable technique of making a coherent fibre bundle. (Reproduced with permission from Vale J, Fundamentals of endoscope design. In: Whitfield HN, Genitourinary Surgery, 4th edn., Vol. 3. Rob and Smith Operative Surgery Series. London: Butterworth-Heinemann, 1994).*

along thin fibres made from a transparent material that has been coated with another transparent material with a lower refractive index. The light then undergoes *multiple total internal reflection* (MTIR).

The problem of retaining the orientation of the fibres to one another has been solved in two ways, the leaching method and the rotating-drum technique. In the leaching method, glass fibres made from high-quality optical glass are coated with glass of a different refractive index. These fibres are then covered with another layer of glass that can be dissolved in acid – it is 'acid-leachable'. These rods are then accurately aligned in a cylinder of acid-leachable glass, heated in a furnace and drawn out to create fibres with a diameter of 8–10 μm and still retain their orientation with each other, as a *coherent* bundle. Both ends of the bundle are fixed, and the acid-leachable glass is then dissolved to leave a flexible fibre-optic bundle (Figure 32.3). The alternative way to produce a *coherent* fibre bundle is to wind a single, very long fibre around a drum. The fibres are then clamped together at one place and accurately divided; subsequently, both ends are polished (Figure 32.4).

The production of a fibre-optic bundle for the transmission of light rather than an image is technically much simpler and cheaper, since the fibres do not have to retain their orientation with each other – this is an *incoherent* bundle.

Instrument design

Lower urinary tract

The earliest cystoscopes consisted basically of just a telescope. Later, a sheath was added, so that instruments could be used in conjunction with the endoscopy; in 1889, Boisseau du Rocher described a sheath through which both the telescope and instruments could be passed. Water was used for irrigation, although the use of air was also described. A mechanism for catheter deflection was introduced by Joachim Albarran in 1896, and the device that bears his name is still in use. At the beginning of the twentieth century, electrocautery was described by several people, and this enabled urologists to treat bladder tumours endoscopically.

When urologists first started to perform endoscopic surgery on the prostate, they were reliant for vision on battery-driven bulbs mounted at the end of the telescope; it reflects well on earlier generations of urologists that they were able to perform any endoscopic surgery on the prostate, given the limitations imposed on them by the available technology. Hugh Young described a cold-punch technique for the removal of obstructing prostatic tissue. The first resectoscope that incorporated electoresection is attributed to Maximillian Stern (1877–1946), but it was Joseph McCarthy who popularized a design that incorporated a lever to move the resectoscope loop. This was widely adopted and forms the basis of the instruments used today.[4]

The principal change that has occurred in the last decade has been the introduction of flexible fibre-optic instruments for both the upper and the lower urinary tracts. Although fibre-optic instruments are more expensive than rigid ones, the expenditure can be justified on the grounds of cost-effectiveness. The majority of diagnostic cystoscopies are now performed on an outpatient basis.[5] This is not the forum in which to join the debate about the relative values of using local anaesthetic rather than just lubricant

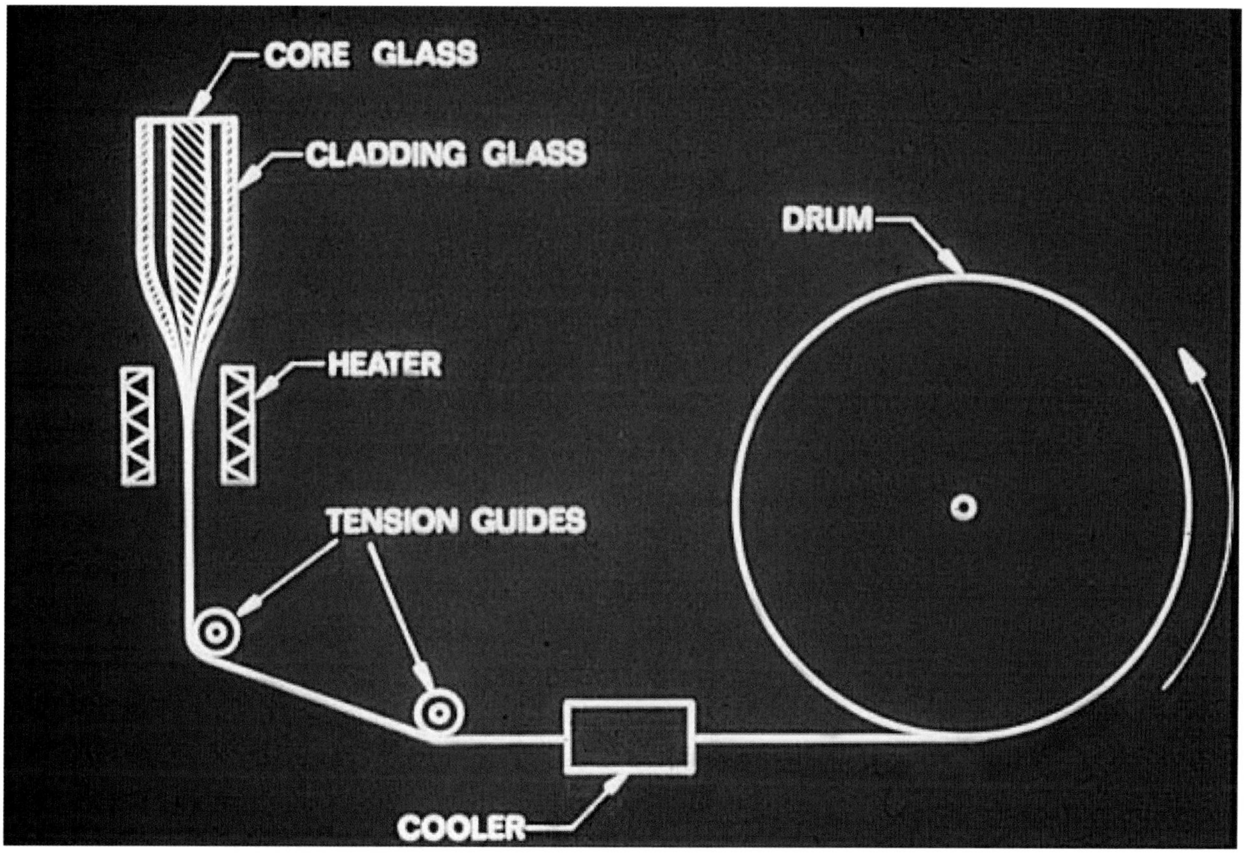

Figure 32.4 *A diagrammatic representation of the drum method of making a coherent fibre bundle (with acknowledgement to Keymed Olympus).*

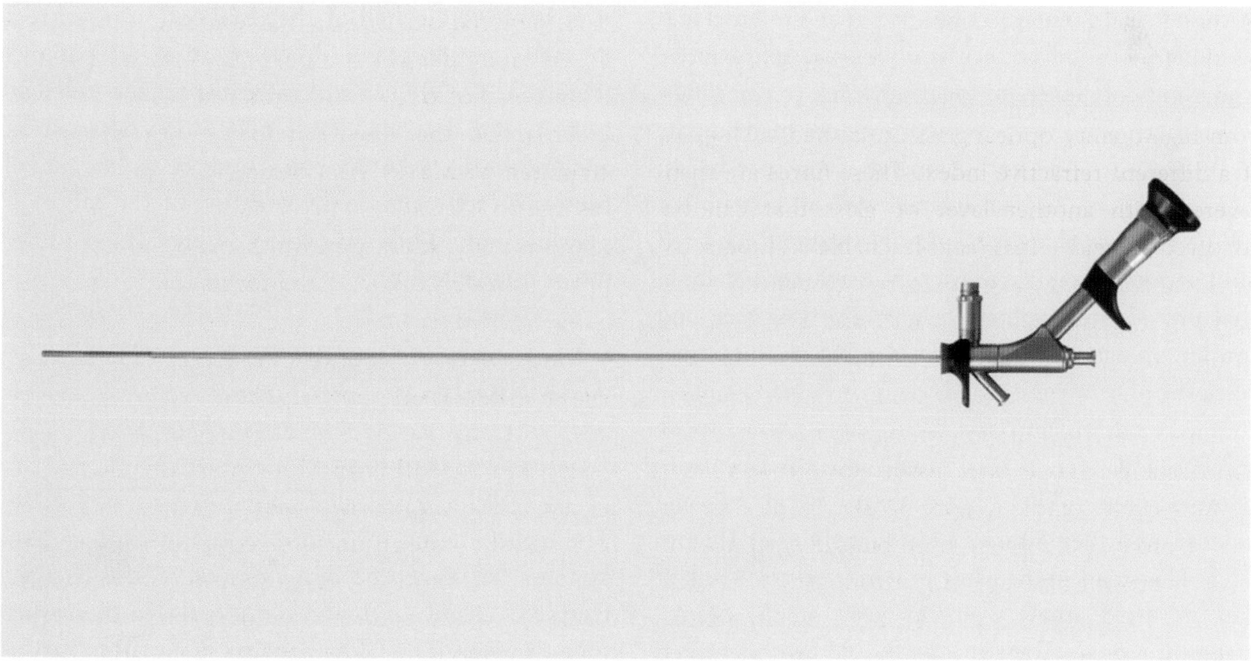

Figure 32.5 *A rigid ureteroscope (with acknowledgement to Keymed Olympus).*

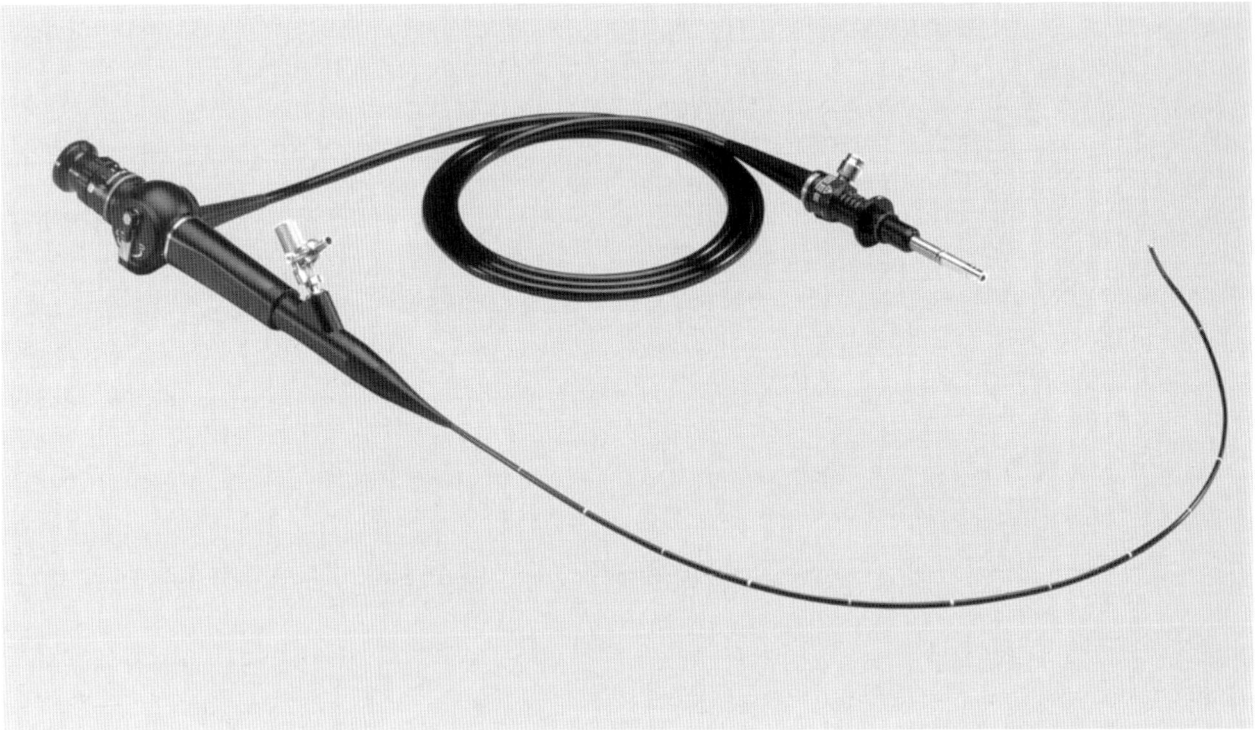

Figure 32.6 *A flexible ureteroscope (with acknowledgement to Keymed Olympus).*

jelly. Suffice it to say that few patients find the procedure more than mildly uncomfortable.

Upper urinary tract

Although rigid ureteroscopes had been designed and used before the advent of the fibre-optic light source, they were only taken up for routine use in the 1980s, when this technology was incorporated. Instruments of various lengths and diameters were produced; most ureters could be inspected with an instrument of 10 Fr, though passing the instrument required skill and patience. There was an instrument channel that provided enough space both for irrigation and for an operating device, often a basket for stone retrieval. Disintegrating devices became available that were safe and effective (see Chapter xxx); biopsy forceps and even a very small resectoscope were manufactured. The instruments have become smaller, and their use correspondingly safer (Figure 32.5) The smallest-diameter ureteroscope is 4 Fr and can be used safely even in very small infants. Ureteroscopy in all age groups should be undertaken with fluoroscopic control.

Fibre-optic technology has had as much influence on the upper as it has on the lower urinary tract. Flexible ureteroscopes with a diameter of 9 Fr that can be angulated 180° in two dimensions have made it possible to view all of the renal collecting system in many patients and much of it in all patients (Figure 32.6). We can not only inspect the pelvicaliceal system but also undertake stone destruction and removal, take biopsies and coagulate small tumours. Appreciating the anatomy of the calices is possible only when renoscopy is performed under image intensification.

CAMERAS

Analogue technology

The technological revolution in the field of camera systems has been the development of the charged couple device (CCD), which has replaced the earlier tube cameras. The CCD consists of small pieces of silicon, called pixels, which are arranged in columns and rows and are sensitive to light. When an image falls on the CCD chip, the optical image is converted into an electronic format. These electronic signals are then reconstructed on the monitor to form the video image. The resolution of a CCD chip is determined by the number of pixels on the sensor. The average chip contains between 250 000 and 380 000 pixels.

A three-chip camera contains three CCD units and offers very high resolution at the expense of significant weight. Most cameras for urological endoscopy (apart from those that are used for laparoscopy) are single chip. The coloured image is obtained by a process of colour separation using a stripe filter. Each stripe represents one of the complementary colours (magenta, green or yellow), and each pixel is assigned to one stripe. In three-chip cameras, the colour separation is achieved with a prism overlying the CCD chips. Each chip receives only one of the three primary colours, and each pixel encodes one colour dot.

Digital technology

The introduction of digital technology has further improved the quality of video imaging. In analogue technology, the images are translated into continuous voltage signals. These signals are susceptible to degradation during transmission, and the quality of the subsequent image may be affected. With digital technology, the signal is converted into a precise number. There is little chance of an error during the processing of these numbers; as a result, the image quality is maintained.[6] These images may be stored on computer hard drives or digital tape drives. They may be modified in different ways, as by highlighting areas of interest. Digital images of endoscopic procedures can be obtained and transmitted to distant sites via telephone lines or over the Internet for teaching, consultation or to seek a second opinion.[7]

In a study where analogue and digital pictures were compared, Berci et al assessed a group of general surgeons, gynaecologists and allied health workers, all of whom were able to identify the superiority of digital over analogue systems in terms of colour definition, image sharpness, contrast and depth of field.[8] The differences that can be observed become particularly relevant when, as in flexible ureterorenoscopy, endoscopic vision is reduced.

Camera systems

For the operating surgeon, it is important to arrange the camera and its monitor in a convenient location. The camera itself must be attached to the eyepiece of the endoscope, either after sterilization or after being covered in a sterile camera drape. The positioning of the monitor screen is important to allow maximum comfort for the surgeon. Research has shown that the height of the monitor should be at or below the eye level of the surgeon. There is added value in having a second monitor screen that allows the anaesthetist and other theatre staff to understand and to monitor the procedure.

All modern cameras can withstand the electrical interference that may arise from cutting and coagulating currents during endoscopic procedures with electrocautery, although it is advisable to mount the camera system and the diathermy unit on separate trolleys.

Light source

A high-intensity light source is essential if the potential of any camera system is to be fulfilled. The two light sources commonly used are xenon and halogen. Although xenon has a more neutral colour, the slightly yellowish light from a halogen bulb can be compensated for by 'white balancing' the camera at the beginning of the procedure. Some light sources come with automatic light-intensity adjustment features that maintain the intensity of light at an optimal level during an endoscopic procedure. This feature is not essential, as most camera systems are provided with automatic shutters that increase or decrease the camera aperture and regulate the amount of light according to need.

Three-dimensional (3-D) imaging

Although the standard video technology provides good-quality imaging, there is a lack of perception of depth. There are two ways to generate a 3-D image. A laparoscope may be used that has two video cameras

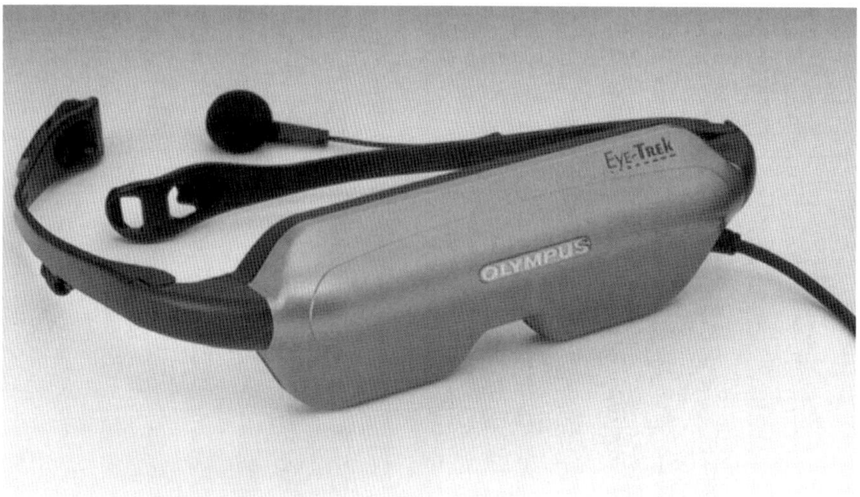

Figure 32.7 *The goggles that are worn to generate a 3-D image in laparoscopy (with acknowledgement to Keymed Olympus).*

mounted at its tip. These capture two slightly different images that are transmitted alternately at a high frequency. Alternatively, a single-lens system may be used with a device that splits the image at the proximal end. The two images, however generated, are sent to a 3-D conversion unit that processes the images and sends them to a high-resolution monitor. 3-D imaging relies on the physiological phenomenon of retinal persistence. The brain fuses two separate off-set images of an object received through both eyes to give a perception of depth; this is called stereopsis.[9] These images, when viewed through optic shutter glasses, appear to be 3-D (Figure 32.7).

This is a useful adjunct in the teaching of laparoscopy where the perception of space and depth is critical. Although there is no evidence that this technology improves the performance of an experienced laparoscopic surgeon, learning laparoscopy will become easier when 3-D imaging is more universally available. Another advance in digital imaging technology is the development of high-definition television (HDTV). The high-resolution image, coupled with HDTV cameras that are extremely sensitive and can be used in low-light conditions, will greatly improve vision and help to improve performance in laparoscopic procedures.[10]

THE FUTURE

The technological evolution is not over. There are already available technologies that even a year or two ago would have been counted as fanciful.

Video endoscopes

Video endoscopes are a new generation of telescopes where the CCD chip camera has been incorporated into the distal end of the telescope just behind the objective lens system.[11] This telescope has no conventional lens system running through its body. The image is captured by the CCD chip and transmitted via cables that run through the telescope directly to the camera. There is minimal loss of information during image transmission. These integrated video endoscopes not only provide superior imaging but also significantly reduce the risks of damage to the telescope and the camera.

Virtual reality

Virtual reality is defined as a computer-generated environment in which detail is faithfully reproduced and the objects within the environment have characteristics akin to their real-life counterparts.[12] This technology was initially developed for military purposes by the US National Aeronautics and Space Administration (NASA), but has more recently been used commercially by the entertainment industry. In endoscopic surgery, the hope and expectation are that surgeons in training will be able to learn and to practise their operative skills by using virtual-reality simulation models in which the operative environment is accurately reproduced. The technology is being refined, so that in addition to visual reality there is also tactile reality. The excit-

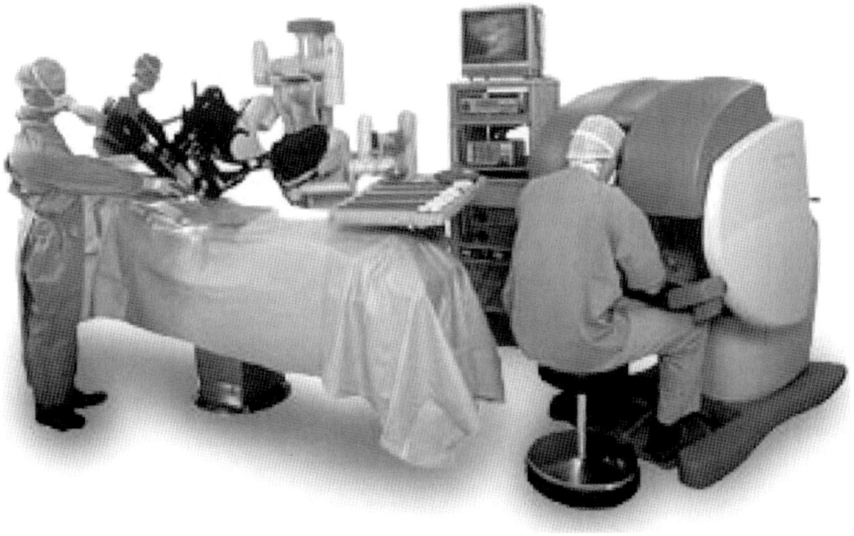

Figure 32.8 *The system for robotic surgery (with acknowledgement to Da Vinci Corporation).*

ing prospect exists that the need to practise on patients may one day be obviated.

Robotic surgery

The technology is now available to enable a surgeon to sit at a console and to operate remotely by 3-D visualization (Figure 32.8). Hand movements are translated into scaled movements of robotic arms that, with seven degrees of motion, can mimic the dexterity of the human hand. Unlike with other 3-D technology, the surgeon does not have to wear goggles. There is a realistic feel to the manipulation of tissues, to suturing and dissecting. The system is expensive, but early indications are that more precise laparoscopic surgery can be performed. The surgeon can sit comfortably, hand tremor is minimized and there is less potential for fatigue. Dual-lens technology is used to create the 3-D image, and the camera-control system allows zooming in and out seamlessly from a macro- to a microview.

CONCLUSIONS

The technology that has been introduced for endoscopic surgery in urology is impressive. There is no doubt that urologists have played a significant part in the developments that have occurred. The increasing complexity of the engineering that is now being employed makes it inevitable that in the future the advances that are made will depend more on the expertise of others. Urologists, however, have always been innovative, and their ideas are likely to be the stimulus for their technological colleagues.

ACKNOWLEDGEMENT

I would like to express my thanks to Ms J Harrison of KeyMed for providing invaluable background technical information and some of the illustrations.

REFERENCES

1. Gorden A. The history and development of endoscopic surgery. In: Sutton C, Diamond MP, eds. Endoscopic Surgery for Gynaecologists. London: WB Saunders, 1993: 3–7
2. Shah J. Endoscopy through the ages. BJU Int 2002; 89: 645–652
3. Hopkins HH, Kapani NS. A flexible fibrescope using static scanning. Nature 1954; 173: 39–41
4. McCarthy JF. A new apparatus for endoscopic plastic surgery of the prostate, diathermy and excision of vesical growths. J Urol 1931; 26: 695
5. Fowler CJ, Boorman LS. Outpatient treatment of superficial bladder cancer. Lancet 1986; 1: 38
6. Kourambas J, Preminger GM. Advances in camera, video and imaging technologies in laparoscopy. Urol Clin North Am 2001; 28: 5–14

7. Moore RG, Adam JB, Partin AW, Docimo HG et al. Telemonitoring of laparoscopic procedures. Surg Endosc 1996; 10: 107–110
8. Berci G, Wren SM, Stain SC, Peters J et al. Individual assessment of visual perception by surgeons observing the same laparoscopic organ with various imaging systems. Surg Endosc 1995; 9: 967–973
9. Zobel J. Basics of three-dimensional endoscopic vision. Endosc Surg 1993; 1: 36–39
10. Durrani AF, Preminger GM. Three dimensional video imaging for endoscopic surgery. Comput Biol Med 1995; 25: 237–247
11. Amory SE, Ford KA, Tsai JL. A new flexible video endoscope for minimal access surgery. Surg Endosc 1993; 7: 200–202
12. Kourambas J, Preminger GM. Advances in camera, video and imaging technologies in laparoscopy. Urol Clin North Am 2001; 28: 5–14

33

Perioperative care of the urological patient

David W Ryan

INTRODUCTION

The range of urological surgery is impressive, covering reconstructive surgery of congenital defects of the urinary tract, malignancy, incontinence, stones, spinal cord injury and impotence. It covers all ranges of patients from the newborn to the adult and often elderly patient with numerous medical problems. Adults only are considered in this chapter. A close working relationship between surgeon and anaesthetist is crucial to the success of the operation phase for any urological patient. The anaesthetist must ensure patient safety and optimization of the medical conditions influencing outcome. In the unfit patient, this may require deferment or further investigation, as well as planning elective high-dependency unit (HDU) or intensive-care unit (ICU) admission. Many patients today are screened in the preadmission outpatient clinic, but it remains a common cause for cancellation in the day-case clinic that a patient arrives for day-case surgery with a recognized but untreated condition such as hypertension. It is also important that conditions that have serious anaesthetic implications, such as sickle-cell disease and malignant hyperpyrexia, or a family history of medical or anaesthetic complications, are referred early and appropriately to the anaesthetist.

MEDICAL HISTORY

A general review of medical health by questionnaire (Figure 33.1) will in many cases identify common risk factors, such as ischaemic heart disease, diabetes mellitus, respiratory illness, and previous problems,

THE NEWCASTLE UPON TYNE HOSPITALS NHS TRUST
FREEMAN HOSPITAL
UROLOGY PRE-ADMISSION CLINIC

AGE
WARD
CONSULTANT
CLINIC DATE
ADMISSION DATE
REASON FOR ADMISSION

<u>PRESENTING SYMPTOMS</u>

FREQ	URGENCY
DYSURIA	URGE INC
NOCTURIA	STRESS INC
POOR FLOW	PMD
HESITANCY	HAEMATURIA
LOIN PAIN	

<u>INVESTIGATIONS/HISTOLOGY</u>

<u>PAST MEDICAL HISTORY</u>

HYPERTENSION	ULCER DISEASE
RHF	MI/IHD
COAD/ASTHMA	CVA
TB	PE/DVT
JAUNDICE	DIABETES
EPILEPSY	PREVIOUS OPS

<u>DRUG HISTORY</u>

ALLERGIES

ANAESTHETIC PROBLEMS

Figure 33.1 *Preoperative systemic questionnaire.*

such as deep-vein thrombosis. Specific items, such as a joint replacement, and a pacemaker, are likely to be volunteered, but subjects such as mouth opening and dentition, nausea and vomiting after procedures are relevant but are unlikely to be asked about. A drug and allergy history needs clear identification, and some patients are unsure of this, so the GP may have to be contacted to clarify medication. Latex allergy is a particular problem, as surgical gloves, catheters, anaesthetic circuits, plastic syringes, IV injection ports and drug vial stoppers all contain latex, and extra care is needed. Most units have a special trolley with latex-free products. A social history of alcohol intake, smoking, and drug dependency and personal circumstances are sometimes less easy to obtain, but they are relevant. Ideally, smoking should be stopped 4–6 weeks prior to surgery, but there is a significant decreased in sputum volume if 1–2 weeks is achieved, and the patient benefits from a reduced carbon monoxide level in the 24 hours preceding operation. A heavy alcohol intake can lead to problems when suddenly stopped; substance withdrawal has similar problems. It is important at this time also to record some simple screening parameters such as pulse, blood pressure, temperature, respiration rate, and weight, as well as an assessment of well-being (Figure 33.2). In the emergency setting, these details may well be incomplete, forgotten or ignored completely.

SYSTEMIC ENQUIRY	
GI	
APPETITE	INDIGESTION
WT LOSS	DYSPHAGIA
ABDO PAIN	BOWEL HABIT
N/V	
CVS/RS	
OEDEMA	CHEST PAIN
WHEEZE	PALPITATIONS
COUGH	SOB
ORTHOPNOEA	WALK TOLERANCE
CNS/MUSCULOSKELETAL	
GENERAL APPEARANCE	
PALLOR	OBESITY
JAUNDICE	CACHEXIA
DEHYDRATED	LYMPHADENOPATHY
BP	PULSE
TEMP	URINALYSIS
WEIGHT	
SOCIAL HISTORY	
SMOKER	COMMUNICATION
ALCOHOL	MOBILITY
DIET	SOCIAL SERVICES
LIVES WITH	OCCUPATION

Figure 33.2 *Systemic enquiry.*

SPECIFIC MEDICAL CONDITIONS

Cardiovascular disease

Symptomatic disease is always relevant, and uncontrolled hypertension, angina, paroxysmal nocturnal dyspnoea and a recent myocardial infarct (MI) are significant conditions indicating that treatment needs to be deferred until they are sorted out. Hypertension is common. Recent guidelines[1] indicate that an acceptable blood pressure is 150/90 mmHg, and above this level, treatment must be commenced along agreed guidelines. The anaesthetic risks are increased in patients with hypertension, myocardial infarct and renal failure[2,3] (Table 33.1). Retention of urine requiring a transurethral resection of prostate

Table 33.1 Conditions identified as carrying a higher operative mortality.[2,3]

Cardiac disease
Hypertension
Heart failure
Renal failure
Obesity
Abdominal surgery
Smoking
COPD*
ASA 3 or more

*Chronic obstructive pulmonary disease

(TURP) following a recent MI is a quite common dilemma – do we operate or wait? The risk is real of a further MI and even perioperative death, but this decreases with time and is generally 50% less at 3 months. Abdominal surgery carries the highest risk. The reinfarction rate is 20–35% in that 3-month window, reducing to 10–15% at 3–6 months and to 6% at 6 months. The death rate after an MI in the general population is normally around 30%, but, importantly, after reinfarction the *mortality rate is doubled*.[4] Sitting with a catheter in situ for weeks does increase concern about the infection rate, and some brinkmanship is needed to balance this out, but veering to a 3-month rule is sensible practice despite domestic pressures. Critical angina is something that cannot be ignored. It represents a medical emergency, and such patients need referral to a cardiologist for stabilization with nitrates, beta blockade and calcium antagonists. Symptomatic but stable cardiac disease carries a 6% mortality compared with 0.1% in the normal population. An echocardiogram is often used to assess left ventricular function, and is mandatory for major cases of heart disease; an ejection fraction of <40% signifies serious disease.

The presence of an abnormal ECG is always indicative of underlying heart disease. The finding of an arrhythmia, of which atrial fibrillation is probably the commonest,[4] is not a contraindication to surgery, providing the patient is well controlled. Similarly, the patient with valvular heart disease requires careful handling and appropriate antibiotic cover, but, providing the condition is stable, the risk has to be accepted. Patients on warfarin need to be converted to IV heparin, and this may take a few days to achieve. Similar planning is required for a patient who has had pulmonary embolism, and a period of 3 months should be allowed before surgery is undertaken. Heart failure also means a limited life expectancy, and the presence of shortness of breath, angina, oedema and poor exercise tolerance must cause one to question the relevance of surgery, as the additional strain on the heart makes outcome unpredictable. Many less than ideal patients will tolerate careful regional or spontaneous anaesthesia for gentle endoscopic surgery, but will not withstand an abdominal operation.[3]

Respiratory disease

Asthma is common. The presence of a wheeze is always significant, and the question has to be asked, can we improve the patient's condition? A simple method of assessment on the ward of obstructive airways disease is peak flow, which correlates well with the forced expiratory volume [in 1 second] (FEV_{-1}). A more sensitive predictor of respiratory reserve is the FEV_1/vital capacity (VC) ratio. Less than 50% of predicted values indicates severe disease and the need for a facility for mechanical ventilation after major surgery.[5,6] Operative procedures therefore must be carefully thought about. Blood gases should be routinely obtained when major surgery is planned. It may well be that optimization with a combination of bronchodilators or steroids will improve matters, and this is best handled by referral to a chest physician. These patients need their surgery timed to be away from the winter flu crisis and into the summer months, and to stop smoking, but these points are too often left to chance. Similar advice applies to chronic bronchitis and bronchiectasis. Chest infections are common in such patients and must be adequately treated before surgery. Planning for such patients who are self-evidently in trouble with their chest conditions allows a preoperative work-up of beneficial chest physiotherapy, bronchodilators and sometimes antibiotics. Ankylosing spondylitis can produce respiratory failure, but it more often presents the anaesthetist with access to the airway problem, which can be resolved only in a hospital with fibre-optic intubating skills.

Metabolic conditions

Diabetes mellitus accounts for 5% of all patients aged over 65 years. Minor surgery can be managed on an outpatient basis, providing the patient is stable, and clear instructions are given regarding omitting medication. These patients should always be undertaken early in the day to allow supervision as eating and medication are reintroduced. Patients with type 1 (insulin-dependent) and the more common type 2 (diet or oral hypoglycaemic drugs) undergoing more complex surgery will require conversion to a glucose-potassium-insulin technique, which achieves easy control in a majority of cases.[7] In the unstable or brittle diabetics, 2 days should be allowed to achieve acceptable blood-glucose levels (5–10 mmol/L). Failure to respect these measures will lead to post-operative hyperglycaemia, ketoacidosis and electrolyte disturbances. Poor wound healing, protein catabolism and an increased infection rate follow. Normally, the management of these cases is protocol led and supervised by the anaesthetist in theatre and the medical team on the ward.[8] The difficulty is always in the emergency case, but, as a rule, abolition of acidosis is the basis of safe practice with rehydration and avoidance of hypoglycaemia. Patients with uncontrolled thyroid disease need to be deferred until this is resolved.

Haematological

Bleeding from the urinary tract is a common presentation of underlying disease. What the anaesthetist usually prefers is a haemoglobin of 10 g/dl, which gives a good reserve of oxygen delivery, but in chronic conditions or emergencies a lower level will be accepted. Particular problems are likely to arise with sickle-cell disease no matter how minor the surgery is, and patients from Africa, the West Indies, Greece and Italy must be screened preoperatively. Thalassaemia carries a similar risk. Regional anaesthesia is often preferred. Polycythaemia is a condition to be wary about, as reactionary haemorrhage often occurs despite the best of planning, and surgery is best avoided unless essential.

Acute and chronic renal failure

The presentation of obstructive urinary disease may result in temporary or irreversible renal failure and is not that uncommon in emergency admissions. It is a high surgical/anaesthetic risk condition.[3] Many patients are elderly and cardiovascular disease is frequent. Rehydration, correction of electrolyte disturbances and reversal of acidosis, including dialysis support in a minority, are requirements before surgery is contemplated. A safe serum potassium level is 5 mmol/L or less. Conversely, a potassium level below 3.5 mmol/L is also to be avoided, as it will result in an increased risk of arrythmias. Vomiting may accompany uraemia and aggravate the electrolyte problems unless resolved. The presence of a fistula or shunt in the arm needs meticulous care in blood sampling and blood-pressure measurement.

Nutrition and obesity

An adequate diet and appropriate body weight are prerequisites for healthy life. Up to 30% of the UK population is now obese, leading to mobility, moving problems and a tendency to venous thrombosis. A hiatus hernia may commonly be present, increasing the pulmonary aspiration risk. Morbid obesity, with a body-mass index of >30 (kg/m^2), often accompanied by sleep apnoea, has the potential for severe post-operative problems, amongst which hypoxia is common. Abdominal surgery, in particular, will aggravate this situation, but even for minor surgery such patients should always have a planned HDU bed for postoperative monitoring and non-invasive ventilation support available.

Diseases of the nervous system

Epileptics need regular anticonvulsant therapy before and after surgery. Demented patients often arrive for catheter changes, and usually a gentle approach is all that is necessary. Paraplegia is a much more complex issue, but the majority of cases are chronic and stable though with a variable nutritional status, psychiatric difficulties, contractures and chronic infections. Most problems involve positioning, temperature and autonomic control during the procedure, and pain, recovery of the cough reflex and respiratory drive with high cord lesions afterwards. Multiple sclerosis and spina bifida patients have similar difficulties. Their needs vary from a simple catheter change to an ileal conduit; therefore, the latter may require a planned HDU bed or even ITU admission. Hypothermia during the procedure can precipitate further demyelination in multiple sclerosis patients. Unlike a myocardial infarct, there is no time-lapse reduction of risk after a stroke. The risk of another stroke is 3%. It is best to wait until after the acute event to ensure recovery and that the patient's blood pressure is normal on aspirin. Heparin increases the risk.

Liver disease

Liver disease patients have multiple problems with impaired coagulation, intolerance of drugs, a tendency to hypoglycaemia and altered conscious state. They are best undertaken in specialized centres and will almost certainly require postoperative HDU or ITU. Special precautions are also required for any patient with hepatitis B or C. Renal failure often accompanies liver disease.

Sepsis

Pyelonephritis, infection accompanying kidney stones and urinary tract infections can vary from mild symptoms to marked pyrexia and rigors. Often an intermediate operation such as a nephrostomy can be helpful in draining pus and allowing time for the patient to recover from the acute condition. This can often be achieved under local anaesthetic. Sepsis is a serious condition and in the presence of hypotension is associated with a high mortality.[9] It should not be underestimated.

ASSESSMENT OF RISK

The anaesthetist is often required to balance the risk of surgery versus medical deterioration. A useful way of doing this is the ASA scale.[10] This grades illness from fit and well to likely to die whatever is done (Figure 33.3). This is a simple scale and gives a good idea of what limitations and expectations can be placed on surgery. It follows that ASA 4 and 5 will require a critical care facility after surgery. The weakness is that disagreement in scoring patients may under- or overestimate the risk. In cardiac disease, the Goldman index is often used and this also allows some prediction of cardiac risk.[11] The recent CEPOD report in relation to urology[12] stresses the importance of a team approach, especially when contemplating radical surgery in the elderly because of their high incidence of medical problems. There is also good correlation with perioperative cardiovascular testing in the elderly and outcome, and this should be used more widely.[13] Forrest et al[3] analysed predicted outcomes for 17 201 surgical cases and found cardiac adverse outcomes for patients with any form of cardiac disease who smoked and underwent abdominal or thoracic surgery. Likewise, adverse respiratory events occurred with patients who smoked, were obese and had respiratory disease when undergoing abdominal or thoracic surgery. The message is clear.

Grade	Description
1	A healthy patient with no systemic disease
2	A patient with mild to moderate illness, with no limitation; for example, small bladder tumours, controlled hypertension, mild diabetes
3	A patient with serious systemic disease from any cause, causing a limitation in activity, such as ischaemic heart disease, or asthma with wheeze
4	A patient with severe systemic disease which is a constant threat to life, such as heart failure, breathless at rest or renal failure on dialysis
5	A patient unlikely to survive 24 hours irrespective of whether surgery is undertaken, as in a leaking aortic aneurysm

Figure 33.3 *ASA grades [modified from reference 10].*

Laboratory tests (Figure 33.4)

Investigations should be directed at relevant pathology. A lot of patients have repeated outpatient cystoscopy, and these investigations do not require repeating each time unless there is cause for concern or a change in circumstances. All patients should have urine analysis to exclude diabetes mellitus, infection and haematuria. Plasma electrolytes ensure that renal and water balance is satisfactory and exclude drug-induced effects. A full blood count excludes anaemia, infection and malignancy. A chest radiograph is indicated only if respiratory or cardiac disease or malignancy is suspected. It is also a useful baseline when major procedures are undertaken because of the patients' propensity to respiratory complications. A cervical spine X-ray should be undertaken in cases of expected airway difficulty as in severe rheumatoid arthritis and ankylosing spondylitis. An ECG should routinely be undertaken in a patient with relevant cardiac pathology. Echocardiography and respiratory function tests may be undertaken in assessment of cardiac and respiratory reserve, respectively. There may also be some special circumstances, such as after bleomycin treatment for testicular malignancy, in which to review the degree of pulmonary fibrosis. Blood gases

INVESTIGATIONS

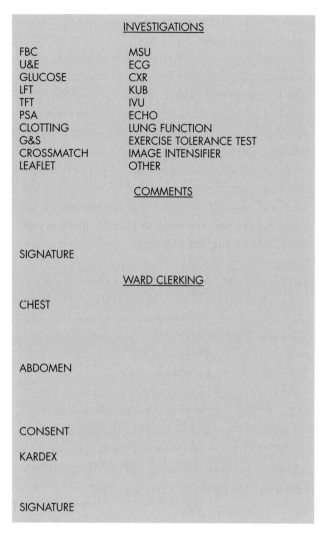

FBC	MSU
U&E	ECG
GLUCOSE	CXR
LFT	KUB
TFT	IVU
PSA	ECHO
CLOTTING	LUNG FUNCTION
G&S	EXERCISE TOLERANCE TEST
CROSSMATCH	IMAGE INTENSIFIER
LEAFLET	OTHER

COMMENTS

SIGNATURE

WARD CLERKING

CHEST

ABDOMEN

CONSENT

KARDEX

SIGNATURE

Figure 33.4 *Summary of investigations performed.*

are helpful in selected cases or respiratory disease. In liver disease, clotting disorders and diabetes mellitus, further specific screening is required.

CLINICAL EXAMINATION AND CONSENT

Fit, healthy patients are just that and do not require a lengthy appraisal. In less well patients, time should be spent checking the airway, mouth opening and teeth, the cardiovascular system and its stability, breathing, chest expansion and ability to cough and checking for any specific neurological deficit. The patient may present with anaemia, cyanosis, jaundice or breathlessness. Clinical signs need to be married to investigations and the whole picture considered as to risk and whether to proceed.

If major surgery is contemplated, factors such as venous access, timing of subcutaneous heparin, consent for a regional block, overnight fluids when laxatives have been given, clotting and blood cross-match need to sorted out at the preoperative visit. Considerations such as the plan for pain control, patient rewarming and blood transfusion need to be explained.

SPECIFIC CONSIDERATIONS

Deep-vein thrombosis prophylaxis[14]

Certain patients are at risk of deep-vein thrombosis (DVT) following surgery (Table 33.2). In the case of major abdominal urological surgery, this has been estimated at 40%, and for endoscopic prostate resection at 10%, with a risk of fatal pulmonary embolism of 0.1–1%. It is appropriate that these patients are given a combination of low-molecular-weight heparin 5000 units at 6 pm the day before the operation, with compression elasticated stockings and intermittent calf pneumatic compression on the day of surgery. The evening timing of heparin permits a safe delay for the institution of a regional blockade on the next day. Epidural anaesthesia should always be considered in abdominal cases, as there is a reduction in the incidence of deep-vein thrombosis,[15] and specifically in open prostatectomy it has been studied and found to benefit the patient.[16]

Table 33.2 Common conditions predisposing to venous thrombosis.[14]

Obesity
Immobility
Pregnancy
Oestrogen-containing contraceptives
History of DVT or thromboembolism
Advanced age
Trauma or surgery to leg, abdomen or pelvis
Malignancy, especially to pelvis or abdomen, or metastasis
COPD
Heart failure
Polycythaemia
Paralysis of lower limb
Recent myocardial infarct

Epidural and spinal blocks

There are two patient groups that will benefit from regional blockade. The epidural is particularly useful for postoperative pain management through a combination of background and intermittent bolus injections. This is normally then supervised by the pain team. An epidural used as the anaesthetic for the operative procedure can provide advantages and a lower mortality to higher risk.[17,18] The obvious advantages are rapid recovery, mobility and less sedation. There are fewer chest complications and reduced cardiovascular problems in properly conducted trials.[17–19] The spinal anaesthetic is useful for unfit patients who, for instance, are breathless and cannot safely be laid flat, and in stable cardiac disease and diabetes requiring endoscopic surgery; it provides 1–2 hours of profound analgesia and paralysis. It requires skilful handling to avoid difficulties. Consent must be obtained prior to the procedure, and a simple booklet of explanation is helpful (Figure 33.5).

Preoperative starvation[20]

Nil by mouth still causes confusion on surgical wards. In fact, elective patients can drink clear fluids up to 2 hours before surgery. Food is normally omitted for 6 hours before surgery. A prolonged period of starvation is hazardous in young children. Milk and fatty foods are a problem if given for breakfast, and up to 8 hours may be needed to ensure an empty stomach electively. I personally *prescribe* all patients a cup of tea or coffee with a splash of milk on the morning of the operation at 7 am with their medication, and ensure that all afternoon patients have a drink and some dry toast. Advice to day patients is normally given by the surgeon, and there is a historical reluctance by anaesthetists to change practice from midnight starvation. The evidence is that there is less nausea and vomiting in patients given sensible oral fluids on the day of surgery.

Drug medication[21,22]

Nil by mouth may mean omission of important medication on the morning of operation. Advice is often far from clear, and Table 33.3 indicates how complex the matter is.

Drugs that need to be *stopped* include anticoagulants, with a planned conversion to heparin for the operative day. Aspirin and non-steroidal drugs can increase bleeding, but unless they are stopped 7–10 days before surgery, little will be gained in terms of platelet recovery. Warfarin is a problem. It needs to be discontinued a few days before surgery, and IV heparin can be substituted for the duration of the operative period. For short operations and in

Table 33.3 Drugs and what to do in the operative period.[17,18]

Drugs to stop	Drugs to continue	Drugs to continue/change dose	Drugs to commence
4 weeks ahead Oestrogen contraceptive HRT *2 weeks ahead* (can vary) MAOIs *Up to 1 week ahead* Aspirin; clopiderol *1 day ahead* Lithium *Day of operation* Oral hypoglycaemics Potassium-sparing diuretics	Antiepileptics Antihypertensives Antianginals Antiarrythmics Drugs for asthma Drugs of dependence Loop diuretics Anxiolytics SSRIs	Increase corticosteroids	Insulin in some diabetics IV heparin for warfarin Antibiotics Antiemetics Analgesics

INTEGRATED RECORD - DAY TREATMENT CENTRE

DAY TREATMENT CENTRE FREEMAN HOSPITAL High Heaton Newcastle upon Tyne NE7 7DN (0191) 284 3111 Fax (0191) 213 1968	Attach addressograph here Patient prefers to be called
Current Medication	Next of Kin Address Telephone
Allergies	Person to contact if different from above: Name Address Telephone
Valuables Yes / No Where stored:.................................. Indemnity form completed Yes / No	Discharge plan: Name of escort home.............................. Telephone.. Transport..

ASSESSMENT (please tick yes or no)

Will you have to go home alone?	❑ YES	❑ NO
Will you be on your own when you get home?	❑ YES	❑ NO
Have you seen and understood the post anaesthetic instructions?	❑ YES	❑ NO
Have you had anything to eat or drink in the last four hours?	❑ YES	❑ NO
Do you have – a cough, cold or runny nose?	❑ YES	❑ NO
Since you were last seen in out patients:-		
Has your general health changed?	❑ YES	❑ NO
Are you taking any new medication?	❑ YES	❑ NO
Have you had any operations or serious illness?	❑ YES	❑ NO
Has the condition requiring treatment today changed significantly?	❑ YES	❑ NO
Have you signed and do you understand your consent form?	❑ YES	❑ NO
For women of child bearing age only:-		
Is there any chance you may be pregnant?	❑ YES	❑ NO

PATIENT's SIGNATURE ....

OBSERVATIONS (ANAESTHETIST)

Temp .... Pulse ....reg/irreg BP .... Weight ....

LMP ☐☐ ☐☐ ☐☐☐☐

ASSESSMENT QUESTIONNAIRE COMPLETED?	❑ YES	❑ NO
INVESTIGATIONS CARRIED OUT?	❑ YES	❑ NO
FIT FOR OPERATION AS A DAY CASE?	❑ YES	❑ NO

PREMED

ANY SIGNIFICANT PROBLEMS?.......................................

POTTS PRINTERS LIMITED NFH/43

Figure 33.5 *Summary of fitness for day-case/outpatient surgery.*

I.D. STICKER	**PRE-OPERATIVE CARE PLAN**

POTENTIAL PROBLEM	NURSING ACTION	EVALUATION
Anxiety	Explain all pre and post operative procedures, giving written information sheets where available.	
Inhalation of vomit	Ensure appropriate nil by mouth period and maintain	
Hazards to safety and well being whilst under anaesthetic	Ensure correct pre-operative preparation	Complete operative check list immediately prior to transfer to theatre.
Other specific problems		

PRE-OP CHECK LIST

	WARD Yes	WARD No	THEATRE Yes	THEATRE No
Identification bracelet in place and details correct?				
Consent form signed and patients understanding checked?				
To accompany patient:- Notes				
X Rays				
Operation site marked if necessary?				
Operation site prepared?				
Removal of the following:- Dentures – Caps or Crowns				
Prosthesis				
Jewellery (rings taped)				
Contact lens/Spectacles				
Make up				
Nail varnish				
Hair grips				
Hearing aid in situ?				
With patient to theatre?				
Allergies (list)				
Bladder empty?				
Pre medication given (enter time)				
Enter date and time patient last had anything to eat				
Enter date and time patient last had anything to drink				
Blood Pressure				
Current Medication				
Ward nurse signature				
Theatre nurse signature				

Figure 33.5 cont'd

ANAESTHETIC RECORD

Date Time Theatre	ASA grade 1 2 3 4 5	Elective Emergency

Anaesthetist (please print)	Surgeon (print)
Operative Procedure (please print)	

Induction	Relaxant	Analgesia	Anti emetic	Inhalation
Propofol mg	Sux mg	Alfent mg	Droperi mg	Enf %
Thio mg	Mivac mg	Fent μg	Prochlor mg	Iso %
Etomidate mg	Atrac mg	Diclof mg	Metoclop mg	Hal %
	Vec mg	Ketor mg	Ondanse mg	Des %
		Atropine mg		Sevo %
	Neostig/Glyc	Glycopy mg		

Respiratory management		
Airway Mask Laryngeal mask size Oral/Nasal:- L/R/ETT mm Tracheostomy mm Type Pre 02 Cuff Pack N.G. Tube Rapid sequence induction Y/N	Circuit Spont resp. Magill Gas flow Bain IPPV Ass resp T piece Ventilator type C02 absorbtion HME Vt mls V mls F mls Ip cms H20	Regional Block Laryngoscopy grade 1/2/3/4

	190		Monitoring
Sa02	180		ECG
ETC02	170		NIPB
	160		Sa02
	150		Fi02
HR	140		ETC02
	130		Vent alarm
BP	120		Other
	110		
	100		IV site
	90		Cannula
	80		Fluids
	70		
	60		
	50		
	40		
Time			Blood loss

POST OPERATIVE INSTRUCTIONS

	Analgesia - Recovery/Ward	Discharge Analgesia
Routine Care Oxygen 1/MIN X Ray hrs	CoCodamol Diclofenac Fentanyl Prochor Metoclop	CoCodamol CoCodamol/Diclofenac Other Sig.

Figure 33.5 cont'd

SURGICAL INSTRUCTIONS TO WARD STAFF

PROCEDURES PERFORMED ....

....

POST OPERATIVE INSTRUCTIONS

1. USUAL ROUTINE CARE [ ]

2. DRAINS — Wound ....
Other (specify) ....
Sutures ....

3. SPECIAL INSTRUCTIONS ....

....

Date ..../..../....   Signature. ....

POST OPERATIVE CARE PLAN

OBSERVATIONS

Time	BP	P	02 Sat	Resp	Temp	Conscious level	Comment

NURSING INTERVENTIONS

Potential problem	Action	Evaluation	Signature
Post operative care	Record BP, pulse		
Haemorrhage	Observe wound site		
Pain	Give appropriate analgesia, monitor effect. Ensure comfortable position.		
Nausea, vomiting	Observe and report Give anti emetics		
Drugs given			
Other problems identified			

DISCHARGE CHECKLIST

Patient mobile	Follow up appointment
Patient voided (if relevant)	District nurse requested and transfer document forwarded to district nurse.
Observations satisfactory	TTO's and dressing (if needed)
Wound checked and satisfactory	Property returned
No nausea or vomiting	Advice given - Verbal / Written
Contact number given	G.P. letter
Named nurse signature	F.U. telephone call

Figure 33.5 cont'd

women on progesterone-only preparations, there is no need to stop medication. Oestrogen-containing contraceptives and hormone replacement therapy are normally stopped several weeks prior to major surgery, and in the former case alternative contraception needs to be discussed. Lithium should be discontinued 24 hours before surgery. Monamine-oxidase inhibitors have a variety of potentially serious interactions, and opinions vary but are often stopped 14 days prior to operation and an alternative chosen. Potassium-sparing diuretics are best discontinued on the morning of the operation to avoid hyperkalaemia.

Drugs that *must not* be stopped include antiepileptics, antihypertensives, antianginals, antiarrythmics, drugs for asthma, steroids, drugs of dependence, immunosuppressants, antiparkinsonian drugs and normal antidepressants.

Drugs requiring *special consideration* include anticoagulants, as already discussed; steroid dosage which is increased for 48 hours after surgery; and oral hypoglycaemics, which are normally withheld on the morning of surgery.[7] A rather ignored problem is recommencement of oral medication. Clearly, if the patient is able to swallow, the oral medication can recommence, but in the event of nausea or vomiting it is problematical. Conversion to IV drugs is not always possible or advisable in a ward environment, and the staff must be alert to the possibility of difficulties. Control of hypertension and angina are particularly common problems and patients can suffer because of omission of their medication.

Premedication

This definition encompasses analgesia and anxiolytics, which today are used only in specific cases. Patients with a history of hiatus hernia will benefit from H2 blocker prophylaxis. Patients with a history of nausea and vomiting are best given oral antiemetics. Antibiotics are indicated for prevention of bacterial endocarditis, when a catheter has been in place for some time, there is a proven infection or bowel surgery is undertaken. The use of laxatives to prepare the bowel can lead to severe dehydration and electrolyte disturbance, and intravenous preoperative fluids overnight can minimize this.

Day-case surgery[23]

A wide range of minor surgical procedures can be carried out, providing the patients are ASA 1 and 2, and it is very desirable, providing there is a responsible adult to take charge of the patient afterwards. Figure 33.6 is an example of a screening questionnaire that can be used to exclude patients. Quite specific written instructions need to be given regarding starvation, medication, time and place, and discharge. The surgery should be straightforward, not overambitious, and unlikely to result in bleeding postoperatively. Surgeon and anaesthetist must be experienced to avoid complications.

SPECIAL SURGICAL CONSIDERATIONS

Prostatectomy

Three types of surgery are undertaken: endoscopic resection, retropubic open prostatectomy and radical open surgery for cancer with clearance of lymph nodes. Endoscopic surgery can be undertaken with either a spontaneously breathing general anaesthetic or spinal anaesthesia. The choice, as already discussed, is directed by the relative fitness of the patient. There is no evidence that one technique is superior to the other in fit patients in terms of myocardial ischaemia[24] and clotting disorders.[25] Blood loss is influenced by duration of operation and the use of a regional technique.[26] Mechanical ventilation results in less irrigation fluid absorption,[27] but this is not usually an issue, providing surgical operating time is limited to 1 hour. Open and radical prostectomy may involve considerable blood loss, and in both an epidural technique is advantageous to the patient postoperatively.

Major complex procedures – such as radical cystectomy and nephrectomy

Major abdominal surgery in what is usually an elderly, smoking and ASA 3 population for 2–8 hours will require careful planning, deep-vein prophylaxis, invasive monitoring, and an epidural

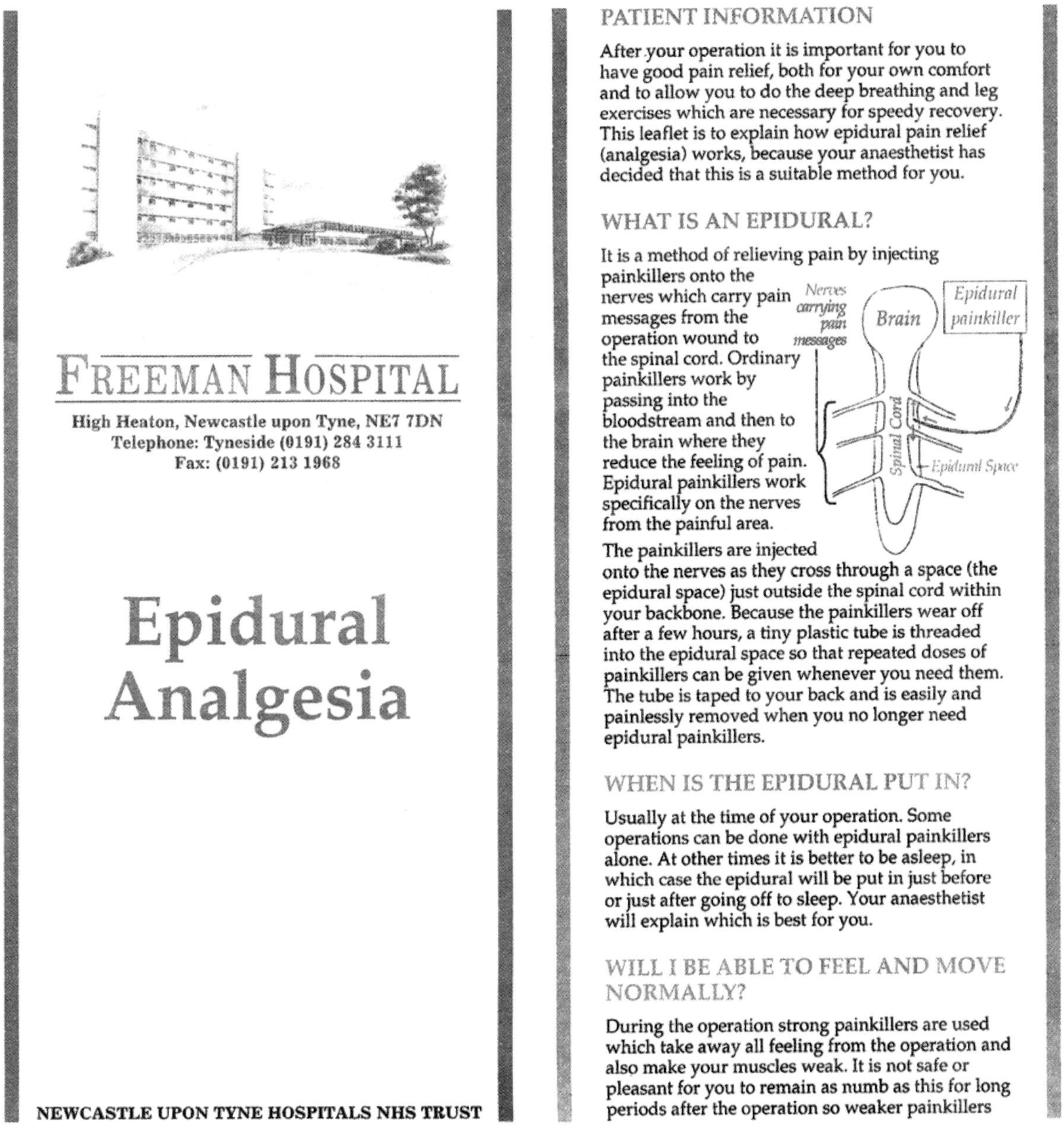

FREEMAN HOSPITAL

High Heaton, Newcastle upon Tyne, NE7 7DN
Telephone: Tyneside (0191) 284 3111
Fax: (0191) 213 1968

Epidural Analgesia

NEWCASTLE UPON TYNE HOSPITALS NHS TRUST

PATIENT INFORMATION

After your operation it is important for you to have good pain relief, both for your own comfort and to allow you to do the deep breathing and leg exercises which are necessary for speedy recovery. This leaflet is to explain how epidural pain relief (analgesia) works, because your anaesthetist has decided that this is a suitable method for you.

WHAT IS AN EPIDURAL?

It is a method of relieving pain by injecting painkillers onto the nerves which carry pain messages from the operation wound to the spinal cord. Ordinary painkillers work by passing into the bloodstream and then to the brain where they reduce the feeling of pain. Epidural painkillers work specifically on the nerves from the painful area.

The painkillers are injected onto the nerves as they cross through a space (the epidural space) just outside the spinal cord within your backbone. Because the painkillers wear off after a few hours, a tiny plastic tube is threaded into the epidural space so that repeated doses of painkillers can be given whenever you need them. The tube is taped to your back and is easily and painlessly removed when you no longer need epidural painkillers.

WHEN IS THE EPIDURAL PUT IN?

Usually at the time of your operation. Some operations can be done with epidural painkillers alone. At other times it is better to be asleep, in which case the epidural will be put in just before or just after going off to sleep. Your anaesthetist will explain which is best for you.

WILL I BE ABLE TO FEEL AND MOVE NORMALLY?

During the operation strong painkillers are used which take away all feeling from the operation and also make your muscles weak. It is not safe or pleasant for you to remain as numb as this for long periods after the operation so weaker painkillers

Figure 33.6 *Patient information booklet on epidural analgesia.*

technique. Selected patients will need HDU/ITU support.[28] Cardiac and respiratory complications are common in these high-risk cases, so careful selection is appropriate.[12]

Percutaneous nephrolithotomy

One of the major advances in renal stone surgery is percutaneous nephrolithotomy (PCN), which is undertaken by a radiologist and a urologist in tandem. It usually lasts between 1 and 2 hours with the patient placed prone. Positioning patients prone and returning them supine requires particular care, and there are risks of pressure sores, nerve and neck injuries, eye damage, removal of lines and extubation during the process. A trolley and table are needed to achieve this. Respiration may be compromised when the patient is prone despite mechanical ventilation unless the diaphragm is allowed free excursion by using pillows.[29] It is unusual that absorption of are used afterwards. For the first hour or two after your operation the strong drugs may still be making your legs numb and weak but this effect will soon wear off. After this, the weaker drugs will treat the pain but should leave you able to feel "touch" and to move normally.

HOW OFTEN ARE THE DRUGS GIVEN?

Usually a continuous infusion ("drip") of painkiller will be given via a pump for the first night after your operation. After this, we often allow you to control the amount of painkiller. Different people need different amounts so this allows you to get it just right for you.

HOW DO I CONTROL IT?

The nurse looking after you will show you how to get a dose of painkiller by pressing a button attached to the epidural pump.

HOW OFTEN SHOULD I USE IT?

Press the button when you feel pain from your operation wound. Do not wait until the pain becomes severe. The painkiller can take 10-20 minutes to "soak in" to the nerves so it is best to press the button as soon as you start to get uncomfortable. The epidural tube is specially positioned beside the nerves from the area of your operation so that it relieves this pain very effectively. It cannot, of course, treat pains elsewhere. If you have any other pains, inform the nurse or doctor and they will arrange suitable treatment. Occasionally, the painkiller spreads more to the nerves on one side of your body. If this happens, the staff will show you how to position yourself with the sore side downwards so that gravity helps the painkiller to spread where it is needed.

CAN I OVERDOSE MYSELF?

The epidural pump is programmed to prevent you giving yourself another dose of painkiller before the previous does has had time to soak in. However, because some people are more sensitive than others to the effects of the painkiller, it is possible to give yourself more than is necessary to relieve your pain. This may make you feel dizzy or make your legs feel weak. If this should happen, call your nurse and the anaesthetist will adjust the dose for you.

WHAT ARE THE SIDE EFFECTS?

Dizziness and heaviness of the legs can occur if too much painkiller is used. This is unusual and is rapidly put right by adjusting the dose.

The epidural may numb the nerves to your bladder and make it more difficult for you to pass urine. Your operation may make it necessary for you to have a tube (catheter) draining your bladder anyway. If you do not have a catheter, the nurses will encourage you to pass urine regularly.

Rarely, a headache can occur for a few days after an epidural.

WHAT ARE THE BENEFITS OF EPIDURAL PAIN RELIEF?

An epidural allows painkillers to be delivered right to the nerves from your operation wound. This usually gives very good pain relief with fewer of the side effects such as drowsiness and sickness which may occur with conventional strong painkillers.

In some people, epidural analgesia is so effective that they feel no pain at all. More commonly, there is a little discomfort at times but overall pain relief is rated as excellent by most patient.

Epidural analgesia improves blood circulation to the legs and is therefore beneficial after certain operations to relieve blocked blood vessels.

HOW LONG WILL I NEED THE EPIDURAL?

Usually for at least 48 hours after your operation. After this, tablets may be sufficient. However, if the pain is still too strong for tablets or if you are unable to take tablets because you have had a stomach operation, the epidural can be continued for up to a week.

Whilst you are having epidural analgesia, you will be visited at least twice daily by the Acute Pain Sister and/or Anaesthetist who will check that you are happy with your pain relief. If you have any further questions about epidural analgesia, they will be happy to answer them.

Figure 33.6 cont'd

excessive irrigation fluid or hypothermia occurs unless the procedure is prolonged. Infection is an ever-present threat.[30]

WHEN IT GOES SUDDENLY WRONG

Myocardial events

These can arise at any phase of the operative day, including preinduction. The most likely serious complications are myocardial infarction, pulmonary oedema and protracted shock. Surgery should be stopped as soon as it is safe to do so. Each individual component requires specific support and admission to a coronary care unit or ICU after stabilization. It is unusual to have an elective patient die on the operating table. Myocardial infarction may be silent and, unless looked for, missed. ECG changes and, specifically, elevated tropinon T should be used to screen high-risk cases, and patients identified within 12 hours should be given thrombolytic therapy.[31]

Pulmonary oedema is often discovered only on awakening the patient; fluid overload from IV or irrigation fluids, and myocardial events are the most likely causes. Institution of mechanical ventilation, diuretics and inotropic support of the heart are required during the acute crises. Persistent shock may result from excessive bleeding or from any of the cardiac events stated above. The implications of a persistent low mean arterial pressure (MAP) of <70 mmHg are cerebral, renal and coronary artery hypoperfusion and hypoxia with potentially irreversible damage. Arrythmias are quite common in theatre and may arise postoperatively, but they may be life-threatening on occasion. Many patients have arrythmias on the operating table, and they are predisposed to them by all types of pre-existing heart disease, electrolyte abnormalites, some medications, such as $\alpha_1$agonists, central lines, chest drains, and anaesthesia and surgery. Infection, hypoxia and shock are common causes of arrythmia after surgery. It is important to distinguish what the actual rhythmn is with a 12-lead ECG and treat as appropriate.[32]

Transurethral resection (TUR) syndrome[33]

Absorption of excessive 1.5% glycine irrigation fluid, which has an osmolality of 220 mOsmol/L, will result in dilutional hyponatraemia and fluid overload. It is most commonly associated with transurethral resection of the prostate. The inclusion of an ethanol marker in the irrigation fluid allows detection of excessive absorption by the exhaled ethanol concentration.[34] Irrigation fluids are electrolyte free, resulting in capillary transfer of fluids, and lead to a low serum sodium level of <120 mmol/L, and glycine is a neuroinhibitor. The results of this are a spectrum of clinical effects, ranging from a confusional state, to cerebral oedema, encephalopathy and grand mal fits. Early measurement of the serum sodium will result in the diagnosis, after which the patient must be transferred to an ICU for mechanical ventilation to support the respiratory and cardiovascular systems and the brain. The use of hypertonic saline to counteract the hyponatraemia is not proven, though case reports exist, and normal saline plus diuretics is just as effective. The aim is to raise the serum sodium slowly until the symptoms disappear.

Respiratory failure (Figures 33.7 and 33.8)

Inadequate reversal of anaesthesia or failure to wake up are matters dealt with in the recovery room. They may, however, lead to difficulties, such as hypoxia and aspiration, which, if unresolved, place the patient's life in jeopardy. These patients will need at the least HDU support while the situation is monitored. The failure to regain a cough reflex must lead

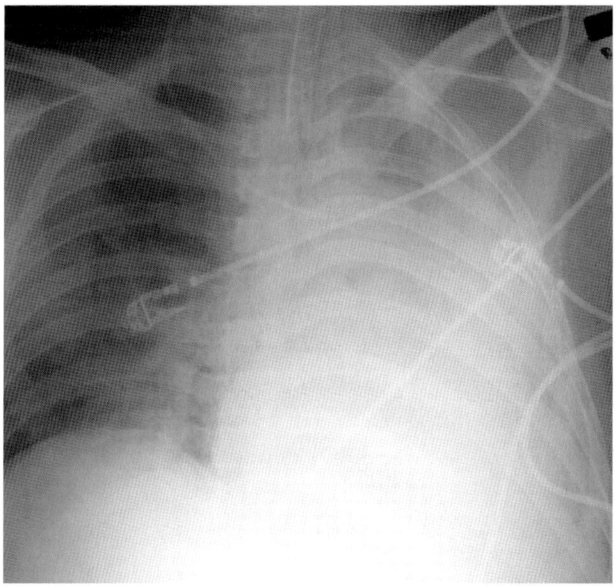

Figure 33.7 *Massive atelectasis. A white-out of the left lung due to a 'plug' of secretions in left main bronchus following major surgery.*

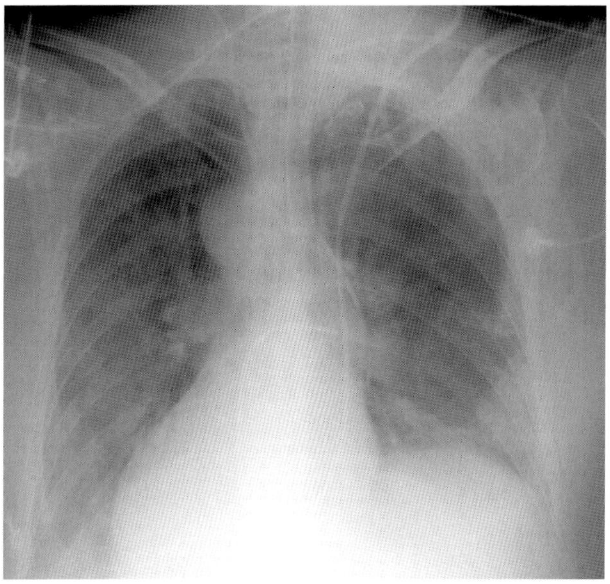

Figure 33.8 *Snowstorm that could be due to pulmonary oedema, infection or acute respiratory distress syndrome (ARDS).*

to reintubation, with a view to early tracheostomy. Aspiration pneumonia is a sinister condition that, if unresolved early, carries a high mortality.[35] Abdominal surgery will result in atelectasis of 50% of the lung in all patients, irrespective of pre-existing lung disease, and in respiratory complications in up to 25%.[36,37] Recovery takes up to 3 days; during this period, pneumonia, atelectasis, and arrythmias precipitated by hypoxia are potential problems.[38] Epidural anaesthesia is beneficial in reducing this incidence.[19] Nursing in an upright position, oxygen, adequate analgesia, careful fluid balance and chest physiotherapy all contribute to the well-rehearsed plan to get the patient safely through this period. Antibiotics should be given as indicated.

Allergic reactions[39]

About 5% of the population is allergic. The risk of developing an allergy from a drug is about 1–3%. The majority of such reactions develop in normal people, are dose dependent and are predictable from the drug's pharmacology. Factors such as overdose, drug toxicity and drug interactions need consideration. Histamine is the main mediator for such reactions. Patients with a history of atopy, asthma and previous reactions are at increased risk. Anaesthesia involves giving in a serial manner a number of drugs with a penchant for histamine release. Blood, colloids, latex, muscle relaxants and antibiotics are common agents implicated in allergic reactions. Clinical features of anaphylaxis may be obscured by anaesthesia, but unexplained cardiovascular collapse, bronchospasm, skin changes, and flushing and oedema are common features of anaphylaxis. The management is to give oxygen, resuscitate with fluids and adrenaline (epinephrine) and then hydrocortisone. About 90% of patients will respond quickly and survive if treated correctly.

Septic shock[40]

Unexplained hypotension following instrumentation may herald the onset of rigors, pyrexia and shock. The features can be non-specific, mild and overlooked. Oxygen, fluids and antibiotics can interrupt the potential downhill course in the majority of cases, but, once established, a 50% mortality rate is predictable.[9] Sepsis is a systemic inflammatory response to infection caused by any class of organisms or their toxins in the bloodstream.[40] Full-blown sepsis picture includes a core temperature of <36°C or >38°C, a white cell count of >12 000 cells/mm^3 or <4000 cells/m^3, a pulse of >90 beats/min, a Pa_{CO_2} of <4.3 kPa or a respiratory rate of >20 breaths per min. A high index of suspicion is needed, as blood cultures are confirmatory in only about 10% of cases. When coupled with a systolic pressure of <90 mmHg despite adequate fluid resuscitation, the risk to the patient's life increases markedly. Septic shock requires transfer to a HDU for invasive monitoring, continued high oxygen administration and aggressive inotropic support with noradrenaline (norepinephrine).[9] ICU transfer is indicated if multiorgan failure develops.

ACKNOWLEDGEMENTS

I have reproduced the routine charts used in our department, and thank the staff who were involved in their production.

REFERENCES

1. Ramsey LE, Williams B, Johnston GD, MacGregor GA et al. British Hypertension Society guidelines for hypertension management 1999: summary. BMJ 1999; 319: 630–635
2. Howell SJ, Sear YM, Yeates D. Risk factors for cardiovascular death after elective surgery under general anaesthesia. Br J Anaesth 1998; 80: 14–19
3. Forrest JB, Rehder K, Cahalan MK, Goldsmith CH. Multicentre study of general anaesthesia. III. Predictors of severe perioperative adverse outcomes. Anesthesiology 1992; 76: 3–15
4. Young Y, Jones GJ. Preoperative evaluation of the patient with cardiovascular disease–risk assessment outcome. In: Prys-Roberts C, Brown BR, eds. International Practice of Anaesthesia. London: Butterworths, 1996: ch. 41
5. Sim K, Morgan C. Pathophysiology of pulmonary disease relevant to anaesthesia. In: Prys-Roberts C, Brown BR, eds. International Practice of Anaesthesia. London: Butterworths, 1996: ch. 64
6. Kroenke K, Laurence VA, Theroux JF, Tuley MR. Operative risk in patients with severe obstructive airways disease. Arch Intern Med 1992; 152: 967–971

7. Drugs in the peri-operative period. II. Corticosteroids and therapy for diabetes mellitus. Drugs Ther Bull 1999; 37: 68–70
8. Bell J, Hockaday TDRC. Diabetes mellitus. In: Weatherill DJ, Ledingham JGG, Warrell DA, eds. Oxford Textbook of Medicine. Oxford: Oxford University Press, 1996: Ch 11.11
9. Ryan DW. Septicaemia and shock. Eur Urol 1999; 35/2 [Curric Urol 2.1: 3–7]
10. American Society of Anesthesiologists. New classification of physical status. Anesthesiology 1963; 24: 111
11. Goldman DL, Caldera DL, Nussbaum SR, Southwick FS et al. Multifactorial index of cardiac risk in non-cardiac patients. N Engl J Med 1977; 297: 845–850
12. Gray AJG, Hoile RW, Ingram GS, Sherry KM. The report of the National Confidential Enquiry into perioperative deaths 1996/1997. London: National CEPOD, 1998: Urology, 75–78
13. Older P, Hall A, Hader R. Cardiopulmonary exercise testing as a screening test for perioperative management of major surgery in the elderly. Chest 1999; 116: 355–362
14. THRIFT Consensus Group. Risk and prophylaxis for venous thromboembolism in hospital patients. BMJ 1992; 305: 567–574
15. Sorenson RM, Pace NL. Mortality and morbidity of regional versus general anaesthesia: a meta-analysis. Anesthesiology 1991; 75: A1053
16. Hendolin H, Mattila MAK, Poikalainen E. The effect of lumbar epidural analgesia on the development of deep vein thrombosis of the legs after open prostatectomy. Acta Chir Scand 1981; 147: 425–429
17. Tuman KJ, McCarthy RJ, March RJ, De Lanria GA et al. Effects of epidural anaesthesia on coagulation and outcome after major vascular surgery. Anesth Analg 1991; 73: 696–704
18. Yeager MR, Glass DD, Neff RK. Epidural anaesthesia and analgesia in high risk surgical cases. Anesthesiology 1987; 66: 729–736
19. Rodgers A, Walker N, Schug S et al. Reduction of postoperative mortality and morbidity with epidural or spinal anaesthesia: results from overview of randomised trials. BMJ 2000; 321: 1493–1497
20. Phillips S, Hutchinson S, Davison T. Preoperative drinking does not affect gastric contents. Br J Anaesthesia 1993; 70: 6–9
21. Drugs in the peri-operative period. III. Hormonal contraceptives and hormone replacement therapy. Drugs Ther Bull 1999; 37: 78–80
22. Drugs in the peri-operative period. I. Stopping or continuing drugs around surgery. Drugs Ther Bull 1999; 37: 62–64
23. Healey TEJ. Baillière's Anaesthesia for day case surgery. Clinical Anaesthesiology. London: Baillière Tindall, 1990: vol. 4
24. Windsor A, French GW, Sear JW, Foex P, Millett SV, Howell SJ. Silent myocardial ischaemia in patients undergoing transurethral prostatectomy. A study to evaluate risk scoring and anaesthetic technique. Anaesthesia 1996; 51: 728–732
25. Smyth R, Cheng D, Asokumar B, Chung F. Coagulopathies in patients after resection of the prostate: spinal versus general anaesthesia. Anesth Analg 1995; 81: 680–685
26. Abrams P, Shah PJ, Bryning K et al. Blood loss during transurethral resection of prostate. Anaesthesia 1982; 37: 71–73
27. Gehring H, Nahm W, Baerwald J et al. Irrigation fluid absorption during transurethral resection of the prostate: spinal vs general anaesthesia. Acta Anaesthesiol Scand 1999; 43: 458–463
28. Ryan DW. Anaesthesia for cystectomy. A comparison of two techniques. Anaesthesia 1982; 37: 554–560
29. Anderton J. The prone position for the surgical patient: a historical review of the principles and hazards. Br J Anaesth 1991; 67: 452–463
30. Artagnan A, Milon D, Corbel L et al. Expérience acquisé en anesthésie et reanimation peri-operatoire dans la nephrolithotomie percutanée. Attitude actuelle dans la traitement endoscopique de la lithiase et de l'anomalie de la jonction pyeloureterale. Prog Urol 1994; 4: 56–62
31. French JK, Williams BF, Hart HH, Wyatt S et al. Prospective evaluation of eligibility for thrombolytic therapy in acute myocardial infarct. BMJ 1996; 312: 1637–1641
32. Atlee JL, Bosnjck ZJ. Mechanisms for cardiac dysrhythmias during anaesthesia. Anesthesiology 1990; 72: 347–374
33. Krane RJ, Siroky MB. Transurethral resection syndrome. In: Fitzpatrick JM, Krane RJ, eds. The Prostate. Edinburgh: Churchill Livingstone, 1989: ch. 21
34. Heide C, Weninger E, Ney L et al. Early detection of TUR syndrome-ethanol measurement in ventilated patients. Anaesth Intensivmed Notfallmed Schmerzther 1997; 32: 610–615
35. Bellingham GJ. Aspiration and inhalation. In: Webb AR, Shapiro MJ, Singer M, Suter PM, eds. Oxford

Textbook of Critical Care. Oxford: Oxford University Press, 1999: 2.61, 79–81
36. Hedenstierna G, Rothen HU. Pulmonary exchange, effects of anaesthesia and of artificial ventilation. In: Prys Roberts C, Brown JR, eds. International Practice of Anaesthesia. London: Butterworths, 1996: ch. 60
37. Pereira ED, Fernandes AL, da Silva Ancao M, de Arauja Pereres C, Attallah AN, Faresin SM. Prospective complications of postoperative pulmonary complications in patients submitted to upper abdominal surgery. Sao Paulo Med J 1999; 117: 151–160
38. Wetterslev J, Hansen EG, Kamp-Jensen M, Roikjaer O, Kanstrup IL. Pa_{O_2} during anaesthesia and years of smoking predict late postoperative hypoxaemia and complications after upper abdominal surgery in patients without preoperative cardiopulmonary dysfunction. Acta Anaesthesiol Scand 2000; 44: 9–16
39. Levy JH. Preoperative considerations of the allergic patient. In: Levy JH, ed. Anaphylactic reactions in anaesthesia and intensive care, 2nd edn. London: Butterworth, 1989: ch. 7
40. American College of Chest Physicians/Society of Critical Care Medicine Consensus Conference. Definitions for septicaemia and organ failure and guidelines for the use of innovative therapies in sepsis. Crit Care Med 1992; 20: 864–874

34

Screening in urology

Nicholas J R George

Screening has been defined as the identification of unrecognized disease or defect by the application of tests, examinations or other procedures that can be applied rapidly. The process may be broadly divided into 'one-shot' screening exercises and procedures applied to chronic diseases or conditions which may be repeated at intervals. The second category may be further subdivided into mass screening, selective screening and case finding. In the context of urological surgery, the debate concerning screening programmes chiefly concerns the search for chronic disease, typically urological neoplasia, usually by means of case finding or, at best, selective screening programmes.

'ONE-SHOT' SCREENING

One-off screening procedures are most frequently employed to detect defects typified by congenital malformation or inherited metabolic disorders, such as phenylketonuria and galactosaemia, for which treatment is available. Screening for disorders which are untreatable has been generally avoided (see Fundamentals of screening, page 609), although this basic concept has recently been challenged.[1] Programmes involving sophisticated tests for rare diseases[2,3] may not, at a superficial glance, seem cost-effective; however, the long-term costs of supporting the patient to adulthood with undetected disease may be the crucial factor in determining public-health policy.

SCREENING FOR CHRONIC DISEASE

Mass screening

Mass screening is the identification of preclinical disease within the population by procedures that have been carefully assessed and validated as part of public health policy.

Mass-screening programmes demand a precise cost–benefit analysis closely linked to the ethical and cultural ethos of the country and government concerned. In general, programmes initiated by the departments of health in the West address only health issues that are both common and, at least in part, preventable, such as heart disease or certain types of neoplasia. Within this politico-medical process, certain groups, such as young women with disease, inevitably attract more political support than other groups such as older men with disease.

Selective screening

In an attempt to boost the effectiveness of screening programmes in relation to cost, the specified test may be directed at selected groups within the overall population. In fact, nearly all programmes are selective in terms of age and sex, as in the case of breast-cancer screening, where high-risk groups of women are targeted in terms of age and menopausal status.

Genetic and racial variables are further examples of factors that may be selectively targeted in screening programmes. Within urology, the risks of prostate cancer are known to be increased in certain families with a history of the disease, and epidemiological studies clearly demonstrate the differing racial incidence of the disease both worldwide and, most dramatically, within the USA itself.

Selective screening may also be undertaken by targeting groups exposed to various industrial or social risks. The lifelong follow-up of workers from aniline dye factories and the association of various diseases with heavy smoking are examples of this type of selectivity.

Case finding

Case finding is widely interpreted as 'screening' by both the general public and the medical profession. In essence, case finding is no more than sporadic attempts by interested doctors and patients to detect disease or establish that disease is not present. As will be described below, chronic urological disease does not, in general, attain criteria sufficient to support full public-health screening programmes. In the absence of such programmes – often interpreted by critics as a 'lack of interest' by the Department of Health – case finding becomes the predominant mode of preclinical disease identification, usually widely, and often inaccurately, reported by both the lay and medical press. Case finding is, however, a genuine and valid attempt by concerned doctors and patients to solve a medical dilemma, but the process should not be confused with scientifically designed and validated mass screening programmes.

In this chapter, the issues and principles of screening will be described in general terms. The process will then be analysed with reference to the generally accepted criteria for screening, and finally the application of these principles to chronic urological disease will be discussed.

LIFETIME EVENTS AND SCREENING TERMINOLOGY

When mass screening programmes for chronic diseases are developed, it is common practice to describe episodes that occur during the patient's lifetime by an accepted terminology which describes and defines the evolving events up to the point of death. These lifetime periods may be illustrated as in Figure 34.1.

Assuming initial health, the first event is the initiation of a biological disease process. This continues until, in the absence of a screening programme, symptoms appear, leading to presentation and eventual clinical diagnosis.

The time from disease initiation to clinical diagnosis is defined as the *total preclinical phase* (TPCP).[4] Clearly, the TPCP is a theoretical concept, as the time at which the disease is initiated can never be known with certainty; indeed, with reference to neoplasia, it is likely that multiple events are required to establish the cancerous process, making it almost impossible to define precisely the start time of the disease.

If a mass screening test has been developed for a disease, it becomes possible to detect its presence

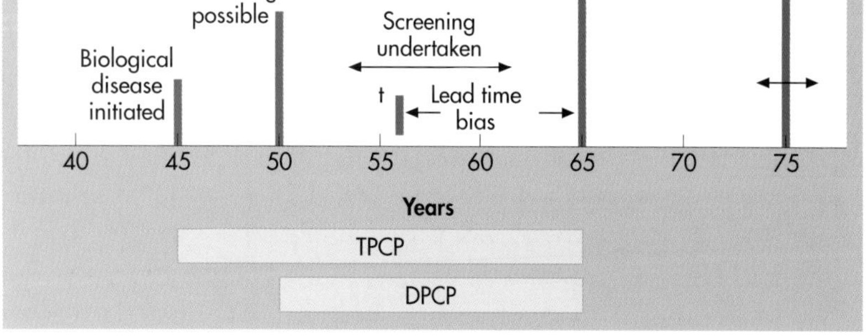

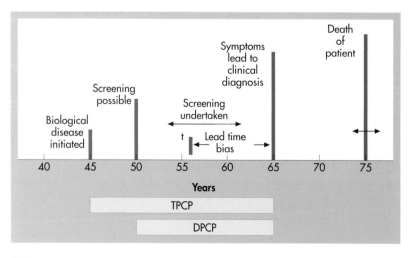

Figure 34.1 *Lifetime events and terminology of screening programmes. DPCP: detectable preclinical phase; TPCP: total preclinical phase. Depending on the sensitivity of the test, screening may be undertaken at any time t during the DPCP. Lead-time bias is defined as the time between the initiation of the test and the time of symptomatic clinical presentation. The death of the patient may occur earlier or later, depending on whether the screening process is harmful or beneficial to the individual.*

during the total preclinical phase. The period between the earliest time at which the disease is detectable by the test and the time at which clinical symptoms become apparent is defined as the *detectable preclinical phase* (DPCP), also known as the 'sojourn time'.[5] Clearly, the length of the DPCP depends on the sensitivity of the screening test, and this is likely to be different for each disease under consideration. It is also apparent that different forms of screening tests for any one disease will be associated with different DPCP times; thus, breast self-examination will have a shorter DPCP than mammography, and digital rectal examination will have a shorter DPCP than a prostate-specific antigen (PSA) screening test. Naturally, the effectiveness of any proposed mass screening programme will be determined by the ratio of DPCP to TPCP – the longer the detectable phase, the more effective the programme. Occasionally, DPCP is mistakenly understood to stand for *precancerous phase*. This is misleading, as a variable portion of the correctly defined DPCP may be related to invasive (that is, not precancerous) yet asymptomatic cancerous growth. Hence, screening for diseases which have a significant invasive asymptomatic period during the DPCP (perhaps breast) is likely to be less effective than screening for diseases with extensive non-invasive periods during the DPCP (perhaps prostate).

The detection of disease during the DPCP by the screening test itself results in difficulties when attempts are made to judge the effectiveness of any single programme. The time between the positive result of the screening test and the time at which clinical symptoms would have appeared is defined as the *lead-time bias*. It will be evident that if treatment for the disease is ineffective, the patient will die at the same point as if it had originally been detected because of clinical symptoms. Survival, however, will apparently have been increased by the amount of time between the positive screening test and the clinical presentation; hence, it is necessary to account for lead-time bias when assessing the efficacy of screening for any particular disease.[6] For severe chronic disease such as cancer, the elimination of lead-time bias is best achieved by randomized, controlled trials of the screening programme, as described below.

The death of the patient is an event which is determined by the severity of the disease and the efficacy of treatment. As noted above, it is necessary to demonstrate that a screening programme results in prolonged survival after lead-time bias and other distortions have been taken into account. It should not be forgotten that screening programmes may also lead to a shortening of the patient's life – if, for instance, death occurs due to septicaemia following transrectal biopsy for presumed prostate cancer suspected on the basis of a screening test, the programme (depending on the frequency of the complication) will be judged as being of questionable value with regard to public health.

A further distortion that may be observed when mass screening for chronic disease is described as *length bias*.[7] In the case of neoplasia, different tumours grow at different rates, and, thus, fast-growing cancers are characterized by a short DPCP. A screening test undertaken during the DPCP will of necessity detect more slow-growing cancers than fast-growing cancers (Figure 34.2); thus, the disease so detected will have a more favourable outcome than the disease detected by standard clinical tests. This length-bias effect may be reduced by repeat screening, but once again it can be seen that improved prognosis in the screening group may not necessarily be related to a real improvement in survival for the disease in question.

It is often difficult to persuade the general public – and occasionally the medical profession – that earlier detection of disease is not automatically associated with a better prognosis. Figures 34.1 and 34.2 well illustrate the complexity of the issues raised when mass screening is undertaken for chronic disease.

FUNDAMENTALS OF SCREENING

Before describing other issues concerned with mass-screening programmes, one should emphasize that there are certain situations in which it is not possible or necessary to offer a screening test.

1. If there is no preclinical phase (TPCP), it is clearly not possible to offer a test which can detect that phase of disease.
2. If there is no possible treatment for the disease, conventional wisdom suggests that screening

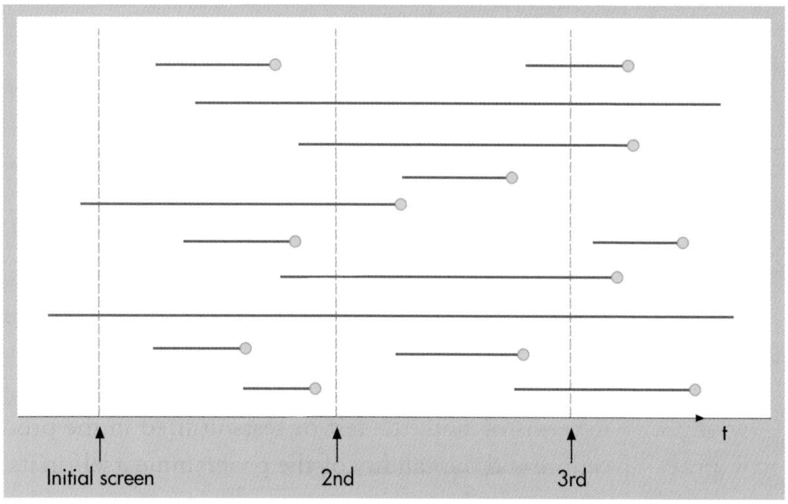

Figure 34.2 *Length bias. Solid lines indicate duration of detectable preclinical phase. Biologically active tumours develop and present more quickly than indolent tumours which progress over long periods of time. Some tumours may never present clinically. Screening events (vertical dotted lines) automatically select a preponderance of the more indolent tumours (see references 20 and 21).*

should not be offered, as, by definition, no improvement in morbidity and mortality will be achieved. Interestingly this principle has recently been questioned in relation to 'single-shot' screening of the newborn for rare inherited disorders. Duchenne's muscular dystrophy is an X-linked lethal disorder of delayed onset with no effective treatment. It has been argued[8] that screening for the disease should be undertaken on the grounds that it would lessen parental distress by alerting them to risks before the disease became apparent in their older children. Clearly, such a proposition raises highly complex ethical arguments which need to be carefully considered before any such programme could be adopted.[1]

3. If it is possible to cure a disease when it presents clinically, there is no need to offer a screening test for the disease. Examples of neoplastic diseases which conform to this definition are clearly few and far between, but testicular tumour might be cited as an example of a cancer curable if efficiently detected in stage one by the patient himself.

ETHICAL CONSIDERATIONS AND ATTITUDES TO SCREENING

It will be realized that in a mass screening programme for disease very different forces are at work which depend on individual expectation of the enterprise. It is often assumed that satisfactory outcomes would, by definition, be acceptable to everybody concerned with the programme. To assess this matter, it is necessary to look at any screening programme from the point of view of both the Department of Health 'the screener', and the individual member of the general public, 'the screenee', who is required to undertake the specified test.

The attitude and perspective of those offering a mass screening programme – usually the Department of Health – are principally influenced by their primary directive to improve the health of the nation as a whole. The screener does *not* promise or imply that every individual screened will be better off as a result of taking the test, although this point is rarely emphasized in the accompanying publicity that suggests that 'screening must be good for you'. In this context, the death of a patient following prostatic biopsy (as noted above) would be an acceptable if regrettable incident were mass screening for prostate cancer to be established as a beneficial programme for the nation as a whole. The individual suffering disadvantage, as inevitably occurs in the best-validated screening programmes, will have a different perspective on the matter. The dichotomy between these two points of view is in part related to the generalized belief noted above that early diagnosis must be good – 'catch the disease early'. It is perhaps understandable how this entrenched view of health and disease may lead to disappointment both for the screener[9] and the screenee who suffers an adverse event following the screening test.

Cost issues are also a major factor for those considering ways of improving the public health. In developing countries, it is by no means certain that screening for certain diseases would be of greater advantage to the population than money put into other aspects of public health such as water supplies and sewage systems. In the West, cost–benefit analysis raises highly complex issues requiring scientific resolution, often in an atmosphere made obscure by the prominent opinions of vested-interest groups. An example, discussed below, is the present controversy surrounding prostate-cancer screening. Critical analysis of mortality figures clearly shows that this disease, compared to others affecting the younger male population, is a relatively insignificant problem, but these economic facts have failed to curtail the debate, which is occupying a significant part of the medical and lay press at the present time.

The expectations and aspirations of those screened are very different. Persons selected by a programme or those who elect to go to their general practitioner naturally hope that disease will *not* be detected. Asymptomatic persons who visit their practitioner do so in the expectation that they will be found to be healthy – what normal person would attend a physician in the expectation that cancer would be found? The screener is looking for disease, but the screenee expects a healthy outcome. These attitudes explain in part the problems that occur when a screening test 'goes wrong' – when either the test induces morbidity or the test reveals disease. Success or failure of the process is a value judgement based on point of view. In practice, of course, the vast majority of people who undergo screening tests are found to be negative (true negative – see below). When diseases are of low prevalence, a negative predictive value is both very accurate and very reassuring for the person concerned. A negative screening test for a rare but serious disease is, in fact, one of the greatest benefits that can accrue from a screening programme.

Ethical considerations in screening programmes are of major importance both to health departments and to the population as a whole. Clinicians readily acknowledge ethical problems in routine medical practice, but in this case the patients have almost invariably sought the help of the physician to deal with their disease. In the case of mass screening, selected people who consider themselves to be healthy have been approached by physicians on behalf of the Department of Health and asked to undertake tests which, as has been seen, will usually, but not necessarily, be of benefit to them. Initiation of the screening process deems that the ethical burden on the screener is as great or greater than that resting on colleagues in clinical medicine.

VALIDITY OF SCREENING

Conventionally, the validity of screening is measured in terms of both the test or tests utilized in the procedure and the validity of the programme itself in its entirety. Each of these aspects may be measured by means of two indicators. Sensitivity relates to the positive identification of preclinical disease, and specificity is associated with establishment of healthy persons within the general population. Naturally, the validity of screening in terms of sensitivity and specificity can be known only if the true disease rate in the population is known – a follow-up diagnostic test is required to confirm or refute the result of the screening test.

The validity of screening tests

In terms of the test, sensitivity is defined as the percentage of persons with a positive test among those who are later found to have the disease. Specificity is defined as the percentage of persons screening negative among people who are genuinely free of disease. The relationship between the indicators and the presence or absence of disease is usually depicted as in Table 34.1. As noted above, the calculations demand that an independent diagnostic test is able to determine which of the screened population has or does not have the disease itself. It has already been seen that application of this diagnostic test may induce significant morbidity in persons who are otherwise genuinely well. Sensitivity is the ratio between true positives and true positives with false negatives. Specificity is the ratio between true negatives and false positives with true negatives.

It is unusual for the screening test itself to demarcate exactly between those with and without disease. Almost invariably, the population groups (healthy and diseased) overlap considerably; hence, variably

Table 34.1 Possible outcomes of screening examinations.

Screening test result	Diagnosis	
	Disease present	Disease absent
Positive	a (True positive)	b (False positive)
Negative	c (False negative)	d (True negative)

Sensitivity = a/a + c; Specificity = d/b + d; Positive predictive value = a/a + b; Negative predictive value = d/c + d.

specified test results will give rise to different levels of calculated sensitivity and specificity.

Conventionally, these difficulties are depicted by means of a bimodal graph, as illustrated in Figure 34.3. The screening test scale is shown on the horizontal axis, and the distribution of the healthy and diseased populations overlaps to a greater or lesser extent. Selection of different discriminant values of the test results (known as the 'cut-off point') demonstrates the *inverse association* between the sensitivity and specificity of the screening test. Selection of cutoff point A determines that the test will have high sensitivity and low specificity – all those with the disease will be identified by the test, but a high proportion without disease will also be identified (false positive). Altering the cutoff point to B results in a test with low sensitivity but high specificity – a small number of persons with the disease are missed (false negative), although the great majority of people without disease are correctly identified as screen negative.

Selection of an appropriate cutoff point and hence particular values of sensitivity and specificity is a complex process involving considerable degrees of subjective judgement related to the disease in question. Some disorders, such as cervical cancer, can afford a high sensitivity for the screening test, as diagnostic clinical confirmation is reliable and relatively inexpensive, while in others, high specificity would be of greater desirability. Value judgements concerning the disease in question, the cost of diagnostic tests and its place in society are required, and the results of such judgements will determine the levels of false-positive and false-negative screening tests that will be tolerated.

Urologists well appreciate the effect a variable cutoff may have on the sensitivity and specificity of disease. Difficulties in calculating effective 'cutoffs' for prostate cancer 'screening' have been widely reported, and the advent of newer, more sophisticated PSA tests ('free and bound') have not lessened the debate on the ideal discriminant value between benign and malignant disease.

A further attempt to refine and optimize values of sensitivity and specificity involves the construction of a receiver operating characteristic (ROC) curve. Such curves can be drawn if the screening test result is both quantitative and variable. Sensitivity on the vertical axis and 1/- specificity on the horizontal axis are plotted for a range of values (Figure 34.4), and the optimal point is that which lies furthest from the diagonal. Although, strictly speaking, ROC curves are difficult to construct for subjective tests such as digital rectal examination, this form of analysis reinforces the impression that PSA is the best predictor of the presence of prostatic carcinoma.[10]

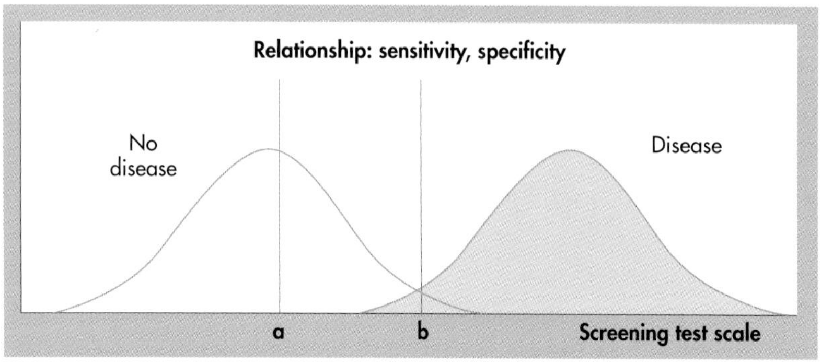

Figure 34.3 *Sensitivity and specificity of a screening test and the effect of variation of the cutoff value. (a) High sensitivity, low specificity; (b) low sensitivity, high specificity.*

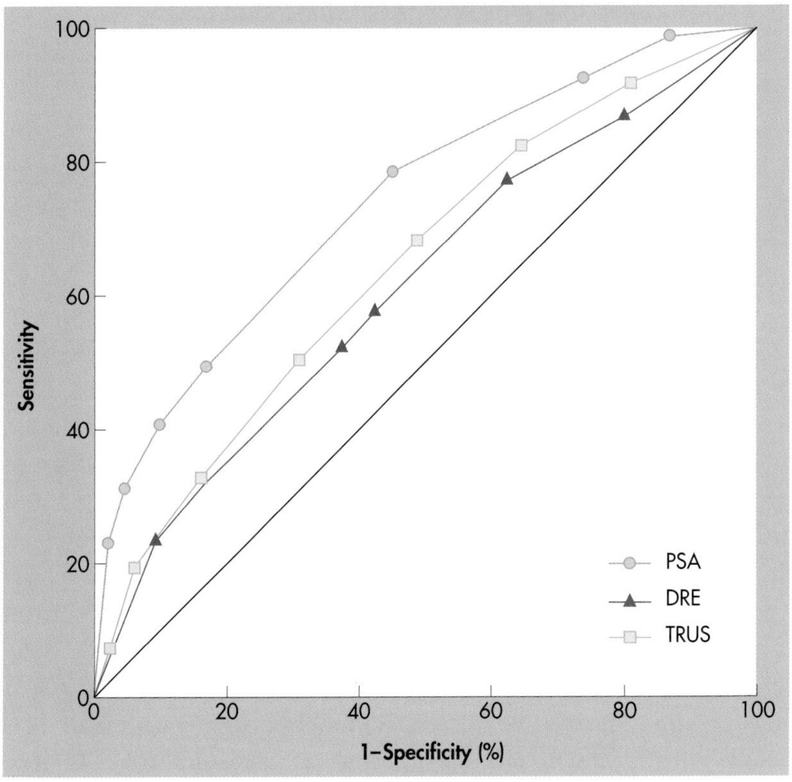

Figure 34.4 *Receiver–operator characteristic curve for serum prostate-specific antigen, transrectal ultrasonography (TRUS) and digital rectal examination (DRE). Data from Ellis et al.*[10]

Checking the sensitivity of a test

The screening test has already been defined as a measurement which is able to identify disease in the preclinical period (DPCP). Unfortunately, because the true prevalence of disease during this stage must, by definition, be unknown, the sensitivity of the test cannot with certainty be calculated. To overcome this problem, screening tests are occasionally tested on populations with known clinical disease. Experience has shown, however, that this may be highly misleading, in that the test may perform exceptionally well when offered such a relatively gross challenge but will perform indifferently in the true DPCP screening situation. Hence, sensitivity and specificity may vary widely according to the stage of the disease.

A further theoretical approach to the problem of defining sensitivity might be to perform a diagnostic test on every person offered the screening test. Clearly, however, the morbidity of the diagnostic test applied to large numbers of asymptomatic people would preclude this approach on ethical grounds alone. The estimation of test sensitivity therefore rests imperfectly with the test itself and the diagnostic measures that are subsequently undertaken to confirm or deny the presence of disease. The emergence of new clinical cases (called in cancer screening programmes 'interval cancers') from a previously screened population, as well as information gathered from rescreening exercises, eventually leads to a reasonable estimate of the sensitivity of a particular screening test. By contrast, the estimation of specificity is less problematical. As the ratio of people with disease to the general population is usually very low, an accurate estimation may be obtained by calculating the proportion of those testing negative to the sum of those with negative or false-positive tests.

The *predictive value* is an important measure of a screening test of interest to both the screener and the screened population (Table 34.1). A positive predictive value is the proportion of those with preclinical disease relative to those with a positive screening test. A negative predictive value is the proportion of persons who are healthy among the population with a negative test. Predictive values vary and relate not only to the validity of the test itself (see above) but also to the prevalence of the disease in the general population. These effects are illustrated in Table 34.2. A high positive predictive value clearly indicates satisfactory test performance, but as disease prevalence declines, so does the positive predictive value until, with a disease of low prevalence, only a very small percentage of those with a positive test actually have preclinical disease – 2% in the example given in Table 34.2. By contrast, under the same circumstances of low prevalence, a negative test clearly indicates that it is very unlikely indeed that the person has the disease. As has been stated above, this is an ideal result from the point of view of screenees, who have attended in the hope that their impression of good health will be supported by the test.

Effect of repeat screening

It might be expected that disease 'pick-up' rates would be maximal during the first screening exercise and reduced thereafter. Table 34.3 illustrates this effect for early studies involving programmes for cervix, breast and lung cancers. More recently, similar effects have been noted during 'screening' for prostate cancer in the USA where, additionally, the incidence of metastatic disease in bone has fallen steadily, perhaps indicating detection of disease earlier in the DPCP.

PROGRAMME VALIDITY

The performance of the screening test itself is naturally but one part of the overall efficacy of any particular screening programme. Other factors which will be crucial to the outcome of the enterprise include the screening request response rate, the interval between screens and the ability accurately to process those people found to be screen positive. Most recently, in the UK, such problems have been vividly illustrated in the case of screening for cervical carcinoma. Allegedly inexperienced and underfunded laboratories have led to significant doubts concerning the interpretation of large numbers of smear tests. Clearly, the efficacy of a programme is no greater than the efficacy of its weakest link.

Overall evaluation of a screening programme depends therefore not only on sensitivity and specificity indicators but on the entire screening infrastructure and most particularly on outcome measures as judged by objectives laid down at the commencement of the programme. Apart from these problems with infrastructure, resources, diagnostic quality control, and so on, it has been noted that screening programmes contain a degree of bias which may significantly affect outcome measures, such that those persons identified with screen-positive disease will almost invariably survive longer than those detected by standard clinical criteria. Some of these biases have already been mentioned

Table 34.2 The effect of preclinical prevalence of disease on positive and negative predictive values.

Prevalence (%)	Predictive value (%)	
	Positive	Negative
10 (high)	68	99.4
1	16	99.9
0.1 (low)	2	99.99

Sensitivity: specificity: 95%

Table 34.3 The effect of repeat screening on the prevalence of disease.

Cancer	Survey	Prevalence (per 10^3)	
		1st pass	2nd pass
Cervix	Females Age 20+ Rescreen <3 years	3.9	1.3
Breast	Females Age 20–64 Rescreen 1 year	2.7	1.5
Lung	Males Age 40–65 Rescreen 6 months	1.0	0.4

Abstracted from Christopherson (1966), Shapiro (1977) and Brett (1968) [22–24].

but are restated below to emphasize their importance in the overall evaluation of screening programmes:

1. *Lead-time bias* is that proportion of the DPCP by which survival will be increased even if the screening programme has no effect on disease mortality.
2. *Length bias* determines that the screening process will naturally select persons with more indolent or biologically inactive disease. Length bias is most pronounced at the initial screen and is in part mitigated by subsequent screening.
3. *Selection bias*. Despite attempts to screen broad sections of the community, the process itself is inevitably voluntary; thus, those who attend screening programmes are generally more interested in their own personal health than those who refuse. As stated above, these health-conscious people expect to be told that they do not have serious disease and to this end have usually spent their lives avoiding risk factors such as unhealthy diets and smoking. Additionally, even if these persons are found to have disease, their attitude to personal health means that it is likely that they will have a better outcome from the disease than those who neglect themselves.
4. *Over-diagnosis bias*. A number of chronic conditions, particularly cancers, may have a semi-indolent phase which may not lead to clinical disease in the natural lifetime of the patient. Over-diagnosis of this form of disease – perhaps best illustrated by the case of prostate cancer – will again lead to false estimates of survival. This bias can be seen to be an extreme form of length bias, as illustrated in Figure 34.2.

These forms of bias, acting individually and together, almost invariably mean that patients with screen-detected disease survive longer than those detected in the normal way. To eliminate effectively the combined influence of these factors requires a *randomized, controlled trial* of the screening process itself.[9] The basic design for such a trial is illustrated in Figure 34.5. It can be seen that not only is the population randomly allocated to a study or control group, but also all cancers are followed whether screen detected or refusal detected. Although it is generally agreed that randomized trials offer the most objective test of a screening process, ethical issues may prevent establishment of a formalized trial structure. While such trials have been established for prostate cancer (see page 594), these issues may cause significant problems for diseases such as breast cancer, where randomization to the control arm may meet with consumer resistance. To circumvent these problems, a number of complex methodologies has been proposed, the details of which are beyond the scope of this account.

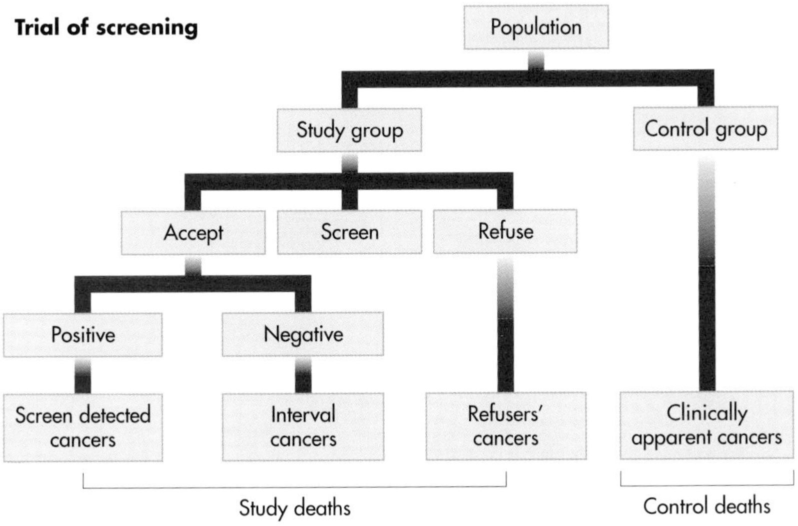

Figure 34.5 *Ideal design of a randomized, controlled trial to evaluate the benefits or otherwise of a screening programme. Refusers: people who refuse to undertake screening tests despite randomization to the screening arm. Interval cancers: cancers arising by conventional clinical symptoms between screening tests.*

SCREENING AND CONTROL OF DISEASE

Screening is but one method of controlling disease in the population. Others include prevention or the application of curative methods once the disease has become manifest. Of these options, screening is a relative newcomer, and its role in the control of mass disease remains somewhat controversial. It is convenient to consider disease control in terms of both mass screening and selective screening.

Encouraged by successes in eliminating chronic inflammatory disease, health departments within the last 25 years have turned their resources towards an attempt to eradicate other chronic diseases such as cancer. However, inspection of mortality-reduction targets shows that screening is expected to contribute only a small proportion of the target total – it has gradually become clear that the complexities and problems involved in mass screening preclude utilization of this methodology as a significant means of disease control.

Several factors underlie this failure to achieve specified goals. The Wilson and Junger criteria (described below) dictate that disease must be common and an important health problem. Yet, careful analysis of mortality data (Figures 34.6 and 34.7) demonstrates clearly that this is often not the case despite public perception to the contrary. Presently, programmes are in place for cervical and breast cancer and certain aspects of cardiovascular disease (hypertension), although organization of programmes varies widely between countries and, within time, in any one country. There remain significant problems related to population compliance. No better example of the discrepancy between expectation and achievement is provided by the prostate cancer 'screening' policy in the USA. Despite enormous publicity and guidelines provided by bodies such as the American Cancer Society, significant screening test take-up rates are to be found only within the Anglo-Saxon population. Take-up within the black community is acknowledged to be low and difficult to achieve. Black men have an incidence of the disease >60% higher than whites and the disease presents at an earlier age,[27] often at a more advanced stage.[28] In a recent study by Catalona investigating high risk populations in Washington, Missouri, only 1200 black men were available to compare with nearly 16,000 whites.[29] It is very clear that, in this group of people, screening is of limited value as a method of disease control.

However, selective screening has been more successful at reducing disease rates in the last few decades. Targeting populations exposed to risk factors such as asbestos and tobacco has been in part successful in reducing disease due to these agents. Nevertheless, prevention strategies are at least as important as a means of disease control. Urine screening of workers who were in the past exposed to aniline dyes continues, but, undoubtedly, the main factor responsible for the reduction in industrial disease-related transitional cell carcinoma is the exclusion of carcinogenic substances from the manufacturing process in the mid-1950s.

In summary, mass screening for chronic disease is effective as a means of disease control in certain carefully defined groups of patients. For the majority, however, other programmes of disease control are required. By contrast, 'single-shot' screening of the newborn is an effective method of disease containment, which, even in the case of rare disease, may prove to be cost-effective in the long term.

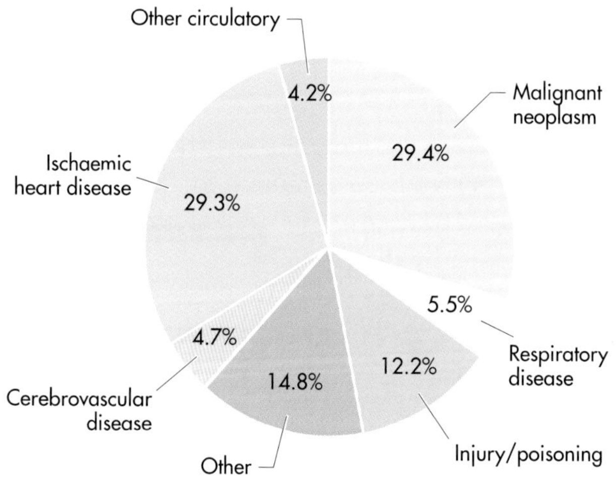

Figure 34.6 *Disease-specific death rates for males in northwest England (1994). In public-health terms, it is observed when viewed in conjunction with Figure 34.7 that mortality due to cardiovascular-related disease far exceeds mortality due to any form of organ-specific cancer. Data from Centre for Cancer Epidemiology, University of Manchester.*

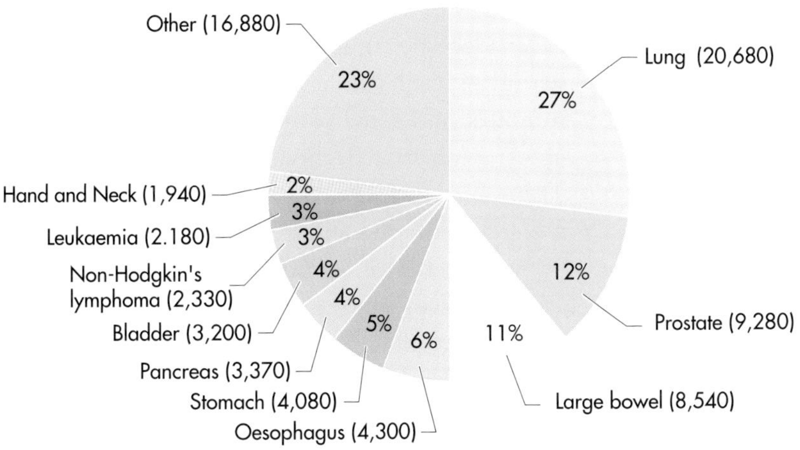

Figure 34.7 *The 10 commonest causes of cancer death in men in the UK (2000). Prostate deaths at any age constitute 12% of the whole. Data from Cancer Research Campaign Factsheet 3, 2002.*[16]

GENERAL PRINCIPLES RELATING SCREENING PROGRAMMES

During the last 30 years, the general principles which underpin a successful screening programme have been analysed and refined. A broad consensus has emerged from individuals and international workshops[11,12] regarding the criteria that should be met to establish a successful screening programme. Of these criteria, the most widely quoted at the present time are those published in the public health papers of the World Health Organization[13] by Wilson and Junger (Table 34.4). It is instructive to discuss each individual principle in turn.

1. *The condition should be an important health problem.* Clearly, this statement refers to the point of view of the health department of the country concerned. Accurate mortality statistics (Figures 34.6 and 34.7) will be required for that country, although these may well reveal that problems considered by the general public to be of major importance may well not be significant in public health terms. Clearly, in the North-West of England, cardiovascular disease is the pre-eminent public-health problem, whereas in males each organ-specific cancer site, with the possible exception of lung, contributes little to the overall picture. For women, breast cancer assumes a significant position in the public-health priority list, not only because of the numbers involved but also because the disease affects younger women whose economic and social lives are important to the nation. By the same token, disorders which affect older men – for example, colorectal and prostate tumours – score less heavily in terms of being an 'important health problem' in the eyes of the Department of Health. The controversy that surrounds prostate cancer screening at the present time is further discussed below.
2. *The natural history of the condition should be adequately understood.* It is naturally very important that the biological progress of the disease should be known with reasonable certainty. This matter is

Table 34.4 Accepted criteria for successful population screening programmes.

1. The condition sought should be an important health problem
2. The natural history of the condition should be adequately understood
3. There should be a detectable latent or preclinical stage
4. A test of suitable sensitivity and specificity should be available
5. There should be an accepted mode of treatment for patients discovered to have the disease
6. Adequate facilities for both diagnosis and treatment should be available
7. The tests must be acceptable to the population
8. The benefits should outweigh any adverse effects of screening
9. The cost of screening must be acceptable in relation to overall medical expenditure
10. Screening for chronic disease is an ongoing process requiring critical analysis and audit of results

From Wilson and Junger (1968).[13]

not always as simple as it might seem. In the case of 'single-shot' antenatal screening for hydronephrosis and urinary tract obstruction, significant numbers of babies with hydronephrosis were detected as the sophistication of interuterine ultrasound increased. Subsequently, it became clear that physiological changes at and after birth restored many of these upper urinary tracts to normal, and it was clear that the 'screening test' was overestimating the incidence of significant pathology in these children. Prostate cancer provides the best example of a chronic condition whose natural history is incompletely understood. Evidence from well-known post-mortem studies from the 1950s indicates that the disease is extremely common in old age – men die 'with' rather than 'of' prostate cancer. The inability to distinguish indolent from aggressive cancers in younger men continues to generate heated debate.

3. *There should be a detectable latent or preclinical stage.* It has already been mentioned that it is impossible, by definition, to perform a screening test on a disease that does not have a detectable preclinical stage. Hence, while cervical dysplasia permits consideration of effective programmes for cervical cancer sputum, cytology and chest X-ray have been found wanting in terms of their ability to reduce mortality from lung cancer.[9]
4. *A test of suitable sensitivity and specificity should be available.* The measures which describe the validity of any particular screening test have been described above, and the difficulties of agreeing an acceptable cutoff point have been emphasized. This problem is particularly well illustrated by reference to PSA and the ability of this marker to distinguish between benign and malignant prostate disease (Figure 34.8). Although 4 ng is generally accepted as an adequate cutoff, significant numbers of men with PSA results under this value are found to have tumours, and some authorities argue that a lower cutoff as illustrated, should be employed.
5. *There should be an accepted mode of treatment for patients discovered to have the disease.* Of course, early diagnosis of an untreatable disease is not a cost-effective public-health policy, although the debate surrounding such conditions as Duchenne's muscular dystrophy has been noted. The proposed treatment should be effective in terms of reducing mortality, and the ideal methodology for evaluation of screening programmes has been described.
6. *Adequate facilities for diagnosis and treatment should be available.* It is self-evident that there is no point in establishing an expensive screening process if facilities to confirm diagnosis and confer treatment are not readily available.
7. *The test must be acceptable to the population.* The poor take-up rate in some screening programmes testifies to the fact that there is a limit to the discomfort which the public is willing to suffer in order to detect asymptomatic disease (from which, in any case, they believe they are not suffering). Mammography is not usually a comfortable procedure, and there is no doubt that in North America the thought of a rectal examination and perhaps transrectal ultrasound is the primary reason for poor attendance at screening sessions by certain segments of society. The paradoxical situation of the Afro-American in the USA has already been mentioned.

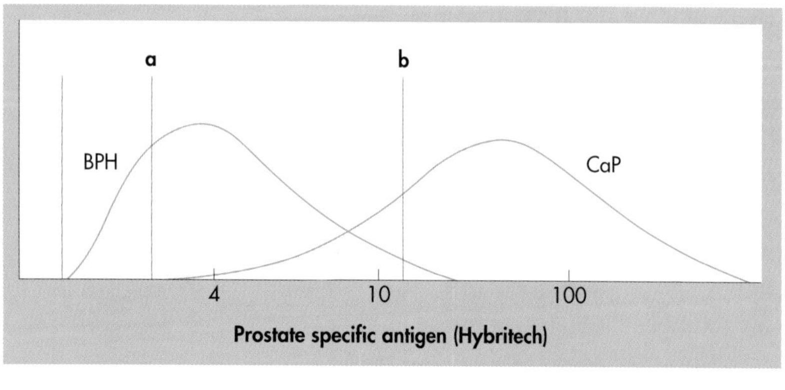

Figure 34.8 *Sensitivity and specificity as applied to prostate-specific antigen testing. Conventionally a cutoff of 4 ng is accepted as the best compromise, although significant numbers of cancers may be identified with PSA values below that level. (a) Theoretical ideal sensitivity, poor specificity; (b) good specificity, unacceptable sensitivity.*

8. *The benefits should outweigh any adverse effect of screening*. 'Benefits' in this context are taken to refer to those as observed from the public-health point of view. Clearly, from the individual standpoint, there may be significant morbidity (and perhaps, rarely, mortality) from a screening test; hence, personally, the individual would be unlikely to recognize any benefit. Judged overall, the benefits to the general population should outweigh the adverse effects within the same population, and outcome measures should indicate a real advantage to the screened populations, ideally in terms of increased survival times.
9. *The cost of screening must be acceptable in relation to overall medical expenditure*. It has been emphasized that screening is but one part of health policy aimed at containing disease. Furthermore, disease containment is but one part of overall medical strategy for the population, and, as such, screening costs have to be considered side by side with all other claims on the health-service purse.
10. *Screening for chronic disease is an ongoing process requiring critical analysis and audit of results*. Self-evidently, disease is an ever-present threat emerging constantly during the life years of the population. Hence, effective screening programmes must be ongoing, as must continuing audit and evaluation of the process.

In general, the Wilson and Junger criteria[13] provide a very good framework for discussion of disease as a matter of public-health policy. The principles are naturally more applicable to some diseases than others, and the opportunity is now taken to discuss screening programmes in terms of organ-based uropathology.

SCREENING FOR UROLOGICAL DISEASE

Single-shot screening

Congenital abnormalities of the urogenital system are relatively common, as such abnormalities are not invariably fatal for the fetus. Within the last 15 years, increasingly sophisticated ultrasound technology has been able to pick up urological abnormalities in utero with increasing confidence. Most normal fetal kidneys are visible before 20 weeks, and hydronephrosis may be detectable as early as 16 weeks. With such technology, the incidence of congenital renal abnormalities has been reported as approximately 1 in 800 live births,[14] which compares favourably with the 1 in 650 reported from autopsy series.[15]

Good-quality pictures may be obtained of both hydronephrosis and hydroureter when present (Figure 34.9a and b). Although not all cases of simple hydronephrosis may need intervention after birth, the screening process undoubtedly identifies at-risk babies, allowing the paediatric service to concentrate its efforts in a cost-effective and efficient manner.

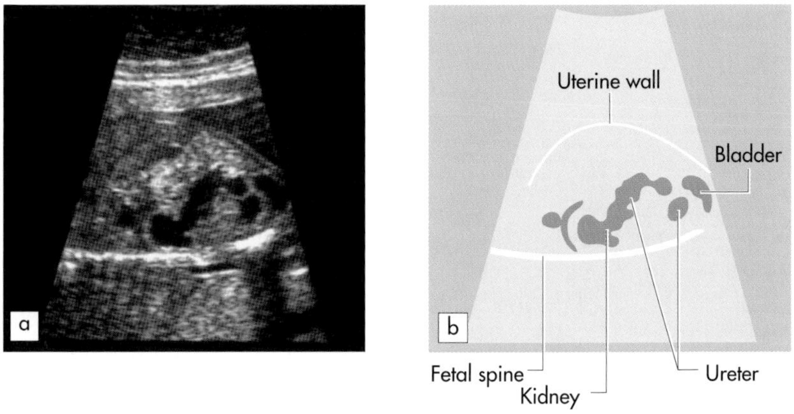

Figure 34.9 *(a) Antenatal ultrasound of a fetus with hydronephrosis and hydroureter but a normal bladder; (b) diagramatic representation to illustrate scan.*

SCREENING FOR CHRONIC UROLOGICAL DISEASE

Screening programmes are directed towards the eradication of serious chronic disease such as cancer (Table 34.5). Therefore, if such programmes are to be applied to the urogenital system, neoplastic disease is most likely to be the target of the enterprise. Serious chronic inflammatory disease, such as tuberculosis, is no longer a significant health problem from a screening point of view. However, as will be seen in terms of numbers, urological cancers, with the possible exception of prostate, do not recommend themselves as ideal subjects for screening protocols.

Renal cancer

Although it is responsible for the most common open operation performed for urological malignancy, kidney cancer is relatively uncommon. This disease, ranking 11th in the UK, was responsible for approximately 3234 deaths in 2001,[16] and the cancer therefore cannot be viewed as a major health problem. Additionally, there is no obvious preclinical phase to detect – most early tumours are discovered by incidental ultrasound examination, which merely identifies relatively small established cancers that have yet to bleed into the renal pelvis. A screening programme therefore would be inappropriate for this disease.

A form of selective screening might apply to patients with von Hippel-Lindau disease, who have multiple abnormalities, including a 30% incidence of renal cell carcinoma. However, the symptoms and signs of the disorder are so characteristic and the association with kidney cancer so strong that the term 'selective screening' is unnecessary for what is in effect a practical clinical surveillance programme.

Bladder cancer

Although more common than kidney cancer, bladder cancer is again not a major public-health problem with 3% (5300) of cancer deaths in 2002.[16] Nevertheless, the debate continues in urological circles as to the diagnostic protocol which should follow the discovery of microscopic haematuria – it is accepted that bleeding usually arises not from a preclinical phase but from established urothelial tumour. Urine cytology is widely utilized as a diagnostic test in those patients who have been discovered to have haematuria, although it is acknowledged that significant false-negative results may occur, particularly in patients with well-differentiated transitional cell tumours. Carcinoma in situ is perhaps a genuine manifestation of the preclinical phase of invasive bladder cancer. Unfortunately, checking this condition against Wilson and Junger criteria reveals that there is little hope of establishing an effective screening programme for the disease. Recent reports have demonstrated the efficacy of detecting bladder cancer by microsatellite analysis of urine DNA.[17] This approach clearly holds out hope for the future, but it should be noted that this work has adopted the questionable technique referred to earlier whereby a potential screening test is evaluated in patients with known clinical disease. As has been emphasized, the real test of such techniques will be when the procedure is applied to a true screening population.

Table 34.5 The benefits and disadvantages of screening for cancer.

Benefits	Disadvantages
Improved prognosis for some cases detected by screening	Longer morbidity for cases whose prognosis is unaltered
Less radical treatment needed to cure some cases	Overtreatment of borderline abnormalities
Reassurance for those with negative test results	False reassurance for those with false-negative results Unnecessary morbidity for those with false-positive results Hazard of screening test
Resource saving	Resource costs

From Provok et al. (1984).[9]

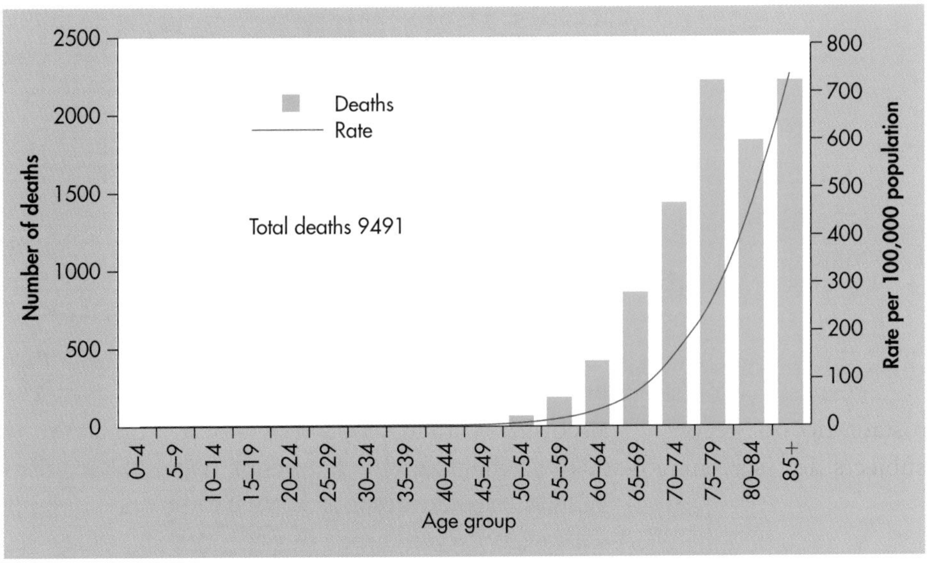

Figure 34.10 *Deaths by age from prostate cancer in the UK (1999). Of 9491 deaths, 743 (8%) occurred in men under 65 years, illustrating the relatively weak impact that the disease in younger men might make on public health policy. Data from Cancer Research Campaign Factsheet 2.4, 2002.*[25]

Prostate cancer

Prostate cancer is acknowledged at the present time as being the second commonest cause of cancer death in males, 9280 patients dying of the disease in 2000. However, from the public-health point of view, these figures are relatively unimpressive. Figures 34.6 and 34.7 show that, taking the northwest of the UK as an example and allowing for the disparity in the data, deaths account for only approximately 3–4% of the regional mortality. Furthermore, Cancer Research Campaign (CRC) figures clearly show (Figure 34.10) that the great majority of these deaths occur in men over 65 years old (92%); hence, from the public-health point of view, deaths from this disease in the 'high political impact' younger age group are a very small proportion of the overall health problem.

Interestingly, data from the CRC for mortality 5 years later in 1999 (Figure 34.7) shows very little change despite active case finding and 'advances' in therapy. On these grounds mass screening is difficult to support from a purely scientific point of view.

Nevertheless public and medical pressure have resulted in a vigorous debate relating to the validity of screening for the disease. The poor performance of current diagnostic modalities – PSA and TRUS – is emphasised by a number of authorities.[30] Variations in diagnostic techniques[31] may carry some advantage but most agree that the essential question relates to whether the accepted radical treatments for the disease can improve survival and quality of life.[30,31] As the arguments continue, relatively large numbers of younger men with biopsy-proven early prostate cancer are being identified, and urologists are struggling to establish rational treatment protocols for the disease thus discovered. It is clear that two basic facets of the debate have emerged, each dependent on the other. Firstly, is screening effective at detecting clinically significant disease and secondly, can the treatments applied reduce mortality? Rational argument would suggest that it is essential to answer the second question before embarking on the first but medical politics may not always allow this to occur. At the present time, as most of the Wilson and Junger criteria cannot be met, both urologists and patients have had to settle for acknowledged over-treatment of detected disease .[18]

Some laudable attempts have been made to determine whether or not a screening programme for early prostate cancer can influence mortality from the disease in the long term. The European randomized study of screening for prostate carcinoma (ERSPC), based in Rotterdam, has adopted the classical approach of a randomized clinical trial (see page 625) to eliminate bias and evaluate the screening programme. The scheme covers 7 countries in Europe and is associated with the PLCO (prostate, lung, colon and ovary) screening study from 10 centres in the USA. Figure 34.11 depicts the screening algorithm for those randomized to the screening

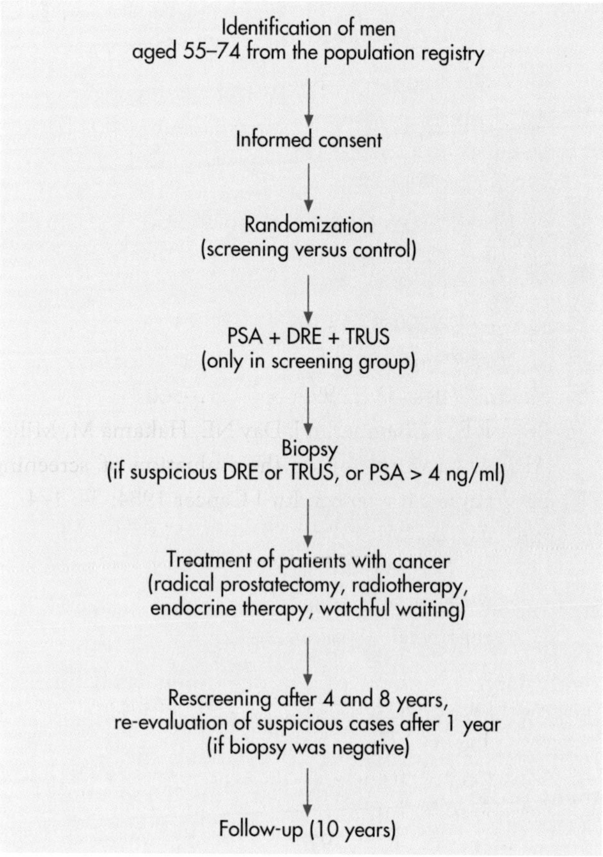

Figure 34.11 *Details of the Rotterdam randomized controlled trial of screening for prostate cancer, taken from Bangma et al.*[19]

group. In this study, screening is by means of PSA, rectal examination and transrectal ultrasound. To-date (2001) recruitment has reached 163,126 men aged 55–69 and could show difference in mortality between the 2 arms by 2007 although many variables may derail these predications.[32] Within this huge enterprise various sub-studies have examined, amongst others, variable cut-off levels (4 vs 3 ng/ml)[33] and comparative data with the American PLCO trial.[34] So far, the reported cancer detection rate is approximately 4.7–5.0 at the differing cut-off points, and 91% of cancers by clinical staging are organ confined.

The problem of establishing the ideal cutoff values is illustrated in Figure 34.12 which demonstrates the previously described reciprocal relation between sensitivity and specificity, and it is clear that determination of the ideal value is problematic. The authors conclude that the answer to this question can be obtained only by making a reasonable effort to detect all cancers in the population and studying the long-term outcomes.[19]

Within the UK the Health Technology Assessment Programme has funded another approach which seeks to answer the second question relating to efficacy of treatment. The ProtecT (prostate testing for cancer and treatment) study is a multicentre trial in which patients with suitable early disease are randomised to radical surgery, radical radiotherapy or watchful waiting (active monitoring).[35] The randomisation and counselling process is reported to take 20 minutes[35] but in practice can last for very much longer, a significant problem which has led to re-evaluation of the processes involved in the trial.[36] This and other trials of therapy such as the Patient Preference Study[37] should eventually determine whether screening for this disease is appropriate and can be regarded as successful public health policy. In the meantime the advice of Schroeder remains aposite.[18]

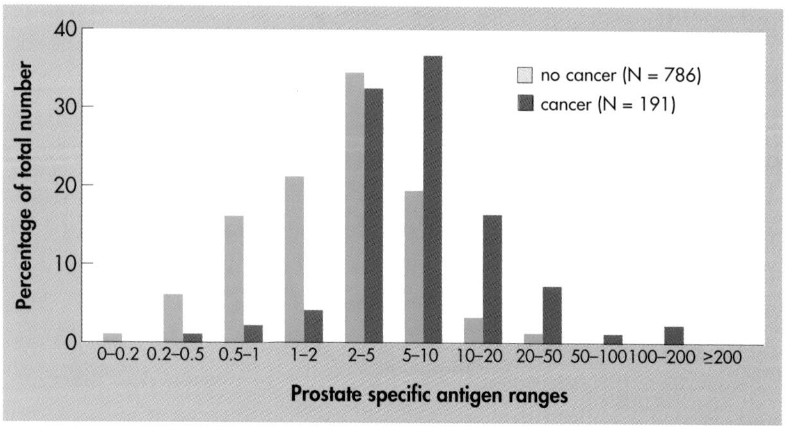

Figure 34.12 *Sensitivity, specificity and cutoff values illustrated by data obtained from the Rotterdam screening study. The extraordinary difficulty of establishing a cutoff between health and disease can be appreciated. Data from Bangma et al.*[19]

Testis cancer

The rarity of this condition precludes a national screening effort, but all urologists will be aware of the importance of self-examination and self-referral in preventing presentation of patients with advanced disease. Publicity about self-examination may be likened to that surrounding breast disease, but, clearly, diagnostic confirmation and treatment are both easier and cheaper for cases of testis cancer, with the added benefit of excellent long-term outcome measures.

CONCLUSION

Screening, as noted above, remains a relatively novel and somewhat unproven mechanism for disease control. With time, the common-sense view that 'it must be good for you' appears to become more rather than less controversial. Recent studies questioning the value of screening for Down's syndrome[38] and cervical cancer[39] have generated heated debate whilst the latest trend of whole body screening with computerised tomography[40] ('the ideal gift for a 50th birthday') has led to accusations of a screening industry feeding off 'simple-minded enthusiasm' – a charge clearly directed at the medical profession as a whole.

Nevertheless the issues are and will remain within the public domain so the urologist must advise according to the evidence taking care to ensure that the patient is not deceived by the apparent simplicity of the available information.

REFERENCES

1. Bowman JE. Screening new-born infants for Duchenne muscular dystrophy. BMJ 1993; 306: 349
2. Bogart MH, Pandian MR, Jones OW. Abnormal maternal serum chorionic gonadotrophin levels in pregnancies with fetal chromosome abnormalities. Prenat Diagn 1987; 7: 623–630
3. Wald NJ, Cuckle HS, Densem JW et al. Maternal serum screening for Down's syndrome in early pregnancy. BMJ 1988; 297: 883–887
4. Cole P, Morrison AS. Basic issues in cancer screening. In: Miller AB, ed. UICC Technical Report Series, 40. Geneva: UICC, 1978: 7
5. Day NE, Walter SD. Simplified models for screening: estimation procedures from mass screening programmes. Biometrics 1984; 40: 1–7
6. Hutchison GB, Shapiro S. Lead time gain by diagnostic screening for breast cancer. JCNI 1968; 41: 665–669
7. Feinleib M, Zelen M. Some pitfalls in the evaluation of screening programmes. Arc Environ Health 1969; 19: 412–417
8. Bradley DM, Parsons PE, Clarke AJ. Experience with screening new-borns for Duchenne muscular dystrophy in Wales. BMJ 1993; 306: 357–360
9. Prorok PC, Chamberlin J, Day NE, Hakama M, Miller AB. UICC workshop on the evaluation of screening programmes for cancer. Int J Cancer 1984; 34: 1–4
10. Ellis WJ, Chetner MP, Preston SD, Brewer MK. Diagnosis of prostatic carcinoma: the yield of serum prostate specific antigen, digital rectal examination and transrectal ultrasonography. J Urol 1994; 152: 1520–1525
11. Whitby LG. Screening for disease: definitions and criteria. Lancet 1974; 2: 819–821
12. Miller AB. Screening in cancer: a report of the UICC workshop in Toronto. UICC Technical Report Series 40. Geneva: UICC, 1978
13. Wilson J, Junger G. Principles and practice of screening for disease. World Health Organization Public Health Paper no. 34, Geneva: WHO, 1968
14. Thomas DFM, Whitaker RH. Prenatal diagnosis. In: Whitaker RH, ed. Current Prospectives in Paediatric Urology. Springer-Verlag, 1989: 45–53
15. Ashleigh DJB, Mostofi FK. Renal agenesis and dysgenesis. J Urol 1960; 83: 211–230
16. Cancer Research UK. Cancer Stats. London: Cancer Research Campaign, 2002
17. Steiner G, Schoenberg MP, Linn JF, Mao L, Sidransky D. Detection of bladder cancer recurrence by microsatellite analysis of urine. Nat Med 1997; 3: 621–624
18. Schröder FH. To screen or not to screen. BMJ 1993; 306: 407–408
19. Bangma CH, Rietbergen JBW, Schröder FH. Prostate specific antigen as a screening test – The Netherlands experience. Urol Clin North Am 1997; 24: 307–314
20. Prorok PC, Connor RJ, Baker SG. Statistical considerations in cancer screening programmes. Urol Clin North Am 1990; 17: 699–708
21. Prorok PC, Connor RJ. Screening for the early detection of cancer. Cancer Invest 1986; 4: 225–238
22. Christopherson WM. The control of cervix cancer. Acta Cytol 1966; 10: 6–10

23. Shapiro S. Evidence on screening for breast cancer from a randomised trial. Cancer 1977; 39: 2772–2782
24. Brett GZ. The value of lung cancer detection by 6 monthly chest radiographs. Thorax 1968; 23: 414–420
25. CRC UK Factsheet. London: Cancer Research Campaign, 2002
26. Ries LAG, Eisner MP, Kosary CL et al. Seer cancer statistics review 1973–1978. Available from HTTP://seer/cancer.gov/publications/CSR19731998/
27. Smith DS, Carvalhal GF, Mager DE et al. Use of lower prostate specific antigen cut-offs for prostate cancer screening in black and white men. J Urol 1998; 160: 1734–1738
28. Powell IJ, Meyskens FL. African-American men and hereditary/familial prostate cancer: intermediate-risk populations for chemo-prevention trials. Urology 2001; 57: 178–181
29. Catalona WJ, Antenor JA, Roehl KA. Screening for prostate cancer in high risk populations. J Urol 2002; 168: 1980–1984
30. Neal DE, Donovan JL. Prostate cancer: to screen or not to screen? Lancet Oncol 2000; 1: 17–24
31. Neal DE, Leung HY, Powell PH et al. Unanswered questions in screening for prostate cancer. Eur J Cancer 2000; 36: 1316–1321
32. de Koning HJ, Liem MK, Baan CA et al. Prostate cancer mortality reduction by screening: power and time frame with complete enrolment in the ERSPC trial. Int J Cancer 2002; 98: 268–273
33. Schroeder FH, Roobol-Bouts M, Vis AN et al. Prostate specific antigen based early detection of prostate cancer – validation of screening without rectal examination. Urology 2001; 57: 83–90
34. de Koning HJ, Auvinen A, Berenguer-Sanchez A et al. Large scale randomised prostate cancer screening trials: programme performances in the ERSPC trial and the PLCO trial. Int J Cancer 2002; 97: 237–244
35. Donovan JL, Frankel SJ, Neal DE, Hamdy FC. Screening for prostate cancer in the UK. BMJ 2001; 323: 763–764
36. Donovan JL, Mills N, Smith M et al. Quality improvement report: improving design and conduct of randomised trials by embedding them in qualitative research: ProtectT. BMJ 2002; 325: 766–770
37. Patient Preference Study. In press, BJUI
38. Wellesley D, Boyle T, Barber J, Howe DT. Retrospective audit of different antenatal screening policies for Down's Syndrome in 8 district general hospitals in one health region. BMJ 2002; 325: 15–19
39. Raffle AE, Alden B, Quinn M, Dabb PJ, Brett MT. Outcomes of screening to prevent cancer: analysis of cumulative incidence of cervical abnormality and modeling of cases and death prevented. BMJ 2003; 326: 901–904
40. Editorial. Screening for cancer with computed tomography. BMJ 2003; 326: 894–895

35

The design, construction and interpretation of clinical trials

Julie A Morris

INTRODUCTION

A clinical trial is defined as a medical experiment on a sample of patients to compare the effects of two or more treatments. The treatments could be, for example, different drugs or surgical techniques, and the measured effects might be symptom severity, recurrence of symptoms, recovery time or death. The results obtained from such a study are then used to make inferences about which treatment should be recommended for a more general population of patients.

Clinical trials are comparative, in that a group of patients given a new treatment is compared with a control group of similar patients receiving either a well-established treatment or no treatment (if no treatment has already been demonstrated to be effective). Furthermore, patients should be assigned randomly to the new or standard treatment to ensure an unbiased evaluation of the effect of the new treatment.

The randomized controlled trial is usually considered the most reliable method of conducting a clinical study.

DRUG TRIALS

The pharmaceutical industry defines four categories of trials: phases I, II, III and IV.

Phase I trials are essentially exploratory trials on healthy human volunteers. They are used to assess the frequency and degree of harmful side-effects (i.e. the toxicity of proposed therapy). Phase II trials determine the level of effectiveness of a particular treatment and further define the non-therapeutic effects (i.e. toxicity). These trials are carried out on patients and are used to decide whether the therapeutic effect of treatment is good enough to warrant further investigation. Phase III trials are definitive studies that are designed to compare a new treatment with an existing established treatment. They are often referred to by the general term 'clinical trials' because they involve the most comprehensive investigation of a new treatment. Phase IV trials are concerned with the monitoring of adverse effects after the drug has been approved for marketing and are basically long-term studies of morbidity and mortality.

In this chapter, only phase III trials (full-scale comparative studies) will be considered in detail, because it is this type of trial that most clinicians outside the pharmaceutical industry come across.

EARLY CLINICAL TRIALS

Treatment evaluation has been attempted as far back as prehistoric times, and there are various reports of studies being carried out in the seventeenth and eighteenth centuries.

An interesting description of a comparative trial of treatments for scurvy carried out in the mid-eighteenth century is given by Lind.[1] Twelve similar patients with scurvy were selected, and divided into six groups of two patients. Each group was given one of the following six treatments in addition to a common diet: a quart of cider a day, 25 gutts of elixir vitriol, two spoonfuls of vinegar, a course of sea water, a nutmeg, or two oranges and a lemon each day. The effects of treatment were evaluated at the end of six days. The men given the oranges and lemons were greatly recovered; one was fit for duty, and the other was appointed nurse to the rest of the sick. Nevertheless, the results of the study were not immediately acted upon. Lind recommended fruit and vegetables as only a secondary priority to 'pure dry air', and it took another 50 years before the British navy supplied lemon juice to its ships.

This study included many of the important aspects of a controlled trial. There was a homogeneous group of patients, equally divided into the various treatment groups, a good description of the differing treatment schedules, and a clear account of the outcome. However, properly conducted clinical trials were not carried out until the late 1940s. The first clinical trial with a properly randomized control group was for streptomycin in the treatment of pulmonary tuberculosis.[2]

PROTOCOLS

An important starting point in designing a study is to write a study protocol. This is a formal document specifying how the clinical trial is to be conducted. It provides detailed information on the various components of the trial, including:

- aims and objectives
- patient selection
- trial design
- treatment schedules
- randomization of patients
- main outcome measures
- required size of study
- planned statistical analysis
- protocol deviations
- adverse events
- patient consent.

It is, in essence, an operating manual giving clear instructions to the members of the clinical trial team as to how the study should be conducted. All clinicians and researchers involved in the study, including a statistician, should be consulted in writing the protocol. A detailed protocol often has to be submitted to ethical committees and funding bodies to provide evidence that the trial is well designed.

TRIAL DESIGN

There are two main types of design: parallel and cross-over. The simplest is the *parallel design*. Two groups of patients are given a different treatment regime over the same period of time. One group receives the new treatment and the other group, acting as the control, receives the standard or placebo treatment. Patients are randomized to one or other of the two groups. This design is most suitable for a study in which the treatment is expected to change the course of the disease and to make an appreciable difference to a patient's condition. The long-term effects of treatment can also be assessed using a parallel design study carrying on over a number of years.

The alternative design is the *cross-over* trial. In its simplest form, each patient receives two treatments, one after the other, and the order of treatments is chosen using a suitable randomization method. Because an assessment of both treatments is made on each patient, a comparison of treatments is calculated 'within-patients'; that is, each patient acts as his or her own control. This allows a more precise comparison because the variability of an outcome measure for a patient recorded at different times will usually be less than that between different patients recorded at the same time. This means that smaller numbers of patients are required in cross-over trials. However, there are a number of disadvantages. A cross-over design is only viable if the evaluation of treatment involves measuring short-term relief of symptoms of a chronic condition. One problem with the design is that the effect of the first treatment may carry over to the second period and hence interfere with the effect of the second treatment. This *carry-over* effect will then bias any comparison between treatments. To overcome this problem, a *wash-out* period should be included between the first and second treatment periods in which no treatment is given. There may also be a greater number of patients who drop out of a cross-over study, simply because a much longer overall treatment period is required. Patients may drop out before receiving the second treatment.

For studies in which the treatment outcome is known fairly quickly, a *sequential design* is sometimes appropriate. This is a parallel group study in which patients are gradually recruited and the data are analysed after each new patient. The trial continues until either a clear difference between treatments emerges or it is considered unlikely that any difference will be shown. The advantage of this design is that the required sample size will be smaller than that of a simple parallel study if the difference between the two treatments is relatively large, and therefore fewer patients will receive the less beneficial treatment.

When two treatments A and B are to be evaluated separately and also in combination against a control, a *factorial design* is used. Patients are then allocated randomly to receive treatment A only, treatment B only, the combination of A and B, or placebo. This design allows clinicians to compare the treatments with placebo, compare the treatments with each other and to assess a possible interaction between them.

RANDOM ALLOCATION

In a parallel design, the treatment given to each patient should be decided by chance – that is, by random allocation. There are various types of randomization.

Simple randomization gives equal probability for each patient to receive one of the treatments. If there are two treatments, labelled A and B, then a simple randomization can be obtained by tossing a coin for each patient, allocating treatment A for heads and treatment B for tails. Alternatively, a table of random numbers can be used, with even numbers indicating treatment A and odd numbers indicating treatment B.

However, this does not ensure that at the end of recruitment, equal numbers of patients receive treatments A and B. This discrepancy can be substantive, particularly for large trials. One way to ensure that equal numbers of patients are allocated to the treatments is to use *blocked randomization*. For every block or group of a specified number of patients, simple randomization is used with the restriction that the block contains an equal allocation of patients. For example, if blocks of size 4 are specified, then a coin can be tossed to allocate the first two or three patients in each block. If the first two patients are allocated to treatment A, then, by default, the next two patients have to be allocated to treatment B. If the first two patients are allocated to treatment A and B respectively, then the third patient in the block is allocated by another toss of the coin. If this patient is allocated to treatment B, then, by default, the fourth patient is allocated to treatment A, and so on.

It is important that the treatment groups in a randomized trial are similar with respect to relevant patient characteristics considered to be significant prognostic factors, for example age or severity of disease. *Stratified randomization* can be used to guard against the possibility of imbalance of these prognostic factors between the different treatment groups. Each prognostic factor is categorized into two or more levels. As an example, suppose age and gender are the relevant factors, with age split into three categories – 'under 40 years', '40 to under 65 years' and '65 years and over'. These two factors define six patient types, or strata:

- male, age < 40
- male, age 40–< 65
- male, age 65 and over
- female, age < 40
- female, age 40–< 65
- female, age 65 and over.

For each of the patient strata, a separate blocked randomization list is prepared. As a patient enters the trial, the stratum to which he or she belongs is identified and the treatment allocation is taken from the appropriate randomization list. The strata should be reasonably low in number because there is a possibility of over-stratification, which may lead to an uneven distribution of patients over the defined strata (some strata may contain no patients at all), and may result in an imbalance in the prognostic factors between the treatment groups.

Note that in a cross-over design, the randomization procedures outlined above are used to randomly allocate the order in which the patients receive the different treatments.

NON-RANDOM AND SYSTEMATIC ALLOCATION

An alternative way of ensuring that the different treatment groups are similar with respect to prognostic factors is to use the *minimization method*. This is a non-random procedure, but provides an acceptable method of allocating patients to treatment. It is particularly suitable for smaller studies with a few key patient characteristics known to be important prognostic factors. The allocation is not prepared in advance but is an ongoing process as patients are recruited. The first patient is given a treatment at random, but for subsequent patients the treatment which would give a better balance of prognostic factors across the treatment groups is determined. This is simply achieved by looking at the numbers of patients with similar prognostic factors who have already been allocated to one of the treatment groups. A weighted randomization (in favour of the treatment which minimizes the imbalance) is then used. The method of minimization only requires a detailed record of the treatment allocations to be kept, which is constantly updated. It can be carried out manually, but is often implemented using a simple computer program.

Systematic allocation of subjects is sometimes used, but is not recommended. Examples of such methods are the alternate allocation of treatment to consecutive patients, or using a patient's date of birth to determine which treatment he or she should receive (e.g. those with even dates receiving treatment A, those with odd dates receiving treatment B). Although these procedures appear to lead to an unbiased allocation of treatment, it is possible for someone with prior knowledge of the assignment method to manipulate the system. For example, a clinician might be reluctant to enter a particular patient into the trial if he or she knows that the patient would be destined to receive a placebo.

HISTORICAL CONTROLS

Some researchers believe that a good control group to compare with current patients on a new treatment would comprise previous patients who had received the standard treatment. These patients are called historical or retrospective controls. The advantage of this approach is that all future patients can be given the new treatment, hence there is no need for randomization of patients and a larger study size can be achieved. The main problem is that the use of the two groups of patients may not lead to a fair comparison. There are many potential sources of bias, which cannot be discounted. Patients in the historical control group are likely to have less well-defined criteria for inclusion, may have come from a different source, and therefore may differ in the type and severity of disease. In addition, ancillary patient care may be much better for the current patients on the new treatment. Therefore, the use of historical controls is not recommended.

BLINDING

It is essential to ensure that the patients randomly allocated to their respective treatments are treated in exactly the same way, otherwise bias may be introduced.

A *double-blind* trial is one in which both the clinician assessing the outcome of treatment and the patient are ignorant of the treatment allocation. This is feasible when, for example, the competing treatments are oral drug therapies. The differing tablets (including a placebo or dummy tablet if used) can be made to look and taste the same.

If it is impracticable to run a double-blind trial (for example if the competing treatments are different surgical procedures to which the clinician cannot be blinded), then the patient alone should be kept ignorant of the treatment. This would then be a *single-blind* trial.

A trial can also be *triple-blind*, that is three groups of individuals are ignorant of the treatment allocation. These could include the patients, the clinicians assessing the outcome and the data analysts.

The maximum degree of blindness that is possible should be used in a clinical trial.

SIZE OF A TRIAL

The number of subjects required in a study is an important consideration and depends on four different factors:

1. Response to the control/standard treatment, e.g. the expected percentage of patients showing relief from symptoms based on experience or previously published data, or the average peak flow rate.
2. Anticipated response to the new treatment.
3. Significance level (α). The quantity α is commonly referred to as the type I error, and is the

probability of detecting a significant difference when the treatments are really equally effective. It is usually set at 0.05. That is, a *p* value of 0.05 (a 5% significance level) is taken as the critical point at which a statistical comparison test of the data will show a significant difference.

4. Power ($1-\beta$). This refers to the power of the study to detect a statistical difference between treatments of size equal to the expected response difference quoted above. The quantity β is commonly called the type II error, and is the probability of not detecting a significant difference between treatments when there really is a difference of this magnitude. In practice, a power of 80% is the lowest level considered acceptable.

The first two factors determine the size of the difference between the effects of the treatments regarded as important (usually denoted by δ). Detailed tables for sample size calculations are given in the book by Machin and Campbell.[3] Alternatively, specialized statistical computer software can be used to determine sample sizes for a wide range of trial designs.

Formulae are given below that correspond to a *two-sided significance level of 5%* and a *power of 80%*. The sample size calculations depend on whether the data are qualitative (e.g. percentages) or quantitative (e.g. continuous measures).

Comparison of proportions

To detect a difference in proportions, $\delta = p_1 - p_2$ (where p_1 is the proportion of successes expected on the standard treatment and p_2 is the proportion of successes on the new treatment), the number of subjects (n) in each group should be at least:

$$n = 7.85[p_1(1 - p_1) + p_2(1 - p_2)]/\delta^2 \qquad (1)$$

Example

In a comparative study of the benefits of radiotherapy versus surveillance in patients with stage I testicular cancer, the expected proportion of patients under surveillance who relapse is 0.25. The investigator believes that a reduction in relapse rate to 0.10 in the radiotherapy group would be clinically important. How many patients should be included in the study for a two-sided significance level of 0.05 and a power of 0.80?

From equation (1), with $p_1 = 0.25$, $p_2 = 0.10$ and $\delta = 0.15$, we obtain $n = 97$ in each of the groups, that is, 194 patients in total.

Comparison of means (unpaired data)

To detect a difference of size $\delta = m_1 - m_2$ (where m_1 and m_2 are the mean responses for the standard treatment and new treatment respectively), the number in each group should be at least:

$$n = 15.7\sigma^2/\delta^2 \qquad (2)$$

where σ is an estimate of the standard deviation of the response measure (assumed to be the same in both treatment groups).

Example

The effects of cimetidine and vitamin C on peak flow rate for patients with benign hypertrophy are to be compared in a randomized parallel trial. The clinician wishes to show a significant improvement of 5 ml/s or more in patients given cimetidine, and believes the standard deviation of peak flow rate in this group of patients will be about 10 ml/s. How many patients should the clinician recruit to the study for a 5% significance level and 80% power?

From equation (2), with $\sigma = 10$ and $\delta = 5$, we obtain $n = 63$ per group, that is, 126 patients in all.

Comparison of means (paired data, e.g. cross-over trial)

To detect a difference between treatments of size δ, and within-subject standard deviation σ_w (i.e. the standard deviation of the paired difference between treatments), the number of subjects in each group should be at least:

$$n = 7.85\sigma_w^2/\delta^2 \qquad (3)$$

It is sometimes difficult to give a suitable value for the within-standard deviation σ_w. A rough approximation can be given by $\sqrt{2}\sigma$ (where σ is the standard deviation of the response measure).

Example

An investigator wishes to compare the effect of a drug having smooth muscle relaxant properties with a placebo on patients with idiopathic detrusor instability using a cross-over trial design. The investigator is looking for a difference in maximum voiding pressure of more than $10\,cmH_2O$ to be significant at the 0.05 level and with a power of 0.80. Previous studies have shown that in the absence of any drug effect, the standard deviation of within-subject maximum voiding pressure is $30\,cmH_2O$. How many patients should the investigator recruit?

From equation (3), with $\sigma_w = 30$ and $\delta = 10$, the investigator would require at least 71 patients in all.

It is important to recognize that studies in which the outcome measures are continuous (and have means as summary statistics) require fewer subjects than those in which the outcome is assessed as simply success or failure. An additional point to remember is that if a fair number of drop-outs is likely during the study, the calculated sample size should be increased accordingly.

SELECTION OF SUBJECTS

If the results of a clinical trial are to be used to make general inferences, it is important that the patients included in the study form a representative sample of all patients with the particular disease. However, in practice, there are restrictions on the eligibility of patients to enter the trial and investigators are limited to patients for whom there is easy access (e.g. in-patients at their own hospital). In addition, it is usually advisable to ensure the variation in the outcome measure in the study group is kept reasonably low (so that the sample size required to show a significant difference between treatments is not prohibitively high), and therefore patients are restricted to those of, for example, a particular age group and severity of disease. It is important to realize that the results of the study will be less able to be generalized the more restrictions are made on the study patients.

PROTOCOL DEVIATIONS

There are a number of ways in which deviations from protocol can occur.

One instance is that in which ineligible patients are included in a trial. Such patients should be excluded from the analysis of the results of the study. The number of ineligible patients can be reduced by using a checklist for eligibility as every patient enters the study, prior to randomization. Another problem occurs when patients do not adhere to their allocated treatment; that is, when they are non-compliant with treatment. This can be reduced, firstly, by ensuring that a detailed explanation of the treatment regime is given to each patient and, secondly, by having frequent checks during the course of treatment. The latter can be achieved by, for example, counting the number of remaining tablets the patient has or by blood/urine tests. The most extreme type of non-compliance occurs when a patient withdraws from the study. This is due either to patient refusal to carry on with the treatment (sometimes unavoidable if the patient moves away from the study area) or to a clinical decision that the treatment for this patient should be changed.

As a general rule, all eligible patients, including non-compliant patients, should be included in the analysis of the results where possible. This approach is sometimes referred to by the term 'analysis by intention to treat', and is considered to lead to a more valid comparison of treatments because it mimics what is likely to happen in clinical practice.

PILOT STUDY

Before carrying out a definitive study involving a large number of subjects, it is sometimes prudent to run a small pilot study. This is used to estimate patient recruitment as well as the level and variability of the outcome measure. The latter information can then be used in the calculation of required sample size for the larger study. The pilot study can also show how questionnaires and assessment scales perform in practice, and whether the planned trial will run smoothly.

MULTICENTRE TRIALS

In some circumstances, it may not be feasible to carry out a trial at a single centre (i.e. one hospital or general practice surgery) because the number of eligible patients available over the study period will be too small. The involvement of a number of different centres in the study should be considered to increase the potential pool of patients. If the clinical trial includes patients and clinicians from a variety of centres, a more broad, representative set of patients will be attained and the results of the study will be more easily generalized. There are, however, a number of disadvantages to running a multicentre trial. A greater cost is involved because the number of staff working on the study and the administration is increased. It is also more difficult to ensure that the study protocol is followed exactly, and that the quality of the data is of a uniformly high standard.

CLINICAL VERSUS STATISTICAL SIGNIFICANCE

If a clinical trial includes a large number of subjects, then even small differences can become statistically significant. For example, suppose in a trial assessing the effects of two drugs on the urinary composition of 1000 patients with enteric hyperoxaluria, the reduction in urinary oxalate excretion output was, on average, 0.01 mmol/24 h greater for one drug compared to the other and that this was found to be a statistically significant result. Because this is such a small difference, it would not be considered as clinically important or significant.

Alternatively, if a clinical trial includes only a small number of subjects, then quite large differences will not be statistically significant. For example, suppose the trial described above involved just ten patients and the difference in reduction in urinary oxalate excretion output was shown to be 0.15 mmol/24 h, but that this difference was not statistically significant. Because a reduction of this magnitude would be clinically important, the result should not be ignored; it provides evidence that a much larger study should be planned.

GUIDELINES FOR THE CRITICAL APPRAISAL OF PUBLISHED CLINICAL TRIAL PAPERS

Studies published in reputable journals are naturally thought to have a sound research basis, with credible results and reliable conclusions. However, this is a mistaken belief. Most journals do have a system of appraisal by independent referees and a number of journals use statisticians as referees, but many low-standard studies still manage to pass through the system and are published. The consequences of misleading results can be serious. A clinician may decide to switch to a new treatment for his or her patients when in actual fact the treatment does not actually have the beneficial effects extolled in the medical article. A researcher may employ time, effort and resources in a fruitless attempt to replicate a study finding. It is therefore important that medical researchers and clinicians are able critically to appraise a paper for themselves.

A summary of the relevant points that need to be considered when reading a clinical trial paper is given below. This closely follows the clinical trials checklist given in Gardner, Machin and Campbell.[4] The list was designed to help the statistical refereeing of papers submitted to the *British Medical Journal*. Note that studies must be judged on the information included in the published paper. A satisfactory answer to a question cannot be assumed if the relevant information is not given.

- *Objective of the study*. Are the aims and objectives of the trial sufficiently described?
- *Study design*. Was a parallel group or cross-over design used? Was the design appropriate for the type of disease and treatment studied? Is the study prospective (that is, a planned study with data to be collected) or retrospective (based on data already collected)? Were concurrent or historical controls used?
- *Criteria for subject eligibility*. Are the diagnostic criteria for entry into the trial specified and the exclusion criteria clearly stated? Are the criteria appropriate?

- *Source of subjects.* How were the subjects recruited? Were they, for example, all hospital in-patients within a specific time frame or consecutive clinic attenders? Was sufficient information given about the health status of the subjects?
- *Treatments.* Were the treatments well defined? Are the treatment periods of reasonable length?
- *Randomization.* Were the subjects randomly allocated to treatment? Is the exact method of randomization (e.g. simple blocked randomization using random number tables or stratified randomization with age and severity of disease defining the strata) described? Is the practical way in which subjects were allocated to treatment (e.g. from a written schedule or sealed envelopes) described? Was there an acceptably short delay between allocation and commencement of treatment?
- *Blindness.* What degree of blindness was used (e.g. double blind, single blind)? How was this achieved? Was the maximum degree of blindness that is possible used in the study?
- *Outcome measures.* Were the outcome measures clearly defined? Are they appropriate? Were they accurately measured and recorded?
- *Prognostic factors.* Were data on important prognostic factors and other relevant patient characteristics recorded?
- *Sample size.* Does the paper report a pre-study calculation of required sample size? Is the study large enough to detect anything other than large (and perhaps unrealistic) differences in the effects of the treatments?
- *Follow-up.* Was there a clearly defined follow-up period? Was a high proportion of subjects followed-up? Did a high proportion of subjects complete their treatment?
- *Drop-outs.* Was the drop-out rate low? Were the drop-outs described for each treatment group separately? Was a comparison of relevant baseline characteristics made between those who dropped out and those who remained in the study?
- *Side-effects.* Were the side-effects of treatment reported?
- *Statistical analysis.* Is there an adequate description of all the statistical procedures used? Are the methods appropriate for the data? Were they applied correctly? If a parametric comparison test has been used (e.g. *t*-test), which requires the data to be Normally distributed, do the data really follow a Normal distribution? Have paired data (e.g. before and after treatment comparisons on the same group of patients) been analysed using an appropriate paired comparison test? Have multiple readings on one subject been treated incorrectly as independent observations? Were the prognostic variables adjusted for in the statistical analysis if there was a clinically significant difference between the treatment groups?
- *Presentation of results.* Is the statistical presentation of data satisfactory? Are the summary statistics given appropriate to the distribution of the data? Note that means and standard deviations should be given for Normally distributed data alone. Are graphs clearly labelled and do they have axes with an unchanging scale? Are confidence intervals presented for the main results?
- *Conclusions.* Are the conclusions drawn from the analysis of the data justified? Are the results of significance tests interpreted correctly? Is a causal relation erroneously implied from an observed association? Are findings wrongly extrapolated to a population of patients not represented in the study sample?

THE CONSORT STATEMENT

A statement called CONSORT (Consolidation of the Standards of Reporting Trials) was published in 1996 by a group of clinical epidemiologists, biostatisticians and journal editors with the aim of improving the standard of written reports of randomized controlled trials.[5] CONSORT includes a checklist of 21 items and a flow diagram that provides a detailed description of the progress of patients through the trial (from the number of eligible patients for inclusion in the trial to the number of trial patients in each treatment group who completed the trial). Most major journals have endorsed the CONSORT statement and have incorporated it as part of the requirements for authors submitting trial reports. It is expected that the CONSORT statement will lead to an improvement in the quality of reporting of randomized controlled trials.

FURTHER READING

A more detailed account of the design and statistical analysis of clinical trials is given by Pocock.[6] Readable introductions to the subject of clinical trials can also be found in Altman[7] and Campbell and Machin.[8] In addition, a very useful broad view of randomized controlled trials and their role in health care is given by Jadad [9].

REFERENCES

1. Lind J. A treatise of the scurvy. Edinburgh: Sands Murray & Cochran, 1753
2. Medical Research Council. Streptomycin treatment of pulmonary tuberculosis. Br Med J 1948; ii: 769–782
3. Machin D, Campbell MJ. Statistical tables for the design of clinical trials. Oxford: Blackwell Scientific Publications, 1987
4. Gardner MJ, Machin D, Campbell MJ. Use of check-lists for the assessment of the statistical content of medical studies. Br Med J 1986; 292: 810–812
5. Begg C, Cho M, Eastwood S, Horton R, et al. Improving the quality of reporting of randomized controlled trials – The CONSORT statement. JAMA 1996; 276: 7–9
6. Pocock SJ. Clinical Trials: A Practical Approach. Chichester: Wiley, 1983
7. Altman DG. Practical Statistics for Medical Research. London: Chapman & Hall, 1991
8. Campbell MJ, Machin D. Medical Statistics: A Commonsense Approach. Chichester: Wiley, 1993
9. Jadad A. Randomised Controlled Trials. BMJ Publishing Group, 1998.

36

Evidence-based medicine for urologists

Mark Emberton

Few urologists will admit to not having felt some kind of emotional response when the term 'evidence-based medicine' was first heard or read. If they are pressed, urologists' responses are probably little different from those of other doctors. Some see it as just another addition to the long list of fashionable ways of thinking about clinical problems – general practitioner fund-holding, quality assurance programmes, total quality management, clinical audit, and critical care pathways – and, typically, championed by a group of enthusiasts keen to promote their novel approach with something approximating evangelical zeal. A certain, but guarded, intellectual inquisitiveness in evidence-based medicine might be allowed – just enough to defend reasonably a position – but no more. For, in the end, evidence-based medicine might be easily dismissed on the grounds that it states the very obvious, yet another term for describing what we already do. Responsible urologists, by definition, practise in a critical and careful way. They keep up to date, go to scientific meetings, discuss cases with their colleagues and give the best care they can to their patients. The question could be posed, 'Who are these people that insist on telling us what we should or should not be doing with men presenting with infertility, benign prostatic hyperplasia or early prostate cancer?'[1–3] 'Surely, with our long specialist training and wealth of clinical experience, we must be best placed to decide what is best for our patients.'

Some urologists will feel increasingly uncomfortable with this position. They may experience guilt about the increasing pile of unread or even unopened journals in their offices. Over two million papers are published in the peer-reviewed literature each year. Urologists will certainly have received numerous notices of new journals, relevant to their field of interest, which have been launched and which they are likely never even to see. They may have felt slight personal frustration at not really being able to get to grips with an important scientific paper because of the assumptions made, the complex design or way the results were analysed and expressed. They may have had the feeling that a recent afternoon spent leafing through some journals was wasted because most of the papers read described studies that were ridiculously too small to be of any consequence, described patients who were quite distinct from their own, or were so badly conceived that they were forced to question the precise role of peer review and editorial discretion. A recent computer literature search might have been equally frustrating: each time the search was altered by introducing a new key word, a different, often mutually exclusive, set of references was generated. All this on top of a nagging feeling that will not go away: just how effective is that new device that was introduced about a year ago? Do the benefits (which seem now to be not as dramatic as they at first appeared) really outweigh the harms (more patients seem to be presenting side-effects than they did at the beginning)?

If you are reading this at all, the chances are that you will recognize some of the frustrations mentioned above. Although sceptical, you may want to know whether understanding what is meant by evidence-based medicine can help you make better clinical decisions. The answers to many of the clinical questions that we all ask are present in the medical literature, but they are not always easy to identify, locate, interpret or implement. Evidence-based medicine is all about searching, interpreting and implementing. This short chapter explains what is meant by evidence-based medicine and tries to say what it is not. The emphasis is on evidence-based medicine as applied to urology, and how it might be used to help in everyday clinical decision making. An appendix is provided, which should help direct the reader to sources of good-quality evidence, both paper-based and electronic. If you see yourself (at least in part) as more of a sceptic than a believer, the author urges you to read on. The aim is to convince you that evidence-based medicine is not just a passing fad, but is an intellectual challenge that is as exacting and demanding as it is rewarding.

THE CASE FOR EVIDENCE-BASED MEDICINE

Urologists do not practise in a vacuum. The work they do is shaped by forces that are influencing the way that all clinicians practise. These forces are now universal. They do not depend on where you practise (developed versus developing countries), they do not depend on how you are paid (salaried versus fee for service), nor do they depend on how the health service is structured (nationally versus locally). There are, broadly, four forces that govern the way we practise medicine. The first is an overwhelming preoccupation with cost control. Second is the increasing trend for health care to be purchased for groups of people that can be easily defined: they might live in a particular area (health authority) or might be members of a particular organization (a health-insurance scheme). Thirdly, those groups who purchase health care are becoming increasingly accountable for their actions. As these groups become distanced from central government, their accountability will increase. The decisions purchasers make will need to be justified. The combination of the decentralization of decision making and increasing accountability will result in a fourth force: a reduction in the freedom offered to clinicians to choose which patient will receive which treatment. It is likely that these rationing decisions will be increasingly shared with the people that purchase health care. Moreover, although it is not yet apparent, the last of these forces will end in a realization by the public, the media and politicians that decisions about rationing health care are becoming increasingly difficult. What is clear is that decisions on who should get what treatment should be explicit and based on the best available evidence. This is where evidence-based medicine can help. In the UK, urologists have seen the beginnings of change through the reforms undertaken in the National Health Service.[4–5] Urologists on both sides of the Atlantic have been sent a number of guidelines that state explicitly how common urological conditions should be managed in the future.[3,6] Evidence-based medicine, or the conscientious, explicit and judicious use of current best evidence when making decisions about the care that patients receive, has been proposed as one solution to the common problems of modern health care.[7]

The forces described above that shape the way we all do our jobs are largely a response to increasingly scarce resources. Resources are only one of three factors that influence the way we treat patients. The other two are evidence and values or opinion. The two urologists with rather polarized opinions presented at the beginning of this chapter represent, in turn, a clinician who values opinion over evidence, followed by a clinician who values evidence over opinion. It is the pressure on resources that will not permit opinion over evidence or presumed benefits over demonstrable benefits. Moreover, we can expect the pressure on resources to increase over the next decade. Individuals who become old will have greater expectations of what they might expect from a urologist than those who are already old: 75-year-old men will no longer accept mild lower urinary tract symptoms as a consequence of ageing. They will expect access to high-quality treatments (which might be new, more expensive technologies), and will be increasingly conversant with systems of redress if dissatisfied. The sector of society with greatest need will, in the future, make greater demands than in the past.

We can therefore expect that opinion will be forced to give way to high-quality evidence. There are plenty of examples in the medical literature that tell us that this is judicious – presumptions that were thought to be correct were shown not to be when put to the test. The example, first used by Sackett, shows that biological plausibility might not necessarily be enough to predict an outcome.[8] Sackett cites two pieces of evidence: first, a study that showed that patients who had ventricular ectopic beats after myocardial infarction were more likely to die; second, that ventricular ectopic beats could be suppressed by certain drugs. It was presumed that administering these drugs would result in fewer deaths after myocardial infarction. This seemed reasonable, but when put to the test the presumption was shown to be wrong. Randomized, controlled trials have since shown that the use of these drugs increased, rather than decreased, the risk of death in this group of patients.[9] As a result, the routine use of these drugs has been strongly discouraged. Good-quality evidence of this kind (appropriately designed and well-conducted studies) is available for many of the things that we clinicians do. Chalmers and his colleagues looked at 226 interventions carried out by obstetricians in the perinatal period. They found that there was evidence of reasonable quality available in about half; 20% were shown to confer some benefit to mothers or neonates; 30% were shown either to confer no benefit or, worse still, to do harm.[10]

WHAT EVIDENCE-BASED MEDICINE INVOLVES

Sackett has described evidence-based medicine as a form of shorthand for five linked ideas,[8] which he outlined as follows. First, the decisions we make on our wards and in our clinics should be based on the best patient, laboratory and population-based evidence. Second, the problem – rather than our habits – should determine where we get our evidence. Third, we need to be able to integrate epidemiological and biostatistical ways of thinking with those derived from pathophysiology and our own personal experience (use of numbers needed to diagnose or likelihood ratios to increase the power of diagnostic information, considering inception cohorts in making prognoses, incorporating meta-analyses of randomized, controlled trials into decisions about therapy, and introducing odds ratios into judgements about iatrogenic disease). Fourth, the conclusions of this search and critical appraisal of evidence are only worthwhile if they are translated into actions that affect patients directly. Fifth, we need continuously to evaluate our performance in applying these ideas. Sackett has summarized these five areas into a description of evidence-based medicine as a 'lifelong process of self-directed learning in which caring for patients creates the need for clinically important information about diagnosis, prognosis, therapy, decision analysis, cost utility analysis and other clinical and heath care issues.' In order to be able to do this, clinicians need to learn or refine some skills. These skills are outlined below, but readers wanting more detailed descriptions should refer to Sackett et al's book.[11]

ASKING THE RIGHT QUESTIONS

This is about formulating questions that have a reasonable chance of being answered.[12] It is an important first step because many hours might be wasted trying to get an answer to a question that is essentially unanswerable. At McMaster University in Canada, where medical students are taught an evidence-based approach to learning medicine, students are encouraged to construct or 'build' questions from 'knowledge gaps' that they become aware of when managing patients. The questions are constructed by first trying to classify the patient or the problem. In other words, one might ask, 'How would I describe a group of patients similar to the one I have just seen?' A concise description might be: fit men, less than 70 years with clinically localized prostate cancer. Once this classification has been made, the question of which cause/prognostic factor/treatment is being considered arises. Would neoadjuvant hormonal cytoreduction be of benefit to this man prior to a radical treatment? This is then followed by consideration of any alternative intervention such as standard therapy alone. The final component of the question building addresses outcome. 'What can I hope to accomplish? Are the benefits of the intervention going to outweigh the risks?' Thus, the elements of question building proposed by advocates of evidence-based medicine are concerned with the patient or problem, the intervention, the comparator and the outcome.[13] This approach, rather than helping frame the perfect question, tends to help find the gaps in our knowledge that we are all too often aware of but too busy to do anything about.

GETTING HOLD OF THE BEST EVIDENCE

This involves tracking down, with the greatest efficiency, the best evidence with which to answer the question posed. This means the best evidence available, not the best evidence possible. In doing this, one should try to classify evidence into one of five broad categories. First (or grade one) evidence refers to systematic reviews of well-conducted randomized trials. This type of study will often contain a meta-analysis of relevant studies. This is the type of study one should aim to find and is becoming more common. Second (or grade two) evidence comes from a randomized, controlled trial. If such a trial has not been conducted or was not possible, grade three evidence should be sought. This group includes studies that were well designed but not randomized. These might include case-control studies and prospective cohort studies. Other non-experimental or uncontrolled studies are labelled as grade four in terms of strength of evidence. These would include the multi-institutional prospectively collected case series. The final category, grade five, is given to expert opinion. Note that single-institution, retrospective case series (probably the most commonly published surgical study) gets no category. As well as the many gaps in our knowledge (Figure 36.1), many areas of clinical urology have to rely on standards of evidence that lie between grades three to five.

Knowing where to look for evidence is half the battle. The dose of a particular drug is best found on the data sheet or from a formulary. But where the source is not so obvious, one needs to know how to look as well as where best to look. It is fair to say that, for most clinical questions, electronic media (which is periodically updated) is replacing written material for searching. Journals are still, and will continue to be, important in alerting clinicians to new important developments, much in the way that newspapers or magazines do. They also provide the reader with what Alan Bennett, the playwright, described as the 'lucky dip' component of learning: stumbling across an article on a subject of no immediate interest but which, on glancing through and on subsequent reading, proves either interesting or useful.

Electronic media have the advantage of being more accessible, better indexed, more up to date and probably cheaper than the paper alternative. Most importantly, electronic media are more easily kept up to date and can offer the searcher an almost infinite number of quickly accessible cross-references. In most hospitals, the medical libraries have become the evidence centres and, as a minimum, should now have access to the World Wide Web; access to bibliographic databases such as MEDLINE, EMBASE or the Cochrane Database of systematic reviews; a well-chosen selection of books and journals; arrangements for getting hold of original articles or published reports; and a good librarian or information manager who can teach clinicians about how best to use the resources and supervise their use of these resources. The main impediment to using such a centre is geography. If evidence is required in a meeting or a clinic, it is usually impractical to get up and leave. It will not be long before the electronic media will be available at the desk through terminals or via

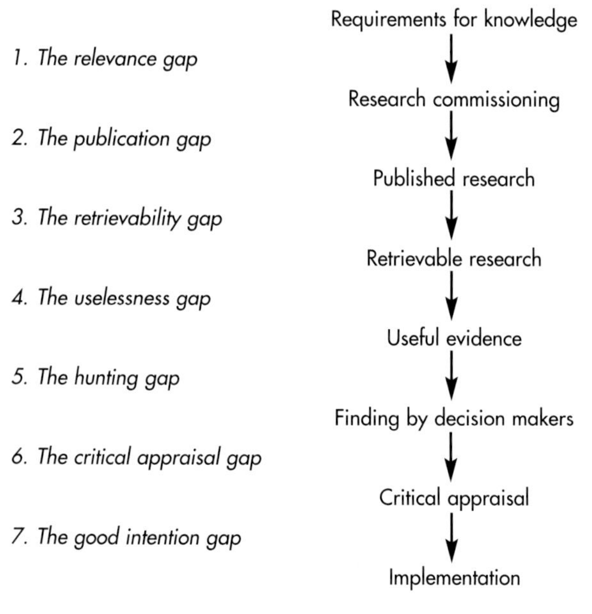

Figure 36.1 *The evidence gaps. (Reproduced by permission of Churchill Livingstone.[7])*

portable, handheld computers. A guide to electronic and other sources is available in the appendix to this chapter.

CRITICAL APPRAISAL

Many patients will be better than their doctors at finding information. Most of us have been faced with patients attending a clinic armed with pages and pages of output from several sources, the Internet being just one. Where we can help our information-seeking patients is in the critical appraisal of the literature. Critical appraisal involves asking two central questions: (1), is this valid or close to the truth?; (2), is this important or potentially useful (often called the 'so what' question)? The terms 'validity' and 'importance' need to be applied differently to different types of evidence. For example, if the validity of evidence regarding a new diagnostic test is being considered, the following questions need to be asked: Was the test compared to a reference standard? Was this done blindly and independently? Was the test evaluated on patients similar to those for whom the test is intended? Was the reference standard applied regardless of the diagnostic test result? In other words, did the investigators forgo applying the reference standard in patients who had a negative result from the diagnostic test in question? For instance, men with negative sextant Tru-cut biopsies of the prostate are unlikely to undergo radical prostatectomy in order to determine whether they are truly free of prostate cancer (true negatives). In evaluating the test, in this case, prostate biopsies, a group of men should be followed up in order to determine the proportion of patients truly free of the target disorder. Failure in any one of these three areas should encourage the reader to call into question the validity of the evidence.

Whether the evidence about a diagnostic test is important requires that another set of questions be asked. The first of these is one that clinicians must ask themselves. What, based on our own clinical experience, are the chances that the patient has the target disorder that we are testing for? These are known as prior or pre-test probabilities. Diagnostic tests that provide big differences between pre-test and post-test probabilities are likely to be useful diagnostic tests.

The next question refers to the ability of the test to distinguish between patients who have the target disorder and patients who do not. This relates to the specificity (the proportion of patients who have the target disorder who test positive) and the sensitivity (the proportion of patients who do not have the target disease who test negative) of the test in question. From the specificity and sensitivity of a test, likelihood ratios, which are becoming the preferred expression, are derived.[14] One reason why likelihood ratios are preferred by devotees of evidence-based medicine is that they are not reliant on a test's being positive or negative, as is the case with specificity and sensitivity. Different levels of a test result produce different changes from pre-test to post-test probabilities.

Although the above is a quick run-through of how one might begin to assess the validity and importance of a paper reporting on a new diagnostic test, techniques of critical appraisal (each addressing validity and importance) need to be applied to other types of report. Papers on prognostic indicators, benefits or adverse effects of new treatments, and proposed guidelines all require a systematic approach, so that the reader can decide whether or not to believe what is being said. Readers wanting details on how to become accomplished at critical appraisal should try David Sackett's book, *Clinical Epidemiology: A Basic Science for Clinical Medicine*, or Trisha Greenhalgh's guide entitled *How to Read a Paper: The Basics of Evidence-Based Medicine*, details of which are given in the appendix. Sackett's well-written guide to critical appraisal was recently serialized in the *British Medical Journal*.[15]

APPLYING EVIDENCE

Going to the trouble of finding evidence on a particular subject and deciding that it was both valid and important is not the end of it. We still have to apply evidence to a particular patient. Remember the mantra: evidence-based medicine must begin and end with patients. In order to apply evidence to a real patient, we need now to ask questions such as, 'Can I apply this *valid* and *important* evidence to a diagnostic test (such as 3% prostate-specific antigen) that I requested for my patient?' or 'Can I apply this valid and important evidence on the prognosis of the patient I saw yesterday in the clinic with superficial bladder cancer?' or 'Can I apply this *valid* and *important* evidence on treatment (such as BCG intravesical immunotherapy for carcinoma in situ of the bladder) for this patient?' or 'Can I apply this *valid* and *important* evidence on harm (such as the long-term complications of ileocystoplasty) for this patient?' These questions are even more relevant when we look at evidence produced by others, such as clinical guidelines, integrated care plans and quality improvement strategies.

Let us review the ways in which we might apply evidence about treatment to an individual patient, a situation we commonly encounter. Sackett et al tell us to ask a series of questions when trying to decide whether evidence can be applied to a particular patient.[11] First, do the results apply to your patient? Rather than rejecting a trial because your patient does not fulfil its entry criteria, for this would exclude most patients we encounter, Sackett et al suggest we rephrase the question in the following way: 'Is my patient so different from those in the trial that the results cannot help me?' Patients may differ genetically, socially and medically. The problem with this is that each clinician's interpretation of this question will differ, as different degrees of biological plausibility are applied. We should be reassured that, historically, the main findings of well-conducted studies have been generally applicable to all patients if applying them made biological sense. There is considerably more risk in applying post hoc subgroup analyses to our particular patient. There has been some notoriously spurious 'evidence' generated from subgroup analysis. The contention that women receiving aspirin would not be protected from transient ischaemic attacks (as opposed to men) was eventually shown to be false when it was looked at prospectively. Equivalence of the treatment may also need to be questioned. Is the treatment under investigation similar to that available locally in terms of skills and resources?

Once direct applicability has been accepted, the second question needs to quantify the amount of benefit that the patient is likely to experience should the treatment be applied. This can be done in two, albeit related, ways: relative benefit and absolute benefit. The former is often expressed as an odds ratio. For a detailed account of how to calculate odds ratios, readers are referred to a statistics manual or the texts cited in the appendix. As a guide, an odds ratio of 1 shows that the treatment has no benefit; less than 1, the treatment has a benefit when compared to the control group; greater than 1, the treatment is less effective than the intervention applied to the control group.

Odds ratios are preferred to the relative risk, which tends to introduce a bias. Readers tend to interpret relative risks as more positive than they genuinely are – a bias called the framing effect. An alternative way of overcoming the framing effect is to calculate the absolute reduction in risk that a treatment will produce. This is an expression of absolute benefit and is most clearly expressed by using the number (of patients) needed to treat (NNT) in order to prevent one event. Put simply, NNTs are the reciprocal of the fraction of patients improved with active treatment minus the fraction improved in the control group. NNTs can summarize complex data remarkably simply and clearly. Some NNTs for cardiac interventions have been generated by the evidence-based medical journal, *Bandolier*.[16] In order to prevent either one myocardial infarction or death in 1 year, 25 patients with unstable angina would need to take aspirin daily for 1 year. On the other hand, 500 healthy American doctors would have to take aspirin over the same period in order to prevent one myocardial infarction or death. As well as expressing the amount of effort that has to be expended in order to prevent a single event, NNTs can be applied to individual patients. This is done by dividing the NNT by the susceptibility of the particular patient to the outcome you want to prevent relative to the susceptibility in the control patients in the trial. If a patient's susceptibility is thought to be twice that of the control group, the NNT would be divided by 2.

Clearly, the decision of whether a man undergoes transurethral resection of the prostate will depend on more than the NNT. Factors such as patient choice, chance, costs and patient preferences are all part of medical or patient decision making. Evidence-based medicine practitioners have made considerable efforts to try to incorporate these important variables into treatment decisions. This is done by using decision analysis, which requires patients to place value on different disease states or outcomes. Decision analyses are time-consuming to conduct but particularly useful when good-quality evidence is missing.

Table 36.1 How evidence-based medicine can help the clinician in a rapidly changing world.

1. Time pressures Meeting the reduction in junior doctors' hours of work has led many to focus on efficiency. Evidence-based medicine can be used to decide which time- and resource-intensive manoeuvres should be dropped and which should be saved.
2. Quality pressures Purchasers of health care will increasingly demand that clinicians are indeed doing 'the right thing right'. Evidence-based medicine will identify clinical acts whose performance is consitient with quality care.
3. Team pressures Increasingly, patients are managed by multidiscipinary teams. Evidence-based medicine provides a common language and rules of evidence by which urologists, oncologists and radiotherapists should be able to agree on who will do what to whom.
4. Teaching pressures Learning evidence-based medicine is the same for undergraduates and postgraduates. It forms an ideal basis for continuous medical education.
5. Financial pressures It is no longer sufficient to provide effective health care – it needs to be cost-effective. Evidence-based medicine will identify those treatments that produce greater improvements in health per pound sterling or dollar spent.
6. Intellectual pressures No one wants to learn facts alone. Evidence-based medicine enables clinicians to keep up to date not only in their own and related fields, but also with the scientific framework within which to identify and answer priority questions about the effectiveness of the treatments they offer their patients.

GETTING STARTED WITH EVIDENCE-BASED MEDICINE

The various ways in which evidence is found, appraised and applied will be of interest to most in that they formalize a process used by all clinicians much of the time. Although learning and applying evidence-based medicine will make it easier for clinicians to cope with many of the changes occurring in health care (Table 36.1), becoming an evidence-based medicine practitioner requires some initial investment, and the learning of the specific techniques. One way of acquiring the necessary knowledge is to read one of the general texts on the subject. However, most find that applying the techniques of evidence-based medicine requires some kind of group work; relevant courses on evidence-based medicine are advertised quite regularly in the medical press. Alternatively, details of courses are held at the Department of Clinical Epidemiology and Biostatistics at McMaster University, Hamilton, Ontario, Canada, and on the World Wide Web site for the Centre for Evidence-Based Medicine in Oxford, UK: http://cebm.jr2.ox.ac.uk/. The courses have evolved from those held initially at McMaster University. They tend to be run as small groups, and to be problem based and centred on actual patients rather than idealized case scenarios. Typically, they last two or three days and should enable participants to be competent in the four key areas of evidence-based medicine outlined above: framing good questions, searching for the best evidence, critical appraisal and applying evidence to everyday practice. In addition, techniques of self-evaluation or self-audit are taught, thereby equipping practitioners to assess whether or not they are applying the techniques of evidence-based medicine optimally.

APPENDIX: GETTING BETTER INFORMATION

Much of the information below was obtained from the very detailed list of sources in Muir Gray's excellent text on the subject.[7]

PUBLISHED EVIDENCE

Bibliographic databases

Primary research (original papers), literature reviews and systematic reviews can all be identified in electronic databases such as MEDLINE or EMBASE. MEDLINE is the National Library of Medicine's bibliographic database, which covers articles published in nearly 4000 biomedical journals since 1966. New journals are not usually included until a number of conditions have been satisfied, such as proof of an adequate peer-review process. Once these conditions have been fulfilled, all issues will be represented. The EMBASE bibliographic database has been produced by Elsevier Science since 1974. It is particularly good for searches in the fields of pharmacology and therapeutics. EMBASE carries more European journals than MEDLINE. There is an increasing number of specialist bibliographic databases. Some of these specialize in nursing issues; others in health economics. HealthSTAR is typical of these. It has been produced since 1975 by the National Library of Medicine/American Hospital Association. It is strong on health services research, health economics and management issues. Many of the articles retrieved on a search conducted on HealthSTAR would not appear on an identical search on MEDLINE or EMBASE.

The Cochrane Library

The Cochrane Library, named after Archie Cochrane, one of the pioneers of evidence-based medicine, was formed in 1995. The library contains a number of databases in electronic format, which currently comprise the Cochrane Database of Systematic Reviews (CDSR), prepared by an international network of people committed to preparing and disseminating high-quality systematic reviews; the York Database of Abstracts of Reviews of Effectiveness (DARE); the Cochrane Controlled Trials Register (CCTR), a useful source of ongoing but as yet unpublished research; and the Cochrane Review Methodology Database (CRMD). Further information on the Cochrane Library can be obtained through Update Software, PO Box 696, Oxford, OX2 7YX, UK; tel. (+44) (0)1865-513902; fax. (+44) (0)1865-516918; email: update@cochrane.co.uk; URL: http://update.co.uk/info.

NHS Centre for Reviews and Dissemination (CRD) reports

The CRD is based at the University of York. It receives commissions from the NHS Executive and Health Departments of Scotland, Wales and Northern Ireland. Through bulletins entitled *Effectiveness Matters*, summaries of high-quality systematic reviews are distributed free of charge to clinicians and other interested parties, including patients. *Effectiveness Matters* tends to concentrate on the assessment of important new interventions. Its most recent publication is based on two separate systematic reviews and addresses prostate cancer screening.[2] More information on publications can be obtained by contacting CRD, University of York, York, YO1 5DD, UK; tel. (+44) (0)1904-433648; fax. (+44) (0)1904-433661; email: revdis@york.ac.uk.

The CRD, in association with the Nuffield Institute for Health at the University of Leeds and Churchill Livingstone, publishes bimonthly magazines on a variety of interventions. These again are distributed free of charge to interested clinicians. Two issues have addressed urological subjects; one addressed the management of subfertility,[1] and the more recent issue addressed the management of prostate cancer.[2]

Other reliable sources

Although using criteria less stringent than the reviews conducted by either CRD or the Cochrane Collaboration, useful reports can be obtained from the Development and Evaluation Committee of the Wessex Regional Health Authority (URL: http://cochrane.epi.bris.ac.uk/rcl/) and from the

NHS Research and Development Programmes, all of which have systematic reviews conducted as part of each initiative (URL: http://libsunt.jr2.ox.ac.uk/a-ordd/index.htm).

Electronic updates have been created in order to keep two recently published textbooks on evidence-based medicine current. The first of these, *Evidence-Based Health Care* by Muir Gray,[7] is continuously updated in the Evidence-Based Healthcare Toolbox (http://www.ihs.ox.ac.uk/ebh.html). The second, *Evidence-Based Medicine*, by David Sackett et al,[11] is also linked in the Toolbox.

Clinical standards advisory group reports

These documents, available through the Department of Health (London: HMSO), address variations in the quality and effectiveness of health care throughout England. The first was produced in 1993 and entitled, 'Access to and availability of specialist services'. No specific urological issues have been addressed since these reports were started.

Epidemiologically based needs assessment reviews

The NHS Executive's District Health Authority Project conducted a series of reviews aimed at assessing the need and demand for health care. These reports were intended to help purchasers plan local services. The reports have been put together in a document published by Radcliffe Medical Publications, Oxford.[17] Two from a total of 20 reports covered urological issues. One addressed the need for prostatectomy, and the other the need for family planning, abortion and fertility services.

Journals of secondary publication

It seems likely that in the future we will see a new type of journal created, the task of which will be to sift through a number of sources of information in order to present edited highlights to a select readership. These journals may limit themselves to subject matter considered relevant to a particular group, such as urologists. Although essentially summarizing papers that have been published elsewhere, they will be of interest to the reader on two counts: the time-consuming process of selection will have been taken care of and, more importantly, the reports will be accompanied by critical commentaries by experts. In urology, clinicians are alerted to articles of interest by a number of journals; *Current Opinion in Urology* (Current Science Ltd, London) is the best known of these, though it is rare for methodological issues to be highlighted, and therefore it is not strictly evidence-based. Another type of journal, rather than limit itself to a certain subject area, defines its selection of papers to be summarized on methodological criteria alone. In November 1995, the BMJ Publishing Group, London (fax: (+44) (0)171 383 6402 or email: bmjsubs@dial.pipex.com), launched the journal *Evidence-Based Medicine*, which reviews bimonthly over 70 international medical journals in order to identify key research papers that are considered by the editorial team to be both scientifically valid and relevant to general medical practice. The abstracts are restricted to one page and are accompanied by commentaries from experts. More recently, reports from *Evidence-Based Medicine* have been compiled onto a CD-ROM, together with the *American College of Physicians (ACP) Journal Club* (January 1991 onwards), called *Best Evidence*. The *ACP Journal Club* is available on CD-ROM from the American College of Physicians, Independence Mall West, Sixth Street at Race, Philadelphia, PA 19106, USA.

One journal, *Bandolier*, has taken secondary publication to new heights. Modern typesetting and a chatty, direct, no-nonsense style have proved very popular with both clinicians and purchasers of health care. The editors make a considerable effort to present the results of randomized clinical trials in ways that will mean something to clinicians. They avoid *P* values where possible, preferring confidence intervals or absolute risk reduction as summary statistics. Where possible, the editors try to calculate meaningful statistics such as numbers needed to treat (NNT) or numbers needed to diagnose (NND). Most health authorities make *Bandolier* available free of charge to health professionals working in the UK. Contact Andrew Moore, Pain Relief Unit, The Churchill, Oxford OX3 7LJ, UK, or by email, andrewmoore%mailgate.jr2@ox.ac.uk, or via the Internet, www.jr2.ox.ac.uk/bandolier.

UNPUBLISHED RESEARCH

Finding out about what research is under way is now possible by using bibliographic databases produced by some of the funding bodies. Finding out about research that was conducted but not finished for whatever reason is much more difficult. The databases that can help identify work in progress are as follows. First, the NHS Research and Development Programme keeps records of all funded projects. An updated list from 1997 is available. More details can be obtained by contacting the Research and Development Directorate, NHS Executive, Quarry House, Leeds LS2 7UE, UK.

The US National Library of Medicine, together with the Association for Health Services Research and the University of North Carolina, keeps an online facility that holds details of current research projects funded by both government agencies and private foundations in the USA (URL: http://www.nlm.gov or the National Library of Medicine, US Department of Health and Human Services, Public Health Service, National Institutes of Health, Bethesda, MD 20894, USA.

COMMUNICATING THE OUTCOMES OF CLINICAL TRIALS

Those who have to read, let alone understand, interpret and apply, the results of clinical trials have for a long time been unhappy with the way that key findings have traditionally been reported. Those involved in evidence-based health care have been trying to find better ways of presenting summary statistics. In other words, they wish to find alternatives to the confusion brought about by use of *P* values, odds ratios, relative risk and its derivatives, relative risk reduction or increase. Since this article was first published, I have been approached by a number of trainees who have wanted to know how to work out more meaningful summary values such as numbers needed to treat (NNT) or perhaps the slightly more appropriate summary value, given that we are surgeons: numbers needed to harm (NNH).

First a definition. NNT is an estimate of the numbers of patients that would have to undergo a given treatment for one of them to achieve a desired outcome who would not have achieved it with a control. Ideally, an NNT should never be quoted on its own. It is only of value if the characteristics of the patients being treated are known, the intervention or the duration of the intervention (as in the case of drug therapy) are explicitly stated, and, finally, the outcome measure being used has been made clear. The most widely known and quoted NNT in urology is the one derived from data from the PLESS Trial of finasteride versus placebo. In the main report, the final summary data were expressed as follows: 14 men need to be treated with finasteride for 3 years in order to prevent one man from going into acute urinary retention or requiring an operation (prostatectomy). One can see immediately that this way of framing a result carries immediate meaning when compared to the other way that the PLESS results were expressed: a 50% risk reduction in the need for surgery or the chances of developing acute urinary retention.

How to calculate an NNT

For a phytotherapy trial, an NNT can be calculated fairly simply.

> NNT = 1/(proportion of men with a >/= 4 point reduction in IPSS with phytotherapy) *minus* (proportion of men with a >/= 4 point reduction in IPSS with placebo)

The following hypothetical data will be used to illustrate the calculation

- 100 patients received the phytotherapy preparation, and 62 reported an IPSS reduction of 4 points or more.
- 103 patients received placebo and 45 reported an IPSS reduction of 4 points or more.

$$\begin{aligned} \text{NNT} &= 1/(62/100) - (45/103) \\ &= 1/0.62 - 0.44 \\ &= 1/0.18 \\ &= 5.5 \end{aligned}$$

Of course, the ideal NNT is 1. All patients who received the treatment benefited, and none of the patients who received the control did. When treatments have NNTs of between 2 and 5, they are thought to be effective, though this is a judgement and will depend on many things; the magnitude of the consequences of doing nothing, the unpleasantness of the treatment and the availability of the resource.

For further reading see Bandolier 55 1998; 5 (9): 6.

ELECTRONIC SOURCES OF INFORMATION

It is worth registering with AMEDEO.COM, which is free of charge. They will email titles and abstracts of any papers from a huge number of journals on a number of subject headings. They provide a weekly service for articles on prostate cancer and are generally strong on oncology, though they have yet to develop a routine service for other areas of urology. The site is sponsored by some of the larger pharmaceutical companies.

WEB SITES WORTH VISITING

TRIP DATABASE (www.gwent.nhs.gov.uk/trip/test-search.html)

This is run by Jon Brassey in Gwent. It is a gateway to a number of useful sites. It gives the user access to Bandolier, DARE, and SIGN (Scottish Intercollegiate Guidelines Network), to name just a few.

DOCTORS NET (www.doctors.net.uk)

This company is led by doctors and aims to improve patient care through modern communication and sound education. All UK registered doctors can register. Again, this site is best used as a portal to medical resources on the Internet. It has an ethical committee overseeing its activities and has been developed in partnership with the department of Health, UK Medical Schools and the Royal Colleges. It is free of charge and offers the following:

- Internet access and email
- forums for discussion and debate
- online jobs service
- library facilities
- bookshop.

TEXTBOOKS ON EVIDENCE-BASED MEDICINE

Greenhalgh T. How to Read a Paper: The Basics of Evidence-Based Medicine. London: BMJ Publications, 1997

Muir Gray J. Evidence-Based Health Care: How to Make Health Policy and Management Decisions. London: Churchill Livingstone, 1997

Sackett DL, Haynes RB, Guyatt GH, Tugwell P. Clinical Epidemiology: A Basic Science for Clinical Medicine, 2nd edn. Boston: Little Brown, 1991

Sackett DL, Richardson W, Rosenberg W, Haynes R. Evidence-Based Medicine: How to Practise and Teach EBM. London: Churchill Livingstone, 1997

Although not in textbook form, a series entitled 'Users' Guides to the Medical Literature' ran in the *Journal of the American Medical Association* from 1993 to 1995. The articles offer detailed accounts of how to interpret and apply different types of medical evidence to clinical situations. They are cited below.

Guyatt G, Sackett D, Cook D. Users' guides to the medical literature. 2. How to use an article about therapy or prevention. What were the results and how will they help me care for my patients? JAMA 1993; 270: 2598–2601

Guyatt G, Sackett D, Sinclair J, Hayward R et al. Users' guides to the medical literature. 9. A method for grading health care recommendations. Evidence Based Medicine Working Group. JAMA 1995; 274: 1800–1804

Hayward R, Wilson M, Tunis S, Bass E et al. Users' guides to the medical literature. 8. How to use clinical practice guidelines. Are the recommendations valid? Evidence Based Medicine Working Group. JAMA 1995; 274: 570–574

Jaeschke R, Guyatt G, Sackett D. Users' guides to the medical literature. 3. How to use an article about a diagnostic test. Are the results of the study valid? Evidence Based Medicine Working Group. JAMA 1994; 271: 389–391

Laupacis M, Wells G, Richardson W, Tugwell P. Users' guides to the medical literature. 5. How to use an article about prognosis. Evidence Based Medicine Working Group. JAMA 1994; 272: 234–237

Levine M, Walter S, Lee H, Haines T et al. Users' guides to the medical literature. 4. How to use an article about harm. Evidence Based Medicine Working Group. JAMA 1994; 271: 1615–1619

Oxman A, Sackett D, Guyatt G. Users' guides to the medical literature. 1. How to get started. JAMA 1993; 270: 2093–2095

Richardson W, Detsky A. Users' guides to the medical literature. 7. How to use a clinical decision analysis. Are the results of the study valid? Evidence Based Medicine Working Group. JAMA 1995; 273: 1292–1295

REFERENCES

1. The management of sub-fertility. Effective Health Care 1992; 3: 1–23
2. Screening for prostate cancer. Effectiveness Matters 1997; 2: 1–4
3. Chamberlain J, Melia J, Moss S, Brown J. Report prepared for the Health Technology Assessment Panel of the NHS Executive on the diagnosis, management, treatment and costs of prostate cancer in England and Wales. Br J Urol 1997; 79(Suppl. 3): 1–32
4. Secretaries of State for Health, England, Wales, Northern Ireland and Scotland. Contracts for services and role of District Health Authorities. London: HMSO, 1989
5. Secretaries of State for Health, England, Wales, Northern Ireland and Scotland. Working for patients. London: HMSO, 1989
6. McConnell J, Barry M, Bruskewitz R. Benign prostatic hyperplasia: diagnosis and treatment. Maryland: Agency for Healthcare Policy and Research, 1994; 8: 1–17
7. Muir Gray J. Evidence-Based Health Care: How to Make Health Policy and Management Decisions. London: Churchill Livingstone, 1997
8. Sackett D, Rosenberg W. The need for evidence-based medicine. J R Soc Med 1995; 88: 620–624
9. Echt D, Liebsen S, Mitchell B. Mortality and morbidity in patients receiving encainide, flecainide, or placebo: the cardiac arrhythmia suppression trial. N Engl J Med 1991; 324: 781–788
10. Chalmers I, Enkin M, Keirse M. Effective Care in Pregnancy and Childbirth. Oxford: Oxford University Press, 1989: 1471–1476
11. Sackett D, Richardson W, Rosenberg W, Haynes R. Evidence-Based Medicine: How to Practise and Teach EBM. London: Churchill Livingstone, 1997
12. Oxman A, Sackett D, Guyatt G. User's guide to the medical literature. 1. How to get started. JAMA 1993; 270: 2093–2095
13. Richardson W, Wilson M, Nishikawa J, Hayward R. The well built clinical question: a key to evidence based decisions. ACP J Club 1995; A12–13
14. Jaeschke R, Guyatt G, Sackett D. User's guide to the medical literature. 6. Are the results of the study valid? JAMA 1994; 271: 389–391
15. Greenhalph T. Statistics for the non-statistician. I. Different types of data need different statistical tests. BMJ 1997; 315: 364–366
16. Moore A, McQuay H, Muir Gray J. NNTs for some cardiac interventions. Bandolier 1995; 17: 7
17. Stevens A, Raftery J. Health Care Needs Assessments: The Epidemiologically Based Needs Assessment Reviews. Oxford: Radcliffe Medical Publications, 1994

Index